The Unstable Shoulder

The Unstable Shoulder

Editors

Russell F. Warren, M.D.

Professor of Surgery
Department of Orthopaedics
Cornell University Medical College; and
Surgeon-in-Chief
Department of Orthopaedics
The Hospital for Special Surgery
New York, New York

Edward V. Craig, M.D.

Professor of Clinical Surgery
Department of Orthopaedics
Cornell University Medical College; and
Attending Surgeon
Department of Orthopaedics
New York Hospital; and
Attending Orthopaedic Surgeon
The Hospital for Special Surgery
New York, New York

David W. Altchek, M.D.

Associate Attending Orthopaedic Surgeon
The Hospital for Special Surgery; and
Assistant Professor
Department of Surgery (Orthopaedics)
Cornell University Medical College
New York, New York

Lippincott - Raven
PUBLISHERS
Philadelphia • New York

Acquisitions Editor: Danette Knopp
Developmental Editor: Juleann Sattinger
Manufacturing Manager: Tim Reynolds
Production Manager: Jodi Borgenicht
Production Editor: Raeann Touhey
Cover Designer: DePinho Graphic Design
Indexer: Susan Lohmeyer
Composition: Maryland Composition

Printed and bound in China

9 8 7 6 5 4 3 2 1

Library of Congress Cataloging-in-Publication Data

The unstable shoulder / editors, Russell F. Warren, Edward V. Craig, David W. Altchek.
p. cm.
Includes bibliographical references and index.
ISBN 0-397-51677-0
1. Shoulder joint—Dislocation. 2. Shoulder joint—Surgery. I. Warren, Russell F. II. Craig, Edward V. III. Altchek, David.
[DNLM: 1. Shoulder Dislocation. WE 810 U59 1999]
RD557.5.U562 1999
617.5′72—dc21
DNLM/DLC
for Library of Congress 98-22298
CIP

Care has been taken to confirm the accuracy of the information presented and to describe generally accepted practices. However, the authors, editors, and publisher are not responsible for errors or omissions or for any consequences from application of the information in this book and make no warranty, expressed or implied, with respect to the contents of the publication.

The authors, editors, and publisher have exerted every effort to ensure that drug selection and dosage set forth in this text are in accordance with current recommendations and practice at the time of publication. However, in view of ongoing research, changes in government regulations, and the constant flow of information relating to drug therapy and drug reactions, the reader is urged to check the package insert for each drug for any change in indications and dosage and for added warnings and precautions. This is particularly important when the recommended agent is a new or infrequently employed drug.

Some drugs and medical devices presented in the publication have Food and Drug Administration (FDA) clearance for limited use in restricted research settings. It is the responsibility of the health care provider to ascertain the FDA status of each drug or device planned for use in their clinical practice.

Dr. Charles Neer has long been a mentor for me both personally and academically, during my shoulder surgery career. My own personal interest in the shoulder started when I suffered a shoulder dislocation that was subsequently repaired by Dr. Neer, and allowed me to return to a number of athletic activities. This was followed by a fellowship with Dr. Neer where I was impressed by the wide range of apthology that can affect the shoulder, and the difficulties of working on shoulder instability.

Dr. Neer has a provided all of us with great insight into these problems. He has developed a number of methodologies for improving treatment, as well as raising a number of questions on the evaluation and management of various instability problems.

Dr. Neer has an inquiring mind and was always open to a different thought and approach to the management of these instability problems. He has provided me throughout the years with opportunities, both in education and research, to answer some of these questions. I have always greatly appreciated his support and confidence. I dedicate this book in his honor.

R.F.W.

I would like to dedicate this book to Dr. Charles Neer. He taught me most of what I know about the shoulder. But he also taught me much more—patience, attention to detail, and responsibility. He taught me to support, yet be demanding of, colleagues, patients, and myself. He taught me about the strength of the bond between surgeon and patient. Most of all, he guided me toward a fascinating and stimulating career. For that I am forever grateful.

E.V.C.

Dr. Russell Warren has served as the mentor to many physicians who have gone on to careers in the field of shoulder surgery. I am one of the many who were fortunate enough to come in contact with his enthusiasm, dedication and drive. For the past decade I have had the extraordinary opportunity of working alongside Dr. Warren. I am continually amazed at how he combines a thorough approach to diagnosis with innovative approaches to treatment. These qualities continue to inspire me on a daily basis. I dedicate this book to one of the true legendary figures in the field of shoulder surgery—my mentor, colleague and friend, Dr. Russell Warren.

D.W.A.

Contents

Contributing Authors

Allen F. Anderson, M.D.
Tennessee Orthopaedic Alliance/The Lipscomb Clinic
4230 Harding Road
Nashville, Tennessee 37205; and
Departments of Orthopaedics and Rehabilitation
Vanderbilt University Medical Center
Nashville, Tennessee 37232

Answorth A. Allen, M.D.
Instructor
Department of Orthopaedics
Cornell University Medical College; and
Assistant Attending
The Hospital for Special Surgery
535 East 70th Street
New York, New York 10021

David W. Altchek, M.D.
Associate Attending Orthopaedic Surgeon
The Hospital for Special Surgery
535 E. 70th Street
New York, New York 10021; and
Assistant Professor
Department of Surgery (Orthopaedics)
Cornell University Medical College
1300 York Avenue
New York, New York 10021

James R. Andrews, M.D.
Clinical Professor
Department of Orthopaedic Surgery
University of Alabama at Birmingham; and
Medical Director
American Sports Medicine Institute
1313 13th Street South
Birmingham, Alabama 35205

Robert A. Arciero, M.D.
Fellowship Director
U.S. Army Joint and Soft-Tissue Trauma Fellowship
Department of Orthopaedics
Keller Army Hospital
Washington Road
West Point, New York 10996

Champ L. Baker, Jr., M.D.
Clinical Assistant Professor
Department of Orthopaedics
Tulane University School of Medicine
New Orleans, Louisiana 70112; and
President and Staff Physician
The Hughston Clinic
6262 Veterans Parkway
Columbus, Georgia 31908

Louis U. Bigliani, M.D.
Professor
Department of Orthopaedic Surgery
Columbia University College of Physicians and Surgeons
630 West 168th Street
New York, New York 10032; and
Chief
The Shoulder Service
Columbia—Presbyterian Medical Center
161 Fort Washington Avenue
New York, New York 10032

Leslie J. Bisson, M.D.
Northtown Orthopaedics
8750 Transit Road
East Amherst, New York 14051

N. Douglas Boardman, M.D.
The Shoulder Service
Center for Sports Medicine and Rehabilitation
4601 Baum Boulevard
Pittsburgh, Pennsylvania 15213

Mark K. Bowen, M.D.
Assistant Professor
Department of Orthopaedic Surgery
Northwestern University
Ward Building, 303 East Chicago
Chicago, Illinois 60611; and
Department of Orthopaedic Surgery
Northwestern Memorial Hospital
250 East Superior Street
Chicago, Illinois 60611-2950

Gregory A. Brown, M.D.
Department of Orthopaedic Surgery
Sports Medicine Division
University of Minnesota
420 Delaware Street Southeast, Box 492
Minneapolis, Minnesota 55455

Wayne Z. Burkhead, Jr., M.D.
Clinical Associate Professor
Department of Orthopaedics
University of Texas—Southwestern Medical School; and
W. B. Carrell Memorial Clinic
2909 Lemmon Ave
Dallas, Texas 75204

Daniel D. Buss, M.D.
Associate Professor
Department of Orthopaedics
University of Minnesota Medical School
422 Delaware Street
Minneapolis, Minnesota 55454; and
Minneapolis Sports Medicine Center
701 25th Street South
Minneapolis, Minnesota 55454

Richard B. Caspari, M.D.
Clinical Professor
Department of Orthopaedics
Medical College of Virginia
P.O. Box 980153, MCV Station
Richmond, Virginia 23298; and
Director
Orthopaedic Research of Virginia
4405 Cox Road, #120
Glen Allen, Virginia 23060

Robert H. Cofield, M.D.
Frank R. and Shari Caywood Professor of Orthopaedics
Department of Orthopaedics
Mayo Medical School; and
Chair
Department of Orthopaedics
Mayo Clinic and Mayo Foundation
200 1st Street, Southwest
Rochester, Minnesota 55905

Daniel E. Cooper, M.D.
W. B. Carrell Memorial Clinic
2909 Lemmon Avenue
Dallas, Texas 75204; and
Attending Physician
Department of Orthopaedics
Baylor University Medical Center
Dallas, Texas 77030

Frank A. Cordasco, M.D.
Assistant Clinical Professor
Department of Orthopaedic Surgery
Columbia University College of Physicians and Surgeons
630 West 168th Street
New York, New York 10032; and
Attending
Department of Orthopaedic Surgery
St. Luke's—Roosevelt Hospital Center
425 West 59th Street
New York, New York 10019

Edward V. Craig, M.D.
Professor of Clinical Surgery
Department of Orthopaedics
Cornell University Medical College
1300 York Avenue
New York, New York 10021; and
Attending Surgeon
Department of Orthopaedics
New York Hospital
525 East 68th Street
New York, New York 10021; and
Attending Orthopaedic Surgeon
The Hospital for Special Surgery
535 East 70th Street
New York, New York 10021

Mark T. Dean, M.D.
W. B. Carrell Memorial Clinic
2909 Lemmon Avenue
Dallas, Texas 75204

Mark C. Diebert, M.D.
Alpine Orthopedic and Sports Medicine
935 Highland Boulevard, Suite 2180
Bozeman, Montana 59715

David M. Dines, M.D.
Associate Clinical Professor
Department of Orthopaedic Surgery
Albert Einstein College of Medicine; and
The Hospital for Special Surgery
535 East 70th Street
New York, New York 10021; and
Chairman
Department of Orthopaedic Surgery
Long Island Jewish Medical Center
935 Northern Boulevard, #201
Great Neck, New York 11021

Paul A. Dowdy, M.D., F.R.C.S.C.
Central Florida Sports Medicine Institute and Central Florida Bone and Joint Institute
1705 Highway 27 North
Davenport, Florida 33837

Jeffrey R. Dugas, M.D.
Chief Resident
Department of Orthopaedic Surgery
The Hospital for Special Surgery
535 East 70th Street
New York, New York 10021

Lucio S. Ernlund, M.D.
Research Fellow
Department of Orthopaedic Surgery
University of Pittsburgh
Center for Sports Medicine
46701 Baum Boulevard
Pittsburgh, Pennsylvania 15213

Gary S. Fanton, M.D.
Director
Sports Orthopedic and Rehabilitation
2884 Sand Hill Road, Suite 110
Menlo Park, California 94025; and
Clinical Professor
Division of Sports Medicine
Stanford University Medical Center
Stanford Health Services
300 Pasteur Drive
Stanford, California 94305

Larry D. Field, M.D.
Co-Director
Upper Extremity Service
Mississippi Sports Medicine and Orthopaedic Center
1325 East Fortification Street
Jackson, Mississippi 39202; and
Clinical Instructor
Department of Orthopaedic Surgery
University of Mississippi Medical Center
2500 North State Street
Jackson, Mississippi 39216

Mark H. Field, M.D.
Fellow
Mississippi Sports Medicine and Orthopaedic Center
1325 East Fortification Street
Jackson, Mississippi 39202

Leesa M. Galatz, M.D.
Chief Orthopaedic Resident
Department of Orthopaedic Surgery
The George Washington University Medical Center
2150 Pennsylvania Avenue, Northwest
Washington, D.C. 20037

Mark H. Getelman, M.D.
Attending Physician
Southern California Orthopedic Institute
6815 Noble Avenue
Van Nuys, California 91405

John R. Green III, M.D.
Assistant Professor
Department of Orthopaedic Surgery
Louisiana State University Medical Center
1501 Kings Highway
P.O. Box 33932
Shreveport, Louisiana 71130-3932

Keith Kenter, M.D.
Assistant Professor
Department of Orthopaedic Surgery
University of Missouri
One Hospital Drive
Columbia, Missouri 65212

Robert F. LaPrade, M.D.
Assistant Professor
Department of Orthopaedic Surgery
Sports Medicine Division
University of Minnesota
420 Delaware Street Southeast, Box 492
Minneapolis, Minnesota 55455

Pierre Mansat, M.D.
Fellow in Adult Reconstruction
Department of Orthopaedics
Mayo Graduate School of Medicine
Mayo Clinic
200 First Street, Southwest
Rochester, Minnesota 55905

George M. McCluskey III, M.D.
The Hughston Clinic
6262 Veterans Parkway
Columbus, Georgia 31908

Raymond J. Meyer, M.D.
Fellow
Minneapolis Sports Medicine Center
701 25th Avenue South, Suite 400
Minneapolis, Minnesota 55454

Robert J. Neviaser, M.D.
Professor and Chairman
Department of Orthopaedic Surgery
George Washington University
2150 Pennsylvania Avenue, Northwest
Washington, D.C. 20037; and
Chairman
Department of Orthopaedic Surgery
The George Washington University Medical Center
901 23rd Street, Northwest
Washington, D.C. 20037

Stephen J. O'Brien, M.D.
Associate Professor of Surgery
Department of Orthopaedics
Cornell University Medical College
525 East 68th Street
New York, New York 10021; and
Associate Attending Orthopaedic Surgeon
Sports Medicine and Shoulder Service
The Hospital for Special Surgery
535 East 70th Street
New York, New York 10021

Peter O'Rourke, M.D.
W. B. Carrell Memorial Clinic
2909 Lemmon Avenue
Dallas, Texas 75204

Michael J. Pagnani, M.D.
Director
Lipscomb Clinic Sports Medicine Fellowship
Tennessee Orthopaedic Alliance/The Lipscomb Clinic
4230 Harding Road, Suite 1000
Nashville, Tennessee 37205; and
Clinical Associate Professor
Departments of Orthopaedics and Rehabilitation
Vanderbilt University Medical Center
Nashville, Tennessee 37232

Helene Pavlov, M.D.
Professor
Department of Radiology
New York Hospital—Cornell University Medical Center
525 East 68th Street
New York, New York 10021; and
Radiologist-in-Chief
Department of Radiology
The Hospital for Special Surgery
535 East 70th Street
New York, New York 10021

David S. Pereira, M.D.
Chief Resident
Department of Orthopaedics
Hospital for Joint Diseases
301 East 17th Street
New York, New York 10003

Hollis G. Potter, M.D.
Associate Professor
Department of Radiology
Cornell University Medical Center
525 East 70th Street
New York, New York 10021; and
Chief
Magnetic Resonance Imaging Division
Department of Radiology
The Hospital for Special Surgery
535 East 70th Street
New York, New York 10021

Edgar K. Ragsdale, M.D.
Department of Orthopaedic Surgery
Southwest Washington Medical Center
400 Northeast Mother Joseph Place
Vancouver, Washington 98688; and
Northwest Surgical Specialists
505 Northeast 87th Avenue, Suite 160
Vancouver, Washington 98664-6440

Felix H. Savoie III, M.D.
Co-Director
Upper Extremity Service
Mississippi Sports Medicine and Orthopaedic Center
1325 East Fortification Street
Jackson, Mississippi 39202; and
Clinical and Associate Professor
Department of Orthopaedic Surgery
University of Mississippi School of Medicine
2500 North State Street
Jackson, Mississippi 39216

Peter T. Simonian, M.D.
Associate Professor
Department of Orthopaedic Surgery
University of Washington
Box 356500
Seattle, Washington 98195

John G. Skedros, M.D.
W. B. Carrell Memorial Clinic
2909 Lemmon Avenue
Dallas, Texas 75204

Stephen J. Snyder, M.D.
Shoulder Team
Southern California Orthopedic Institute
6815 Noble Avenue
Van Nuys, California 91405

Kevin P. Speer, M.D.
Associate Professor
Duke Division of Orthopedic Surgery
Duke University Medical Center
Box 3371
Durham, North Carolina 27710

William C. Standeffer, Jr., M.D.
Tennessee Orthopaedic Alliance/The Lipscomb Clinic
4230 Harding Road, Suite 1000
Nashville, Tennessee 37205; and
Departments of Orthopaedics and Rehabilitation
Vanderbilt University Medical Center
Nashville, Tennessee 37237

Michael E. Torchia, M.D.
Mayo Clinic and Mayo Foundation
200 First Street, Southwest
Rochester, Minnesota 55905

Michael S. Wall, M.D.
Sports Orthopaedic and Rehabilitation
2884 Sand Hill Road, Suite 110
Menlo Park, California 94025; and
Division of Sports Medicine
Stanford University Medical Center
Stanford Health Services
300 Pasteur Drive
Stanford, California 94305

Jon J.P. Warner, M.D.
Visiting Associate Professor
Department of Orthopaedic Surgery
Harvard Medical School; and
Chief
Harvard Shoulder Service
Department of Orthopaedic Surgery
Massachusetts General Hospital
55 Fruit Street
Boston, Massachusetts 02114

Russell F. Warren, M.D.
Professor of Surgery
Department of Orthopaedics
Cornell University Medical College
1300 York Avenue
New York, New York 10021; and
Surgeon-in-Chief
Department of Orthopaedics
The Hospital for Special Surgery
535 East 70th Street
New York, New York 10021

Kevin E. Wilk, P.T.
Adjunct Assistant Professor
Department of Physical Therapy
Marquette University
Milwaukee, Wisconsin 53201; and
National Director Research and Clinical Education
Healthsouth Rehabilitation Corporation
1201 Eleventh Avenue, South, # 100
Birmingham, Alabama 35205

Stephen J. Zabinski, M.D.
Assistant Clinical Professor
Department of Orthopaedic Surgery
Thomas Jefferson University
850 Walnut Street
Philadelphia, Pennsylvania 19107; and
Department of Orthopaedic Surgery
Shore Memorial Hospital
1 East New York Avenue
Somers Point, New Jersey 08224

Joshua M. Zimmerman, M.D.
W. B. Carrell Memorial Clinic
2909 Lemmon Avenue
Dallas, Texas 75204

Joseph D. Zuckerman, M.D.
Professor
Department of Orthopaedic Surgery
New York University School of Medicine
550 1st Avenue
New York, New York 10016; and
Chairman
Department of Orthopaedic Surgery
Hospital for Joint Diseases
301 East 17th Street
New York, New York 10003

Preface

Shoulder instability is one of the more complex and difficult conditions of the shoulder requiring treatment. Considerable progress has been made in our understanding of the pathophysiology of shoulder instability, making treatment more precise and appropriate. With this volume, we have attempted to organize the tremendous amount of available information concerning shoulder instability on the basis of etiology and methods of treatment.

The authors were selected based on their specific area of interest. The chapters address a number of issues, such as pathologic findings of shoulder instability, methods of addressing acute trauma instability, multidirectional instability, and the role of arthroscopy. Surgical techniques both arthroscopic and open are highlighted, and new techniques, such as capsular shrinkage are addressed. Shoulder instability procedures may have complications or result in failure. These issues are clearly discussed with treatment approaches illustrated.

We wish to thank every author for their diligent work in organizing and presenting the information for their area of interest in a concise format. We believe we have reached our original goal of providing the reader with methods for a better understanding of shoulder instability, and successful treatment algorithms.

Russell F. Warren, M.D.
Edward V. Craig, M.D.
David W. Altchek, M.D.

Section 1

Basic Science

The Unstable Shoulder,
edited by R.F. Warren, E.V. Craig, and D.W. Altchek.
Lippincott–Raven Publishers, Philadelphia © 1999.

CHAPTER 1

Introduction and Historical Aspects

Michael J. Pagnani

Those who cannot remember the past are condemned to repeat it

Santayana

Our current understanding of the unstable shoulder has resulted from an evolutionary process that dates back to antiquity. We have experienced a relative explosion in clinical and scientific information regarding shoulder instability during the past two decades, but we remain indebted to concepts that were promulgated long ago. The highlights of the historical evolution of principles of pathology, diagnosis, and treatment of shoulder instability are presented. In looking back toward the past, it is fascinating to find ideas that were put forth and then forgotten, only to be rediscovered in a different context centuries later.

THE UNSTABLE SHOULDER BEFORE THE BIRTH OF ORTHOPEDICS

Antiquity

The dislocated shoulder was recognized as a distinct affliction long before Nicolas Andry coined the term *l'orthopedie* in 1741. The Edwin Smith Papyrus, written around 1600 B.C., indicates that the ancient Egyptians were well versed in the treatment of fractures and dislocations of the shoulder (1). The tomb of the Egyptian sculptor Ipuy, constructed during the 12th century B.C., is adorned with an illustration that has been interpreted as representing the Kocher method of shoulder reduction (2) (Fig. 1).

The *Corpus Hippocrates* was composed by students of the Greek physician Hippocrates; it may be the remains of an ancient library of medical learning. Hippocrates lived in the 5th century B.C.; he was a contemporary of Socrates, Plato, and Aristotle. The classic "Hippocratic method" of shoulder reduction is described in the section On Articulations (3). This technique involved placement of the caretaker's heel in the patient's axilla to provide countertraction to a longitudinal force on the arm. Several other ways to facilitate reduction were mentioned as well. One method involved the use of the ambe, a piece of wood covered with soft cloth that was applied to the axilla to help relocate the humeral head. Other techniques included positioning of the shoulder over the rung of a ladder and the use of a chair as an adjunct to reduction. Hippocrates advocated passage of a hot iron through the inferior portion of the axilla to treat recurrent instability of the shoulder. The cautery was intended to induce scar formation over the anteroinferior shoulder. This is the earliest example of operative treatment for the unstable shoulder. Apparently all the dislocations that Hippocrates had encountered were "into the armpit," although it was admitted that they could possibly occur in other directions. Differentiation was made between traumatic and atraumatic instability. The writings stress that direct (rather than rotatory) forces should be used to reduce the shoulder, as rotatory forces were not natural. The teachings of Hippocrates remained the cornerstone of the treatment of the dislocated shoulder until the 18th century.

Contemporary advances in the other sciences in ancient Greece and Rome were applied to the treatment of shoulder instability. According to the Latin author Celsus, Heraclides of Tarentum was the first to adapt the reduction of dislocations to the mechanical inventions of Archimedes around the year 230 B.C. (4). The ancient Egyptians, Greeks, and Romans were not alone in their knowledge of techniques of shoulder reduction. The people of ancient India may have developed proficiency in the art of reduction before the Hippocratic era, and the Talmud also refers to the reduction of dislocations (5).

M. J. Pagnani: Tennessee Orthopaedic Alliance/The Lipscomb Clinic, Nashville, Tennessee 37205; and Departments of Orthopaedics and Rehabilitation, Vanderbilt University Medical Center, Nashville, Tennessee 37232.

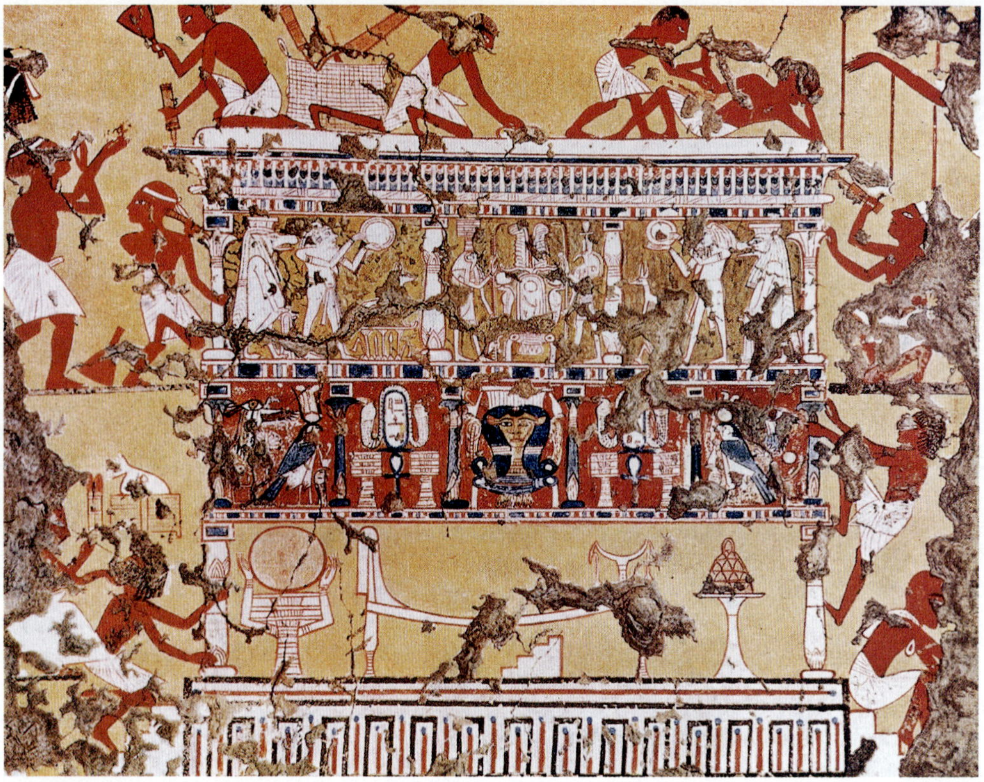

FIG. 1. The tomb of the Egyptian sculptor Ipuy. Artwork on the structure has been interpreted as representing the Kocher method of shoulder reduction. Constructed in the 12th century B.C., note the two figures in the upper right. (From Hussein M. Kocher's method is 3000 years old. *J Bone Joint Surg [Br]* 1968;50:669, with permission.)

The Middle Ages and Renaissance

Although little progress was made in Western medicine during the Dark Ages, an increase in medical knowledge occurred in the Middle East and in the Far East. The Arab physician Albucasis (936–1013) did not use machines to reduce dislocations, instead preferring the heel-in-axilla method. He noted that the shoulder could dislocate in three different directions (inferior, inward, and superior), but he believed that posterior dislocation was not possible. Like Hippocrates, he advocated treatment with cautery in some cases (6).

As a result of prohibitions regarding postmortem examination of the body, investigation into the pathoanatomy of the unstable shoulder was limited until relatively recent times. However, it has been reported that Roger (Ruggiero) of Palermo taught that capsular rupture was the primary lesion in acute dislocation in the 13th century (7).

Ambroise Pare, the French military surgeon who served during the 16th century under King Francois I, described several methods and devices for reduction of the dislocated shoulder. He was an advocate of the use of pulleys to achieve a mechanical advantage during reduction. Pare noted four directions of dislocations, but was not familiar with the posterior type (8,9). Woodcuttings from the era illustrate the methods of shoulder reduction of Pare and his contemporaries (10) (Fig. 2). Advances in the understanding and treatment of the unstable shoulder were relatively minor in the 2,000 years encompassing the eras of Hippocrates and Pare. The emergence of experimental science, anatomical dissection, and radiography, and the critical evaluation of treatment have led to a relative explosion of knowledge within the past 200 years.

DESCRIPTION OF TYPES OF INSTABILITY

Direction of Instability

Anterior dislocation of the shoulder was a recognized entity in the ancient world. Superior and inferior dislocations were apparently known to Albucasis and Pare. Langier is commonly credited with the first report of superior dislocation in 1839 (7,11) and Middledorf and Scharm with the first description of inferior dislocation in 1859 (7,12,13). However, Chelius provided what appears to be a clear description of the luxatio erecta associated with inferior dislocation in 1847. He wrote, ''In dislocation inwards, the elbow stands out from the trunk, and is inclined a little backwards; the direction of the arm corresponds to the middle of the collar bone. . . . Beneath the greater pectoral muscle is felt the protuberance of the head. . . .'' (14).

Malgaigne (15) stated that posterior dislocation was first reported in 1804). Sedillott presented a posterior dislocation in the English literature in 1834 (16,17), and Sir Astley Cooper described a posterior dislocation that occurred after an ep-

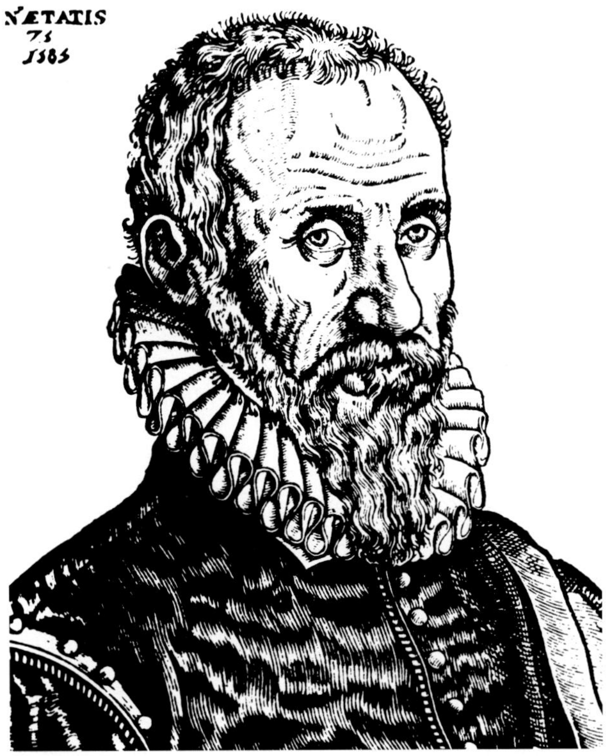

A

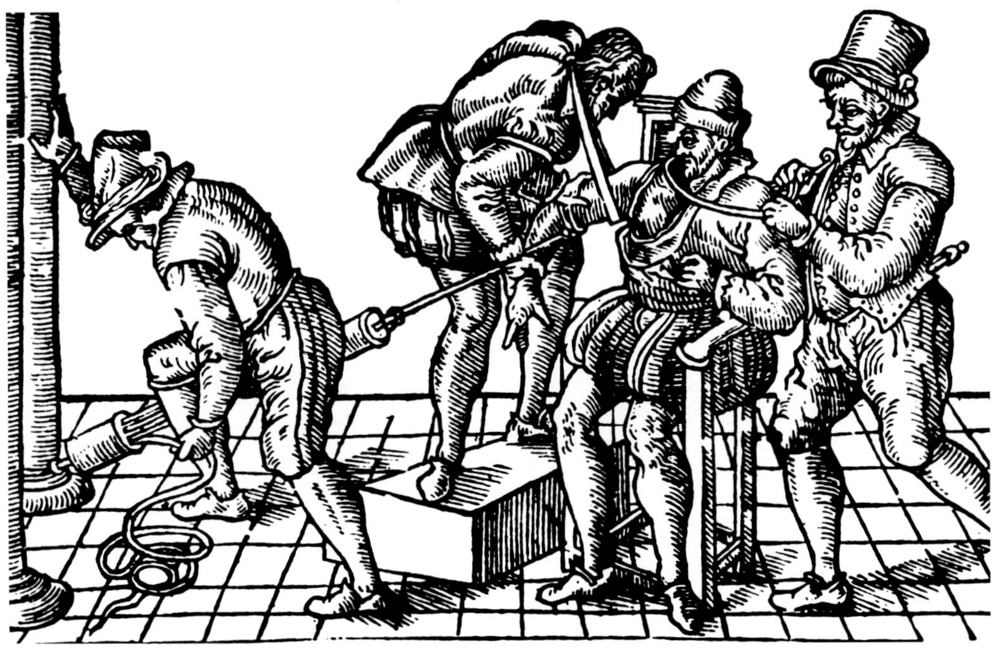

B

FIG. 2. A: Ambroise Pare. **B:** Woodcutting illustrating Pare's use of pulleys to facilitate reduction. (From Brockbank W, Griffiths D. Orthopaedic surgery in the sixteenth and seventeenth centuries. 1. Luxations of the shoulder. *J Bone Joint Surg [Br]* 1948;30B:365, with permission.)

ileptic seizure in 1839 (18). Malgaigne (15), in 1855, collected 37 cases of posterior dislocation. This series remains the largest of its type in the literature. In 1904, Moullin and Keith (19) reported a posterior dislocation that occurred when a patient made a backhand stroke in tennis. This case may be the first report of sports-related posterior instability.

Bateman (20), in 1972, described a group of patients with both anterior and posterior instability that was voluntary in character. In 1978, he expanded his description of this ''important but uncommon'' type of instability and noted that it was characterized by ''marked instability, with luxation occurring on a voluntary basis both anteriorly and posteriorly . . . the most important change is the downward drop of the humeral head in relation to the glenoid. The weight of the arm produces a definite furrow below the acromion as the arm sags at the side. Often both shoulders are involved . . . '' (21). Two years later, Neer and Foster (22) identified involuntary multidirectional instability as a separate entity that required alternative methods of diagnosis and treatment.

Atraumatic and Voluntary Instability

The fact that shoulder instability could occur in some patients without antecedent trauma was noted in the ancient world. In fact, the *Corpus Hippocrates* differentiated between traumatic and atraumatic instability (3). However, this differentiation was not stressed until Tavernier (23) distinguished atraumatic instability as a separate subtype in 1930. Rowe (24), in 1956, re-emphasized this concept and detailed its prognostic and therapeutic significance.

Volitional control of the unstable shoulder has important ramifications for treatment. According to Genovesi (25), Portal described a case of voluntary dislocation in 1722. In 1923, Reischauer (26) discussed voluntary dislocators in detail. Rowe et al. (27) renewed interest in this phenomenon in a 1973 paper.

Subluxation

Cooper (28) mentioned ''partial dislocation'' during the 1820s. Moseley (29), DePalma (30), and Bateman (31), in their books published in the 1940s and 1950s, reintroduced the concept of anterior subluxation and discussed posterior subluxation as well. Blazina and Saltzman (32) as well as LeClerc (33) brought attention to phenomenon of anterior subluxation in 1969. Rowe and Zarins (34) described the ''dead-arm'' syndrome associated with anterior subluxation in 1981. Hawkins et al. (35) and Fronek et al. (36) reported on two series of patients with recurrent posterior subluxation during the 1980s.

PATHOLOGY

True understanding of the pathologic basis of shoulder instability was greatly dependent on the postmortem examination of the shoulder. As a result of cultural and religious prohibitions, the dissection of human cadavers was not widely practiced in medical schools until the time of Vesalius during the 16th century (37). There is no evidence of the formal dissection of human specimens in the *Corpus Hippocrates.* During the late 1700s, Bonn was one of the first individuals to perform cadaveric dissections on shoulder dislocations (38,39). In ensuing years, several theories were developed regarding the primary pathologic lesion in the unstable shoulder.

Pathoanatomy of Anterior Instability

Capsular Tears and Excess Capsular Volume

Two prominent physicians made significant observations with regard to the pathology of the unstable shoulder during the first half of the 19th century. Sir Astley Cooper, surgeon to the English King George IV and a student of John Hunter, dissected a cadaveric specimen with a recent dislocation and found that the capsular ligament was torn on whole length of inner side of glenoid cavity and that ''the tendon of the subscapularis was also extensively torn'' (28) (Fig. 3A, B). Joseph-Francois Malgaigne of France suggested that dislocation was combined with complete or near-complete rupture of the capsule and that recurrence was due to enlargement of

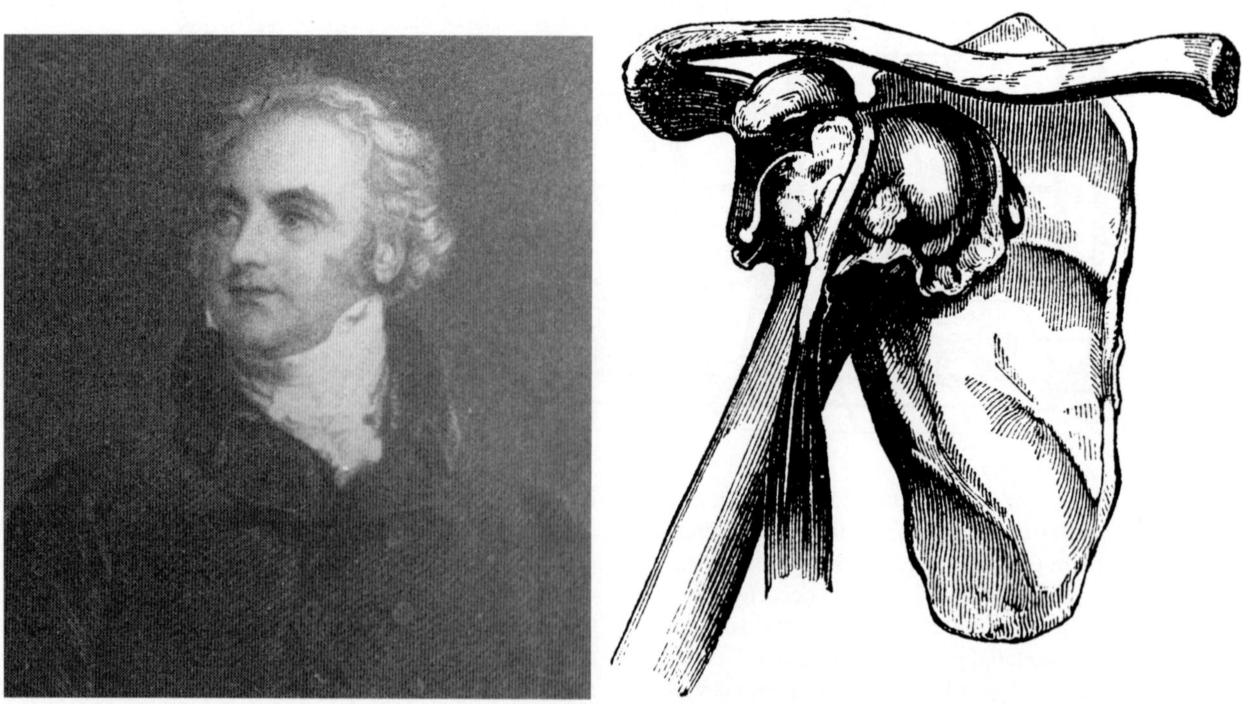

A B

FIG. 3. A: Sir Astley Cooper. **B:** Illustration from Cooper's dissection of a dislocated shoulder showing capsular rupture. (From Cooper A. *Treatise on dislocations and on fractures in the joints.* 1822, with permission.)

the joint cavity after the healing of a capsular tear (15). Malgaigne believed that, on occasion, the capsule was capable of extraordinary stretch without rupture. During the same era, Chelius of Germany wrote that damage was "for the most part restricted to tearing of the capsular ligament" (14). In 1883, supporting the leading theory of the age, Popke (40) believed that capsular tearing from the glenoid was the inciting event in recurrent dislocation.

In 1874, Joessel (41,42) proposed that a capsular tear at the insertion of the supraspinatus and infraspinatus tendons was the essential lesion in recurrent anterior instability. He hypothesized that tearing of rotator cuff insertion allowed increased excursion of the humeral head upon the glenoid. Joessel also noted marked increases in capsular volume in cases of dislocation.

Perthes (43), in 1906, held that Joessel's finding of disruption of the capsule near the rotator cuff insertion was consistent with one of two major mechanisms of shoulder dislocation. He noted that these types of capsular tears were often associated with a tear of the rotator cuff or with avulsion of the greater tuberosity. These findings are suggestive of a posterior mechanism of dislocation that is seen more commonly in association with fractures.

Thomas of Philadelphia wrote a series of articles between 1909 and 1925 (44–47) that stressed that the primary pathologic entity was capsular tearing, with resultant laxity in the capsule caused by scar formation at the site of the rent. He was able to simulate anterior dislocations in cadavers and invariably found a tear in the anterior and lower part of the capsule. Thomas disagreed with the hypothesis that a capsular tear at the humeral attachment of the rotator cuff was an important cause of recurrent instability.

Shearing of the lateral capsule from the humeral neck was described by Nicola (48) in 1942. Bach et al. (49) reported similar findings in 1988, and noted that simple closure of the defect restored stability to the shoulder.

Stripping of the Capsule and Labrum from the Anterior Glenoid Neck

In 1880, Eve (50) made several important observations after examining a postmortem specimen derived from a patient with previously normal shoulder function who had sustained a dislocation in a train accident. Although he stated that he had "been unable to find on record a single case of dislocation of the humerus in which the joint was not opened," Eve found that capsular rupture was not present in his case. Instead, he noted that the capsule was stripped off the anterior border of the glenoid but remained continuous with the periosteum (50,51). In 1881, Stimson (52) reported another case of a dislocation without capsular rupture. Citing Eve's report in 1887, Caird (51) argued that an anterior dislocation could be intracapsular in some cases and not always associated with capsular tearing.

Broca and Hartmann (53), in 1890, reported their finding of capsular-periosteal separation at the anterior glenoid neck and labral detachment in an autopsy specimen (Fig. 4). In this report, they concurred with Eve and Caird in stating that, contrary to earlier beliefs, the pathologic lesion occupied an intracapsular position. Perthes (1906) considered separation of the anterior capsule from the glenoid to be one of two major mechanisms of anterior dislocation, noting that it was rare for the glenohumeral ligaments to tear completely (54,55) (Fig. 5).

The importance of the anterior capsular stripping in relation to the labrum and the bony glenoid was stressed in the English literature by A.S. Blundell Bankart (1879–

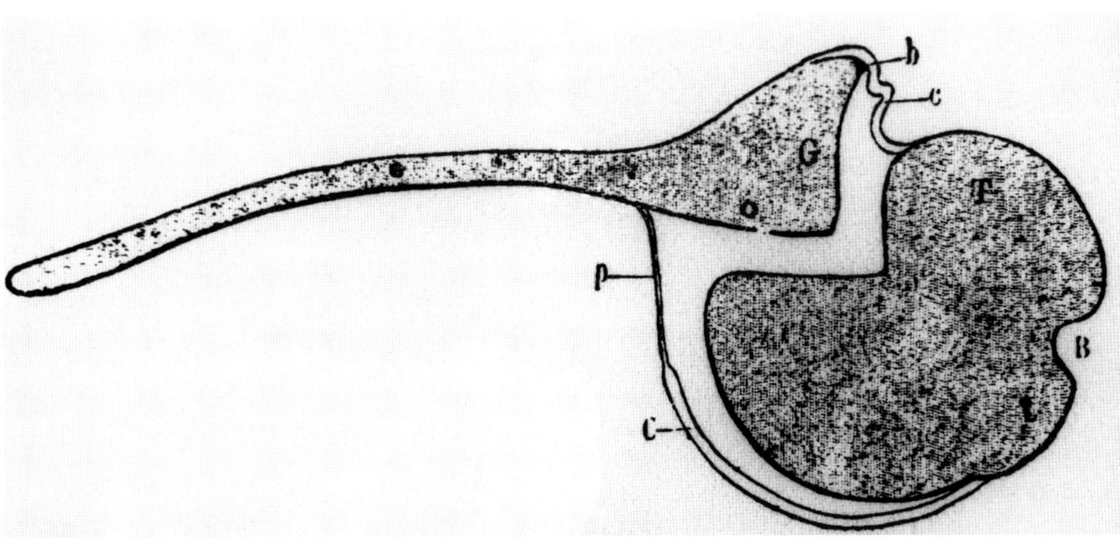

FIG. 4. Drawing from Broca and Hartmann's paper showing stripping of the anterior capsule from the glenoid. p,periosteum; c,capsule. (From Broca A, Hartmann H. Contribution a l'etude des luxations de l'epaule [luxations dites incompletes, decollements periostiques, luxationes directes et luxationes indirectes]. *Bull Soc Anat Paris* 1890;ixv:312–336, with permission.)

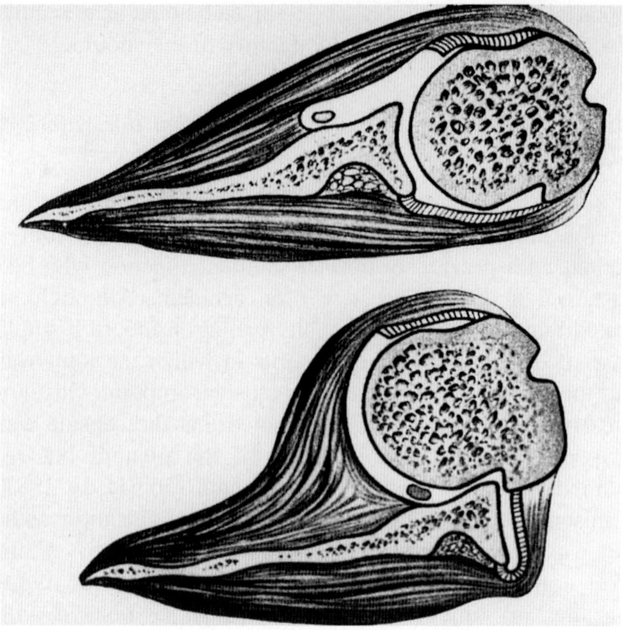

FIG. 5. Illustration from Perthes' papers demonstrating detachment of the anterior glenoid and labrum in association with an anterior dislocation. (From Perthes G. Ueber operationen der habituellen Schulterluxation. *Dtsch Z Chir* 1906;85:199, with permission.)

1951) of London, beginning in 1923 (56–59) (Fig. 6). Several investigators have interpreted Bankart's description of the essential lesion in recurrent anterior instability as being detachment of the glenoid labrum. However, in his first article on recurrent anterior dislocation (56), he stated that the essential feature is the detachment of the capsule from the fibrocartilaginous glenoid ligament. In this context, he appears to refer to the labrum as the glenoid ligament and, contrary to the interpretations of earlier writers, he is noting that capsular detachment from the labrum is the essential defect. He later reiterated (58) that "The only abnormal laxity that is encountered is due to the fact that the capsule is detached from the glenoid margin," and then stated in 1948 that "it may be that in the past I have laid too much stress upon the role of the fibrocartilage or glenoid labrum. This may be torn from bone or the capsule may be torn from it" (59).

Bost and Inman (60), Moseley and Overgard (61), Jakobsson (62), and Townley (63) subsequently showed that detachment of the labrum was insufficient to cause anterior instability unless it was accompanied by disruption of the anterior capsule. Lippett et al. (64) recently showed that resection of the anterior labrum reduced resistance to anterior translation by 20% in shoulders that had been subjected to a compressive load.

The Glenohumeral Ligaments

The discovery of the glenohumeral ligaments and the coracohumeral ligament has been attributed to Schlemm (65). Schlemm (1853) examined the ligaments in cadavera by approaching the joint from posterior and resecting the humeral head. Fick (66), in 1904, proposed that these ligaments were important for joint stability. Six years later, Delorme (67) made a detailed anatomical description of the glenohumeral ligament system based on cadaveric experiments in which he induced dislocations (Fig. 7). He noted that the inferior glenohumeral ligament tightened with external rotation and abduction of the humerus, preventing further translation of the humeral head upon the glenoid. Delorme also considered the middle glenohumeral ligament an important stabilizer in the midrange of abduction. Many years later, Turkel et al. (68), of the Hospital for Special Surgery (HSS) in New York, found the inferior glenohumeral ligament to be the primary static restraint against anterior instability in the abducted shoulder. O'Brien et al. (69), also of the HSS, have shown that the inferior glenohumeral ligament is a complex structure with functionally disparate anterior and posterior bands. Other investigators have noted that the middle ligament is an important secondary stabilizer in the midrange of abduction.

Muscular Forces

The belief that the pathoanatomy of shoulder instability was largely confined to the capsule was by no means a universal one. As mentioned earlier, Joessel (41,70) and Perthes (43,54) implicated tears of the rotator cuff as an

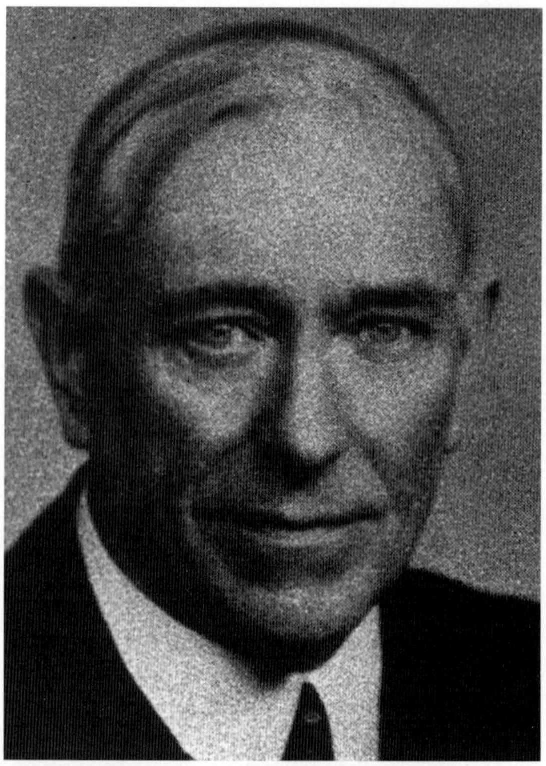

FIG. 6. A.S. Blundell Bankart.

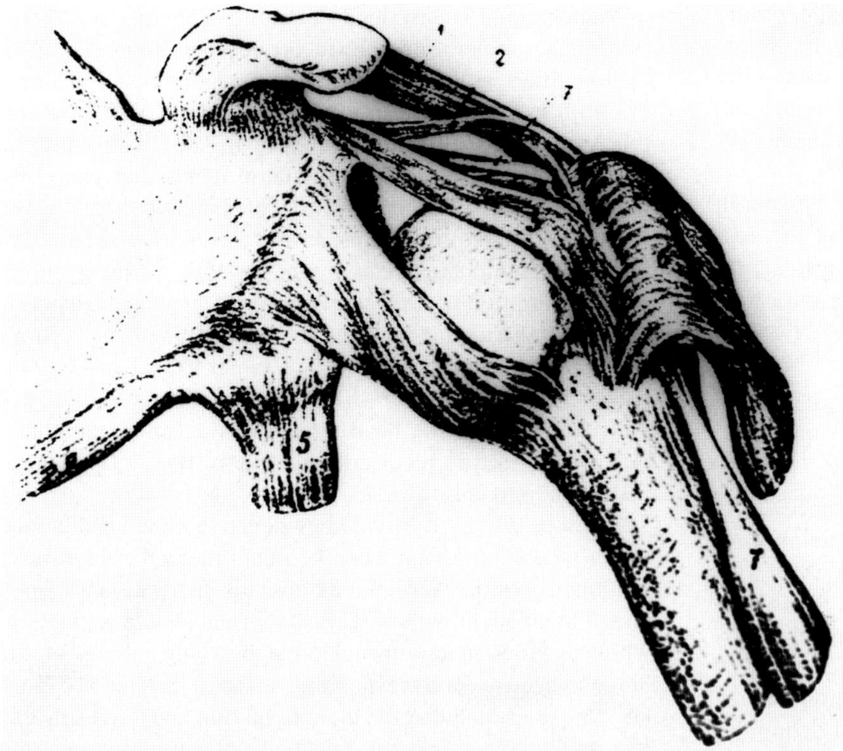

FIG. 7. Drawing of the glenohumeral ligaments from Delorme's paper: *1*, coracohumeral ligament; *2*, superior glenohumeral ligament; *3*, middle glenohumeral ligament; *4*, inferior glenohumeral ligament. (From Delorme. Die Hemmungsbander des Schultergelenks und ihre Bedeutung fur die Schulterluxation. *Arch Klin Chir* 1910;92:79–101, with permission.)

etiologic factor during the late 19th and early 20th centuries (Fig. 8). This mechanism is consistent with dislocations that occur in older patients in whom associated cuff tears are frequent. More recently, Jobe (71) has described damage to the rotator cuff in throwers with instability.

In 1921, Sever of Boston wrote, ''It is well recognized that the capsule is insignificant'' (72). Sever believed that dislocation was due to ''muscle imbalance.'' Stevens, also of Boston, echoed these sentiments in 1926 when he stated that the surgeon should ''disregard the capsule of the joint, because the capsule is a loose bag'' (73). DePalma (1950) attributed a central role to the subscapularis muscle and tendon that he believed were disrupted during dislocation. In his words, ''This writer is of the opinion that capsular, labral lesions and humeral head defects are not the primary causative agents of recurrent dislocations. . . . Neuromuscular imbalance, chiefly of the short rotator muscles, is the most important single caus-

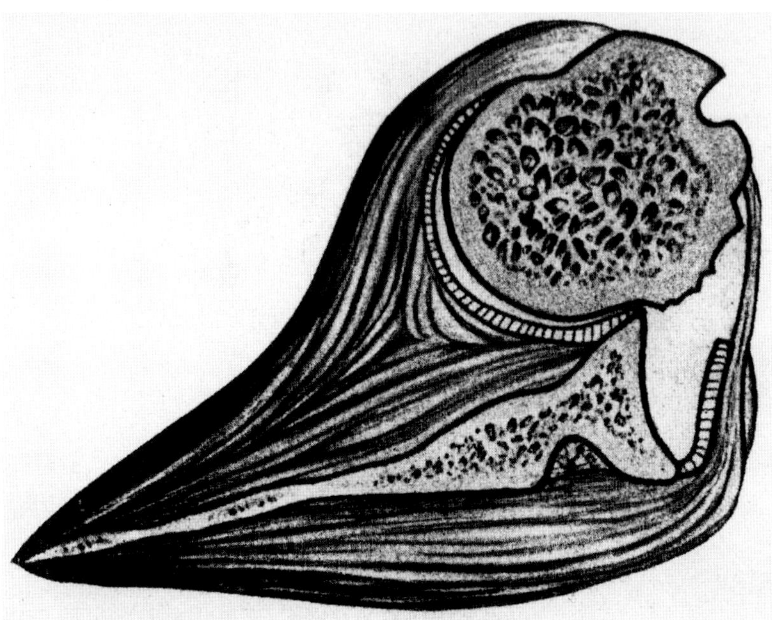

FIG. 8. Illustration from Perthes' papers demonstrating detachment of the anterior glenoid and labrum in association with an anterior dislocation. (From Perthes' G. Ueber operationen der habituellen Schulterluxation. *Dtsch Z Chir 1906;85:199, with permission*)

ative factor'' (30). Jens (1964) implicated an abnormally proximal insertion site of the subscapularis tendon as the primary lesion in selected cases of anterior instability (74). Symeonides, in 1972, considered lengthening and laxity of the subscapularis muscle to be the dominant factor in most cases of anterior instability (75).

Cain and McKernan and their associates in Pittsburgh have recently shown that simulated contraction of the posterior rotator cuff reduces strain in the anterior capsule (76–78). However, these investigators note that the cuff may not be sufficient to prevent instability in the face of extensive capsulolabral damage.

Negative Intra-articular Pressure

Humphry (79), in 1858, recognized the importance of the relative vacuum within the joint space in maintaining joint stability. Humphry credited Weber and Weber (80) with performing the first experiments that confirmed the role of atmospheric pressure in the stabilization of synovial joints. Aeby (81), in 1876, and Fick (66), 1904, also called attention to this phenomenon. In recent years, attention has returned to the role of atmosphere pressure in stabilizing the shoulder and to the effect of capsular venting on translation patterns (82–85).

Bony Alignment and Defects of the Humeral Head

Some investigators have proposed that inherent abnormalities in the bony structures of the shoulder may predispose to instability. Saha of India examined the influence of glenoid size, tilt, and version and humeral torsion on shoulder instability during the late 1950s and 1960s (86–89).

Malgaigne (15) described flattening of the posterior portion of the humeral head in recurrent dislocators and cited Denonvilliers as being the first to note this lesion. Calandriello has credited Curling with the earliest description of this lesion in 1837 (90). Flower (91), in 1861, noted defects in posterolateral portions of humeral heads that were obtained from 41 specimens of dislocated shoulders that were housed in London museums. In his words, ''. . . where the head of the humerus rests upon the edge of the glenoid fossa, absorption occurs, and a groove is evacuated, usually between the articular head and the greater tuberosity.'' Similar bony defects were found by Cramer (92), Kraske (93), Kuster (94), and Popke (40). At the time, some investigators believed that the head defect was a genetic anomaly that predisposed to recurrent dislocation. Bazy (95) continued to support this view in 1918.

In 1880, Eve (50) provided evidence that the head defect was a secondary lesion when he noted the defect in a fresh specimen obtained 12 h after a traumatic dislocation was sustained in a patient with previously normal shoulder function who was killed in a train accident. Observing a defect in the humeral head and a corresponding lesion of the glenoid, Lobker (96) suggested that the glenoid margin had a wearing effect on the posterior surface of the head caused by pressure erosion as the humeral head dislocated anteriorly. In 1887, Caird (51) was able to produce the head defect by causing forceful dislocations in cadaveric specimens (Fig. 9). He believed that subcoracoid dislocation was ''always associated with an indentation fracture of the head of the humerus caused by the dense, hard lip of the glenoid.'' Hermodsson (97), in 1934, noted that the head defect was seen in primary as well as recurrent dislocations. He reiterated that the defect was the compressive result, not the cause, of instability. Townley (63), in 1950, showed that an isolated humeral head defect

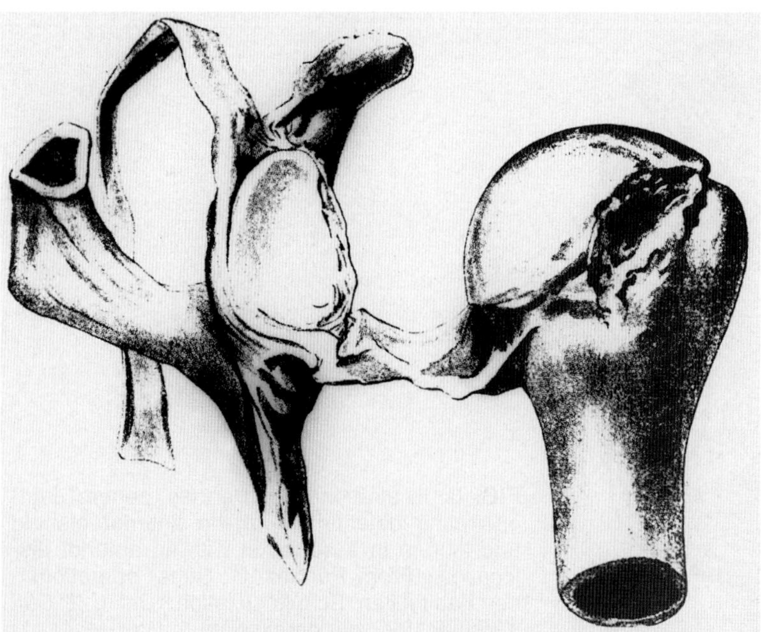

FIG. 9. Caird's depiction of a defect in the humeral head produced by a forceful dislocation in a cadaveric specimen. (From Caird F. The shoulder joint in relation to certain dislocations and fractures. *Edinb Med J* 1887;32:708, with permission.)

was insufficient to cause instability unless it was accompanied by disruption of the anterior capsule.

Pathoanatomy of Posterior Instability

Reports regarding the pathological basis of posterior instability are much less common. T.T. Thomas implicated excessive capsular volume in its pathogenesis in the early 20th century (47). M.A. Thomas (98), in 1937, described an impaction fracture of anteromedial head in association with posterior dislocation. Rowe and Yee (99), in 1944, found posterior capsular-periosteal separation in two patients during operative stabilization for posterior instability. Warren et al. (100), in 1984, showed that the posterior and anterosuperior capsule were the primary static restraints against posterior instability. These findings were confirmed by the work of Oveson and Nielson (101).

Pathoanatomy of Inferior Instability

In 1942, Pettersson published an arthrographic study in which he noted anteroinferior capsular dilation in recurrent dislocators (39). During the 1950s, Bateman (31) and Moseley (29) recognized that capsular laxity was present in some unstable shoulders. In their description of multidirectional instability, Neer and Foster (22) implicated abnormal capsular volume in the production of the inferior component of instability. Two years earlier, Bateman (21) had reported on a group of patients in whom ''. . . the usual capsular signs are not present, but rather there is a total laxity frontward, backward, and downward.''

Basmajian and Bazant (102), in 1959, had implicated the importance of the superior capsule and coracohumeral ligament in preventing ''downward'' translation of the adducted shoulder. Oveson and Nielson (103) reported similar findings in 1985. Recently, Warner, Bowen, and co-workers found that the superior glenohumeral ligament was the primary static restraint against inferior translation in the adducted arm (85,104,105). In the abducted arm, the inferior glenohumeral ligament became the primary restraint against inferior subluxation.

The Rotator Interval

The term ''rotator interval'' was introduced by Neer (106) in 1970 to indicate the space between the supraspinatus and subscapularis tendons. Nobuhara and Ikeda (107) of Japan, in 1987, noted that the capsule in this region was sometimes absent, creating an abnormally large space in the anterosuperior capsule. These investigators implicated such a lesion in the etiology of excessive inferior translation. Earlier, Rowe and Zarins (34) had found that a similar lesion was associated with anterior instability. Recently, Harryman et al. (108) found that the rotator interval played a significant role in preventing both inferior and posterior translation.

Summary

As these historical developments are reviewed, the comments made by Dickson et al. (109) in 1953 provide a wry assessment of the existing literature regarding the pathology of the unstable shoulder: ''Much of the confusion that exists on this subject arises from the fact that many authors have dogmatically limited themselves to consideration of one particular pathologic change as the sole cause of recurrent dislocation of the shoulder.'' With time, it became apparent that no single ''essential lesion'' was responsible for all cases of shoulder instability.

OPERATIVE TREATMENT

During the Middle Ages, practitioners of surgery held a much lower status than their contemporaries, the Doctors of Physick. Doctors of Physick generally were university-trained masters of the classical languages in which medical knowledge from the past had been preserved. Surgery was not studied in medieval universities in part because of prohibitions on the shedding of blood and also because its manual nature made it less dignified.

During the 16th century in Great Britain, practitioners of surgery were organized into a guild of Barber-Surgeons with a distinction within the guild prohibiting the barber from acting as surgeon and forbidding surgeons from shaving anyone. During the 17th century, a formal period of surgical training was required. Not until 1745 did the surgeons manage to secede from the barbers.

Reduction Methods

Until the latter part of the 19th century, an ''operation'' for shoulder instability usually consisted of an attempt at closed reduction that was performed by the ''surgeon.'' Techniques of reduction became quite sophisticated and were widely discussed among practitioners as the art of ''surgery.'' Hugh Owen Thomas of Liverpool (1834–1891) came from a family of reputable bone-setters and combined this knowledge with formal surgical training to become the leader of orthopedic surgery in Great Britain (110). In the words of Thomas, ''[in the] period before anaesthetics were commonly used during the reduction of dislocations of the shoulder-joint, injury to the axillary artery, the formation of traumatic aneurism [sic], injury to the axillary plexus of nerves and consequent palsy of the upper extremity and fracture of the humerus were not uncommon mishaps, that followed after attempts to reduce dislocations of the shoulder'' (111). The old literature is replete with reports of axillary artery and vein damage after reduction of the dislocated shoulder (16,112). Stimson (112) reviewed the literature in 1885 and found dozens of reported cases of iatrogenic damage to the axillary vessels during attempts at shoulder reduction.

Attempts at reduction could also result in the loss of limb or life. Guerin of France reported that when four assistants applied traction to the elbow with "a simultaneous jerk, the forearm was pulled out of the elbow and remained in the hands of the assistants" (16,29). South (44), in 1847, provided a revealing insight into the primitive means available for assistance with a difficult reduction during the preanesthetic era:

> The two great auxiliaries in reducing dislocations are bleeding and nauseating doses of tartar emetic. The bleeding should always be made in a large stream from one or both arms, according to [the patient's] apparent strength, and whilst the patient stands upright, till he feels faint, which is best determined by his bursting into a cold, clammy sweat, and unless carefully noticed he drops on the floor before the surgeon is aware. . . . Frequently the excitement of pain revives him, and it is then advisable to give him a grain of tartar emetic every ten minutes, so as to keep him in a constant state of nausea till reduction is effected. If the dislocation be of long standing it is well to reduce the patient's strength by spare diet and purging for two or three days previous to the operation; and on the same morning to give him nauseating doses of tartar emetic for some hours prior to the extension. . . .

Even the introduction of chloroform did not spare the physician from occasional mishaps. A Mr. Taylor of Victoria injured his arm in an accident on May 12, 1883. The next day, his pain had largely resolved, but he continued to complain of stiffness of the shoulder. His physicians made the diagnosis of a fracture-dislocation. The following account was taken from the *New Zealand Herald* and reprinted in the *New York Medical Journal* on October 6, 1883:

> An attempt at reduction of the dislocation by pulley extension at the wrist and countertraction in the axilla was made, the patient being under the influence of chloroform. After extension had been made for some time the tissues in the axilla gave way; the wound thus made was sewed up; haemorrhage then occurred, that was controlled by pressure, but next day the limb was found to be gangrenous and was amputated; death occurred within twenty-four hours. A coroner's inquest was held on the case, and a verdict of "death from misadventure, no blame being attached to the doctors" was returned.

The Techniques of Hippocrates and Pare

As discussed earlier, the reduction methods of Hippocrates dominated the scene for 2,000 years and were mimicked by Pare. Cooper, (28), in 1822, continued to advocate the heel-in-axilla method in most cases of dislocation. Cooper occasionally used the ambe and pulleys, although he did not recommend them for general use. Hugh Owen Thomas (111) designed a special chair that he used to facilitate the reduction of dislocated shoulders (Fig. 10). Hippocrates had described a similar use of a chair 2,000 years earlier.

Overhead Reduction Techniques

In 1762, Charles White of Manchester, England, described the use of overhead traction and pulleys to suspend the body in the air and facilitate reduction (113). Malgaigne

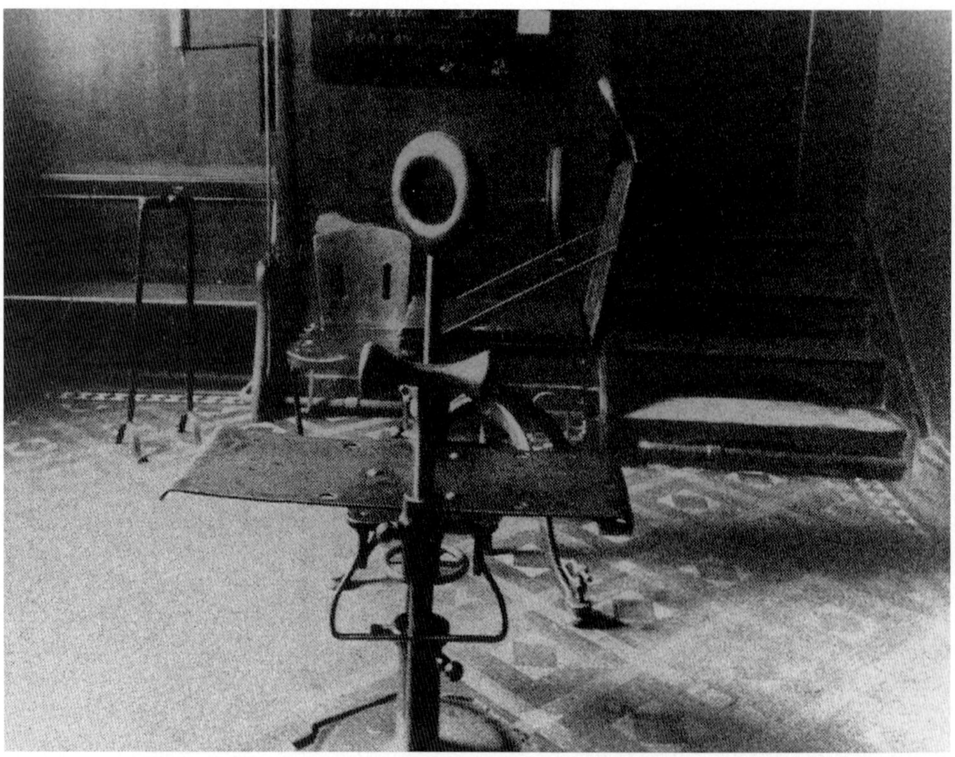

FIG. 10. Chair used by H.O. Thomas to facilitate reduction. (From Aitken D. *Hugh Owen Thomas: his principles and practice.* London: Oxford University Press, 1935;81–82, with permission.)

(114), in 1832, advocated a less traumatic method of overhead reduction that was originally described by LeMothe during the late 18th century. Milch (115) of New York, in 1938, reported on a technique of reduction that featured overhead abduction and external rotation. This method has also been attributed to Sir Robert Jones, who was the nephew of Hugh Owen Thomas (116).

Gravity Reduction Techniques

South, in 1847, mentioned a technique of gravity reduction that involved "tiring the opposing muscles, by attaching a trifling weight for some hours" (14). He attributed the technique to Henry Cline (the son of Sir Astley Cooper's mentor).

Lewis Stimson (117) of New York credited Cole, a house officer at the Chambers Street Hospital, for coming up with the gravity method of reduction that now bears Stimson's name. Stimson's son Henry was the American Secretary of War under Franklin Roosevelt during World War II.

Rotational Techniques

The classic Hippocratic teachings have proscribed rotational forces in attaining closed reduction, and such forces were apparently avoided until Emil Theodur Kocher of Switzerland described a leverage technique for reduction in 1870 (118) (Fig. 11). This method featured forward flexion of the externally rotated arm, followed by internal rotation of the humerus. Kocher based his method on cadaveric studies that showed that the coracohumeral ligament relaxed with flexion of the arm, allowing the humeral head to be returned to the glenoid fossa.

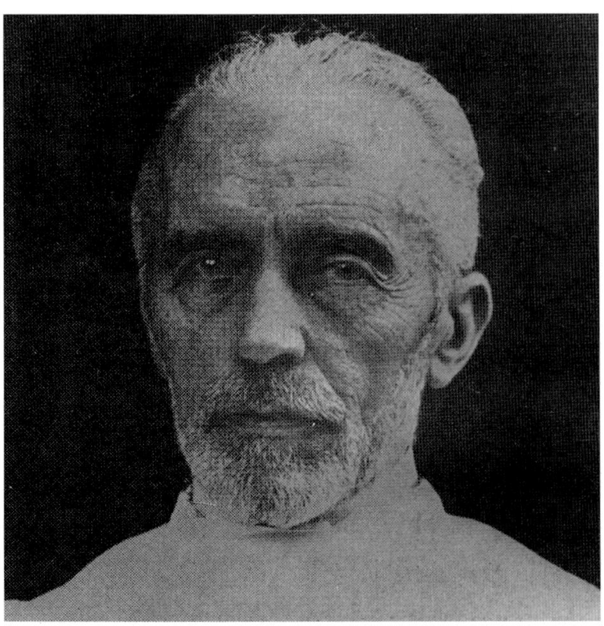

FIG. 11. Emil Theodur Kocher

Scapular Rotation

Kuhn (119) described manipulation of the scapula to facilitate reduction in *Paris Medicale* in 1876. In 1982, Anderson et al. (120) reintroduced the concept of scapular rotation. In this technique, the vertebral border of the scapula is lifted away from the thorax to create scapular winging. This manuever changes the apparent version of the glenoid, allowing the humeral head to reduce.

Operative Procedures for Anterior Instability

Early Attempts

As mentioned earlier, Hippocrates and Albucasis attempted to induce scar formation and stability in recurrent dislocators by placing a cautery in the region of the anterior capsule. Weinhold and Dieffenbach performed subcutaneous anterior tenotomy to aid in the reduction of chronic dislocations during the early 1800s. Malgaigne (15) practiced subcutaneous capsulotomy in hopes of inducing an inflammatory contraction of the capsule to stop recurrent dislocation a few decades later.

In general, invasive surgery had few successes before the mid-19th century. The advancement of anesthesia (with the administration of ether and chloroform during the 1840s) and the introduction of principles of antisepsis by Pasteur and Lister during the 1860s led to a more invasive approach to the surgical treatment of shoulder instability. Albert of Vienna performed arthrodesis of the shoulder for recurrent instability around 1880 (121,122). During the same period, Cramer (92), Kuster (94), and Popke (40) described resection of the humeral head in the treatment of recurrent dislocation. Popke (40) reported that Volkmann also advocated head resection.

Capsulorraphy (Fig. 12 A, B)

In 1883, Arpad Gerster (123), a Hungarian-born surgeon who was trained in Austria and who practiced in New York, attempted capsulorraphy on a 20-year-old patient named Jennie. The patient had sustained a traumatic dislocation that was reducible but unstable despite 5 weeks of cast immobilization. Gerster removed a 1½-inch-wide, semielliptical piece of anterior capsule and then reapproximated the capsule. The patient apparently became septic shortly after surgery, and the wound was treated in an open fashion after removal of the sutures. Fortunately, Gerster (124) reported that Jennie's movements promised to become normal during the postoperative period. Bardenheuer performed capsulorraphy in 1886. He reported no postoperative recurrence after 4 months.

Ricard (125) of France is often credited with the first capsulorraphy procedure, which he reported during the early 1890s. He believed that the most important pathologic factor was enlargement of the capsule. He did not open the joint. Instead, he determined the integrity of intra-articular

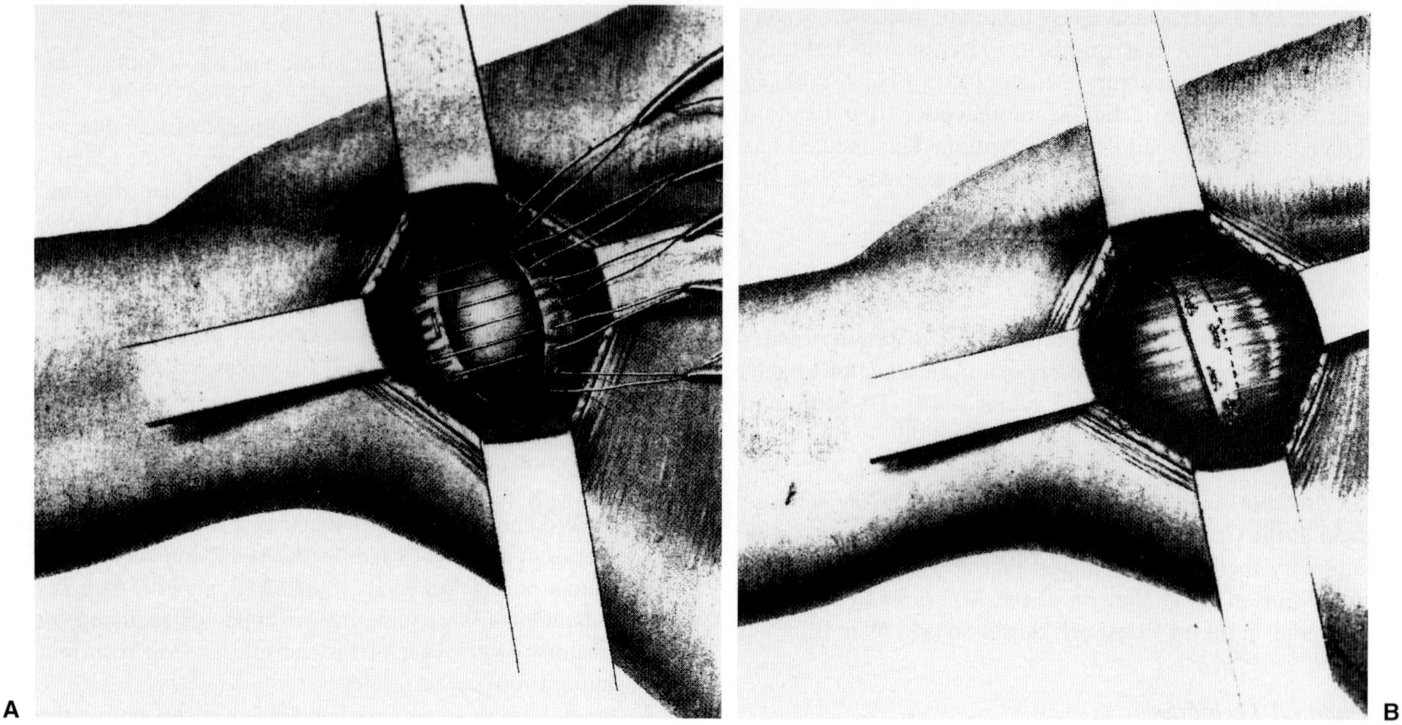

FIG. 12. A, B: Capsulorraphy as performed in the early 20th century. (From MacAusland W. Recurrent dislocation of the shoulder with report of cases. *Surg Gynecol Obstet* 1924;38:739–747, with permission.)

structures by palpation and then plicated the capsule. Burrell and Lovett (126) of Boston popularized capsulorraphy in the United States with their report of six cases in 1897. Their technique was similar to that described by Gerster. Samter (127), in 1900, devised a technique of capsular exposure that involved division of the subscapularis tendon before capsulorraphy. Other investigators had simply reefed the inferior capsule or had lifted the subscapularis tendon from the capsule without dividing it.

Thomas of Philadelphia strongly argued for repairs aimed at the capsule during the second and third decades of the 20th century (44–47). He approached the capsule through an axillary incision that he preferred to the deltopectoral approach. He reported postoperative recurrence occurred in 8 of 18 shoulders in epileptic patients and in 11 of 33 shoulders in nonepileptics. Thomas believed that recurrence postoperatively was not necessarily a bad thing, as it resulted in further scar formation. Interestingly, Paul B. Magnuson, one of the architects of the Magnuson-Stack operation, served as an intern under Thomas during this period. Magnuson did not share Thomas's optimistic outlook with regard to capsular repairs. Looking back in 1945, Magnuson stated that plication of the capsule was apparently not very successful (128). Henderson (129) of the Mayo Clinic abandoned capsulorraphy shortly after reporting a 50% recurrence rate in 1921.

Interest in capsulorraphy was renewed by the concept of inferior capsular shift for multidirectional instability as described by Neer and Foster (22) in 1980. Whereas Neer and Foster advocated shift of the lateral side of the capsule, Warren devised a T-plasty medial capsular shift. Rockwood (7) has advocated a central capsular plication similar to that performed by Gerster more than 100 years ago.

Procedures that involve Division, Shortening, or Transfer of Muscle

Muller (130), in 1898, shortened the external rotators in an attempt to prevent recurrent anterior dislocation. Clairmont and Ehrlich (131), in 1909, developed a myoplasty for anterior instability in which they passed the posterior part of deltoid muscle beneath the subcapital part of the humeral shaft and reattached the muscle to the coracoid process (Fig. 13A-C). According to Armour (132), Sir Robert Jones performed a similar procedure during the same time period. Ollerenshaw (133) described a muscle flap like the Clairmont-Ehrlich procedure in the English literature in 1920.

In 1913, Young (134) of the University of Pennsylvania, attributing instability to "deforming muscle forces," transferred the pectoralis major to the deltoid and sectioned the latissimus dorsi. He credited Allis with suggesting this operation. An alternative muscle transfer was performed by Finsterer (135) who, in 1917, brought part of the biceps and the coracobrachialis from coracoid and transferred

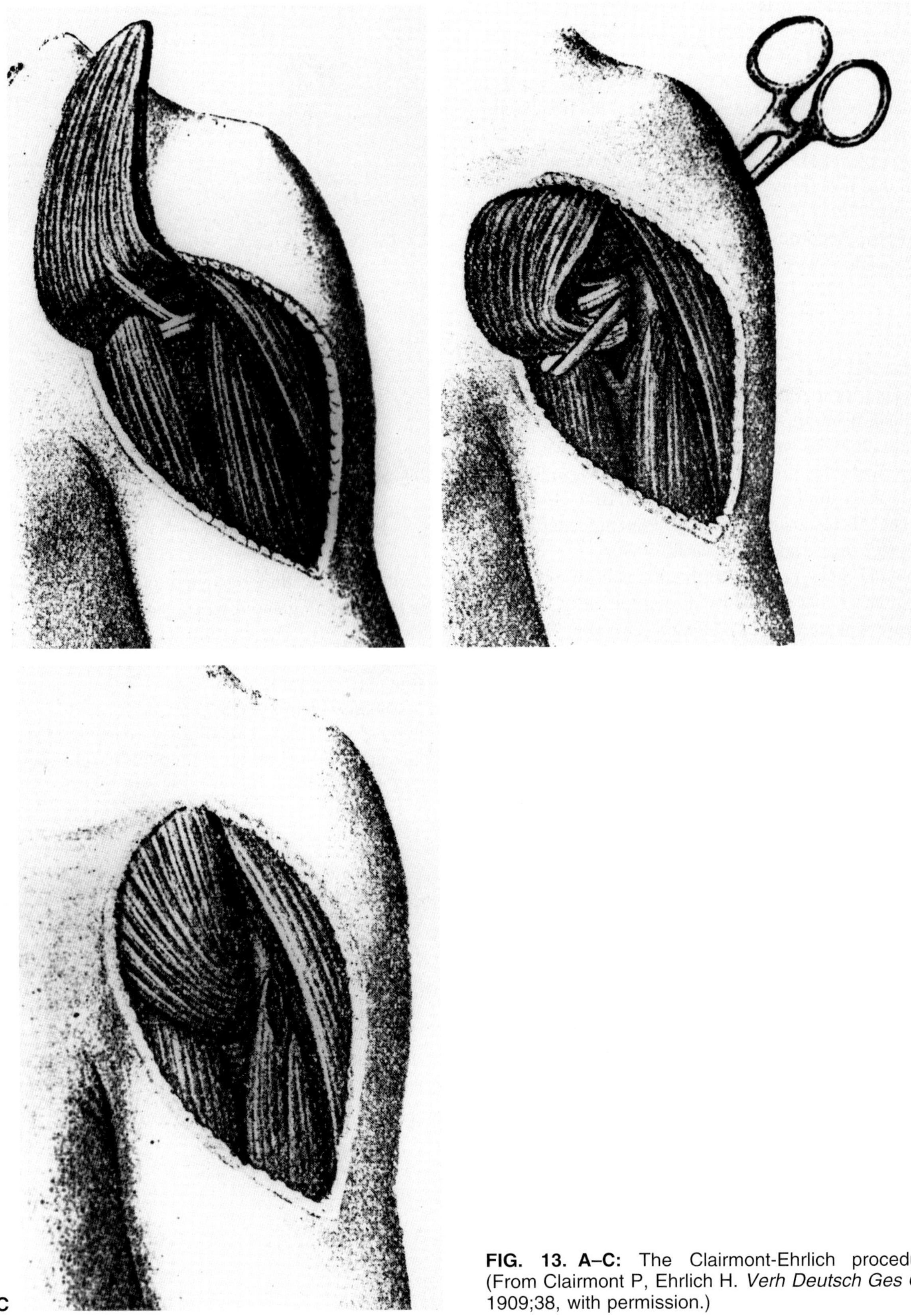

FIG. 13. A–C: The Clairmont-Ehrlich procedure. (From Clairmont P, Ehrlich H. *Verh Deutsch Ges Chir* 1909;38, with permission.)

them posteriorly. Saha of India, in 1956, designed the latissimus dorsi transfer (posteriorly to infraspinatus insertion) for the treatment of patients with recurrent anterior dislocation and normal bony anatomy (86–89). Connolly (136) also described infraspinatus transfer for the treatment of patients with large defects in the humeral head.

In 1912, Roepke (137) reefed the subscapularis tendon for the prevention of instability. Stevens (73) reefed the subscapularis, infraspinatus, and teres minor in a procedure described in 1926. According to Osmond-Clarke (138), the Putti-Platt procedure was developed independently by Vittorio Putti of Italy (1923) (Fig. 14) and Henry Platt of England (1925) (Fig. 15). Neither Putti nor Platt described the technique in the literature. In this procedure, the lateral stump of a transected subscapularis tendon is attached to soft tissues and capsule anterior to the glenoid, and the medial stump is fixed to the lateral stump, shortening the subscapularis (Fig. 16A-C). Codivilla, who was Putti's teacher, may have been the first to perform this procedure (7). Matti (139), a Swiss surgeon, reported a similar technique in 1936. Brav (140), in 1955, presented his results with the Putti-Platt procedure and noted a 10% recurrence rate at 2-year follow-up.

Magnuson and Stack (141) described transfer of the subscapularis to the greater tuberosity during the early 1940s. This procedure was favored by DePalma (30) (Fig. 17).

Repair of the Capsule and Labrum to the Glenoid

Perthes (43), in 1906, stressed that operative treatment should be directed at restoration of abnormal anatomy. He described a procedure designed to repair the separated capsule to the bony glenoid when capsular stripping was noted intraoperatively. The capsule was reattached with nails or with wires passed through drill holes (Fig. 18). In 1925, Perthes (101) reported that repair of the capsule or labrum to the bony glenoid had been performed in six patients without postoperative recurrence. Perthes also advocated repair and nailing of the rotator cuff insertion when the

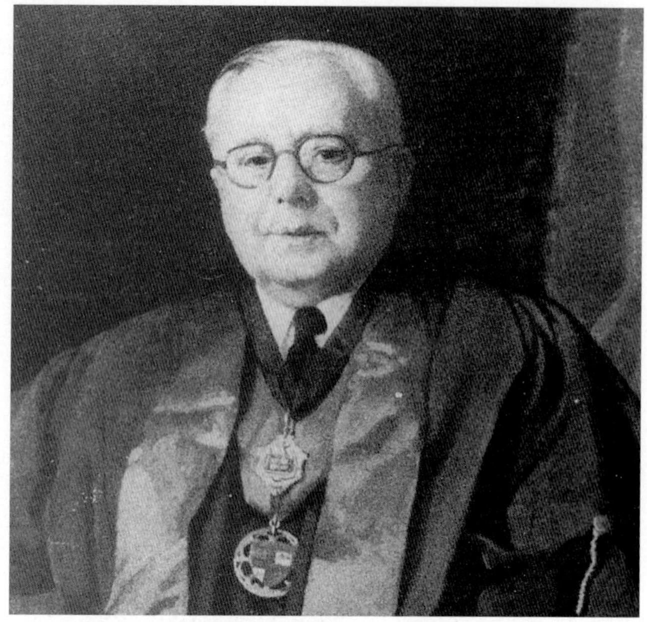

FIG. 15. Henry Platt.

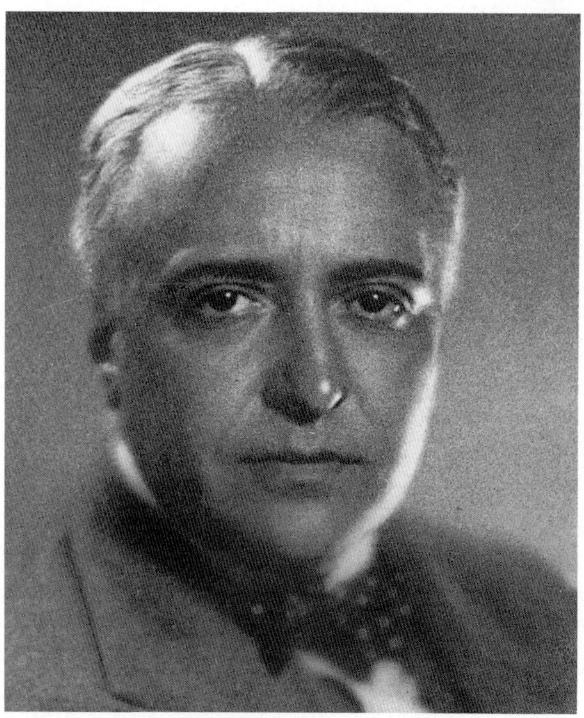

FIG. 14. Vittorio Putti.

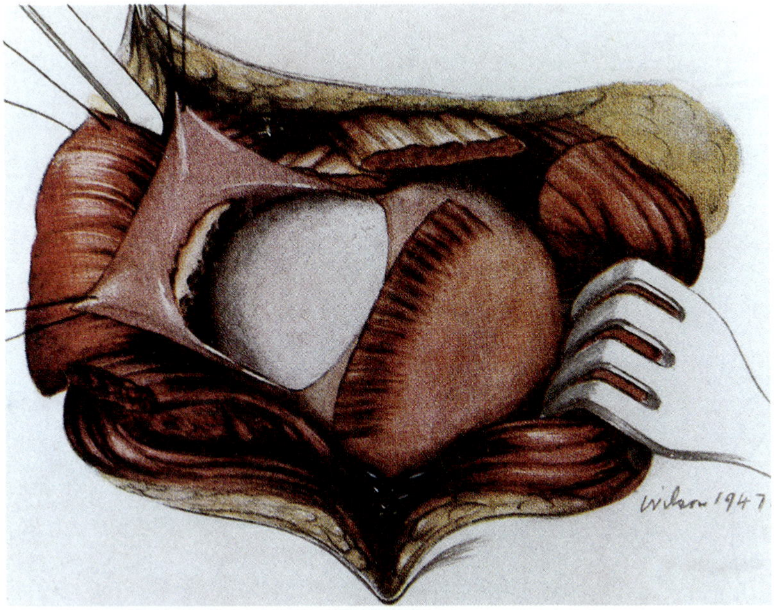

A

FIG. 16. A–C: The Putti-Platt procedure. (From Osmond-Clarke H. Habitual dislocation of the shoulder: the Putti-Platt operation. *J Bone Joint Surg [Br]* 1948;30B:19–25, with permission.)

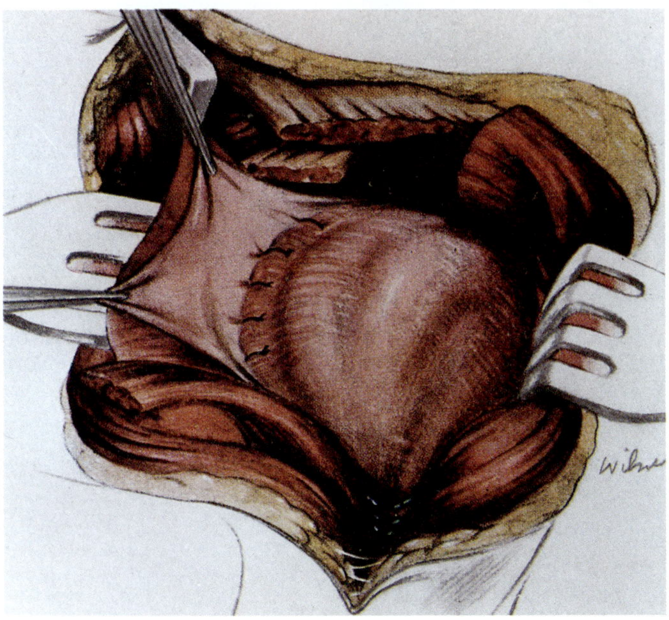

B

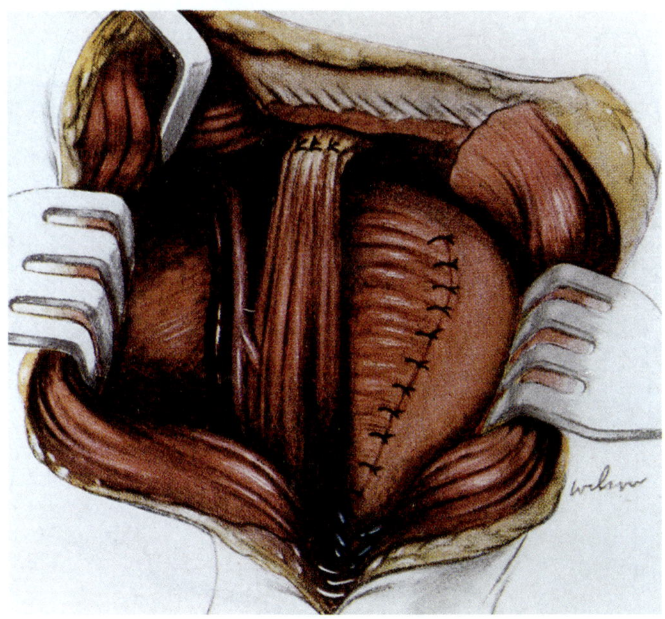

C

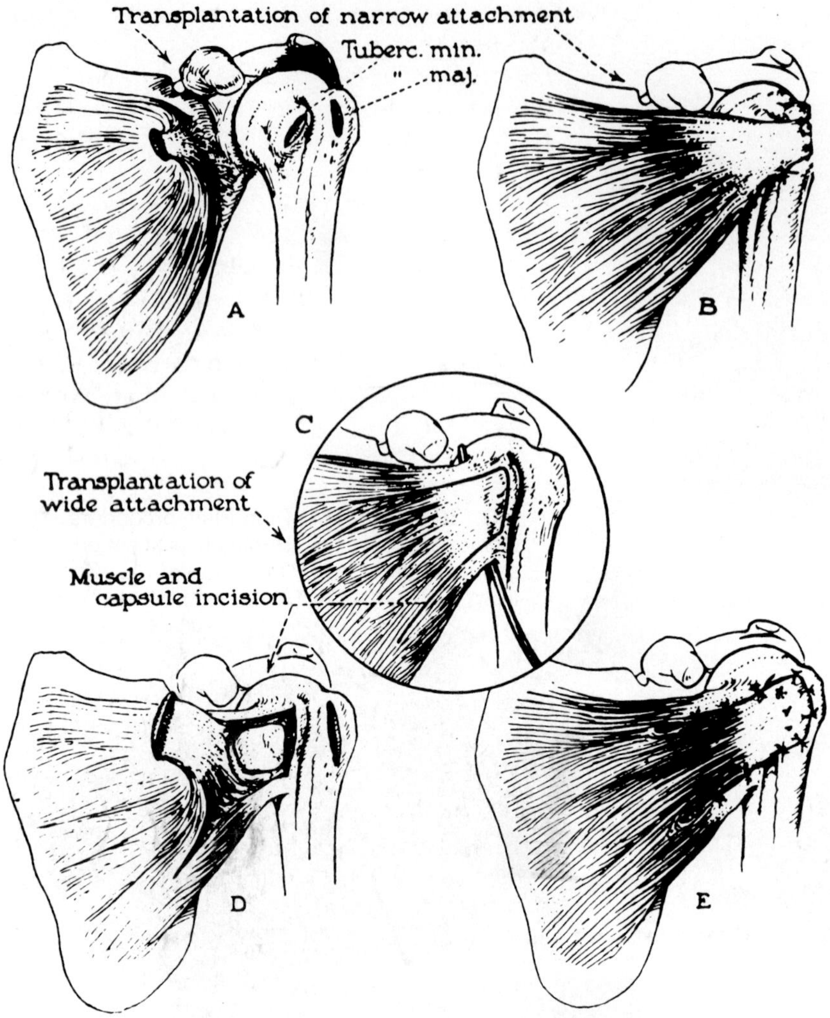

FIG. 17. The Magnuson-Stack procedure. (From Magnuson P. Treatment of recurrent dislocation of the shoulder. *Surg Clin North Am* 1945;25:14–20, with permission.)

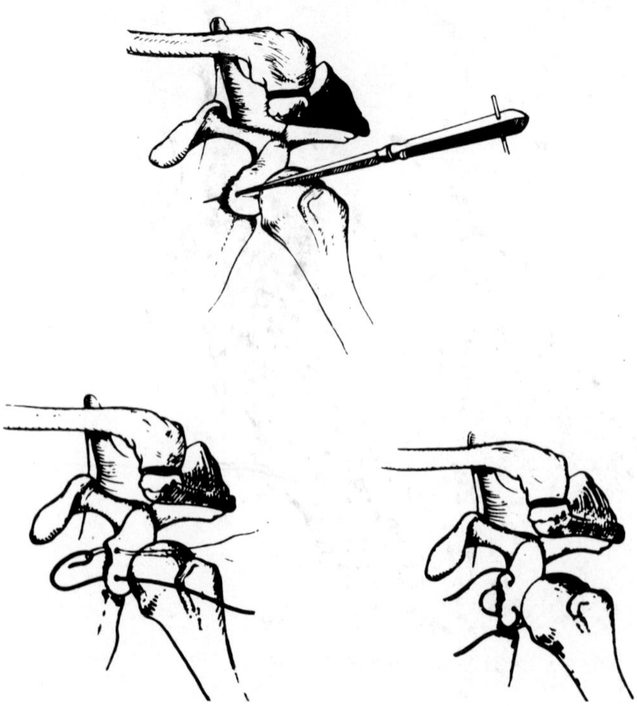

FIG. 18. Perthes technique. (From Perthes G. Ueber Ergebnisse der Operationen bei habitueller Schulterluxation, mit besonderer Berucksichtigung unseres Verfahrens. *Dtsch Z Chir* 1925;194:1, with permission.)

insertion was damaged since he believed that the primary pathologic lesion was located laterally in some cases. He reported no recurrences in five cases treated by this alternate method.

In 1923, Bankart (56) introduced the concept of capsulolabral repair to the English literature, when he wrote that the "only rational treatment is to reattach the fibrous capsule to the glenoid ligament whence it has been torn. . . ." He later added that, "Capsular plication and Clairmont procedures are based on erroneous principles of pathology" (57–59). Bankart believed that plication of a more lateral part of the capsule and operations of the Clairmont-Ehrlich type could prevent instability only at the expense of shoulder motion. His technique required the passage of sutures through drill holes in the bony glenoid for reattachment of the capsule and labrum (Fig. 19A,B). Dickson and Devas (142) reported on 50 patients operated upon by Bankart and his colleagues between 1925 and 1954. Only 2 of the 50 patients developed postoperative instability. Excellent long-term results of the Bankart procedure were also reported by Rowe et al. (143) in 1978.

Fouche in South Africa (144) and Delitalia (145), who was Putti's successor in Italy, used staples to perform Bankart-type procedures during the early 1930s. Downing and Myers (146) described stapling techniques in the English literature in 1946. du Toit and Roux reported their results with this method in 1956 (144). Metcalfe (147), in 1947, used a one-hole plate in order to perform the Bankart procedure without drill holes in the glenoid. Luckey (148), in 1949, and Viek and Bell (149), in 1959,

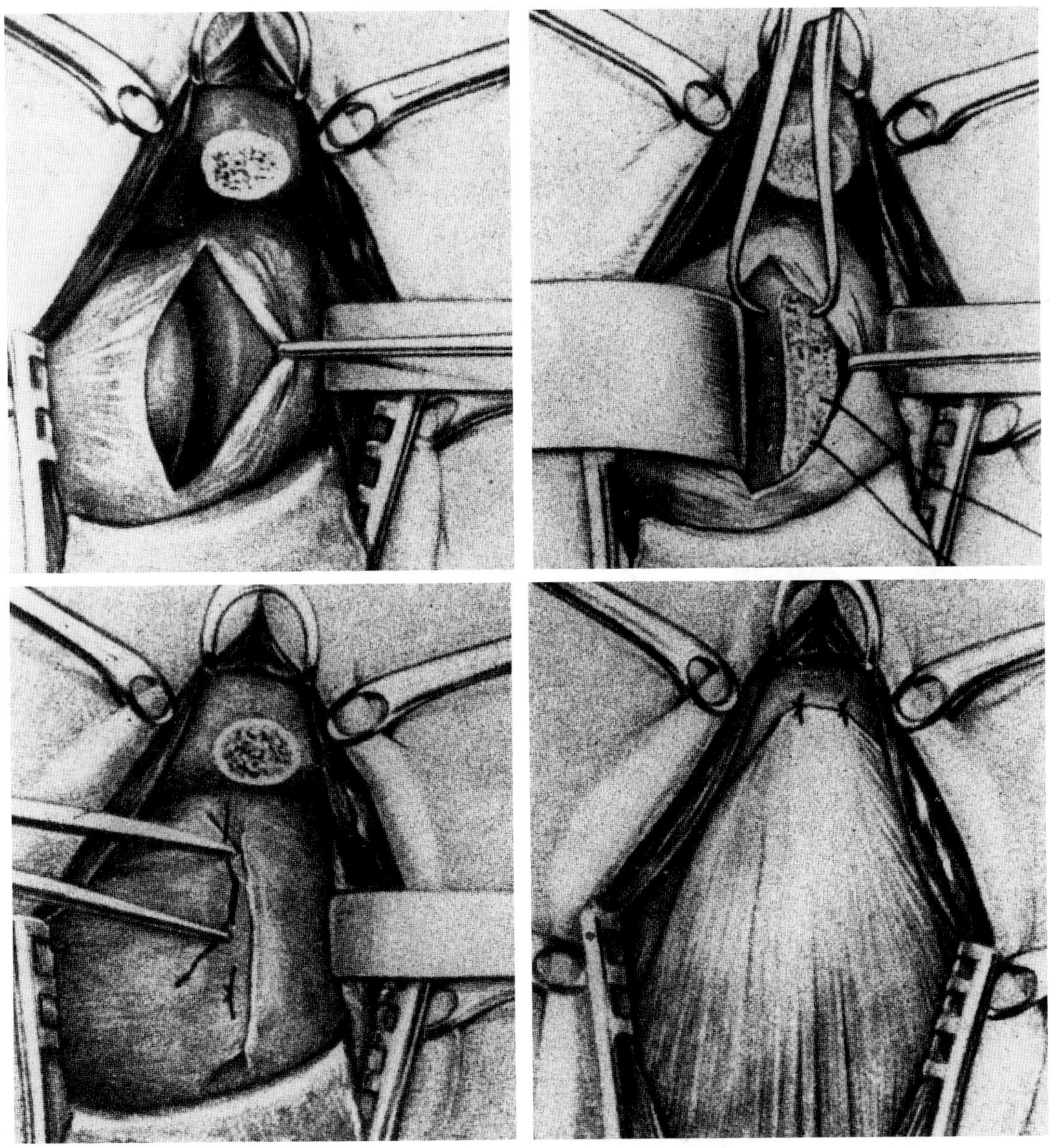

A

B

FIG. 19. A, B: Bankart's technique. (From Bankart A. The pathology and treatment of recurrent dislocation of the shoulder-joint. *Br J Surg* 1938;26:23–29, with permission.)

described the use of pull-out sutures to facilitate the Bankart procedure. Suture anchors were developed during the late 1980s to facilitate placement of intraosseous sutures (150). Johnon (151) developed an arthroscopic technique of Bankart repair using metal staples during the early 1980s. Caspari, Morgan, and Warren modified the pull-out suture method for arthroscopic transglenoid suture stabilization shortly thereafter (152). Subsequently, biodegradable implants (153,154) and suture anchors (155) have become available as potential methods of arthroscopic reattachment of soft tissues to the glenoid.

Tenosuspension, Fascial Grafts, and Check Ligaments

In 1903, Carl Beck (156), a German-born surgeon who practiced in New York, stabilized a dislocating shoulder by connecting the humeral head and the acromion with wires. The wire was passed through drill holes and was removed after 5 weeks. Beck reported a "perfect result" after 6 months. Seidel (157) of Dresden used a fascial flap to cover the anterior joint after he performed a capsulorraphy in 1913. Schultze (158) performed a similar procedure in 1914. Joseph (159), in 1917, pioneered "tenosuspension" for shoulder stabilization by passing a fascia lata graft through drill holes in the acromion and greater tuberosity. Plummer and Potts (160) described a similar fascial graft in the English literature in 1925. Loeffler (161), in 1920, devised a fascial sling that ran from the acromion, passed under the humeral head, and was then placed around the clavicle.

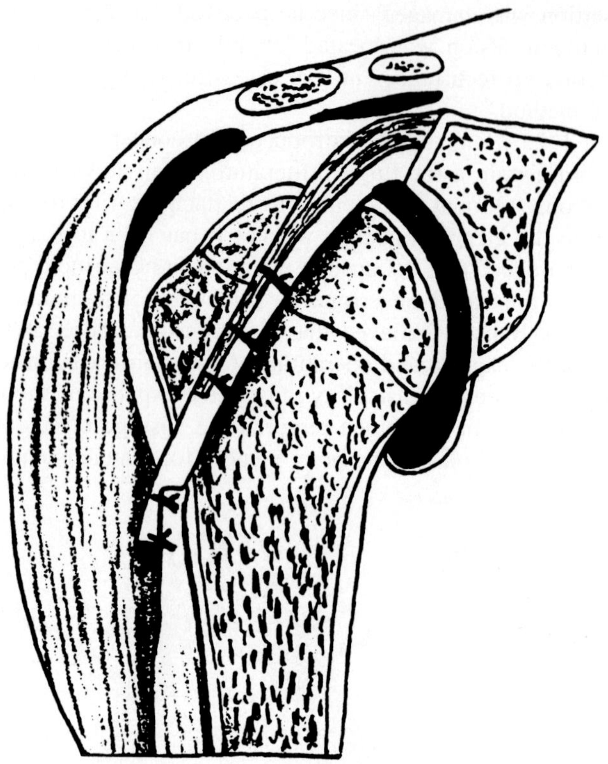

FIG. 21. Nicola procedure.

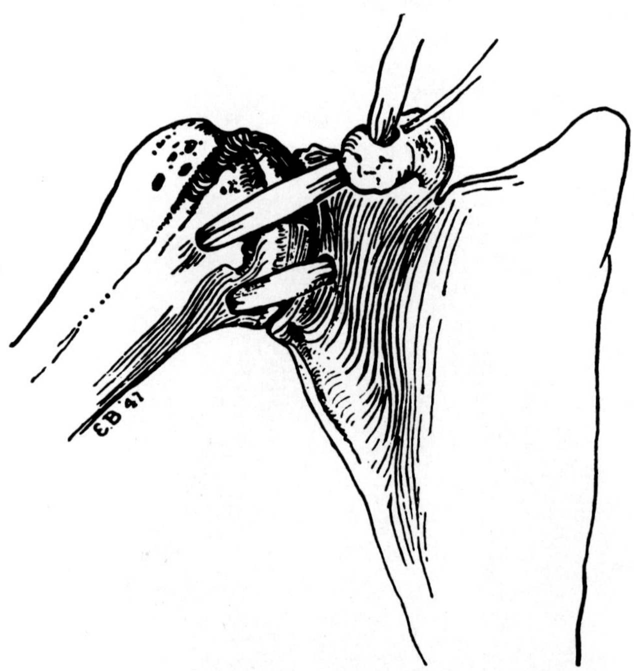

FIG. 20. Fascial graft as described by Gallie and LeMesurier (From Gallie W, LeMesurier A. Recurring dislocation of the shoulder. *J Bone Joint Surg [Br]* 1948;30B:9–18, with permission.)

Henderson (129), of the Mayo Clinic, unhappy with the results of capsulorraphy and of the Clairmont-Ehrlich procedure, adopted a tenosuspension method that used a free peroneus longus tendon graft passed through the greater tuberosity and the acromion in 1926. Rich (162) devised a silk check ligament consisting of a double band of silk ligatures between the scapula and the humerus in 1917. He also interlaced bone grafts to produce a functional arthrodesis. A silk check ligament was also used by Spitzy (163) of Vienna. Gallie and LeMesurier (164) of Canada, in 1927, used a fascial transplant as a check ligament in an attempt to block abduction between the scapula and the humerus (Fig. 20). In 1948, these investigators reported a 4% recurrence rate with this procedure (165). Bateman (20,21) continued to use the Gallie method into the 1970s.

Rupp (166) and Heymanowitsch (167), in separate 1926 papers, placed the long head of the biceps through a canal in the humeral head to stabilize the shoulder. In 1929, this procedure was modified by Toufick Nicola of the Hospital for the Ruptured and Crippled (later, the Hospital for Special Surgery) in New York (48,168) (Fig. 21). In 1948, Adams (169) reported that the results of the Nicola procedure were inferior to those of the Putti-Platt or Bankart procedures.

Bony Procedures

In 1901, Hildebrand (170) reported an attempt to prevent recurrent dislocation by deepening the glenoid fossa with sharp curette. Eden (171), in 1917, transferred a corticocancellous bone block from the tibia to the scapular neck to act as an extended buttress of the anterior glenoid to compensate for erosion of the anterior glenoid. The same year, Hybbinette, a Swede, reportedly performed a similar procedure using an iliac crest bone graft (172, 173). Speed (11) of Chicago described Eden's technique in the English literature in 1927. Speed noted that Phemister had also used Eden's method. The Eden-Hybbinette procedure became especially popular in the Scandinavian countries (62,173).

Oudard, a Frenchman, created an osseous prop over the anterior glenoid by sawing off the tip of the coracoid and placing a transplanted bone block from the tibia between the sawed-off tip and the base of the coracoid (174–176) (Fig. 22A, B). Oudard, in later years, incorporated shortening of the subscapularis tendon into his procedure. Noesske (177) broke the base of the coracoid and directed it inferiorly to act as a bony buttress. These procedures were reported in 1924. Tavernier (23) advocated Oudard's technique in 1930. Jinnaka (178), in 1939, and Iwahara (179), in 1954, both of Japan, developed modifications of Oudard's procedure.

In 1938, Boicev (180) described the transfer of the divided coracoid through a tunnel between the anterior capsule and the subscapularis and the reattachment of the coracoid to the base with a screw or silk suture. Variations of these procedures were devised by Trillat (181), Laterjet (182, 183), and Helfet (184) and reported during the 1950s. Helfet designated his technique the ''Bristow procedure,'' in honor of his former chief, Rowley Bristow (184). Bristow himself probably never performed the procedure (7).

Meyer-Burgdorff (185) attempted a cuneiform osteotomy of the posterior glenoid and scapular neck for recurrent anterior dislocation in 1933. The procedure was intended to retrovert the glenoid and to increase the prominence of its anterior margin. In 1961, Saha and Das (88) discussed anterior opening wedge osteotomy of the scapular neck to achieve the same goal.

Rotational humeral osteotomy was performed by Weber (Swiss) in 1964 for the treatment of recurrent anterior dislocation associated with a large Hill-Sachs lesion (186). Saha advocated rotational humeral osteotomy at about the same time.

The Controversy over Technique in Anterior Stabilization

During the late 1940s and 1950s, controversy erupted between advocates of Bankart-type repairs and proponents of procedures designed to limit external rotation of the arm such as the Putti-Platt and Magnuson-Stack. Osmond-Clarke (187) and Adams (169) noted that the Bankart was a technically difficult procedure. DePalma (30) was of the opinion that the surgeon should adopt the simplest procedure that limited external rotation. This argument was best summed up by the statements made by

A

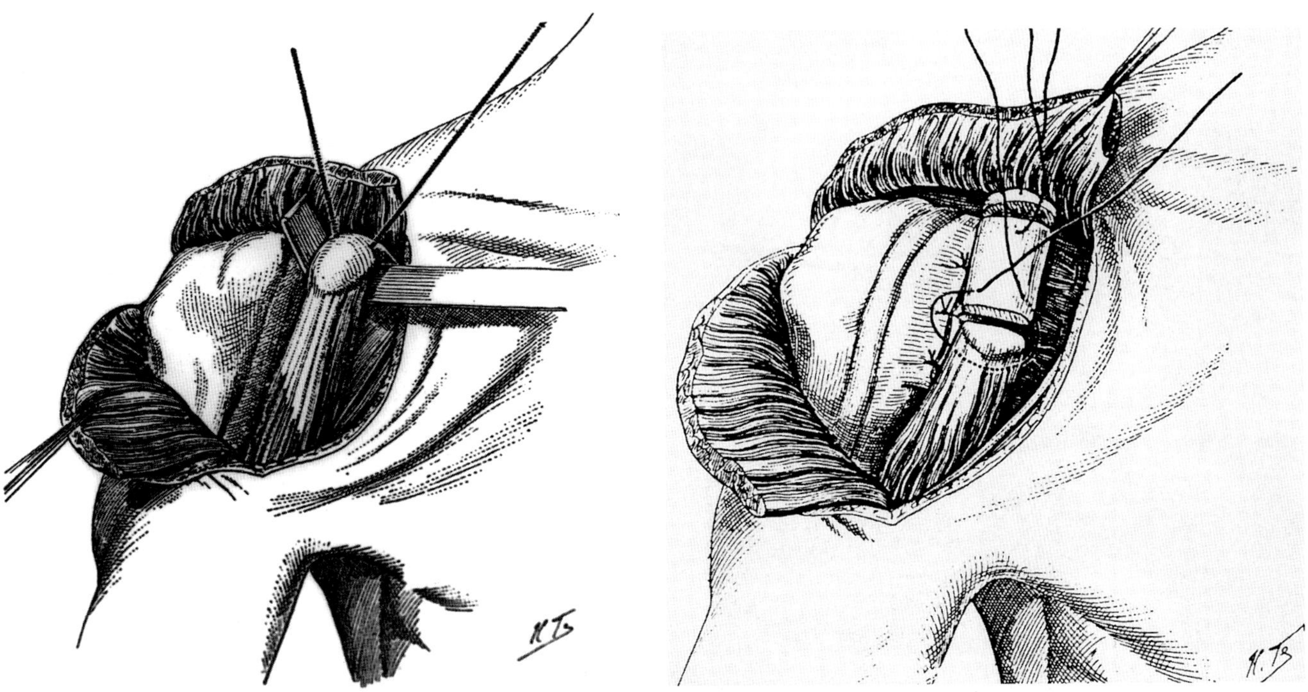

B

FIG. 22. A, B: Oudard's technique. (From Oudard P. La luxation recidivante de l'epaule [variete anterinterne] procede operatoire. *J Chir* 1924;23:13–25, with permission.)

Carr (188) in 1956: "I wish to emphasize that completely normal scapulohumeral motion should not be the requirement for an excellent result. . . . Restriction of movement is the price paid willingly for stability and full confidence in the shoulder."

The supporters of the Bankart repair countered with results that showed low recurrence rates with superior maintenance of function (143,144). In Rowe's words, "Our experience with Bankart operation is that it is not necessary to limit external rotation to prevent recurrence" (143). The desire to maximize function while providing stability has become a cornerstone in the current treatment of the unstable shoulder.

Operative Procedures for Posterior Instability

Most of the procedures described for posterior instability were modifications of those previously discussed in the treatment of anterior instability. According to MacAusland, Dehner performed a posterior capsulorraphy for posterior dislocation in 1899 (189,190). Thomas, during the 1920s, reported on three operative cases for posterior recurrence that were treated with a posterior capsulorraphy (47) (Fig. 23).

Rocher (191) described use of a posterior bone block derived from the tibia in 1931. Kaplan (192) devised a reversed Clairmont-Ehrlich procedure for posterior dislocations during the 1930s. May (193) developed a modification of the Nicola procedure for posterior dislocation and reported on it in 1943. Rowe and Yee (99), in 1944, recommended a posterior Bankart-type repair for traumatic posterior instability. Moseley (194) developed a vitallium prosthesis for the glenoid margin to facilitate capsular repair for posterior dislocations in epileptics.

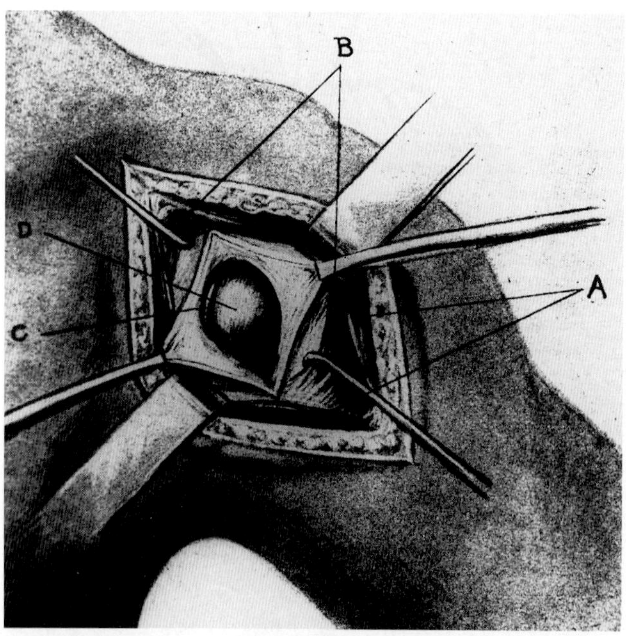

FIG. 23. Posterior capsulorraphy as described by Thomas in the 1920s. (From Thomas T. Recurrent dislocation of the shoulder joint. *JAMA* 1925;85:1202, with permission.)

Wilson and McKeever (195), in 1949, favored the use of transfixation wires from the humerus into the acromion in cases of old, unstable posterior dislocation. Soon afterward, McLaughlin (196,197) described subscapularis transfer into the humeral head defect for fixed posterior dislocation. He advocated capsular plication and bone block for recurrent posterior instability that was not chronic or fixed.

In 1967, Scott (198) reported on glenoid osteotomy for the surgical treatment of recurrent posterior dislocation.

In recent years, Neer (22) has proposed a posterior capsular shift for the treatment of posterior instability. Fronek et al. (36) have devised a posterior T-plasty capsulorraphy for these cases (36). Norris and Brems (199) have advocated an anterior approach for the treatment of posterior instability.

RADIOGRAPHIC FINDINGS

The use of ionizing radiation was pioneered in 1895 by the physicist Roentgen who termed his discovery the x-ray because he did not know what it was. Walter Bradford Cannon, a Harvard medical student, revealed that internal parts of the human body could be revealed with x-rays. According to Hermoddsen (97), Francke first mentioned the radiographic changes of the humeral head associated with dislocation. Steinhausen made a radiographic analysis of motion at the shoulder joint in 1899 (39,200). In his classic 1906 paper, Perthes (54) discussed radiographic findings in two of his patients.

Schultze (158), in 1914, presented a detailed study of the radiographic changes associated with instability. Pilz (201), in 1925, noted the head defect and stressed the need for an angled projection to view the defect properly. Didiee (202) advocated his popular projection technique in 1930. Hermodsson (97), in 1934, suggested internal rotation and tangential views to see the defect. Hill and Sachs (203), in 1940, stressed the radiographic finding of the head defect in the English literature, hence the term "Hill-Sachs lesion."

The axillary view was described by Lawrence (204) in 1915. Roukos et al. (205), in 1972, designed a modification of the axillary view (the West Point view) to facilitate visualization of the anterior rim of the glenoid.

Bennett (206), in 1941, described another lesion that he found exclusively in the shoulders of professional baseball pitchers. He wrote, "Because of the extensive use of the arm and the tremendous pull on the posterior capsule and triceps tendon, there develops on the posterior inferior border of the glenoid fossa a deposit of bone strikingly similar to the osteoarthritic deposit that one sees in older patients." Similar lesions have been noted in patients with recurrent posterior subluxation (36). To achieve better visualization of these bony deposits, Bennett and his x-ray technician,

W. Ross Mitchell, devised a special view to show the posterior aspect of the glenoid.

Using ideas expressed by William S. Stryker, Hall et al. (207), in 1959, designed a special view to visualize the "notch" in the posterolateral portion of the head. Although these investigators stated that they wished to avoid eponymous designation, this projection has come to be known as the "Stryker notch view." This view has been shown to be extremely helpful in detecting Hill–Sachs lesions that have not been noted on standard views (208).

SUMMARY

The shoulder surgeon of today benefits greatly from the insights and discoveries of earlier investigators of the unstable shoulder. Many of the recent discoveries in the understanding and treatment of shoulder instability are based on concepts that were promulgated long ago, but that were then cast aside or forgotten. The older literature has provided a solid base for further advancements in the field, and we are indebted to those individuals whose ideas have raised our level of knowledge.

REFERENCES

1. Breasted J. *The Edwin Smith surgical papyrus*. Chicago: University of Chicago Press, 1930:354–357.
2. Hussein M. Kocher's method is 3000 years old. *J Bone Joint Surg [Br]* 1968;50B:669.
3. Adams F. *The genuine works of Hippocrates*. New York: William Wood & Co., 1849:85–96.
4. Libby W. *The history of medicine in its salient features*. Boston: Houghton Mifflin, 1922:54.
5. Castiglioni A. *A history of medicine*. New York: Alfred A. Knopf, 1947:90–91.
6. Brown A. *Old masterpieces in surgery*. Omaha, NE: Privately Printed, 1928:25.
7. Rockwood C. Fractures and dislocations of the shoulder. In: Rockwood C, Green D, eds. *Fractures in adults*. Philadelphia: JB Lippincott, 1983:722–859.
8. Malgaigne J. *Surgery and Ambroise Pare*. Hamby WB, translator. Norman, OK: University of Oklahoma Press, 1965:280.
9. Pare A. *Dix livres de la chirurgie*. Johnson T, translator. London: 1678.
10. Brockbank W, Griffiths D. Orthopaedic surgery in the sixteenth and seventeenth centuries. 1. Luxations of the shoulder. *J Bone Joint Surg [Br]* 1948;30B:365.
11. Speed K. *Fractures and dislocations*. Philadelphia: Lea & Febiger, 1942.
12. Lynn F. Erect dislocation of the shoulder. *Surg Gynecol Obstet* 1925;39:51–55.
13. Middledorpf M, Scharm B. *De Nova Humeri Luxations Specie. Clinique Europenne*, vol. II. Dissert Inag. Breslau 1859;.
14. Chelius J. *A system of surgery*. South JF, translator. Philadelphia: Lea & Blanchard, 1847.
15. Malgaigne J. *Traite des fractures et des luxations*. Paris: JB Bailliere, 1855:.
16. Hamilton F. *Treatise on fractures and dislocations*. Philadelphia: Henry C. Lea's Son & Co., 1880:635–674.
17. Sedillott. *Am J Med Sci* 1834.
18. Cooper A. On the dislocation of the os humeri upon the dorsum scapula, and open fractures of the shoulder joint. *Guys Hosp Rep* 1839;4:265–284.
19. Moullin C, Keith A. A case of backward dislocation of the humerus caused by muscular action. *Lancet* 1904;96.
20. Bateman J. *The shoulder and neck*. Philadelphia: WB Saunders, 1972:411–412.
21. Bateman J. *The shoulder and neck*. Philadephia: WB Saunders, 1978:515–519.
22. Neer C II, Foster C. Inferior capsular shift for involuntary inferior and multidirectional instability of the shoulder: a preliminary report. *J Bone Joint Surg [Am]* 1980;62A:897–908.
23. Tavernier L. The recurrent luxation of the shoulder. *J Bone Joint Surg* 1930;12:458–461.
24. Rowe C. Prognosis in dislocations of the shoulder. *J Bone Joint Surg [Am]* 1956;38A:957–977.
25. Genovesi A. Contributo allo conoscenza della lussaziona volontaria della spalla. *Arch Putti* 1962;17:142–147.
26. Reischauer F. Ueber willkurliche Schulterverrenkungen (rein willkurliche, habituell willkurliche, und Pendel-Luxationen) und "Schnappende Schulter." *Arch Orthop Unfall Chir* 1923;22:45–80.
27. Rowe C. Voluntary dislocation of the shoulder: a preliminary report on a clinical, electromyographic, and psychiatric study of twenty-six patients. *J Bone Joint Surg [Am]* 1973;55A:445–460.
28. Cooper A. *Treatise on dislocations and on fractures in the joints*. 1822.
29. Moseley H. *Shoulder lesions*. New York: Paul B. Hoeber, 1953.
30. DePalma A. *Surgery of the shoulder*. Philadelphia: JB Lippincott, 1950:236.
31. Bateman J. *The shoulder and environs*. St. Louis: CV Mosby, 1955: 498–521.
32. Blazina M, Saltzman J. Recurrent anterior subluxation of the shoulder in athletics—a distinct entity. *J Bone Joint Surg [Am]* 1969;51A: 1037–1038.
33. LeClerc J. Chronic subluxation of the shoulder. *J Bone Joint Surg [Am]* 1969;51B:778.
34. Rowe C, Zarins B. Recurrent transient subluxation of the shoulder. *J Bone Joint Surg [Am]* 1981;63A:863–872.
35. Hawkins R, Koppert G, Johnston G. Recurrent posterior instability (subluxation) of the shoulder. *J Bone Joint Surg [Am]* 1984;66A: 169–174.
36. Fronek J, Warren R, Bowen M. Posterior subluxation of the glenohumeral joint. *J Bone Joint Surg [Am]* 1989;71A:205–216.
37. Boorstin D. *The discoverers: a history of man's search to know his world and himself*. New York: Vintage Books, 1985:351–360.
38. Bonn. *Abhandlung von der Verrunkung des Oberarms*. 1783.
39. Pettersson G. Rupture of the tendon aponeurosis of the shoulder joint in anterior inferior dislocation. *Acta Chir Scand 1942;77*[Suppl]:1–187.
40. Popke L. Zur Kasuistik und Therapie der Inverterirten und Habituellen Schulterluxation. *Zentralbl Chir* 1883;10:28.
41. Joessel D. Anatomische Beitrage zur Kentnisse der Humerusluxation mit Fraktur der Tuberkul. *Dtsch Z Chir* 1874;4:124.
42. Jobe F, Giangarra C, Kvitne R, Glousman R. Anterior capsulolabral reconstruction of the shoulder in athletes in overhead sports. *Am J Sports Med* 1991;19:428–434.
43. Perthes G. Ueber operationen der habituellen Schulterluxation. *Dtsch Z Chir* 1906;85:199.
44. Thomas T. Habitual or recurrent anterior dislocation of the shoulder. I. Etiology and pathology. *Am J Med Sci* 1909;137:237–246.
45. Thomas T. Recurrent anterior dislocation of the shoulder. *JAMA* 1910;54:834.
46. Thomas T. A common mechanism for most injuries to the shoulder region. *JAMA* 1914;63:1018.
47. Thomas T. Recurrent dislocation of the shoulder joint. *JAMA* 1925;85:1202.
48. Nicola T. Anterior dislocation of the shoulder: the role of the anterior capsule. *J Bone Joint Surg [Am]* 1942;24A:614–616.
49. Bach B, Warren R, Fronek J. Disruption of the lateral capsule of the shoulder: a cause of recurrent dislocation. *J Bone Joint Surg [Br]* 1988;70B:274–276.
50. Eve F. A case of subcoracoid dislocation of the humerus, the formation of an indentation on the posterior surface of the head, the joint being unopened; with remarks on the mode of production of the fracture of the anatomical neck, with dislocation. *Med Chir Trans Soc Lond* 1880;63:317–321.
51. Caird F. The shoulder joint in relation to certain dislocations and fractures. *Edinb Med J* 1887;32:708.

52. Stimson L. Shoulder joint dislocation without rupture of the capsule. *NY Med Rec* 1881;19:24.
53. Broca A, Hartmann H. Contribution a l'etude des luxations de l'epaule (luxations dites incompletes, decollements periostiques, luxationes directes et luxationes indirectes). *Bull Soc Anat Paris* 1890;312–336.
54. Perthes G. Ueber Ergebnisse der Operationen bei habitueller Schulterluxation, mit besonderer Berucksichtigung unseres Verfahrens. *Dtsch Z Chir* 1925;194:1.
55. Perthes G. Habitual dislocation of the shoulder. *JAMA* 1926;86:589.
56. Bankart A. Recurrent or habitual dislocation of the shoulder-joint. *BMJ* 1923;1132–1133.
57. Bankart A. Dislocations of the shoulder-joint. In: *The Robert Jones birthday volume*. 1928:307–314.
58. Bankart A. The pathology and treatment of recurrent dislocation of the shoulder-joint. *Br J Surg* 1938;26:23–29.
59. Bankart A. Discussion of recurrent dislocation of the shoulder. *J Bone Joint Surg [Br]* 1948;30B:46–48.
60. Bost F, Inman V. The pathological changes in recurrent dislocation of the shoulder: a report of Bankart's operative procedure. *J Bone Joint Surg* 1942;24:595–613.
61. Moseley H, Overgard B. The anterior capsular mechanism in recurrent dislocation of the shoulder: morphological and clinical studies with special reference to the glenoid labrum and the glenohumeral ligaments. *J Bone Joint Surg [Br]* 1962;44B:913–927.
62. Jakobsson A. On recurrent dislocation of the shoulder joint. *Acta Orthop Scand* 1949;18:283–318.
63. Townley C. The capsular mechanism in recurrent dislocation of the shoulder. *J Bone Joint Surg [Am]* 1950;32A:370–380.
64. Lippitt S, Vanderhooft E, Harris S, Sidles J, Harryman D II, Matsen F III. Glenohumeral stability from concavity-compression: a quantitative analysis. *J Shoulder Elbow Surg* 1993;2:27–35.
65. Schlemm F. Ueber die Verstarkungsbander am Schultergelenk. *Arch Anat Physiol Wissenschaft Med* 1853;45.
66. Fick R. *Handbuch der Anatomie und Mechanik der Gelenke*, vol. 2, part I. Jena: Gustav Fisher, 1904:163–199.
67. Delorme. Die Hemmungsbander des Schultergelenks und ihre Bedeutung fur die Schulterluxation. *Arch Klin Chir* 1910;92:79–101.
68. Turkel S, Panio M, Marshall J, Girgis F. Stabilizing mechanisms preventing anterior dislocation of the glenohumeral joint. *J Bone Joint Surg [Am]* 1981;63A:1208–1217.
69. O'Brien S, Neves M, Arnoczky S, Rozbruch S, DiCarlo E, Warren R, Schwartz R. The anatomy and histology of the inferior glenohumeral ligament complex of the shoulder. *Am J Sports Med* 1990;18:449–456.
70. Joessel D. Ueber die Recidine der Humerus-Luxationen. *Dtsch Z Chir* 1880;4:167–184.
71. Jobe F, Kvitne R. Shoulder pain in the throwing athlete: the relationship of anterior instability and rotator cuff impingement. *Orthop Rev* 1989;18:963–975.
72. Sever J. Recurrent dislocation of the shoulder joint: a mechanical consideration of its treatment. *JAMA* 1921;76:925–927.
73. Stevens J. Dislocation of the shoulder. *Ann Surg* 1926;83:84–103.
74. Jens J. The role of the subscapularis muscle in recurrent dislocation of the shoulder. *J Bone Joint Surg [Br]* 1964;46B:780–781.
75. Symeonides P. The significance of the subscapularis muscle in the pathogenesis of recurrent dislocation of the shoulder. *J Bone Joint Surg [Br]* 1972;54B:476–483.
76. Cain P, Mutschler T, Fu F, Lee S. Anterior stability of the glenohumeral joint: a dynamic model. *Am J Sports Med* 1987;15:144–148.
77. McKernan D, Mutschler T, Rudert M, Luo L, Harner C, Fu F. Significance of a partial and full Bankart lesion: a biomechanical study. Presented at the Annual Meeting of Orthopaedic Research Society, Las Vegas, 1989.
78. McKernan D, Mutschler T, Rudert M, Klein A, Victorino G, Harner C, Fu F. The characterization of rotator cuff muscle forces and their effect on glenohumeral joint stability: a biomechanical study. *Orthop Trans* 1990;14:237–238.
79. Humphry G. *A treatise on the human skeleton (including the joints)*. Cambridge: Macmillon, 1858.
80. Weber W, Weber E. *Mechanik der menschlichen genverkzenge*. University of Gottingen: 1836.
81. Aeby C. Beitrage zur Kenntnisse der Gelenke. I. Ueber Form und Mechanik des Schultergelenkes beim Menschen. *Dtsch Z Chir* 1876;6:354–378.
82. Browne A, Hoffmeyer P, An K, Morrey B. The influence of atmospheric pressure on shoulder stability. *Orthop Trans* 1990;14:259.
83. Gibb T, Sidles J, Harryman D, McQuade K, Matsen F. The effect of capsular venting on glenohumeral laxity. *Clin Orthop* 1991;268: 120–127.
84. Kumar V, Balasubramianium P. The role of atmospheric pressure in stabilizing the shoulder: an experimental study. *J Bone Joint Surg [Br]* 1985;67B:719–721.
85. Warner J, Deng X, Warren R, Torzilli P, O'Brien S, Altchek D. Superior-inferior translation in the intact and vented glenohumeral joint. Presented at the Annual Meeting of American Shoulder and Elbow Surgeons, Anaheim, 1991.
86. Saha A. *Theory of shoulder mechanism*. Springfield, IL: Charles C Thomas, 1961.
87. Saha A. Anterior recurrent dislocation of the shoulder. *Acta Orthop Scand* 1967;68:479–493.
88. Saha A, Das A. Recurrent anterior dislocation of the shoulder. *Indian J Orthop* 1967;1:132–137.
89. Saha A. Dynamic stability of the glenohumeral joint. *Acta Orthop Scand* 1971;42:491–505.
90. Calandriello B. The pathology of recurrent dislocation of the shoulder. *Clin Orthop* 1961;20:33–39.
91. Flower W. On the pathological changes produced in the shoulder-joint by traumatic dislocation; as derived from an examination of all the specimens illustrating this injury in the museums of London. *Trans Pathol Soc Lond* 1860–61;12:179–200.
92. Cramer F. Resection des Oberamkopfes wegen Habitueller Luxation (Nach einem im Artzlichen Verein zu Wiesbaden gehaltenen Vortage). *Berl Klin Wochenschr* 1882;19:21–25.
93. Kraske. Discussion of Ueber habituelle Schulterluxation. *Verh Dtsch Gesell Chir* 1882;11:112–114.
94. Kuster E. Ueber Habituelle Shulterluxation. *Verh Dtsch Gesell Chir* 1882;11:112–114.
95. Bazy L. Les lesiones de la tete humerale dans les luxations recidivantes de l'epaule. *Bull Soc Chir Paris* 1918;44:1961–1964.
96. Lobker K. Einige Praparate von habitueller Shulterluxation. *Arch Klin Chir* 1887;34:658–667.
97. Hermodsson I. Rontgenogische Studien uber die traumatischen und und habituellen Schultergelenkeverrenkungen nach vorn und nach unten. Thesis Stockholm. *Acta Radiol* 1934;20[Suppl]:1–173.
98. Thomas M. Posterior subacromial dislocations of the head of the humerus. *AJR* 1937;27:767–773.
99. Rowe C, Yee L. A posterior approach to the shoulder joint. *J Bone Joint Surg* 1944;26:580–584.
100. Warren R, Kornblatt I, Marchand R. Static factors affecting posterior shoulder stability. *Orthop Trans* 1984;8:89.
101. Oveson J, Nielson S. Posterior instability of the shoulder: a cadaver study. *Acta Orthop Scand* 1986;57:436–439.
102. Basmajian J, Bazant F. Factors preventing downward dislocation of the adducted shoulder joint. *J Bone Joint Surg [Am]* 1959;41A: 1182–1186.
103. Oveson J, Nielson S. Experimental distal subluxation in the glenohumeral joint. *Arch Orthop Trauma Surg* 1985;104:78–81.
104. Bowen M, Warren R. Ligamentous control of shoulder stability based on selective cutting and static translation. *Clin Sports Med* 1991;15:757–782.
105. Warner J, Deng X, Warren R, Torzilli P. Static capsuloligamentous constraints to superior-inferior translation of the glenohumeral joint. *Am J Sports Med* 1992;20:675–685.
106. Neer C II. Displaced proximal humeral fractures. Part II. Treatment of three-part and four-part displacement. *J Bone Joint Surg [Am]* 1970;52A:1077–1103.
107. Nobuhara K, Ikeda H. Rotator interval lesion. *Clin Orthop* 1987;223: 44–50.
108. Harryman D, Sidles J, Harris S, Matsen F. Role of the rotator interval capsule in passive motion and stability of the shoulder. *J Bone Joint Surg [Am]* 1992;74A:53–66.
109. Dickson J, Humphries A, O'Dell H. *Recurrent dislocation of the shoulder*. Baltimore: Wilkins & Wilkins, 1953.
110. Aitken D. *Hugh Owen Thomas: his principles and practice*. London: Oxford University Press, 1935:81–82.
111. Thomas H. *Fractures, dislocations, diseases, and deformities of the*

bones of the trunk and upper extremities. London: HK Lewis, 1887: 57.
112. Stimson L. Injuries of the main blood-vessels in the axilla caused by efforts to reduce dislocations of the shoulder. *NY Med J* 1885;41: 658–663.
113. White C. A new method for reducing shoulders without the use of the ambe. *Med Obs Inqu* 1762;2:373.
114. Malgaigne J. Les luxationes scapulohumerales. Nouveau moyen de les distinguer des fracturs du col de l'humerus. Nouvelle methode de reduction. Experiences faites a l'hotel Dieu. *Gaz Med Paris* 1832;3:506–508.
115. Milch H. Treatment of dislocations of the shoulder. *Surgery* 1938;3: 732–740.
116. Watson-Jones R. Robert Jones traction. In: *Fractures and joint injuries*. Baltimore: Williams & Wilkins, 1943:460–461.
117. Stimson L. An easy method of reducing dislocation of the shoulder and hip. *NY Med Rec* 1900;57:356–357.
118. Kocher E. Eine neue Reductions methode fur Schulterverrenkung. *Berl Klin Wochnschr* 1870;7:101–105.
119. Kuhn. New method of reducing dislocations of the shoulder. *Paris Med* 1876.
120. Anderson D, Zuirbulis R, Ciullo J. Scapular manipulation for reduction of anterior shoulder dislocation. *Clin Orthop* 1982;164:181–183.
121. Albert E. Arthrodese bei habitueller Schulterluxation. *Int Klin Rundschau* 1888.
122. Albert E. Arthrodese bei einer Habituellen Luxation der Schultergelenkes. *Klin Rundschau* 1898;2:281–283.
123. Gerster A. Subcoracoid dislocations of the humerus; paralyses of the serratus magnus; arthrotomy. *NY Med J* 1884;39:390.
124. Bardenheuer. Die Verletzungen der oberen extremitaten. *Dtsch Chir* 1886;63:268.
125. Ricard. Traitement des luxations recidivantes de l'epaule par la suture de la capsule articulare on arthrorrophie. *Gaz Hop* 1894;49:179.
126. Burrell H, Lovett R. Habitual or recurrent dislocation of the shoulder. *Am J Med Sci* 1897;114:166–179.
127. Samter. Zur operativen Behandlung der habituellen Schulterverrenkung. *Arch Klin Chir* 1900;62:115–125.
128. Magnuson P. Treatment of recurrent dislocation of the shoulder. *Surg Clin North Am* 1945;25:14–20.
129. Henderson M. "Tenosuspension" for habitual dislocation of the shoulder. *Surg Gynecol Obstet* 1926;43:18–25.
130. Muller W. Ueber habituellen Schulterluxation. Presented at the twenty-seventh chirurgcongres, Berlin, 1898.
131. Clairmont P, Ehrlich H. Ein Neues Operationsverfahren zur Behandlung der Habiltuellen Schulterluxation mittels Muskelplastik. *Verh Dtsch Ges Chir* 1909;38:79–103.
132. Armour. *Liverpool Med J* 1914;34:100.
133. Ollerenshaw J. Habitual dislocation of the shoulder joint. *J Orthop Surg* 1920;18:255–264.
134. Young J. Recurrent dislocation of the shoulder joint. *Ann Surg* 1916;63:375.
135. Finsterer. Die Operative Behandlung der Habituellen Schulterluxation. *Dtsch Z Chir* 1917;141:354.
136. Connolly J. Humeral head defects associated with shoulder dislocations: their diagnostic and surgical significance. In: ed. *Academy of Orthopaedic Surgeons Instructional Course Lectures*. St. Louis: Mosby, 1972:42–54.
137. Roepke. *Verh Dtsch Gesell Chir Berl* 1912;42:351.
138. Osmond-Clarke H. Habitual dislocation of the shoulder: the Putti-Platt operation. *J Bone Joint Surg [Br]* 1948;30B:19–25.
139. Matti H. Zur operativen Behandlung der habituellen Luxation des Schultergelenks. *Zentralbl Chir* 1936;63:3011–3018.
140. Brav E. An evaluation of the Putti-Platt reconstruction procedure for recurrent dislocation of the shoulder. *J Bone Joint Surg [Am]* 1955;37A:731–741.
141. Magnuson P, Stack J. Recurrent dislocation of the shoulder. *JAMA* 1943;123:889–892.
142. Dickson J, Devas M. Bankart's operation for recurrent dislocation of the shoulder. *J Bone Joint Surg [Br]* 1957;39B:114–119.
143. Rowe C, Patel D, Southmayd W. The Bankart procedure: a long-term end-result study. *J Bone Joint Surg [Am]* 1978;60A:1–16.
144. du Toit G, Roux D. Recurrent dislocation of the shoulder: a twenty-four year study of the Johannesburg staple operation. *J Bone Joint Surg [Am]* 1956;38A:1–12.
145. Delitalia. Le base anatome patologica della lussazione abituale di spalla. *Giorn Ven Sci Med* 1937;6:3809.
146. Downing F, Myers O. A simplfication of Bankart's capsulorraphy for recurrent instability of the shoulder. *J Bone Joint Surg* 1946;28: 250–252.
147. Metcalfe J. The Bankart operation for recurrent dislocation of the shoulder. *US Navy Med Bull* 1947;47:672–675.
148. Luckey C. Recurrent dislocation of the shoulder. Modification of the Bankart capsulorraphy. *Am J Surg* 1949;77:220–222.
149. Viek P, Bell B. The Bankart shoulder reconstruction. The use of pull-out wires and other practical details. *J Bone Joint Surg [Am]* 1959;41A:236–242.
150. Richmond J, Donaldson W, Fu F, Harner C. Modification of the Bankart reconstruction with a suture anchor: report of a new technique. *Am J Sports Med* 1991;19:343–346.
151. Johnson L. Symposium on arthroscopy. Presented at the Annual Meeting of Arthroscopy Association of North America, San Francisco, 1986.
152. Moran M, Warren R. Development of a synovial cyst after arthroscopy of the shoulder. A brief note. *J Bone Joint Surg [Am]* 1989;71A:127–129.
153. Warner J, Warren R. Arthroscopic Bankart repair using a cannulated, absorbable fixation device. *Oper Tech Orthop* 1991;1:192–198.
154. Warner J, Pagnani M, Warren R, Kavanaugh J, Montgomery W. Arthroscopic Bankart repair with an absorbable, cannulated fixation device. *Orthop Trans* 1991;15:761–762.
155. Wolf E, Wilk R, Richmond J. Arthroscopic Bankart repair using suture anchors. *Oper Tech Orthop* 1991;1:184–191.
156. Beck C. Humeroacromial suture for habitual dislocation of the shoulder. *NY Med J* 1903;78:64.
157. Seidel. Ueber die Operation der habituellen Schulterluxation. *Zentralbl Chir* 1913;34:1344.
158. Schultze E. Die habituellen Schulterluxation. Klinischer und experimenteller Beitrag. *Arch Klin Chir Berl* 1914;104:138.
159. Joseph E. Eine neue Operation zur Verhutung der habituellen Schulterverrenkung. *Berl Klin Wochnschr* 1917;54:525.
160. Plummer W, Potts F. Two cases of recurrent anterior dislocation of the shoulder. *J Bone Joint Surg* 1925;7:190–198.
161. Loeffler F. Die Behandlung der habituellen Schulterluxation durch Bildung eines extraartikularen Hemmungsbandes. *Zentralbl Chir* 1920;47:324–326.
162. Rich E. Dislocations of the shoulder. *Northwest Med* 1917;16:114.
163. Spitzy H. Stabilization of the shoulder joint for habitual dislocation. *Surg Gynecol Obstet* 1928;46:256–257.
164. Gallie W, LeMesurier A. An operation for the relief of recurring dislocation of the shoulder. *Trans Am Surg Assoc* 1927;45:392–398.
165. Gallie W, LeMesurier A. Recurring dislocation of the shoulder. *J Bone Joint Surg [Br]* 1948;30B:9–18.
166. Rupp F. Ueber ein Vereinfachtes Operationverfahren bei Habitueller Schulterluxation. *Dtsch Z Chir* 1926;198:18–25.
167. Heymanowitsch Z. Ein Beitrag zur Operativen Behandlung der Habituellen Schulterluxation. *Zentralbl Chir* 1926;53:2229.
168. Nicola T. Operation for the relief of recurrent dislocation of the shoulder. *Am J Surg* 1931;11:119–121.
169. Adams J. Recurrent dislocation of the shoulder. *J Bone Joint Surg [Br]* 1948;30B:26–38.
170. Hildebrand O. Zur Operativen Behandlung der Habituellen Schulterluxation. *Arch Klin Chir* 1902;66:360.
171. Eden R. Zur operativen behandlung der habituellen schulterluxation unter mitteilung, eines neuen verfahrens bei abriss am inneren pfannenrande. *Dtsch Z Chir* 1918;144:269.
172. Hybbinette S. De la transplatation d'un fragment ossex pour remedier aux luxations recidivantes de l'epaule; constatations et resultats operatiores. *Acta Orthop Scand* 1932;71:411–445.
173. Thomasen E. Habitual dislocation of the shoulder: a study on the nature and treatment of the disease including remarks on traumatic dislocation. *Acta Orthop Scand* 1944;15:206–246.
174. Oudard P. La luxation recidivante de l'epaule (variete anter-interne) procede operatoire. *J Chir* 1924;23:13–25.
175. Oudard P. Le traitement de la luxation recidivante de l'epaule. *Rev Chir* 1943;81:113.
176. Oudard P. Le traitement de la luxation recidivante de l'epaule (variete antero-interne par la butee osseuse). *Rev Med* 1946;1:305.
177. Noesske. *Zentralbl Chir* 1924;43:2402.

178. Jinnaka S. Modification of Oudard's operation. *Geka* 1939;3:1–5.
179. Iwahara T. Modification of Oudard's operation. *Shujitsu* 1954;8: 393–399.
180. Boicev B. Solla lussazione abituale della spalla. *Chir Org Mov* 1938;23:354.
181. Trillat A. Traitement de la luxation recidivante de l'epaule. Considerations. Techniques. *Lyon Chir* 1954;49:986.
182. Laterjet M. A propos du traitement des luxations recidivante de l'epaule. *Lyon Chir* 1954;49:994–997.
183. Laterjet M. Technique de la butee coracoidienne preglenoidienne dans le traitement des luxations recidivantes de l'epaule. *Lyon Chir* 1958;54:604–607
184. Helfet A. Coracoid transplantation for recurring dislocation of the shoulder. *J Bone Joint Surg [Br]* 1958;40B:198–202.
185. Meyer-Burgdorff H. Die behandlung der habituellen Schulterluxation. *Zentralbl Chir* 1933;60:827.
186. Weber B, Simpson L, Hardegger F. Rotational humeral osteotomy for anterior dislocation of the shoulder associated with a large Hill–Sachs lesion. *J Bone Joint Surg [Am]* 1984;66A:1443–1450.
187. Osmond-Clarke H. Discussion of recurrent dislocation of the shoulder. *J Bone Joint Surg [Br]* 1948;30B:46–48.
188. Carr C. Discussion of prognosis in dislocations of the shoulder. *J Bone Joint Surg [Am]* 1956;38A:977.
189. Dehner H. Ueber habituelle Schulterluxation und ihre Radikaloperation. *Muenchen Med Wochenschr* 1899;5:165.
190. MacAusland W. Recurrent dislocation of the shoulder with report of cases. *Surg Gynecol Obstet* 1924;38:739–747.
191. Rocher H. Butee glenoidienne posterieure par graffen costal dans une subluxation habituelle de l'epaule. *Rev Tech Chir (Paris Chir)* 1931;23:33–43.
192. Kaplan A. Zur Frage de Operativen Behandlung habitueller Schultergelenkluxation nach hinten. *Arch F Kiln Chir* 1933;174:579–582.
193. May H. Nicola operation for posterior subacromial dislocation of the humerus. *J Bone Joint Surg* 1943;25:78–84.
194. Moseley H. The use of a metallic glenoid rim in recurrent dislocation of the shoulder. *Can Med Assoc J* 1947;56:320–321.
195. Wilson J, McKeever F. Traumatic posterior dislocation of the shoulder. *J Bone Joint Surg [Am]* 1949;31A:160–172.
196. McLaughlin H. Posterior dislocation of the shoulder. *J Bone Joint Surg [Am]* 1952;34A:584–590.
197. McLaughlin H. Posterior dislocation of the shoulder. *J Bone Joint Surg [Am]* 1962;44A:1477.
198. Scott D. Treatment of recurrent posterior dislocations of the shoulder by glenoplasty. Report of three cases. *J Bone Joint Surg [Am]* 1967;49A:471–476.
199. Brems J. Anterior approach to posterior instability. *J Shoulder Elbow Surg* 1993;2[Suppl]:S26.
200. Steinhausen. *Arch Anat Physiol* 1899;23:403.
201. Pilz W. Zur Roentgenuntersuchung der habituellen Schulterverrenkung. *Arch Klin Chir* 1925;135:1–22.
202. Didiee J. Le radiodiagnostic dans la luxation recidivante de l'epaule. *J Radiol Electrol* 1930;14:209–218.
203. Hill H, Sachs M. Groved defect of the humeral head; a frequently unrecognized complication of dislocation of the shoulder joint. *Radiology* 1940;35:690–700.
204. Lawrence W. New position in radiographing the shoulder joint. *AJR* 1915;2:728–730.
205. Roukos J, Feagin J, Abbott H. Modified axillary roentgenogram: a useful adjunct in the diagnosis of recurrent instability of the shoulder. *Clin Orthop* 1972;82:84–86.
206. Bennett G. Shoulder and elbow lesions of the professional baseball pitcher. *JAMA* 1941;117:510–514.
207. Hall R, Isaac F, Booth C. Dislocations of the shoulder with special reference to accompanying small fractures. *J Bone Joint Surg [Am]* 1959;41A:489–494.
208. Pavlov H, Warren RF, Weiss CB Jr., Dines DM. The roentgenographic evaluation of anterior shoulder instability. *Clin Orthop* 1985;194:153–158.
209. Asplund G. Ein operierter Fall von willkurlicher (habituell-willkurlicher) hinterer Schultergelenkluxation. *Acta Chir Scand* 1942;87: 103–112.
210. Baas J. *Outlines of the history of medicine*. Henderson HE, translator. Huntington, NY: 1971:205–209.
211. Campbell E, Colton J. *The surgery of Theodoric*. New York: Appleton-Century-Crafts, Inc., 1955:209–210.
212. Deuerlich R. Ueber die Complication der luxation humeri mit Fractur des tuberculum majus. Thesis, University of Gottingen, 1874.
213. Flood V. Discovery of a new ligament. *Lancet* 1827;671.
214. Francke G. Dislocations of the shoulder. *Dtsch Z Chir* 1898;48:399.
215. Lobker K. Einige Praparate von habitueller Schulterluxation. *Verh Dtsch Gesell Chir* 1886;210–219.
216. Malgaigne J. Luxations de l'articulation scapulo-humerale. *J Prog Sci Inst Med* 1830;III.
217. Moseley H. *Recurrent dislocation of the shoulder.* Montreal: McGill University Press, 1961.
218. Myers O. Experience with capsulorraphy for recurrent dislocation of the shoulder. *J Bone Joint Surg* 1946;28:253–261.
219. Nicola T. Recurrent anterior dislocation of the shoulder: a new operation. *J Bone Joint Surg* 1929;11:128–132.
220. O'Brien S, Schwartz R, Warren R, Torzilli P. Capsular restraints to anterior/posterior motion of the shoulder. *Orthop Trans* 1988;12:143.
221. Roser. Uber die pathologische Anatomieder Oberarmluxationen. *Arch Physiol Heilkd Stutt* 1842;1:401–420.
222. Speed K. Recurrent anterior dislocation at the shoulder: operative cure by bone graft. *Surg Gynecol Obstet* 1927;44:468–477.
223. Stimson L. *A practical treatise on fractures and dislocations*. New York: Lea Brothers, 1907.
224. Tyrrell F. *The lecture notes of Sir Astley Cooper on the practice of surgery with additional notes and cases.* Boston: Lilly & Wait, 1831: 195–234.

The Unstable Shoulder,
edited by R.F. Warren, E.V. Craig, and D.W. Altchek.
Lippincott–Raven Publishers, Philadelphia © 1999.

CHAPTER 2

Gross and Microscopic Anatomy of the Shoulder

Jeffrey R. Dugas, Daniel E. Cooper, and Stephen J. O'Brien

OSTEOLOGY

The scapula and clavicle serve as a means to attach the upper extremity to the trunk of the human body. This articular arrangement affords the upper extremity a unique and vast range of motion that allows for near-universal positioning of the terminal aspect of the upper extremity in space.

Scapula

The scapula is a triangular bone that lies on the dorsolateral surface of the thoracic cage, spanning the second through the seventh ribs with the base of the triangle facing medially. The medial border (also called the *base*) is closer to the midline at its most superior portion, and angles slightly away from the midline more distally. From the scapula project three processes: the spine, the acromion, and the coracoid (Fig. 1). The scapula also possesses three borders, including superior, medial, and lateral, as well as three angles, including superior, inferior, and lateral. The glenoid fossa is set upon the expanded aspect of the lateral angle. The costal surface, or subscapular fossa, of the body of the scapula is concave and smooth over the lateral one-third of the surface, whereas the medial portion is marked by oblique ridges that serve as the site of origin for the subscapularis muscle. The dorsal surface is convex and is divided by the projecting spine into the supraspinous and infraspinous fossae (Fig. 2). The supraspinous fossa is the smaller of the two cavities and is concave, smooth, and wider at the medial border than it is toward the lateral side. The infraspinous fossa is much larger, providing an area for the origin for the infraspinatus muscle. The origin of the muscle is over the medial two-thirds of the bone, whereas the lateral third is merely traversed by the muscle without attachment to it. The lateral, or axillary, border of the scapula, extending from the inferior angle to the inferior glenoid, exhibits a flattened area along its course, where the teres major, teres minor, and long head of the triceps originate. The medial border is the longest border of the bone and provides the attachment site for the levator scapulae and two rhomboideus muscles on the dorsal side, as well as the serratus anterior on the costal side. The superior border is the shortest in length and thinnest in breadth. In some cases, the inferior angle may serve as a site of origin for a small number of fibers from the latissimus dorsi muscle. The suprascapular notch is a small indentation in the lateral aspect of the superior border of the bone near the base of the coracoid through which passes the suprascapular nerve. In some instances, this tunnel may be completely enclosed with bone.

The glenoid cavity is an irregularly shaped oval with the cranial (superior) portion narrower than the bulbous caudal (inferior) portion. The cavity has also been described as being shaped like a comma (Fig. 3) On the basis of studies conducted by Saha (1,2), the average height of the adult glenoid is 35 mm, and the average width from anterior to posterior is 25 mm. The line that divides the superior and inferior portions of the fossa corresponds to the transepiphyseal line, which is present before fusion of the two ossification centers that form the glenoid (Fig. 4). Saha also demonstrated that the glenoid cavity may be either anteverted or retroverted in relation to the body of the scapula (3). In 75% of specimens, the glenoid was retroverted an average of 7.4 degrees. In the remaining 25%, the glenoid

J. R. Dugas: Department of Orthopaedic Surgery, The Hospital for Special Surgery, New York, New York 10021.

D. E. Cooper: W.B. Carrell Memorial Clinic, Dallas, Texas 75204; and Department of Orthopaedics, Baylor University Medical Center, Dallas, Texas 77030.

S. J. O'Brien: Department of Orthopaedics, Cornell University Medical College, New York, New York 10021; and Sports Medicine and Shoulder Service, The Hospital for Special Surgery, New York, New York 10021.

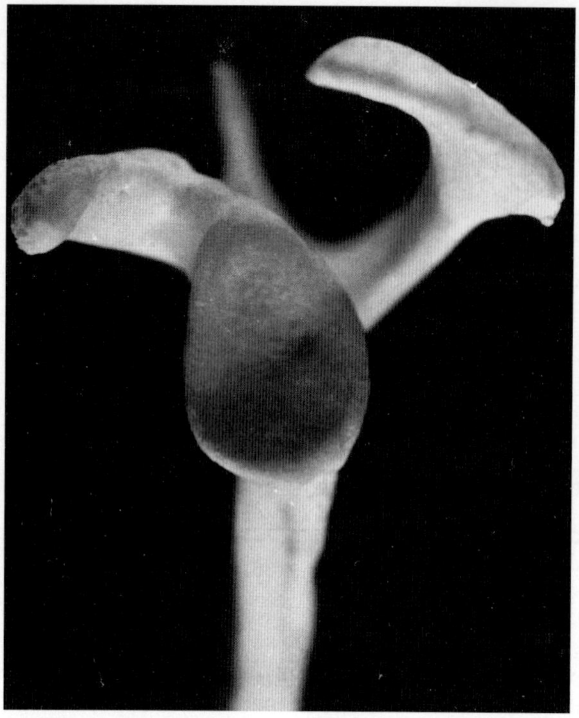

FIG. 1. Three processes of scapula. The acromion is a lateral and superior extension of the spine of the scapula. The coracoid is wide at its base and narrows as it projects anteriorly and then superolaterally. The glenoid fossa is the laterally projecting area that articulates with the humeral head. (From Jenkins DB, ed. *Hollinshead's functional anatomy of the limbs and back*. Philadelphia: WB Saunders, 1991:69, with permission.)

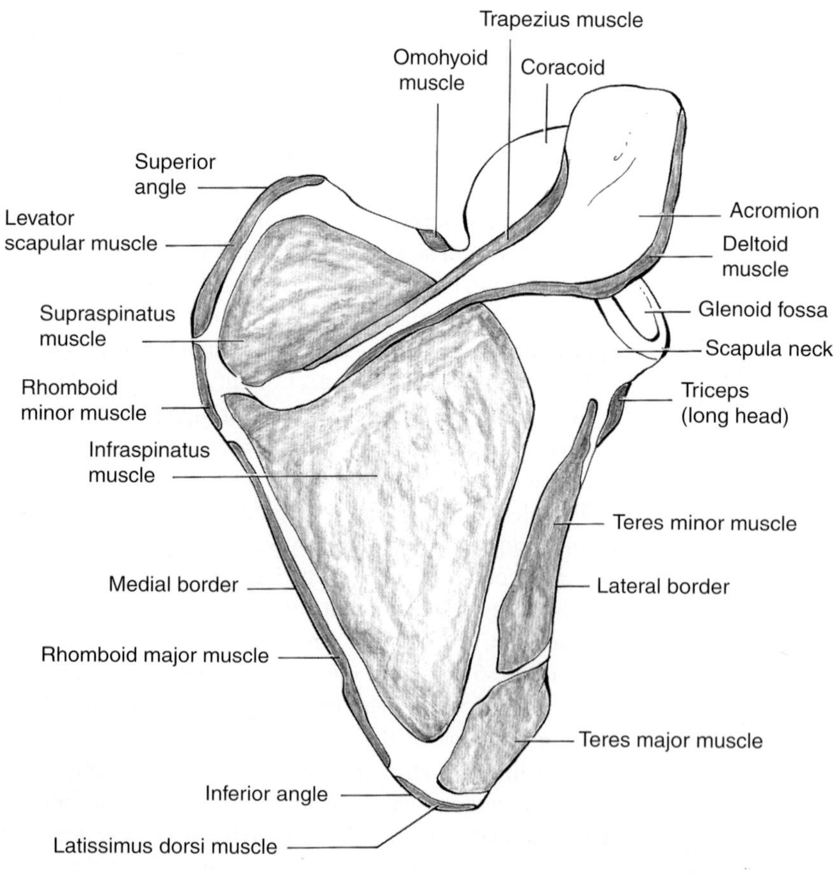

FIG. 2. Dorsal surface of scapula. Note that scapular spine divides the surface into supra- and infraspinous fossae. The supraspinatus and infraspinatus muscle bellies do not take origin from the entire surface of the fossae. Rather, their origin is chiefly from the more medial aspect of the bone, the lateral aspect of the fossae being traversed by muscle fibers.

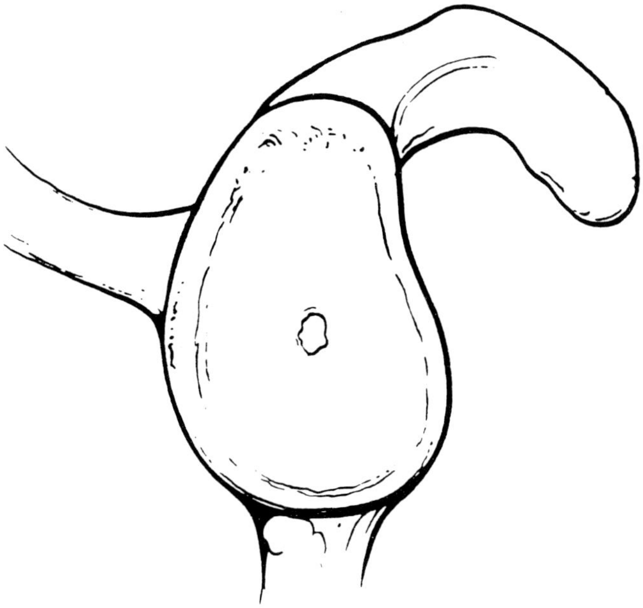

FIG. 3. Glenoid fossa viewed from lateral side. Note the similarity to inverted comma. The average height in the adult is 35 mm, the average width 25 mm. (From O'Brien SJ, Arnoczky SP, Warren RF, Rozbruch SR. Developmental anatomy of the shoulder and anatomy of the glenohumeral joint. In: Rockwood CA, Matsen FA, eds. *The Shoulder.* Philadelphia: WB Saunders, 1990:11–33, with permission.)

was anteverted from 2 to 10 degrees. The glenoid is also tilted from superomedial to inferolateral an average of 15 degrees (Fig. 5). At the very superior margin of the glenoid, there is a small elevation in the lateral projection of the scapula called the supraglenoid tubercle, from which the long head of the biceps arises.

Clavicle

The clavicle is an S-shaped tubular bone that forms the anterior portion of the shoulder girdle. It contains no medullary cavity, but rather is composed mostly of trabecular bone with a thin shell of compact bone surrounding. It is positioned at the upper anterior part of the thorax just above the first rib. By its medial and lateral articulations (one with the axial skeleton and one with the scapula), it functions to keep the upper extremity free and away from the trunk. The most medial aspect of the bone is slightly flared and seats poorly into the indentation in the manubrium of the sternum (Fig. 6). The lateral articulation is oval-shaped and tilted slightly downward for articulation with the acromion. The curvature of the clavicle is best described as *convex* anteriorly at the medial (sternal) aspect, and *concave* anteriorly at the lateral (acromial) portion (Fig. 7). The medial two-thirds are roughly triangular in cross section. The bone takes on a more flattened cross section lateral to the coracoid process. The undersurface of the medial clavicle is notable for a small oval-shaped projection called the costal tubercle, from which arises the costoclavicular ligament. Laterally, the upper surface is flattened and rough and is the site of attachment for the deltoid anteriorly and the trapezius posteriorly. The undersurface contains the conoid tubercle and trapezoid line, which give rise to the two cor-

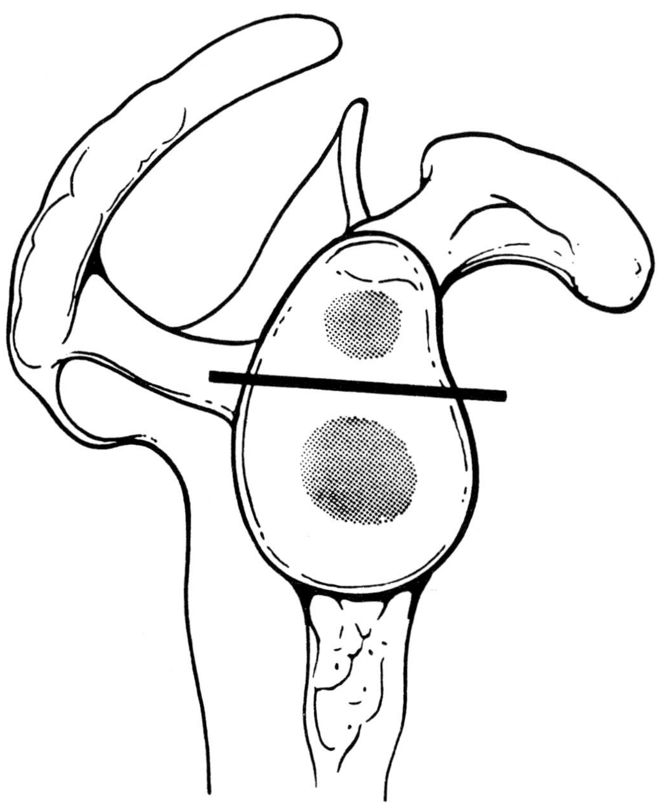

FIG. 4. Superior and inferior ossification centers that join to form the adult glenoid. Note the transepiphyseal line, thought to represent the location of the joining of the two centers of ossification. (From O'Brien SJ, Arnoczky SP, Warren RF, Rozbruch SR. Developmental anatomy of the shoulder and anatomy of the glenohumeral joint. In: Rockwood CA, Matsen FA, eds. *The Shoulder.* Philadelphia: WB Saunders, 1990: 11–33, with permission.)

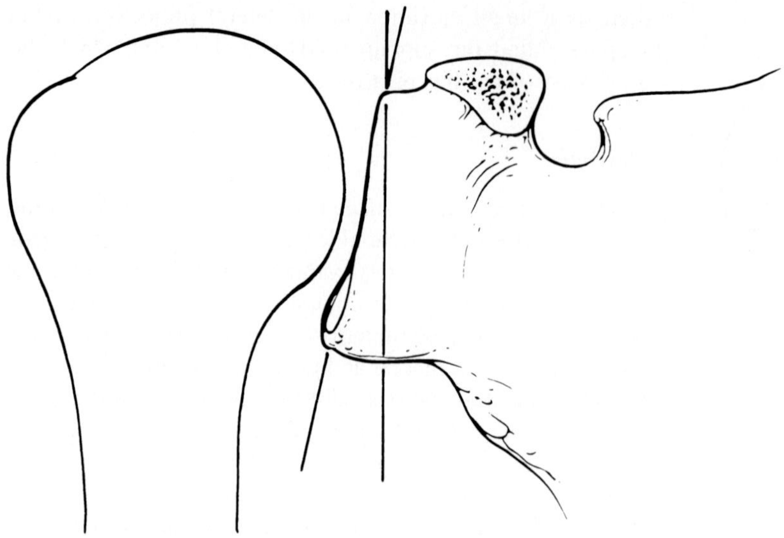

FIG. 5. Normal version and tilt of glenoid surface. Note that 75% have retroverted glenoid, while the other 25% are anteverted. Average retroversion is 7.4 degrees, anteversion ranges from 2 to 10 degrees. The glenoid is tilted 15 degrees, superomedially to inferolaterally.

acoclavicular ligaments that bear the same names. Between these medial and lateral undersurface projections lies a shallow groove into which the subclavius muscle inserts. The lateral superior surface is confluent with the medial superior border that separates the anterior and posterior medial surfaces. The subclavian border separates the inferior surface from the posterior surface medially.

In females, the clavicle is generally shorter and smoother and possesses less radius of curvature than that of the male clavicle. People who perform heavy manual labor may have markedly thickened, roughened clavicles.

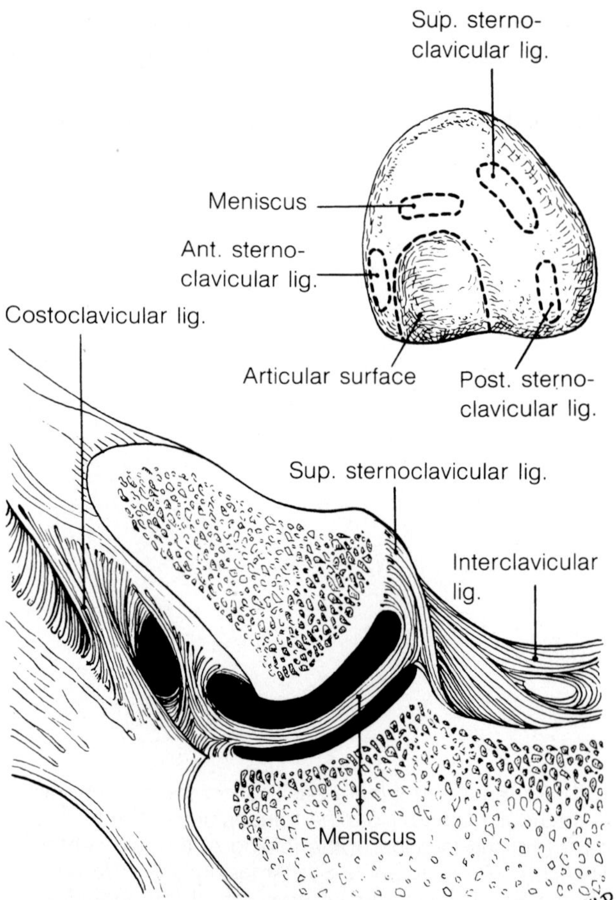

FIG. 6. Medial articulation of the clavicle. There is relative incongruence of the articulation with the manubrium.

Humeral Head

The humerus is the long tubular bone of the upper extremity that has at its proximal end a slightly flared metaphysis with a short neck and nearly hemispherical articular head. The articular surface is retroverted from 20 to 30 degrees in relation to the shaft of the humerus, and is inclined from 130 to 150 degrees (Fig. 8). The bicipital groove lies on the anterolateral surface of the head, and is

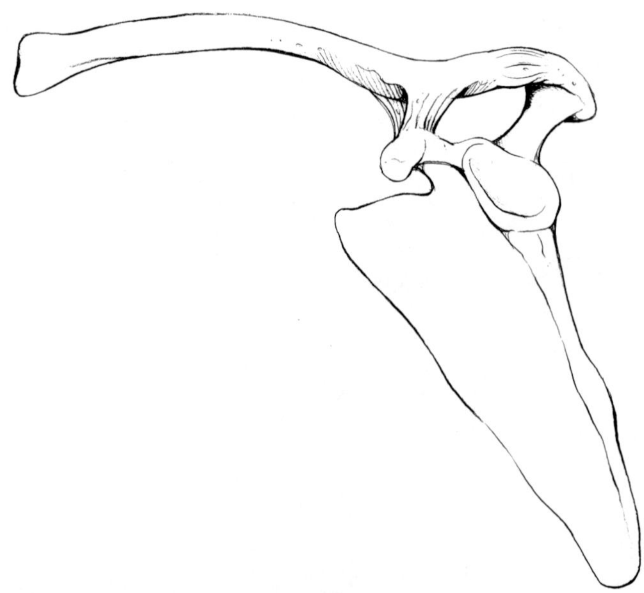

FIG. 7. AP view of clavicle. Note the insertion sites of the conoid and trapezoid ligaments. The thickened capsule surrounding the lateral articulation with the acromion provides stability in the anteroposterior plane.

offset 30 degrees in relation to a line drawn from the shaft of the humerus through the center of the head. This groove is formed as the base of the area between the lesser and greater tuberosities. The *anatomic* neck is an indentation at the base of the head where the capsule of the shoulder joint inserts. The *surgical* neck is the area just below the tuberosities and is a frequent location of fractures (Fig. 9). The greater tuberosity represents the most lateral bony aspect of the shoulder and is situated with its uppermost portion lateral to the articular surface of the head and its most medial border forming the lateral aspect of the bicipital groove. The uppermost portion is divided by two ridges into three facets, where three of the four rotator cuff tendons insert: supraspinatus, infraspinatus, and teres minor. The lesser tuberosity, although smaller in breadth, is more prominent than the greater tuberosity. The peak of the lesser tuberosity is directed anteromedially, and serves as the insertion point of the subscapularis muscle (fourth tendon of the rotator cuff). The tendon of the long head of the biceps brachii is seated in the groove formed by the two tuberosities.

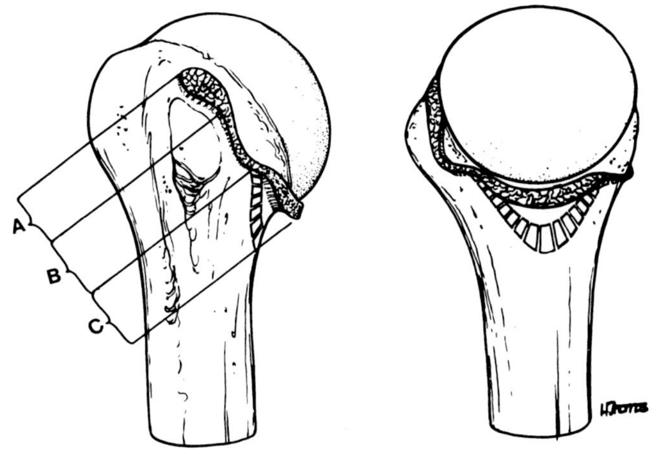

FIG. 9. Surgical and anatomic neck of humerus. Note insertion of joint capsule at the neck in a V pattern. (From Rockwood CA Jr, Matsen FA, eds. *The shoulder.* Philadelphia: WB Saunders, 1990, with permission.)

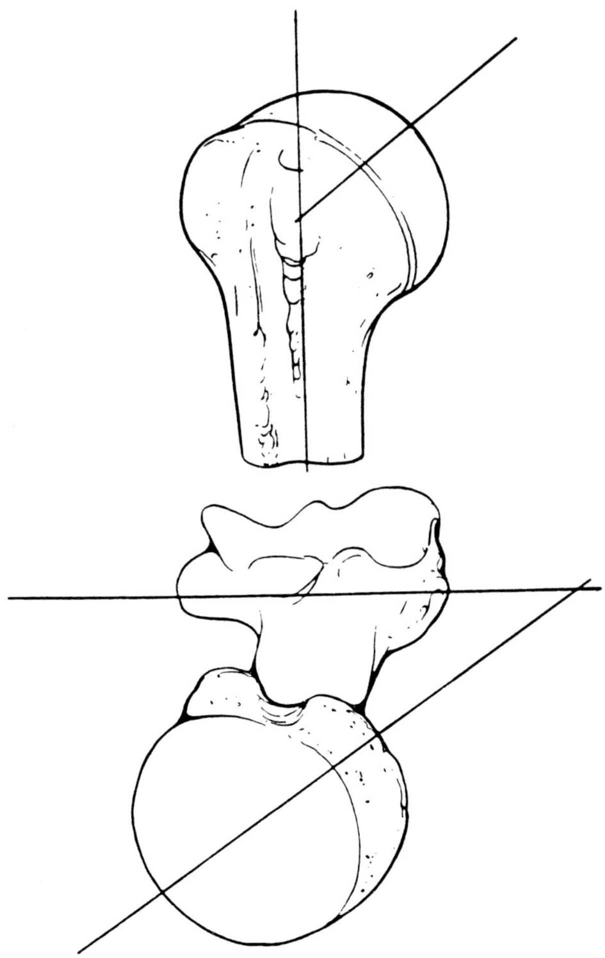

FIG. 8. Normal version of humeral head. The range of normal humeral head retroversion is 20 to 30 degrees. The normal articular surface is inclined approximately 130 to 150 degrees. (From O'Brien SJ, Arnoczky SP, Warren RF, Rozbruch SR. Developmental anatomy of the shoulder and anatomy of the glenohumeral joint. In: Rockwood CA, Matsen FA, eds. *The Shoulder.* Philadelphia: WB Saunders, 1990: 11–33, with permission.)

Acromion Process

The acromion process is the lateral terminal projection of the spine of the adult scapula. It forms the so-called "roof" over the head of the humerus. Descriptively, the acromion is a roughly triangular shaped, oblong process, which is directed laterally at its base but curves anteriorly toward its most distal portion. The acromion is thicker at its base and thinner toward its terminal portion. The upper surface is convex and roughened, and provides for the origin of some fibers of the deltoid muscle (Fig. 10). The

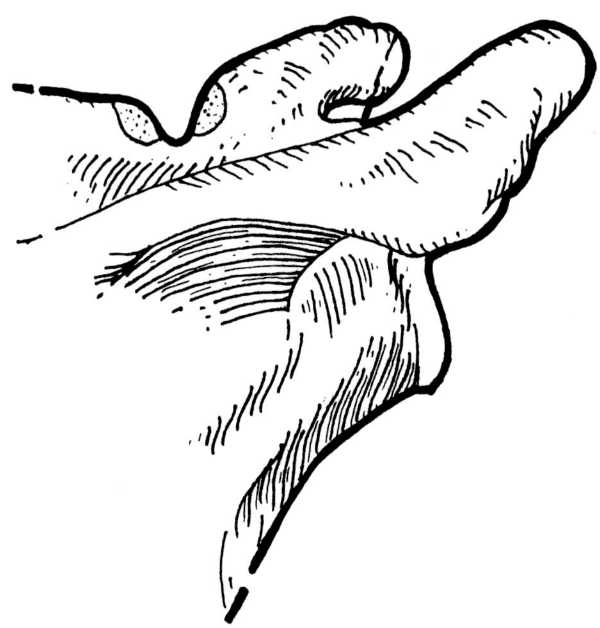

FIG. 10. Acromion process. The roughened superior surface serves as origin for a portion of the deltoid. The undersurface is covered by the coracoacromial ligament.

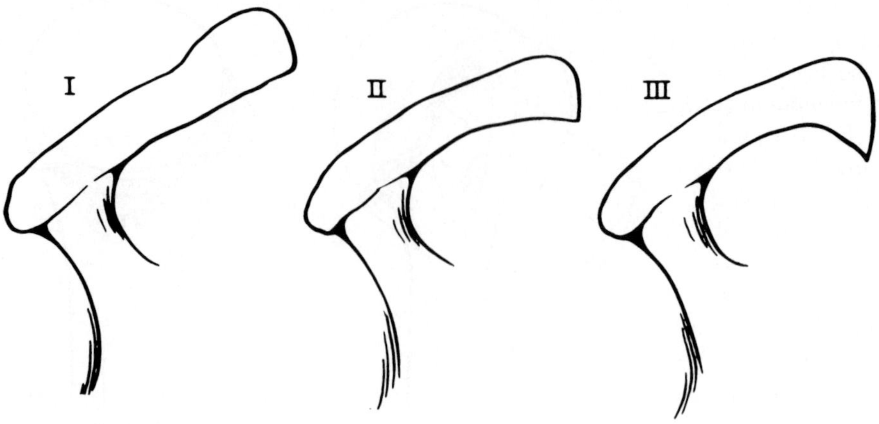

FIG. 11. Drawing of three types of acromion as originally described by Bigliani et al. (82). Type I has a flat undersurface along the entire anteroposterior course, type II is gently curved from front to back, and type III has an anterior "hook."

undersurface is smooth and concave, and closely opposed by the subacromial bursa. At the medial aspect of the most anterior portion of the acromion, there is a small concave facet that serves to articulate with the lateral clavicle. The inner margin of the process is concave in contradistinction to the outer convex margin. This inner margin serves as an attachment site for a portion of the trapezius muscle. The apex of the acromion process anteriorly serves as the site of attachment of the coracoacromial ligament.

Bigliani et al. (4) described three variations on the orientation of the acromion. In the type I acromion, the undersurface is flat, while the type II acromion is curved, and the type III acromion contains an anterior ''hook'' (Fig. 11).

Coracoid Process

The coracoid is a thick, curved, hook-shaped process that arises from the superior aspect of the neck of the scapula. From its broad base, it takes off in an upward direction before decreasing in breadth and turning anteriorly and outward (Fig. 12). The anterior border of the process is smooth at its base, providing a floor for the passage of the subscapularis muscle. The medial edge of the distal process is roughened, serving as an attachment site for the pectoralis minor muscle. The apex of the process serves as the origin of the conjoined tendon, which is made up of the short head of the biceps and the coracobrachialis muscles.

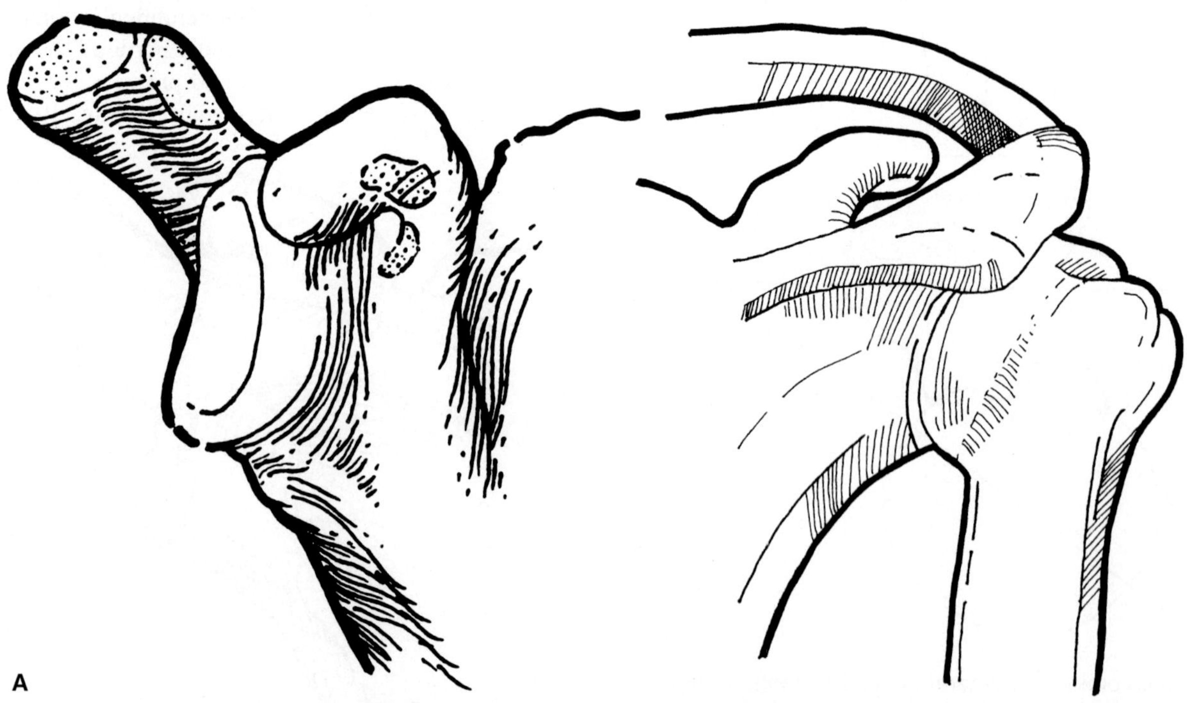

FIG. 12. A, B: Coracoid process. **A:** AP view. The coracoid process arises from the superior surface of the scapula and narrows as it proceeds away from the scapula in an anterior and lateral direction. The pectoralis minor muscle inserts onto the medial border of the distal coracoid. The anterior surface serves as the site of origin for the conjoined tendon of the short head of the biceps and the coracobrachialis.

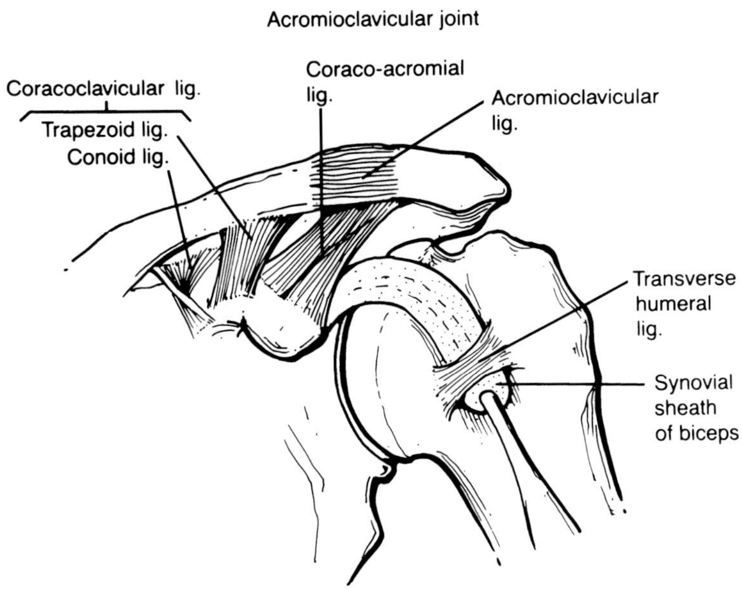

FIG. 13. Diagrammatic view of the acromioclavicular articulation and the coracoclavicular ligaments (conoid and trapezoid). These two ligaments arise from the medial border of the coracoid near its base. Note the course of the coracoacromial ligament from the lateral aspect of the coracoid to the anterior undersurface of the acromion.

The coracoclavicular ligaments insert along the medial surface closer to the base of the coracoid, and the coracoacromial ligament takes its origin from a roughened surface on the distal lateral aspect of the process (Fig. 13).

ARTICULAR SURFACE ANATOMY

The glenohumeral articulation is a synovial joint with very little inherent stability, owing to the shape and contour of the articular surfaces. The articular surface of the humeral head has an average height of 48 mm with a 25-mm radius of curvature, and the average width of the articular surface is 45 mm, with a radius of curvature measuring 22 mm (5). As noted previously, the average width of the glenoid fossa is 25 mm, while the average height is 35 mm. Saha (1) performed contact studies in 20 cadaveric shoulders in which he described three variations in articular anatomy. In type A articulations, the radius of curvature of the humeral head is smaller than that of the glenoid. In these situations, the area of articulation is small and circular and is centered in the glenoid cavity. Type B articulations are characterized by similar radii of curvature leading to a larger circular area of contact. The type C articulations are notable for a humeral head with a larger radius of curvature than the glenoid, leading to a peripheral, ring-shaped area of articulation (1) (Fig. 14).

Throughout the range of glenohumeral motion, only 25% to 30% of the humeral head is covered by the glenoid (6–8). Saha described a measure of this relative uncovering as the *glenohumeral index*, which is determined by the formula

$$\frac{\text{Maximum diameter of the glenoid}}{\text{Maximum diameter of the humeral head}}$$

In the original study, this ratio was determined to be 0.75 in the sagittal plane and 0.60 in the transverse plane (3). Several years after the original paper by Saha, the same measurements were again taken and found to be very similar at 0.86 in the sagittal plane and 0.58 in the transverse plane (9). As noted above, there may be slight variation in the anatomy of this articulation that may predispose certain individuals to instability, although this has not been proved to date.

The glenoid cavity has a limited amount of depth in both the transverse and the sagittal planes. In the superior-to-inferior direction, the depth of the glenoid averages 9.0 mm, while in the transverse plane the average depth is only 2.5 mm

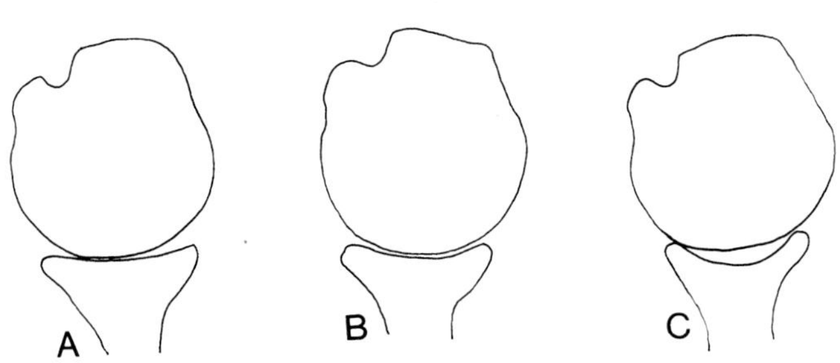

FIG. 14. Types of glenohumeral articulations as described by Saha (80). Type A shows a head smaller than the glenoid, type B has a similar radius of curvature, and type C demonstrates a humeral head larger than the glenoid. (From Saha AK. Dynamic stability of the glenohumeral joint. *Acta Orthop Scand* 1971:42;491, with permission.)

(10). A small bare area is also commonly found in the central portion of the glenoid just below the equator. This area has been shown to be more consistently present in older individuals, perhaps suggesting a degenerative etiology for the lack of cartilage in this location (11). Several factors tend to secure the head in its place. In addition to the soft-tissue structures, a negative pressure that exists in the glenohumeral joint tends to maintain joint congruity. Arthrotomy of the shoulder capsule eliminates this vacuum and leads to inferior migration of the head, even without disrupting any of the soft-tissue envelope about the joint (12).

LABRUM

Whereas the fibrocartilagenous menisci of the knee has been a well-studied anatomic structure for many years, the glenoid labrum had received little attention until relatively recent years. The labrum is a triangular structure composed of dense fibrous tissue rather than cartilage (11). Cooper et al. (13) have demonstrated the existence of a narrow ''transition zone'' between the articular surface of the glenoid and the true labrum, which is fibrocartilagenous histologically.

The blood supply to the labrum has been shown to arise from branches of the suprascapular, circumflex scapular, and posterior humeral circumflex vessels. These sources combine to form an arborizing network of vessels that penetrate the tissue in a radial pattern. Branches from the capsular and periosteal blood supply also support the labrum (13). No vascular supply is afforded by the underlying glenoid bone. Like the menisci of the knee, the vascularity of the labrum is limited to the periphery near its attachment to the joint capsule. The periosteal and capsular supply to the peripheral labrum are constant throughout the circumference of the structure; however, the superior and anterosuperior portions of the labrum have been shown to be less vascular as compared with the posterior and inferior labrum (13).

Morphologically, the labrum varies considerably from region to region. The attachment superiorly is looser and more elastic than the inferior attachment, which is more of a rounded extension of the articular surface and relatively inelastic. At the most superior portion of the labrum (12 o'clock), the labrum inserts firmly into the biceps tendon lateral to the actual insertion of the biceps onto the supraglenoid tubercle. This superior area is unique in that the articular surface extends proximally over the superior lip of the glenoid for a short distance into a recess created by the slightly offset insertion of the biceps tendon. This small recess is approximately 5 mm in depth. In addition to the biceps tendon, the labrum serves as the attachment site for the superior, inferior, and middle glenohumeral ligament complexes in most people (Fig. 15). Little variation exists between the anterior and posterior labrum inferiorly, although in some instances the anterior tissue may be slightly thicker.

Several anatomic variations have been described in regard to the anterior attachment of the labrum to the glenoid rim. In the study by Cooper et al. (13), 4 of 11 specimens

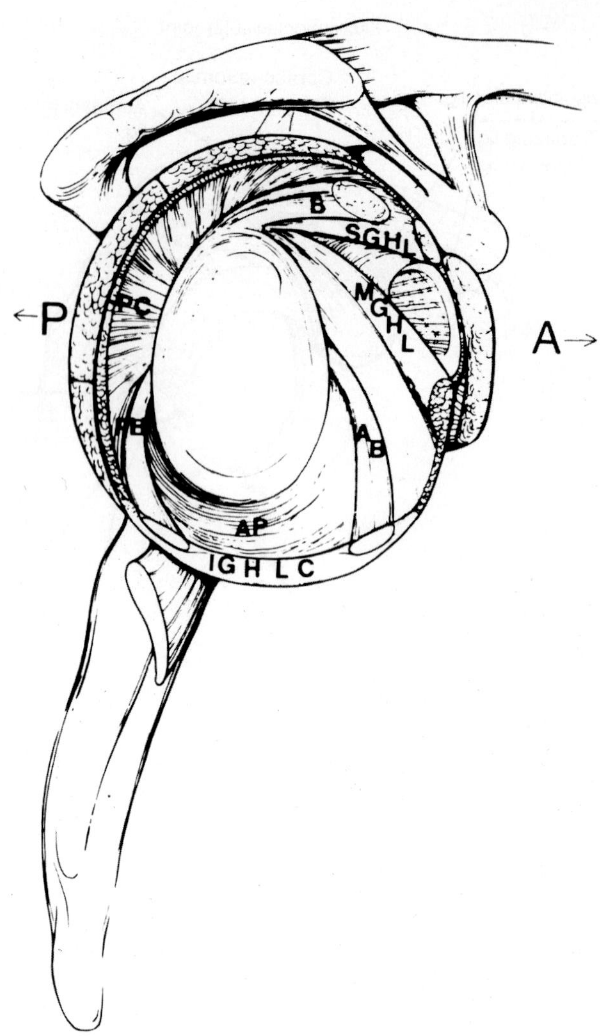

FIG. 15. Relationship of glenoid labrum to glenohumeral ligaments. *A*, anterior; *P*, posterior; *B*, biceps tendon; *MGHL*, middle glenohumeral ligament; *SGHL*, superior glenohumeral ligament; *AP*, axillary pouch; *PB*, posterior band; *PC*, posterior capsule. (From O'Brien SJ, Neves MC, Arnoczky SP, et al. The anatomy and histology of the inferior glenohumeral ligament complex of the shoulder. *Am J Sports Med* 1990;18:449, with permission.)

contained an area where there was no attachment at the 2 o'clock position. This sublabral foramen (Fig. 16) provided direct access to the subscapularis recess beneath the free edge of the labrum. In another 5 of 11 specimens, there was a loose capsular attachment of the labrum to the glenoid at this location. It is important to recognize that this sublabral foramen is not a pathologic condition.

The thought that the labrum functions as a static stabilizer of the glenohumeral joint has been well documented (14,15). As noted above, the average depth of the articular surface of the glenoid in the transverse plane is 2.5 mm. Howell and Galinat believed that the labrum serves to deepen the glenoid by an additional 2.5 mm both anteriorly and posteriorly, adding to the static stability of the joint (10). The variation in regional anatomy of the labrum has

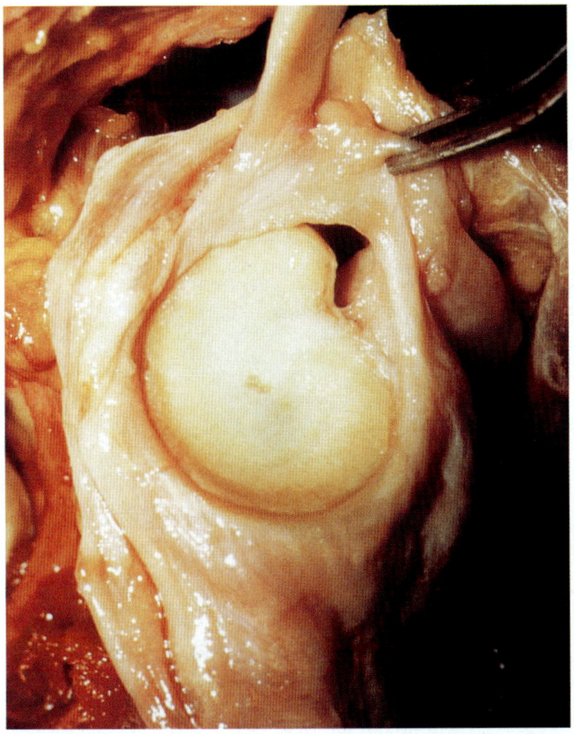

FIG. 16. Photograph of the sublabral foramen. This normal variant of labral anatomy should not be confused with a labral detachment.

suggested the possibility that it may function at least in part as not only a deepening of the glenoid, but also as a mobile extension of the glenoid surface superiorly.

LIGAMENTOUS ANATOMY

Glenohumeral Ligaments

Although recently receiving much attention in the orthopedic literature, the glenohumeral ligaments were written about as early as 1853 by Schlemm and described in 1934 by Codman as "slightly firmer portions of the capsular ligaments" (16).

The superior glenohumeral ligament (SGHL) has been shown to be present in 90% to 97% of shoulders in cadaveric studies (11,17). It is the most constant of the glenohumeral ligaments. There are three well-documented anatomical variations of the SGHL (Fig. 17). These include a common origin with the biceps tendon, origin from the labrum just anterior to the biceps tendon, or arising in common with the middle glenohumeral ligament (11). The SGHL inserts into the fovea capitis of the humerus near the tip of the lesser tuberosity, along with a portion of the coracohumeral ligament. The ligament may vary in thickness from definite robust ligamentous tissue to a whispy thickening of the superior capsule. A study conducted by O'Brien, Schwartz and colleagues (18) in 1988 concluded that the SGHL contributed little to the static stability of the glenohumeral joint in the anteroposterior plane. However, in a more recent study, the SGHL was shown to be the primary restraint to inferior translation of the humeral head in the adducted shoulder (19). In the abducted shoulder, the SGHL becomes slack (see Fig. 20).

The middle glenohumeral ligament (MGHL) demonstrates the greatest variability in both size and presence. In the classic study by DePalma (11), the MGHL was considered well formed in only 71% of specimens, poorly formed in 17%, and absent in the remaining 12%. In the later study by O'Brien, the MGHL was found to be absent in 27% of specimens (17). As with the SGHL, the middle glenohumeral ligament varies from a well-defined ligamentous structure measuring up to 2.0 cm in width and 4.0 mm in thickness, to a whispy thickening of the anterior capsule (20). It originates from the labrum just beneath the superior glenohumeral ligament or from the neck of the glenoid at the same level. Its insertion is on the humerus just medial to the lesser tuberosity, deep and closely opposed to the

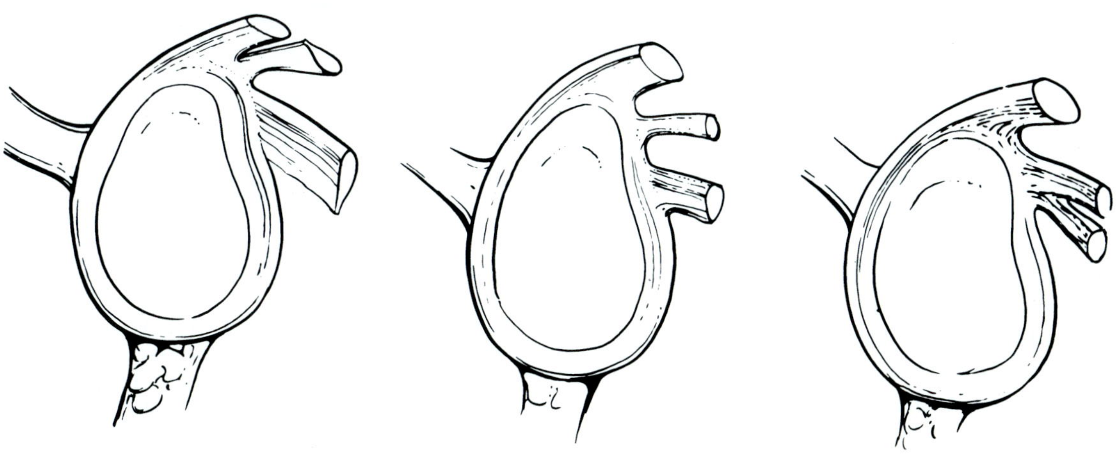

FIG. 17. Diagram of the variation in normal anatomy of the SGHL as described by DePalma et al. (8). The SGHL originates in one of three ways: (i) it may begin in common with the biceps tendon, (ii) it may take origin from the labrum just anterior to the biceps anchor, or (iii) it may arise in common with the MGHL.

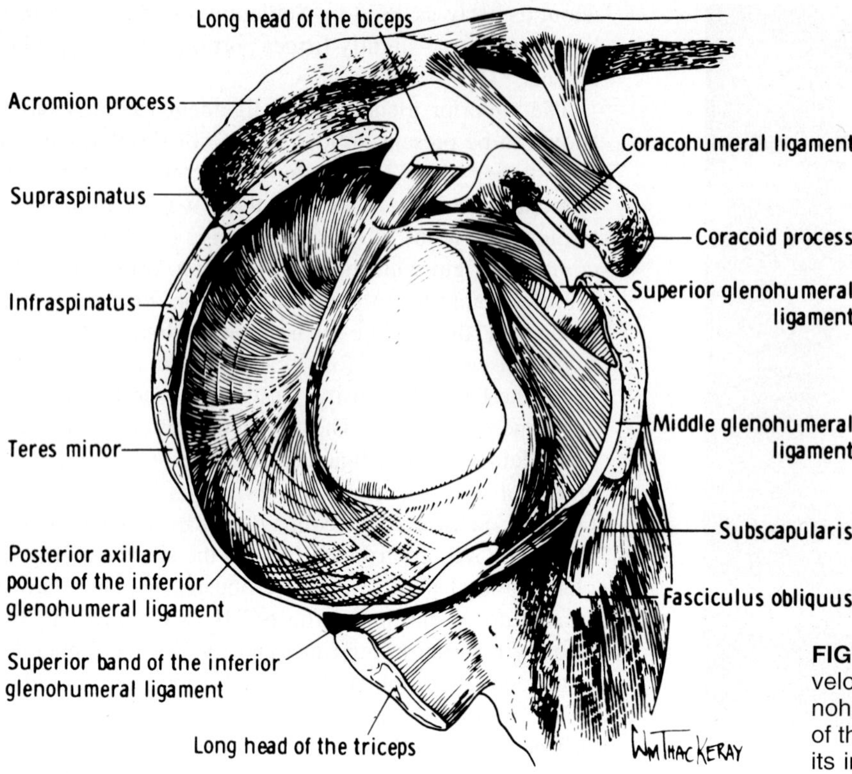

FIG. 18. Diagram of the soft-tissue envelope immediately surrounding the glenohumeral articulation. Note the joining of the MGHL with the subscapularis near its insertion onto the humerus.

subscapularis tendon (21). It joins the subscapularis tendon approximately 2 cm medial to its insertion (Fig. 18). When well developed, the MGHL functions as a significant restraint to inferior translation with the shoulder in adduction and external rotation (19). It has also been shown to function as a secondary stabilizer to anterior translation if the anterior portion of the inferior glenohumeral ligament is injured (18). It also resists external rotation of the adducted shoulder. In instances in which the ligament is poorly formed, it can be noticed as a pair of parallel thickenings in the capsule without a distinct attachment site on the glenoid or labrum. The ligament becomes increasingly taut in the extremes of internal and external rotation.

The inferior glenohumeral ligament (IGHL) complex is composed of both an anterior band (AB) and a posterior band (PB), as well as a capsular ''hammock'' between the two bands forming the axillary pouch (Fig. 19). The anterior and posterior bands take origin from either the labrum or the adjacent glenoid neck, and insert onto the anatomic neck of the humerus. The anterior band has been shown to originate between the 2 o'clock and 4 o'clock positions, and the posterior band between the 7 o'clock and 9 o'clock positions (17). On the humeral side, the complex inserts in either a 90-degree arc (see Fig. 9) just lateral to the inferior articular surface, or in a V-shaped insertion with the AB and PB inserting near the articular surface and the axillary pouch extending further lateral (see Fig. 9). Early investigators determined that the anterior superior aspect of the ligament was particularly thickened in some specimens, calling it the ''superior band.'' These studies were per-

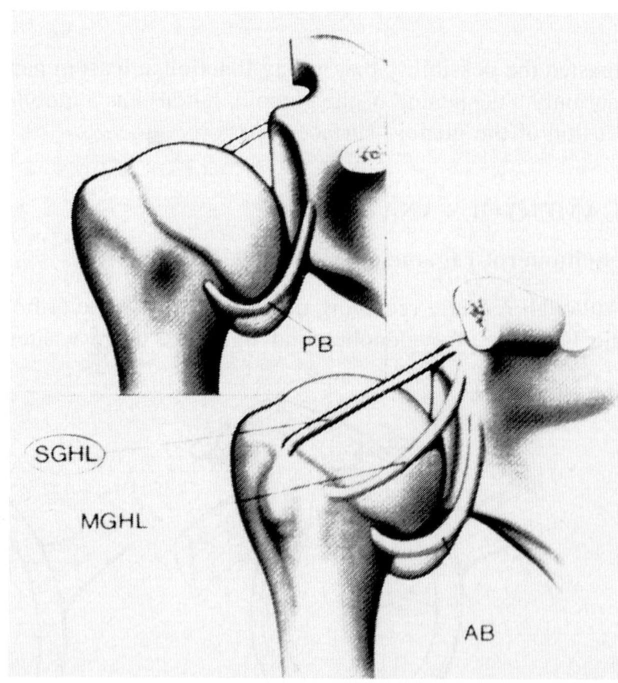

FIG. 19. Inferior glenohumeral ligament. This tissue forms a "hammock" beneath the humeral head. This illustration shows the humerus in adduction and neutral rotation. The SGHL is the primary restraint to inferior translation. *SGHL*, superior glenohumeral ligament (the anterior and posterior bands of the IGHL are relatively lax in this position); *AB*, anterior band; *PB*, posterior band; *MGHL*, middle glenohumeral ligament. (From Bowen MK, Warren RF. Ligamentous control of shoulder stability based on selective cutting and static translation experiment. *Clin Sports Med* 1991;10:757–782, with permission.)

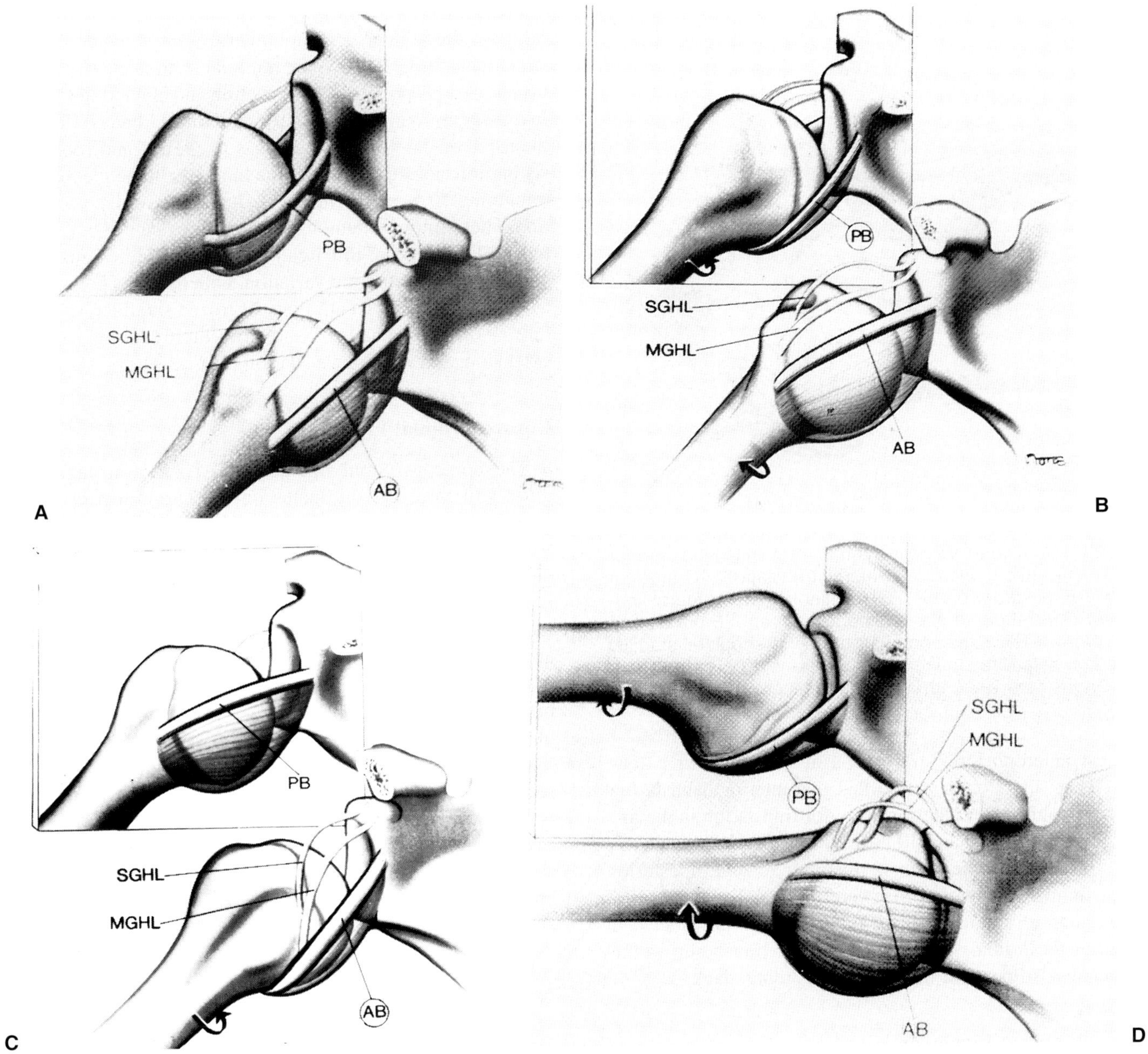

FIG. 20. Function of the IGHL to restrain anterior and posterior motion of the humeral head within the glenoid with the shoulder in 45 degrees of abduction and **(A)** neutral rotation. External rotation moves the AB anterosuperiorly, and the posterior band resists inferior translation of the humeral head **(B)**. In internal rotation **(C)** the anterior band moves inferiorly resisting inferior translation. Note that in 45 degrees of abduction the SGHL is relatively lax. With the arm in 90 degrees of abduction and external rotation **(D)**, the posterior band moves inferiorly to resist inferior translation. *(figure continues)*

formed by disarticulating the humerus or by approaching the joint by a posterior arthrotomy. More recently, arthroscopic examination has led to a better understanding of the IGHL complex as we understand it today (17). The AB is thicker than the PB and the anterior capsule, and is generally easier to distinguish than the PB because of its higher origin from the glenoid rim. When comparing the various portions of the IGHL complex, the length of the anterior band, axillary pouch, and posterior band are all similar at around 43 mm (22). In this study, Ticker et al. (22) showed that the portions of the IGHL complex are thicker medially toward their glenoid insertions than they are laterally. On the basis of their study, these investigators also concluded that both the anterior band and axillary pouch function to restrain the humeral head against rapid anterior displacement.

The IGHL is the primary static restraint to anterior and posterior translation of the humeral head in the abducted shoulder (Fig. 20A-E). In a cadaveric study by O'Brien et al. (18), the abducted shoulder was shown to have the

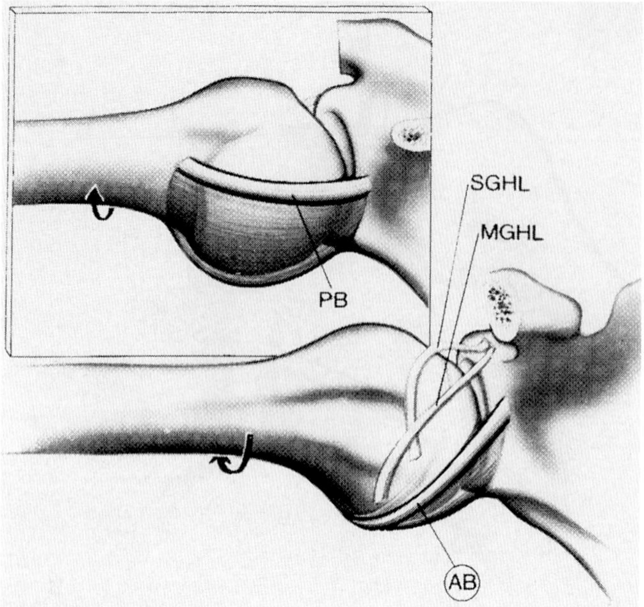

E

FIG. 20. *Continued.* While in internal rotation **(E)** the anterior band moves inferiorly to resist inferior translation. *AB*, anterior band; *PB*, posterior band; *MGHL*, middle glenohumeral ligament; *SGHL*, superior glenohumeral ligament. (From Bowen MK, Warren RF. Ligamentous control of shoulder stability based on selective cutting and static translation experiment. *Clin Sports Med* 1991;10:757–782, with permission.)

greatest anteroposterior translation at 0 degrees of extension. They also demonstrated that the anterior band is the primary stabilizer to anterior-posterior translation in the abducted shoulder in 0 and 30 degrees of extension, while the posterior band is the primary restraint to anteroposterior translation in 30 degrees of forward flexion. The IGHL also offers support against inferior translation of the head and becomes the primary restraint to inferior translation in the abducted position with the SGHL becoming slack.

Coracohumeral Ligament

As with other ligamentous structures about the shoulder, little attention had been paid to the coracohumeral ligament (CHL) until recently. In a study by Cooper et al. (23), three anatomic variations were noted. In the first group, which included 9 of 12 specimens, the CHL was in fact a fold in the anterior superior capsule that could be enhanced by inferior migration of the humeral head. These findings were confirmed histologically, with no discrete collagen bundles forming a true ligament. The second group, which included only 2 of 12 specimens, was similar to the first group, except that the fold was incomplete anteriorly. In only one specimen, the third type, was a discrete ligamentous structure encountered. The CHL originates on the coracoid process of the scapula and travels laterally in the interval between the subscapularis and supraspinatus, converging with the SGHL near its insertion point on the lesser tuberosity.

Previously thought to contribute to superior-inferior stability of the adducted glenohumeral joint, Cooper demonstrated that the CHL provided minimal or no suspensory function in various positions of adduction and abduction (23,24). In a study by Warner et al. (19) involving 11 cadaveric specimens, 1 of the 11 ligaments was thickened and robust resisting inferior translation of the humerus in the glenoid; the remaining 10 were essentially insignificant in size and function. These findings demonstrate the wide range of both structure and function of this ligament and should be considered part of normal anatomic variation. Other studies have implicated the CHL in the pathology of frozen shoulder. Contracture of the CHL has been shown to limit external rotation, extension, and inferior translation (25).

Coracoacromial Ligament

The coracoacromial ligament (CAL) is a strong triangular structure that originates on the lateral aspect of the coracoid and inserts just in front of the articular surface of the clavicle on the acromion and continues along the undersurface of the anterior acromion (Fig. 21). Laterally, it is continuous with the deep deltoid fascia. The CAL is directly confluent with the inferior capsule of the AC joint in approximately 60% of individuals (26). The ligament ranges in length from 3 to 5 cm, and from 0.95 to 2.8 cm in width. The insertion of the ligament on the undersurface of the acromion is in the shape of a "T", with one-half of the fibers inserting anteromedially and the other half inserting anteroinferiorly. Few fibers reach the posterior aspect of the acromion (26).

Biomechanically, the CA ligament has been shown to be a vital structure in the stability of the AC joint. In sectioning studies, release of the CA ligament was mandatory in

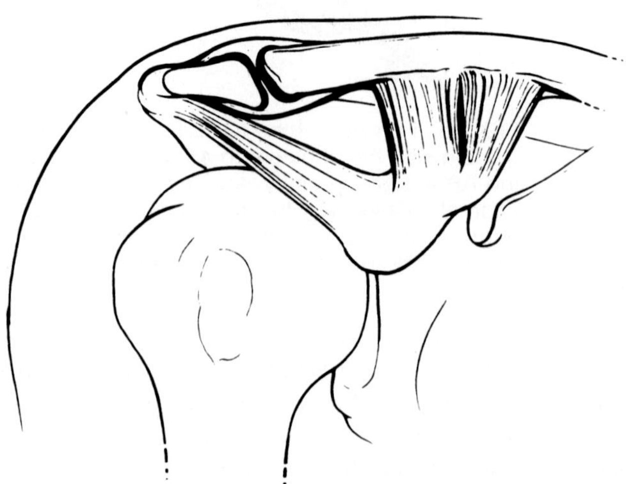

FIG. 21. Ligaments arising from the coracoid process. The coracoacromial ligament originates on the lateral aspect of the coracoid process and traverses the undersurface of the acromion before becoming confluent with the deep deltoid fascia laterally. The conoid ligament arises slightly posterior and medial to the trapezoid ligament.

order to disarticulate the joint (26). The subacromial bulk of the CA ligament has been proposed as a buffer protecting the rotator cuff tendons from impingement. Thickening or hypertrophy of the ligament has also been implicated as a possible etiology of impingement.

Coracoclavicular Ligaments

The conoid and trapezoid ligaments (coracoclavicular ligaments) are short, broad ligaments that take their origin from the superior aspect of the proximal coracoid process just behind the insertion of the pectoralis minor, and insert on the undersurface of the clavicle (Fig. 21). The conoid ligament arises slightly posterior and medial to the trapezoid ligament on the coracoid process. The trapezoid ligament inserts along the oblique line of the clavicle, which is the ridge on the undersurface mentioned above (Fig. 7). The conoid ligament is cone-shaped, inserting onto the conoid tubercle of the clavicle more laterally, but also giving fibers to the oblique line as well. The anterior border of the trapezoid ligament is free; the posterior border blends with the conoid ligament. These ligaments are extra-articular, but they serve to maintain the clavicle in its position of articulation with the acromion process. They are the strongest of the static stabilizers of the acromioclavicular joint. This is of clinical importance in that with increasing severity of AC joint injury, the likelihood of coracoclavicular ligament rupture also increases (34a).

Studies by Salter et al. (26) have demonstrated that the length of the trapezoid ligament may vary from 0.85 to 2.50 cm in length and from 0.80 to 2.50 cm in width. The conoid ligament measured 0.70 to 2.50 cm in length and 0.40 to 0.95 cm in width. The approximate distance between the undersurface of the clavicle and the upper border of the coracoid process is 1.3 cm (27,28).

Mechanically, these ligaments serve to join the actions of glenohumeral flexion and abduction to the motions of the scapula against the thorax. The clavicle has been noted to rotate about its longitudinal axis during glenohumeral abduction. With increasing abduction, the clavicle rotates through an arc of approximately 45 degrees in a counterclockwise direction (29). The coracoclavicular ligaments limit this rotation, and therefore also have some control over scapular motion by virtue of their attachment to the coracoid process (30). Numerous studies have demonstrated the role of the coracoclavicular ligaments in stabilizing the acromioclavicular articulation. Urist (31) provided evidence that complete acromioclavicular dislocation could occur without disruption of the coracoclavicular ligaments. Urist showed that the clavicle could be dislocated either anteriorly or posteriorly with sectioning of the acromioclavicular ligament and joint capsule along with detachment of the deltoid and trapezius muscles. However, superior or inferior complete dislocation could not be achieved without sectioning of the coracoclavicular ligaments (31). Rockwood and colleagues (32,33) later repeated the studies of Urist and obtained similar findings. Individual ligament contribution to the stability of the acromioclavicular articulation was studied by Fukuda et al. (34). These investigators determined that, at low levels of displacement, the acromioclavicular ligament was the primary restraint to both superior and posterior translation. However, at higher levels of displacement, the conoid ligament became the primary restraint to superior translation, while the acromioclavicular ligament remained the primary restraint to posterior movement. The function of the trapezoid ligament was shown to be restraint of acromioclavicular joint compression at both low- and high-level stresses (34). From these studies, it can be concluded that the coracoclavicular ligaments are the primary restraint to superior clavicular dislocation.

CAPSULE AND SYNOVIUM

The shoulder is a diarthrodial joint surrounded by a joint capsule lined with synovium. The capsule of the shoulder joint comprises three distinct layers of collagen in various orientations (Fig. 22). The inner and outer layers are similar in that the fibers of these layers are oriented along the coronal axis extending from the humerus to the glenoid neck. The fibers of the middle layer differ in that they are ori-

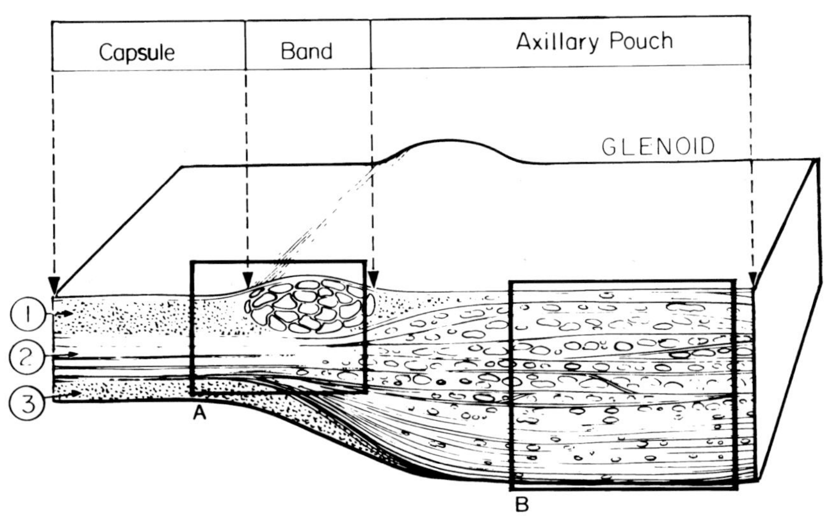

FIG. 22. Diagram of histologic appearance of shoulder joint capsule. The inner and outer layers are similar histologically with collagen fibers oriented from the humerus to the glenoid. The fibers of the middle layer *(2)* are oriented perpendicular to the other layers. In the region of the inferior axillary pouch *(B)* the layers become somewhat confluent. *1*, inner layer; *2*, middle layer; *3*, outer layer; *A*, posterior band; *B*, axillary pouch. (From O'Brien SJ, Neves MC, Arnoczky SP, et al. The anatomy and histology of the inferior glenohumeral ligament complex of the shoulder. *Am J Sports Med* 1990;18:449, with permission.)

ented in the sagittal plane in a direction approximately perpendicular to the fibers of the other two layers (35). The capsule extends from the glenoid neck to the anatomic neck of the humerus, being more closely opposed to the articular surface of the humerus superiorly.

The dimensions and characteristics of the shoulder capsule are variable depending on the location in relation to the glenohumeral joint. The capsule anterior to the inferior glenohumeral ligament complex is relatively thicker than the capsule posterior to the inferior glenohumeral ligament complex. This is caused primarily by the relative increase in thickness of the middle layer of collagen anteriorly. The anterior band of the inferior glenohumeral ligament is a thickened portion of the inner layer of the capsule. This finding is confirmed histologically, as the anterior band is seen as an area of well-organized, coarse collagen bundles. The posterior band is a similar thickening of the inner layer, except that the transition from normal capsule to posterior band is more marked than the transition anteriorly. This difference, which can only be appreciated histologically, may be attributable to the fact that the posterior capsule is relatively thinner than the anterior capsule, making the transition to the thicker ligamentous structure more prominent. This is represented schematically in Figure 22. As noted above, the posterior capsule is quite thin. The outer layer is least prominent posteriorly, where it blends with the loose areolar tissue surrounding the capsule.

The axillary pouch, which is the joint capsule between the anterior and posterior bands of the inferior glenohumeral ligaments, demonstrates a more gradual transition. The outer layer is nearly nonexistent in the axillary pouch. The coarse fibers of the inner layer blend gradually with the perpendicularly oriented fibers of the middle layer. Looking further anterior, the three layers again become distinct toward the anterior band. The capsule is relatively thickened anterior to the anterior band, with intermingling of the fibers between the middle and outer layers.

The shoulder joint capsule is sensitive to changes in its environment. For example, heating of the joint capsule beyond 65°C has been shown to cause shrinking of the collagen bundles (36). This may become an important means of increasing stability to a previously unstable shoulder. Currently, studies are under way using an arthroscopic heat probe in an effort to cause contraction of the joint capsule at selected sites based on patient needs. Upon application of the probe, and heating to approximately 67°C, the tissue becomes gradually caramelized and shrinks.

The increase in the total volume of the joint capsule has been implicated as a possible etiology of instability. In 1968, Reeves (37) published data that demonstrated the volume of the shoulder joint capsule. He noted that normal values were 16 to 20 ml, and that persons with instability had increased volumes. These studies were performed using arthrography; however, intra-articular pressure was not taken into account in this study. In 1994, Sperber and Wredmark (38) performed a study using arthroscopic injection after measuring intra-articular pressure and body surface area. They found no correlation between joint volume and body surface area, and there was no difference in volume between shoulders that had previously dislocated and normal shoulders in the same patient. They concluded that no irreversible capsular stretching occurs at the time of dislocation. Speer and Moorman (personal communication, 1993) demonstrated that, in a shoulder that has been subjected to anterior dislocation, the vacuum effect is lost as a result of an increase in compliance of the joint capsule.

The shoulder capsule has been shown to have innervation arising from the axillary, subscapular, musculocutaneous, suprascapular, and possibly radial nerves (39–41). More specifically, the scapular side of the shoulder joint capsule is supplied by the axillary and musculocutaneous articular branches that terminate in the anterior and superior capsule. The middle anterior portion of the capsule is supplied by a branch from the subscapular nerve. The inferior, anterior, and posterior capsule are all supplied by an articular branch of the axillary nerve. On the humeral side, the capsule is supplied by the same nerves, except that there is no contribution from the subscapular nerve. In the region of the capsule surrounding the labrum, mechanoreceptors have been identified that are part of a synergistic reflex arc that may play a role in shoulder stability (42,43).

BURSAE, NORMAL RECESSES, AND SPACES

Several bursae positioned about the glenohumeral joint are of clinical significance. These include the subacromial bursa and the subscapular bursa (Fig. 23). Another bursa may exist between the joint capsule and the tendon of the infraspinatus muscle (infraspinatus bursa). Additionally, in some cases there may exist a bursa between the conoid and trapezoid ligaments.

The subacromial bursa is a synovium-lined space that lies between the superior surface of the rotator cuff and the undersurface of the deltoid muscle. The bursa extends from the musculotendinous junction of the rotator cuff medially to the humeral shaft beyond the tuberosities where the rotator cuff inserts. In the normal state, this bursa is only 1 to 2 mm thick. In the diseased state this tissue may become massively enlarged and irritated, generally as a result of subacromial impingement.

The subscapularis bursa is an oblong structure lying between the scapular neck and the subscapularis muscle and tendon. There is a communication between this bursa and the joint between the superior and middle glenohumeral ligaments. The bursa serves to protect the subscapularis muscle and tendon as it passes over the neck of the scapula and under the coracoid process. In cases of synovitis of the shoulder, it is frequently in this region where the most intense proliferation is found.

There are a number of recesses about the shoulder that are variable in presence, size, and shape. DePalma (11) described six variations of recesses in the anterior capsule alone. These

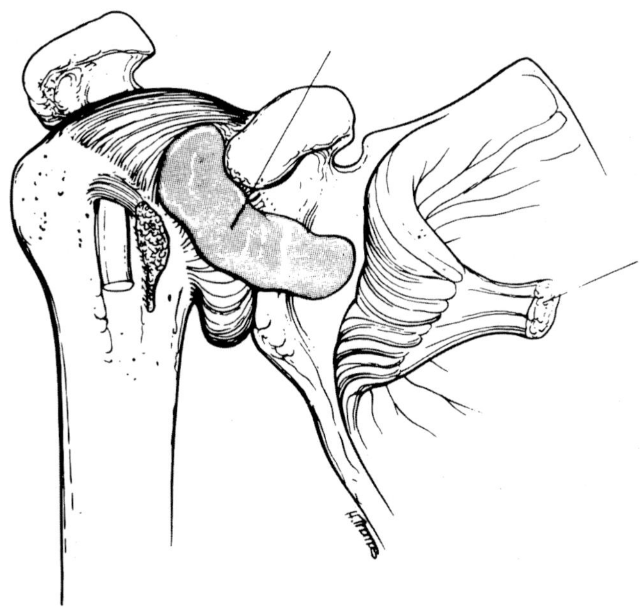

FIG. 23. Diagram of the subscapularis bursa. This bursa lies between the scapular neck and the subscapularis. There is a communication between the bursa and the glenohumeral joint between the superior and middle glenohumeral ligaments. (From O'Brien SJ, Arnoczky SP, Warren RF, Rozbruch SR. Developmental anatomy of the shoulder and anatomy of the glenohumeral joint. In: Rockwood CA Jr, Matsen FA III, eds. *The shoulder*. Philadelphia: WB Saunders, 1990:11–33, with permission.)

variations were very much dependent on the anatomy of the glenohumeral ligaments and the subscapularis bursa. Type I, found in 30.2% of specimens, has one synovial recess immediately above the middle glenohumeral ligament. Type II (2%) has one synovial recess immediately below the middle glenohumeral ligament. Type III (40.6%) has one recess immediately above and one recess immediately below the middle glenohumeral ligament. Type IV (9%) has one synovial recess directly above the anterior band of the inferior glenohumeral ligament and no middle glenohumeral ligament. Type V (5.1%) has two small folds of synovium in the place of the middle glenohumeral ligament. Type VI (11.4%) has no synovial recesses at all, but very well-defined glenohumeral ligaments (Fig. 24). DePalma's studies led him to conclude that, in the presence of well-defined synovial recesses, thinning of the anterior capsule occurred, which would predispose a person to instability.

ROTATOR INTERVAL

The rotator interval is a triangular area of tissue, with its base at the coracoid process and its apex at the insertion of the coracohumeral ligament laterally on the humerus. It is bordered superiorly by the anterior edge of the supraspinatus tendon and inferiorly by the superior edge of the subscapularis tendon (Fig. 25). In normal persons, this space is occupied by capsular tissue, which is thickened by both

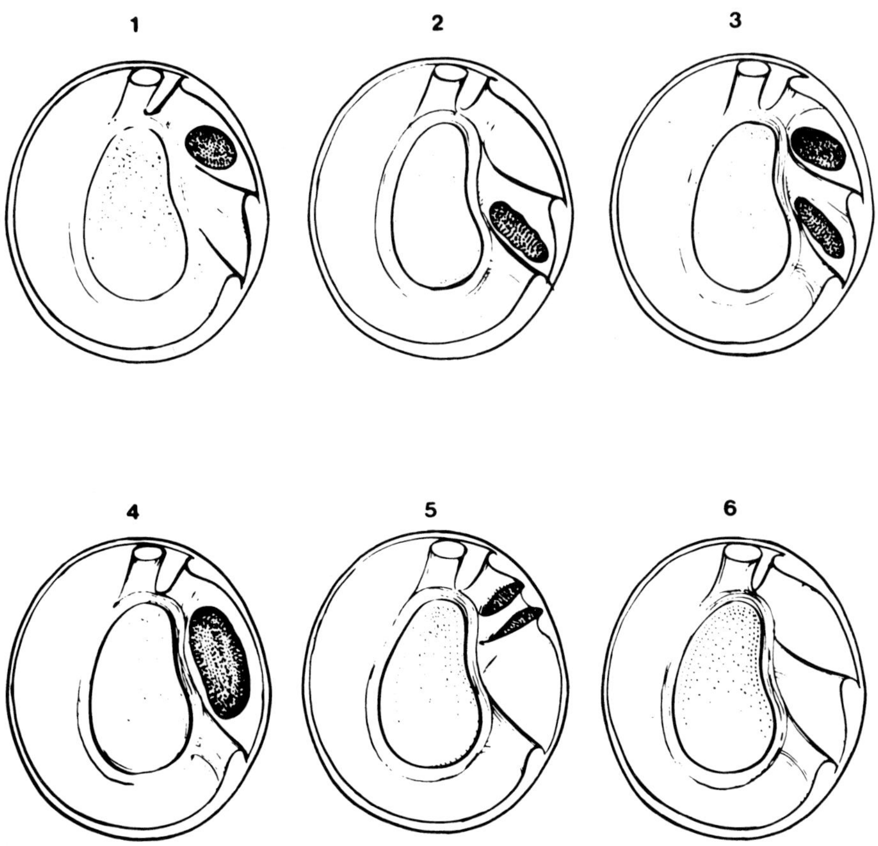

FIG. 24. Variation in shoulder anatomy with regard to recesses and spaces as described by DePalma et al. (8). See text for details.

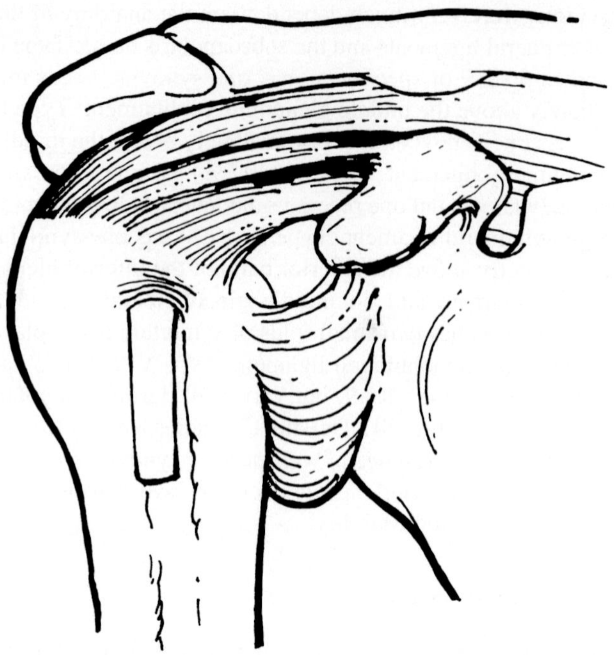

FIG. 25. Diagram of the rotator interval, bordered anteriorly by the superior aspect of the subscapularis muscle and tendon and posteriorly by the supraspinatus muscle and tendon. This "space" is usually occupied by capsular tissue. (Redrawn from O'Brien SJ, Arnoczky SP, Warren RF, Rozbruch SR. Developmental anatomy of the shoulder and anatomy of the glenohumeral joint. In: Rockwood CA Jr, Matsen FA III, eds. *The shoulder.* Philadelphia: WB Saunders, 1990: 11–33, with permission.)

the superior glenohumeral ligament and the coracohumeral ligament (35). The base of this triangular interval is its greatest dimension.

The characteristics of the rotator interval and its contribution to glenohumeral stability have been described in a cadaveric model by Harryman et al. (44). These investigators demonstrated that sectioning of the rotator interval permitted increased glenohumeral translation in the anterior, posterior, and inferior directions. Operative imbrication of the interval tissue then led to less translation than had been observed in the intact state in the posterior and inferior directions. Operative release of the rotator interval tissue to regain motion and operative closure or plication of the rotator interval for instability have been described both in combination with other procedures and in isolation (45–47). In clinical studies, posterior laxity has not been encountered after isolated sectioning of the rotator interval (45,47). This may be attributable to either inadequacy of the model used for the cadaver studies or a dynamic stabilizing force that is present in the live model. By contrast, the inferior and anterior translation noted in the cadaveric studies were reproduced in the clinical studies.

Defects in the capsular tissue of the rotator interval have been well described in the orthopedic literature (6,45–51). The etiology of these defects remains undetermined. Traumatic dislocation of the shoulder is unlikely because most patients in the clinical studies describing this lesion had not sustained an acute traumatic event. Recurrent subluxation inducing cumulative microtrauma has been postulated as a cause of these defects, but this possibility lacks clinical support at this time. Field et al. (47) postulated a congenital basis for these defects that predisposes those patients to increased humeral head translation and subsequently to later complaints because of the enlargement of the defect and clinically significant instability.

ROTATOR CUFF

The rotator cuff is a sheath of tissue composed of the tendinous portions of the subscapularis, supraspinatus, infraspinatus, and teres minor muscles. Together they surround the glenohumeral joint, humeral head, and joint capsule forming a nearly continuous sleeve around these structures (Fig. 26). Figure 18 nicely depicts the relationship of the rotator cuff tendons to the remainder of the soft-tissue envelope.

In general, tendons of the rotator cuff are composed largely of water (55% of wet weight) and collagen (85%

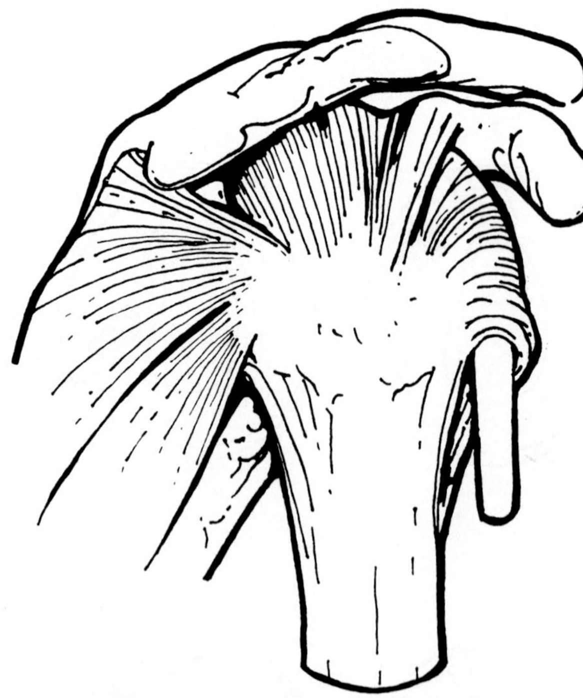

FIG. 26. The rotator cuff forms a "sleeve" around the anterior, superior, and posterior aspect of the humeral head and glenoid. Note also the coracohumeral ligament arising from base of the coracoid and traveling between the subscapularis and supraspinatus. (Redrawn from O'Brien SJ, Arnoczky SP, Warren RF, Rozbruch SR. Developmental anatomy of the shoulder and anatomy of the glenohumeral joint. In: Rockwood CA Jr, Matsen FA III, eds. *The shoulder.* Philadelphia: WB Saunders, 1990:11–33, with permission.)

dry weight). Type I collagen predominates, but trace amounts of type III and type XII collagen are consistently present. The proportion of type III collagen increases with age, rotator cuff tear, and degeneration (52–56). Glycosaminoglycan concentration is higher in rotator cuff tendons than in other tendons (57). Nearly 50% of the glycosaminoglycan content is hyaluronic acid, which is a significantly higher proportion than is seen in other tendons (57).

Before considering the combined anatomy and function of the rotator cuff, it is worthwhile to discuss the anatomic features of each portion of the rotator cuff individually.

Subscapularis

The subscapularis is a large triangular muscle that takes its origin over a broad area of the medial subscapular fossa of the scapula. Although muscle tissue occupies the entire fossa, the fibers originate along ridges located only along the medial two-thirds (58). Several fibers also arise from the lower two-thirds of the groove on the axillary border of the bone. The muscle fibers pass laterally, converging to terminate in a tendon, which inserts onto the lesser tuberosity of the humerus (Fig. 27). The fibers that originate on the axillary border of the scapula insert onto the neck of the humerus for a distance of approximately 2 cm. The tendinous portion of the muscle lies just anterior to the anterior joint capsule and becomes intimately attached to it before insertion on the humerus. The muscle belly runs below the coracoid process, and is separated from its base by a large bursa (subscapularis bursa; see Fig. 23). The muscle is innervated by branches of the fifth and sixth cervical nerve roots through the upper and lower subscapular nerves. The primary action of the subscapularis is internal rotation of the arm (59). Itoi et al. (60) demonstrated that the subscapularis is the least important contributor to anterior stability in the intact shoulder.

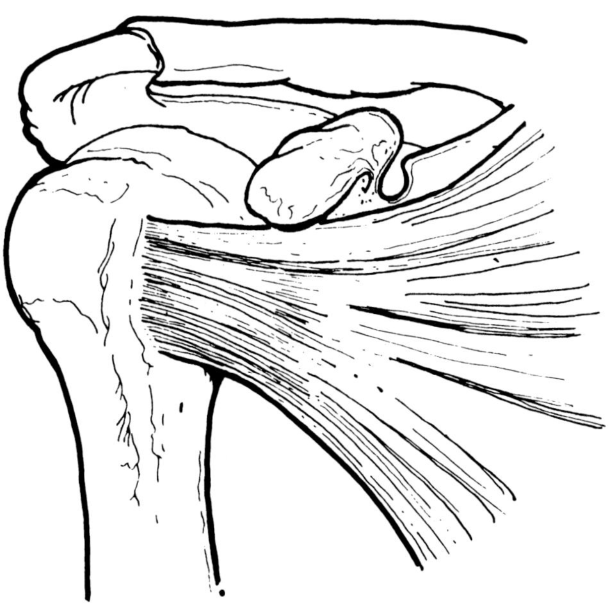

FIG. 27. Subscapularis muscle and tendon, inserting onto lesser tuberosity.

The tendinous portion of the subscapularis is composed of four to six bundles of collagen fibers that extend from the myotendinous junction to the lesser tuberosity. Toward the anterior surface of the tendon, the bundles are tightly packed, whereas on the undersurface they are separated by loose connective tissue (61). Fibers from the subscapularis join a few fibers from the supraspinatus to form the floor of the bicipital groove. A zone of fibrocartilagenous tissue is present at the insertion of the tendon.

Supraspinatus

The supraspinatus muscle occupies the entire supraspinatus fossa of the scapula. The muscle takes its origin from the medial two-thirds of a thick fascia that lines the entire fossa. The fibers of the muscle run from medial to lateral and terminate in a thick tendon that inserts onto the highest of three facets of the greater tuberosity of the humerus (Fig. 28). Near its insertion on the humerus, several fibers join with those of the subscapularis to form the floor of the bicipital groove. The supraspinatus is innervated by the suprascapular nerve, and serves to abduct the humerus.

Clark and Harryman (61) divided the supraspinatus and infraspinatus tendons into five distinct layers on the basis of their dissections (Fig. 29). Layer I (1 mm thick) is composed of fibers of the coracohumeral ligament that are oriented obliquely in relation to the muscle axes. Large arte-

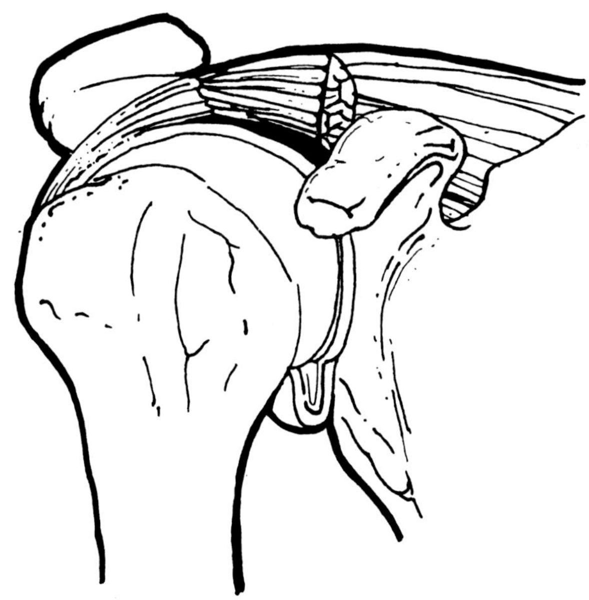

FIG. 28. Supraspinatus muscle and tendon with insertion onto greater tuberosity. (Redrawn from O'Brien SJ, Arnoczky SP, Warren RF, Rozbruch SR. Developmental anatomy of the shoulder and anatomy of the glenohumeral joint. In: Rockwood CA Jr, Matsen FA III, eds. *The shoulder.* Philadelphia: WB Saunders, 1990:11–33, with permission.)

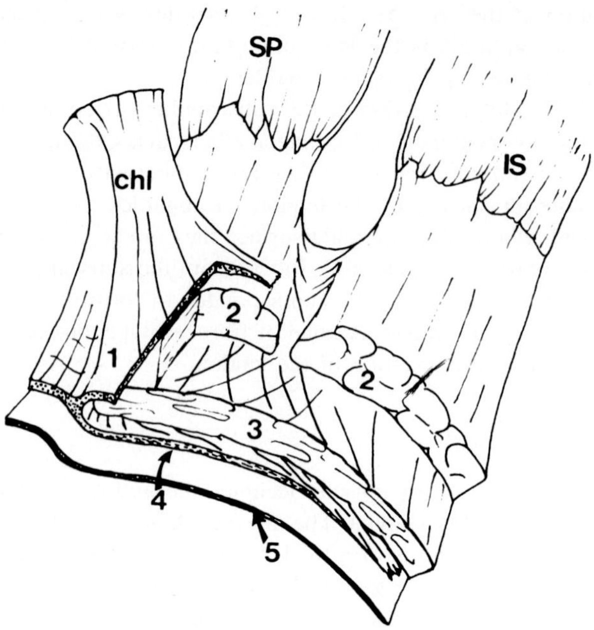

FIG. 29. Five microscopic layers of supraspinatus and infraspinatus as described by Clark and Harryman (61). See text for details.

rioles are contained in this layer. Layer II (3–5 mm thick) is composed of closely packed bundles of tendon fibers that extend directly from the muscle belly of either the supraspinatus or infraspinatus to the tuberosity. Fibers from this layer are also seen lining the floor of the bicipital groove. This layer is supplied by arterioles from layer I, which have crossed into layer II between fascicles. Layer III (3 mm thick) contains smaller tendinous bundles as compared with layer II. These bundles lack uniform orientation, with fibers crossing one another at 45-degree angles. Smaller arterioles are present in this layer. Layer IV is predominantly loose connective tissue in which there are thick bands of collagen. Layer V (1.5 to 2 mm thick) is the deepest layer, composed of a sheet of interwoven collagen fibrils. This layer extends from the glenoid labrum medially to the humerus laterally. Interdigitation of fibers near the insertion on the humerus is predominantly seen in layer III (61).

In a study by Itoi et al., performed at the Mayo Clinic, the tendon was divided into anterior, middle, and posterior bands. These investigators found that the posterior portion was significantly thinner in cross section than the anterior and middle sections (62,63). They also demonstrated that the modulus of elasticity and ultimate load was greater in the anterior and middle portions than the posterior portion. They concluded that the anterior portion is the strongest and bears most of the stress. The bursal-side portion of the tendon has been shown to have a lower modulus of elasticity than the articular-side portion. The bursal-side portion also has a higher ultimate stress and strain (64).

Several studies have demonstrated that the supraspinatus serves to reduce the required deltoid force necessary to abduct the humerus by around 30% (65,66). The absence or paralysis of the supraspinatus decreases the power of active abduction to 80% of normal at takeoff from the side, and to nearly zero at 90 degrees of abduction (67).

Infraspinatus

This thick triangular muscle occupies most of the infraspinous fossa of the scapula, taking its origin from the medial two-thirds of the fossa. Along its medial inferior border, it is in direct contact with the teres minor muscle, which lies below it. The fibers are oriented from medial to lateral and terminate in a tendinous portion that travels over the posterior capsule and posterior aspect of the glenohumeral joint to insert onto the middle facet of the greater tuberosity of the humerus. The infraspinatus is supplied by the suprascapular nerve.

The infraspinatus is the primary external rotator of the humerus. In addition, the infraspinatus has also been shown to be an abductor of the arm and to play an important anterior stabilizing role in the mechanics of the glenohumeral joint (3,68–72).

Teres Minor

This narrow, elongated muscle arises from the dorsal surface of the axillary border of the scapula. The fibers of the muscle travel superolaterally and terminate in a tendon that inserts onto the inferior facet of the greater tuberosity of the humerus. Similar to the subscapularis, several fibers insert along the proximal two centimeters of the neck of the humerus. Like the deltoid, it is innervated by the axillary nerve.

The teres minor functions as an external rotator of the humerus, but not to the same extent as the infraspinatus. Like the infraspinatus, the teres minor acts as a stabilizer against anterior translation, particularly with the arm in abduction.

Vascular Supply

Six arteries provide the blood supply to the rotator cuff muscles and tendons. These include the suprascapular artery, anterior humeral circumflex artery, posterior humeral circumflex artery, thoracoacromial artery, suprahumeral artery, and subscapular artery. Table 1 shows the frequency of contribution on the basis of dissection and flow studies (73).

Several large anastamoses exist between the posterior humeral circumflex artery and the suprascapular artery. These constitute the predominant supply to the infraspinatus and teres minor. The anterior humeral circumflex artery is the major supply to the subscapularis muscle and tendon (Fig. 30). It anastamoses with the posterior humeral circumflex just over the tendon of the long head of the biceps. The anterior humeral circumflex artery is also the major blood supply to the humeral head (Fig. 30). A large branch of the artery enters the head via the bicipital groove. Branches

TABLE 1. *Frequency of contribution from various arterial branches to the rotator cuff tendons of the shoulder*

Artery	Frequency (%)
Suprascapular	100
Anterior humeral circumflex	100
Posterior humeral circumflex	100
Thoracoacromial	76
Suprahumeral	59
Suscapular	38

from the thoracoacromial artery supply the supraspinatus muscle and tendon, and often anastamoses with both humeral circumflex vessels.

A hypovascular region of the rotator cuff has been found in two-thirds of specimens in the tendinous portion of the supraspinatus just medial to its insertion. A similar hypovascular region is also noted in 37% of infraspinatus and in 7% of subscapularis tendons. This area of hypovascularity was first noticed by Codman (7) in 1934. Several studies since then have supported his findings (74,75,77a). Rathburn and Macnab (76) noted that these areas may be present at birth but that they also correspond to regions that are probably subject to increased stress and wear over time. Rathburn and Macnab also noted that the "critical zone" of the supraspinatus tendon received less blood flow with the arm held in adduction because of the compression effect

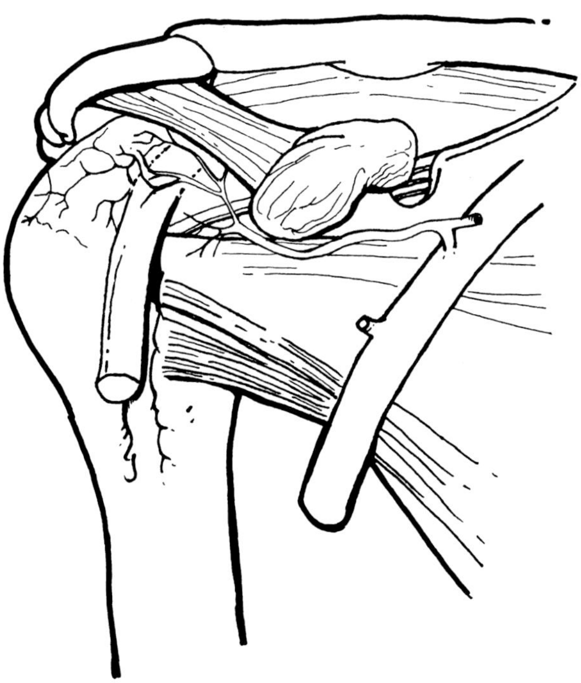

FIG. 30. The anterior humeral circumflex artery is the second of three branches of the third portion of the axillary artery. It provides most of the blood supply to the humeral head.

of the humeral head. Brooks et al. (77) noted that the distal 15 mm of both the supraspinatus and infraspinatus were equally hypovascular.

BICEPS TENDON

The biceps muscles (short and long heads) are the primary flexors of the elbow and the strongest supinator of the forearm. The short head arises with the coracobrachialis in a broad flat tendon from the apex of the coracoid process of the scapula. The long head had been thought to arise solely from the supraglenoid tubercle, but this notion has recently been challenged. The biceps tendon is surrounded by a synovial sheath during its intra-articular course over the anterior portion of the humeral head. The tendon then passes through a special opening in the joint capsule, which allows the passage of synovial fluid to the tendon. The tendon travels through the bicipital groove created by the greater and lesser tuberosities before joining the muscle belly. The bicipital groove is covered with a fibrous extension of the pectoralis major tendon, which serves to maintain the biceps tendon in the bicipital groove.

Recent studies concerning the biceps tendon have demonstrated that the origin of the tendon may not be solely from the supraglenoid tubercle. Pal et al. (78) demonstrated in a 1991 study that 70% of adult human cadaver specimens had a deficiency of the posterosuperior labrum, where the biceps tendon crosses over it. They also showed that the major origin of the tendon of the long head of the biceps was from the supraglenoid tubercle in only 25% of specimens. The remainder took origin from a crescentic ridge or accessory facet at the posterosuperior glenoid (78). In another study from 1995, Gigis et al. (79) stated that the origin of the biceps extends over nearly the whole periphery of the glenoid labrum except at a small area near the supraglenoid tubercle, which may be the area of deficiency described earlier by Pal. In yet another large cadaveric study, Vangsness et al. (80) determined that approximately 50% of the long head of the biceps tendon arises from the supraglenoid tubercle, and the remaining 50% arises directly from the labrum. From their dissections, they were able to describe four basic types of biceps tendon takeoff from the labrum, which are depicted in Figure 31.

In addition to flexion of the elbow and forearm supination, the biceps tendon provides several functions intrinsic to the shoulder joint. The proximal tendon of the long head of the biceps contributes to anterior stability of the glenohumeral joint in the overhead position of abduction and external rotation (81). The same study demonstrated that the biceps tendon also helps reduce some of the load borne by the inferior glenohumeral ligament complex. A more recent biomechanical study performed at our institution demonstrated that contraction of the tendon of the long head of the biceps resulted in significantly less translation of the humeral head in the glenoid, with a more pronounced effect in lower levels of humeral elevation (82).

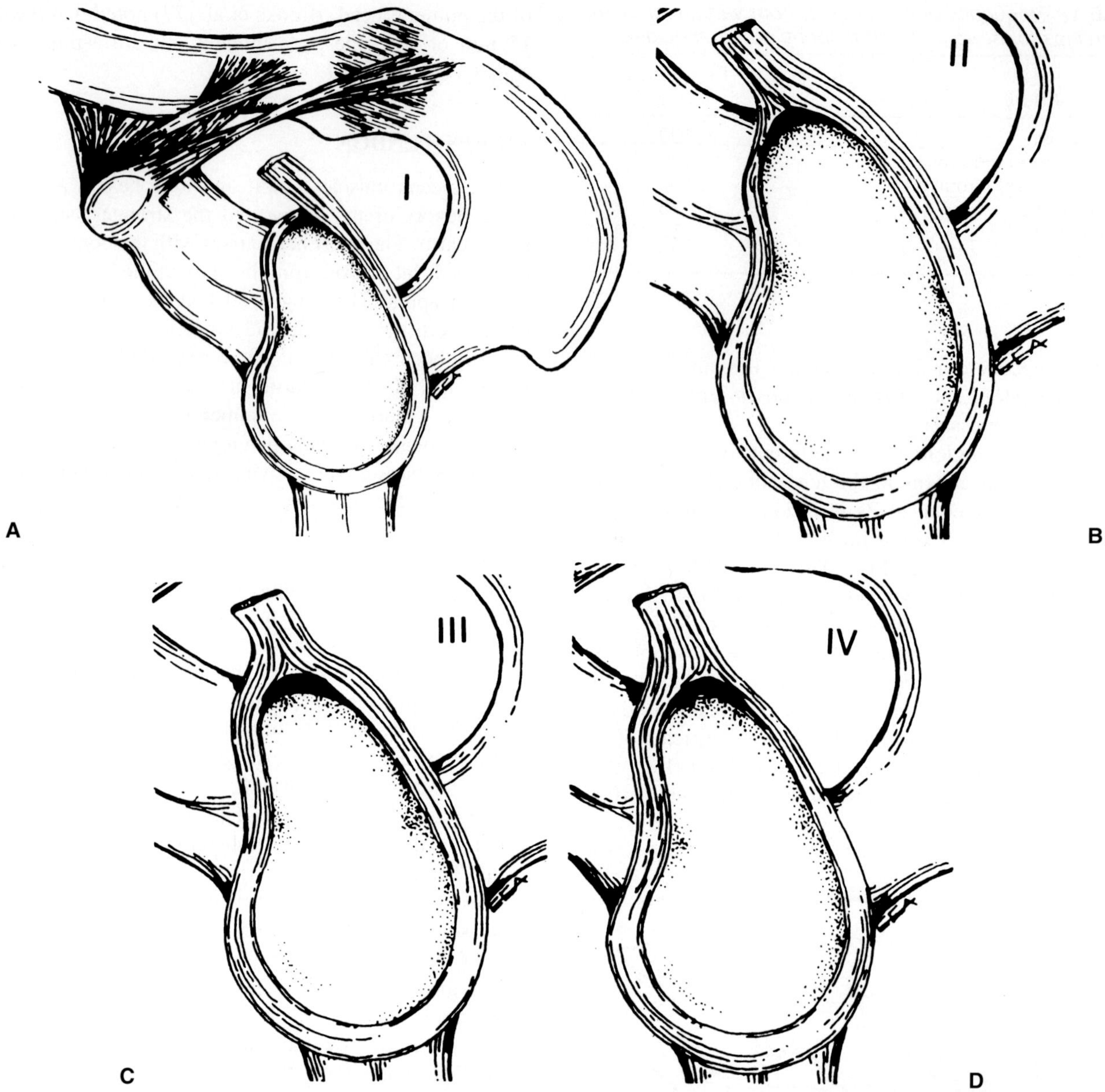

FIG. 31. A–D: Variations in the type of biceps tendon origin from the superior labrum and glenoid as described by Vangsness et al. (80). In type I, the biceps arises entirely from the posterior labrum with no anterior contribution. In type II, most of the labral contribution is from posterior, with a small amount from anterior. Type III has equal contributions from the anterior and posterior labrum. In type IV, most of the labral contribution arises from anterior, with a small amount from posterior. Relative frequencies of the four types: I, 22%; II, 33%; III, 37%; IV, 18%.

INTERACTIONS OF ROTATOR CUFF AND LIGAMENTS

Complete understanding of the shoulder and its function requires thorough knowledge of the surgical anatomy of the joint. At the very basic level, knowledge of the various layers that comprise the soft-tissue envelope about the shoulder is mandatory for surgeons. There are essentially four layers of soft tissue surrounding the glenohumeral joint on its anterior, lateral, and posterior borders with a distinct plane separating each layer (83) (Fig. 32) The outermost layer includes the deltoid and pectoralis major muscle bellies and the overlying deltopectoral fascia and epimysium. Layer II is broken down into anterior and posterior components. Anteriorly, layer II contains the clavipectoral fascia, the conjoined tendon of the coracobrachialis and the short head of the biceps brachii muscles, and the coracoacromial ligament. Posteriorly, layer II contains the fascia overlying the infraspinatus and teres minor; this is continuous with the clavipectoral fascia anteriorly. Beneath layer II is the subdeltoid bursa, which is present on the

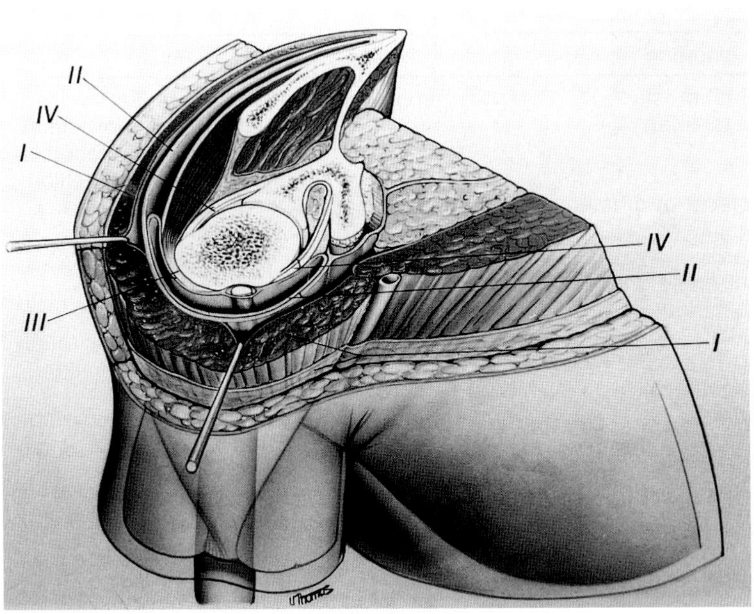

FIG. 32. Pictorial diagram of the four layers comprising the soft-tissue envelope about the shoulder as described by Cooper et al. (83). See text for details.

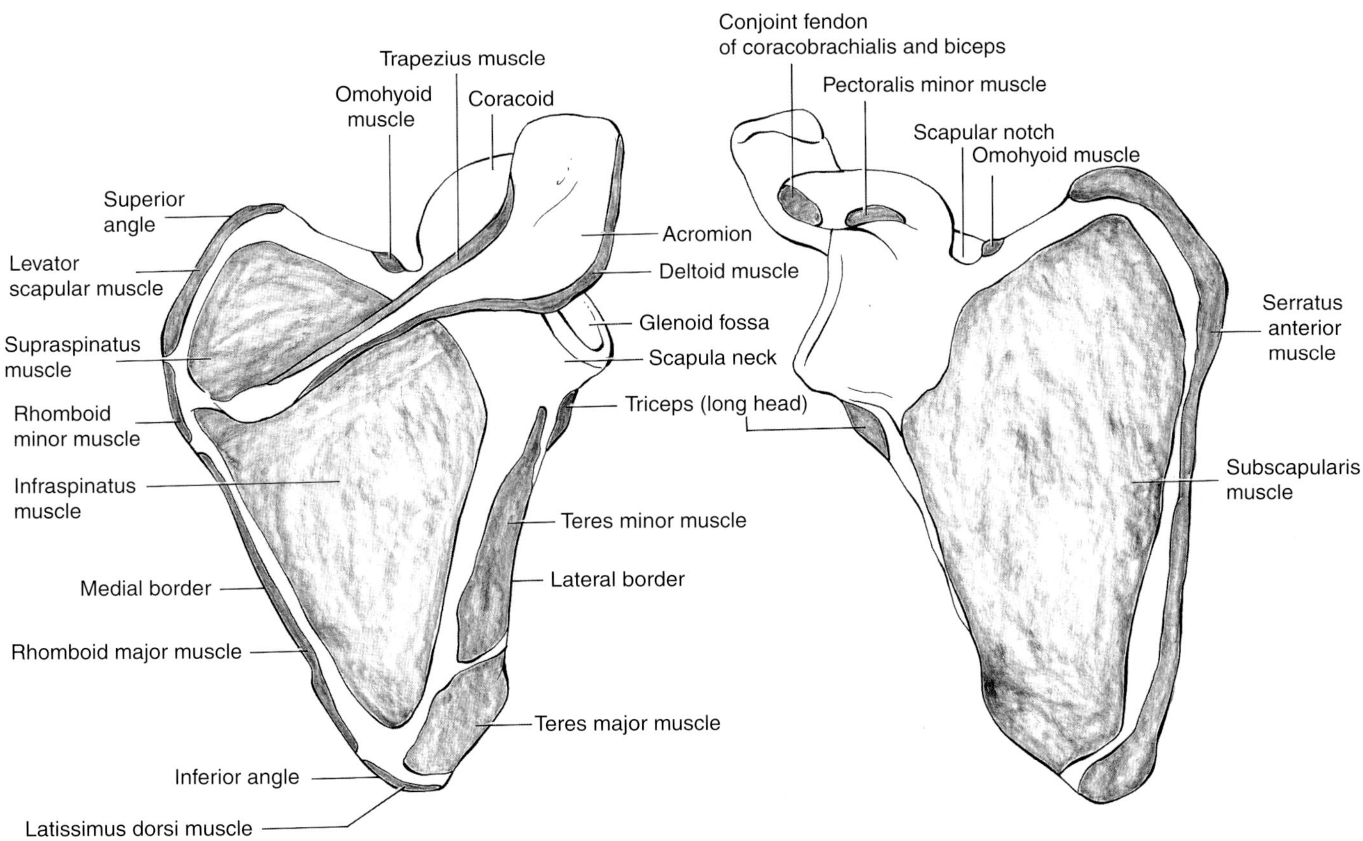

FIG. 33. The origins, insertions, and innervation of muscles about the scapula. (From Jenkins DB, ed. *Hollinshead's functional anatomy of the limbs and back.* Philadelphia: WB Saunders, 1991, with permission. Note the corresponding information provided in Table 3.)

TABLE 2. *Muscles surrounding the shoulder*

Muscle	Origin	Insertion	Innervation	Action
Deltoid	Lateral third of clavicle, acromion, spine of scapula	Deltoid tuberosity on humeral shaft	Axillary nerve	Anterior fibers; flexion/int. rotation; posterior fibers: extension/ext. rotation; middle fibers: abduction
Infraspinatus	Medial two-thirds of infraspinatus fossa	Middle facet of greater tuberosity of humerus	Suprascapular nerve	Strongest external rotator of humerus
Latissimus dorsi	Spinous processes of lower six thoracic and all lumar/sacral vertebrae, posterior iliac crest	Superior angle and upper border of scapula	Thoracodorsal nerve	Scapular elevation
Pectoralis major	Sternum, medial two-thirds of clavicle, costal cartilages 1–6	Greater tubercle of humerus	Medial pectoral nerve	Internal rotation and adduction of arm; some flexion and extension of arm
Pectoralis minor	Ribs 3–5	Coracoid process	Medial pectoral nerve	Downward rotation of scapula, shoulder depression
Rhomboid major	Spinous processes of T2–T5	Medial border of scapula	Dorsal scapular nerve	Scapular elevation and retraction, rotates glenoid downward
Rhomboid minor	Lower aspect of ligamentum nuchae, spinous processes of C7 and T1	Medial border of scapula at base of spine	Dorsal scapular nerve	Same as rhomboid major
Serratus anterior	Anterior ribs 1–8	Medial border of scapula, inferior angle	Long thoracic nerve	Holds medial border of scapula against chest wall (prevents winging), upward rotation of glenoid
Subscapularis	Subscapular fossa	Lesser tubercle of humerus	Upper and lower subscapular nerves	Internal rotation of arm
Supraspinatus	Supraspinatus fossa of scapula	greater tubercle of humerus	Suprascapular nerve	Arm abduction
Teres major	Inferior angle of scapula	Medial lip of intertubercular groove of humerus	Lower subscapular nerve	Adduction, internal rotation, extension
Teres minor	Upper two-thirds of lateral border of scapula	Greater tubercle of humerus	Axillary nerve	External rotation of scapula
Trapezius	External occipital protuberance, spinous processes C7–T12	Spine of scapula, lateral one-third of clavicle, acromion	Accessory nerve	Scapular elevation, depression, retraction, and rotation

anterior, superior, lateral, and in some cases posterior portions of the space. Layer III includes the deep layer of the subdeltoid bursa and the rotator cuff tendons and muscles. Layer IV is simply the glenohumeral joint capsule and investing ligaments. Variation within these layers is greatest in the deep layer and pertains mostly to the glenohumeral ligaments.

The structures about the shoulder that contribute to its unique mobility and purposeful positioning of the distal upper extremity have been described above (Table 2 and Fig. 33). Individually, most of these structures are incapable of supporting the arm or positioning it in space. However, as a result of specific contributions of both the dynamic and static actions and restraints of the bones and soft tissues that make up the shoulder, mobility and stability are achieved. These dynamic and static restraints are listed in Table 3.

Combinations of interactions of these various contributors provide for variations in stability of the glenohumeral joint. For instance, posterior dislocation in an intact cadaver shoulder is only possible with sectioning of the anterior capsule from the 1 to 3 o'clock positions in addition to the entire posterior capsule (84).

TABLE 3. *Static and dynamic stabilizers of the glenohumeral joint*

Static restraints	Dynamic restraints
Bony structures	Rotator cuff muscles/tendons
Labrum	Biceps tendon/muscle
Glenohumeral ligaments	Deltoid muscle
Joint capsule	
Negative joint pressure	

Interactions of various structures about the shoulder continues to be a well-researched area in orthopedics. Our understanding of the mechanics of motion and stability of the shoulder has vastly increased in recent years leading to improved diagnostic capacity, as well as better treatment options and more successful return to activity. Only through continued attention to the very basic anatomy and its variations will continued advances be possible.

REFERENCES

1. Saha AK. *Theory of shoulder mechanism: descriptive and applied.* Springfield: Charles C Thomas, 1961.
2. Saha AK. Mechanism of shoulder movements and a plea for the recognition of "zero position" of the glenohumeral joint. *Clin Orthop* 1983;173:11.
3. Saha AK. Dynamic stability of the glenohumeral joint. *Acta Orthop Scand* 1971;42:491.
4. Bigliani LU, Morrison DS, April EW. The morphology of the acromion and rotator cuff impingement. *Orthop Trans* 1986;10:228.
5. Iannotti JP, Gabriel JP, Schneck SL, Evans BG, Misra S. The normal glenohumeral relationships. *J Bone Joint Surg* 1992;744:491.
6. Bost FC, Inmann VTG. The pathological changes in recurrent dislocation of the shoulder. *J Bone Joint Surg* 1942;24:595.
7. Codman EA. *The shoulder.* Boston: Thomas Todd, 1934.
8. Steindler A. *Kinesiology of the human body under normal and pathological conditions.* Springfield, IL: Charles C Thomas, 1955.
9. Maki S, Gruen T. Anthropometric study of the glenohumeral joint. Paper presented at the Twenty-second Annual Orthopaedic Research Society, New Orleans, January 28–30, 1976.
10. Howell SM, Galinat BJ. The containment mechanism: the primary stabilizer of the glenohumeral joint. Presented at the annual meeting of the American Academy of Orthopaedic Surgeons, San Francisco, January 23, 1987.
11. DePalma AF, Callery G, Bennett GA. Variational anatomy and degenerative lesions of the shoulder joint. *AAOS Instruct Course Lect* 1949;6:225.
12. Kumar VP, Balasubramaniam P. The role of atmospheric pressure in stabilizing the shoulder: an experimental study. *J Bone Joint Surg [Br]* 1985;67B:719.
13. Cooper DE, Arnoczky SP, O'Brien SJ, Warren RF, DiCarlo E, Allen AA. Anatomy, histology and vascularity of the glenoid labrum: An anatomic study. *J Bone Joint Surg [Am]* 1992;74A:46–52.
14. Bankart ASB. The pathology and treatment of recurrent dislocation of the shoulder. *J Bone Joint Surg* 1938;26:23–29.
15. Townley CO. *J Bone Joint Surg [Am]* 1950;32A:370.
16. Codman EA. The capsular mechanism in recurrent dislocation of the shoulder. *The shoulder.* Boston: Thomas Todd & Co., 1934:12.
17. O'Brien SJ, Neves MC, Arnoczky SP, et al. The anatomy and histology of the inferior glenohumeral ligament complex of the shoulder. *Am J Sports Med* 1990;18:449.
18. O'Brien SJ, Schwartz RS, Warren RF, et al. Capsular restraints to anterior-posterior motion of the abducted shoulder: a biomechanical study. *J Shoulder Elbow Surg* 1995;4:298.
19. Warner JP, Xiang-Hua D, Warren RF, Torzilli PA. Static capsuloligamentous restraints to superior-inferior translation of the glenohumeral joint. *Am J Sports Med* 1992;20:675.
20. DeLorme D. die Hemmungs bander des Schultergelenks and ihre Deductung fur die Schulter Luxationen. *Arch Klin Chir* 1910;92:79.
21. Turkel SJ, Panio MW, Marshall JL, Girgis FG. Stabilizing mechanisms preventing anterior dislocation of the glenohumeral joint. *J Bone Joint Surg [Am]* 1981;63A:1208.
22. Ticker JB, Bigliani LU, Soslowsky LJ, et al. Inferior glenohumeral ligament: geometric and strain-rat dependent properties. *J Shoulder Elbow Surg* 1996;5:269.
23. Cooper DE, Warner JP, O'Brien SJ, et al. Anatomy, histology, and function of the coracohumeral ligament: an anatomic and biomechanical study. *J Bone Joint Surg [Br]* 1992;74B(Suppl):9–10.
24. Basmajian JV, Bazant FJ. Factors preventing downward dislocation of the adducted shoulder joint. *J Bone Joint Surg* 1959;41A:1182.
25. Neer CS II, Satterlee CC, Dalsey RM, Flatow EL. The anatomy and potential effects of contracture of the coracohumeral ligament. *Clin Orthop* 1992;280:182.
26. Salter GE, Nasca RJ, Shelle BS. Anatomical observations on the acromioclavicular joint and supporting ligaments. *Am J Sports Med* 1987;15:199.
27. Bearden JM, Hughston JC, Whatley GS. Acromioclavicular dislocation: method of treatment. *Am J Sports Med* 1973;1 (4):5–17.
28. Bosworth BM. Complete acromioclavicular dislocation. *N Engl J Med* 1949;241:221.
29. Inman VT, McLaughlin HD, Neviaser J, Rose C. Treatment of complete acromioclavicular dislocation. *J Bone Joint Surg [Am]* 1962;44A:1008.
30. Kennedy JC, Cameron H. Complete dislocation of the acromioclavicular joint. *J Bone Joint Surg [Br]* 1954;36B:202.
31. Urist MR. Complete dislocation of the acromioclavicular joint: the nature of the traumatic lesion and effective methods of treatment with an analysis of 41 cases. *J Bone Joint Surg* 1946;28:813.
32. Rockwood CA Jr. Injuries to the acromioclavicular joint. In: Rockwood CA Jr, Green DP, eds. *Fractures in adults*, vol. 1. Philadelphia: JB Lippincott, 1984:860–910.
33. Rockwood CA Jr, Young DC. Disorders of the acromioclavicular joint. In: Rockwood CA Jr, Matsen FA, Williams GR Jr. eds. *The shoulder*, 2nd ed. Philadelphia: WB Saunders, 1998:483–553.
34. Fukuda K, Craig EV, An KN, Cofield RH, Chao EYS. Biomechanical study of the ligamentous system of the acromioclavicular joint. *J Bone Joint Surg [Am]* 1986;68A:434.

34a. Williams GR, Rockwood CA Jr. Injuries to the acromioclavicular joint, the sternoclavicular joint, clavicle, scapula, coracoid, sternum, and ribs. In Delee JC, Drez D, eds. *Orthopaedic sports medicine.* Philadelphia: WB Saunders, 1994:481–579.

35. O'Brien SJ, Arnoczky SP, Warren RF, Rozbruch SR. Developmental anatomy of the shoulder and anatomy of the glenohumeral joint. In: Rockwood CA, Matsen FA, eds. *The shoulder.* Philadelphia: WB Saunders, 1990:16.
36. Hayashi K, Thabit G III, Massa KL, et al. The effect of thermal heating on the length and histologic properties of the glenohumeral joint capsule. *Am J Sports Med* 1997;25:107.
37. Reeves B. Arthrography of the shoulder. *J Bone Joint Surg [Br]* 1966;48B:24.
38. Sperber A, Wredmark T. Capsular elasticity and joint volume in recurrent anterior shoulder instability. *J Arthrosc Relat Surg* 1994;10:598.
39. Gardner E. The innervation of the shoulder joint. *Anat Rec* 1949;102:1–18.
40. Rudinger N. *Die Gelenknerven des menschlichen korpers.* Erlangen: Verlag von Ferdinand Enke, 1857.
41. Wrete M. The innervation of the shoulder joint in man. *Acta Anat* 1949;7:173.
42. Murakami M, Kojima Y, Maeda T, et al. Sensory nerve endings in the shoulder joint capsule of the monkey as sensors of dynamic stabilizing system. *Transactions of the Combined Meeting of the ORS of USA, Japan, and Canada 1991.* 1991:315.
43. Guanche C, Knatt T, Solomonow M, Lu Y, Baratta R. The synergistic action of the capsule and shoulder muscles. *Am J Sports Med* 1995;23:301.
44. Harryman DT, Sidles JA, Harris SL, et al. The role of the rotator interval capsule in passive motion and stability of the shoulder. *J Bone Joint Surg [Am]* 1992;74A:53.
45. Nobuhara K, Ikeda H. Rotator interval lesion. *Clin Orthop* 1987;223:44–50.
46. Rowe CR, Zarins B, Ciullo JV. Recurrent transient subluxation of the shoulder. *J Bone Joint Surg [Am]* 1981;63A:863.
47. Field LD, Warren RF, O'Brien SJ, Altchek DW, Wickiewicz TL. Isolated closure of rotator interval defects for shoulder instability. *Am J Sports Med* 1995;23:557.
48. Altchek DW, Dines DM. The surgical treatment of anterior instability: selective capsular repair. *Oper Techn Sports Med* 1993;1:285.
49. Moseley HF, Overgaard B. The anterior capsular mechanism in recurrent anterior dislocation of the shoulder. *J Bone Joint Surg* 1962;44B:913.
50. Rowe CR, Zarins B, Ciullo JV. Recurrent anterior dislocation of the shoulder after surgical repair. *J Bone Joint Surg [Am]* 1984;66A:159.
51. Speer KP. Anatomy and pathomechanics of shoulder instability. *Oper Techn Sports Med* 1993;1:252.
52. Kumagai J, Sarkar K, Uhthoff HK. The collagen types in the attachment zone of rotator cuff tendons in the elderly: an immunohistochemical study. *J Rheumatol* 1994;21:2096.

53. Rodeo SA, Arnoczky SP, Torzilli PA, et al. Tendon healing in a bone tunnel: A biomechanical and histological study in the dog. *J Bone Joint Surg [Am]* 1993;75A:1795.
54. Tomonaga A, Hamada K, Gotoh M, et al. Localization of mRNA of procollagen {ALPHA} 1 type III in torn supraspinatus tendons by in situ hybridization. *J Shoulder Elbow Surg* 1995;4:69.
55. Viidik A. Structure and function of normal and healing tendons and ligaments. In: Mow VC, Ratcliffe A, Woo SL-Y, eds. *Biomechanics of diarthrodial joints*, vol. 1. New York: Springer-Verlag, 1990.
56. Blevins FT, Djurasovic M, Flatow EL, Vogel KG. Biology of the rotator cuff tendon. *Orthop Clin North Am* 1997;28:1.
57. Berenson MC, Blevins FT, Plaas AHK, et al. Proteoglycans of human rotator cuff tendons. *Trans Orthop Res* 1996;21:766.
58. Gray H. *Gray's anatomy.* Pick TP, Howden R, eds. New York: Crown, 1977.
59. Jenkins DB. In: *Hollinshead's functional anatomy of the limbs and back.* Philadelphia: WB Saunders, 1991.
60. Itoi E, Newman SR, Kuechle DK, Morrey BF, An KN: Dynamic anterior stabilizers of the shoulder with the arm in abduction. *J Bone Joint Surg [Br]* 1994;76B:834.
61. Clark JM, Harryman DT. Tendons, ligaments, and capsule of the rotator cuff. *J Bone Joint Surg [Am]* 1992;74A:713.
62. Itoi E, Berglund LJ, Grabowski JJ, et al. Tensile properties of the supraspinatus tendon. *J Orthop Res* 1995;13:578.
63. Soslowsky LJ, Carpenter JE, Bucchieri JS, Flatow EL. Biomechanics of the rotator cuff. *Orthop Clin North Am* 1997;28:17.
64. Nakajima T, Rokuuma N, Hamada K, et al. Histologic and biomechanical characteristics of the supraspinatus tendon: reference to rotator cuff tearing. *J Shoulder Elbow Surg* 1994;3:79.
65. Sharkey NA, Marder RA. The rotator cuff opposes superior translation of the humeral head. *Am J Sports Med* 1995;23:100.
66. Thompson WO, Debski RE, Boardman ND III, et al. A biomechanical analysis of rotator cuff deficiency in a cadaveric model. *Am J Sports Med* 1996;24:286.
67. Bechtol CO. Biomechanics of the shoulder. *Clin Orthop* 1980;146:37.
68. Inman VT, Saunders JB, Abbott LC. Observations on the function of the shoulder joint. *J Bone Joint Surg* 1944;26:1.
69. Poppen NK, Walker PS. Forces at the glenohumeral joint in abduction. *Clin Orthop* 1978;135:165.
70. Cain PR, Mucschler TA, Fu FH, Lee SK. Anterior stability of the glenohumeral joint: a dynamic model. *Am J Sports Med* 1987;15:144.
71. McKernan DJ, Mutschler TA, Rudert MJ, et al. The characterisation of rotator cuff muscle forces and their effect on glenohumeral joint stability: a biomechanical study. *Orthop Trans* 1990;14:237.
72. Otis JC, Jiang CC, Wickiewicz TL, Peterson MG, Warren RF, Santner TJ. Changes in the moment arms of the rotator cuff and deltoid muscles with abduction and rotation. *J Bone Joint Surg [Am]* 1994;76A:667.
73. Chansky HA, Iannotti JP. The vascularity of the rotator cuff. *Clin Sports Med* 1991;10:807.
74. Rothman RH, Parke WW. The vascular anatomy of the rotator cuff. *Clin Orthop* 1965;41:176.
75. Lohr JF, Uhthoff HK. The microvascular pattern of the supraspinatus tendon. *Clin Orthop* 1990;254:35.
76. Rathburn JB, Macnab I. The microvascular pattern of the rotator cuff. *J Bone Joint Surg [Br]* 1970;52B:540.
77. Brooks CH, Revell WJ, Heatley FW. A quantitative histological study of the vascularity of the rotator cuff tendon. *J Bone Joint Surg [Br]* 1992;74B:151.

77a. Moseley HF, Goldie I. The arterial pattern of the rotator cuff of the shoulder. *J Bone Joint Surg [Br]* 1963;45B:780.

78. Pal GP, Bhatt RH, Patel VS. Relationship between the tendon of the long head of the biceps brachii and the glenoidal labrum in humans. *Anat Rec* 1991;229:278.
79. Gigis P, Natsis C, Polyzonis M. New aspects on the topography of the tendon of the long head of the biceps brachii muscle. One more stabilizer factor of the shoulder joint. *Bull Assoc Anat* 1995;79:9.
80. Vangsness CT Jr, Jorgenson SS, Watson T, Johnson DL. The origin of the long head of the biceps from the scapula and glenoid labrum: an anatomical study of 100 shoulders. *J Bone Joint Surg [Br]* 1994;76B:951.
81. Rodosky MW, Harner CD, Fu FH. The role of the long head of the biceps muscle and superior glenoid labrum in anterior stability of the shoulder. *Am J Sports Med* 1994;22:121.
82. Pagnani MJ, Deng XH, Warren RF, Torzilli PA, O'Brien SJ. Role of the long head of the biceps brachii in glenohumeral stability: a biomechanical study in cadavera. *J Shoulder Elbow Surg* 1996;5:255.
83. Cooper DE, O'Brien SJ, Warren RF. Supporting layers of the glenohumeral joint. *Clin Orthop* 1993;289:144.
84. Warren RF, Kornblatt IB, Marchand R. Static factors affecting posterior shoulder stability. *Orthop Trans* 1984;8:89.

The Unstable Shoulder,
edited by R.F. Warren, E.V. Craig, and D.W. Altchek.
Lippincott–Raven Publishers, Philadelphia © 1999.

CHAPTER 3

Anatomy, Biomechanics, and Pathophysiology of Glenohumeral Instability

Jon J. P. Warner and N. Douglas Boardman III

HISTORICAL OBSERVATIONS

Traditionally, much of our understanding of shoulder instability had come from clinical and pathologic observations (1–40). These observations led to empirically devised clinical approaches for the management of the unstable shoulder (2,3,7,41–56). More recently, our clinical perceptions of shoulder instability have been modified by numerous anatomic and biomechanical studies. These new objective approaches to this challenging clinical problem represent the result of exciting collaborative work between clinicians, biomechanical engineers, chemists, and other basic scientists. From these investigations, we have obtained a greater appreciation of the unique anatomic arrangement of the glenohumeral joint—a minimally constrained articulation permitting an extreme range of motion while balancing mobility and stability.

Both static and dynamic factors function to allow maximum glenohumeral rotation, while limiting excessive translation of the humeral head on the glenoid. Saha (57, 58) emphasized articular components and dynamic factors, DePalma et al. (12) and Symeonides (39) emphasized the role of the subscapularis muscle, and Moseley and Overgaard (29), Townley (40), and Turkel et al. (59) stressed the importance of static capsuloligamentous restraints. Recent clinical and experimental work has also shown that the glenohumeral joint maintains stability through negative intra-articular pressure (60–64), adhesion-cohesion (65), concavity-compression (through dynamic muscle contraction) (66—72), coordinated rotator cuff contraction (73–87), labral function (71,88–94), and coordinated scapulothoracic–glenohumeral motion (86,95–103).

Numerous pathologic lesions have been implicated as causes of glenohumeral instability. These include labral detachment (3,51,71,88,92,93,104–109), congenital or acquired capsular laxity (4,43,45,48,49,71,110–122), abnormal glenoid and humeral version (7,13,22,44,53–56,113, 124–128), loss of glenoid bone through fracture (1,72), glenoid hypoplasia (129–136), posterior humeral head defect (Hill-Sachs) (9,14,21,137), rotator cuff dysfunction or tear (12,17,39, 67,69,75,78,83,85,107,138–149), lateral capsular avulsion (150), and loss of normal scapulothoracic function (100,103). We now know that no single factor alone maintains glenohumeral joint stability and no single lesion results in instability. Rather, clinical instability is an individualized problem, with static and dynamic factors playing a complex and interdependent role in maintaining stability. Furthermore, these factors are modified by age, exposure to trauma, and congenital variations in the anatomy of both osseous and soft tissues. This chapter attempts to define these factors and clarify their interdependence and relative importance to stability of the shoulder. Such an understanding is crucial to the orthopedic surgeon's clinical strategy for management of glenohumeral instability.

THE SPECTRUM OF INSTABILITY

Instability and *laxity*—two descriptive terms frequently applied to the shoulder—must be clearly differentiated from one another. *Laxity* defines asymptomatic translation of the humeral head on the glenoid, which may be demonstrated in normal shoulders and represents a necessary feature of the soft tissues about the shoulder required for normal glenohumeral rotation. *Instability* is a clinical diagnosis manifest as excessive translation of the humeral head on the glenoid occurring during active shoulder rotation in asso-

J. J. P. Warner: Department of Orthopaedic Surgery, Harvard Medical School, Boston, Massachusetts 02114; and Department of Orthopaedic Surgery, Massachusetts General Hospital, Boston, Massachusetts 02114.

N. D. Boardman III: The Shoulder Service, Center for Sports Medicine and Rehabilitation, Pittsburgh, Pennsylvania 15213.

ciation with symptoms. A spectrum of instability exists that represents increasing degrees of injury to those dynamic and static factors that normally function to contain the humeral head in the glenoid. *Dislocation* is defined as complete separation of the articular surfaces, whereas subluxation is broadly defined as symptomatic increased humeral head translation beyond that permitted by normal tissue laxity, but without complete separation of articular surfaces. As both clinical and experimental studies have demonstrated a wide range of normal ''play'' in the glenohumeral joint, clinical subluxation requires increased translation in association with symptoms (61,64,71,110,114,115,117,121, 122,151–159).

More recently, use of the arthroscope has suggested the existence of smaller degrees of symptomatic subluxation, and Altchek et al. (88) have termed this *microsubluxation*. This group appears to include athletes in whom symptomatic labral tears develop as a result of failure of humeral head containment during throwing motions. Glenohumeral translation is less than that detectable on physical examination as clinical subluxation but is sufficient to cause excessive edge loading or shearing stress to the labrum (88, 91,93,160).

DIRECTION OF INSTABILITY

The primary direction of instability may be anterior, posterior, or inferior and, although 95% of all instability has been observed to be anterior, there is often a secondary multidirectional component. This secondary component may manifest itself during examination under anesthesia as seemingly excessive posterior translation of the humeral head on the glenoid in a patient with documented anterior instability (110,121,152,154,161). This phenomenon is explained by the ''circle concept'' and by the ''load-sharing concept'' of glenohumeral instability (162). These concepts are discussed in depth in the following text but, in general terms, we now know that capsular injury or laxity must occur on both sides of the joint when there is either an anterior or posterior dislocation (Fig. 1). Moreover, contributions of specific capsuloligamentous structures to joint stability depend on both shoulder position and direction of applied force.

History and physical examination define the primary direction of instability, and examination under anesthesia confirms the diagnosis. These techniques are discussed in Chapters 5 and 8. In general, instability is classified by the direction of greatest humeral head translation, and a significant component of inferior translation is considered the hallmark of the clinical syndrome of multidirectional instability (43,48,49,110,116,151,154,156,159,163).

THE ROLE OF TRAUMA: THE SUSCEPTIBILITY EQUATION

Considerable individual variation exists in terms of capsuloligamentous structures, inherent normal shoulder laxity, conditioning and strength of dynamic muscular stabilizers of the glenohumeral joint (11,110,112,114,117,119,121, 122,152,154,156,158,159,164–170). Moreover, there appears to be a complex interactive stabilizing mechanism between capsular and muscular factors mediated through proprioception, and certain pathologic conditions may affect this mechanism (171–175). Both athletic and nonathletic people subject their shoulders to varying degrees of stress, depending on sports and work activity. For example, repetitive overhead motions in throwing and swimming place the shoulder at greater risk of instability than do sports not requiring overhead use of the arm. In broad terms, one may formulate a *susceptibility equation* for risk of glenohumeral instability:

$$P_I = A_R + S_S + D_S$$

where:

P_I = probability of instability
A_R = risk activity
S_S = quality of static stabilizers
D_S = strength and conditioning of dynamic stabilizers

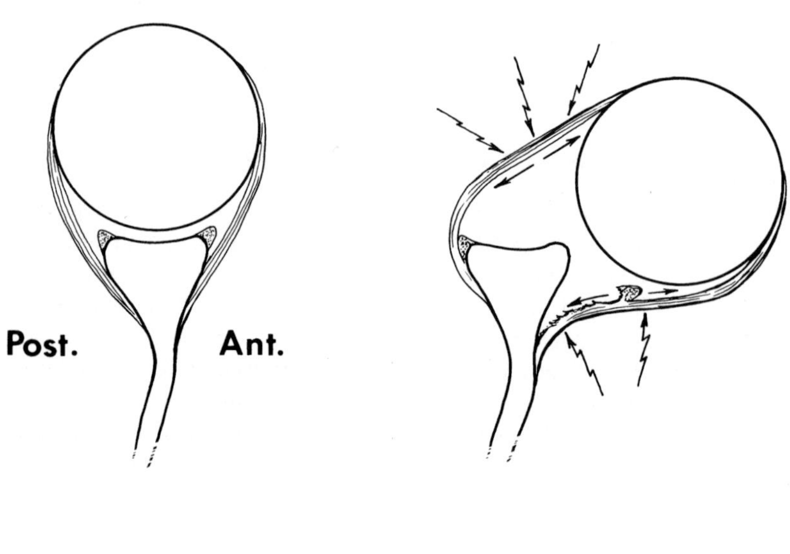

FIG. 1. Circle concept of shoulder instability. Anterior dislocation requires injury on both anterior and posterior sides of the joint.

So, an individual with deficient capsuloligamentous structures, or one with poor strength and conditioning of the rotator cuff muscles, might theoretically be at greater risk of glenohumeral instability, especially if he or she participates in overhead sports (176). Conversely, even an individual with well-developed ligaments and excellent conditioning and strength of the rotator cuff muscles might sustain a traumatic dislocation from a sudden force that exceeds the ultimate failure strength of these ligaments.

The force causing clinical instability may take the form of a single stress applied in such a way as to exceed the ultimate strength of the ligamentous tissues, as may occur with a fall onto an abducted and externally rotated arm. Instability may also develop gradually with accumulated "microtrauma" in the form of repetitive submaximal loads that stretch the ligaments, causing plastic deformation (71,111,119). Repetitive overhead motions with fatigue and failure of the dynamic stabilizers to contain the humeral head in the glenoid might produce excessive translation sufficient to plastically deform the capsuloligamentous structures (122). Proprioceptive feedback from ligaments coordinates the protective effect of dynamic stabilizers during shoulder motion, and fatigue, capsular injury, or congenital laxity may interfere with this protective mechanism (59,171–175). In clinical practice, "microtrauma" from such recurrent injury leading to clinical subluxation seems to be a more common mechanism of glenohumeral instability.

In contrast to traumatic glenohumeral instability, involuntary, atraumatic instability occurs in an entirely separate group of individuals. In these people, varying degrees of symptoms develop in the setting of congenital ligamentous laxity, rather than acquired laxity (116,120, 121,153,161) (Fig. 2). In these cases, pain or instability often develops with less stressful activities, such as reaching into a closet or tossing a ball. Distinguishing this group and those with a traumatic etiology constitutes the first step in any therapeutic approach. Matsen et al. (106) have provided a useful clinical classification in the form of two mnemonics that not only reflect etiology and pathology but also help direct treatment. The "TUBS" group defines those individuals who have a *t*raumatic etiology of instability. The problem is usually *u*nilateral, patients often have a *B*ankart lesion, and they generally require a *s*urgical solution of the problem. By contrast, the "AMBRI" group includes those patients with an *a*traumatic etiology. These people usually have *m*ultidirectional instability, *b*ilateral symptoms, and most often respond to a physician-directed *r*ehabilitation program (177). In the event of failure of conservative treatment, an *i*nferior capsular shift is the procedure that best manages the excessive capsular volume found in these patients. Although this classification offers a useful general approach, in our experience there is often an overlap of patient groups, such that in a person with ligamentous laxity, traumatic instability may develop in association with a Bankart lesion (110).

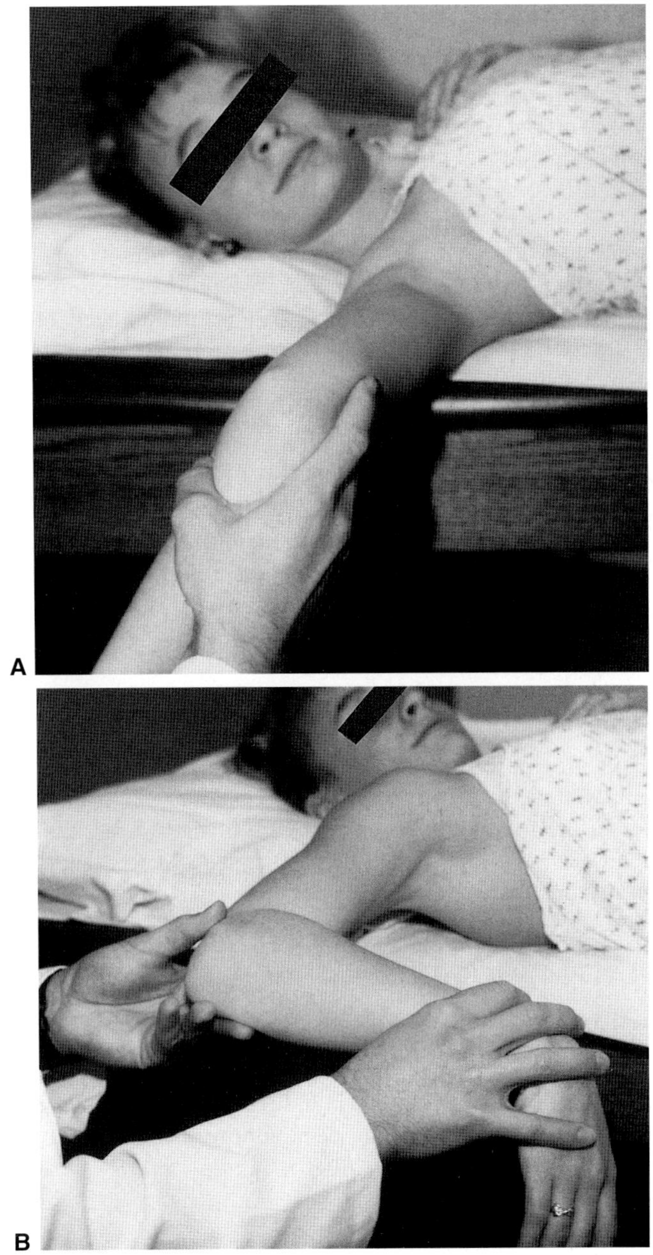

FIG. 2. A, B: A 14-year-old swimmer with hyperlaxity of the shoulder.

Voluntary instability comprises a separate category considered in detail in Chapter 25. In general, these patients have the ability either to selectively contract portions of their shoulder musculature or to selectively position the arm so as to dislocate or subluxate the glenohumeral joint (147, 161). Although excessive capsular laxity is a necessary component of their instability, it is a secondary feature relative to the volitional control of dynamic muscle forces about the joint.

NATURAL HISTORY OF SHOULDER INSTABILITY

The clinical implications of an initial episode of instability for risk of recurrence are discussed in Chapter 26; however, several biologic and biomechanical factors should be emphasized. Clinical experience has shown that age is the most important risk factor for recurrence of instability after an initial traumatic dislocation (18,178–180). This is thought to result from failure of healing of the Bankart lesion, even if the arm is immobilized (18, 37,50,51,108,109,142,178,179,181). Unfortunately, no objective experimental data appear in the literature to validate this assumption, and we now know that, when a dislocation occurs, the capsular tissue stretches even if a Bankart lesion is created (71,111,119,182). Older patients appear to have a lower rate of recurrence of instability after traumatic dislocation, attributed to healing of capsular injury or avulsed greater tuberosity but, again, there is no objective experimental validation of this assumption (18,27,36,105,142,146,183).

COMPONENTS OF SHOULDER STABILITY

As previously stated, the complex interaction of static and dynamic restraints maintains glenohumeral joint stability. In the following discussion, each of these restraints is reviewed individually, and the consequences of deficiency of any one component presented.

STATIC RESTRAINTS

Articular Anatomy

Evolutionary changes have led to unique adaptations of the scapulohumeral complex in order to facilitate prehensile activity and the large range of motion available to the human shoulder. Detailed consideration of these evolutionary adaptations is beyond the scope of this text and has been well described elsewhere (97). It is important to realize, however, that the shoulder complex represents an intercalated arrangement between the scapula, clavicle, and humerus, and that the scapula in humans is suspended by muscles alone. The coordinated scapulothoracic–glenohumeral motion relationship is a critical component of normal shoulder function.

Orientation (Version)

The glenohumeral joint in the adult is formed by the humeral head and the glenoid surface of the scapula. The geometric relationship of these two joint surfaces allows for the large range of motion which is normally available to this articulation. Both arthrographic and radiographic studies have been used to characterize this relationship, though considerable controversy remains concerning the relative importance of articular geometry to shoulder stability. In a resting position with the arm hanging at the side, the scapula faces 30 degrees anteriorly on the chest wall and tilts 3 degrees upward relative to the transverse plane and 20 degrees forward relative to the sagittal plane (167)(Fig. 3). Saha (13,58) was among the first to define glenoid orientation using axillary and anteroposterior (AP) radiographs (Fig. 4). Saha reported a wide range of normal, with 75% of cases averaging about 7 degrees of retroversion and 25% having anteversion of 2 to 10 degrees. Both Saha (57,58) and Basmajian and Bazant (95) observed that the glenoid averages a superior tilt of 5 degrees, although neither reported a range of normal for this value. Although other factors have been shown to contribute to inferior stability of the glenohumeral joint, recent biomechanical work has validated the concept of scapular inclination as an important factor controlling inferior stability (98,105,184).

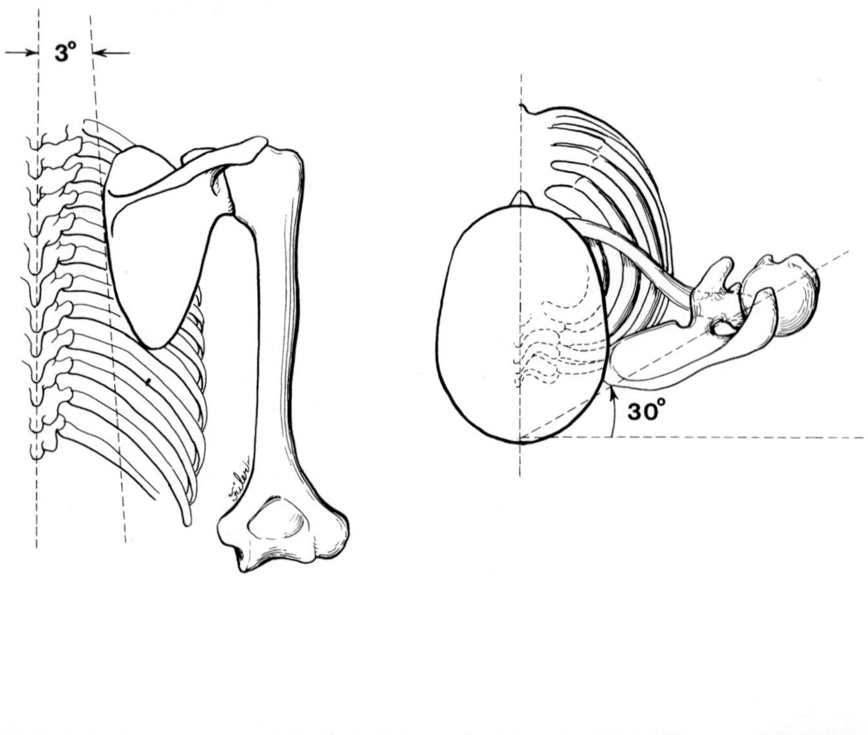

FIG. 3. Scapular orientation on the chest wall is 30 degrees anterior and three degrees upward. (From Warner JJP. The gross anatomy of the joint surfaces, ligaments, labrum, and capsule. In: Matsen FA, Fu FH, Hawkins RJ, eds. *The shoulder: a balance of mobility and stability.* Rosemont, IL: American Academy of Orthopaedic Surgeons, 1993:7–27, with permission.)

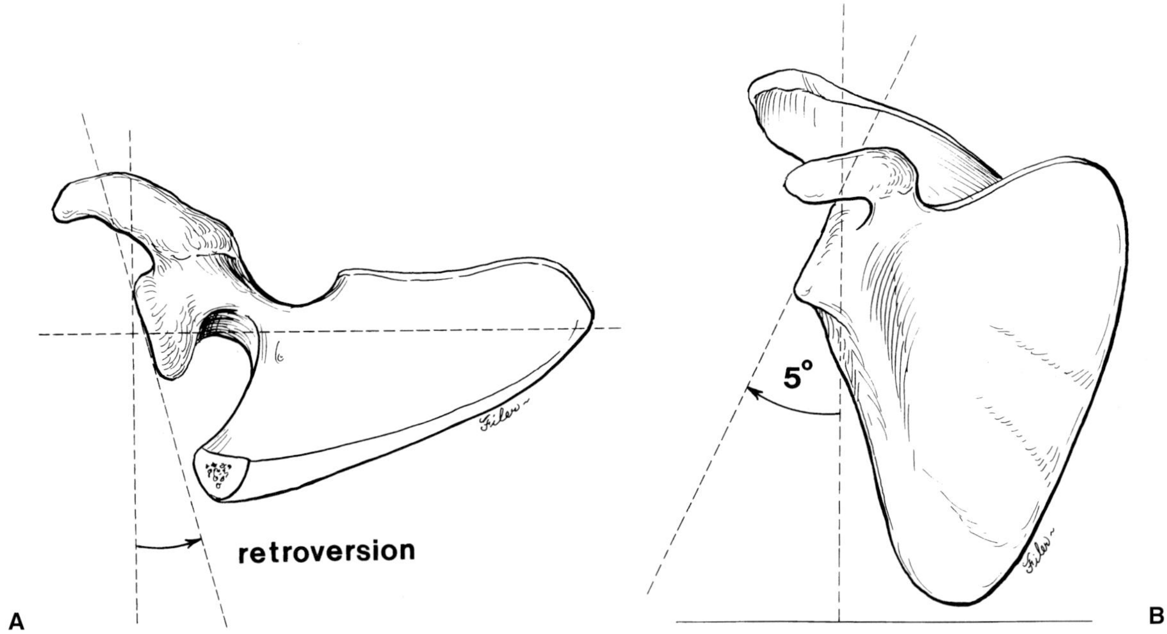

FIG. 4. Glenoid version averages. **A:** A 7-degree retroversion. **B:** A 5-degree superior tilt. (From Warner JJP. The gross anatomy of the joint surfaces, ligaments, labrum, and capsule. In: Matsen FA, Fu FH, Hawkins RJ, eds. *The shoulder: a balance of mobility and stability.* Rosemont, IL: American Academy of Orthopaedic Surgeons, 1993:7–27, with permission.)

Other investigators have reported on radiographic or computed tomography (CT) studies demonstrating that lesser or greater degrees of glenoid version are associated with instability (22,44,53,123,124). Within this context, Saha and colleagues (13), Scott (53), Brewer et al. (124), and others (22,44) have made a case for glenoid osteotomy to manage shoulder instability; however, their measurements of version involved the use of two reference axes that may lack reproducibility. Moreover, recent CT studies by Randelli and Gambrioli (128) and Hurley et al. (44) have provided further conflicting data on this subject.

The articular surface of the humeral head has been described by Inman et al. (97) to have evolved into an arrangement with dorsal inclination and retrotorsion. Although these workers explained the teleologic necessity for this evolutionary anatomic arrangement as a key feature of prehensile activity in humans, they did not specifically report values for these parameters. Saha (57,58) used radiographic studies, including a special modified axillary view, to show that the neck-shaft angle averages 130 to 140 degrees and that retroversion averages 30 degrees relative to the transepicondylar line, although he did not report ranges of normal (Fig. 5). Randelli and Gambrioli (128) studied normal volunteers with CT and reported the range of humeral retrotorsion to be 25 to 30 degrees. They then compared this value with that of a group of patients with recurrent anterior instability and found no significant difference. More recently, Kronberg et al. (125,126) used a modified radiographic technique to study shoulders of normal volunteers and individuals with recurrent anterior instability. In dominant and nondominant shoulders of normal volunteers, humeral retrotorsion measured 33 ± 9.3 degrees and 29 ± 8.4 degrees, respectively. This was significantly greater than the respective values of 26 ± 4.3 degrees and 23 ± 10.9 degrees observed in shoulders of patients with recurrent anterior instability. Therefore, it appears that further study is required to resolve this continued controversy over the importance of humeral retrotorsion to shoulder stability.

Glenohumeral Surface Area and Articular Contact

At the glenohumeral joint, a large spherical humeral head articulates with the smaller glenoid surface. Historically, articular geometry at the glenohumeral joint was believed to constitute a less important stabilizing factor than at other joints, such as the hip. This conclusion was based on (a) the small area of the glenoid relative to the humeral head (57,58), and (b) the relative shallowness or larger radius of curvature of the glenoid compared with the humeral head (139,185).

The glenoid surface is shaped like an inverted comma, with a superior portion that is narrow and an inferior portion that is broad. Its average vertical and transverse dimensions are 35 mm and 25 mm, respectively, whereas the vertical and transverse dimensions of the humeral articular surface average 48 mm and 45 mm, respectively (167). This surface area mismatch may also be expressed by the glenohumeral index (GH_I):

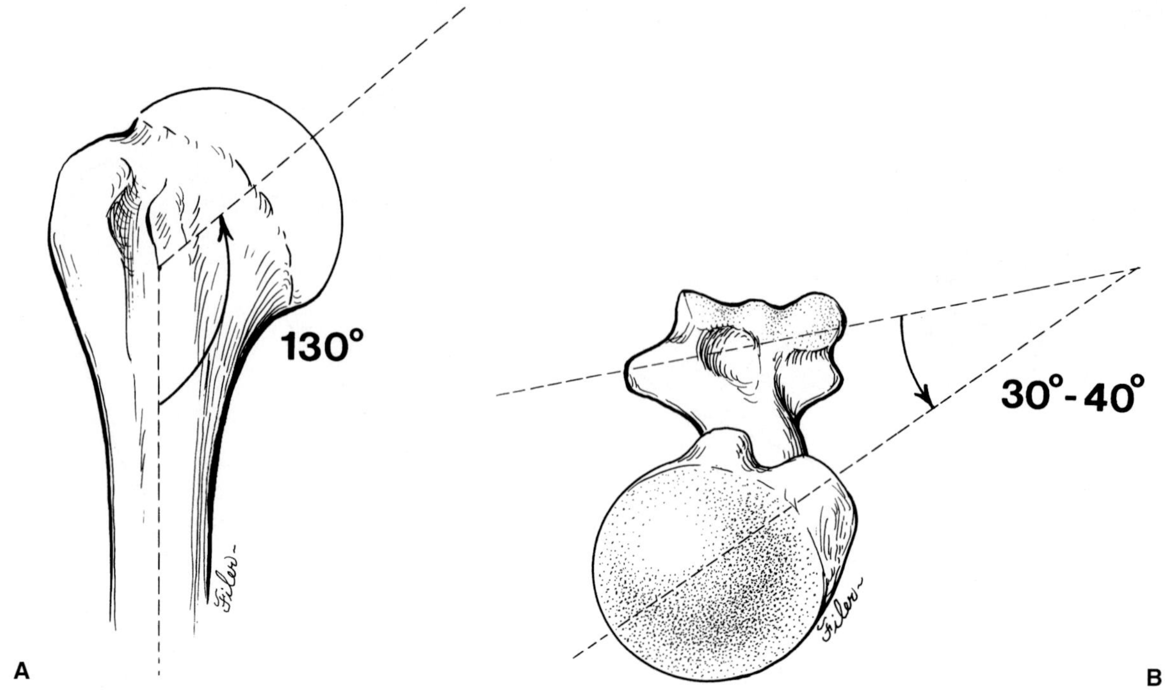

FIG. 5. Humeral articular orientation averages **(A)** 130-degree neck-shaft angle, and **(B)** 30 to 40 degrees of retroversion. (From Warner JP, Caborn DNM. Overview of shoulder instability. *Crit Rev Phys Rehabil Med* 1992;4:145–198, with permission.)

$$GH_I = \text{maximum glenoid diameter/maximum humeral head diameter}$$

Saha (57,58) and others (117,159) have calculated this index to be 0.75 and 0.76 in the sagittal and transverse planes, respectively. Historically, investigators have described the glenohumeral joint variously as analogous to a "ball and socket" (68) or to a "golfball sitting on a tee" (37). These conclusions led to several biomechanical models and clinical approaches to instability. Currently, it remains controversial as to whether the humeral head articulates in the glenoid fossa with a perfect conforming fit. Saha (57) described three types of articulations: type A glenoid radius of curvature larger than that of humeral head, type B matching radii of curvature, and type C glenoid radius of curvature smaller than that of humeral head. In a similar anatomic study, Sarrafian (38) found glenoid and humeral surfaces to have matching radii of curvature. Recent observations on joint conformity, using magnetic resonance imaging (MRI) and CT studies, tend to confirm Sarrafian's conclusion that the type B articulation of Saha represents the most common morphology. Yet, plane radiographic studies may give the impression that the glenoid is flatter, as the radiolucent glenoid articular cartilage adds concavity to the relatively flat subchondral bone surface (Fig. 6).

Soslowsky et al. (186,187) recently clarified this concept using stereophotogrammetric techniques to define the three-dimensional anatomy of the glenohumeral articulation. These investigators found the articular surfaces to be almost perfectly matched, with deviations of less than 1% of the radius of curvature, and congruent to within 3 mm of each other in all cases studied. These studies provided a more quantitative measure of the GH_I, with only 25% to 30% of the humeral head contacting the glenoid in any position of rotation. In addition, this work also assessed cartilage thickness over the entire joint. Glenoid cartilage was found to be thickest at the periphery (mean, 3.8 mm) and thinnest centrally (mean, 1.2 mm). Conversely, humeral articular cartilage was thickest centrally (mean, 2.0 mm) and thinnest peripherally (mean, 0.6 mm). Moreover, the head was observed to maintain relatively uniform contact on the glenoid surface throughout shoulder motion (188) (Fig. 6).

These observations are difficult to reconcile with those biomechanical studies that have shown a coupled translation during glenohumeral rotation, as a perfectly congruent joint would be expected to rotate without significant translation (114,115,155,189). Bowen et al. (185) used Fuji film to demonstrate glenohumeral contact in cadaver shoulders subjected to 50 and 100 lb of joint compression. In the adducted joint, glenohumeral contact was found to be nonconforming, with the humeral head contacting the glenoid centrally in the area of thinner cartilage. This is the "bare area" previously described by DePalma (11) as an acquired area of cartilage thinning. Histologic section of the glenoid showed that subchondral trabecular bone density is greater here, supporting the observation that this is the contact point of the humeral head on the glenoid in the adducted shoulder. Recent studies by Muller-Gerbl (190) using CT-osteodensitometry have confirmed increased subchondral bone density centrally on the glenoid.

A

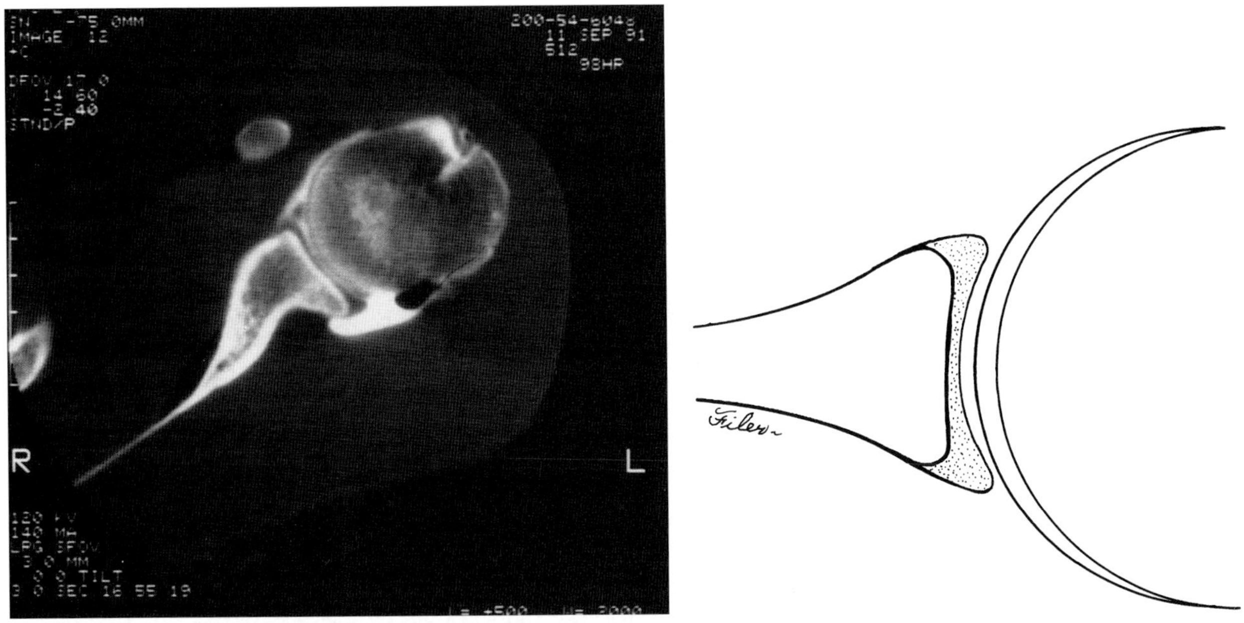

B

FIG. 6. The bony glenoid is relatively flat; however, the concave articular cartilage enhances conformity with the humeral head. **A:** Computed tomography arthrogram demonstrates conformity of articular surfaces. **B:** Illustration demonstrating how articular cartilage match results in conformity despite relatively flat osseous glenoid. (From Warner JJP, Schulte KR, Imhoff AB. *Current concepts in shoulder instability. Advances in operative orthopaedics*, vol. 3. St. Louis: Mosby–Year Book, 1995:217–248, with permission.)

However, recent biomechanical models employed to examine glenohumeral motion in the laboratory have in fact demonstrated nearly ''ball-and-socket'' kinematics (108, 191). By applying loads to the rotator cuff and deltoid tendons to produce glenohumeral motion in cadavera, both Kelkar et al. (188) and Thompson et al. (191) found only minimal translation accompanying rotation. The results of such investigations appear to coincide with the stereophotogrammetric findings of Soslowsky et al. (186,187)that glenohumeral articulation is quite conforming. Thus, surface area mismatch, rather than lack of conformity, may contribute to the potential for glenohumeral instability.

Glenoid Labrum

Although numerous studies have evaluated the anatomy of the glenoid labrum, until recently there was only a limited understanding of its morphologic variability and its role in glenohumeral stability (88–90,94). The labrum is a fibrous structure that forms a ring around the periphery of the glenoid and acts as an anchor point on the glenoid for the capsuloligamentous structures. It attaches to the glenoid articular cartilage through a narrow fibrocartilaginous transition zone but is essentially fibrous throughout its structure. It has been likened to the meniscus of the knee; Howell and Galinat (68) demonstrated that it contributes functionally to stability by increasing the depth of the glenoid socket. These investigators measured a series of cadaver glenoids and observed that the depth of the sockets averaged 9 mm and 5 mm in the superoinferior and AP planes, respectively, and that loss of the glenoid labrum decreased depth of the socket by 50% in either direction. They proposed that the stabilizing effect of the labrum was analogous to that of a ''chock block,'' preventing the wheel of a tractor from rolling down a hill (Fig. 7). Experimental work by Soslowsky et al. (186,187) and by Bowen et al. (185) has suggested that the labrum may also contribute to stability by increasing surface area and acting as a load-bearing structure for the humeral head. Moreover, Lippitt et al. (70), Vahey et al. (72), and Bowen et al. (192) have shown that the labrum plays a significant stabilizing role when the humeral head is compressed into the glenoid even when ligaments are cut or lax (Fig. 6).

Cooper et al. (89) demonstrated significant anatomic variability in the labrum around the periphery of the glenoid. In its superior portion above the equator of the glenoid, the labrum quite frequently loosely attaches and may therefore function more as a mobile extension of the glenoid surface than as a rigid ''chock block'' (Fig. 8). It is below the equator of the glenoid that the labrum consistently attaches to articular cartilage. Therefore, labral detachments below the equator of the glenoid more likely indicate instability while a loosely attached labrum above the equator more likely represents a normal anatomic variant.

Capsuloligamentous Structures

Historically, the glenohumeral ligaments were first described as thickenings in the capsule of the shoulder joint (8,11,15,33,38,183). Most subsequent studies have at-

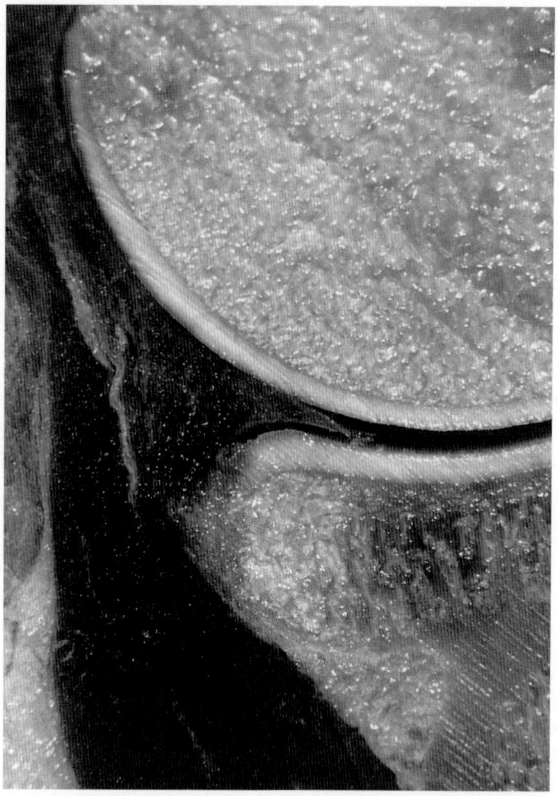

A

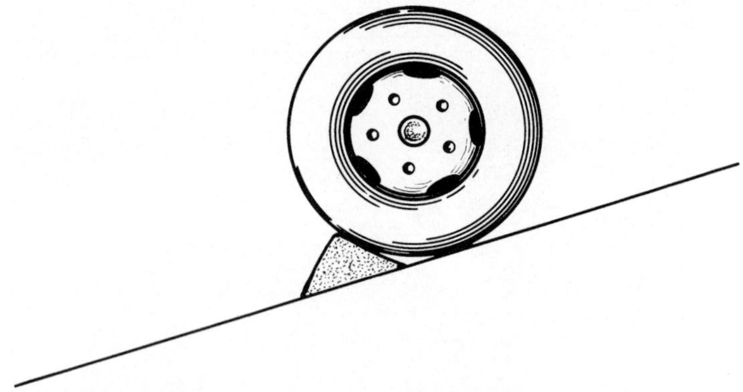

B

FIG. 7. A: The inferior glenoid labrum forms a triangular wedge that both deepens the glenoid cavity and forms an attachment for the inferior glenohumeral ligament. (From Cooper DE, Arnoczky SP, O'Brien SJ, Warren RF, DiCarlo EF, Allen AA. Anatomy, histology, and vascularity of the glenoid labrum. *J Bone Joint Surg [Am]* 1992;74A:46–52, with permission.) **B:** The labrum also prevents translation in a manner analogous to a "chock-block," preventing a wheel from rolling down a hill. (From Warner JJP. The gross anatomy of the joint surfaces, ligaments, labrum, and capsule. In: Matsen FA, Fu FH, Hawkins RJ, eds. *The shoulder: a balance of mobility and stability.* Rosemont, IL: American Academy of Orthopaedic Surgeons, 1993:7–27, with permission.)

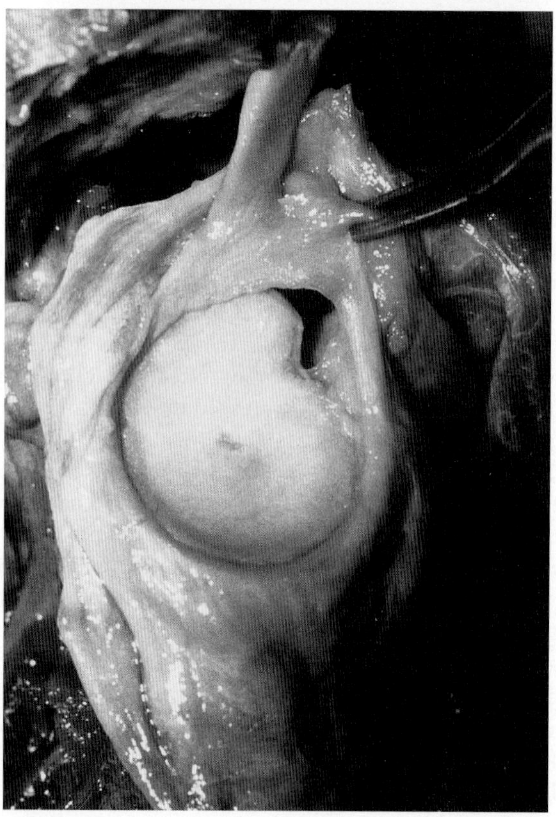

FIG. 8. The glenoid labrum may be loosely attached above the glenoid equator. (From Cooper DE, Arnoczky SP, O'Brien SJ, Warren RF, DiCarlo EF, Allen AA. Anatomy, histology, and vascularity of the glenoid labrum. *J Bone Joint Surg [Am]* 1992;74A:46–52, with permission.)

tempted to elucidate capsuloligamentous anatomy by qualitative clinical observations at arthroscopy or arthrotomy (4,5,16,26,28–31,37,50,104,105,109,165,168) or by cadaveric dissections (10,38,164,165). More recent experimental investigations have sought to define anatomy and function of these ligaments through selective cutting and biomechanical testing (65,74,114,115,117,118,151,155,159,162,193–196) and analysis of structural and material properties (111,116,119,182,183,197–199). Several investigators have also attempted to elaborate on the interrelationships of the rotator cuff and capsule (169,200,201).

DePalma (11) was one of the first investigators to point out the wide variability of glenohumeral capsular anatomy and described six common variants based on the pattern of synovial recesses encountered on dissection. He believed that these patterns might correlate with the risk of developing an unstable joint. Others have suggested that ligament anatomy correlates with instability (26,148,168). Turkel et al. (59) were the first to perform anatomic radiographic studies to clarify the orientation and position of the ligaments during shoulder abduction. Warner et al. (169) performed a similar study, using simulated rotator cuff contraction to move the glenohumeral joint. Moreover, both clinical experience and experimental studies have recognized the usefulness of arthroscopic visualization of capsular anatomy through small incisions that do not distort the ligamentous relationships (26,117,147,159,168–170) (Fig. 9). The following discussion considers each ligament or area of the capsule according to these historic concepts of anatomy.

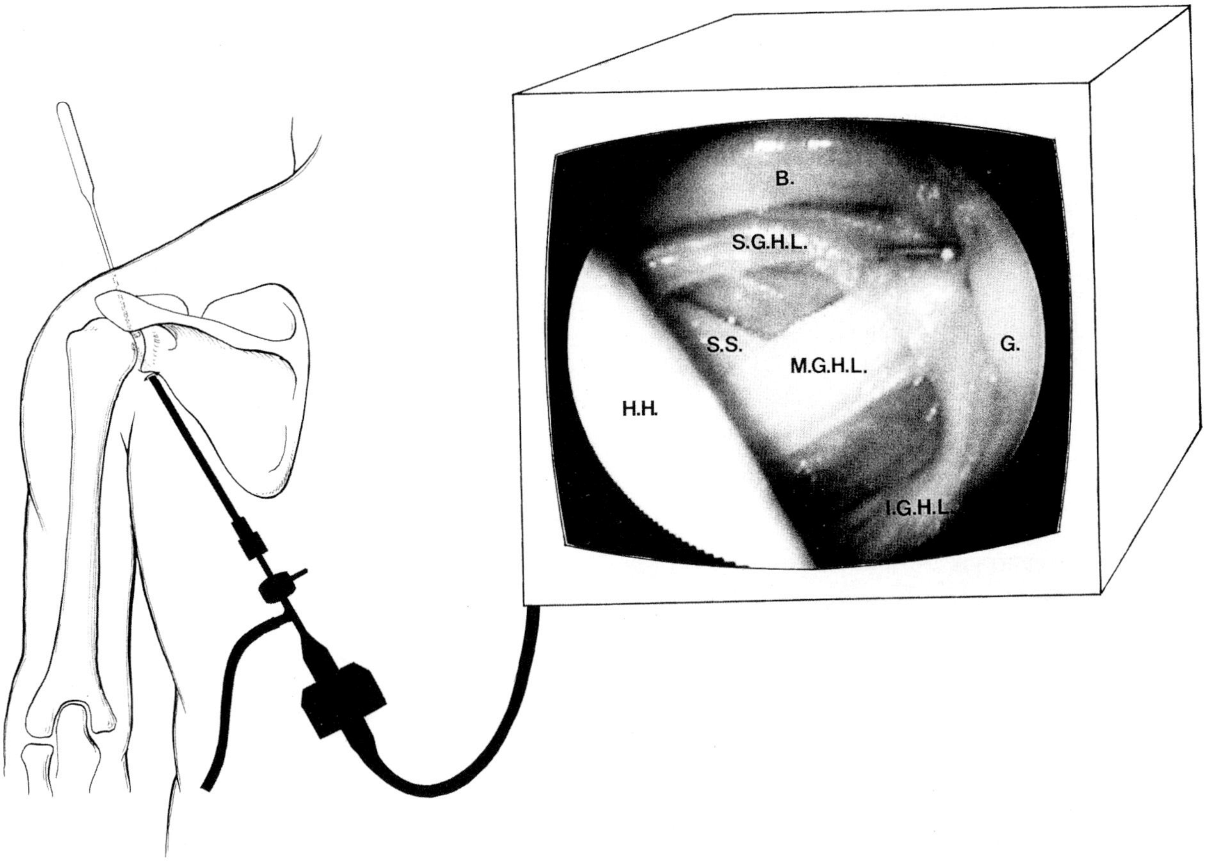

FIG. 9. Arthroscopic capsuloligamentous anatomy, posterior to anterior view. The superior glenohumeral ligament (SGHL) is a well-developed band in this shoulder. The middle glenohumeral ligament (MGHL) is cord-like and well developed. The anterior band of the inferior glenohumeral ligament complex (IGHLC) is similarly well developed. *B*, biceps tendon; *G*, glenoid; *HH*, humeral head; *SS*, subscapularis. (From Warner JJP, Caborn DNM, Berger R, Fu FH, Seel M. Dynamic capsulologamentous anatomy of the glenohumeral joint. *J Shoulder Elbow Surg* 1993;2:115–133, with permission.)

"Rotator Interval:" Superior Glenohumeral and Coracohumeral Ligaments

The "rotator interval" comprises that region between the anterior border of the supraspinatus tendon and the superior border of the subscapularis tendon. The ligamentous components of this region include the superior glenohumeral ligament (SGHL) and the coracohumeral ligament (CHL) (155, 167,201,202). Historically, the CHL has been considered the main structural component in this area, whereas the SGHL was seen as playing only a small role in stability (31,32,95, 194,195,203,204). Classic descriptions of the CHL have it as a dense fibrous structure originating on the lateral surface of the coracoid and inserting into the greater and lesser tuberosities adjacent to the bicipital groove (11,167,203)(Fig. 10). Some investigators have suggested that it may represent an accessory insertion of the pectoralis minor (167). Recent gross anatomic and histologic work by Cooper et al. (205) has demonstrated that the CHL is usually a thin capsular fold without ligamentous form, coursing from the coracoid process to the greater tuberosity of the humerus, forming a "pup tent" of capsule bridging this area.

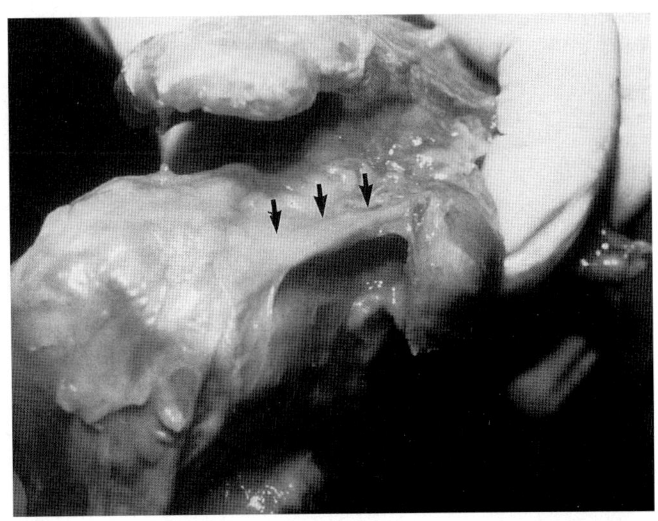

FIG. 10. The coracohumeral ligament *(arrows)* runs from the coracoid process to the greater and lesser tuberosities. (From Warner JJP, Schule KR, Imhoff AB. *Current concepts in shoulder instability. Advances in operative orthopaedics*, vol. 3. St. Louis: Mosby–Yearbook, 1995:217–248, with permission.)

The SGHL has received comparatively less consideration in the literature than the CHL which it parallels and underlies. DePalma (12) and others (117,151,159,166,169, 205) have found it to be present, although significantly variable in size and course, in more than 90% of cases. It originates from the superior glenoid just inferior to the biceps tendon and inserts onto the lesser tuberosity of the humerus. It is almost always visible during arthroscopy (159,168,169) (Fig. 9). O'Brien et al. (117,166,167) concluded that it plays little role in shoulder stability because of its variable and small size. Contrary to this position, Cooper et al. (203) demonstrated that it is consistently present as a ligamentous structure and, unlike the CHL, has collagen bundles organized in a longitudinal fashion. Warner et al. (122) have suggested that the SGHL plays a major role in inferior stability, whereas Warren et al. (220) have suggested that it may also play a role in posterior stability of the shoulder. Because the SGHL and CHL parallel one another, we may surmise that they have a similar role in providing stability by limiting inferior translation and external rotation of the adducted arm. Both clinical (32) and experimental studies (155,159,204) have shown that deficiency or injury to the rotator interval may result in multidirectional instability, whereas contracture in this region may limit glenohumeral motion (202,206).

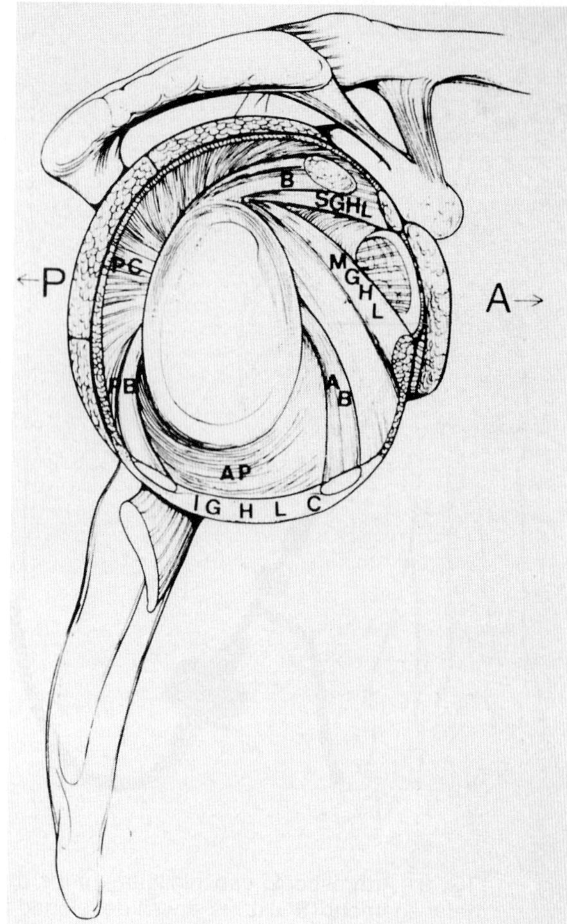

FIG. 12. Capsuloligamentous anatomy. The humeral head has been removed. The inferior glenohumeral ligament complex (IGHLC) consists of the anterior band *(AB)*, posterior band *(PB)*, and axillary pouch *(AP)*. *A*, anterior; *B*, biceps; *P*, posterior; *PC*, posterior capsule. (From O'Brien SJ, Neves MC, Arnoczky SP, Rozbruck SR, DiCarlo EF, Warren RF, Schwartz R, Wickiewicz TL. The anatomy and histology of the inferior glenohumeral ligament complex of the shoulder. *Am J Sports Med* 1990;18:579–589, with permission.)

A

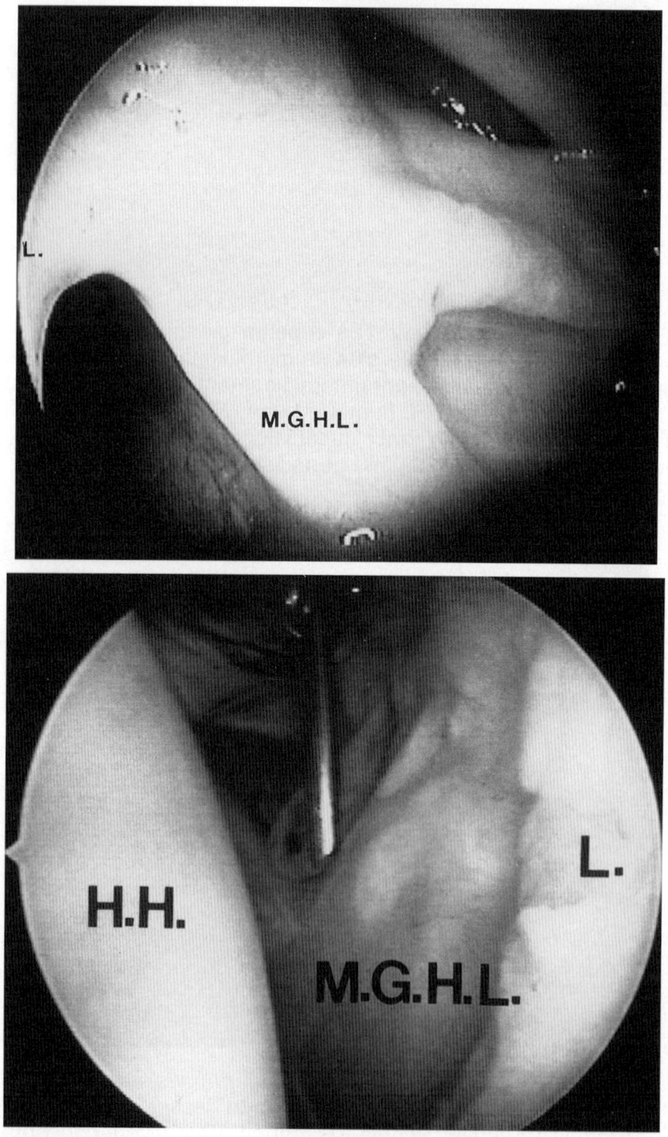

B

FIG. 11. Arthroscopic view of the middle glenohumeral ligament (MGHL). **A:** Cord-like variation. **B:** Sheet-like variation. *L*, labrum; *HH*, humeral head.

Middle Glenohumeral Ligament

DePalma (11) and others (117,159,166–169) have observed that the middle glenohumeral ligament (MGHL) has the greatest variation in size of all the ligaments of the shoulder. It is absent in up to 30% of cases and is poorly defined in another 10%. When present, it usually originates from the superior glenoid just inferior to the SGHL, slightly medial to the labrum. It has two morphologic variations: (a) sheet-like and confluent with the anterior band of the inferior glenohumeral ligament, or (b) cord-like with a foraminal separation between it and the anterior band of the inferior glenohumeral ligament (Fig. 11). It has been identified as a secondary restraint to anterior and inferior instability; some investigators believe that it plays a greater protective role for anterior stability when its morphology is cord-like (165,168).

Inferior Glenohumeral Ligament Complex

This portion of the shoulder capsule was originally described by DePalma et al. (11) as a triangular-shaped structure running from the labrum to the humeral neck between the subscapularis and the triceps. Turkel et al. (59) modified this anatomic description by defining a thickening in its anterior edge, which they termed the superior band. Others have observed this superior band to be a consistent ligamentous structure (165,168,169). Using arthroscopic inspection and gross and histologic dissection, O'Brien et al. (166) have recently redefined this structure as an inferior glenohumeral ligament complex (IGHLC) with a three-component nature. They found evidence of discrete anterior and posterior bands with an interposed thinner axillary pouch (Fig. 12). On the basis of their observations, O'Brien's group suggested that this complex functions in a fashion analogous to a hammock supporting the humeral head in the glenoid during abduction and rotation of the joint (Fig. 13). Other biomechanical and arthroscopic studies have supported their observations (117,151,159,169). However, Bigliani et al. (111) recently studied this portion of the capsule and, although they found the anterior band to be consistently present and to represent the thickest area of this region (mean 2.8 mm), they found no evidence of a discrete posterior ligamentous band.

Posterior Capsule

O'Brien et al. (166,167) defined this region as that part of the capsule superior to the posterior band of the IGHLC, whereas Warren et al. (122) pointed out that there is little

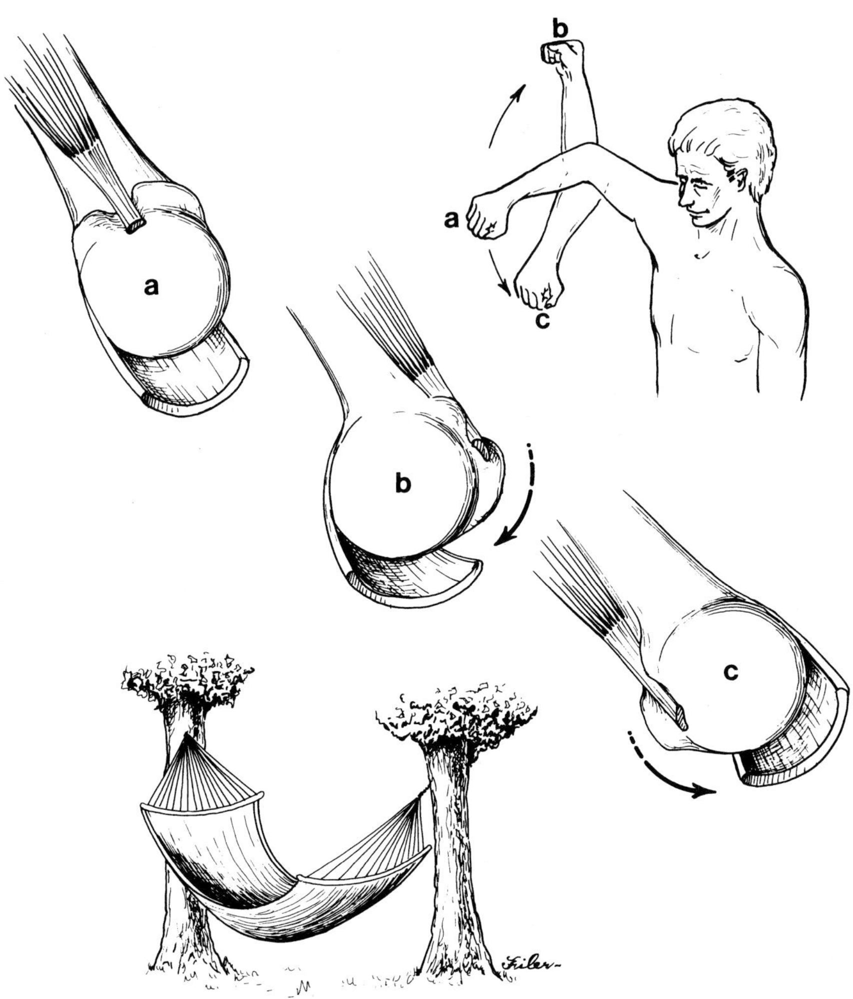

FIG. 13. The inferior glenohumeral ligament complex supports the humeral head like a hammock *(a)*. Reciprocal tightening *(b)* external rotation and *(c)* internal rotation provides a barrier to anterior and posterior instability, respectively. (From Warner JP, Caborn DNM. Overview of shoulder instability. *Crit Rev Phys Rehabil Med* 1992;4:145–198, with permission.)

anatomic information aside from that in studies addressing its biomechanical contribution to stability of the shoulder (162,195,207). It has been shown to be the thinnest part of the capsule (111) (Fig. 14).

Material Properties

Consideration of the normal anatomy of the glenohumeral joint must include information on the size of the capsular ligaments, as well as their tensile properties. Relatively few investigations have examined the structural and material properties of the glenohumeral ligaments until recently (20–22). The capsule is, in fact, quite redundant, having a surface area twice that of the humeral head (139). It is composed of types I, II, and III collagen and is similar in composition to other joint capsules. Reeves (183) and Kaltsas (199) found that the ultimate tensile load of the anteroinferior capsule in cadaveric shoulders averaged 2,000 N, with decreasing ability to withstand load evident after age 50. The capsules of older specimens exhibited predominantly midsubstance failures, whereas those in younger specimens failed most often by avulsion off the glenoid.

Bigliani et al. (111) have recently measured thickness, width, length, and tensile properties of the IGHLC. They found that the superior portion of the IGHLC had the greatest thickness (2.8 mm) and the posterior region the least (1.7 mm). No discrete posterior band was identified, and no significant differences were found for resting length or width. The ultimate stress or tensile strength of the IGHLC was found to be 5.5 MPa, much lower than the values reported for the ligaments of the knee 35 to 80 MPa (208,209). Failure occurred at the glenoid insertion in 40%, at the humeral insertion in 25%, and in the midsubstance of the ligament complex in 35%. They also demonstrated significant plastic deformation of the IGHLC before tensile failure, concluding that laxity may be acquired without actual disruption of the ligament attachment. Before this study, only subjective evidence of congenital laxity existed (143). In an investigation of the tensile properties of the SGHL and CHL, Boardman et al. (197) demonstrated significantly greater stiffness and ultimate load in the CHL than in the SGHL, with the latter possessing tensile properties similar to those of the IGHLC.

Morrey and Chao (85) calculated the anterior shear force in the maximally abducted and externally rotated shoulder to be 60 kg (Fig. 15). This force must be resisted by both capsule and rotator cuff. Contraction of the rotator cuff, especially the external rotators with the arm in this position, has been shown to reduce stress in the anterior capsule (75). Thus, under extreme loading conditions where the anterior shear force is greater than the capsular tensile strength, or if the cuff does not effectively contract, the ligaments may fail. Such a situation might occur, for example, with a forceful fall onto the abducted and externally rotated arm or a seizure, where asynchronous muscle contraction produces a posterior shear force. Proprioceptive interaction between ligaments and muscles may function to mediate this protective mechanism (171–174,210).

In older patients, there appears to be an age-related attrition of strength in rotator cuff tissues, which is greater than that in capsular tissues, so an anterior dislocation commonly results in a rotator cuff tear with or without capsular rupture (183). This phenomenon has been termed the ''posterior mechanism'' of shoulder dislocation (138).

Rotator Cuff Bulk

Bulk effect of rotator cuff muscles about the shoulder was originally thought to contribute to limiting translation and rotation (63,162,194,195,207,211). However, recent work by Motzkin and coworkers (212) has shown that passive muscle bulk contributes little to glenohumeral joint stability.

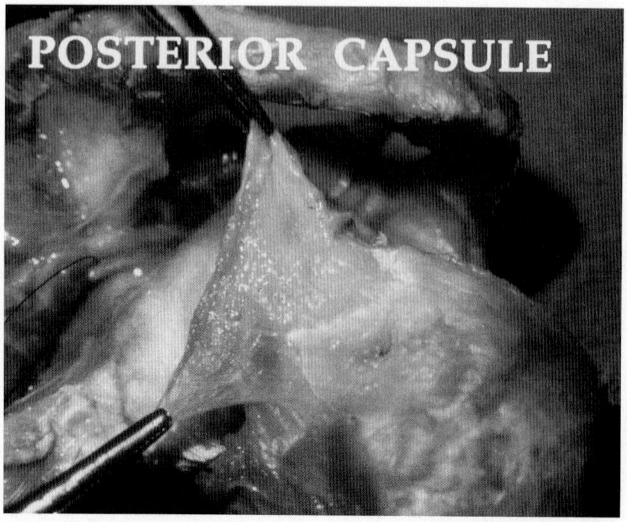

FIG. 14. Shoulder specimen demonstrating thin posterior capsule.

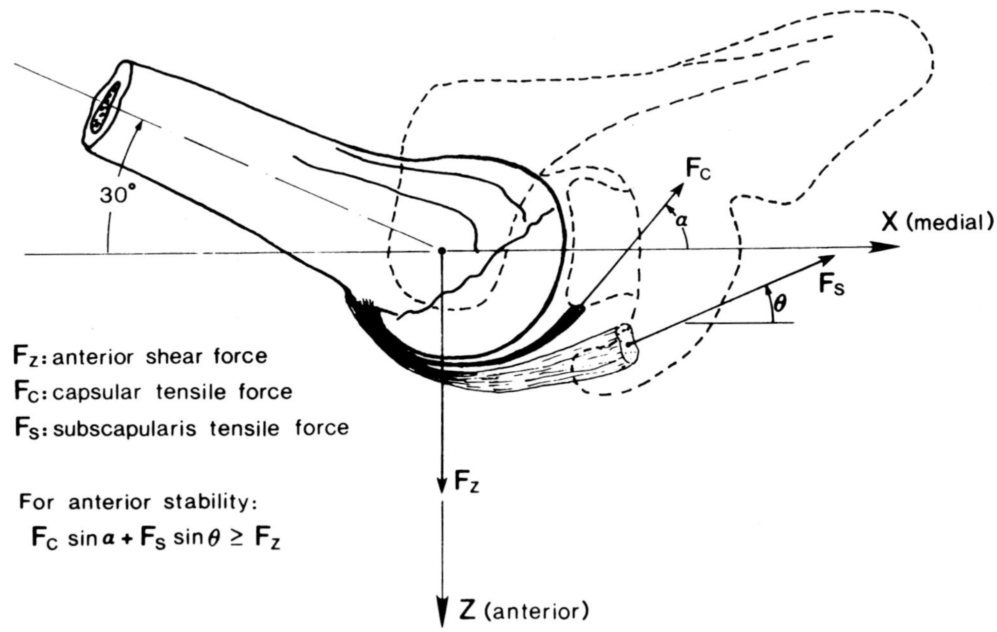

FIG. 15. Vector diagram of forces across the shoulder in abduction and external rotation. Anterior shear force *(F_z)* must be resisted by combined tensile force *(F_s)*. (From Morrey BF, Chao EYS. Recurrent anterior dislocation of the shoulder: clinical and anatomic considerations. In: Black J, Dumbleton JH, eds. *Clinical biomechanics: a case history approach.* New York: Churchill Livingstone, 1981:24–46, with permission.)

DYNAMIC RESTRAINTS

The rotator cuff and long head of the biceps function dynamically during shoulder motion to contain the humeral head in the glenoid by the following mechanisms: (a) joint compression, (b) coordinated contraction to steer the humeral head into the glenoid, and (c) dynamization of glenohumeral ligaments through cuff attachments. Other important dynamic factors include coordinated scapulothoracic rhythm, negative intra-articular pressure, and adhesion-cohesion.

Joint Compression

Compression of the articular surface provided by contraction of the rotator cuff and long head of the biceps brachii enhances joint stability by enhancing the conforming fit of the humeral head into the glenoid (68,70,145,192, 213–217) (Fig. 6). Experimental studies by Bowen et al. (192) and Lippitt et al. (70) have shown that the magnitude of this stabilizing effect greatly exceeds that of the static capsuloligamentous factors. Recently, Vahey et al. (72) introduced the concept of scapulohumeral balance to illustrate that glenoid geometry coupled with joint compression provides a major stabilizing force. Howell and Galinat (68) originally described this effect as the "containment concept" and have suggested that this mechanism of dynamic stability is more important than a coordinated and balanced functioning rotator cuff. They observed that selective nerve block of the supra- and infraspinatus muscles of patients with anterior instability did not result in clinical instability or loss of humeral head containment on uniplanar radiographic studies during transverse plane rotation.

We agree that this effect is an important stabilizing mechanism of the glenohumeral joint, although we do believe that coordinated rotator cuff and biceps function also play a significant role through all ranges of shoulder motion. Radiographic studies by Poppen and Walker (101) and others (96,148,149) have demonstrated that rotator cuff tears can result in superior translation of the humeral head during scapular plane abduction, although the kinematic investigations of Thompson et al. (191) have demonstrated the maintenance of normal glenohumeral motion in the presence of rotator cuff tears as long as the force couple provided by the subscapularis and infraspinatus/teres minor remains functionally intact.

Coordinated Rotator Cuff Contraction/Steering Effect

Poppen and Walker (101) used a simplified two-dimensional model to examine the magnitude and direction of the forces across the glenohumeral joint during abduction. Inman et al. (97) and others (96,139,148,183) have also studied two-dimensional forces across the glenohumeral joint by planar vector analysis; more recently, Bassett et al. (73) have assessed three-dimensional orientation of the muscles across the abducted shoulder. These observations support the complex role of the rotator cuff in controlling shoulder motion and stability.

Forces at the glenohumeral joint have a magnitude and direction and can therefore be subjected to a vector analysis (Fig. 16). If the resultant vector (**R**) is calculated, it will be oriented in one of three directions relative to the glenoid surface: (a) within the confines of the glenoid (Fig. 16A), (b) outside the glenoid (Fig. 16B), or (c) away from the glenoid (Fig. 16C). These represent joint compression, joint shear, and joint distraction, respectively.

When the resultant force vector **R** falls within the confines of the glenoid, the resultant load is shared only by the glenoid-labrum surface (Fig. 16A). This is probably the case through most rotations of the humeral head on the glenoid. If the resultant force vector R falls outside the glenoid, the resulting load is shared by the labrum, capsuloligamentous structures, and rotator cuff (Fig. 16B). This effect is probably greatest at extremes of rotation. If the resultant force vector **R** is directed away from the glenoid, as occurs with distraction of the humeral head out of the glenoid during follow-through when throwing, bony anatomy plays little role in stability (Fig. 16C). In this situation, rotator cuff contraction and ligament tension probably resist further displacement and act as the mechanism to keep the joint surfaces coapted. From this analysis, one may extrapolate to a clinical situation in which rotator cuff injury or dysfunction may result from overloading or strain from repeated attempts to decelerate and contain the humeral head during throwing motions (121). Negative intraarticular pressure and adhesion-cohesion mechanisms may play a role in humeral head containment, though probably only at low forces across the joint, and are discussed further in the following text.

Electromyographic (EMG) studies conducted by Glousman et al. (78) and others (84) have shown abnormal patterns of rotator cuff activity in shoulders of overhead athletes with instability, and Warner et al. (121) have demonstrated altered rotator cuff strength patterns in patients with anterior instability. Moreover, experimental studies have also demonstrated that contraction of portions of the rotator cuff and long head of the biceps reduces strain in the IGHL when the arm is placed into a position of abduction and external rotation (25,169). Clinically, we know that asynchronous contraction of portions of the rotator cuff in patients with voluntary instability can cause subluxation or dislocation of the shoulder (51). All these studies support the concept of a very important protective role for the rotator cuff and biceps to prevent instability, and loss of normal patterns of muscle activity may compromise this mechanism.

Ligament "Dynamization"

Through much of the range of glenohumeral rotation the capsuloligamentous structures remain quite lax, although Warner et al. (159,169) and others (117,118,151, 167,196) have shown that, at the extremes of rotation, these static structures function in a load-sharing manner

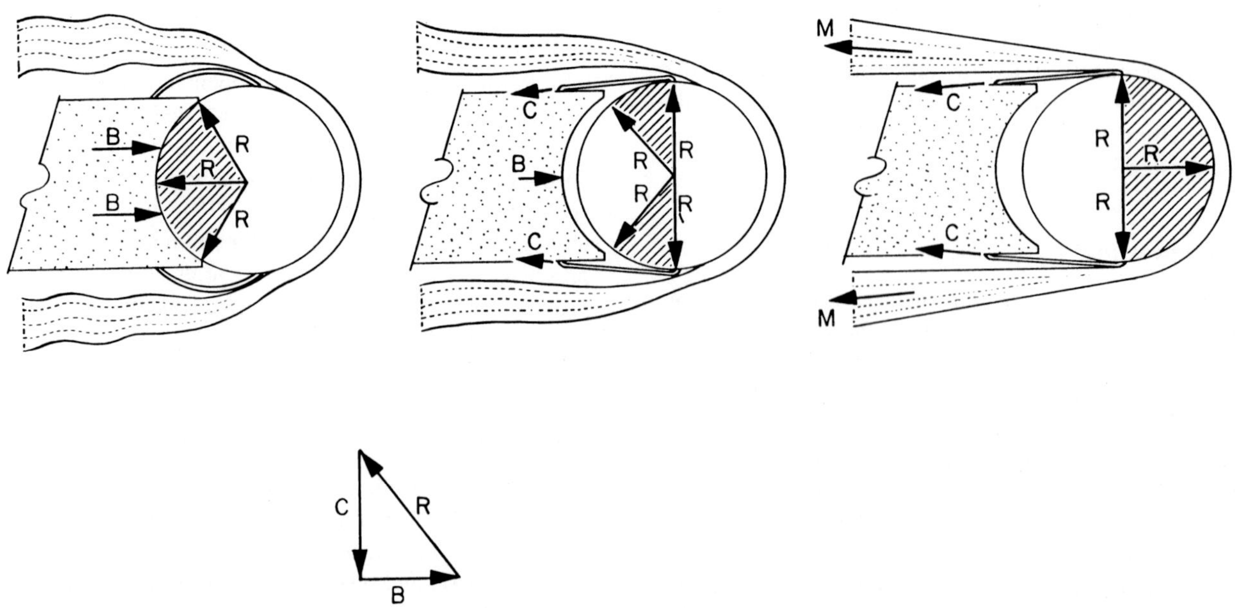

FIG. 16. Force diagram of stability of the glenohumeral joint. (From Warren RF, MD, personal communication) **A:** With pure joint compression, all joint reactive force *(R)* is contained within the articular surfaces *(B)*. **B:** With shear force, the tendency for the humeral head to move out of the glenoid must be resisted by a force *(R)* within the soft tissues. This is achieved through both the joint surfaces *(B)* and the capsular soft tissues *(C)*. **C:** With distraction force, stability must be maintained purely by capsular *(C)* and muscle forces *(M)* as the resultant force is away from the glenoid *(R)*.

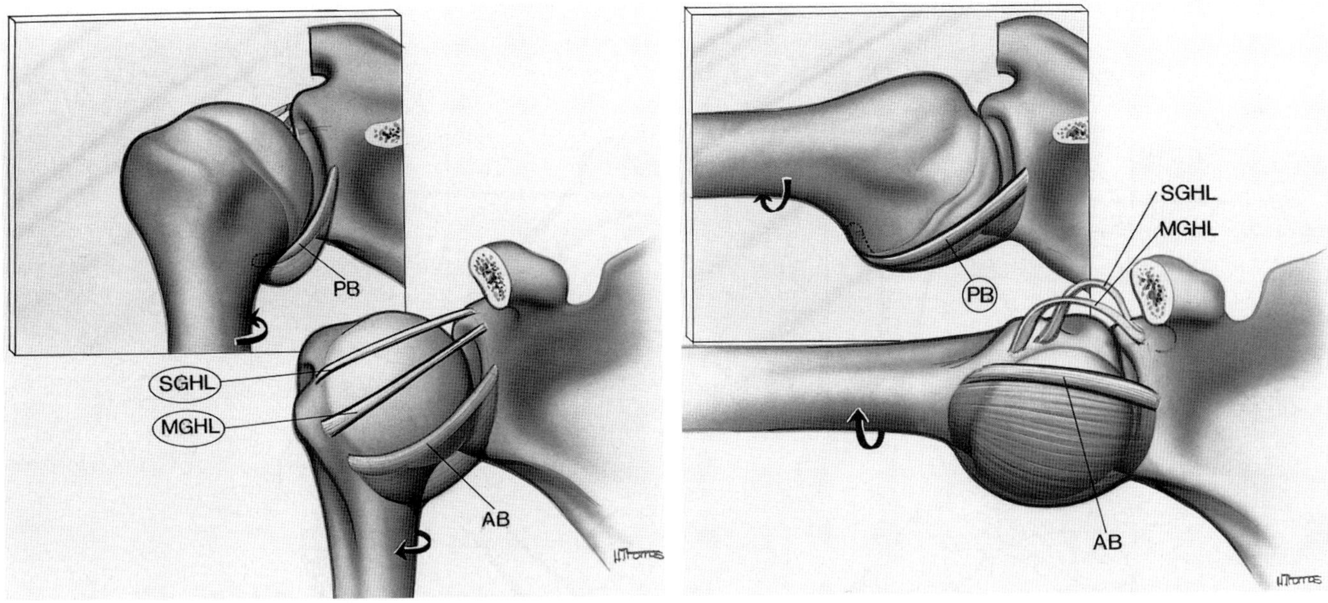

A B

FIG. 17. Function of the glenohumeral ligaments. The glenohumeral capsule is enhanced by ligamentous thickenings, which are relatively consistent. These ligaments tighten and loosen, depending on arm position. **A:** With the shoulder in adduction and external rotation, the superior *(SGHL)* and middle *(MGHL)* glenohumeral ligaments are maximally lengthened, whereas the anterior band *(AB)* and posterior band *(PB)* of the inferior glenohumeral ligament complex are lax. **B:** With the arm in abduction and external rotation, the *AB* and *PB* of the inferior glenohumeral ligament complex tighten underneath the humeral head, whereas the *SGHL* and *MGHL* become lax.

to prevent excessive translation and rotation (Fig. 17). Clark et al. (200) and others (164) have demonstrated that the rotator cuff tendons are attached to the humerus directly through portions of the capsule and ligaments and have proposed the possibility that rotator cuff contraction causes tension in the ligaments, thereby ''dynamizing'' these structures during active glenohumeral rotation. Work by Warner et al. (169) using a dynamic shoulder model has indicated that ligament orientation is indeed affected by rotator cuff contraction, lending further support to this dynamization theory.

Kinematics: Effect of Scapulothoracic Motion

Normal shoulder function requires a coordinated glenohumeral: scapulothoracic motion relationship. Since Codman (8) first introduced the concept of ''scapulohumeral rhythm,'' others have recognized that these two articulations function in an intercalated manner to maintain joint stability (57,95,98,103). Although there is some variation in the glenohumeral-to-scapulothoracic motion ratio, in the early stages of abduction, it averages about 2:1 (96,194). Clinical and radiographic studies have confirmed that patients with shoulder instability have abnormal scapulothoracic motion (99,100,103). Moreover, EMG studies of the axioscapular muscles (trapezius, serratus anterior) have demonstrated that fatigue of these muscles may lead to poor scapulothoracic control (78,87, 218). Such scapulothoracic weakness might produce varying degrees of scapular winging, with a biomechanical consequence of failure to provide a stable glenoid platform for the humeral head during shoulder motion (Fig. 18). This failure in turn might result in greater strain on the glenohumeral ligaments and an increased tendency for instability. Herein lies the rationale for shoulder rehabilitation programs to strengthen the axioscapular muscles as well as the rotator cuff.

Negative Intra-articular Pressure and Adhesion-Cohesion

Kumar and Balasubramaniam (63) were the first to observe that venting the joint capsule of a cadaveric shoulder resulted in marked inferior translation of the adducted arm. On the basis of this observation, they concluded that capsular structures play little role in joint stability when the arm is in this position. Basmajian and Bazant (95) and others (13,23,57,58,159) have suggested that superior glenoid tilt stabilizes the glenohumeral joint against inferior instability; however, the radiographic studies of Poppen and Walker (101) and others (96,148) have shown that in the adducted, unloaded shoulder, the glenoid faces slightly downward in most people. Because the rotator cuff is not contracting when the arm is hanging at the side, negative intra-articular pressure constitutes a major mechanism preventing inferior subluxation in this position.

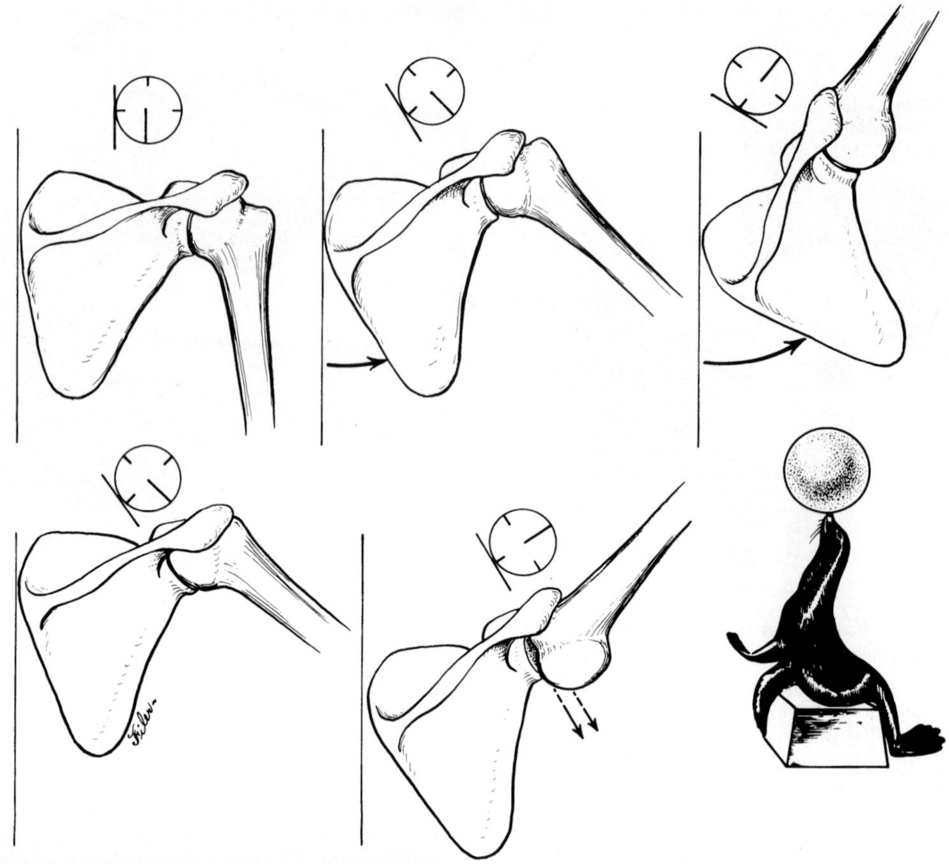

A

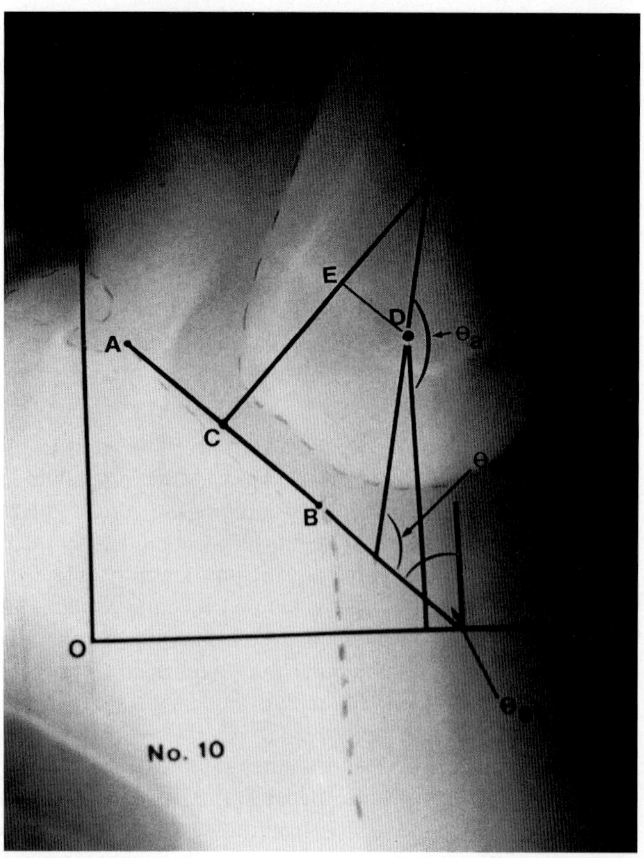

B

FIG. 18. A: Top row: Normal scapulothoracic motion positions the glenoid underneath the humeral head so that it is a stable platform. **Bottom row:** Failure of the scapula to properly rotate, as in winging, unbalances the joint by placing the glenoid in a position where it is not directly beneath the humeral head. This is analogous to a seal balancing a ball on its nose. (From Warner JP, Caborn DNM. Overview of shoulder instability. *Crit Rev Phys Rehabil Med* 1992;4:145–198, with permission.) **B:** Radiographic measurements of a patient with inferior subluxation of the humeral head who has abnormal scapulothoracic motion during abduction. Glenohumeral rotation *(gh)* is much greater than scapulothoracic rotation *(st)*; therefore, at maximum abduction of the arm *(a)*, the glenoid is subluxated inferiorly. The center of the glenoid is marked by a line *(CE)* bissecting a line *(AB)* tangential to the glenoid surface. The center of the humeral head *(D)* is inferior to this line. (From Warner JJP, Flatow EL. Anatomy and biomechanics. In: Bigliani LU, ed. *The unstable shoulder*. Rosemont, IL: American Academy of Orthopaedic Surgeons. 1997:1–20, with permission.)

Browne et al. (60) demonstrated the average intra-articular pressure in an adducted cadaver shoulder to be −42 cm H_2O, and the application of a 25-N inferior force caused the pressure to drop to −82 cm H_2O. This negative pressure most likely results from high osmotic pressure in interstitial tissues, causing water to be drawn out of the glenohumeral joint (106). Simkin (65) has suggested that the articular surface may gain stability through an adhesion-cohesion effect analogous to water between two glass microscope slides, preventing them from being pulled apart.

The biomechanical explanation for the negative pressure effect is presented diagrammatically in Figure 19. In simple terms, the glenohumeral joint consists of a closed compartment surrounded by an elastic diaphragm (joint capsule and cuff). Distraction of the articular surfaces produces a negative pressure in this closed compartment. This "suction effect" resists further displacement of the joint surfaces. Glenohumeral capsular laxity, large joint volume, or a capsular tear will decrease negative pressure for any given amount of displacement of the articular surface. In other words, the "suction effect" will be less. Patients with congenital ligamentous laxity, a rotator interval lesion, or a capsular tear from dislocation or fracture might lose the stabilizing effect of negative intra-articular pressure.

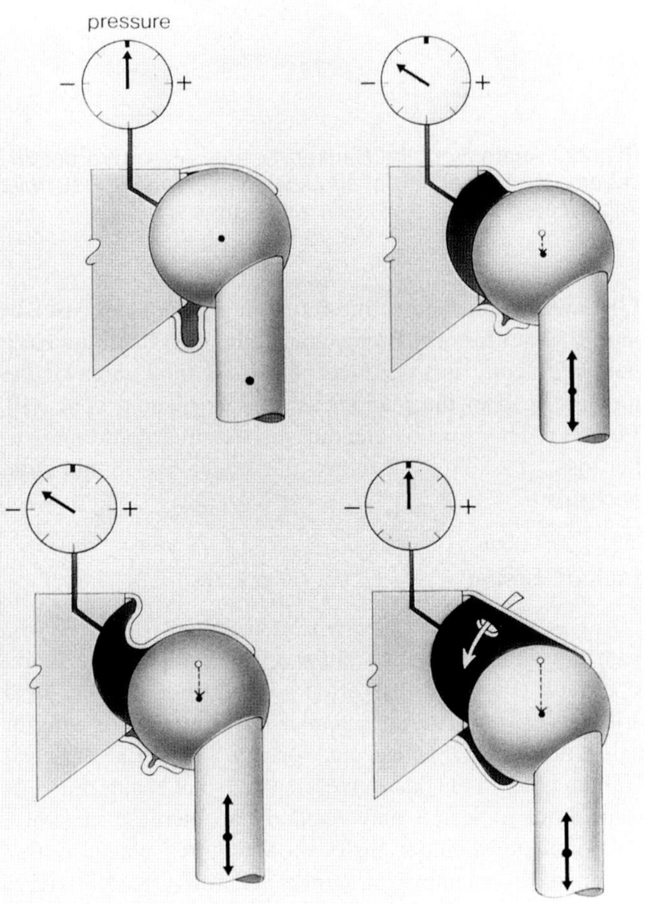

FIG. 19. Role of negative intra-articular pressure in stability of the glenohumeral joint. **Top left and right:** In a normal shoulder, the closed compartment of the joint creates a vaccum effect of a negative pressure relative to atmosphere as the weight of the arm tends to subluxate the humeral head inferiorly. **Bottom left and right:** In an abmormally lax shoulder or one with an actual defect in the capsule, the negative pressure or vacuum effect is lessened or eliminated. Thus, there is greater inferior subluxation of the humeral head (From Pagnani MJ, Warren RF, eds. The pathophysiology of anterior shoulder instability. *Sports Med Arthrosc Rev* 1993;1:177–189, with permission.)

Although the magnitude of the negative pressure effect in multiple planes of arm motion has not yet been clarified, recent experimental studies have suggested that ligament tension and muscle contraction are more important stabilizing mechanisms (61,64). Warner et al. (64) showed that in the adducted shoulder venting of the joint capsule resulted in a wide-ranging increase in inferior translation with application of an inferior force of 50 N. This range of translation appeared to be attributable to the variable morphology of the SGHL. In positions of greater abduction, the pressure effect was markedly diminished, such that at 90 degrees of abduction, venting the joint capsule produced only a few millimeters of inferior translation with loading. Furthermore, application of joint compression eliminated the effect of venting. On the basis of these observations, it was concluded that negative intra-articular pressure plays a significant stabilizing role only with the arm at rest in adduction, and even in this position acts in concert with the SGHL. Muscle contraction or tension in the ligaments during active motion of the joint have a much greater role in stability.

PATHOANATOMY

Glenoid Dysplasia

In rare cases, developmental hypoplasia or dysplasia of the glenoid can contribute to instability by reducing the glenohumeral index or by disrupting the concavity-compression effect of the convex humeral head fitting within the concave glenoid (Fig. 20). In these instances, the glenoid may be either flatter or smaller than in normal individuals. Morrey and Janes (47) encountered a dysplastic glenoid in 3% of 223 surgically treated cases, whereas the literature has reported approximately 50 cases (46,129–135). In our experience, 1% to 3% of patients with shoulder instability have radiographic evidence of glenoid dysplasia, and we generally avoid surgical procedures in these patients.

Glenoid Fractures or Bony Bankart

Aston and Gregory (1) reported on glenoid fracture accompanying anterior shoulder dislocation. Rowe (37,51, 109) suggested that loss of up to one-third of the glenoid was inconsequential for shoulder function, as long as the

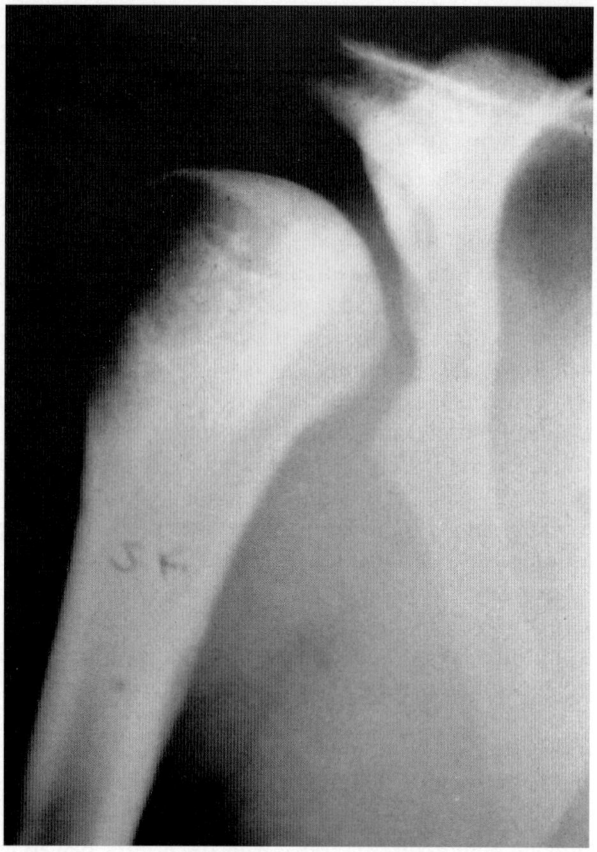

FIG. 20. Example of a patient with glenoid dysplasia. (From Warner JP, Caborn DNM. Overview of shoulder instability. *Crit Rev Phys Rehabil Med* 1992;4:145–198, with permission.)

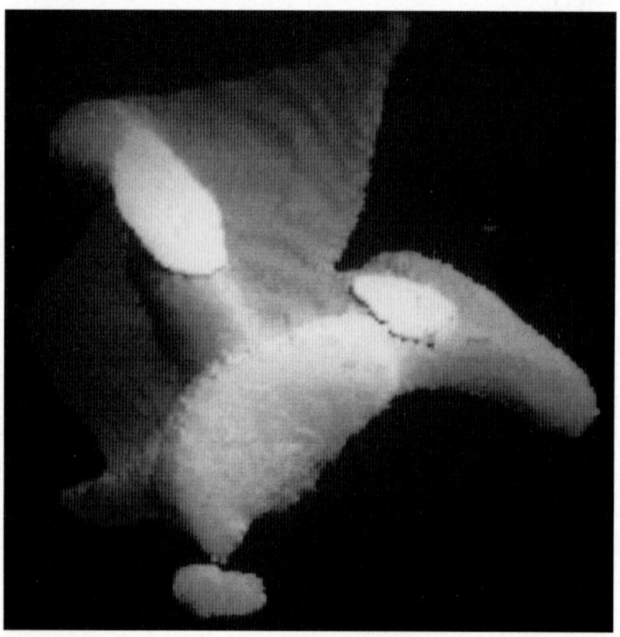

FIG. 21. Three-dimensional reconstruction of glenoid in a patient with recurrent instability. Computed tomography shows fracture involving the anterior one-third of the glenoid. (From Warner JJP, Schulte KR, Imhoff AB. *Current concepts in shoulder instability. Advances in operative orthopaedics*, vol. 3. St. Louis: Mosby–Year Book, 1995:217–248, with permission.)

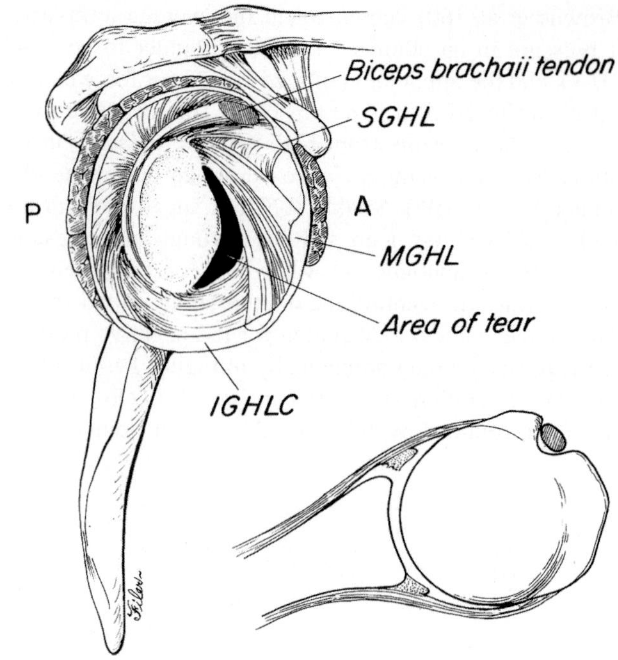

FIG. 22. Anatomy of the Bankart Lesion. (From Warner JP, Caborn DNM. Overview of shoulder instability. *Crit Rev Phys Rehabil Med* 1992;4:145–198, with permission.)

IGHL was reattached to the remaining glenoid in cases of bony Bankart lesions. Biomechanically, the effect of a large glenoid fracture is to reduce both the contact area of the humeral head in the glenoid as well as glenoid concavity (Fig. 21). This loss of glenoid surface area contributes to the loss of stability through the concavity-compression mechanism.

Bankart Lesion

A Bankart lesion represents detachment of the IGHL from the glenoid through either glenoid fracture or labral separation (Fig. 22). It is often accompanied by periosteal stripping off the anterior scapular neck in cases of anterior dislocation (2,3,5,17). Recent work by Speer et al. (71) and Bigliani et al. (111) has shown that an isolated anterior soft-tissue Bankart lesion may result in an increase in laxity, but complete shoulder dislocation requires plastic deformation of ligamentous structures as well (182,198) (Fig. 23).

Hill-Sachs Lesion

The Hill-Sachs lesion represents an impression fracture of the posterolateral margin of the humeral head created by anterior displacement of the head over the glenoid rim with anterior dislocation (9,14,16,20,21) (Fig. 23). It may accompany, in varying degrees of severity, more than 80% of anterior dislocations and 25% of anterior subluxations (219). Hermodsson (20) observed that this humeral head defect is larger with dislocations of greater duration, recurrent dislocation, and anterior inferior dislocation. Rowe (37, 109) and others (6,110,161) generally consider this lesion to have little consequence for anterior stability as long as an adequate anterior soft-tissue reconstruction is performed. Tension in the anterior capsule with external rotation may produce obligate posterior translation, which will prevent the humeral head from coming forward and falling out anteriorly through the Hill-Sachs lesion (189) (Fig. 24). However, when the Hill-Sachs lesion comprises greater than 30% of the humeral articular surface, it may contribute to anterior instability, even if an adequate anterior repair is performed, although there is no objective experimental evidence to support this (37,109) (Fig. 25). Concern over this potential loss of stability has formed the rationale for a variety of reconstructive procedures, including infraspinatus tendon transfer (77,109), humeral neck rotational osteotomy (55,56), segmental allograft reconstruction (Gerber C, personal communication, 1997) and humeral head hemiarthroplasty. Nonetheless, our experience parallels Rowe's, in that anterior capsular reconstruction appears to suffice without addressing the Hill-Sachs lesion in most cases.

Capsular Injury

Since the 13th century, the lesion of anterior dislocation was thought to be capsular rupture (35,36), although subsequent observations by Flower (16) and others (2,3,5,9,37,

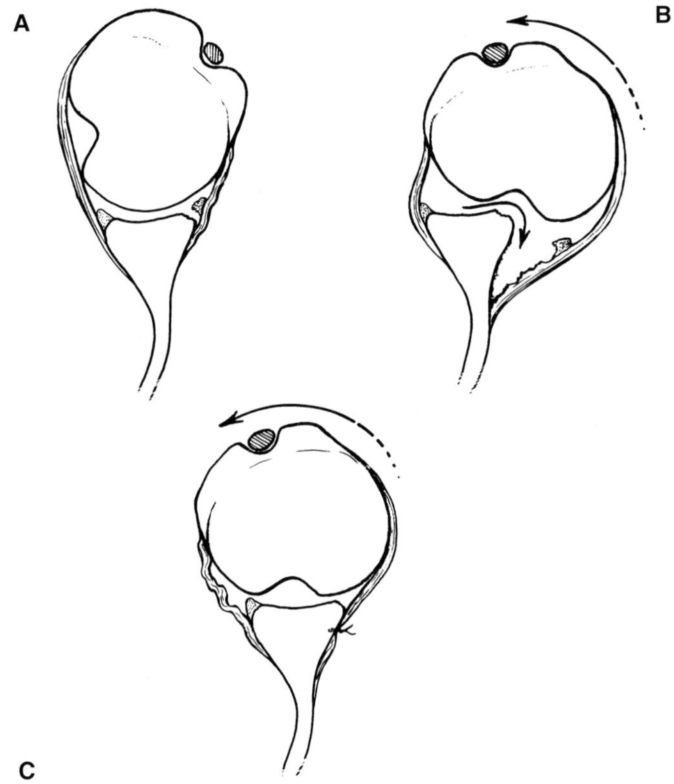

FIG. 24. A: Biomechanics of a Hill-Sachs lesion. **B:** External rotation produces anterior translation caused by Bankart lesion, and humeral head dislocates through the Hill-Sachs lesion. **C:** Bankart repair prevents anterior translation with external rotation, and Hill-Sachs lesion remains contained on glenoid. (From Warner JP, Caborn DNM. Overview of shoulder instability. *Crit Rev Phys Rehabil Med* 1992;4:145–198, with permission.)

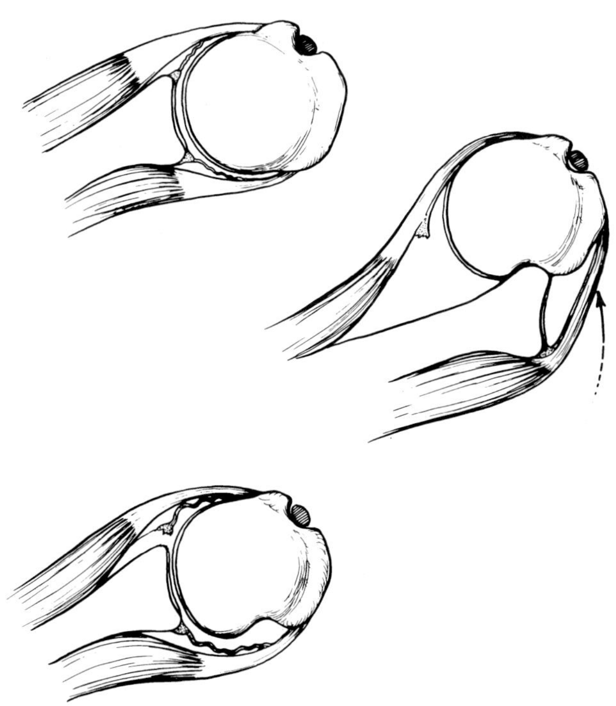

FIG. 23. Anterior glenohumeral dislocation results in labral tear with stripping of soft tissue off scapular neck. Impaction of the posterior head on the anterior glenoid produces a Hill-Sachs lesion. (From Warner JP, Caborn DNM. Overview of shoulder instability. *Crit Rev Phys Rehabil Med* 1992;4:145–198, with permission.)

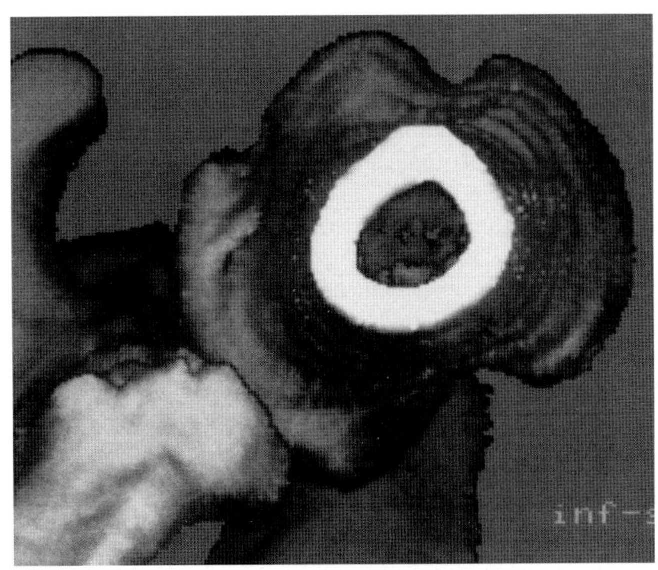

FIG. 25. Three-dimensional scan of patient with huge Hill-Sachs lesion and loss of one-third of glenoid. (From Warner JJP, Schulte KR, Imhoff AB. Current concepts in shoulder instability. *Advances in operative orthopaedics*, vol. 3. St. Louis: Mosby–Year Book, 1995:217–248, with permission.)

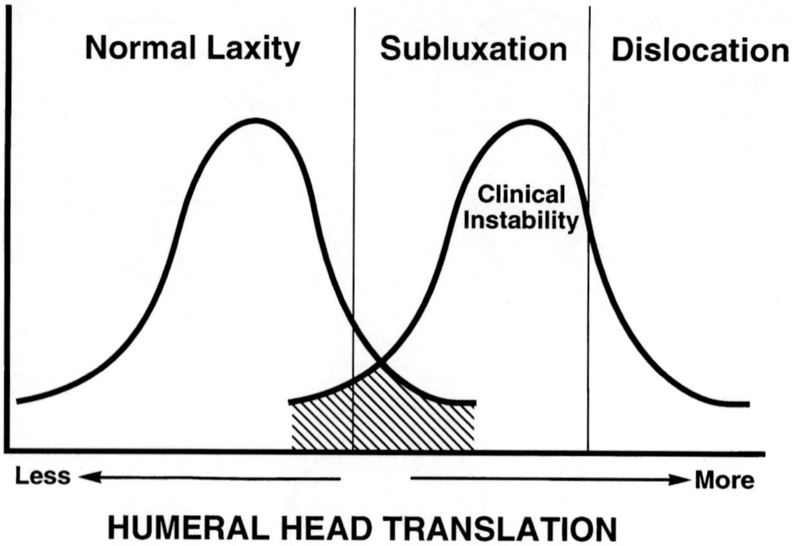

FIG. 26. Graphic representation of range of normal laxity versus instability. See text for explanation.

51,109) claimed that the principal lesion of anterior instability consisted of stripping of capsular soft tissue off the scapula as a result of dislocation. In 1968, Reeves (35) demonstrated capsular rupture by arthrogram in 55% of the anterior dislocations he treated. In 1972, Symeonides (39) observed that 7 of 45 patients undergoing surgery for recurrent instability had rupture of the anterior capsule with labral detachment. In 1991, Johnson (104) reported that of 121 who underwent shoulder arthroscopy after anterior dislocation, 54% had torn glenohumeral ligaments. Both Neer and Foster (48) and Altchek et al. (110) have observed combined Bankart lesions and capsular laxity in patients with anterior inferior multidirectional instability. Recent experimental studies of glenohumeral motion and material properties of glenohumeral ligaments have confirmed that humeral head translation cannot occur to the point of dislocation without plastic deformation or capsular rupture (71,111).

The concept of combined labral detachment and ligament laxity has clinical implications for therapy, as it suggests that some degree of capsular shift must accompany traditional Bankart repairs in order to re-establish normal ligament tension relationships. The laboratory work of Bigliani et al. also implicates lateral capsular avulsion in addition to capsular laxity and labral injury as a contributing mechanism in the pathogenesis of instability (111). Addressing the Bankart lesion alone would fail to take into account the capsular injury and could result in surgical failure.

Excessive Capsular Laxity

As previously discussed, there appears to exist a continuum between normal and pathologic laxity (instability) of the shoulder (114,115,153,156,158). Emery (164) has shown that normal adolescents have a large degree of inherent hyperlaxity of the shoulder; O'Driscoll (220) has demonstrated a high incidence of subsequent instability in contralateral shoulders in individuals having surgery for shoulder instability. Although it is unclear as to whether laxity of the glenohumeral joint predisposes to clinical instability, there is probably an overlap between normal and abnormal populations (Fig. 26). We believe that pathologic capsular laxity may be either congenital or acquired from cumulative microtrauma, such as in the case of an adolescent swimmer performing thousands of strokes during workouts, although we acknowledge that no definitive proof exists to date.

Rotator Cuff and Subscapularis Injury

The association of rotator cuff tear with anterior shoulder dislocation was first reported by Joessel in 1880 (23). Subsequently, Neviaser et al. (146) and others (17,18,27,39,139, 228) have observed disruption of the supra- and infraspinatus, as well as the subscapularis in association with anterior dislocation. Whereas greater tuberosity avulsion fracture has been associated with a low rate of recurrent instability following initial dislocation, subscapularis tears are associated with a greater risk of recurrent instability (29). Moseley and Overgaard (29) and DePalma et al. (12) observed subscapularis laxity or rupture in 25 and 38 cases, respectively. Hauser (17) and Symeonides (39) also found subscapularis injury in association with anterior instability, although Gerber and Krushell (140) have reported isolated subscapularis tears in the absence of instability. In our experience, significant subscapularis injury only occasionally accompanies anterior dislocation in patients older than 50 years of age and may, in these cases, be associated with recurrence of instability.

OVERALL CONCEPT OF STABILITY/ INSTABILITY

Successful management of shoulder instability requires a thorough knowledge of all factors responsible for stability

58. Saha AK. Mechanics of elevation of the glenohumeral joint: its application in rehabilitation of flail shoulder in upper brachial plexus injuries and poliomyelitis and in replacement of the upper humerus by prosthesis. *Acta Orthop Scand* 1973;44:668–678.
59. Turkel SJ, Panio MW, Marshall JL, Girgis FG. Stabilizing mechanisms preventing anterior dislocation of the glenohumeral joint. *J Bone Joint Surg [Am]* 1981;63A:1208–1217.
60. Browne AO, Hoffmeyer P, An KN, Morrey BF. The influence of atmospheric pressure on shoulder stability. *Orthop Trans* 1990;14: 259.
61. Gibb TD, Sidles JA, Harryman DT II, Matsen FA III. The effect of capsular venting on glenohumeral laxity. *Clin Orthop* 1991;268:120–127.
62. Helmig P, Sojberg JO, Sneppen O, et al. Glenohumeral movement patterns after puncture of the joint capsule: an experimental study. *J Shoulder Elbow Surg* 1993;2:209–215.
63. Kumar VP, Balasubramaniam P. The role of atmospheric pressure in stabilising the shoulder: an experimental study. *J Bone Joint Surg [Br]* 1985;67B:719–721.
64. Warner JJP, Deng X, Warren RF, Torzilli PA. Superior-inferior translation of the intact and vented glenohumeral joint. *J Shoulder Elbow Surg* 1993;2:99–105.
65. Simkin PA. Structure and function of joints. In: Schumacher HR, ed. *Primer in the rheumatic diseases,* 9th ed. Atlanta Arthritis Foundation, 1988.
66. Galinat BJ, Howell SM. The containment mechanism: the primary stabilizer of the glenohumeral joint. *Orthop Trans* 1987;11:458.
67. Howell SM, Galinat BJ, Renzi AJ, Marone PJ. Normal and abnormal mechanics of the glenohumeral joint in the horizontal plane. *J Bone Joint Surg [Am]* 1988;70A:227–232.
68. Howell SM, Galinat BJ. The glenoid-labral socket: a constrained articular surface. *Clin Orthop* 1989;243:122–125.
69. Howell SM, Kraft TA. The role of the supraspinatus and infraspinatus muscles in glenohumeral kinematics of anterior shoulder instability. *Clin Orthop* 1991;263:128–134.
70. Lippitt SB, Vanderhooft JE, Harris SL, Sidles JA, Harryman DT II, Matsen FA III. Glenohumeral stability from concavity-compression: a quantitative analysis. *J Shoulder Elbow Surg* 1993;2:27–35.
71. Speer KP, Deng X, Borrero S, Torzilli PA, Altchek DA, Warren RF. Biomechanical evaluation of a simulated Bankart lesion. *J Bone Joint Surg [Am]* 1994;76A:1819–1826.
72. Vahey J, Lippitt SB, Matsen FA III. Scapulohumeral balance: the limits of angular stability provided by glenoid geometry. Presented at the Annual Meeting of the American Academy of Orthopaedic Surgeons, San Francisco, February 1993.
73. Bassett RW, Browne AO, Morrey BF, An KN. Glenohumeral muscle force and moment mechanics in a position of shoulder instability. *J Biomech* 1990;23:405–415.
74. Blasier RB, Guldberg RE, Tothman ED. Anterior shoulder stability: contributions of rotator cuff forces and the capsular ligaments in a cadaveric model. *J Shoulder Elbow Surg* 1992;1:140–150.
75. Cain PR, Mutschler TA, Fu FH, et al. Anterior stability of the glenohumeral joint: a dynamic model. *Am J Sports Med* 1987;15:144–148.
76. D'Alessandro DF, Jobe FW, Perry J, Glousman RE, Pink M. Dynamic stabilizers of the glenohumeral joint: an anatomic and electromyographic analysis. Presented at the Annual Meeting of the American Shoulder and Elbow Surgeons, New Orleans, February 1990.
77. deLuca CJ, Forrest WJ. Force analysis of individual muscles acting simultaneously on the shoulder joint during isometric abduction. *J Biomech* 1973;6:385.
78. Glousman R, Jobe F, Tibone J, et al. Dynamic electromyographic analysis of the throwing shoulder with glenohumeral instability. *J Bone Joint Surg [Am]* 1988;70A:220–226.
79. Gowan ID, Jobe FW, Tibone JE, Perry J, Moynes DR. A comparative electromyographic analysis of the shoulder during pitching: professional versus amateur pitchers. *Am J Sports Med* 1987;15:586–590.
80. Jobe FW, Tibone JE, Perry J, Moynes D. An EMG analysis of the shoulder in throwing and pitching: a preliminary report. *Am J Sports Med* 1983;11:3–5.
81. Kronberg M, Nemeth G, Brostrom LA. Muscle activity and coordination in the normal shoulder: an electromyographic study. *Clin Orthop* 1990;257:76–85.
82. Kronberg M, Brostrom LA, Nemeth G. Difference in shoulder muscle activity between patients with generalized joint laxity and normal controls. *Clin Orthop* 1991;269:181–192.
83. Malicky DM, Blasier RB, Guldberg RE, Borodtin JL, Palmer ML, Soslowsky LJ. Anterior glenohumeral stabilization efficiency in a biomechanical model combining ligamentous and muscular constraints. *Trans Orthop Res Soc* 1993;39:314.
84. McMahon PJ, Jobe FW, Pink MM, Brault JR, Perry J. Comparative electromyographic analysis of shoulder muscles during planar motions: anterior glenohumeral instability versus normal. *J Shoulder Elbow Surg* 1996;5:118–123.
85. Morrey BF, Chao EYS. Recurrent anterior dislocation of the shoulder: clinical and anatomic considerations. In: Black J, Dumbleton JH, eds. *Clinical biomechanics: a case history approach.* New York: Churchill Livingstone, 1981:24–46.
86. Moseley BJ, Jobe FW, Perry J, Tibone JE. EMG analysis of the scapular rotator muscles during a baseball rehabilitation program. Presented at the Annual Meeting of the American Shoulder and Elbow Surgeons, New Orleans, February 1990.
87. Nuber GW, Jobe FW, Perry J, Moyes DR, Antonelli D. Fine wire electromyographic analysis of muscles of the shoulder during swimming. *Am J Sports Med* 1986;14:7–11.
88. Altchek DW, Warren RF, Wickiewicz TL, Ortiz G. Arthroscopic labral debridement: a three-year follow-up study. *Am J Sports Med* 1992;20:702–706.
89. Cooper DE, Arnoczky SP, O'Brien SJ, Warren RF, DiCarlo EF. Anatomy, histology, and vascularity of the glenoid labrum: an anatomical study. *J Bone Joint Surg [Am]* 1992;74A:46–52.
90. Hata Y, Nakatsuchi Y, Saitoh S, Husuka M, Uchiyama S. Anatomic study of the glenoid labrum. *J Shoulder Elbow Surg* 1992;1:207–214.
91. Kohn D. The clinical relevance of glenoid labrum lesions. *Arthroscopy* 1987;3:223–230.
92. McKernan DJ, Mutschler TA, Rudert MJ, Luo L, Fu FH, Harner CD. Significance of a partial and full Bankart lesion: a biomechanical comparison. *Trans Orthop Res Soc* 1989;35:231.
93. Pappas AM, Goss TP, Kleinman PK. Symptomatic shoulder instability due to lesions of the glenoid labrum. *Am J Sports Med* 1983;11:279–288.
94. Prodromos CC, Ferry JA, Schiller AL, Zarins B. Histological studies of the glenoid labrum from fetal life to old age. *J Bone Joint Surg [Am]* 1990;72A:1344–1348.
95. Basmajian JV, Bazant FJ. Factors preventing downward dislocation of the adducted shoulder joint: an electromyographic and morphological study. *J Bone Joint Surg [Am]* 1959;41A:1182–1186.
96. Freedman L, Munro RR. Abduction of the arm in the scapular plane: scapular and glenohumeral movements: a roentgenographic study. *J Bone Joint Surg [Am]* 1966;18A:1503.
97. Inman VT, Saunders JB, Abbott LC. Observations on the function of the shoulder joint. *J Bone Joint Surg* 1944;26:1–30.
98. Itoi E, Motzkin NE, An K-N, Morrey BF. Scapular inclination and inferior instability of the shoulder. *J Shoulder Elbow Surg* 1992;1: 131–139.
99. Leffert RD, Gumley G. The relationship between dead arm syndrome and thoracic outlet syndrome. *Clin Orthop* 1987;223:20–31.
100. Ozaki J. Glenohumeral movements of the involuntary inferior and multidirectional instability. *Clin Orthop* 1989;238:107–111.
101. Poppen NK, Walker PS. Forces at the glenohumeral joint in abduction. *Clin Orthop* 1978;58:165.
102. Poppen NK, Walker PS. Normal and abnormal motion of the shoulder. *J Bone Joint Surg [Am]* 1976;58A:195–201.
103. Warner JJP, Micheli LJ, Arslanian LE, Kennedy J, Kennedy R. Scapulothoracic motion in normal shoulders and shoulders with glenohumeral instability and impingement syndrome: a study using Moire topographic analysis. *Clin Orthop* 1992;285:191–199.
104. Johnson LL. Diagnostic arthroscopic findings in traumatic anterior dislocation of the shoulder. Presented at the Closed Meeting of the American Shoulder and Elbow Surgeons, Seattle, September 1991.
105. Kinnett JG, Warren RF, Jacobs B. Recurrent dislocation of the shoulder after age fifty. *Clin Orthop* 1980;149:164–168.
106. Matsen FA III, Thomas SC, Rockwood CA Jr. Anterior glenohumeral instability. In: Rockwood CA Jr, Matsen FA III, eds. *The shoulder.* Philadelphia: WB Saunders, 1990:526–622.

107. Rodosky MW, Rudert MJ, Harner CD, Luo L, Fu FH. Significance of a superior labral lesion of the shoulder: a biomechanical study. *Trans Orthop Res Soc* 1990;36:276.
108. Rowe CR, Zarins B. Recurrent transient subluxation of the shoulder. *J Bone Joint Surg* 1981;63A:863–871.
109. Rowe CR, Zarins B, Ciullo JV. Recurrent dislocation of the shoulder after surgical repair: apparent causes of failure and treatment. *J Bone Joint Surg [Am]* 1984;66A:159–168.
110. Altchek DW, Warren RF, Skyhar MJ, Ortiz G. T-plasty modification of the Bankart procedure for multidirectional instability of the anterior and inferior types. *J Bone Joint Surg [Am]* 1991;73A:105–112.
111. Bigliani LU, Pollock RG, Soslowsky LJ, Flatow EL, Pawluk RJ, Mow VC. Tensile properties of the inferior glenohumeral ligament. *J Orthop Res* 1992;10:187–197.
112. Fronek J, Warren RF, Bowen M. Posterior subluxation of the glenohumeral joint. *J Bone Joint Surg [Am]* 1989;71A:205–216.
113. Galinat BJ, Howell SM, Kraft TA. The glenoid-posterior acromion angle: an accurate method of evaluating glenoid version. *Orthop Trans* 1988;12:727.
114. Harryman DT II, Sidles JA, Clark JM, McQuade KJ, Gibhb TD, Matsen FA III. Translation of the humeral head on the glenoid with passive glenohumeral motion. *J Bone Joint Surg [Am]* 1990;72A:1334–1343.
115. Harryman DT II, Sidles JA, Harris SL, Matsen FA III. Laxity of the normal glenohumeral joint: a quantitative in-vivo assessment. *J Shoulder Elbow Surg* 1992;1:66–76.
116. Hawkins RJ, Abrams JS, Schutte J. Multidirectional instability of the shoulder: an approach to diagnosis. *Orthop Trans* 1987;11:246.
117. O'Brien SJ, Schwartz RS, Warren RF, Torzilli PA. Capsular restraints to anterior-posterior motion of the abducted shoulder: a biomechanical study. *J Shoulder Elbow Surg* 1995;4:298–308.
118. O'Connell PW, Nuber GW, Mileski RA, Lautenschlager E. The contribution of the glenohumeral ligaments to anterior stability of the shoulder. *Am J Sports Med* 1990;18:579–589.
119. Ticker JB, Flatow EL, Pawluk RJ, Soslowsky LJ, Hepler MD, Bigliani LU. The inferior glenohumeral ligament: a correlative biomechanical, biochemical, and histological investigation. *Trans Orthop Res Soc* 1993;39:313.
120. Uthoff H, Piscopo M. Anterior capsular redundancy of the shoulder: congenital or traumatic? *J Bone Joint Surg [Br]* 1985;67B:363–366.
121. Warner JJP, Micheli LJ, Arslanian LE, Kennedy D, Kennedy R. Patterns of flexibility, laxity, and strength in normal shoulders and shoulders with instability and impingement. *Am J Sports Med* 1990;18:366–375.
122. Warren RF, Kornblatt IB, Marchand R. Static factors influencing posterior shoulder stability. *Orthop Trans* 1984;8:89.
123. Bestard EA, Schoene HR, Bestard EH. Glenoplasty in the management of recurrent shoulder dislocation. *Contemp Orthop* 1986;12:47–55.
124. Brewer BJ, Wubben RC, Carrera GF. Excessive retroversion of the glenoid cavity: a cause of non-traumatic posterior instability of the shoulder. *J Bone Joint Surg [Am]* 1986;68A:724–730.
125. Kronberg M, Brostrom LA. Humeral head retroversion in patients with unstable humeroscapular joints. *Clin Orthop* 1990;260:207–211.
126. Kronberg M, Brostrom LA, Soderlund V. Retroversion of the humeral head in the normal shoulder and its relationship to the normal range of motion. *Clin Orthop* 1990;253:113–117.
127. Mallon WJ, Brown HR, Vogler JB III, Salutario M. Radiographic and geometric anatomy of the scapula. *Clin Orthop* 1992;277:142–154.
128. Randelli M, Gambrioli PL. Glenohumeral osteometry by computed tomography in normal and unstable shoulders. *Clin Orthop* 1986;208:151–156.
129. Kozlowski K, Colavita N, Morris L, Kittle K. Bilateral glenoid dysplasia: report of 8 cases. *Aust Radiol* 1985;29:174–177.
130. Kozlowski K, Scougall J. Congenital bilateral glenoid hypoplasia: a report of four cases. *Br J Radiol* 1987;60:705–706.
131. Lintner DM, Sebastianelli WJ, Hanks GA, Kalenak A. Glenoid dysplasia: a case report and review of the literature. *Clin Orthop* 1992;283:145–148.
132. McClure JG, Raney RB. Anomalies of the scapula. *Clin Orthop* 1975;110:22–31.
133. Owen R. Bilateral glenoid hypoplasia: report of five cases. *J Bone Joint Surg [Br]* 1953;35B:262.
134. Pettersson H. Bilateral dysplasia of the neck of the scapula and associated anomalies. *Acta Radiol Diagn* 1981;22:81–84
135. Resnick D, Walter RD, Crudale AS. Bilateral dysplasia of the scapular neck. *AJR* 1982;139:387–389.
136. Thomas PS, Reid M, McCurdy A. Pelvis-shoulder dysplasia. *Pediatr Radiol* 1977;5:219.
137. Hawkins RJ, Angelo RL. Glenohumeral osteoarthrosis: a late complication of the Putti-Platt repair. *J Bone Joint Surg [Am]* 1990;72A:1193–1197.
138. Craig EV. The posterior mechanism of acute anterior shoulder dislocations. *Clin Orthop* 1984;190:212–216.
139. Deutsch A, Altchek DW, Schwartz E, Otis JC, Warren RF. Radiologic measurement of superior displacement of the humeral head in impingement syndrome. *J Shoulder Elbow Surg* 1996;5:186–193.
140. Gerber C, Krushell RJ. Isolated rupture of the tendon of the subscapularis muscle: clinical features in 16 cases. *J Bone Joint Surg [Br]* 1991;73B:389–394.
141. Grauer JD, Paulos LE, Smutz WP. Biceps tendon and superior labral injuries. *Arthroscopy* 1992;8:488–497.
142. Hawkins RJ, Bell RH, Hawkins RH, Koppert GJ. Anterior dislocation of the shoulder in the older patient. *Clin Orthop* 1986;206:192–195.
143. Himeno S, Tsumuro H. The role of the rotator cuff as a stabilizing mechanism of the shoulder. In: Baterman JE, Welsch RP, eds. *Surgery of the shoulder.* Philadelphia: Decker, 1989:17–21.
144. Howell SM, Imobersteg AM, Seger DH, Marone PJ. Clarification of the role of the supraspinatus muscle in shoulder function. *J Bone Joint Surg [Am]* 1986;68A:398.
145. Itoi E, Motzkin NE, Morrey BF, An K-N. Stabilizing function of the long head of the biceps in the hanging arm position. *J Shoulder Elbow Surg* 1994;3:135–142.
146. Neviaser RJ, Neviaser TJ, Neviaser JS. Concurrent rupture of the rotator cuff and anterior dislocation of the shoulder in the older patient. *J Bone Joint Surg [Am]* 1988;70A:1308–1311.
147. Rowe CR, Pierce DS, Clark JG. Voluntary dislocation of the shoulder: a preliminary report on a clinical, electromyographic, and psychiatric study of twenty-six patients. *J Bone Joint Surg [Am]* 1973;55A:445–460.
148. Warner JJP, Paletta G, Warren RF. Biplanar roentgenographic evaluation of glenohumeral instability and rotator cuff tears. Presented at the Annual Meeting of the American Academy of Orthopaedic Surgeons, Anaheim, CA, March 1991.
149. Weiner DS, MacNab I. Superior migration of the humeral head: a radiological aid in the diagnosis of tears of the rotator cuff. *J Bone Joint Surg [Br]* 1970;52B:524–527.
150. Bach BR, Warren RF, Fronek J. Disruption of the lateral capsule of the shoulder: a case of recurrent dislocation. *J Bone Joint Surg [Br]* 1988;70B:274–276.
151. Bowen MK, Deng X, Warren RF, et al. The role of the inferior glenohumeral ligament complex in limiting inferior translation of the glenohumeral joint. *Trans Orthop Res Soc* 1992;38:497.
152. Cofield RH, Irving JF. Evaluation and classification of shoulder instability with reference to examination under anesthesia. *Clin Orthop* 1987;223:32–43.
153. Emery RJH, Mullaji AB. Glenohumeral instability in normal adolescents: incidence and significance. *J Bone Joint Surg [Br]* 1991;73B:406–408.
154. Gerber C, Ganz R. Clinical assessment of instability of the shoulder with special reference to anterior and posterior drawer tests. *J Bone Joint Surg [Br]* 1984;66B:551–556.
155. Harryman DT II, Sidles JA, Harris SL, Matsen FA III. The role of the rotator interval capsule in passive motion and stability of the shoulder. *J Bone Joint Surg [Am]* 1992;74A:53–66.
156. Hawkins RJ, Schutte JP, Janda DH, Huckell GH. Translation of the glenohumeral joint with the patient under anesthesia. *J Shoulder Elbow Surg* 1996;5:286–292.
157. Kuboyama M. The role of soft tissue in downward stability of the glenohumeral joint: an experimental study in fresh cadavers. Presented at the Fourth International Shoulder Surgery Conference, New York, October 1989.
158. Lippitt SB, Harris SL, Harryman DT II, Sidles J, Matsen FA III. In

vivo quantification of the laxity of normal and unstable glenohumeral joints. *J Shoulder Elbow Surg* 1994;3:215–233.
159. Warner JJP, Deng X, Warren RF, Torzilli PA. Static capsuloligamentous restraints to superior-inferior translation of the glenohumeral joint. *Am J Sports Med* 1992;20:675–685.
160. Garth WP, Allman FL, Armstrong WS. Occult anterior subluxations of the shoulder in noncontact sports. *Am J Sports Med* 1987;15:579–585.
161. Warren RF. Subluxation of the shoulder in athletes. *Clin Sports Med* 1983;2:339–354.
162. Ovesen J, Nielsen S. Anterior and posterior shoulder instability: a cadaver study. *Acta Orthop Scand* 1986;57:324–327.
163. Cooper RA, Brems JJ. The inferior capsular-shift procedure for multidirectional instability of the shoulder. *J Bone Joint Surg [Am]* 1992;74A:1516–1521.
164. Ferrari DA. Capsular ligaments of the shoulder: anatomical and functional study of the anterior-superior capsule. *Am J Sports Med* 1990;18:20-24.
165. Morgan CD, Rames R, Snyder S. Arthroscopic assessment of anatomic variations of the glenohumeral ligaments associated with recurrent anterior shoulder instability. Presented at the Annual Meeting of the American Shoulder and Elbow Surgeons, Washington, DC, February 1993.
166. O'Brien SJ, Neves MC, Arnoczky SP, et al. The anatomy and histology of the inferior glenohumeral ligament complex of the shoulder. *Am J Sports Med* 1990;18:449–456.
167. O'Brien SJ, Arnoczky SP, Warren RF, Rozburch SR. Developmental anatomy of the shoulder and anatomy of the glenohumeral joint. In: Rockwood CA Jr, Matsen FA III, eds. *The shoulder*. Philadelphia: WB Saunders, 1990:1–33.
168. Rames RD, Moynes CD, Snyder SJ. Anatomic variations of the glenohumeral ligaments. Presented at the Annual Meeting of the American Academy of Orthopaedic Surgeons, Anaheim, CA, March 1991.
169. Warner JJP, Caborn DNM, Berger R, Fu FH, Seel M. Dynamic capsuloligamentous anatomy of the glenohumeral joint. *J Shoulder Elbow Surg* 1993;2:115–133.
170. Warner JJP, Janetta-Alpers C, Miller MD. Correlation of glenohumeral laxity with arthroscopic ligament anatomy. *J Shoulder Elbow Surg* 1994;3:S32.
171. Blasier RB, Carpenter JE, Huston LJ. Shoulder proprioception: effect of joint laxity, joint position, and direction of motion. *Orthop Rev* 1994;23:45–50.
172. Carpenter JE, Blasier RB, Pellizzon GG. The effect of muscular fatigue in shoulder proprioception. *Trans Orthop Res Soc* 1993;39:311.
173. Kocher MS, Lephart SM, Warner JJP, Winge S, Fu FH. Proprioception in patients with shoulder instability. *Trans Orthop Res Soc* 1993;39:312.
174. Lephart SM, Warner JJP, Borsa PA, Fu FH. Proprioception of the shoulder joint in healthy, unstable, and surgically repaired shoulders. *J Shoulder Elbow Surg* 1994;3:371–380.
175. Warner JJP, Lephart S, Fu FH. Role of proprioception in pathoetiology of shoulder instability. *Clin Orthop* 1996;330:35–39.
176. Mow VC, Bigliani LU, Flatow EL, et al. Material properties of the inferior glenohumeral ligament and the glenohumeral articular cartilage. In: Matsen FA III, Fu FH, Hawkins RJ, eds. *The shoulder: a balance of mobility and stability*. Rosemont, IL: American Academy of Orthopaedic Surgeons, 1993;29–67.
177. Burkhead WZ Jr, Rockwood CA Jr. Treatment of instability of the shoulder with an exercise program. *J Bone Joint Surg [Am]* 1992;74A:890–896.
178. Ehgartner K. Is the duration of cast fixation after shoulder dislocation an influence in the frequency of recurrent dislocation? *Arch Orthop Unfallchir* 1977;89:187–190.
179. Hovelius L. Anterior dislocation of the shoulder in teenagers and young adults: five-year prognosis. *J Bone Joint Surg [Am]* 1987;69A:393–399.
180. Simmonet WT, Cofield RH. Prognosis in anterior shoulder dislocation. Presented at the Annual Meeting of the American Orthopaedic Society for Sports Medicine, Homestead, VA, March 1983.
181. Arciero RA, Wheeler JH, Ryan JB, et al. Arthroscopic Bankart repair versus nonoperative treatment for acute, initial anterior shoulder dislocations. *Am J Sports Med* 1994;22:589–594.
182. Ticker JB, Bigliani LU, Soslowsky LJ, Pawluk RJ, Flatow EL, Mow VC. Inferior glenohumeral ligament: geometric and strain rate dependent properties. *J Shoulder Elbow Surg* 1996;5:269–279.
183. Reeves B. Experiments on the tensile strength of the anterior capsular structures of the shoulder in man. *J Bone Joint Surg [Br]* 1968;50B:858–865.
184. Klein AH, Luo L, Harner CD, Fu FH. The Bankart lesion of the shoulder: a biomechanical analysis following repair. *Trans Orthop Res Soc* 1992;38:290.
185. Bowen MK, Deng X, Hannafin JA, Arnoczky SP, Warren RF, Warner JJP, Hashimoto J. An analysis of the patterns of glenohumeral joint contact and their relationship to the glenoid bare area. *Trans Orthop Res Soc* 1992;38:496.
186. Soslowsky LJ, Flatow EL, Bigliani LU, Mow VC. Articular geometry of the glenohumeral joint. *Clin Orthop* 1992;285:181–190.
187. Soslowsky LJ, Flatow EL, Bigliani LU, Pawluk RJ, Ateshian GA, Mow VC. Quantitation of in-situ contact area at the glenohumeral joint: a biomechanical study. *J Orthop Res* 1992;38:524–534.
188. Kelkar R, Newton PM, Armengol J, et al. Three-dimensional kinematics of the glenohumeral joint during abduction in the scapular plane. *Trans Orthop Res Soc* 1993;39:136.
189. Bowen MK, Deng X, Warner JJP, Warren RF, Torzilli PA. Coupled translation: rotation of the glenohumeral joint. Presented at the Annual Meeting of the American Academy of Orthopaedic Surgeons, Washington, DC, February 1992.
190. Muller-Gerbl M, Putz R, Hodapp N, Schuitte E, Wimmer B. Computed tomography-osteoabsorptiometry for assessing the density distribution of subchondral bone as a measure of long-term mechanical adaptation in individual joints. *Skel Radiol* 1989;18:507–512.
191. Thompson WO, Debski RE, Boardman ND III, et al. A biomechanical analysis of rotator cuff deficiency in a biomechanical model. *Am J Sports Med* 1996;24:286–292.
192. Bowen MK, Deng X, Warner JJP, Warren RF, Torzilli PA. The effect of joint compression on stability of the glenohumeral joint. *Trans Orthop Res Soc* 1992;38:289.
193. Blasier RB, Soslowsky LJ, Malicky DM, Guldberg RE, Borodkin J, Palmer ML. Anterior glenohumeral stabilization efficiency in a biomechanical model combining ligamentous and muscular constraints. *J Shoulder Elbow Surg* 1994;3:S23.
194. Ovesen J, Nielsen S. Experimental distal subluxation in the glenohumeral joint. *Arch Orthop Trauma Surg* 1985;104:78–81.
195. Ovesen J, Nielsen S. Posterior instability of the shoulder: a cadaver study. *Acta Orthop Scand* 1986;57:436–439.
196. Terry GC, Hammon D, France P, et al. The stabilizing function of passive shoulder restraints. *Am J Sports Med* 1991;19:26–34.
197. Boardman ND III, Debski RE, Warner JJP, et al. Tensile properties of the superior glenohumeral and coracohumeral ligaments. *J Shoulder Elbow Surg* 1996;5:249–254.
198. Hara H, Ito N, Iwasaki K. Strength of the glenoid labrum and adjacent shoulder capsule. *J Shoulder Elbow Surg* 1996;5:263–268.
199. Kaltsas DS. Comparative study of the properties of the shoulder joint capsule with those of other joint capsules. *Clin Orthop* 1983;173:20–26.
200. Clark JM, Sidles JA, Matsen F III. The relationship of the glenohumeral joint capsule to the rotator cuff. *Clin Orthop* 1990;254:29–34.
201. Clark JM, Harryman DT II. Tendons, ligaments and capsule of the rotator cuff: gross and microscopic anatomy. *J Bone Joint Surg [Am]* 1992;74A:713–725.
202. Neer CS II, Satterlee CC, Dalsey RM, et al. The anatomy and potential effects of contracture of the coracohumeral ligament. *Clin Orthop* 1992;280:182–185.
203. Edelson JG, Taitz C, Grishkan A. The coracohumeral ligament: anatomy of a substantial but neglected structure. *J Bone Joint Surg [Br]* 1991;73B:150–153.
204. Helmig P, Sojberg JO, Kjaersgaard-Andersen P, Nielsen S, Ovesen J. Distal humeral migration as a component of multidirectional shoulder instability: an anatomical study in autopsy specimens. *Clin Orthop* 1990;252:139–143.
205. Cooper DE, O'Brien SJ, Arnoczky SP, Warren RF. The structure and function of the coracohumeral ligament: an anatomic and microscopic study. *J Shoulder Elbow Surg* 1993;2:70–77.
206. Ozaki J, Nakagawa Y, Sakurai G, Tumai S. Recalcitrant chronic adhesive capsulitis of the shoulder: role of contracture of the coracohumeral ligament and rotator interval in pathogenesis and treatment. *J Bone Joint Surg [Am]* 1989;71A:1511–1515.

207. Ovesen J, Sojberg JO. Lesions in different types of anterior glenohumeral dislocation. An experimental study. *Arch Orthop Trauma Surg* 1986;105:216–218.
208. Woo SL-Y, Gomez MA, Seguchi Y, Endo CM, Akeson WH. Measurement of mechanical properties of ligament substance from a bone–ligament–bone preparation. *J Orthop Res* 1983;1:22–29.
209. Woo SL-Y, Newton PO, MacKenna DA, Lyon RM. A comparative evaluation of the mechanical properties of the rabbit medial collateral and anterior cruciate ligaments. *J Biomech* 1992;25:377–386.
210. Jerosch J, Clahsen H, Grosse-Hackmann A, et al. Effects of proprioceptive fibers in the capsule tissue in stabilizing the glenohumeral joint. *Orthop Trans* 1992;16:773.
211. Ovesen J, Sojberg JO. Transposition of the coracohumeral ligament to the humerus in treatment of vertical shoulder joint instability: clinical applicability of experimental technique. *Arch Orthop Trauma Surg* 1987;106:323–326.
212. Motzkin NE, Itoi E, Morrey BF. Contribution of bulk tissues and deltoid to inferior stability of the shoulder. *Trans Orthop Res Soc* 1992;38:494.
213. Itoi E, Newman SR, Kuechle DK, Morrey BF, An K-N. Stabilising function of the biceps in stable and unstable shoulders. *J Bone Joint Surg [Br]* 1993;75B:546–550.
214. Itoi E, Newman SR, Kuechle DK, Morrey BF, An K-N. Dynamic anterior stabilisers of the shoulder with the arm in abduction. *J Bone Joint Surg [Br]* 1994;76B:834–836.
215. Pagnani MJ, Deng X, Warren RF, Torzilli PA, O'Brien SJ. Role of the long head of the biceps brachii in glenohumeral stability: a biomechanical study in cadavera. *J Shoulder Elbow Surg* 1996;5:255–262.
216. Rodosky MW, Harner CD, Fu FH. The role of the long head of the biceps muscle and superior glenoid labrum in anterior stability of the shoulder. *Am J Sports Med* 1994;22:121–130.
217. Warner JJP, McMahon PJ. The role of the long head of the biceps brachii in superior stability of the glenohumeral joint. *J Bone Joint Surg [Am]* 1995;77A:366–372.
218. Bearn JG. An electromyographic study of the trapezius, deltoid, pectoralis major, biceps, and triceps muscles during static loading of the upper limb. *Anat Rec* 1961;140:103–107.
219. Pavlov H, Warren RF, Weiss CB Jr, Dines D. The roentgenographic evaluation of anterior shoulder instability. *Clin Orthop* 1985;194:153–158.
220. O'Driscoll SW, Evans DC. Contralateral shoulder instability following anterior repair: an epidemiological investigation. *J Bone Joint Surg [Br]* 1991;73B:941–946.
221. Pettersson G. Rupture of the tendon aponeurosis of the shoulder joint in antero-inferior dislocation: a study on the origin and occurrence of the ruptures. *Acta Chir Scand* 1942;77(Suppl):1–187.
222. Janevic J, Craig EV, Hsu KC, Engebretisen L, Lew WD. Biomechanics of repair of glenohumeral instability. *Trans Orthop Res Soc* 1992;38:495.
223. MacDonald PB, Hawkins RJ, Fowler PJ, Miniaci A. Release of the subscapularis for internal rotation contracture and pain after anterior repair for recurrent anterior dislocation of the shoulder. *J Bone Joint Surg [Am]* 1992;74A:734–737.

The Unstable Shoulder,
edited by R.F. Warren, E.V. Craig, and D.W. Altchek.
Lippincott–Raven Publishers, Philadelphia © 1999.

CHAPTER 4

Instability Mechanisms in the Throwing Athlete

James R. Andrews and Leslie J. Bisson

The act of throwing produces tremendous demands on the glenohumeral joint. It requires extremes of motion, coordinated movement, and synchronized firing of multiple muscle groups, all at high velocity. The supranormal ranges of motion necessary for the throw, as well as the extraordinary number of times the athlete throws in practice and in games, tend to stress repetitively, and ultimately lengthen, the glenohumeral ligaments, specifically the anterior inferior band. Attenuation of these static stabilizers leaves the thrower dependent on the dynamic stabilizers to prevent instability. Excessive dependence on the dynamic stabilizers such as the rotator cuff leaves the athlete susceptible to glenohumeral instability if these dynamic stabilizers are fatigued or injured.

To date, research has focused primarily on instability mechanisms and treatment in the baseball pitcher; the bulk of the material reviewed in this chapter involves this athlete. Although much of the knowledge gained from the study of the baseball pitcher can be applied to athletes involved in other overhead sports, certain differences are peculiar to each sport. These are addressed separately at the end of this discussion.

PATHOGENIC MECHANISM IN OVERHEAD ATHLETES

Before beginning a discussion of the various causes of instability in the throwing and overhead athlete, it is first necessary to understand the sequence of events that take place during an overhand throw. Although a throw occurs as a continuous motion, it has been divided into various phases by several investigators to simplify analysis and description (1–6). This chapter describes the six phases that occur in an overhand throw: windup, stride, arm cocking, arm acceleration, arm deceleration, and follow-through (1, 3,6) (Fig. 1). The baseball throw is used as a model, and the differences pertaining to other sports are described in the sections on each sport.

The *windup* (Fig. 1A, B) begins the throw, and the objective is to gently place the thrower in an appropriate starting position. It begins with the first motion of the thrower and ends when the ball leaves the gloved hand (or when there is maximum lift of the "lead" leg—the leg opposite the throwing arm). This phase is characterized by low joint loads, minimal torques, and little electromyographic (EMG) activity in the throwing arm.

The *stride* phase (Fig. 1C–F) generates linear velocity toward the target by driving the lead foot in the direction of the throw (7). This phase begins when the lead foot initiates motion toward the target and the arm starts to separate, and it ends when the lead foot contacts the ground. Both shoulders abduct during this phase, and the throwing shoulder externally rotates. At foot contact, the throwing shoulder is abducted and externally rotated, and the elbow is flexed. The magnitudes of stride length, elbow flexion, and shoulder external rotation vary among different sports, but shoulder abduction usually approximates 90 degrees (1, 2,8–11). During this phase, the deltoid and supraspinatous abduct the arm; the rotator cuff positions the humeral head within the glenoid fossa; and the scapular rotators (specifically the trapezius and serratus anterior) position the glenoid for the humeral head (12).

Arm cocking begins with lead foot contact and ends with maximal external rotation of the shoulder (Fig. 1F–H; see also Fig. 4). Arm cocking produces a tense, forceful unit that is ready for accelerated release. The shoulder remains abducted approximately 90 degrees in the coronal plane

J. R. Andrews: Department of Orthopaedic Surgery, University of Alabama at Birmingham; and American Sports Medicine Institute, Birmingham, Alabama 35205.

L. J. Bisson: Northtown Orthopaedics, East Amherst, New York 14051.

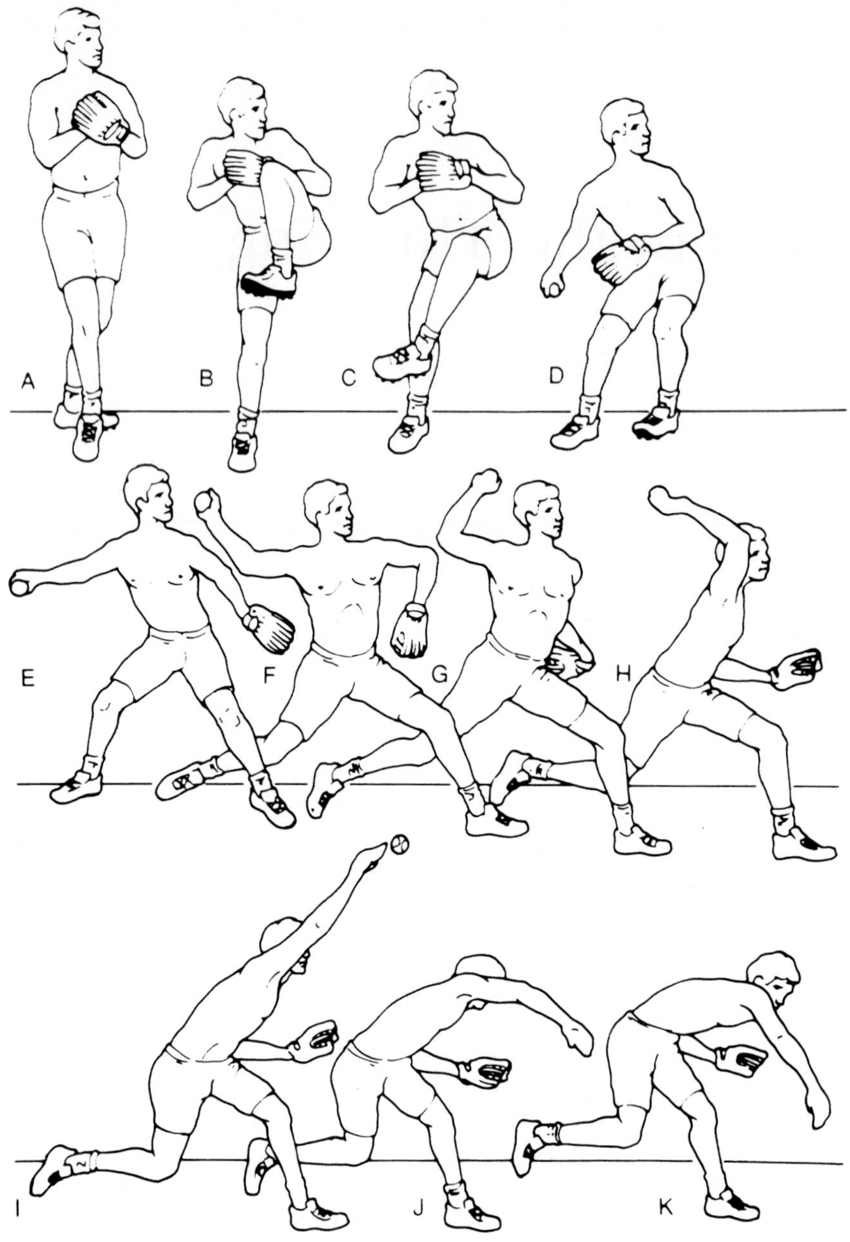

FIG. 1. A–K: Sequence of positions in throwing. (From Dillman CJ, Fleisig GS, Andrews JR. Mechanics of throwing. In: Hawkins RJ, Misamore GW, eds. *Shoulder injuries in the athlete.* New York: Churchill Livingstone, 1996:23–30, with permission.)

throughout this phase (1). In the horizontal plane, the shoulder moves from 30 degrees of abduction (at foot contact) to 15 degrees of adduction (at maximum external rotation) (1). At the end of the cocking phase the shoulder is externally rotated between 150 and 180 degrees (measured with respect to the trunk) (1,2,6,8,9) (Fig. 2). The scapular stabilizing muscles (levator scapulae, serratus anterior, trapezius, rhomboids, and pectoralis minor) act during this phase to position the glenoid under the humeral head. The muscles of the rotator cuff fire to control glenohumeral distraction, and the internal rotators (pectoralis major, latissimus dorsi, anterior deltoid, teres major, and subscapularis) fire eccentrically to decelerate external rotation (2,3,13).

The *arm acceleration* phase (Fig. 1H, I) occurs from maximal external shoulder rotation to ball release. The energy stored during the previous phases is now transferred to the ball. The shoulder once again remains abducted approximately 90 degrees throughout this phase, implying that this is a preferred position for shoulder function (7). In the horizontal plane the shoulder moves from 15 degrees of adduction to neutral (1). External rotation changes from 180 degrees to 90 degrees at a rate of 6,000 to 7,500 degrees per second (1,2,8,14,15) (Fig. 3). The internal rotators of the shoulder concentrically contract during this time, helping to produce this high internal rotation velocity (12, 13,16,17). The rotator cuff muscles and scapular stabilizers are also active during acceleration (13). The supraspinatus and teres minor show approximately 50% of the EMG activity created during a manual maximum test, while infraspinatus activity is approximately 30% (13).

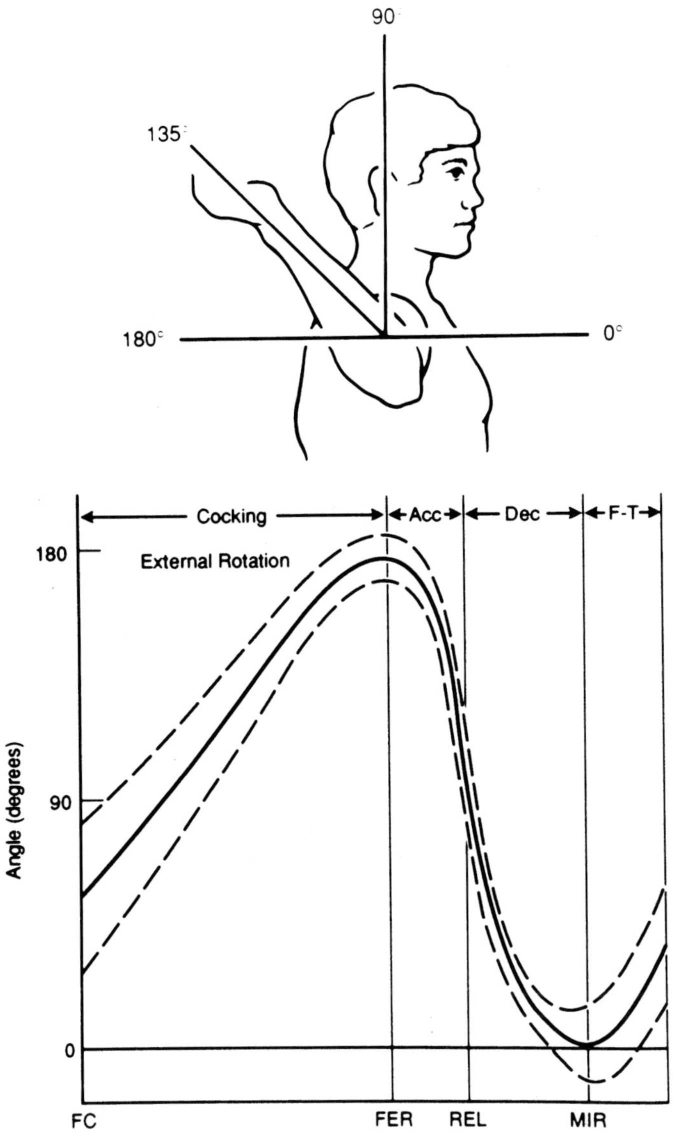

FIG. 2. External and internal rotation of the arm about the shoulder in throwing. *Solid line*, average angular displacement for 29 highly skilled subjects throwing at an average velocity of 85 mph. *Dotted line*, ± 1 SD. (From Dillman CJ, Fleisig GS, Andrews JR. Mechanics of throwing. In: Hawkins RJ, Misamore GW, eds. *Shoulder injuries in the athlete*. New York: Churchill Livingstone, 1996:23–30, with permission.)

Arm deceleration takes place from the moment of ball release to the point of maximum internal rotation of the shoulder (Fig. 1I, J; see also Fig. 5). Large compressive forces are necessary to prevent distraction of the shoulder joint, as the arm is literally thrown toward the target. The shoulder remains abducted about 90 to 100 degrees in the coronal plane, and moves from neutral to 35 degrees of adduction in the horizontal plane. The shoulder internally rotates from 90 degrees of external rotation at ball release to 0 degrees of external rotation at the end of deceleration. It is thought that a long arc of deceleration reduces the potential for injury (18). Eccentric contraction of the infraspinatus, supraspinatus, teres major and minor, latissimus dorsi, and posterior deltoid produce a posterior force to resist anterior humeral translation (12,13,19,20). Superior humeral translation and shoulder abduction are resisted by the teres major, latissimus dorsi, and posterior deltoid (3).

The final phase in the overhead throw is the *follow-through* phase (Fig. 1K), which starts with maximal internal rotation of the shoulder and ends when the throwing arm finishes its movement across the body and the athlete is in a balanced position. The body moves forward with the arm during this phase to decrease the distraction force at the glenohumeral joint. The shoulder adducts slightly in the coronal plane during this phase (about 10 degrees) and continues adducting in the horizontal plane to end at about 60 degrees. The posterior shoulder muscles continue to be active, decelerating the horizontally adducting arm, and the middle trapezius and rhomboids eccentrically act to slow scapular protraction (13).

Anterior Instability

Glenohumeral *laxity* is defined by the amount that the humeral head can be passively translated on the glenoid (21) and exhibits a considerable amount of variation, both between individuals and between the dominant and nondominant arm of a given thrower. Glenohumeral *instability* is a clinical condition in which excessive humeral translation on the glenoid results in symptoms (21).

As can be seen from the discussion on throwing mechanics, the throwing motion requires supranormal glenohumeral external rotation during the cocking and early acceleration phases. External rotation to such a degree is necessary in order to generate the hand velocity required for the throw. The anterior band of the inferior glenohumeral ligament is the primary static restraint to anterior translation when the shoulder is abducted 90 degrees (22), and a substantial amount of plastic deformation can occur in this ligament complex before failure (23). As the thrower repeatedly assumes a position of hyper-external rotation at 90 degrees of abduction during practice and in games, it is an inevitable consequence that the static stabilizers of the glenohumeral joint that serve to resist anterior and inferior translation (i.e., the anterior band of the inferior glenohumeral ligament) will become chronically attenuated. Chronic attenuation of the static stabilizers is one reason high-level throwers exhibit excessive translation of the humeral head on the glenoid when compared to nonathletes, and such laxity must be exhibited if the player is to perform high-performance throwing activities. The relative loss of contribution to stability resulting from attenuation of the static stabilizers necessitates an increased contribution by the dynamic stabilizers such as the rotator cuff. Symptom-free throwing in the face of excessive laxity of the static stabilizers is possible due to dynamic control of shoulder stability by the rotator cuff. Rotator cuff contraction on both sides of the joint supplements the static restraints, and to-

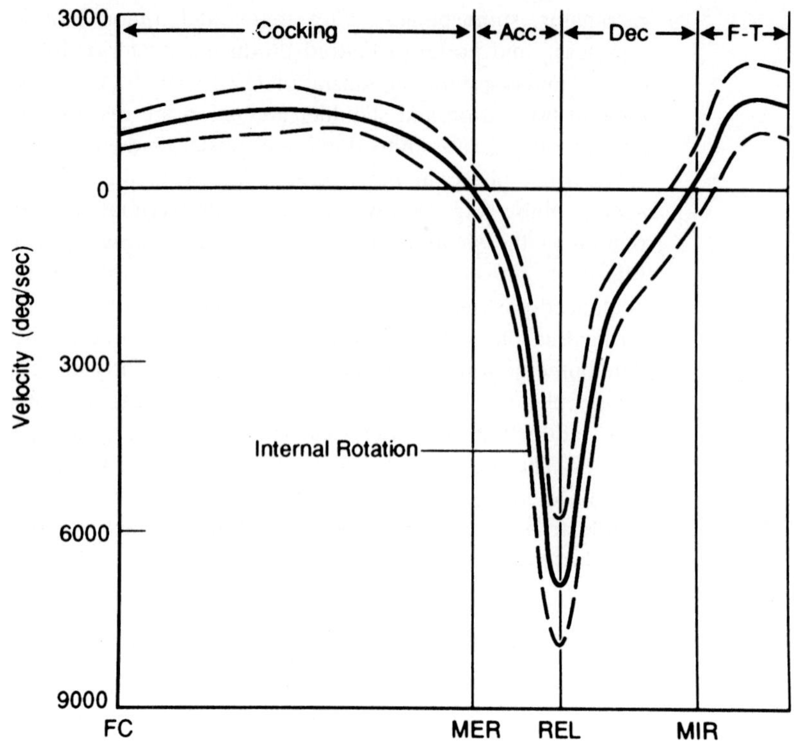

FIG. 3. Average angular velocity for internal and external rotation of arm about shoulder in throwing. Based on 29 highly skilled subjects throwing an average speed of 85 mph. (From Dillman CJ, Fleisig GS, Andrews JR. Mechanics of throwing. In: Hawkins RJ, Misamore GW, eds. *Shoulder injuries in the athlete.* New York: Churchill Livingstone, 1996:23–30, with permission.)

gether the static and dynamic restraints provide sufficient stability. The increased dependence of throwers on dynamic stabilizers predisposes them to overuse musculotendinous injuries to the rotator cuff. Instability occurs when an alteration in dynamic stability renders the rotator cuff muscles unable to control the humeral head motion within the glenoid during the throwing motion. Failure of the dynamic stabilizers may occur as a result of injury, overuse, or pain.

Avulsion

The anterior band of the inferior glenohumeral ligament is the primary restraint to anterior translation of the humeral head on the glenoid with the arm in 90 degrees of abduction (22). Traumatic avulsion of the origin of this ligament from the anterior glenoid produces the Bankhart lesion, and this commonly results in recurrent anterior instability. Avulsion of the glenohumeral ligaments from the humeral insertion (the HAGL lesion) occurs less commonly, but it also leads to recurrent instability. Mid-substance tears of the ligament are least frequent, but lead to a similar clinical situation. These lesions are usually caused by a single discrete episode of trauma rather than repetitive overuse and are not a primary mechanism of instability in overhead athletes unless they happened to have sustained a single traumatic episode as a result of their sport.

A more frequent type of avulsion injury in the thrower or overhead athlete involves the biceps attachment at the superior aspect of the glenoid, referred to as a SLAP lesion (for superior labral anterior and posterior to the biceps tendon). During the deceleration and follow-through phases of throwing, the biceps acts at the elbow to slow arm extension. The forces generated in the biceps tendon during this activity are transmitted across the glenohumeral joint to the biceps anchor and an avulsion tear of the biceps/labrum complex can result (24). Snyder et al. (25) have classified SLAP lesions into four types: type I, labral fraying with no detachment; type II, detachment of the superior labrum at the biceps anchor; type III, a bucket-handle tear of the labrum with an intact biceps anchor; and type IV, a tear similar to type III, but extending into the biceps tendon.

Other types of labral tears are a result of abnormal translations of the humeral head on the glenoid. During the phases of throwing, the humeral head moves from anterior to posterior on the glenoid, and large compressive, shear, and distractive forces are generated (Figs. 4 and 5). Failure of the static and dynamic stabilizers to control these humeral head translations can lead to degenerative tearing of the labrum, and these tears may actually reflect a primary instability of the glenohumeral joint (26). It is therefore mandatory to evaluate the shoulder for an underlying instability when a labral tear is present.

Posterior Traction

The deceleration phase of the throw is the most violent of the phases, and requires large contractions of the posterior shoulder muscles in order to resist distraction of the glenohumeral joint, as well as internal rotation and horizontal adduction. The compressive forces necessary to re-

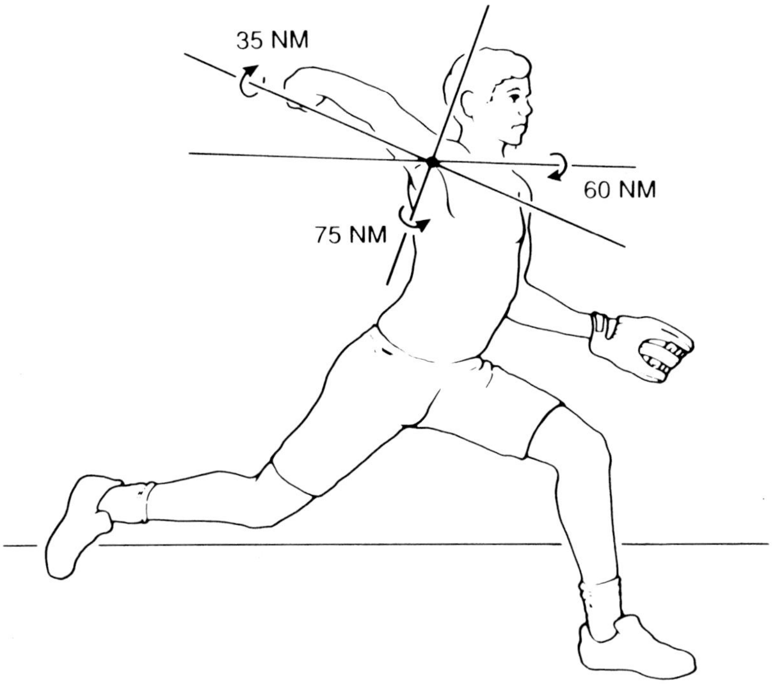

FIG. 4. Average maximum resultant torques acting about the shoulder as the arm is approaching maximal external rotation. Based on 29 highly skilled throwers. 60 nm, internal rotation torque; 75 nm, horizontal adduction torque; 35 nm, shoulder abduction torque. (From Dillman CJ, Fleisig GS, Andrews JR. Mechanics of throwing. In: Hawkins RJ, Misamore GW, eds. *Shoulder injuries in the athlete.* New York: Churchill Livingstone, 1996:23–30, with permission.)

sist glenohumeral distraction can approach body weight (3). A large posterior shear force is required in order to prevent excessive anterior humeral translation, and a horizontal abduction torque slows the horizontally adducting arm. The significant forces generated during this phase control the arm following ball release, and may cause the posterior rotator cuff muscles to fail under tension. This may be one mechanism for the production of undersurface tears of the rotator cuff. An imbalance between strength of the anterior and posterior muscles, with the posterior muscles being relatively weaker, may exacerbate the problem.

The tension applied to the posterior cuff muscles during deceleration is also transmitted to the posterior capsule, and may lead to posterior capsulitis and posterior capsular laxity. Warren et al. (27) have described the circle concept of shoulder instability, whereby capsular laxity is required both anteriorly and posteriorly in order to result in instability (Fig. 6). The posterior capsular laxity produced dur-

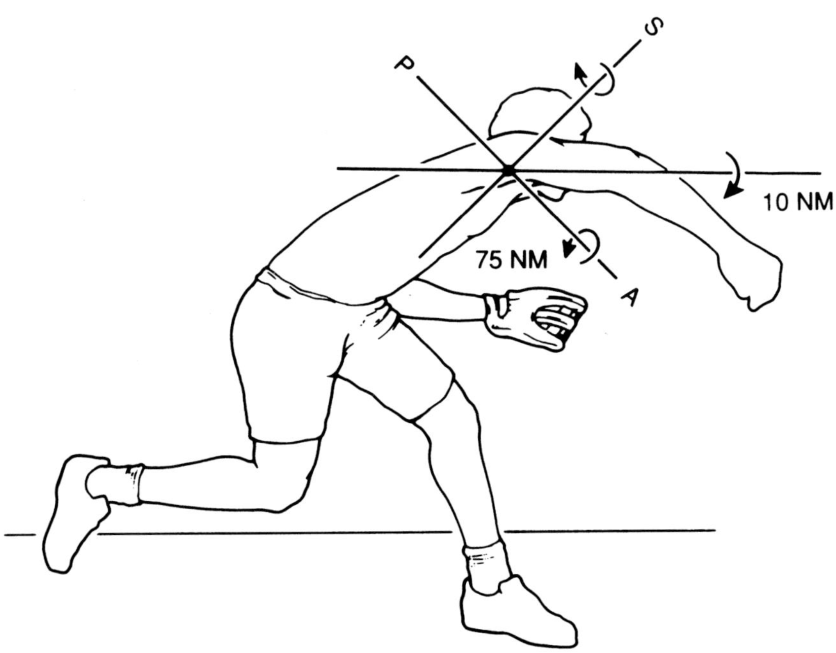

FIG. 5. Average (n = 29) maximum resultant torques occurring during the arm deceleration phase of throwing. 75 nm, shoulder adduction torque; 80 nm, horizontal abduction torque; 10 nm, internal rotation torque. (From Dillman CJ, Fleisig GS, Andrews JR. Mechanics of throwing. In: Hawkins RJ, Misamore GW, eds. *Shoulder injuries in the athlete.* New York: Churchill Livingstone, 1996:23–30, with permission.)

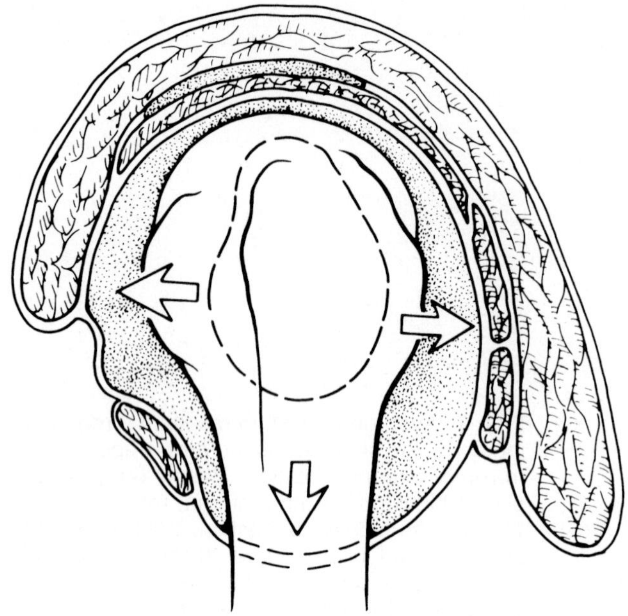

FIG. 6. Circle concept of shoulder instability. (From Hawkins RJ, Misamore GW. Overview of glenohumeral instability. In: Hawkins RJ, Misamore GW, eds. *Shoulder injuries in the athlete.* New York: Churchill Livingstone, 1996:137, with permission.)

ing repeated deceleration may therefore contribute to anterior instability.

Rotator Cuff Pathology

Because of the chronic attenuation of the static stabilizers with repeated overhead activity in high-level athletes, increased importance is placed on the dynamic stabilizers, such as the rotator cuff. Action of the rotator cuff is necessary to compress the humeral head into the glenoid fossa, and it is this compression that provides stability during many overhead athletic activities. The high demands placed on the rotator cuff during these activities can result in progressive muscle fatigue, overload, inflammation, and ultimately tendon failure.

The site of rotator cuff tendonitis in the thrower commonly involves the undersurface of the posterior half of the supraspinatus and the superior half of the infraspinatous (28). This injury is caused by excessive tensile forces generated in the cuff muscles as they eccentrically contract in order to resist shoulder distraction, internal rotation, and horizontal adduction during arm deceleration (3,13).

An underlying glenohumeral instability may also contribute to rotator cuff injury. Any component of glenohumeral instability which allows excessive anterior translation of the humerus during the throwing motion can cause impingement of the undersurface of the posterior rotator cuff muscles against the posterior surface of the glenoid, the so-called ''internal impingement'' lesion (29). Repeated internal impingement, attributable to either abnormal capsular laxity, muscle weakness, or fatigue, may be another cause of undersurface rotator cuff fraying and posterior labral tears.

External compression of the rotator cuff against the undersurface of the acromion can also result in rotator cuff and bicipital tendinitis. This may be a primary pathology in the presence of a hooked acromion, os acromionale, or degenerative acromial spurs, or it may occur in the presence of poor throwing mechanics. During the deceleration phase of throwing, a substantial adduction torque and inferior force are produced at the shoulder (3). Failure to generate sufficient forces and torques can cause superior translation of the humerus. Because the arm is horizontally adducted, internally rotated, and abducted during the deceleration phase, superior translation leads to repeated abrasion of the rotator cuff muscles and biceps tendon against the inferior acromion and coracoacromial ligament.

Scapula Versus Glenohumeral Joint

The scapula is the proximal base supporting the upper extremity, and plays an important role in the overhead athlete. Coordinated scapular motion allows maintenance of a constant length-tension relationship for optimum rotator cuff muscle function during the overhead activity (30). The stability afforded by the large periscapular muscles allows the deltoid and rotator cuff muscles to exert their forces on the humerus, rather than on the scapula.

The muscles controlling the scapula can be divided into elevators, depressors, protractors, retractors, upward rotators, and downward rotators. Protractors move the scapula lateral and anterior on the thorax, while retractors move the scapula toward the vertebral column. Upward rotation involves lateral and forward motion of the inferior angle of the scapula, thus orienting the glenoid upward, and downward rotation occurs in the opposite direction. Elevation of the scapula is accomplished by contraction of the upper trapezius, levator scapulae, and rhomboideus minor and major. Depression is through action of the latissimus dorsi, lower trapezius, lower serratus anterior, and pectoralis minor. Protractors include the serratus anterior and the pectoralis minor and major, and retractors include the trapezius (especially the middle part) and rhomboideus minor and major. Upward scapular rotation is initiated by the middle portion of the trapezius, and the serratus anterior pulls the inferior angle forward at 45 degrees of abduction. The upper trapezius assists by elevating the lateral scapula while the lower trapezius depresses the base of the scapular spine. Downward rotation is accomplished by elevation of the medial scapula via the levator scapulae and rhomboids, while the pectoralis minor, lower pectoralis major, and latissimus dorsi depress the lateral scapula. Normal arm elevation involves upward scapular rotation of 60 degrees, 15 cm of lateral gliding, and elevation of 10 to 12 cm (31).

Several investigators have demonstrated the importance of the scapular muscles in controlling forces and providing stability at the glenohumeral joint during shoulder motion (32–34). During the windup and cocking phases of throwing, the trapezius and rhomboids maximally retract the scapula. This may act to pre-tension the anterior muscles, allowing full release of the stored energy during acceleration and follow-through. Full retraction is also required to perform swimming strokes such as the crawl with maximum effectiveness. Inability to achieve full retraction can cause an increase in stress on the structures resisting anterior humeral translation due to ''antetilting'' of the glenoid (33). Upward scapular rotation takes place during the cocking phase of the throw, and occurs via the action of the serratus anterior and upper and middle trapezius. This rotates the acromion superiorly, preventing the humerus from impinging on the undersurface of the acromion. Scapular protraction and downward rotation take place during the acceleration phase, and result from concentric contraction of the serratus anterior and pectoralis major and minor. The rhomboids contract eccentrically during this phase to stabilize the medial border of the scapula during acceleration (13). The scapula follows the humeral head and arm during acceleration and follow-through, providing a stable joint and protecting the capsule and rotator cuff from tensile injury (33). The large scapular stabilizing muscles also help dissipate the forces on the upper extremity by contracting eccentrically during the follow-through phase of the throw (33,34).

Fatigability Relationships to Training

It can be seen that the act of throwing requires a precise synchronization of activity between the muscles controlling the scapula and those controlling the humerus. This precise firing pattern may be altered secondary to poor mechanics, fatigue of certain muscles, or injury to one component of the kinetic chain. Injuries are often attributed to overuse, which may be associated with fatigue. As a player tires and physiologic limits are reached, an alteration in mechanics may be used to compensate. Fatigue is believed to cause altered arm position during arm cocking and arm acceleration. This change in pitching mechanics may lead to changes in stresses on the body. Chen et al. (35) have shown that fatigue of the rotator cuff–deltoid complex results in altered humeral translation with abduction in normal volunteers. Loss of the centering ability of the rotator cuff as a result of fatigue may lead to abnormal glenohumeral translation and subsequent injury.

Poor mechanics are believed to increase stress on the shoulder (as well as the elbow) and are implicated in injury patterns. Four kinematic parameters have been correlated with increased shoulder force (36): placement of the lead foot toward the open side, pointing of the lead toe toward the open side, and increased or decreased shoulder rotation at the moment of lead foot contact. Delayed external rotation of the shoulder was associated with an increased compressive force, while early external rotation was associated with an increased anterior force at the glenohumeral joint. It should be noted, however, that the increases in load from any one of these mechanisms was small. The risk of injury may therefore be increased when several of these improper mechanisms are in effect.

Kinetic Chain

The principle of the kinetic chain is that energy and momentum are transferred sequentially through adjoining body segments via coordinated motion, resulting in maximum transfer to the terminal segment (37–39). In the activity of throwing, the kinetic chain is comprised of the legs and hips, trunk, shoulder, upper arm, forearm, and hand, with the ball serving as the terminal segment (40–43). Use of all of the components of the kinetic chain allows the thrower to attain maximum performance without causing undue overload of the shoulder and elbow. Conversely, failure or fatigue of one or more components of the kinetic chain places increased demands on the remainder of the chain, increasing the potential for injury.

Role of Training and Conditioning in Prevention

Clearly, all components of the kinetic chain must be kept working, to lessen the risk of overuse injuries caused by fatigue of one portion of the chain. The use of a conditioning program that focuses on increasing the strength and endurance of each component of the kinetic chain, as well as drills designed to enhance the coordinated transfer of energy from one part of the chain to the next, would be expected to result in a decrease in the number of injuries sustained to the terminal segments of the chain (i.e., the wrist, shoulder, and elbow), where comparative strength is weakest and energy transfer is highest.

Although single joint exercises done using relatively heavy resistance over limited ranges of motion are useful during certain stages of rehabilitation, exercises performed at high speed involving multiple joints moving in multiple directions (e.g., rubber tubing exercises and plyometrics) should be emphasized in the thrower's exercise program. The regimen should also emphasize eccentric forms of conditioning, as this is the predominant form of muscle activity during throwing.

SPORTS-SPECIFIC MECHANISMS

Baseball Thrower

The preceding discussion has focused primarily on the mechanisms of instability, using the baseball thrower as a model, but several important points are worth repeating. The act of pitching a baseball requires extreme external rotation of the shoulder with the arm abducted 90 degrees.

Angular velocities at the shoulder during acceleration can exceed 7,000 degrees per second. Anterior translation forces on the glenohumeral joint can reach one-half body weight, and distractive forces can approach body weight. In the high-level baseball thrower, the static stabilizers of the glenohumeral joint will exhibit chronic laxity as a result of the repetitive stresses placed on them by the throwing activity, and the thrower is therefore excessively dependent on the action of the dynamic stabilizers to provide a stable joint. The glenohumeral laxity that allows a player to throw a baseball greater than 90 mph places him in a position susceptible to instability if optimum function of the rotator cuff is interrupted. This should be contrasted with the non-athlete, who does not exhibit symptoms of instability in the face of pathology of the rotator cuff. Breakdown of the dynamic stabilizers in a baseball thrower secondary to any cause leads to symptoms referable both to the rotator cuff and to instability. Both tensile and compressive rotator cuff disorders can indirectly result from this instability. Jobe et al (44,45) have created a classification based on the underlying disorder in an attempt to clarify the management of the baseball thrower with shoulder pain:

Group I: Throwers with pure impingement
Group II: Throwers with instability secondary to anterior ligament and labral injury with secondary impingement
Group III: Throwers with instability secondary to hyperelasticity with secondary impingement
Group IV: Throwers with pure instability

We have found a somewhat different system to be quite helpful in the evaluation of the thrower (Fig. 7). Rotator cuff disease is classified as primary or secondary, and tensile or compressive. Athletes with stable or unstable shoulders may experience repetitive microtrauma to the rotator cuff as a result of throwing, leading to dynamic failure of the rotator cuff. Primary tensile cuff disease (PTCD) is caused by repetitive deceleration forces and occurs in stable shoulders. Arthroscopically, a partial undersurface tear of the posterior/superior rotator cuff is observed. Primary compressive cuff disease (PCCD) also occurs in stable shoulders, but the cuff pathology occurs first on the bursal side of the cuff. PCCD is caused by the inability of the rotator cuff to produce sufficient adduction torques and inferior forces during the deceleration phase of throwing, leading to superior translation of the humerus. Athletes with compromise of the subacromial space due to acromial spurs or hooks, os acromionale, coracoid or coracoacromial ligament hypertrophy, or acromioclavicular joint hypertrophy are at increased risk of PCCD. Secondary tensile cuff disease (STCD) and secondary compressive cuff disease (SCCD) occur in the thrower with pre-existing instability. As a consequence of their instability, these individuals subject the rotator cuff to excessive loads during the throwing act. The rotator cuff injury is therefore secondary to the underlying instability. The rotator cuff lesions seen arthroscopically in secondary tensile disease and secondary compressive disease are similar to their primary counterparts. The common end point in this classification scheme is acquired instability due to rotator cuff microtrauma.

Both classification systems attempt to draw lines across a spectrum of injuries. There is usually a combination of instability and rotator cuff disease in the thrower, and most players have symptoms and findings indicative of both problems.

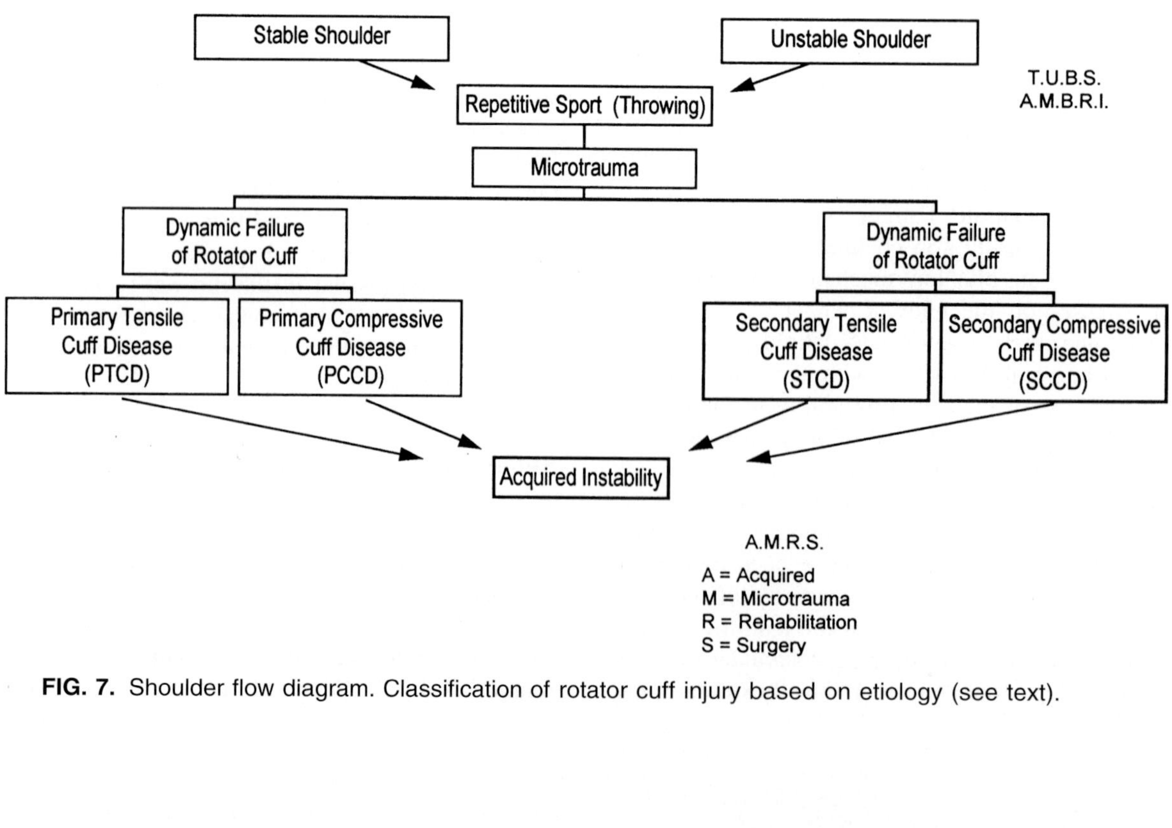

FIG. 7. Shoulder flow diagram. Classification of rotator cuff injury based on etiology (see text).

Football Thrower

Whereas the mechanism of the football throw is basically similar to the baseball pitch, it does have some important differences. Because of the greater mass of the football (426 g vs 142 g), a passer cannot generate the internal rotation velocity of 6,000 degrees per second that the pitcher can (8,11). Therefore, shoulder external rotation occurs earlier, allowing more time for internal rotation to take place. A passer also has larger magnitudes of horizontal shoulder adduction and elbow flexion (8,11), referred to as "leading with the elbow." The passer also has less contribution of the trunk and legs to the throw, being manifest as a shorter stride, a more erect posture, and less pelvis and upper torso velocity than a pitcher (8). Finally, the follow-through motion is abbreviated, because of both lower force and torque magnitudes at the shoulder and elbow as well as the need to prepare for impact from an opposing player at the completion of the pass.

Pure glenohumeral instability is much less common in the football thrower than in the baseball thrower. This is probably attributable to fewer throws (both per game and over the course of the season), as well as lower torques and forces generated with each throw. Rotator cuff disease, however, is not uncommon among football throwers. The rotator cuff may become trapped between the coracoacromial arch and the greater tuberosity of the humerus and cause shoulder pain. Bony prominences, fibrosis of the subacromial bursa, and altered biomechanics of the shoulder due to joint laxity or muscle weakness may restrict motion of the soft tissues and present as rotator cuff pathology. Anterior capsular laxity or posterior capsular tightness can result in upward and anterior translation of the humerus with arm elevation (46). Also, relative contracture of the levator scapulae and rhomboids can result in diminished upward scapular rotation with failure of acromial elevation during acceleration (47). This can lead to impingement of the rotator cuff against the undersurface of the acromion.

Tennis and Racquet Sports

Most shoulder injuries in tennis players are due to overuse and involve the rotator cuff and biceps tendon (48). Tensile overload of the posterior rotator cuff as a result of its function as a shoulder decelerator, as well as anterior instability of the glenohumeral joint, have been implicated as primary mechanisms in shoulder overuse injuries in overhead athletes (49–51). Repetitive overhead activities such as the tennis serve (typically performed at extreme ER in 90 degrees of abduction) can result in progressive attenuation of the static stabilizers of the shoulder joint, with the consequence of an increased load being placed on the dynamic stabilizers such as the rotator cuff. This increased load can lead to microtraumatic injury to the tendons and resultant symptomatic instability.

The serve involves a programmed sequence of muscle activation that is similar to the baseball throw and, like the baseball throw, can be divided into multiple phases. These include windup, cocking, acceleration, deceleration, and follow-through (52,53) (Fig. 8). Windup occurs from initiation of the serving stance to ball toss, and is characterized by minimal EMG activity. Cocking, like that in the baseball throw, terminates at maximal external rotation and involves moderately high activity in the rotator cuff, biceps, and serratus anterior (3). As compared with the baseball throw, less activity of the deltoid is necessary during cocking because trunk rotation contributes to arm abduction. External rotation of 154 degrees during cocking has been reported (54). Acceleration begins with maximal external rotation and ends at ball impact. High EMG activity occurs in the internal rotators (pectoralis major, latissimus dorsi, and subscapularis) and serratus anterior (55). Angular velocities of up to 2,300 degrees per second in internal rotation have been measured in professional tennis players during the acceleration phase of the serve (54). Deceleration is from ball impact to maximal internal rotation, and follow-through follows maximal internal rotation. Moderately high activity is noted in the posterior rotator cuff, serratus anterior, biceps, deltoid, and latissimus dorsi during deceleration.

The ranges of motion necessary to perform the tennis serve, along with the velocities and forces produced at the glenohumeral joint, have important implications for shoulder injury. Repeated stressful external rotation in abduction may cause attenuation of the anterior capsule and resultant anterior laxity of the shoulder. It has been noted in several studies that skilled tennis players exhibit diminished internal and increased external rotation of the shoulder in abduction when the dominant is compared with the nondominant extremity (56–58). This is most likely due to anterior capsular laxity with posterior capsular contracture. Laxity of the anterior capsule may lead to anterior translation in the abducted, externally rotated position, and relative contracture of the posterior capsule can cause impingement of the humeral head against the undersurface of the acromion with forward elevation (59). Several investigators have also documented an increase in strength of the internal rotators of the dominant arm without a concomitant increase in the strength of the external rotators (57,60,61). In an athlete with chronic attenuation of the static stabilizers of the shoulder, such an imbalance of the dynamic stabilizers may predispose the player to subluxation and to attritional damage to the rotator cuff.

Because of the overall similarities to the baseball throw, a conditioning program used for pitchers may be applied to the tennis player. Once again, emphasis should be placed on high-speed, multi-joint, multidirectional conditioning of the rotator cuff and scapular stabilizer muscles in an eccentric fashion.

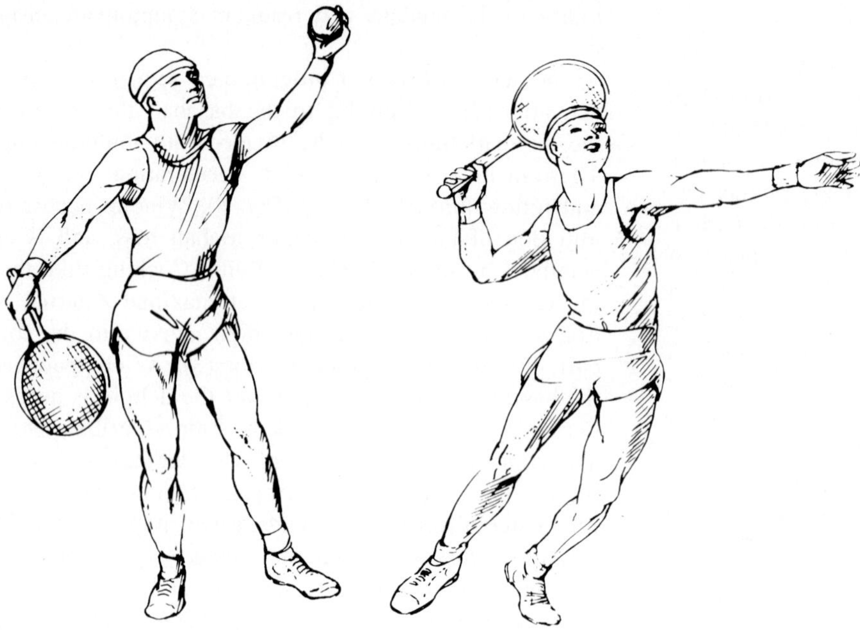

A,B

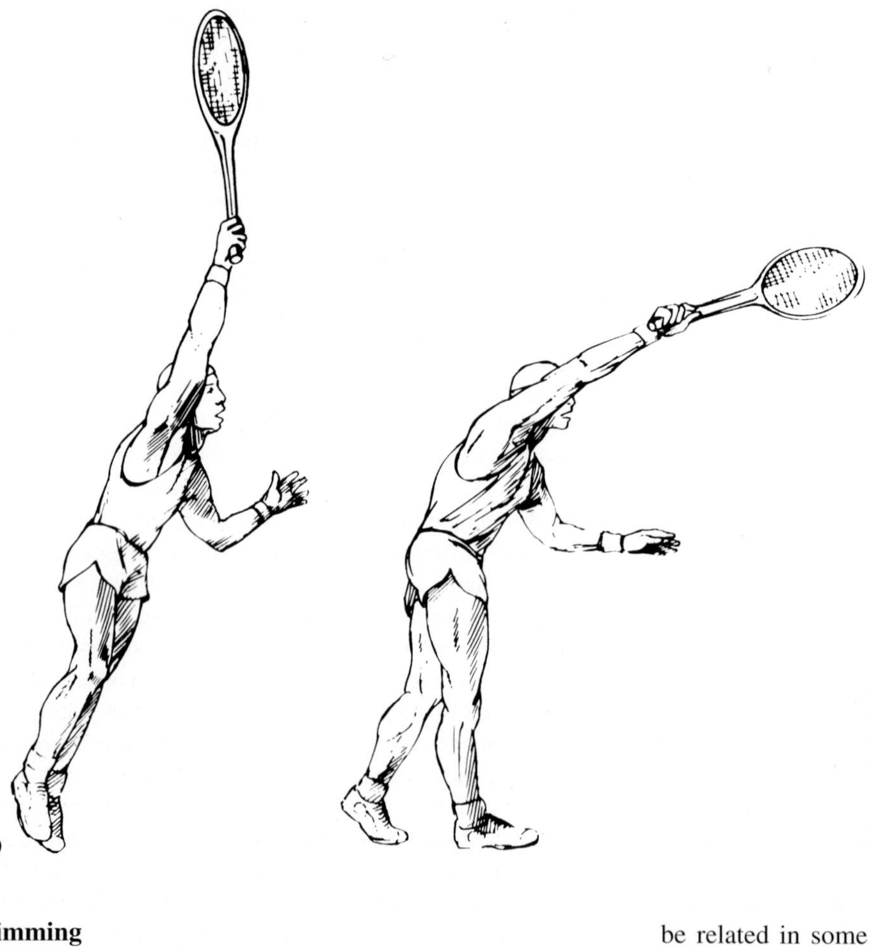

C,D

FIG. 8. A–D: Sequence of the tennis serve. **A:** Windup. **B:** Cocking. **C:** Acceleration. **D:** Deceleration and follow-through. (From Field LD, Altchek DW. Tennis injuries. In: Hawkins RJ, Misamore GW, eds. *Shoulder injuries in the athlete.* New York: Churchill Livingstone, 1996:403–416, with permission.)

Swimming

Several investigators have estimated that 40% to 60% of competitive swimmers experience shoulder pain severe enough to interrupt their training regimen (62–68). Because of the emphasis on the free-style in the training routine, most of the shoulder problems in swimmers are thought to be related in some way to this stroke (69). To understand the mechanisms responsible for injury in the swimmer's shoulder, one must first be familiar with the mechanics of the swimming stroke.

Swimming strokes have been broken down into *pull-through* and *recovery* phases by Richardson, Jobe, and Collins (70) (Fig. 9). The pull-through phase supplies the pro-

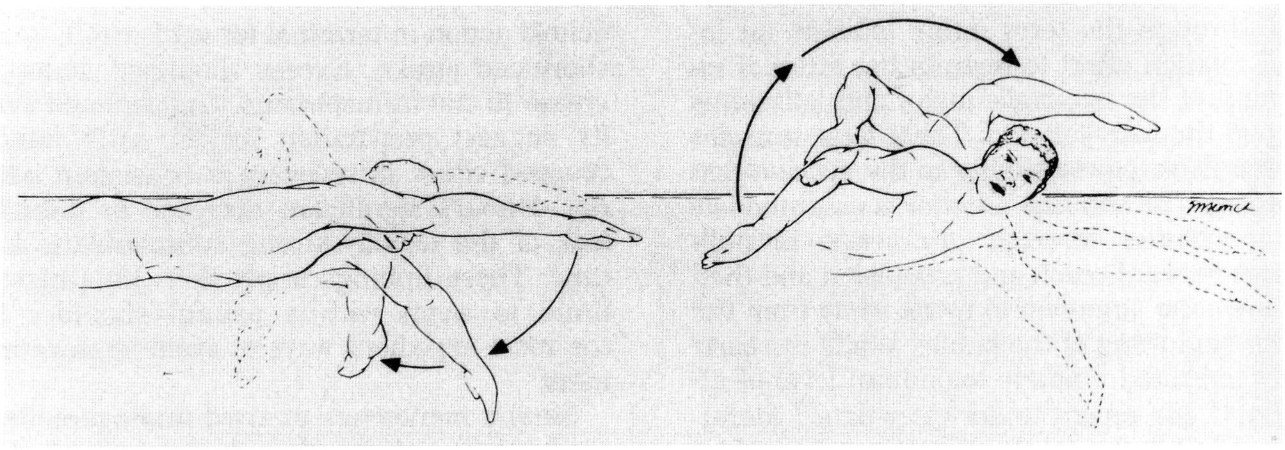

FIG. 9. Phases of the freestyle stroke. **Left:** Pull-through. **Right:** Recovery. (From Perry J, Glousman RE. Biomechanics of throwing. In: Nicholas JA, Hershman EB, eds. *The upper extremity in sports medicine*, 2nd ed. St. Louis: CV Mosby, 1995:713, with permission.)

pulsive force of the stroke by a combination of shoulder extension, internal rotation, and adduction. It begins with entry of the hand into the water (the catch) and ends when the shoulder has reached maximal internal rotation and adduction. This phase takes up about 65% of the stroke cycle. During pull-through the pectoralis major and latissimus dorsi muscles provide the internal rotation forces necessary to pull the body through the water. This internal rotation force is resisted by the teres minor. The serratus anterior is continuously active during both phases of stroke, contributing to forward propulsion via scapular protraction during pull-through, and allowing the acromion to rotate away from the humerus during recovery (71). Fatigue of the serratus anterior may lead to asynchronous humeral abduction and scapular rotation, resulting in subacromial impingement.

The remaining 35% of the stroke cycle consists of the recovery phase, which functions to position the arm in an optimal position to begin pull-through. The recovery phase begins with elbow lift as the shoulder begins abduction and external rotation; this phase ends as the hand enters the water. It is believed that the shoulder must reach the mid-position of external rotation by the middle of recovery to avoid subacromial impingement (69). Delayed external rotation of the humerus during recovery results in abduction of the internally rotated humerus, trapping the rotator cuff under the coracoacromial arch. The recovery phase is characterized by intense activity of the supraspinatus and subscapularis (and the infraspinatus, to a lesser degree) as these muscles assist the deltoid in lifting and advancing the arm in preparation for the next pull-through (72). The rhomboid and trapezius muscles retract the scapula during recovery to assist in clearing the arm from the water. The abduction, extension, and internal rotation of the arm during this phase, as well as the forward reach that takes place as the hand enters the water, all place the arm at risk of subacromial impingement. Humeral head depression by the rotator cuff and the long head of the biceps tendon (when the shoulder is flexed/abducted) (73) minimize the amount of subacromial impingement that takes place during recovery.

Although excessive laxity of the glenohumeral joint is not an infrequent finding in many swimmers, it seems to have a predilection for specialists in the backstroke (62,63, 66,68). At the beginning of pull-through, when the hand enters the water (the catch), the backstroker's shoulder is maximally externally rotated, forward flexed, and horizontally abducted. Realizing that this is a provocative position for anterior glenohumeral instability, it is not surprising to find that an athlete who assumes this position between 2,400 and 4,000 times per arm per 10,000-m training session (69) will often develop symptomatic anterior laxity from attenuation of the anterior inferior glenohumeral ligament.

Gymnastics

Injuries to the shoulder represent 0.7% to 16.7% of gymnastics injuries (74). These injuries are more often related to overuse than due to acute trauma, and they are more frequent in male rather than female competitors (75). The preponderance of shoulder injuries seen in males is thought to reflect the higher stresses placed on the male's shoulders in events such as the rings (particularly during the iron cross and dislocate maneuvers), pommel horse, high bar, and parallel bars, where routines are designed to emphasize power and strength (75). The use of the doweled grip to enhance grip strength during the routine permits performance of higher velocity and more frequent swinging maneuvers, placing additional stress on the upper extremity.

The most common injuries to the gymnast's shoulder involve overuse injuries of the rotator cuff and biceps tendon (76). The athlete complains of pain while swinging on the rings or bar, or while performing handstands. It is likely that these injuries are due in part to a subclinical instability of the glenohumeral joint which results in subacromial edema and inflammation, as primary rotator cuff degeneration in this age group is rare. For this reason, the emphasis on strengthening of the dynamic glenohumeral joint stabilizers is important from both a preventative and therapeutic standpoint.

True instability complaints in the absence of impingement do occur, most frequently of the anterior and inferior type (76). Selection of the most flexible athletes to perform the sport and the performance of routines that require the shoulder to operate at the extremes of the range of motion place the gymnast at risk of the development of symptomatic instability. Because of the hyperlaxity needed for performance, there is relative incompetence of the static stabilizers (e.g., the anterior inferior glenohumeral ligament), and the gymnast must rely on the dynamic stabilizers of the glenohumeral joint to control their mobility. Proximal stability during maneuvers such as the iron cross is afforded by the serratus anterior, and the rotator cuff muscles are balanced by the rhomboids, levator scapulae, and the lower trapezius (76). Because of the high degree of muscle performance, debilitating instability is unusual (76). However, lesser degrees of translation that occur as a result of fatigue failure of the dynamic stabilizers or ineffective muscle recruitment patterns can lead to abrasion of the humeral head against the anterior or posterior labrum, causing a symptomatic labral tear.

REFERENCES

1. Dillman CJ, Fleisig GS, Andrews JR. Biomechanics of pitching with emphasis upon shoulder kinematics. *J Orthop Sports Phys Ther* 1993;18:402–408.
2. Feltner M, Dapena J. Dynamics of the shoulder and elbow joints of the throwing arm during a baseball pitch. *Int J Sport Biomech* 1986;2: 235–259.
3. Fleisig GS, Andrews JR, Dillman CJ, Escamilla RG. Kinetics of baseball pitching with implications about injury mechanisms. *Am J Sports Med* 1995;23:233–239.
4. Jobe FW, Jobe CM. Painful athletic injuries of the shoulder. *Clin Orthop* 1983;173:117–124.
5. Sisto DJ, Jobe FW, Moynes DR. An electromyographic analysis of the elbow in pitching. *Am J Sports Med* 1987;15:260–263.
6. Werner SL, Fleisig GS, Dillman CJ, Andrews JR. Biomechanics of the elbow during baseball pitching. *J Orthop Sports Phys Ther* 1993;17:274–278.
7. Fleisig GS, Barrentine SW, Escamilla RF, Andrews JR. Biomechanics of overhand throwing with implications for injuries. *Sports Med* 1996;21:421–437.
8. Fleisig GS, Escamilla RF, Andrews JR, Matsuo T, Sattershite Y, Barrentine SW. Kinematic and kinetic comparison between baseball pitching and football passing. *J Applied Biomech* 1996;12:207–224.
9. Sakurai S, Ikegami Y, Okamota A, et al. A three-dimensional cinematographic analysis of upper limb movement during fastball and curveball baseball pitches. *J Appl Biomech* 1993;9:47–65.
10. Elliott B, Grove JR, Gibson B, et al. Three-dimensional cinematographic analysis of the fastball and curveball pitches in baseball. *Int J Sport Biomech* 1986;2:20–28.
11. Rash GS, Shapiro R. A three-dimensional dynamic analysis of the quaterback's throwing motion in American football. *J Appl Biol* 1995;1:443–459.
12. Bradley JP. Electromyographic analysis of muscle action about the shoulder. *Clin Sports Med* 1991;10:789–805.
13. DiGiovine NM, Jobe FW, Pink M, Perry J. An electromyographic analysis of the upper extremity in pitching. *J Shoulder Elbow Surg* 1992;1:15–25.
14. Pappas AM, Zawacki RM, McCarthy CR. Rehabilitation of the pitching shoulder. *Am J Sports Med* 1985;13:223–235.
15. Vaughn RE. Three dimensional kinematics of the baseball pitch. In: Terauds J, Barham JN, eds. *Biomechanics in sports*. II. Proceedings of ISBS. Del Mar, CA: Research Centre for Sports, 1985:72–78.
16. Gowan ID. Comparative electromyographic analysis of the shoulder during pitching. *J Sports Med* 1987;15:586–590.
17. Moynes DR. Electromyography and motion analysis of the upper extremeity in sports. *Phys Ther* 1986;66:1905–1911.
18. Dillman CJ, Gleisig GS, Werner SL, Andrews JR. Biomechanics of the shoulder in sports: throwing activities. In: Matsen FA, ed. *The shoulder: a balance of mobility and stability*. Rosemont, IL: American Academy of Orthopaedic Surgeons, 1993:621–633.
19. Jobe FW, Tibone JI, Perry J, Moynes D. An EMG analysis of the shoulder in throwing and pitching: a preliminary report. *Am J Sports Med* 1983;11:3–5.
20. Jacobs P. The overhand baseball pitch: a kinesiological analysis and related strength-conditioning programming. *National Strength and Conditioning J* 1987;9:5–13.
21. Matsen FA 3d, Harryman DT 2d, Sidles JA. Mechanics of glenohumeral instability. *Clin Sports Med* 1991;10:783–788.
22. O'Brien SJ, Neves MC, Arnoczky SP, et al. The anatomy and histology of the inferior glenohumeral ligament complex of the shoulder. *Am J Sports Med* 1990;18:449.
23. Pollack RG, Bigliani LU, Flatow EL, et al. The mechanical properties of the inferior glenohumeral ligament. Presented at the Annual Meeting of the American Shoulder and Elbow Surgeons, New Orleans, LA, 1990.
24. Andrews JR, Carson WG. The arthroscopic treatment of glenoid labrum tears in the throwing athlete. *Orthop Trans* 1984;8:44.
25. Snyder SJ, Karzel RP, Del Pizzo W, Ferkel RD, Friedman MJ. SLAP lesions of the shoulder. *Arthroscopy* 1990;6:274–279.
26. Pappas AM, Gross TD, Kleinman PK. Symptomatic shoulder instability due to lesions of the glenoid labrum. *Am J Sports Med* 1983;11: 279–288.
27. Warren RF, Kornblatt IB, Marchand R. Static factors affecting posterior shoulder stability. *Orthop Trans* 1984;8:89.
28. Andrews JR, Angelo RL. Shoulder arthroscopy for the throwing athlete. *Tech Orthop* 1988;3:75–81.
29. Walch G, Boileau P, Noel E, Donell ST. Impingement of the deep surface of the supraspinatous tendon on the posterosuperior glenoid rim: an arthroscopic study. *J Shoulder Elbow Surg* 1992;1:238–245.
30. Andrews JR, Wilk KE. Shoulder injuries in baseball. In: Andrews JR, Wilk KE, eds. *The athlete's shoulder*. New York: Churchill Livingstone, 1994.
31. Kapandji IA. *The physiology of the joints*, 5th ed, vol. 1. New York: Churchill Livingstone, 1982.
32. Kibler WB, Shapiro RL, Chandler TJ, et al. Posterior shoulder muscle firing patterns in tennis players. AOSSM Interim Meeting, New Orleans, 1990.
33. Kibler WB. Role of the scapula in the overhead throwing motion. *Contemp Orthop* 1991;22:525–532.
34. Glousman RE, Jobe FW, Tibone JE, Moynes D, Antonelli D, Perry J. Dynamic electromyographic analysis of the throwing shoulder with glenohumeral instability. *J Bone Joint Surg* 1988;70:220–226.
35. Chen S, Wickiewicz TL, Otis JC, Warren RF. Glenohumeral kinematics in a muscle fatigue model: a radiographic study. *Orthop Trans* 1995;18:1126.
36. Fleisig GS, Dillman CJ, Escamilla RF, Andrews JR. Kinetics of baseball pitching with implications about injury mechanisms. *Am J Sports Med* 1995;23:233–239.
37. Kreighbaum E, Barthels K. *Biomechanics: a qualitative approach for studying human movement*. New York: Macmillan, 1990.
38. Norkin CC, Levangie PK. *Joint structure and function: a comprehensive analysis*. Philadelphia: FA Davis, 1983.
39. Steindler A. *Kinesiology of the human body under normal and pathological conditions*. Springfield: Charles C Thomas, 1955.
40. Dillman CJ. Proper mechanics of pitching. *Sports Med Update* 1990;5:15–18.
41. Elliott B, Marsh T, Overheu P. A biomechanical comparison of multisegment and single unit topspin forehand drives in tennis. *Int J Sport Biomech* 1989;5:350–364.

42. Feltner ME, Dapena J. Three-dimensional interactions in a two-segment kinetic chain. Part I. General model. *Int J Sport Biomech* 1989;5: 403–419.
43. Feltner ME, Dapena J. Three-dimensional interactions in a two-segment kinetic chain. Part II. Application to the throwing arm in baseball pitching. *Int J Sport Biomech* 1989;5:420–450.
44. Jobe FW, Tibone JE, Jobe CM, Kvitne RS. The shoulder in sports. In: Rockwood CA, Matsen FA (eds). *The shoulder*. Philadelphia: WB Saunders, 1990:961–990.
45. Jobe FW, Glousmann RE. Anterior capsulolabral reconstruction. *Tech Orthop* 1985;3:29.
46. Turkel SJ, Panio MW, Marshall DVM, Girgis FG. Stabilizing mechanisms preventing anterior dislocation of the glenohumeral joint. *J Bone Joint Surg [Am]* 1981;63A:1208–1217.
47. Seto JL, Brewster CE, Shields CL Jr. Shoulder injuries in football. In: Andrews JR, Wilk KE, eds. *The athlete's shoulder*. New York: Churchill Livingstone, 1994.
48. Reece LA, Fricker PA, Maguire KF. Injuries to elite young tennis players at the Australian Institute of Sport. *Aust J Sci Med Sport* 1986;18:11.
49. Jobe FW, Kvitne RS. Shoulder pain in the overhand or throwing athlete: the relationship of anterior instability and rotator cuff impingement. *Orthop Rev* 1989;18:963–975.
50. Andrews JR, Kupferman SP, Dillman CJ.abral tears in throwing and racquet sports. *Clin Sports Med* 1991;10:901–911.
51. Nirschl RP. Shoulder tendinitis. *Upper extremity injuries in athletes*. American Academy of Orthopaedic Surgeons Symposium, Washington, DC. St. Louis: CV Mosby, 1986.
52. Morris M, Jobe FW, Perry J, Pink M, Healy BS. Electromyographic analysis of elbow function in tennis players. *Am J Sports Med* 1989;17:241–247.
53. Ellenbecker TS. Shoulder injuries in tennis. In: Andrews JR, Wilk KE, eds. *The athlete's shoulder*. New York: Churchill Livingstone, 1994.
54. Dillman CJ. Presentation on the upper extremity in tennis and throwing athletes. United States Tennis Association National Meeting, Tucson, Arizona, March 1991.
55. Rhu KN, McCormick J, Jobe FW, Moynes DR, Antonelli DJ. An electromyographic analysis of shoulder function in tennis players. *Am J Sports Med* 1988;16:481–485.
56. Chandler TJ, Kibler WB, Uhl TL, Wooten B, Kiser A, Stone E. Flexibility comparisons of junior elite tennis players to other athletes. *Am J Sports Med* 1990;18:134–136.
57. Ellenbecker TS. Shoulder internal and external rotation strength and range of motion of highly skilled junior tennis players. *Isokinet Exerc Sci* 1992;2:1.
58. Chinn CJ, Priest JD, Kent BE. Upper extremity range of motion, grip strength, and girth in highly skilled tennis players. *Phys Ther* 1974;54: 474.
59. Matsen FA III, Arntz CT. Subacromial impingement. In: Rockwood CA Jr, Matsen FA III, eds. *The shoulder*, 1st ed. Philadelphia: WB Saunders, 1990.
60. Ellenbecker TS. A total arm strength isokinetic profile of highly skilled tennis players. *Isokinet Exerc Sci* 1991;1:9–21.
61. Koziris LP, Kraemer WJ, Triplett NT, et al. Strength imbalances in women in tennis players. *Med Sci Sports Exerc* 1991;23:253(abst).
62. Johnson JE, Sim FH, Scott SG. Musculoskeletal injuries in competitive swimmers. *Mayo Clin Proc* 1987;62:289.
63. Kennedy JC, Craig AB, Schneider RD. Swimming. In: Schneider RC, Kennedy JC, Plant ML, eds. *Sports injuries: mechanisms, prevention and treatment*. Baltimore: Williams & Wilkins, 1985.
64. McMaster WC. Painful shoulder in swimmers: a diagnostic challenge. *Phys Sports Med* 1986;14:108.
65. McMaster WC. Diagnosing swimmer's shoulder. *Swimming Tech* 1987;(Feb–Apr):17.
66. Falkel JE. Swimming injuries. In: Sanders B, ed. *Sports physical therapy*. Norwalk, CT: Appleton & Lange, 1990:477.
67. Nuber GW, Jobe FW, Perry J, Moynes DR, Antonelli D. Fine wire electromyography analysis of muscles in the shoulder in swimming. *Am J Sports Med* 1986;14:7–11.
68. Falkel JE, Murphy TC. Swimming injuries. In: Malone T, ed. *Sports injury management series*. Baltimore: Williams & Wilkins, 1988.
69. Murphy TC. Shoulder injuries in swimming. In: Andrews JR, Wilk KE, eds. *The athlete's shoulder*. New York: Churchill Livingstone, 1994.
70. Richardson AB, Jobe FW, Collins HR. The shoulder in competitive swimming. *Am J Sports Med* 1980;81:159–163.
71. Pink M, Jobe FW, Perry J, Kerrigan J, Browne A, Scovazzo ML. The normal shoulder during the butterfly stroke. *Clin Orthop* 1993;288: 48–59.
72. Pink M, Perry J, Browne A, Scovazzo ML, Kerrigan J. The normal shoulder during freestyle swimming: an electromyographic cinematographic study of twelve muscles. *Am J Sports Med* 1991;19 (6):569–576.
73. Richardson AB. The biomechanics of swimming: the shoulder and knee. In: Cuillo JV, ed. Swimming. *Clin Sports Med* 1986;5:103.
74. Meeusen R, Borms J. Gymnastic injuries. *Sports Med* 1992;13:337.
75. Weiker GG. Upper extremity gymnastic injuries. In: Nicholas JA, Hershman EB, eds. *The upper extremity in sports medicine*, 2nd ed. St. Louis: CV Mosby, 1994.
76. Helmsley KP. Shoulder injuries in gymnastics. In: Andrews JR, Wilk KE, eds. *The athlete's shoulder*. New York: Churchill Livingstone, 1994.

Section 2

Diagnostic Considerations

The Unstable Shoulder,
edited by R.F. Warren, E.V. Craig, and D.W. Altchek.
Lippincott–Raven Publishers, Philadelphia © 1999.

CHAPTER 5

Clinical Evaluation of the Unstable Shoulder

Answorth A. Allen

The anatomy of the glenohumeral articulation is unique in that it allows the most motion of any joint in the body and is stable throughout the range of motion. However, excessive glenohumeral translation can be pathologic and may compromise function and patient comfort. Instability is one of the most common problems in the glenohumeral joint. Glenohumeral instability encompasses a spectrum of disorders ranging from a dislocated shoulder, in which the instability pattern is obvious to more subtle instability problems such as shoulder subluxation, in which the instability pattern may not be clear. For the purposes of this chapter, it is important to define commonly used terms in the instability vernacular such as *laxity*, *subluxation*, and *dislocation*.

Laxity is defined as *asymptomatic* passive translation of the humeral head relative to the glenoid. The operative words are *asymptomatic* and *passive translation*. Patients do not usually complain of shoulder laxity. Glenohumeral joint laxity is usually a bilateral condition, and ''excessive shoulder'' laxity is often seen within the context of generalized ligamentous laxity. The degree of laxity is assessed with the physical examination and is usually associated with increased passive translation (i.e., increased ''play in the joint'').

Instability is defined as excessive *symptomatic* translation of the humeral head relative to the glenoid articular surface during *active* motion. Here the operative words are *symptomatic* and *active motion*. Patients will complain of shoulder instability symptoms. The spectrum of glenohumeral joint instability is represented clinically by shoulder *subluxation* and shoulder *dislocation*. Glenohumeral subluxation is symptomatic translation of the humeral head relative to the glenoid articular surface without complete separation of the articular surfaces. Glenohumeral dislocation is increased translation of the humeral head relative to the glenoid articular surface to the point of complete separation of articular surfaces.

A. A. Allen: Department of Orthopaedics, Cornell Medical College; and The Hospital for Special Surgery, New York, New York 10021.

The purpose of this chapter is to discuss clinical evaluation of the unstable shoulder. Emphasis is placed on the classification of instability patterns and the history and physical examination. Radiographic evaluation is discussed in Chapter 6.

CLASSIFICATION OF GLENOHUMERAL JOINT INSTABILITY

The objective of a classification system is to provide some insight and understanding of the pathogenesis and natural history of the problem. It can also be used as a guide for management and as an indicator of prognosis. Several classification systems have been proposed for instability of the glenohumeral joint, generally based on the mechanism of injury and the direction and frequency of instability (1–7). The traditional classification of glenohumeral instability is shown in Table 1 (8).

This chapter focuses on three broad categories of instability patterns: anterior instability (Table 2), posterior instability (Table 3), and multidirectional instability (Table 4). Superior and inferior dislocations (luxatio erecta) and instability after prior surgery will also be discussed.

HISTORY

In general, a careful detailed history that considers the classification of shoulder instability is the first step in the diagnosis of glenohumeral instability. The chief complaint, age, circumstances surrounding the onset of the problem, and details of any therapeutic interventions should be elicited. Any progression of the problem and the type and frequency of sports activity are also important considerations. Family history and handedness should also be documented. The specifics of the history in patients with different instability patterns are described below.

TABLE 1. *Shoulder instability classification*

- Frequency
  - Acute
  - Recurrent
  - Fixed (chronic)
- Cause
  - Traumatic event (macrotrauma)
  - Atraumatic event (voluntary, involuntary)
  - Microtrauma
  - Congenital condition
  - Neuromuscular condition (Erb's palsy, cerebral palsy, seizures)
- Direction
  - Anterior
  - Posterior
  - Inferior
  - Multidirectional
- Degree
  - Dislocation
  - Subluxation
  - Microtrauma (transient)

TABLE 2. *Classification of anterior instability*

1. Traumatic, acute dislocation (subcoracoid, subglenoid, subclavicular, intrathoracic)
2. Traumatic, acute subluxation
3. Recurrent anterior instability
   a. Chronic recurrent anterior dislocation
   b. Chronic recurrent anterior subluxation
4. Fixed (locked) anterior dislocation

TABLE 3. *Classification of posterior instability*

1. Traumatic acute dislocation (subacromial, subglenoid, subspinous)
2. Traumatic acute subluxation
3. Recurrent posterior instability
   a. Recurrent posterior dislocation
   b. Recurrent posterior subluxation
4. Voluntary (atraumatic subluxation/dislocation)
   a. Positional type
   b. Muscular type
5. Chronic (locked) dislocation (size of reversed Hill-Sachs lesion)
   a. <25% of the articular surface
   b. 25–40% of the articular surface
   c. <40% of the articular surface

TABLE 4. *Classification of multidirectional instability*

Type	Description
I	Global instability: atraumatic multidirectional instability
II	Anterior/inferior instability: acute macrotraumatic episode in the setting of underlying hyperlaxity
III	Posterior/inferior instability: repetitive microtraumatic episodes in the setting of underlying hyperlaxity
IV	Anterior/posterior instability

ANTERIOR INSTABILITY

Acute Anterior Dislocations

Most cases of glenohumeral instability are anterior. The clinical presentation ranges from the obvious anterior dislocation to the more subtle shoulder subluxation. The glenohumeral joint is the most commonly dislocated joint in the body and most of these dislocations are anterior (9–18). Cave et al. (19) evaluated 1,600 cases of shoulder injuries and found that approximately 25% were dislocations, 84% of which were anterior glenohumeral dislocations. A major traumatic event is usually associated with an acute anterior dislocation. In a series of 500 cases of anterior dislocations reported by Rowe (20), almost 80% of the dislocations were anterior and 96% were caused by a major traumatic event. In a recent series of 57 patients with documented anterior shoulder dislocation reported by Baker et al. (21), 76% of the dislocations occurred during athletic activity.

Although major trauma is usually involved in an acute anterior dislocation, the shoulder does not usually dislocate as a result of a direct blow. The mechanism involves a combination of forces that stresses the abducted, extended and externally rotated arm resulting in excessive forces to the anterior capsule, glenohumeral ligaments and rotator cuff. The humeral head is forced anteriorly and out of the glenoid fossa. In the athletic population, this frequently occurs during the second decade during sports activities such as wrestling, tackling during a football game, rebounding in basketball, and sliding into base during baseball or softball. In the general population, motor vehicle accidents, falls, and altercations are also frequent etiologies of traumatic anterior glenohumeral dislocations.

An alert patient is usually aware that the shoulder is "out," and this is confirmed by an excruciatingly painful deformity of the glenohumeral joint. The most common type of anterior dislocation is the *subcoracoid* dislocation. Here the humeral head is anterior to the glenoid and inferior to the coracoid process. With the *subglenoid dislocation*, the head of the humerus is anterior and below the glenoid fossa. The head of the humerus lies medial to the coracoid process at the inferior border of the clavicle in a *subclavicular* dislocation. Significant trauma is usually associated with an *intrathoracic* dislocation. The head of the humerus lies between the ribs and the thoracic cavity. There is huge potential for pulmonary, vascular, and neurologic complications (11,22). The different types of anterior dislocations are usually confirmed by radiographic appearance.

Acute Anterior Subluxation

During the past decade, practitioners have developed more awareness of the more subtle patterns of shoulder instability. Unlike the acutely dislocated shoulder, for which the diagnosis is usually obvious from the history, physical examination, and radiographs, patients with subluxation may not necessarily recall the specifics of the instability episode, and the clinical presentation can be variable.

Acute anterior glenohumeral subluxation usually occurs as a result of a mechanism similar to anterior dislocation, in which the externally rotated, extended, and abducted arm is stressed by forces inadequate to cause a complete separation of the articular surfaces. This can result in varying degrees of labral and capsular injury. In some cases, the joint may dislocate and reduce spontaneously and the patient may present with subsequent subluxation or dislocation episodes.

Acute anterior subluxation episodes can occur with all the activities that can cause an anterior shoulder dislocation, such as wrestling, tackling during football, and rebounding during basketball. Acute anterior subluxation can also occur while weight lifting, specifically with the bench and military press. The patient may present with acute shoulder pain, a perception of instability, or transient neurologic symptoms. They will often feel that they are at risk of dislocation of the joint and will learn to avoid the activities that reproduces the symptoms. The development of recurrent anterior subluxation is dependent on the degree of injury to the capsulolabral structures and the patient's activity level.

Recurrent Anterior Dislocation

After a traumatic acute anterior dislocation, recurrent anterior dislocation appears to be the rule rather than the exception. In fact, recurrent anterior instability is the most common complication after anterior glenohumeral dislocations (20,23–26). In cases that are managed nonoperatively, the re-dislocation rate appears independent of duration and type of immobilization but is directly correlated to the patient's age at the time of the initial dislocation (27–30).

The mechanism of injury in patients with recurrent anterior dislocation of the glenohumeral joint is usually similar to those that cause the index dislocation, although the force required may be significantly less. Typically, an indirect force is involved to the abducted, extended, and externally rotated arm. In some patients, the shoulder may redislocate with relatively minor activities such as sneezing, getting dressed, and sleeping. Patients with recurrent anterior dislocations caused by routine activities of daily living are more likely to be candidates for surgery. It is important to determine whether the patient is able to reduce the shoulder themselves or if assistance is required. Any history of neurologic or rotator cuff injuries associated with previous dislocation episodes should be noted. The nature and type of the rehabilitation efforts should be documented. Any previous surgical intervention should be noted.

Recurrent Anterior Subluxation

Patients with chronic recurrent anterior glenohumeral subluxation may present a diagnostic dilemma. Although some patients may present with a sense of shoulder instability or apprehension with the arm abducted and externally rotated, shoulder pain is often the primary complaint. In some patients, recurrent anterior shoulder subluxation may develop after one specific traumatic episode; others will have a gradual onset of shoulder instability symptoms from repetitive activity. A distinct perception of the shoulder sliding in and out of the joint may be present. Others may present with transient neurological symptoms such as numbness and tingling in the fingers. Often the only complaint is reproducible shoulder pain with certain activities or arm position. Patients with anterior instability may complain of pain on the posterior aspect of the shoulder joint, presenting a confusing clinical picture. Overhead athletes with occult glenohumeral instability may also present with impingement-type symptoms (i.e., anterolateral shoulder pain with activities above the horizontal). This represents a secondary non-outlet impingement and may be related to inflammation of the rotator cuff and capsule, which are stressed or overused during the subluxation episodes. The pattern of shoulder subluxation is usually directly related to the sport and arm position during the sport. In throwers, pain during phase 1 of the throwing motion is usually consistent with recurrent anterior shoulder subluxation. Reaching for a rebound or side arm tackling are both provocative positions which can elicit symptoms. Recurrent anterior subluxation may progress to a frank dislocation (31–33).

Fixed (Locked) Anterior Dislocations

Chronic locked anterior dislocations are only encountered if the diagnosis of an acute anterior dislocation was initially missed or not treated. This usually occurs in the setting of a major trauma, in which the patient is debilitated from other injuries or in the setting of a convulsive disorder or electroshock therapy, in which the patient is not aware that the shoulder was dislocated. Patients usually present with loss of motion or a nonpainful deformity of the shoulder. The differential diagnosis includes a frozen shoulder; the diagnosis is usually confirmed by the physical examination and an axillary radiograph.

POSTERIOR INSTABILITY

Posterior glenohumeral instability occurs less frequently than anterior instability. In the clinical series of 581 shoulder dislocations reported by McLaughlin (34), there were 22 cases of posterior dislocations or subluxations representing an incidence of 4%. The diagnosis of posterior dislocation may be missed at the initial presentation in up to 50% to 80% of patients (35,36), generally because of an inadequate history and physical examination.

The classification of posterior instability is shown in Table 3. It is based on the degree, frequency, direction, and etiology of instability. Clinically isolated posterior instability is rare as there is frequently an inferior component to the instability pattern. There is some overlap with multidirectional instability(type III MDI).

Acute Posterior Dislocation

The diagnosis of posterior instability is based on a careful detailed history, an appropriate level of suspicion, and a thorough physical examination. An acute dislocation can result from either direct or indirect force to the glenohumeral joint. A dislocation can result from a direct force if the patient sustains a direct blow to the anterior aspect of the glenohumeral joint. A fall on the outstretched adducted arm can generate an axial force on the humerus and cause a posterior displacement of the humeral head relative to the glenoid (37). Acute posterior dislocation or subluxation can also result from the same combination of forces in an offensive lineman. When blocking, the arm is flexed, adducted, and internally rotated, and a direct axial load from the opponent may cause a posterior subluxation or dislocation of the humeral head.

Dislocations can also result from forceful muscular contractions from a seizure or electric shock. Although anterior dislocations can occur, usually activation of the stronger adductors and internal rotators (lattisimus dorsi, pectoralis major, subscapularis, and teres majors) will cause adduction, flexion, and internal rotation of the humerus with resultant dorsal and posterior displacement of the humeral head relative to the glenoid (38–40).

In many cases, posterior dislocations or subluxations will reduce spontaneously; it is often unclear to the patient that a dislocation or subluxation episode occurred sustained. In some cases, the humerus may remain posterior to the glenoid. The most common location is in the *subacromial* region (i.e., behind the glenoid and beneath the acromion). Other possibilities include a *subspinous* dislocation with the head of the humerus medial to the acromion and beneath the spine of the scapula, and the *subglenoid* dislocation where the head is behind and beneath the glenoid.

There can be associated fractures of the proximal humerus and posterior glenoid rim as well as rotator cuff ruptures with a traumatic posterior glenohumeral joint dislocation (41–43).

Acute Posterior Subluxation

An acute posterior subluxation occurs with a mechanism similar to acute posterior dislocations. In this scenario, the forces are usually not adequate to cause a dislocation. Frequently, there is associated chondral and labral injuries. Patients usually present with posterior shoulder pain and mechanical symptoms such as painful clicking or locking with certain activities or arm positions (35,36,44).

Recurrent Posterior Instability (Dislocation/Subluxation)

Patients with recurrent posterior instability have significant injury to the posterior capsulolabral structures from a major traumatic event or from repetitive microtrauma (34, 35,37). Patients in the latter group will have an insidious onset of symptoms and will usually have an inferior component to the instability pattern. Patients with posterior instability will usually present with a sense of looseness/instability or perceptible posterior dislocation of the shoulder when performing activities with the arm flexed, adducted and internally rotated. Activities such as the follow-through phase of pitching (phase 3), bench pressing, rowing, the pull-through phase of swimming, and rowing can all elicit these symptoms (35,36). The location of the pain can be quite variable and may be localized to the posterior joint line, the anterior aspect of the shoulder, or the anterolateral aspect of the arm. In patients with posterior subluxation who continue to participate in the inciting activity, a progression of symptoms can result.

Voluntary Posterior Instability

Patients with voluntary posterior instability have the ability to reproduce the subluxation or dislocation episodes. They can be divided into two groups: ''positional'' and ''muscular.'' Those patients with muscular control of their instability will often have some underlying emotional or character problems and will often use their disability for a secondary gain. This is an extremely difficult group of patients to treat. They are not surgical candidates and should receive counselling. Patients with positional control of their posterior instability will have symptoms when the arm is placed in certain positions. By avoiding these positions, they are usually asymptomatic. They can be taught to avoid these positions but, if significant disability exists, they may be candidates for surgical intervention (4,6,35).

Chronic (Locked) Posterior Dislocations

Locked posterior dislocation will often occur in alcoholics or demented persons in whom the initial injury was missed. Usually these patients are unaware that the shoulder was ever dislocated. They will usually hold the arm in adduction and internal rotation. External rotation of the arm is often limited beyond zero degrees. Forward elevation is often less than 90 degrees. They are frequently misdiagnosed with a frozen shoulder. A history of seizure disorder, excessive alcohol use or electroshock therapy should alert the examiner to this possibility. The correct diagnosis is based on a good history, a thorough examination, and radiographs, specifically the axillary view. The degree of articular surface involvement and the duration of the dislocation are important prognostic factors (37).

MULTIDIRECTIONAL INSTABILITY

A consistent feature of multidirectional instability is excessive capsular laxity resulting in abnormal glenohumeral translation in more than one direction. Recurrent glenohumeral subluxations or dislocations may occur with relatively little trauma. In the original description by Neer and Foster (4), the presence of inferior instability is a prerequisite for the diagnosis. Symptomatic presentation includes pain, a perception of instability, or neurologic symptoms.

In the classification system described by Pagnani and Warren (45), patients with *type I MDI* have global instability with subluxation or dislocation anteriorly, posteriorly, and inferiorly. They often have generalized ligamentous laxity and a family history of generalized ligamentous laxity. There may be an underlying connective tissue disorder such as Marfan's syndrome or Ehlers-Danlos syndrome with the potential for underlying cardiac and ophthalmologic abnormalities.

Type II MDI patients have anterior and inferior instability. Typically they sustain a single traumatic event in the context of an underlying asymptomatic multidirectional laxity. They will frequently have a Bankart lesion and are best managed surgically with repair of the Bankart lesion and a capsular shift procedure to decrease the capsular redundancy.

The third group of patients, *type III MDI*, have posterior and inferior instability of the glenohumeral joint. They usually develop progressive capsular laxity from repetitive microtrauma from activities such as competitive swimming, gymnastics, and pitching. These patients with progressive capsular stretching from repetitive microtrauma can also develop global capsular laxity or an anterior-inferior instability. The authors (45) also describe the *type IV MDI*, where the instability pattern is anterior and posterior with no inferior instability. I have not seen this in my clinical experience.

The clinical presentation of patients with multidirectional instability can be vague and confusing. Patients may present with shoulder pain, a sense of instability in the shoulder, and neurologic symptoms. From the history there is often some clue as to the predominant instability pattern. Patients who present with symptoms in the overhead position with the arm abducted and externally rotated usually have a predominantly anterior and inferior component of their instability patterns and those who have symptoms with the arm adducted, flexed, and internally rotated usually have a posterior and inferior pattern of instability. There can also be a voluntary component in patients with MDI. Again, this can be positional or muscular; in the latter group, the possibility of underlying psychiatric and emotional problems should be considered when the history is taken.

INFERIOR DISLOCATIONS (LUXATIO ERECTA)

Luxatio erecta or inferior dislocation of the glenohumeral joint occurs infrequently and is usually secondary to significant trauma to the shoulder (46–48). The humeral head is dislocated inferior to the glenoid fossa. The humerus is usually locked below the glenoid in the position between 110 and 160 degrees of abduction, and the head of the humerus may be palpable along the lateral aspect of the chest wall. The patient is in severe pain and there is an obvious deformity of the proximal humerus. There are usually significant soft-tissue injuries including avulsion of the supraspinatus, pectoralis major, and teres minor muscles. Proximal humerus fracture and tuberosity avulsions are not uncommon.

SUPERIOR DISLOCATIONS

With a superior dislocation, the humeral head lies above the superior glenoid rim. Because very little is written on superior dislocations in the contemporary literature, it is reasonable to assume that this injury is extremely rare (48, 49). In 1912, Stimson reviewed 14 cases of superior glenohumeral joint dislocations (49). The usual mechanism of injury is a direct blow to the posterior aspect of the shoulder directed forward and upward on the abducted arm. The humerus is displaced upward, resulting in significant soft-tissue injury to the capsule and musculotendinous structures. Fractures of the acromion, clavicle, coracoid process, or humeral tuberosities may occur. The patient is usually in extreme pain and the humeral head lies above the level of the acromion while the arm is foreshortened and abducted to the side. A careful neurovascular examination should be performed, as neurovascular injuries are not uncommon. Motion of the shoulder is usually restricted and very painful.

DIFFERENTIAL DIAGNOSIS

The diagnosis of shoulder instability requires a careful history. Most patient will have traumatic anterior instability, and the diagnosis may be obvious. The more subtle instability patterns frequently occur in patients with atraumatic instability. Clinical presentation includes pain, a perception of instability, or neurologic symptoms. Other causes of these symptoms should be considered in the differential diagnosis. If the dislocation is the result of a seizure disorder the patient should have a complete neurologic evaluation to rule out a primary neurologic condition and to make sure that the disorder is well controlled. Patients with shoulder subluxation and mechanical symptoms may have a labral tear, which can result in "functional instability" of the glenohumeral joint (50). Superior labral anteroposterior lesions (SLAP) may be a source of shoulder pain. Partial rotator cuff tears, acromioclavicular joint problems, chondral injuries, loose bodies, early degenerative joint disease, suprascapular nerve injury, long thoracic nerve injuries, and snapping scapula should all be considered in the differential diagnosis. Another cause of shoulder pain with the arm in maximum flexion, abduction, and external rotation is posterosuperior (''*internal*'') impingement, described by Walch et al. (51). Pain results from direct impingement of the under surface of the rotator cuff against the posterosuperior rim of the glenoid when the shoulder is maximally flexed and externally rotated.

PHYSICAL EXAMINATION

The purpose of the physical examination is to determine the predominant direction and degree of instability. Although most of the emphasis is on the specific test for shoulder instability, a general impression of the patient should be obtained and the cervical spine and upper extremity should be evaluated. Examination of the shoulder should be complete and systematic. The history usually gives the clinician a definitive sense of the mechanism of injury, direction, frequency, and type of instability pattern that may be present. The physical examination should confirm the suspected instability pattern derived from the history.

Similar to other musculoskeletal examinations, inspection, palpation, range of motion, strength testing, and neurovascular examination should all be done in a methodical fashion. The presence of generalized ligamentous laxity should also be assessed. Specific tests for shoulder instability include apprehension testing (31,32), relocation testing (52,53), sulcus sign (4), the load-and-shift test (drawer testing) (54), the posterior stress test, and the Jerk test (55). Before the examination begins, the patient should disrobe to permit access to both shoulders and the upper torso. The sequence of the examination should be logical. I prefer to perform specific maneuvers with the patient standing initially, then sitting, and finally supine. The contralateral extremity should be examined first to gain the patient's trust and confidence.

Acute Anterior Dislocation

As discussed previously, most cases of acute anterior glenohumeral joint dislocations will result from a major traumatic injury. In the athletic population, this can result from such sports as football, hockey, downhill skiing, and wrestling. The acute anterior shoulder dislocation is extremely painful, and the patient usually presents with the arm in slight abduction and internal rotation. In many cases, the patient is aware that the shoulder is ''out,'' and the affected arm is grasped with the opposite hand to keep the shoulder stable. The patient tends to lean to the affected side (Fig. 1). The shoulder should be inspected for obvious deformity, swelling, abrasions, or lacerations.

A careful neurovascular examination should be performed to rule out concomitant brachial plexus and vascular injury. The incidence of nerve injury may be as high as 35% in a first-time dislocator, and the axillary nerve is most frequently involved (56). Examination of cutaneous sensitivity over the lateral aspect of the shoulder in the distribution of the axillary nerve should be performed. In the acute situation, this test may be unreliable and electromyographic (EMG) evaluation may be necessary (56). Axillary artery injury (57,58) can also occur at the time of acute dislocation, and peripheral pulses should be checked. In cases involving significant trauma that has caused an intrathoracic or subclavicular dislocation, the possibility of a neurovascular or pulmonary injury is increased. The shoulder should be palpated for crepitation and point tenderness. The acromioclavicular and sternoclavicular joints should also be palpated and inspected. A posterior sternoclavicular joint dislocation can result in serious vascular injuries and is potentially life-threatening. Although unlikely in a young athlete, the possibility of an associated proximal humerus fracture should be considered. In the older patient population if there is any suspicion of a fracture, a radiograph should be obtained before a reduction maneuver is attempted. Although passive range of motion of the shoulder may be attempted, the patient will usually resist any attempt to move the extremity. The specific tests for a shoulder instability are usually not indicated in the acutely anteriorly dislocated shoulder.

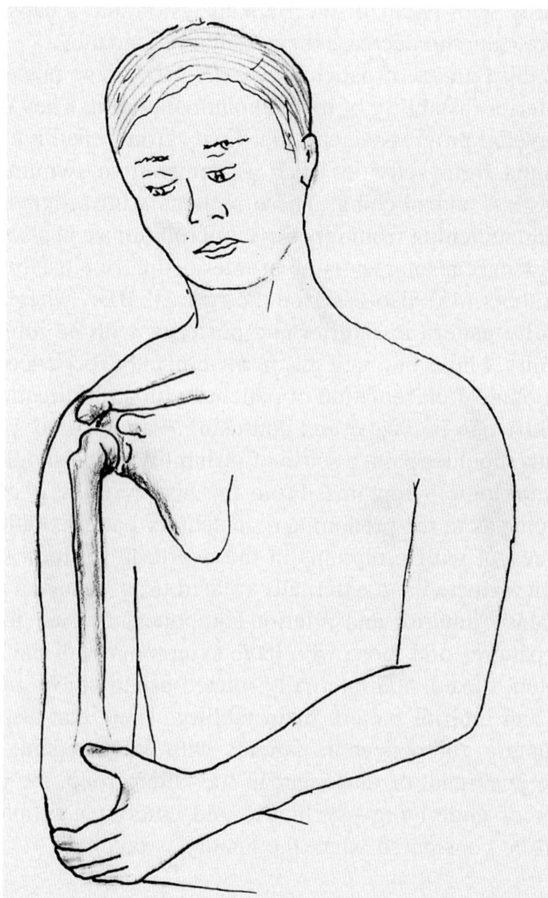

FIG. 1. Anterior shoulder dislocation. Usual presentation of a patient with anterior shoulder dislocation. The patient tends to lean toward the affected side and the arm is held by the contralateral extremity in abduction and internal rotation.

Recurrent Anterior Instability

Before the shoulder is examined, the patient should be partially disrobed to allow access to the shoulder and the scapula. The examination is begun with the patient standing. The cervical spine should be examined first. The spinous processes should be palpated and the neck placed through a range of motion. Axial loading and lateral bending of the cervical spine should be performed to screen for an underlying cervical spine problem. Generalized ligamentous laxity should be assessed by thumb hyperabduction, with the wrist volar-flexed, index metacarpal extension, elbow hyperextension, and knee hyperextension (59, 60).

The shoulder examination begins with inspection of the deltoid, trapezius, rotator cuff muscles, and the muscles of the upper arm. Excessive atrophy of the deltoid and rotator cuff muscles may be secondary to injuries to the axillary and suprascapular nerves, respectively. The acromioclavicular and sternoclavicular joints should be inspected and palpated. The supraclavicular fossa should be palpated for tenderness and masses. Active range of motion should be observed to assess scapula rhythm and to rule out scapula winging. Shoulder elevation, external rotation, abduction, and internal rotation are assessed at the side and at 90 degrees of abduction. The shoulder should be taken through a passive range of motion. The presence of pain and any discrepancy between active and passive range of motion should be noted as well as any arm position that causes shoulder pain. In the throwing athlete, it is especially important to document external and internal rotation with the arm abducted. Cross-chest adduction should be performed to assess the degree of posterior capsular tightness.

Muscle strength testing should be done for the rotator cuff and the deltoid muscles. The supraspinatus muscle can be isolated with the arm at 90 degrees of scapula elevation and 45 degrees of internal humeral rotation. For the infraspinatus, muscle strength testing is done with the arm externally rotated at 0 degrees of scapula elevation and -45 degrees of humeral rotation. The subscapularis muscle is assessed with the arm internally rotated using the Gerber push with force as described by Kelly et al. (61). Elbow flexion and extension strength testing should be done to assess the biceps and coracobrachialis muscles and the triceps muscle. A shoulder shrug test should also be performed to assess the trapezius and to ensure there is no evidence of spinal accessory nerve injury. The patient is placed in the supine position and the specific test for anterior shoulder instability is then performed.

The apprehension test is the most widely used test for anterior glenohumeral instability (Fig. 2). A positive test is represented by an expression of apprehension as the humeral head is placed in a position that causes subluxation or impending dislocation. The patient is usually placed in the supine position with the shoulder toward the edge of the bed. With the arm in 90 degrees of abduction, the elbow

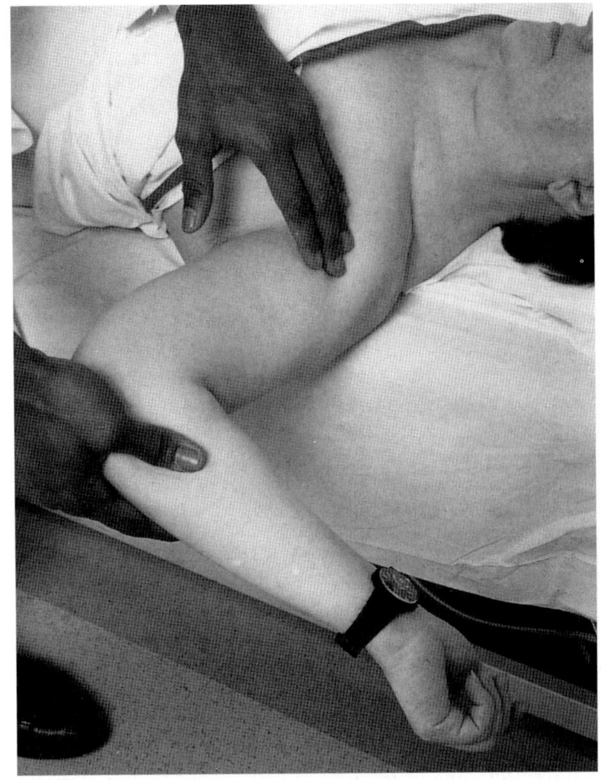

FIG. 2. Apprehension test. The patient is supine and the shoulder is placed in 90-degree abduction. The arm is externally rotated until the patient expresses apprehension with verbal cues, facial expression or reflex muscular contraction.

is grasped with one hand and the arm is slowly externally rotated. The other hand is placed at the level of the joint to guard against any sudden instability episodes. The test is considered positive if the patient expresses *apprehension* that the shoulder will dislocate from further external rotation by verbal communication, facial expression, or by reflex contracture of the shoulder muscles. It has been suggested that shoulder *pain* with the arm in the apprehension position in the overhead athlete is consistent with underlying glenohumeral instability even if *apprehension* is absent (52). Clinically, pain with apprehension testing may also be seen in patients with shoulder impingement.

The relocation test can be used to differentiate between anterior instability and impingement (52,53). It is usually performed at the same time as the apprehension test while the patient is in the supine position (Fig. 3). With the arm in abduction and external rotation—the apprehension position—a posteriorly directed force is applied to the proximal humerus. If there is a resultant decrease in apprehension, the patient may allow further external rotation of the arm. Diminished apprehension or pain with the posteriorly directed force is consistent with a positive relocation test. It has been demonstrated that the relocation test is not specific for shoulder instability (62). Patients with rotator cuff tendinitis or partial rotator cuff tears may obtain relief of

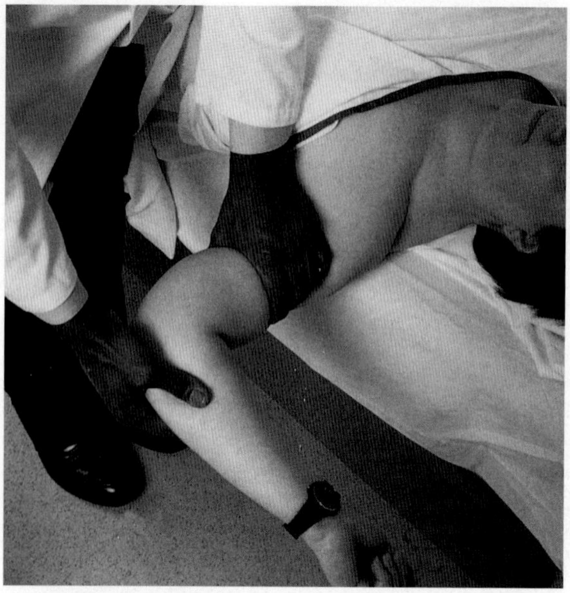

FIG. 3. Relocation test. With the arm in the apprehension position, a posteriorly directed force is applied. A diminished sense of apprehension signifies a positive relocation test.

pain with the relocation test. With the arm abducted and externally rotated, the under surface of the tendon may impinge on the posterosuperior glenoid rim resulting in internal impingement. When a posteriorly directed force is applied, the rotator cuff is directed away from the posterosuperior glenoid rim, resulting in pain relief. A positive relocation test, in which apprehension is eliminated, appears to be a more specific test for anterior instability than a relocation test in which pain is eliminated because this response can be seen in patients with instability and rotator cuff disease.

The load-and-shift (drawer) test can be used to establish the degree of symptomatic translation of the humeral head relative to the glenoid and to assess whether this translation is adequate to reproduce the patient's symptoms. The test can be performed in a seated or supine position (Fig. 4). The examiner stands behind the patient and places one hand over the acromion and scapula to stabilize the shoulder, while the other hand cups the proximal humerus with the thumb on the posterior joint line and the index finger on the anterior aspect of the shoulder to assess the degree of translation in the posterior and inferior directions, respectively. The humeral head is *loaded* by pushing it into the glenoid fossa and is moved relative to the glenoid in the AP direction *(shifting)*, while the degree of translation is recorded. Any pain, crepitation, and apprehension should also be noted.

I prefer to perform this test with the patient in the supine position (Fig. 5). It is imperative that the patient be relaxed for the test to be clinically useful. The contralateral extremity is examined first to gain the patient's confidence. The arm is initially abducted to approximately 45 degrees in the scapular plane and neutral rotation. The scapula should be grasped with one hand while the other hand cups the elbow. An axial load is applied to the humerus with the hand grasping the elbow to compress the humeral head into the glenoid fossa *(loading)*. The hand that was initially on the scapula is then moved to the proximal humerus, and the humeral head is *shifted* relative to the glenoid marking the degree of translation and the reproduction of crepitation or pain.

The humerus can also be placed in flexion, adduction, and internal rotation, and loaded posteriorly, to assess whether there is any excessive translation or crepitation or pain with this maneuver. The degree of translation with the load-and-shift test can be graded (63):

Grade I: Increased translation relative to the contralateral side, to the glenoid rim, but not over the glenoid edge
Grade II: Translation over the glenoid rim with spontaneous reduction when the force is removed
Grade III: Translation beyond the glenoid rim, but no spontaneous reduction when the pressure is removed corresponding to glenohumeral joint dislocation

The Sulcus sign test is performed with the patient standing. It is routinely performed in patients with shoulder instability and provides a clinical assessment of inferior capsular laxity. The test is performed by standing in front of the

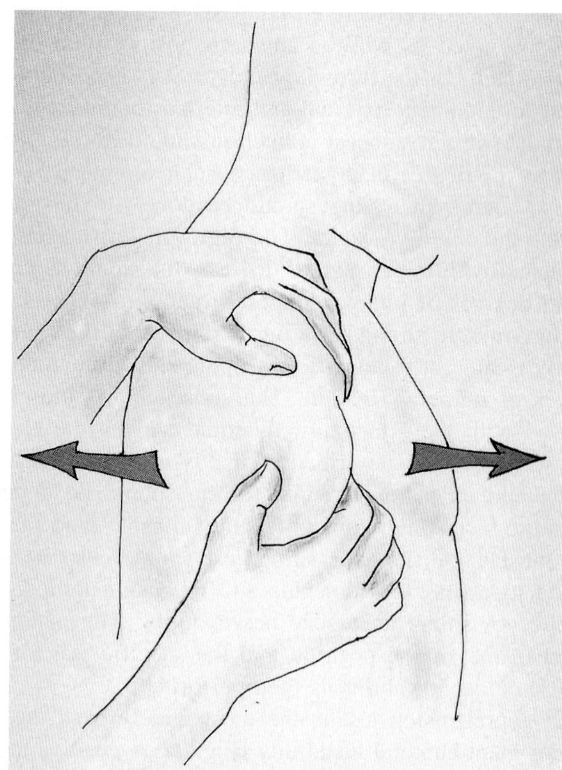

FIG. 4. Load-and-shift test. The patient is usually seated or standing. Translation in the posteroanterior plane is assessed with the thumb and index fingers on the humeral head. The humeral head is loaded by centering it into the glenoid fossa before translation (shifting).

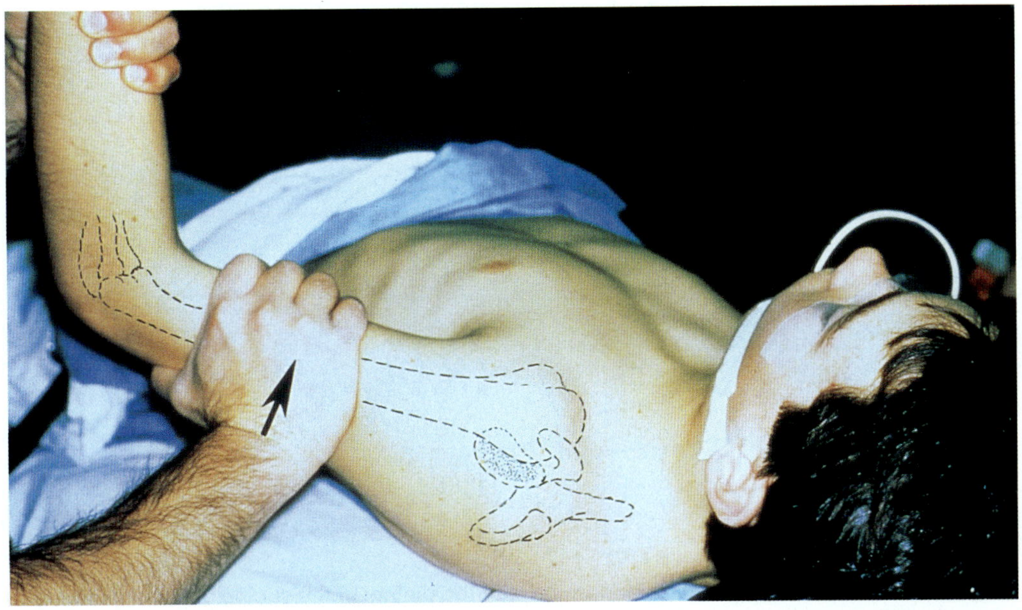

FIG. 5. Drawer testing in the supine position. (Courtesty of Jon J. P. Warner, M.D.)

patient and simultaneously applying a downward traction force to both extremities; that is, the examiner grasps both forearms of the patient and applies an axial load down the arm (Fig. 6). In patients with excessive inferior capsular laxity, there is increased translation between the lateral border of the acromion and the top of the humeral head; i.e., a sulcus develops. The degree of translation can be graded clinically. Less than 1 cm is equivalent to a 1+ sulcus, 1 to 2 cm is equivalent to a 2+ sulcus, and more than 2 cm is consistent with a 3- sulcus. It has been suggested that a 3+ sulcus is pathognomonic of multidirectional instability (64).

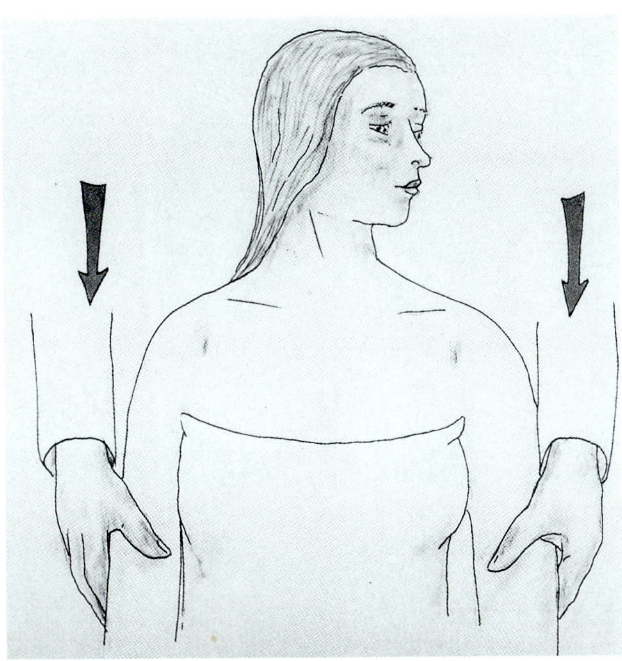

FIG. 6. Sulcus sign. The patient is usually standing, and a longitudinal traction is applied to the arm. A sulcus or dimpling at the lateral border of the acromion is consistent with a positive test.

Fixed (Locked) Anterior Dislocation

The diagnosis of a locked anterior dislocation is usually made by examining the patient posteriorly and noting the absence of the prominence of the deltoid. There may be a fullness and deformity in the anterior aspect of the joint. Patients may have surprisingly good function with activities of daily living. There may some limitation of rotation. In older patients, the possibility of a chronic rotator cuff tear should be considered. The diagnosis is usually confirmed by radiographs.

Acute Posterior Dislocations/Subluxation

Most cases of acute posterior dislocations or subluxation will reduce spontaneously. These patients will have some tenderness to palpation of the posterior joint and are usually reluctant to move the arm. Passive range of motion is usually normal. There may be some weakness of external rotation. The posterior stress test and the Jerk test may be positive. If the dislocation is locked, there is relative flattening of the anterior aspect of the shoulder with posterior prominence and rounding of the posterior aspect of the shoulder as compared with the contralateral extremity. When viewed from the front, there is frequently anterior prominence of the coracoid. External rotation of the arm beyond the neutral position is usually not possible. The pos-

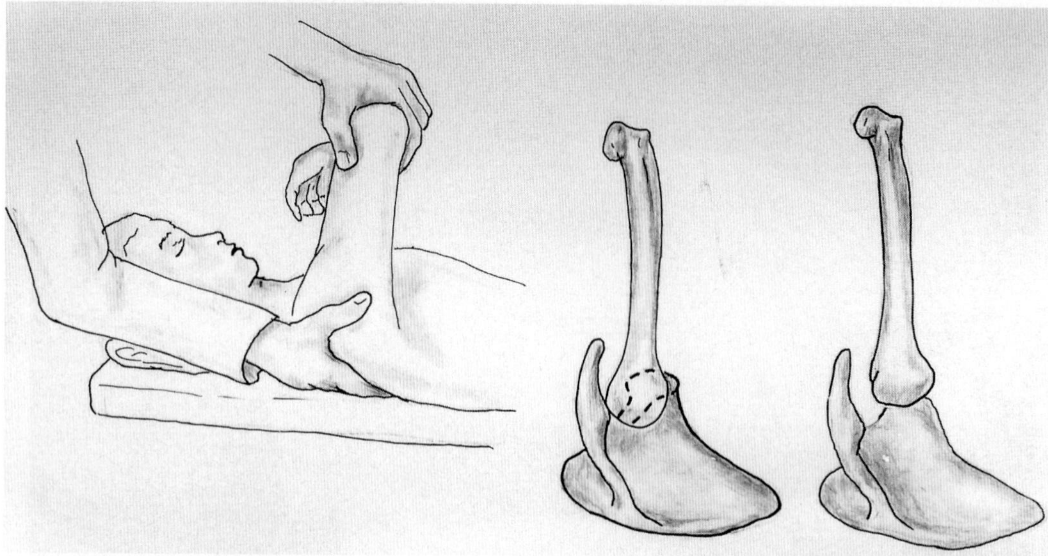

FIG. 7. Posterior stress test. The test is performed with the patient in the supine position. A positive test is confirmed with palpable luxation of the humeral head over the glenoid rim. (From Warner JJP, Caborn DN. Overview of shoulder instability. *Crit Rev Phys Rehabil Med* 1992;4:145–198, with permission.)

sibility of a concomitant injury to the lesser tuberosity proximal humerus and rotator cuff should also be considered.

Recurrent Posterior Instability

In general, patients with chronic posterior subluxation or recurrent posterior dislocations will have more subtle clinical findings. There is usually no obvious deformity, but there can be some atrophy of the external rotators. Posterior joint line tenderness may be the result of posterior synovitis. Crepitation along the posterior joint line may be consistent with a labral or chondral injury. Range of motion and strength testing are often normal, although some patients may have weakness in external rotation. Patients are often able to reproduce their symptoms by placing the arm in forward elevation, adduction and internal rotation. Specific tests to assess posterior instability include the posterior stress test (Fig. 7) and the Jerk test. The posterior stress test is usually performed with the patient in the supine position. The arm is placed in approximately 90 degrees of forward flexion and then internally rotated while a posterior force is applied down the shaft of the humerus. A positive test corresponds to pain, crepitation, or an audible clunk as the humeral head shifts over the glenoid. This is similar to the Jerk test, which is performed with the patient's arm placed in flexion and internal rotation, while the elbow is flexed to 90 degrees; a posterior force is applied down the shaft of the humerus by pushing on the flexed elbow. The shoulder is then brought into extension beyond the plane of the scapula and a palpable and often painful audible shift will occur as the humeral head reduces over the glenoid rim and into the glenoid fossa from a subluxed position. The load-and-shift (drawer) test can also be used to assess a posterior instability. With posterior drawer testing with the arm abducted and internally rotated, instability, pain and crepitation can occur with reproduction of the patient's symptoms.

Fixed (Chronic) Posterior Dislocations

The hallmark of a chronic locked posterior dislocation is limited external rotation (less than zero degrees) and limited

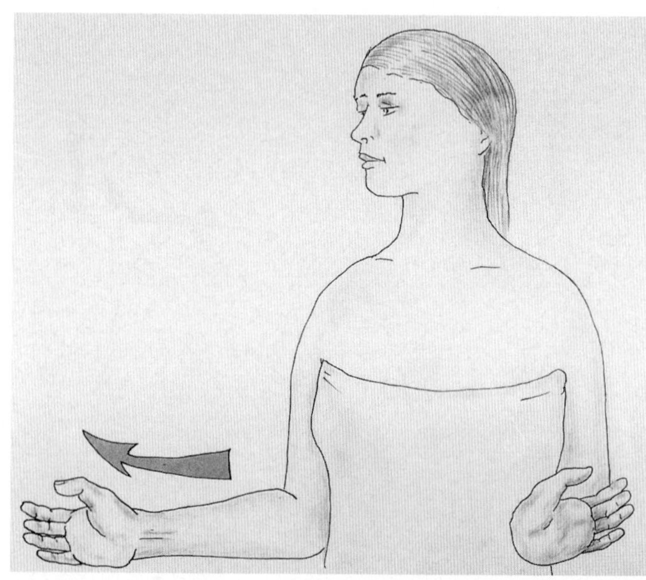

FIG. 8. Patient with chronic (locked) posterior dislocation. The patient is unable to rotate the arm externally, and the shoulder appears shorter on the left, as compared with the right.

active forward flexion of the arm (less than 100 degrees) (Fig. 8). As in the acute locked posterior dislocation, there is relative flattening of the anterior aspect of the shoulder with posterior prominence and rounding of the posterior aspect of the shoulder, as compared with the contralateral extremity. When viewed from the front, there is often anterior prominence of the coracoid. The possibility of concomitant to the lesser tuberosity, proximal humerus, and rotator cuff tears should be considered. The size of the anteromedial humeral head defect and chronicity of the injury are important prognostic factors (34,37).

PRIOR SURGERY

Historically, many of the reconstructive procedures for glenohumeral instability emphasized a nonanatomic approach and resulted in significant complications (65–70). Current techniques of shoulder stabilization are based on an anatomic approach designed to restore normal anatomy by addressing the specific anatomic problem in a given situation. Recurrent anterior instability is the most common complication after anterior shoulder stabilization. Recurrence rates for arthroscopic and open anterior stabilization can range from 0% to 50% (48,71). Common causes of recurrent instability include an incorrect initial diagnosis and subsequent inadequate or inappropriate surgical procedures. Another common complication is loss of motion, usually external rotation with the arm at the side or in abduction. Excessive unidirectional overtightening may cause increased articular forces and subsequent glenohumeral joint arthritis (72–74).

In patients with failed posterior instability repair, the usual causes include trauma, incorrect diagnosis, and inappropriate patient selection. Patients with uncontrolled seizures, voluntary dislocators with character, and emotional disorders are poor candidates for surgery. Glenohumeral arthritis may also develop after excessively tight posterior repairs. Patients with posterior instability repairs are more likely to have capsulorraphy arthritis than those with anterior instability repairs (75).

The history should be detailed; it should document the circumstances and symptoms surrounding the initial instability episodes and the nature of the treatment rendered. In cases in which surgery has been performed, obtaining the operative records and medical reports documenting the preoperative and postoperative care can be extremely helpful. If possible, a history should be obtained from the patient's previous surgeon and physical therapist. A detailed history should be obtained from the patient regarding the onset of instability after the initial surgery. Patients with recurrent traumatic instability will often recall a specific event that caused the instability episode. This is often a similar mechanism to the index dislocation.

In patients with atraumatic onset of instability symptoms, the patient's complaints and clinical symptoms may be more subtle. It is important to compare the patient's current symptoms with those experienced before the index operation. What specific activities tend to cause the current symptoms? How often do these episodes occur? Are there certain arm positions that duplicate these symptoms? Has there been any use of orthotic devices? Do these devices help prevent the instability episodes?

The issue of patient motivation and secondary gain should also be considered when obtaining the history. Workers compensation claims, pending litigation, and emotional and character problems may be significant counfounding variables. Other causes of the patient's symptoms that were missed at the initial evaluation, such as underlying neurologic conditions, should also be considered.

Physical Examination

The physical examination should be thorough, proceeding in the same manner described for anterior and posterior shoulder instability. The cervical spine should be examined, and the patient should be assessed for generalized ligamentous laxity. The uninvolved shoulder should be examined first to gain the patient's confidence and to provide a baseline for comparison. Upon evaluation of the involved shoulder, the type and location of the previous incision should be noted. This can provide some clues as to the type of procedure that was attempted. The character of the scar should also be documented. Excessively wide scars may suggest an underlying connective tissue or collagen disorder. There is always some degree of muscle atrophy after instability surgery. The deltoid and the infraspinatus muscles should be examined carefully. If there is any suggestion of an axillary nerve or suprascapular nerve injury, an EMG and neurologic consultation should be obtained before any further surgical intervention.

Systematic palpation of the acromioclavicular joint, sternoclavicular joints, the tuberosities, biceps tendon, and joint line should be performed.

Active and passive ranges of motion of the involved and uninvolved extremities are compared. Forward elevation and internal and external rotation with the arm at the side and in abduction are recorded. Range of motion should be recorded in all planes and any limitation, as compared with the contralateral extremity, noted. Motion may be limited in specific planes. Excessive tightening of the anterior or posterior capsule can lead to posterior and anterior subluxation of the humeral head, respectively, resulting in symptomatic subluxation of the shoulder. It is also important to observe the shoulder as the arm is brought through a range of motion. In patients with posterior instability, flexion, abduction, and internal rotation may cause spontaneous audible posterior subluxation or dislocation of the shoulder. It is important to observe the patient's reaction to any subluxation or dislocation of the joint.

Muscle strength testing is then performed. There is often

some relative weakness after instability surgery. Profound muscle weakness may be associated with nerve injury or tendon rupture.

The specific tests for glenohumeral instability are then performed. Apprehension testing, relocation testing, drawer testing, and sulcus sign testing are the usual tests for anterior glenohumeral instability. Patients with posterior instability are evaluated with the posterior stress test, drawer test, and the Jerk test. The Sulcus sign should also be performed to screen for occult multidirectional instability.

COMPLICATIONS

Anterior Dislocations

The most common complication after traumatic anterior glenohumeral dislocation is recurrent dislocation. The primary factor that influences the redislocation rate is the age of the patient at the time of the initial dislocation. It has been suggested that in patients younger than 20 years of age, the redislocation rate is 80% to 92% (24). In patients older than 40 years of age, the dislocation rates drop to 10% to 15%. Hovelius (29) and Simonet and Cofield (27) also observed an increased recurrence rate in younger patients with decreasing recurrence as the patient's age increases. The incidence of recurrence appears to be independent of the type and duration of immobilization (30).

Rotator cuff injuries occur relatively frequently after an anterior glenohumeral dislocation. The incidence of rotator cuff tears appears to be age related. In patients older than 40 years of age, the incidence is approximately 30% (76, 77); by age 60, the incidence exceeds 80% (76,78). Rotator cuff tears can also occur in the younger population and are often seen in the context of high-energy trauma to the shoulder, as in skiing accidents and motor vehicular accidents. In these circumstances, the possibility of a subscapularis tendon rupture should also be considered. Sometimes the presence of an axillary nerve injury can make the diagnosis of a rotator cuff tear confusing. When nerve injury or rotator cuff injury is suspected, appropriate electromyographic and imaging studies should be obtained.

Nerve injuries occur frequently after traumatic anterior glenohumeral instability. The incidence may be as high as 35% (56). Although the axillary nerve is most frequently injured, brachial plexopathy and isolated injuries to the musculocutaneous, radial, ulnar, and median nerves can also occur. Blom and Dahlback (56) reported a 35% incidence of axillary nerve injuries in 73 patients with anterior dislocation or fracture of the humeral neck. The incidence of nerve injury appears to be influenced by the age of the patient at the time of the dislocation, the extent of trauma responsible for the dislocation, and the duration of time before the shoulder is reduced.

Although vascular injuries are often seen in the context of fracture-dislocations of the shoulder, they are highly unusual in patients with anterior shoulder dislocations. It appears that older patients with relatively fragile vessels and a previous history of dislocations are more susceptible to vascular injuries (57,58).

Anterior glenoid rim fractures and proximal humerus fractures can also occur after a traumatic anterior glenohumeral dislocation. Nondisplaced greater tuberosity fractures are not uncommon after dislocations in younger patients. In older patients, there is a greater possibility of a proximal humeral fracture, and radiographs should be obtained before a reduction maneuver is attempted.

Posterior Dislocation

Posterior glenoid rim fractures and proximal humerus fractures occur relatively frequently in patients with traumatic posterior dislocations of the shoulder (34,37). Posterior glenoid rim occurs as the humerus is forced out of the glenoid fossa. Compression fractures of the anteromedial aspect of the proximal humeral head are characteristic of a traumatic posterior dislocation. This is called a reverse Hill-Sachs lesion. In locked posterior dislocations, the posterior rim of the glenoid is impacted into the anteromedial head of the proximal humerus. Avulsion of the lesser tuberosity is often seen in patients with posterior dislocations caused by contraction of the subscapularis tendon.

Although rotator cuff tears are not usually seen with shoulder dislocations, ruptures of the supraspinatus tendon after posterior dislocations have been found under experimental conditions (41,42). Neurovascular injury is not a consistent feature of posterior shoulder dislocations.

REFERENCES

1. Gerber CH, Ganz R. Clinical assessment of instability of the shoulder with special reference to anterior and posterior drawer tests. *J Bone Joint Surg [Br]* 1984;66B:551–556.
2. Lippitt S, Matsen F. Mechanism of glenohumeral joint stability. *Clin Orthop* 1993;291:20.
3. Mallon WJ, Speer KP. Multidirectional instability: current concepts. *J Shoulder Elbow Surg* 1995;4:54.
4. Neer CS, Foster CR. Inferior capsular shift for involuntary and multidirectional instability of the shoulder. *J Bone Joint Surg [Am]* 1980;62A:897.
5. Rowe CR, Zarins B. Chronic unreduced dislocations of the shoulder. *J Bone Joint Surg [Am]* 1982;64A:494.
6. Rowe CR, Pierce DS, Clark JG. Voluntary dislocation of the shoulder. *J Bone Joint Surg [Am]* 1973;55A:445.
7. Sillman JF, Hawkins RJ. Classification and physical diagnosis of instability of the shoulder. *Clin Orthop* 1993;291:7.
8. Warner JJP, Caborn DN. Overview of shoulder instability. *Crit Rev Phys Rehabil Med* 1992;4:145–198.
9. Gold AM. Fractured neck of the humerus with separation and dislocation of the humeral head (fracture-dislocation of the shoulder, severe type). *Bull Hosp Joint Dis* 1971;32:87–99.
10. Mosley HF. The basic lesions of recurrent anterior dislocation. *Surg Clin North Am* 1963;43:1631–1634.
11. Patel MR, Pardee ML, Singerman RC. Intrathoracic dislocation of the head of the humerus. *J Bone Joint Surg [Am]* 1963;45A:1712–1714.
12. Saxena K, Stavas J. Inferior glenohumeral dislocation. *Ann Emerg Med* 1983;12:718–720.
13. West EF. Intrathoracic dislocation of the humerus. *J Bone Joint Surg [Br]* 1949;31B:61–62.

14. Symeonide PP. The significance of the subscapularis muscle in the pathogenesis of recurrent anterior dislocation of the shoulder. *J Bone Joint Surg [Br]* 1972;54B:476–483.
15. Bankart AS. Recurrent or habitual dislocation of the shoulder joint. *BMJ* 1923;2:1132–1133.
16. Bankart AS. The pathology and treatment of recurrent dislocation of the joint. *Br J Surg* 1938;26:23–29.
17. Reeves B. Arthrography in acute dislocation of the shoulder. *J Bone Joint Surg [Br]* 1966;48B:182.
18. Moseley HF, Overgaard B. The anterior capsular mechanism in recurrent anterior dislocation of the shoulder: morphological and clinical studies with special reference to the glenoid labrum and the glenohumeral ligaments. *J Bone Joint Surg [Br]* 1962;48B:913–927.
19. Cave EF, Burke JF, Boyd RJ. *Trauma management*. Chicago: Year Book, 1974.
20. Rowe CR. Prognosis in dislocations of the shoulder. *J Bone Joint Surg [Am]* 1956;38A:957–977.
21. Baker CL, Uribe JW, Whitman C. Arthroscopic evaluation of acute initial anterior shoulder dislocations. *Am J Sports Med* 1990;18:25–28.
22. Glessner JR. Intrathoracic dislocation of the humeral head. *J Bone Joint Surg [Am]* 1961;42A:428–430.
23. Caird FM. The shoulder joint in relation to certain dislocations and fractures. *Edinb Med J* 1887;32:708.
24. McLaughlin HL, Cavaliaro WU. Primary anterior dislocation of the shoulder. *Am J Surg* 1950;80:615–621.
25. Adams JC. Recurrent dislocation of the shoulder. *J Bone Joint Surg [Br]* 1948;30B:26,38.
26. Rowe CR. Instabilities of the glenohumeral joint. *Bull Hosp Joint Dis* 1978;39:180–186.
27. Simonet WT, Cofield RH. Prognosis in anterior shoulder dislocation. *Orthop Trans* 1983;8:70.
28. Aronen JG, Regan K. Decreasing the incidence of occurrence of first time anterior dislocations with rehabilitation. *Am J Sports Med* 1984;12:283–291.
29. Hovelius L. Anterior dislocation of the shoulder in teenagers and young adults: five-year prognosis. *J Bone Joint Surg [Am]* 1987;69A: 393–399.
30. Hovelius L, Akermark C, Albrektsson B, et al. Bristow-Latarjet procedure for recurrent anterior dislocation of the shoulder: a 2-5 year follow-up study on the results of 112 cases. *Acta Orthop Scand* 1983: 54:284–290.
31. Blazina ME, Satzman JS. Recurrent anterior subluxation of the shoulder in athletics: a distinct entity. *J Bone Joint Surg [Am]* 1969;51A: 1037–1038.
32. Protzman RR. Anterior instability of the shoulder. *J Bone Joint Surg [Am]* 1980;62A:909–918.
33. Rowe CR, Zarins B. Recurrent transient subluxation of the shoulder. *J Bone Joint Surg [Am]* 1981;63A:863–872.
34. McLaughlin HL. Posterior dislocation of the shoulder. *J Bone Surg [Am]* 1952;34A:584.
35. Fronek J, Warren RF, Bowen M. Posterior subluxation of the glenohumeral joint. *J Bone Joint Surg [Am]* 1989;71:205–216.
36. Bowen MK, Warren RF. Surgical approaches to posterior instability of the shoulder: operative technique. *Sports Med* 1993;1:301–310.
37. Hawkins RJ, Neer CS II, Pianta RM, et al. Locked posterior dislocation of the shoulder. *J Bone Joint Surg [Am]* 1987;69A:9–18.
38. Ahlgren O, Lorentzon R, Larsson SE. Posterior dislocation of the shoulder associated with general seizures. *Acta Orthop Scand* 1981;52:694–695.
39. Nobel W. Posterior traumatic dislocation of the shoulder. *J Bone Joint Surg [Am]* 1962;44A:523–538.
40. Hill NA, McLaughlin HL. Locked posterior dislocation simulating a "frozen shoulder." *J Trauma* 1963;3:225–234.
41. Ovesen J, Nielsen S. Anterior and posterior instability: a cadaver study. *Acta Orthop Scand* 1985;57:324–338.
42. Ovesen J, Sojbjerg JO. Posterior shoulder dislocation: muscle and capsular lesions in cadaver experiments. *Acta Orthop Scand* 1986;57: 535.
43. Moeller JC. Compound posterior dislocation of the glenohumeral joint: case report. *J Bone Joint Surg [Am]* 1975;57A:1006–1007.
44. Rockwood CA Jr. Subluxation of the shoulder: the classification, diagnosis, and treatment. *Orthop Trans* 1979;3:306.
45. Pagnani MJ, Warren RF. Multidirectional instability: medial T-Plasty and selective capsular repairs. *Sports Med Arthrosc Rev* 1993;1:249–258.
46. Roca LA, Riamos-Vertiz JR. Luxacion erecta de hombro. *Rev San Mil Arg* 1962;61:135.
47. Peiro A, Ferrandis R, Correa F. Bilateral erect dislocation of the shoulders. *Injury* 1975;6:294–295.
48. Matsen FA III, Thomas SC, Rockwood CA Jr. Anterior glenohumeral instability. In: Rockwood CA Jr, Matsen FA III, eds. *The shoulder*. Philadelphia: WB Saunders, 1990:526–622.
49. Stimson LA. *A practical treatise on fractures and dislocations*, 7th ed. Philadelphia: Lea & Febiger, 1912.
50. Pappas AM, Goss TP, Kleinman PK. Symptomatic shoulder instability due to lesions of the glenoid labrum. *Am J Sports Med* 1983;11: 279.
51. Walch G, Bioleau P, Noel E, Donnell ST. Impingement on the deep surface of the supraspinatus tendon on the posterosuperior glenoid rim: an arthroscopic study. *J Shoulder Elbow Surg* 1992;1:238–245.
52. Jobe FW, Bradley JP. The diagnosis and nonoperative treatment of shoulder injuries in athletes. *Clin Sports Med* 1989;8:419.
53. Kvitne RS, Jobe FW. The diagnosis and treatment of anterior shoulder instability in the throwing athlete. *Clin Orthop* 1993;291:107.
54. Hawkins RJ, Schutte JP, Huckle GH. The assessment of glenohumeral translation using manual and fluoroscopic techniques. *Orthop Trans* 1988;12:727.
55. Pollock RG, Bigliani LU. Recurrent posterior shoulder instability. Diagnosis and treatment. *Clin Orthop* 1993;291:85–96.
56. Blom S, Dahlback LO. Nerve injuries in dislocations of the shoulder joint and fractures of the neck of the humerus: a clinical and electromyelographic study. *Acta Chir Scand* 1970;136:461–466.
57. Baratta JB, Lim V, Mastromonaco E, et al. Axillary artery disruption secondary to anterior dislocation of the shoulder. *J Trauma* 1983;23: 1009–1011.
58. Curr JF. Rupture of the axillary artery complicating dislocation of the shoulder: report of a case. *J Bone Joint Surg [Br]* 1970;52B:313–317.
59. Beighton P, Grahame R, Bird H. Assessment of hypermobility. In: Beighton P, Grahame R, Bird H, eds. *Hypermobility of joints*. Heidelberg: Springer-Verlag, 1983:9–24.
60. Beighton P, Solomon L, Soskolne CL. Articular mobility in an African population. *Ann Rheum Dis* 1973;32:413–416.
61. Kelly BT, Kadimas WR, Speer KP. The manual muscle examination for rotator cuff strength. *Am J Sports Med* 1996;24:581–588.
62. Speer KP, Hannafin JA, Altchek DW, et al. An evaluation of the shoulder relocation test. *Am J Sports Med* 1994;22:177–183.
63. Altchek DW, Warren RF, Skyhar MJ, et al. T-plasty modification of the Bankart procedure for multidirectional instability of the anterior and inferior types. *J Bone Joint Surg [Am]* 1991;73:105–112.
64. Norris TR. Diagnostic techniques of shoulder instability. *AAOS Course Lectures* 1985;34:239.
65. Morrey BF, Janes JM. Recurrent anterior dislocation of the shoulder: long-term follow-up of the Putti-Platt and Bankart procedures. *J Bone Joint Surg [Am]* 1976;58A:252.
66. Miller LS, Donohue JR, Good RP, et al. The Magnuson-Stack procedure for recurrent glenohumeral dislocation. *Am J Sports Med* 1984;12:133.
67. Brav EA. An evaluation of the Putti-Platt reconstruction procedure for recurrent dislocation of the shoulder. *J Bone Joint Surg [Am]* 1985;37A:731.
68. Ferlic DC, DiGiovine NM. A long-term retrospective study of the modified Brislow procedure. *Am J Sports Med* 1988;16:469.
69. Laterjet M. A propos du traitment des luxations recidivantes de l'épaule. *Lyon Clin* 1954;49:994.
70. Torg JS, Balduini FC, Bonci C, et al. A modified Bristow-Helfet-May procedure for recurrent dislocation and subluxation of the shoulder: report of two hundred and twelve cases. *J Bone Joint Surg [Am]* 1987;69A:904.
71. Matsen FA III, Thomas SC. Glenohumeral instability. In: Evarts CM, ed. *Surgery of the musculoskeletal system*. New York: Churchill Livingstone, 1990:1439.
72. Harryman DT II, Sidles JA, Clark JM, et al. Translation of the humeral head on the glenoid with passive glenohumeral motion. *J Bone Joint Surg [Am]* 1990;72A:1334.

73. Matsen FA III, Harryman DT II, Sidles JA, Lippitt SL. *Practical evaluation and management of the shoulder*. Philadelphia: WB Saunders, 1994.
74. Angelo RL, Hawkins RJ. Osteoarthritis following an excessively tight Putti-Platt repair. *Orthop Trans* 1988;12:728.
75. Samilson RL, Prieto V. Dislocation arthropathy of the shoulder. *J Bone Joint Surg [Am]* 1983;65A:456.
76. Pettersson G. Rupture of the tendon aponeurosis of the shoulder joint in antero-inferior dislocation: a study on the origin and occurrence of the ruptures. *Acta Chir Scand* 1942;77(Suppl):1–187.
77. Hawkins RJ, Bell RH, Hawkins RH, Koppert GJ. Anterior dislocation of the shoulder in the older patient. *Clin Orthop* 1986;206:192.
78. Neviaser RJ, Neviaser TJ, Neviaser JS. Concurrent rupture of the rotator cuff and anterior dislocation of the shoulder in the older patient. *J Bone Joint Surg [Am]* 1988;70A:1308.

The Unstable Shoulder,
edited by R.F. Warren, E.V. Craig, and D.W. Altchek.
Lippincott–Raven Publishers, Philadelphia © 1999.

CHAPTER 6

Radiographic Assessment of Shoulder Instability

X-ray and Computed Tomography Scan

Helene Pavlov

The radiographic examination of the shoulder demonstrates bony integrity and alignment and has the potential for documenting evidence of a prior subluxation and/or dislocation, post-traumatic arthritic changes, loose bodies, and/or periarticular calcification and/or ossification. The radiographic examination of the shoulder should be tailored according to the patient's age, symptoms, and suspected clinical concern.

PATIENTS YOUNGER THAN AGE 40

In a patient younger than 40 years of age with an acute dislocation or suspected fracture, or both, the following three radiographic views provide the most cost-efficient maximum diagnostic yield: a *posterior oblique view with the humerus in internal rotation*; a *transcapular "Y" view*; and an *axillary view*. Ideally, the posterior oblique view and transcapular views are performed with the patient standing or sitting as opposed to supine. The posterior oblique view is obtained tangential to the glenohumeral joint performed with the posterior aspect of the affected shoulder rotated 30 to 45 degrees toward the cassette, using either a straight central x-ray beam (the Grashey view) or preferably with the beam angled 20 degrees caudad or 45 degrees caudad, the apical oblique view (1–9) (Fig. 1A). On the posterior oblique view, the anterior and posterior glenoid rims are superimposed and the humeral head and glenoid do not overlap. Overlap of the humeral head and the glenoid on this view suggests a posterior dislocation. The posterior oblique view is distinguished from the routine frontal anteroposterior (AP) view of the shoulder, performed with the patient positioned flat against the cassette, on which there is 50% to 75% overlap of the humeral head with the glenoid (Fig. 1B).

H. Pavlov: Department of Radiology, New York Hospital—Cornell University Medical Center; and Department of Radiology, The Hospital for Special Surgery, New York, New York 10021.

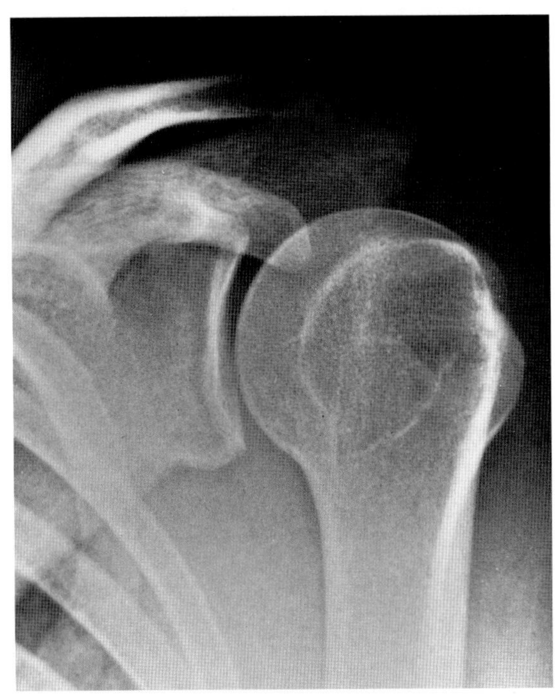

A

FIG. 1. Apical oblique view of the shoulder **(A)** demonstrates the glenohumeral joint in tangent.

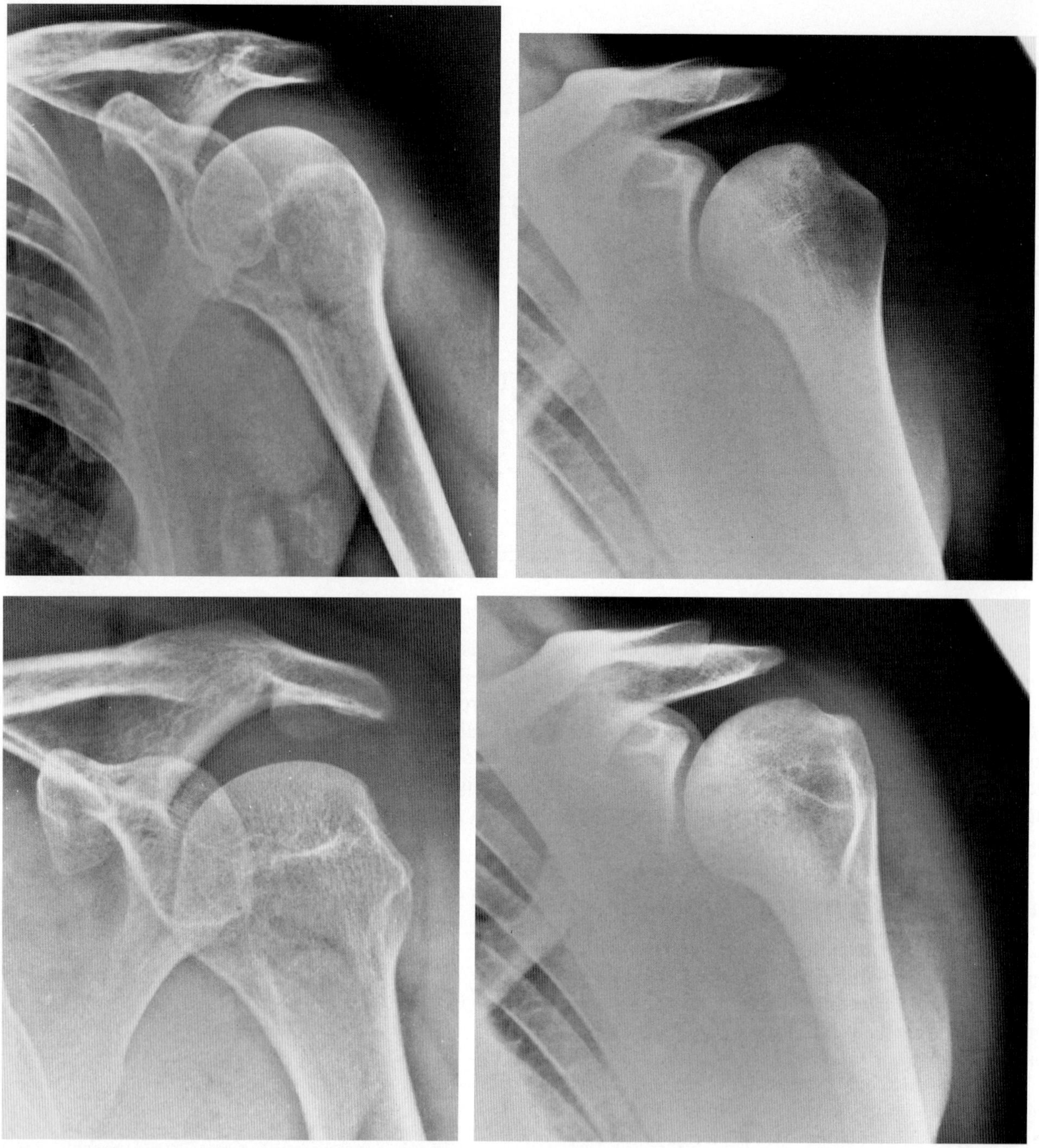

B C D E

FIG. 1. *Continued.* AP view of the shoulder **(B)** demonstrates the glenoid fossa en face with normal overlap of the humeral head and the glenoid by approximately 75%. With the humerus in internal rotation **(A,B)**, the normal humeral head has a round contour like a light bulb . A Hill-Sachs defect is identified as a notched defect **(C)** or as an area of flattening at the posterolateral aspect of the humeral head **(D).** With the humerus in external rotation **(E)** the greater tuberosity is seen in profile.

Internal Rotation

With the humerus in internal rotation, the humeral head has a round ''light bulb'' contour and the greater tuberosity is superimposed on the humeral head (Fig. 1A, B). Internal rotation of the humeral head is sensitive for identifying a Hill-Sachs defect (Fig. 1C, D). When the humerus is in external rotation, the greater tuberosity is visualized in profile (Fig. 1E). External rotation of the humerus is not recommended immediately after reduction of a shoulder dislocation as it places the patient at risk of a redislocation (10).

Transcapular or ''Y'' View

The transcapular or ''Y'' view is obtained with the anterior aspect of the affected shoulder rotated approximately 30 to 45 degrees toward the cassette and the central ray directed through the scapular blade, perpendicular to the x-ray cassette (11–16). On this view, the coracoid process and acromium process intersect with the scapular blade to form a ''Y.'' The glenoid is at the point of intersection and normally the humeral head is superimposed on the glenoid (Fig. 2A). An anterior or posterior dislocation is confirmed on this view by the

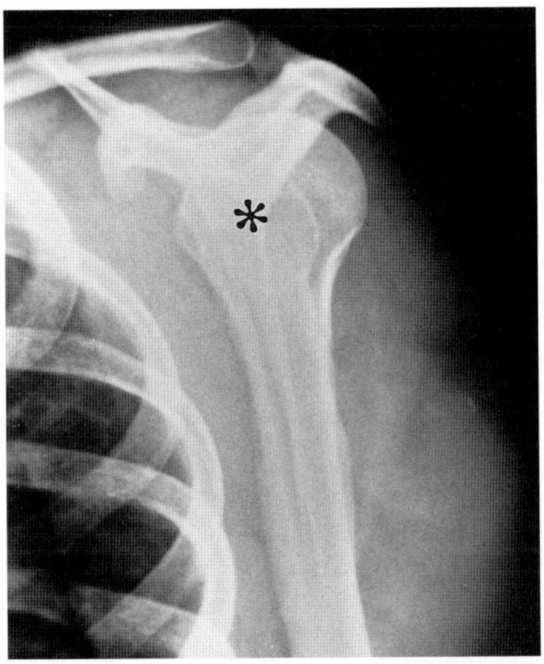

A

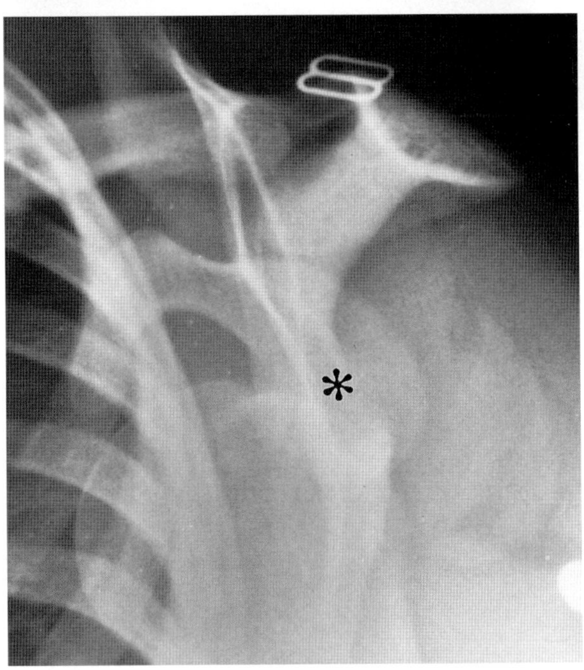

B

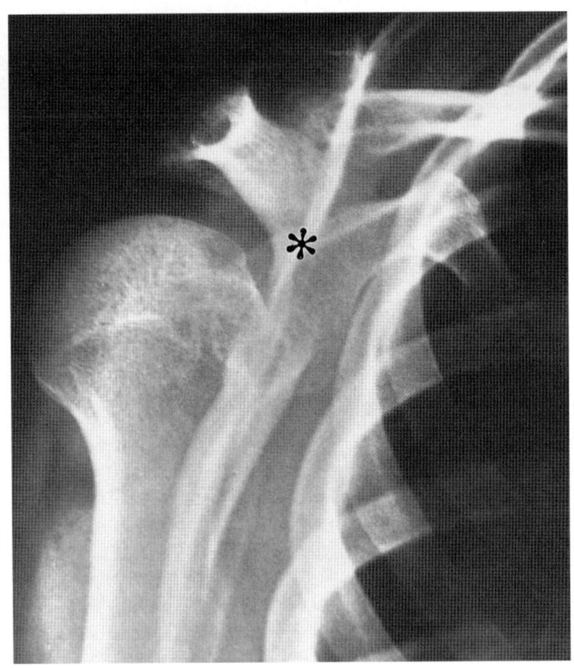

C

FIG. 2. A: Normal transcapular view of the shoulder demonstrates the coracoid process and the acromium process intersecting with the scapular blade at the glenoid (*). The intersection of the coracoid process, the acromium process and the scapular blade form a Y, referred to as a "Y" view. Normally, the humeral head is superimposed on the glenoid. **B:** An anterior dislocation is identified by the position of the humeral head beneath the coracoid process. **C:** A posterior dislocation identified by the position of the humeral head beneath the acromium process.

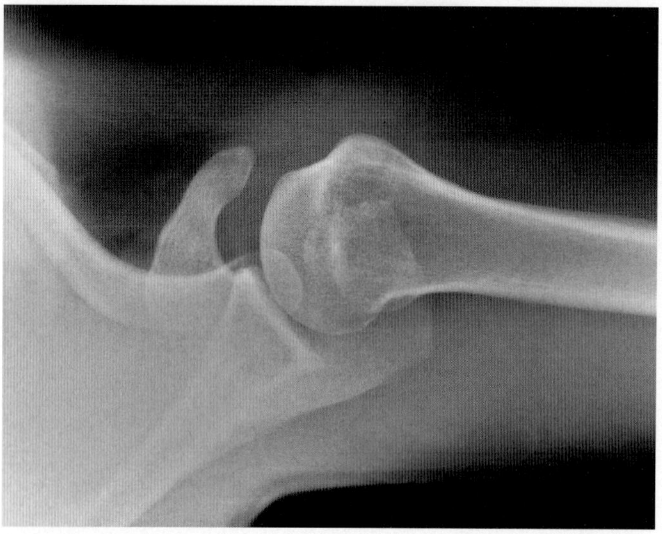

FIG. 3. Axillary view demonstrates the humeral head to be anterior subluxed; the anterior aspect of the glenoid is normal and superimposed on the clavicle.

location of the humeral head either beneath the coracoid process (anterior dislocation) (Fig. 2B) or beneath the acromium process (posterior dislocation) (Fig. 2C).

Axillary View

The axillary view is performed with the patient supine and the shoulder abducted 90 degrees and the central ray directed cephalad to the medial aspect of the joint with the cassette placed superior to the shoulder, perpendicular to the table (17). The arm must never be forcibly abducted in a patient with a recent dislocation as this position repeats the mechanism of injury and the shoulder is easily vulnerable to repeat dislocation (18). This view is difficult to obtain because a patient with shoulder instability or recent dislocation typically will resist arm abduction and also because technical expertise is required to obtain a diagnostic examination. However, this view is sensitive for identifying anterior or posterior subluxation and an osseous Bankart lesion (Fig. 3).

A

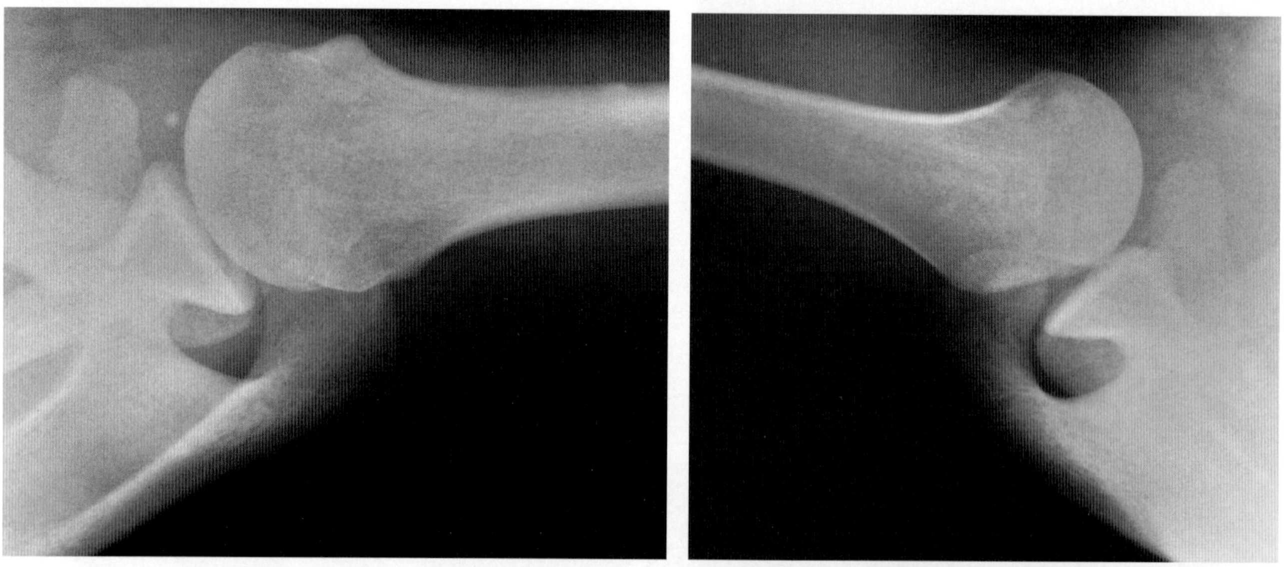

B

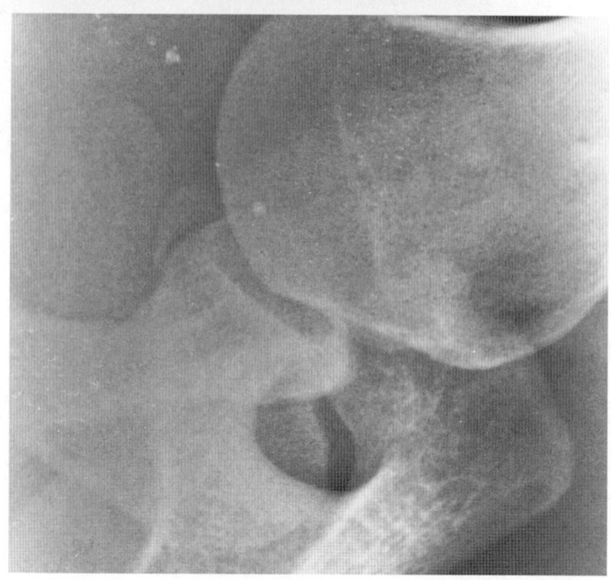

C

FIG. 4. A: The West Point view demonstrates normal glenohumeral joint alignment. The anterior aspect of the glenoid is normal and is not superimposed on bone. **B:** Bankart fracture demonstrated by truncation of an anterior glenoid and anterior subluxation of the humeral head. **C:** An osseous Bankart fracture is identified as a small triangular shaped corticated bony fragment at the anterior aspect of the glenoid. A Hill-Sachs defect is also present in this patient and in 4**B**. (From Pavlov H, Warren RF, Weiss CB, et al. The roentgenographic evaluation of anterior shoulder instability. *Clin Orthop* 1985;194:153–158, with permission.)

PATIENTS YOUNGER THAN AGE 35 TO 40

In a patient under 35 to 40 years of age with chronic instability, the recommended radiographic views are the *posterior oblique view with the humerus in internal rotation, the West Point axillary view and the Stryker Notch view.* The West Point view is performed as a modified prone axillary view as described by Rokous et al. and is obtained with the shoulder abducted 90 degrees with the elbow bent and the arm hanging over the tableside. The hand and arm are positioned so the anterior humeral surface faces the floor (4,17). The x-ray beam is directed cephalad and medially centered inferior and medial to the acromioclavicular joint. The cassette is placed above the shoulder, perpendicular to the table. The West Point view is sensitive for identifying anterior or posterior subluxation and an osseous Bankart lesion (Fig. 4A-C).

The Stryker Notch view is performed with the patient supine and the arm elevated over the head with the palm supporting the back of the head (3,4,20). Technically, the

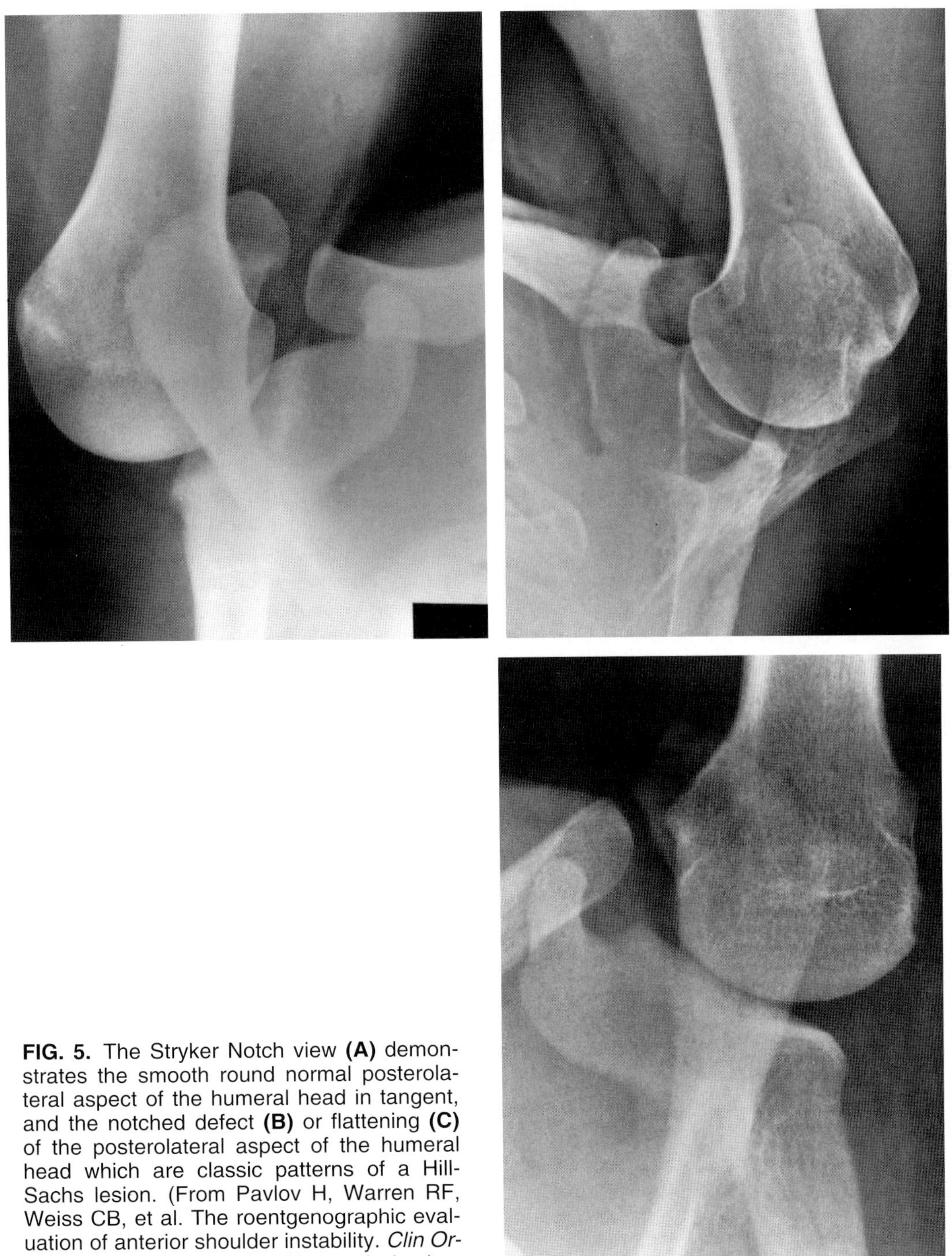

FIG. 5. The Stryker Notch view **(A)** demonstrates the smooth round normal posterolateral aspect of the humeral head in tangent, and the notched defect **(B)** or flattening **(C)** of the posterolateral aspect of the humeral head which are classic patterns of a Hill-Sachs lesion. (From Pavlov H, Warren RF, Weiss CB, et al. The roentgenographic evaluation of anterior shoulder instability. *Clin Orthop* 1985;194:153–158, with permission.)

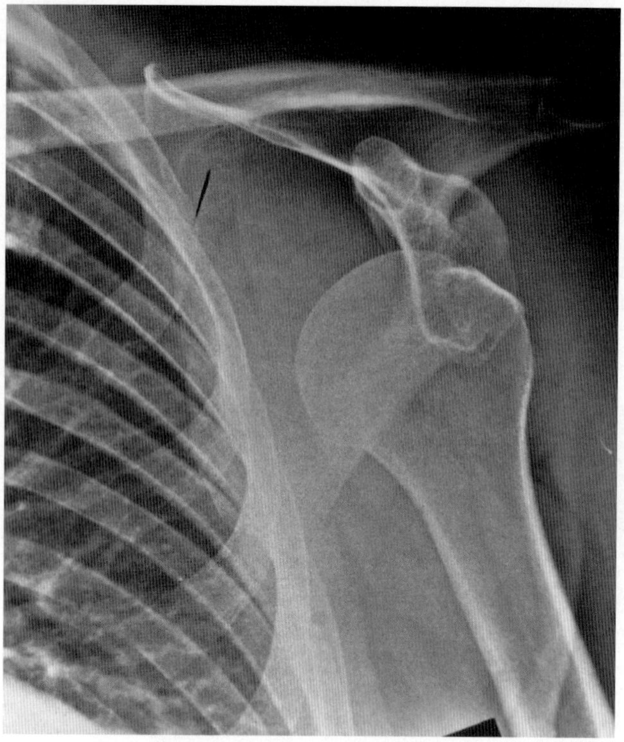

FIG. 6. Anterior subcoracoid dislocation.

critical factor for obtaining a Stryker Notch view is that the humerus is parallel to the longitudinal axis of the body, with the elbow pointing toward the ceiling. On the Stryker Notch view, the posterolateral aspect of the humeral head is seen in tangent and is normally round and smooth and is sensitive for identifying a Hill-Sachs defect (Fig. 5A-C).

Approximately 95% to 97% of all glenohumeral dislocations are anterior (6,11) (Fig. 6). Anterior dislocations occur secondary to forces applied with the shoulder in abduction and external rotation. With an anterior dislocation, the humeral head is displaced inferior to the coracoid or clavicle or, less commonly, the glenoid and rarely intrathoracic, where the humeral head can be trapped between two ribs (19,21). Greater tuberosity fractures are frequent with anterior dislocations and surgical neck fractures with intrathoracic dislocations (21).

Roentgen evidence of a prior anterior dislocation is dependent on the presence of a Hill-Sachs and/or Bankart lesion. The Hill-Sachs defect is a result of the posterolateral aspect of the humeral head impacted against the anterior glenoid rim (22). An indentation, flattening, or notch at the posterolateral aspect of the humeral head is pathognomonic of a Hill-Sachs defect (11,23,24) (Figs. 1C, D and 5B, C). The sensitivity for identifying a Hill-Sachs lesion is 92% on either the frontal view with the humerus in internal rotation or on the Stryker Notch view (4). A Hill-Sachs lesion can be overlooked if the humerus is incompletely internally rotated such that the greater tuberosity projects beyond the posterior lateral contour of the humeral head (4,24).

Incidence of a Hill-Sachs defect is reported at 27% associated with acute anterior dislocation and 50% to 100% (25) or 74% with recurrent anterior dislocations (22). Differences in reported incidences of identifying the Hill-Sachs defect presumably are related to patient selection, available radiographic interpretation and accuracy of interpretation (20). In a study comparing various cohorts of patients, the Hill-Sachs lesion was present in 77% of patients with shoulder instability, with specific incidence of 66% in patients with subluxation; 77% in patients with documented dislocation and 86% in patients with a combination of symptoms (4). Approximately 40% of anterior dislocations are recurrent with increased incidence of recurrences associated with a younger initial onset (26). The Hill-Sachs lesion is reported to be larger when there is a history of recurrent anterior dislocation and/or in association with anteroinferior rather than pure anterior dislocations. There is also reported to be a predilection to redislocation in patients with a Hill-Sachs lesion (18) and increased incidence of dislocation in older patients with a large Hill-Sachs lesion (27).

The Bankart lesion is a fracture of the anterior glenoid rim that occurs at the time of the anterior dislocation (28). Reportedly, approximately 15% of patients with anterior dislocations and 20% of patients with instability incur a Bankart lesion (4,20,29,30). Analysis of specific cohorts of patients showed the incidence of an osseous Bankart lesion to be 40% in patients with subluxation, 15% in patients with documented dislocation, and 20% in patients with both subluxation and dislocation (4). An osseous Bankart lesion is typically evident on the West Point and axillary views; however, a small osseous Bankart lesion may be more readily identified on the West Point view, as compared with the axillary view, because the anterior glenoid is not superimposed on other osseous structures (7,8) (Fig. 4B, C). A large osseous Bankart lesion may be evident on the posterior oblique view (Fig. 7A), Stryker Notch view (Fig. 7B), and even occasionally on the routine frontal view of the shoulder (29) (Fig. 7C).

Posterior glenohumeral dislocations account for only 2% of all glenohumeral dislocations (18); however, more than 50% are overlooked in the initial clinical evaluation (6,31–33). Posterior dislocations occur as a result of an electric shock or epileptic convulsions and can be bilateral (34,35). Clinically, fixed internal rotation with the inability to externally rotate and/or decreased abduction suggests a posterior dislocation (36). Radiographic diagnosis of a posterior dislocation depends on recognition that the humeral head overlaps the glenoid on the posterior oblique view of the glenohumeral joint (Fig. 8A)

FIG. 8. Posterior dislocation identified by the overlap of the humeral head with glenoid on the apical oblique view **(A)** or by the lack of sufficient overlap of the humeral head with the glenoid on the routine AP view **(B)**. Note the associated flattening of the medial aspect of the humeral head. (From Pavlov H, Freiberger RH. Fractures and dislocations about the shoulder. *Semin Roentgenol* 1978;13:85–96, with permission.)

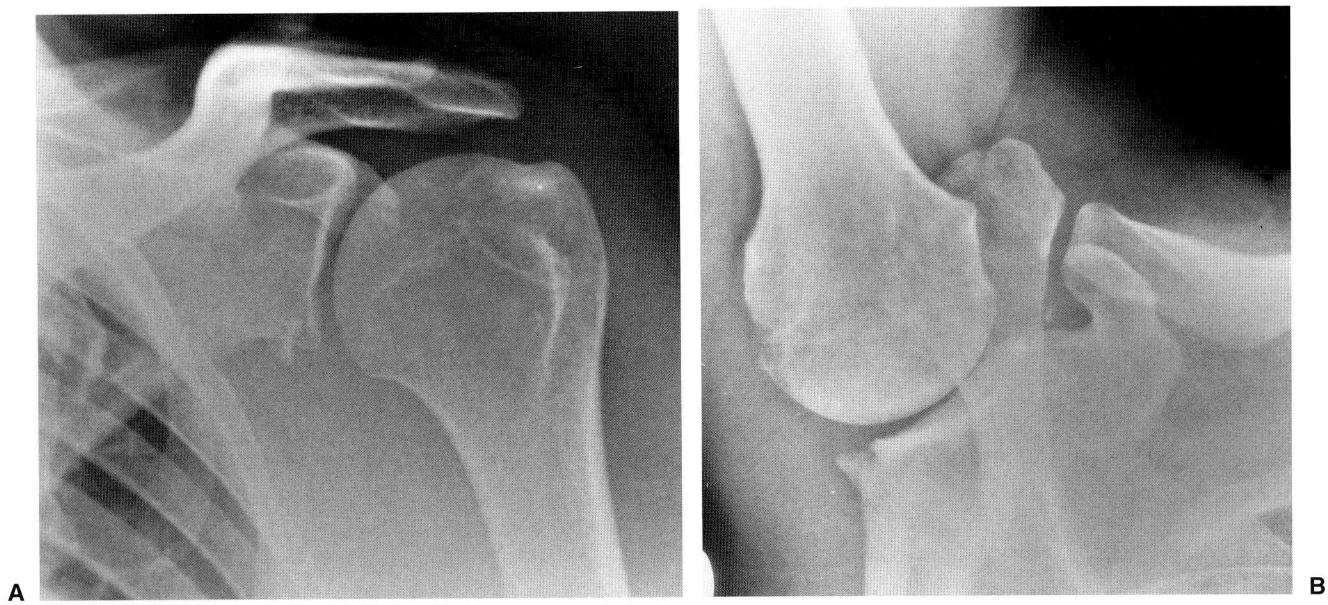

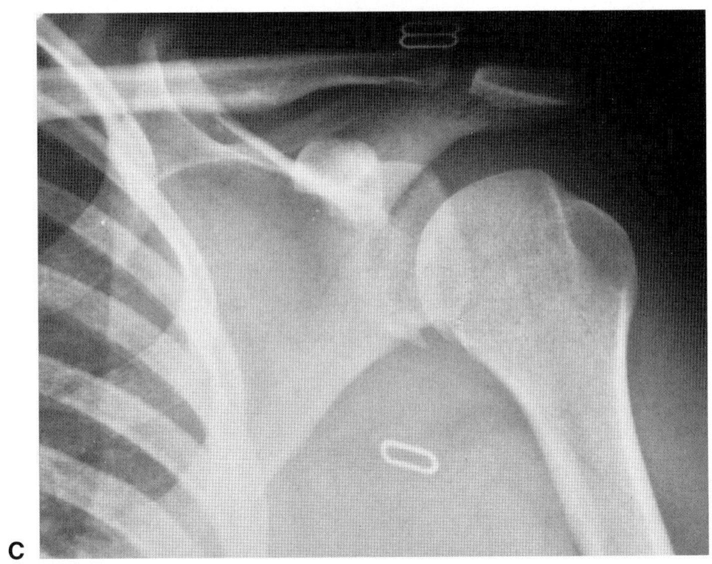

FIG. 7. A large osseous Bankart fracture that extends to the inferior aspect of the anterior glenoid can be identified on the posterior oblique view **(A),** the Stryker Notch view **(B)** and occasionally also on the frontal view of the shoulder **(C)**. Note the associated Hill-Sachs deformities **(B,C)**.

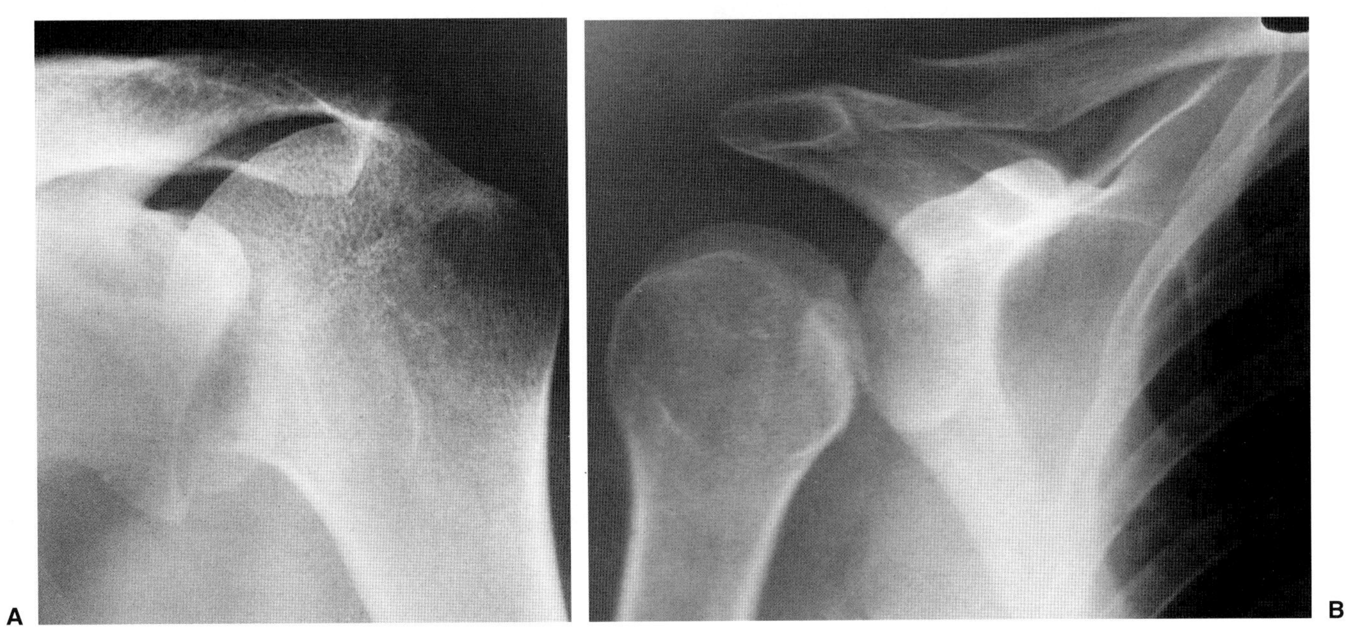

and barely overlaps the glenoid on the routine anteroposterior (AP) view of the shoulder, as opposed to the normal 50% to 75% overlap (Fig. 8B). Unfortunately, if the AP and/or posterior oblique view are not obtained correctly, the degree of overlap can be difficult to assess and identification of a posterior subluxation is also difficult. The West Point, axillary, and transcapular views are excellent projections for diagnosing a suspected posterior dislocation or subluxation.

The *transthoracic view* of the shoulder can also be used in the diagnosis of a posterior dislocation. On this view, there is normally a smooth arch, Maloney's arch, formed by the lateral margin of the scapula and glenoid and inferiomedial margin of the humeral cortex (19). With anterior dislocation, the humeral head disrupts the arch, and with posterior dislocation, the arch forms an acute angle. Overlap of the rib cage and lung parenchyma, however, limits interpretation to the untrained eye, and this view is best used to evaluate the position of proximal humeral shaft fractures as opposed to diagnosing a dislocation (11) (Fig. 9).

Radiographic evidence of a prior posterior dislocation includes flattening of the medial aspect of the humeral head (Fig. 8B) or a *trough sign* (33) (Fig. 10A). The trough sign is formed by the presence of two articular surfaces at the medial aspect of the humeral head secondary to the impaction of the anterior aspect of the humeral head against the posterior aspect of the glenoid (Fig. 10B).

The most common complication of a glenohumeral dislocation is a fracture of the greater or lesser tuberosity; approximately 15% of anterior dislocations are associated with greater tuberosity fractures and, similarly, approximately 15% of posterior dislocations are associated with lesser tuberosity fractures (33). A fat fluid level on the upright (sitting or standing) film confirms an intraarticular fracture (Fig. 11). Isolated lessor tuberosity fractures are rare (37,38). In the skeletally immature patient, especially the adolescent, an isolated fracture may represent an avulsion injury which can usually be identified on the axillary or West Point view or the Stryker Notch view. Additional complications of glenohumeral dislocation include avascular necrosis of the humeral head (39), adhesive capsulitis, periarticular fibrosis, rotator cuff tears, myositis ossificans, or periarticular heterotopic ossifications (39) and/or intraarticular loose bodies (11,40). Heterotopic ossification and avascular necrosis are uncommon and primarily associated with fracture dislocations (19). Avascular necrosis of the humeral head is diagnosed by increased density along the articular suface of the humeral head with the absence of joint space narrowing. Nonunion of a fractured tuberosity is a rare complication, identified by corticated fracture margins obliterating the marrow cavity. Intra-articular osteochondral loose bodies on plain films are typically identified in the bicipital tendon sleeve or axillary recess. Degenerative arthritis results from prior dislocation especially associated with posterior dislocation possibly secondary to delayed diagnosis (41).

Voluntary glenohumeral dislocations occur in adolescents and may be anterior, posterior, or multidirectional. Typically, patients can dislocate and reduce voluntarily.

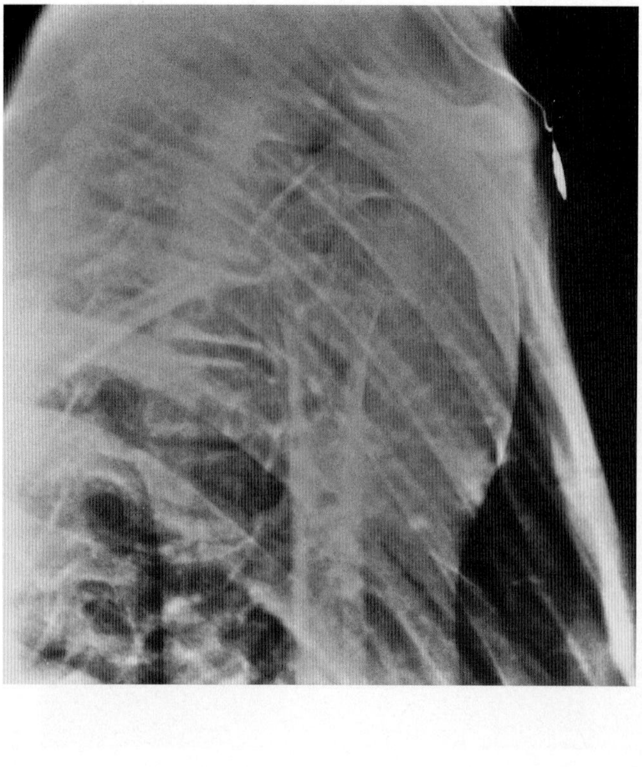

FIG. 9. Normal Maloney's arch as seen on the transthoracic view.

The radiographic findings are the same as those resulting from traumatic dislocations (42).

In addition to anterior and posterior subluxations or dislocations, there are several other glenohumeral malalignments. A *luxatio erecto* (2,43) is an uncommon dislocation in which the patient presents with the arm fixed and elevated over the head and cannot lower his/her arm (Fig. 12). A fracture of the acromium process or of the inferior glenoid may be associated with this lesion.

A *pseudo-subluxation* is evident on upright frontal views when the humerus is inferiorally located with respect to the glenoid. It is termed a pseudo subluxation because the humerus will return to a normal glenoid position without surgical involvement or manipulation in most patients (11,44,45). A pseudo-subluxation results from blood, pus, or fluid in the joint which, when removed or absorbed, causes the humerus to return to normal location. This finding is typically identified in patients who have had an intra-articular fracture.

Superior migration of the humeral head with respect to the glenoid occurs secondary to a rotator cuff tear. Superior migration is best determined by evaluating the superior as-

A

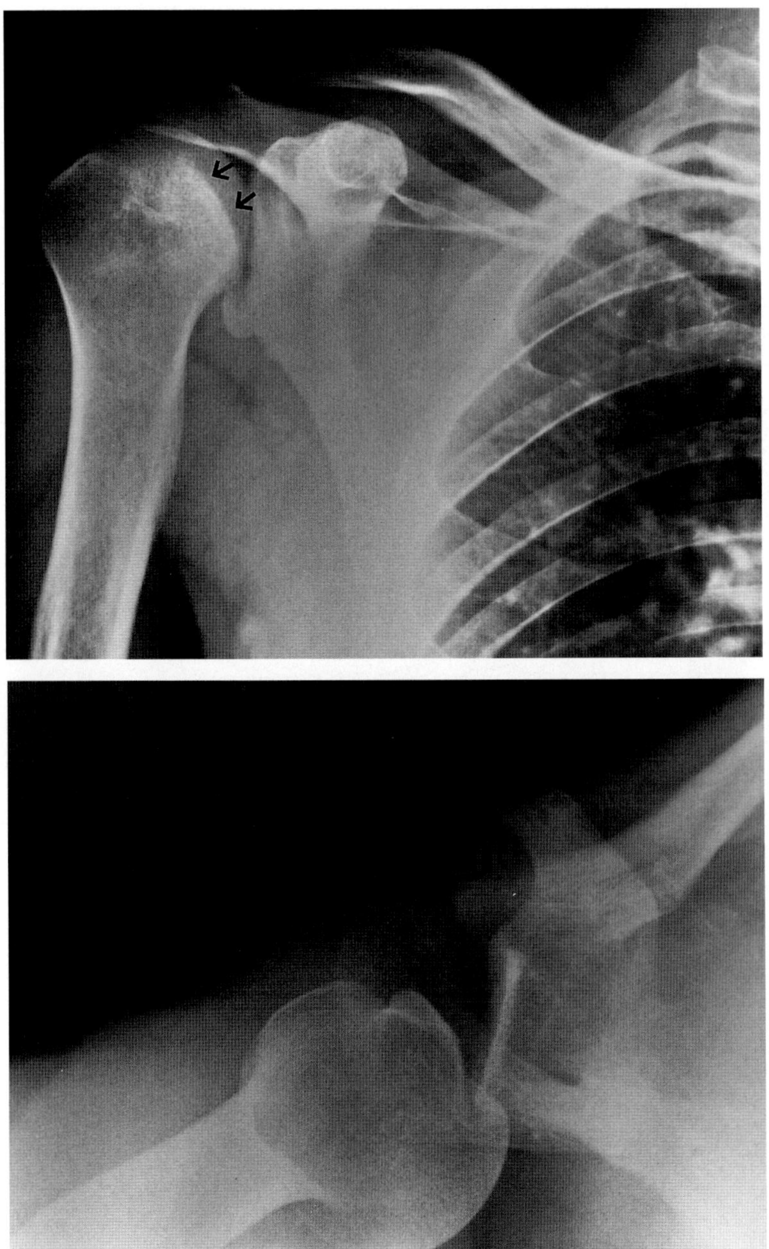

B

FIG. 10. A posterior dislocation is demonstrated on the posterior oblique view **(A)** by the overlap of the glenoid and humerus. There is a prominent trough sign *(arrows)*. As seen on the axillary view **(B)**, the trough results secondary to impaction of the posterior aspect of the glenoid with the anterior aspect of the humeral head.

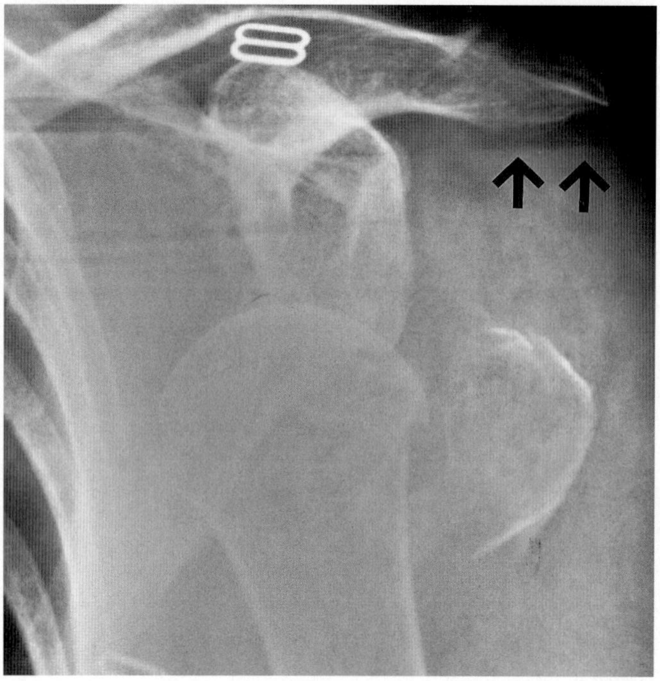

FIG. 11. Anterior subcoracoid fracture dislocation. The greater tuberosity is fractured and displaced. A fat fluid level *(arrows)* inferior to the acromium process is evident. (From Pavlov H, Freiberger RH. Fractures and dislocations about the shoulder. *Semin Roentgenol* 1978;13:85–96, with permission.)

pect of the humeral head with that of the glenoid as opposed to the distance between the humeral head and the undersurface of the acromium as this latter distance may be widened or narrowed according to the central x-ray beam angulation. A concavity on the undersurface of the acromium process congruent to that of the humeral head confirms chronic superior migration and is indicative of a chronic rotator cuff tear (11). Patients with a chronic rotator cuff tear, superior subluxation, and sudden onset of shoulder pain may have an acromium stress fracture that can occur in the absence of trauma. This injury is best identified on the axillary projection and should not be mistaken for an os acrominale (46).

PATIENTS OLDER THAN AGE 40

In a patient older than 40 years of age, the radiographic evaluation optimally consists of a *posterior oblique projection with the humerus in internal rotation*, an *AP view of the shoulder with the humerus in external rotation*, an *axillary view*, and an *outlet view*. With acute shoulder pain, an examination of the shoulder obtained with the humerus in internal and external rotation is indicated to exclude an isolated greater tuberosity fracture or calcific tendonitis or bursitis. An anterior dislocation in these patients is fre-

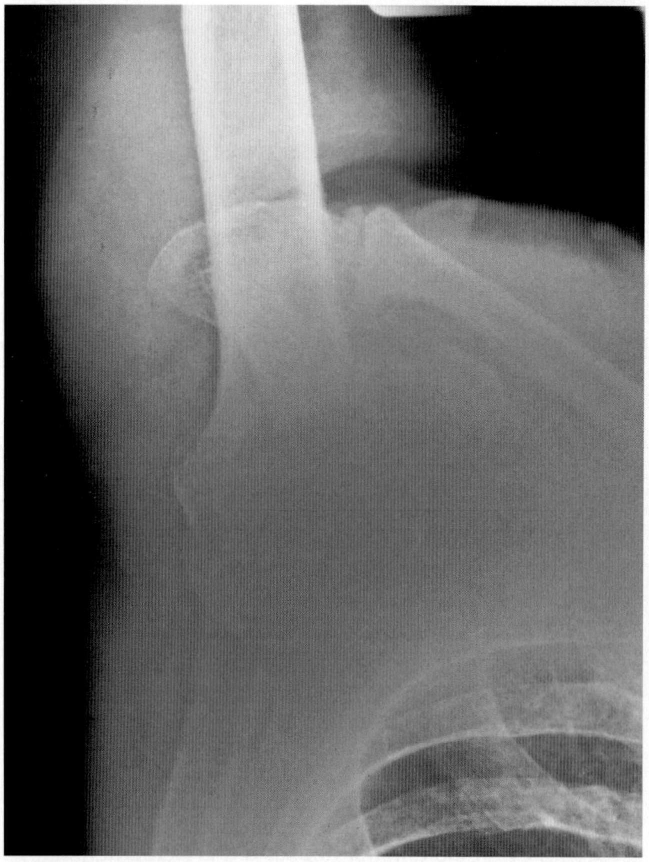

FIG. 12. A luxato erecto in which the humerus is fixed in an upright position.

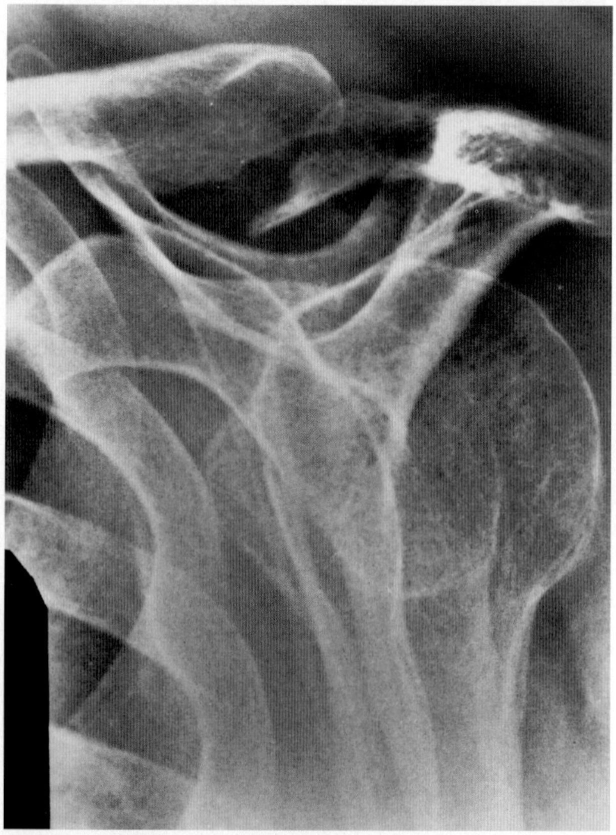

FIG. 13. Outlet view demonstrating a large hook spur on the undersurface of the anterior aspect of the acromium process.

quently complicated by a rotator cuff tear (47). Without a history of trauma, pain in this patient group is more likely related to rotator cuff pathology, calcific tendonitis or bursitis or an arthritic process, rather than instability. The outlet view is useful to evaluate the undersurface of the acromium process, which can contribute to rotator cuff pathology (Fig. 13).

Evaluation of the shoulder by computed tomography (CT) is indicated when a humeral or glenoid fracture is suspected clinically but plain films are either not diagnostic or equivocal or the demonstration of the injury is inadequate for surgical planning (48,49). The CT examination is extremely beneficial to confirm the extent of injury, the location and/or position of fracture fragments, and glenohumeral alignment. Anterior or posterior subluxation (Fig. 14A), a Hill-Sachs fracture secondary to an anterior dislocation, a trough lesion secondary to a posterior dislocation (33), and an osseous Bankart lesion are easily diagnosed on the CT examination (Fig. 14B, C).

In 80% of cases, fracture fragments of the humeral head are not displaced; however, when there is severe communication, CT is helpful to determine the exact position and rotation of fracture fragments and the integrity of the articular surface (50). In following fracture healing, CT can help detect early signs of malunited fragments that may interfere with rotation (50). CT demonstrates the position of fracture fragments in the axial plane and the relationship with the glenoid; the longitudinal fracture fragment relationship is best evaluated on plain radiographs or on CT sagittal and/ or coronal reconstruction.

As both shoulders are evaluated simultaneously, comparison of one side to the other is a distinct advantage of CT imaging over plain films (51,52). The CT study of the shoulder is ideally performed with the patient supine and the arms in neutral rotation, i.e., hands by the patient's sides with the palms resting on the sides of the thighs with the thumbs facing the ceiling. Three or four slices through the glenohumeral joint are usually sufficient for gross evaluation of the glenohumeral alignment (Fig. 14D). Because there may be superior or inferior migration of the humeral head, with respect to the glenoid on one side versus the other, the number of slices can be adjusted according to

A

B

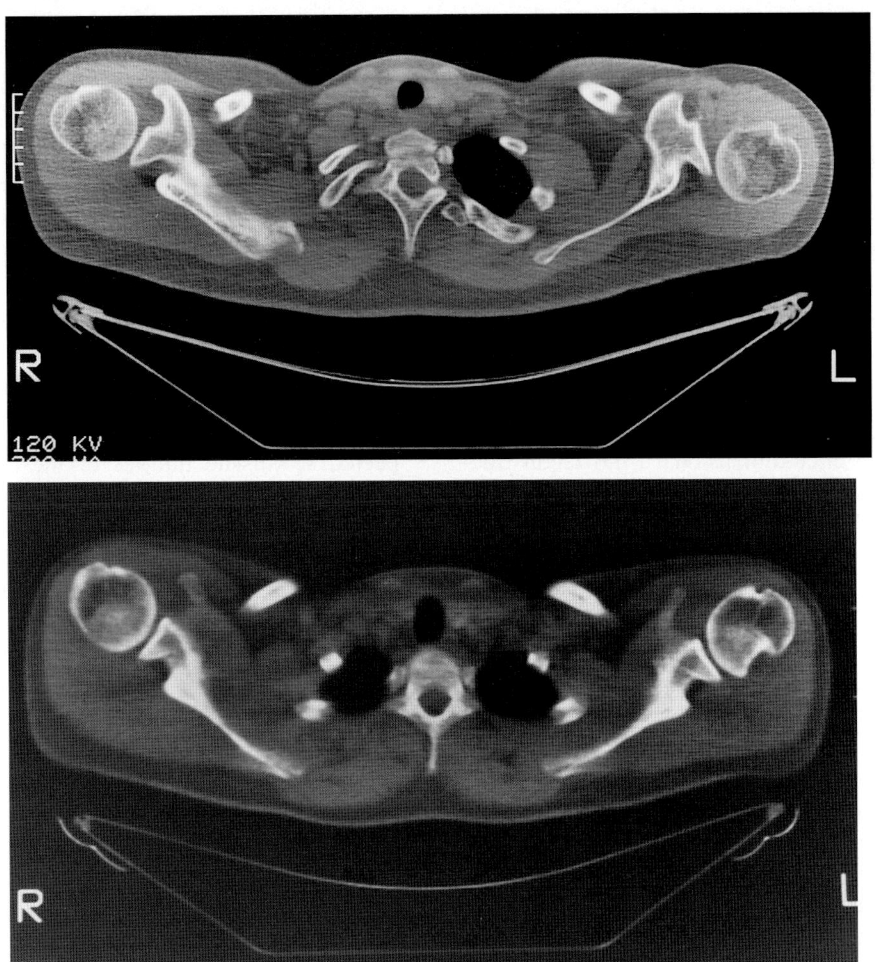

FIG. 14. A: Axial computed tomography (CT) image demonstrates a posterior subluxation on the left. **B:** Axial CT image demonstrates a large Hill-Sachs deformity on the left. The glenohumeral alignment is anatomic bilaterally. *(figure continues)*

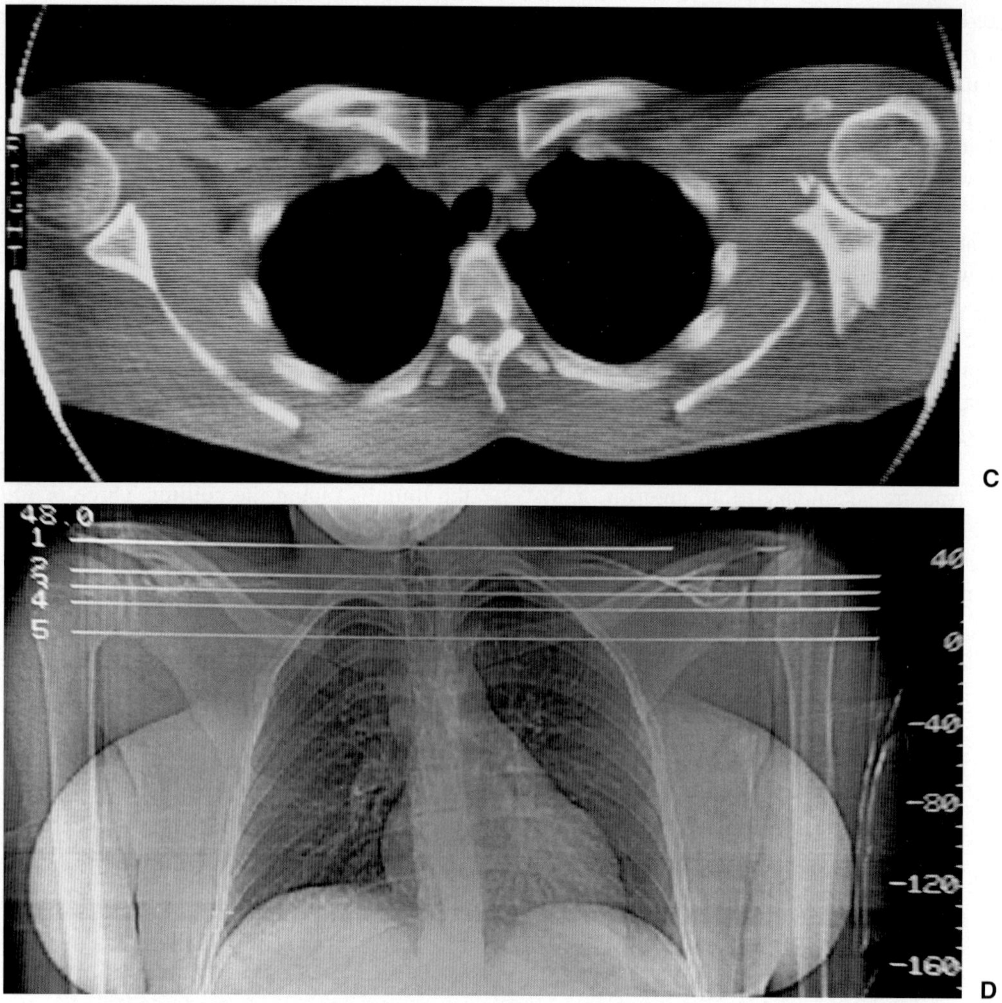

FIG. 14. *Continued.* **C:** An axial CT slice at the level of the inferior aspect of the glenohumeral joint demonstrates a Bankart fracture on the left. **D:** Scout localizer identifies appropriate levels for axial slices.

the scout localizer. If three-dimensional (3D) reconstruction is required for surgical planning, multiple thin axial images are required. The value of the 3D images is debatable and is usually considered more useful to the orthopedic surgeon than to the radiologist as an aid for visually localizing a lesion or position of fracture fragments (Fig. 15A, B).

Evaluation of the articular cartilaginous surface of the humeral head and glenoid labrum, or localization of intra-articular chondral loose bodies, is limited on the CT examination. Double-contrast arthrography and tomography, for example, arthrotomography or CT arthrography (a CT examination performed after the intra-articular injection of 2 to 3` ml of radiographic contrast and 6 to -10 cc of room air) can be used to evaluate nonosseous Bankart and/or capsular lesions secondary to dislocation (53–58) (Fig. 16). Only minimal coating with contrast is necessary for evaluation of articular cartilage lesions. In general, arthrotomography and CT arthrography to disclose suspected soft-tissue injuries of the capsule and glenoid labrum have been replaced by magnetic resonance imaging (MRI) because the arthrogram is an invasive study requiring a needle stick and introduction of contrast into the joint which has the potential, albeit rare, for allergic reaction and/or infection (53–58). Because MRI is a non-invasive study that provides enhanced definition of the joint capsule, intra-articular structures and surrounding muscles, MRI is a more appropriate cost-effective examination. Arthrotomography or CT arthrography, however, is useful in the patient who is claustraphobic, has a pacemaker and/or other contraindication to an MRI examination, or if the MRI is not accessible.

In conclusion, plain films and, when necessary, CT, provide valuable information in the work-up of a patient with shoulder instability. In order to maximize diagnostic yield per radiographic cost, time and radiation exposure, the plain film examination should be tailored for the suspected diagnosis and the patient's age. In patients with acute dislo-

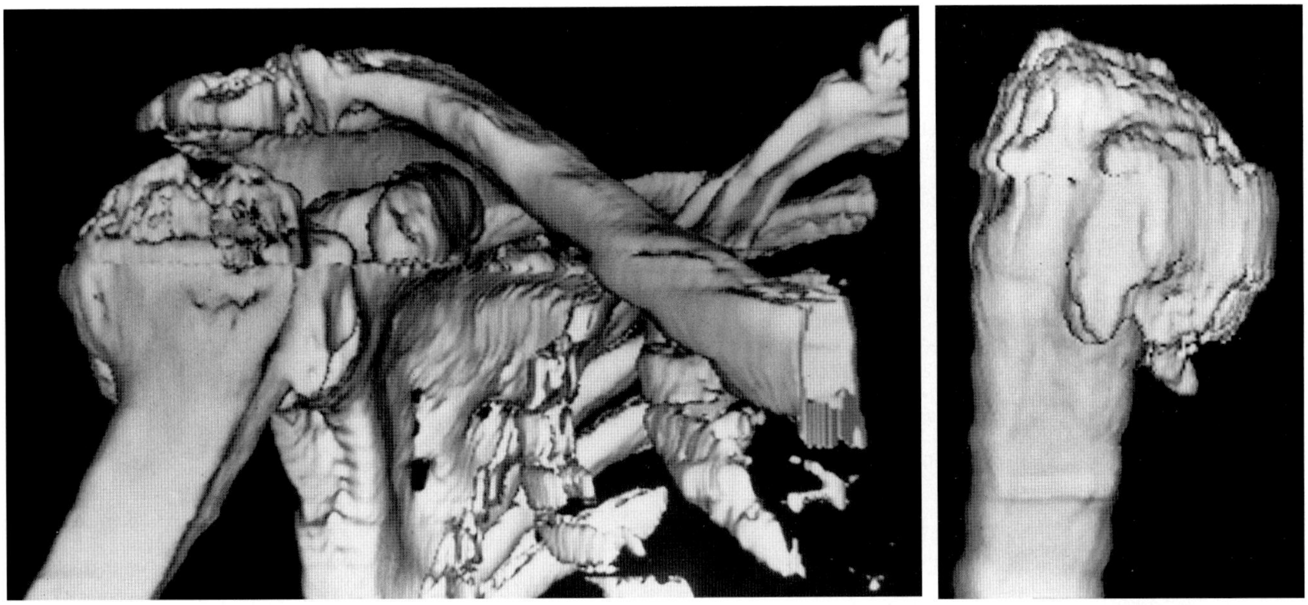

A B

FIG. 15. Three-dimensional (3D) computed tomography of the shoulder demonstrates severe glenohumeral degenerative osteoarthritis. **A:** The shoulder is displayed from the front with the humerus in internal rotation; the bicipital groove is medially located. **B:** The 3D display of the humerus in external rotation, with the joint removed, confirms the extent of proliferative osteophytes around the humeral head and tuberosities.

cation and/or trauma, a posterior oblique projection tangential to the glenohumeral joint with the humerus in internal rotation, a transcapular "Y" view, and an axillary view are recommended. In a patient with chronic instability who is younger than 40 years of age, the posterior oblique projection with the humerus in internal rotation, a West Point axillary view, and a Stryker Notch view are indicated. In patients over forty years of age with pain and without history of trauma, a posterior oblique projection with the humerus in internal rotation, a frontal view of the shoulder with the humerus in external rotation, and an axillary or outlet view to evaluate the undersurface of the acromium process are most helpful. The plain film radiographs are ideal to determine the glenohumeral alignment and evidence of previous anterior and/or posterior dislocation. Plain films and CT are limited, however, for assessment of the regional soft tissues of the shoulder. Although arthrotomography and CT arthrotomography can be used to assess the intracapsular structures and glenoid labrum, they have in most instances been replaced by MRI.

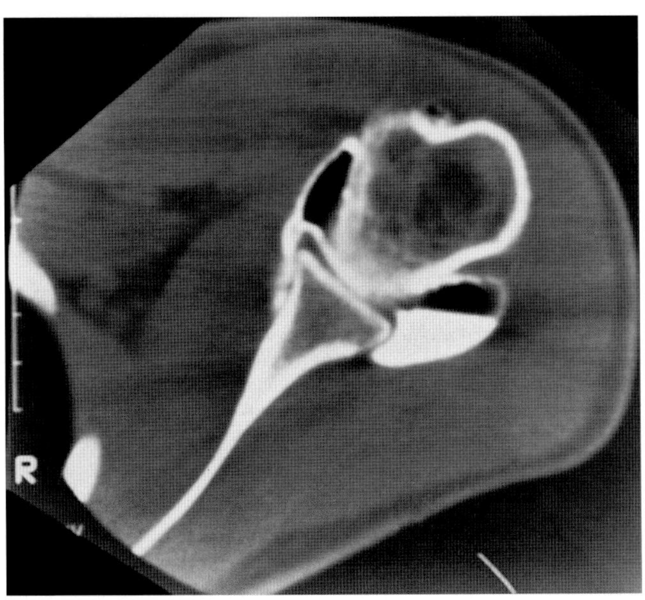

FIG. 16. Computed tomography axial image following a double-contrast arthrogram demonstrates the articular cartilage overlying the anterior and posterior glenoid labrum outlined by contrast. The cartilage is smooth and normal. Contrast is also present in the bicipital groove, confirming the normal position of the biceps tendon.

REFERENCES

1. Merrill V. *Atlas of roentgenographic positions*, 3rd ed, vol 1. St. Louis: CV Mosby, 1967.
2. Rockwood CA. Fracture and dislocations about the shoulder. In Rockwood CA, Green DP, eds. *Fractures*. Philadelphia: JB Lippincott, 1975.
3. Engebretsen L, Craig EV. Radiologic features of shoulder instability. *Clin Orthop* 1993;291:29–44.
4. Pavlov H, Warren RF, Weiss CB, et al. The roentgenographic evaluation of anterior shoulder instability. *Clin Orthop* 1985;194:153–158.
5. Lewis RW. *The joints of the extremities: a radiographic study*. Springfield, IL: Charles C Thomas, 1955.
6. Rogers LF. The shoulder and humeral shaft. In: *Radiology of skeletal trauma*. 2nd ed. New York: Churchill Livingtone, 1992:653–748.
7. Garth WP Jr, Sappery CE, Ochs CW. Roentgenographic demonstration of I instability of the shoulder: the apical oblique projection. *J Bone Joint Surg* 1984;66A:1450.
8. Kornbuth PI, Salazar AM. The apical oblique view of the shoulder: its usefulness in acute trauma. *AJR* 1987;149:113.
9. Richardson JB, Ramsay A, Davidson JK, Kelly IG. Radiographs in shoulder trauma. *J Bone Joint Surg* 1988;70B:457.
10. Gusmer PB, Potter HG. Imaging of shoulder instability. *Clin Sports Med* 1995;14:777–795.
11. Pavlov H, Freiberger RH. Fractures and dislocations about the shoulder. *Semin Roentgenol* 1978;13:85–96.
12. DeSmet A. Anterior oblique projection in radiography of the traumatized shoulder. *AJR* 1980;134:515.
13. Flinn RM, MacMillan CL Jr, Campbell DR, Fraser DB. Optimal radiography of the acutely injured shoulder. *J Can Assoc Radiol* 1983;34:128.
14. Harris JH Jr, Harris WH. *The radiology of emergency medicine*. Baltimore: Williams & Wilkins, 1975:112.
15. Horsfield D, Renton P. The other view in the radiography of shoulder trauma. *Radiography* 1980;549:213.
16. Rubin SA, Gray RL, Green WR. The scapular Y: a diagnostic aid in shoulder trauma. *Radiology* 1974;10:725.
17. Rokous JR, Feagin JA, Abbott HG. Modified axillary roentgenograms, a useful adjunct in the diagnosis of recurrent instability of the shoulder. *Clin Orthop* 1972;82:84.
18. Richards RD, Sartoris DJ, Pathria MN, et al. Hill-Sachs lesions and normal humeral groove: MR features allowing their differentiation. *Radiology* 1994;190:665–668.
19. Neer CS II, Rockwood CA Jr. Fractures and dislocations of the shoulder. In: Rockwood CA Jr, Green DP, eds. *Fractures*. Philadelphia: JB Lippincott, 1975.
20. Hall RH, Isaac F, Booth CR. Dislocations of the shoulder with special reference to accompanying small fractures. *J Bone Joint Surg* 1959;41A:489.
21. West EF. Intrathoracic dislocation of the humerus. *J Bone Joint Surg* 1949;31B:61.
22. Hill HA, Sachs MD. The grooved defect of the humeral head. A frequently unrecognized complication in dislocations of the shoulder joint. *Radiology* 1940;35:696–700.
23. Danzig LA, Greenway G, Resnick S. The Hill-Sachs lesion. *Am J Sports Med* 1980;8:328.
24. Rowe CR, Zarins B. Recurrent transient subluxation of the shoulder. *J Bone Joint Surg* 1981;63A:863.
25. Rowe CR. Prognosis in dislocations of the shoulder. *J Bone Joint Surg* 1956;38A:957.
26. Rowe CR, Sakellarides HT. Factors related to recurrences of anterior dislocations of the shoulder. *Clin Orthop* 1961;20:40.
27. Hovelius L. Anterior dislocation of the shoulder in teenagers and young adults. *J Bone Joint Surg* 1987;69A:393.
28. Bankart ASB. Recurrent or habitual dislocation of the shoulder joint. *BMJ* 1923;2:1132–1133.
29. Astor JW Jr, Gregory CF. Dislocation of the shoulder with significant fracture of the glenoid. *J Bone Joint Surg* 1973;55A:1531.
30. MacDonald FR. Intra-articular fractures in recurrent dislocation of the shoulder. *J Can Assoc Radiol* 1962;13:1.
31. Schulz TJ, Jacobs B, Patterson RL Jr. Unrecognized dislocations of the shoulder. *J Trauma* 1969;9:1009.
32. Rowe CR, Zarins B. Chronic unreduced dislocations of the shoulder. *J Bone Joint Surg* 1982;64A:494.
33. Cisternino SJ, Rogers LF, Stufflebam BC, Kruglik GD. The trough line: a radiographic sign of posterior shoulder dislocation. *AJR* 1978;130:951.
34. McLaughlin HL. Posterior dislocation of the shoulder. *J Bone Joint Surg* 1952;34A:584.
35. Shaw JL. Bilateral posterior fracture-dislocation of the shoulder and other trauma caused by convulsive seizures. *J Bone Joint Surg* 1971;53A:1437.
36. Dimon JH III. Posterior dislocation and posterior fracture-dislocation of the shoulder. A report of 25 cases. *South Med J* 1967;60:661.
37. Ross GJ, Love MB. Isolated avulsion fracture of the lesser tuberosity of the humerus: report of two cases. *Radiology* 1989;172:833.
38. Shibuya S, Ogawa K. Isolated avulsion fracture of the lesser tuberosity of the humerus. *Clin Orthop* 1986;211:215.
39. Neer CS. Displaced proximal humeral fractures. *J Bone Joint Surg* 1970;52A:1077.
40. Killoran PJ, Marcove RC, Freiberger RH. Shoulder arthrography. *AJR* 1968;103:658–668.
41. Samilson RL, Prieto V. Dislocation arthropathy of the shoulder. *J Bone Joint Surg* 1983;65A:456.
42. Braunstein EM, Martel W. Voluntary glenohumeral dislocation. *AJR* 1977;129:911.
43. Lynn PS. Erect dislocation of the shoulder. *Surg Gynecol Obstet* 1921;39:51.
44. Cotton F. Subluxation of the shoulder downward. *Boston Mod Surg J* 1921;185:405.
45. Laskia RS, Schreiker S. Inferior subluxation of the humeral head: the drooping shoulder. *Radiology* 1971;98:585.
46. Dennis DA, Ferlic DC, Clayton ML. Acromial stress fractures associated with cuff-tear arthropathy. *J Bone Joint Surg* 1986;68A:937.
47. Johnson JR, Bayley JIL. Early complications of acute anterior dislocation of the shoulder in the middle-aged and elderly patient. *Injury* 1982;13:431.
48. Seltzer SE, Wiessman BN. CT findings in normal and dislocating shoulders. *J Can Assoc Radiol* 1985;36:41.
49. Danzig L, Resnick D, Greenway G. Evaluation of unstable shoulders by computed tomography. A preliminary study. *Am J Sports Med* 1982;10:138–141.
50. Castagno AA, Shuman WP, Kilcoyne RF, et al. Complex fractures of the proximal humerus: role of CT in treatment. *Radiology* 1987;165:759.
51. Blasier RBM, Burkus J. Management of posterior fracture dislocation of the shoulder. *Clin Orthop* 1988;232:197–204.
52. Hawkins RJ, Neer CS II, Pianta RM, Mendoza FX. Locked posterior dislocation of the shoulder. *J Bone Joint Surg* 1987;69A:9.
53. Ghelman B, Goldman AB. The double contrast shoulder arthrogram: evaluation of rotator cuff tears. *Radiology* 1977;124:251–254.
54. Goldman AB, Ghelman B. The double contrast shoulder arthrogram: a review of one hundred and fifty eight cases. *Radiology* 1978;127:655–663.
55. Mink JH, Richardson A, Grant TT. Evaluation of glenoid labrum by double-contrast shoulder arthrography. *AJR* 1979;133:883.
56. Deutsch AL, Resnick D, Mink JH, et al. Computed and conventional arthrotomography of the glenohumeral joint: normal anatomy and clinical experience. *Radiology* 1984;153:603–609.
57. Rafii M, Firooznia H, Golimbu C, Minkoff J, Bonamo JJ. CT arthrography of capsular structures of the shoulder. *AJR* 1986;46:362.
58. Rafii M, Firooznia H, Bonamo JJ, Minkoff J, Golimbu C. Athlete shoulder injuries: CT arthrographic findings. *Radiology* 1987;62:559.

The Unstable Shoulder,
edited by R.F. Warren, E.V. Craig, and D.W. Altchek.
Lippincott–Raven Publishers, Philadelphia © 1999.

CHAPTER 7

Radiographic Assessment of Shoulder Instability

Magnetic Resonance Imaging

Hollis G. Potter

Diagnostic assessment of the unstable shoulder requires a detailed patient history, comprehensive physical examination, initial plain radiographic assessment, and, in a select group of cases, more advanced diagnostic imaging techniques. The glenohumeral joint permits a diverse range of motion at varying loads but is inherently unstable, as the articular surface of the glenoid is considerably smaller than that of the humerus. A thorough radiographic assessment requires assessment of the ligamentous, cartilaginous, and capsular structures that provide the static stabilizing forces of the glenohumeral joint, as well as the dynamic constraints, including the rotator cuff tendons.

The indications for performing advanced imaging studies in the setting of shoulder instability include establishing the primary diagnosis, if left in question by physical and plain radiographic assessment, detecting associated soft-tissue (cartilaginous, tendinous, and capsular) abnormalities in patients with documented osseous trauma, and assisting in preoperative planning for those patients deemed surgical candidates. Because of its superior soft-tissue contrast over computed tomography (CT), as well as its direct multiplanar capabilities, magnetic resonance imaging (MRI) has replaced conventional CT arthrography at many centers as the primary modality for assessment of the unstable shoulder, following routine radiography. Advantages of MRI include a lack of ionizing radiation and the ability to detect subtle alterations in injured soft tissue without the use of either intravenous or intra-articular contrast agents. As patients with clinical instability may sustain trauma to articular cartilage, fibrocartilage, the capsular ligamentous complex, osseous structures, and the rotator cuff, MRI is ideal in that differential contrast is seen between all these structures, because of their inherent magnetic properties.

A complete MR assessment of the unstable shoulder requires three planes of imaging, including axial, oblique sagittal, and oblique coronal. Oblique coronal images are required because of the oblique orientation of the rotator cuff tendons; specifically, the supraspinatus, infraspinatus, and teres minor tendons are best viewed in the oblique coronal plane, which is performed parallel to the long axis of the glenohumeral joint. The oblique sagittal sequence is perpendicular to the oblique coronal and provides a survey view of the cuff muscles, which is helpful in assessing for subtle nerve injuries and denervation effect that may be sustained at the time of the translational episode. The subscapularis and biceps tendons, capsule, and capsular labral complex are best seen on axial images. As MR images are digitized, spatial resolution, or the ability to depict two lines as separate structures, is a function of the picture element or pixel. Small pixels, acquired by a diminished field of view and increased size of the imaging matrix, impart an ability to depict the capsule and glenohumeral ligaments as discrete structures (Fig. 1).

PRINCIPLES OF MAGNETIC RESONANCE IMAGING

Signal acquired from the MR unit is a function of the nuclear spin of atoms, and clinical units exploit the magnetic properties of hydrogen atoms. The inherent magnetic

H. G. Potter: Department of Radiology, Cornell University Medical Center, New York, New York 10021; and Magnetic Resonance Imaging Division, Department of Radiology, The Hospital for Special Surgery, New York, New York 10021.

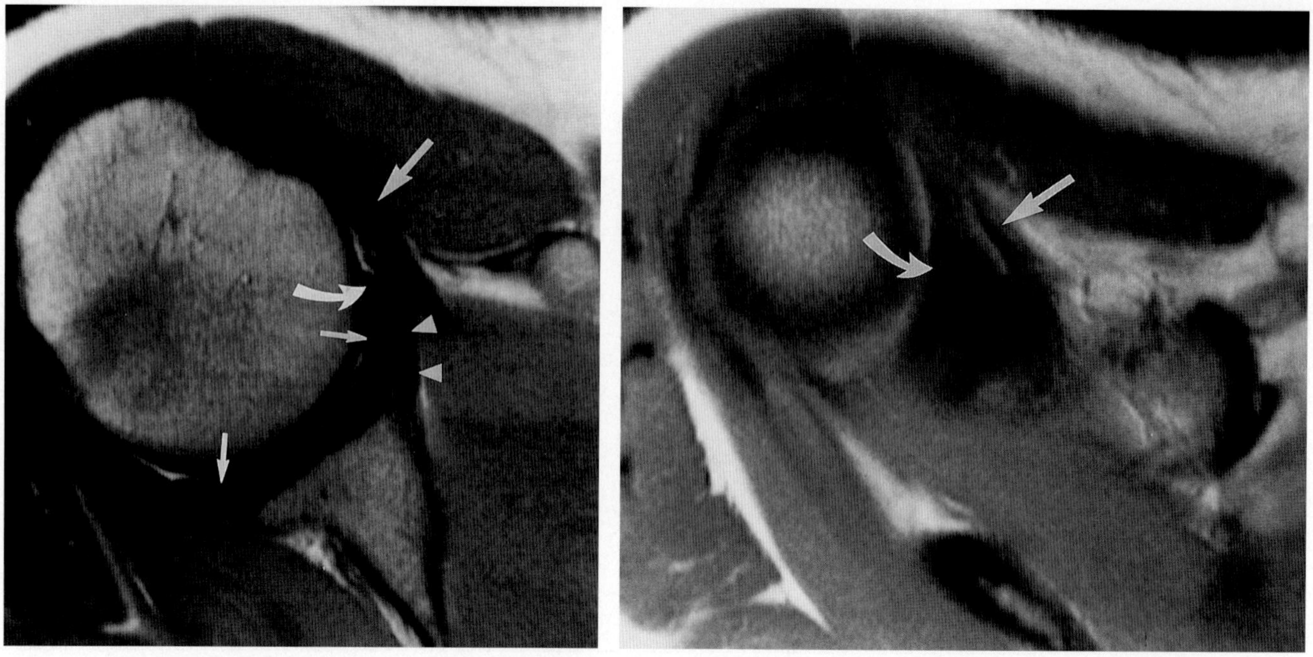

A B

FIG. 1. A: High-resolution axial fast spin-echo sequence through the right shoulder of an asymptomatic 18-year-old woman. Axial image through the level of the midlabrum demonstrates an intact anterior capsule *(arrowheads)* noted just deep to the subscapularis tendon *(long straight arrow)*. Note the intact middle glenohumeral ligament *(curved arrow)*, as well as the intact anterior and posterior labrum *(short straight arrows)*. The capsule is clearly depicted by virtue of differential signal characteristics of high signal intensity fluid, and the low signal intensity capsule. Note the intermediate signal intensity of the articular cartilage. **B:** Axial fast spin-echo sequence at a more cephalad level demonstrates the biceps anchor *(curved arrow)*, as well as the superior glenohumeral ligament *(straight arrow)*.

properties and electrical charge of the hydrogen atom produce a spin. When placed in a high-strength external magnetic field, these hydrogen protons align with a discrete vector quantity according to the axis of the external magnetic field (Bo). A series of nuclear-selective imparted radiofrequency (RF) pulses disturb the energy state of these protons. When the disturbing RF pulse is turned off, thermal equilibrium is once again regained, releasing electromagnetic energy. This energy then induces an electrical current in the surrounding coil, and this electrical current represents the MR signal. Once the raw signal is spatially encoded, an anatomic image with differential soft-tissue contrast is obtained.

The RF pulses are delivered at specific frequencies, flipping the spinning protons from the vertical plane (parallel to Bo) into the transverse plane. The excited hydrogen atoms, existing at a higher energy state, eventually return to their steady state, and the rate at which the longitudinal recovery is achieved is known as T1 relaxation. As fat protons, seen in both subcutaneous and marrow fat, restore this equilibrium quickly, fat has a short T1 relaxation time and therefore yields bright signal on a T1-weighted sequence.

T2-weighted sequences exploit the inherent decay that exists with the excited protons in the transverse plane, which occurs as a result of inherent field inhomogeneities. Despite attempts to create a perfect, homogeneous external field, inherent inhomogeneities exist, including air, calcium, hemoglobin degradation products, orthopedic instrumentation, and system eddies in the surrounding field. Because of these inherent field inhomogeneities, rapid decay of transverse magnetization occurs, and the vector of individual hydrogen atoms dephase relative to each other in the transverse plane. The rate at which this latter process occurs is known as T2 relaxation time and may be described as a decay function. By altering the repetition rate of the imparted RF pulses (TR), and the time interval between the incident RF pulse and when signal is recorded (TE), one can create differential contrast between tissues that have subtle differences in histologic composition.

A T1-weighted imaging sequence uses a short TR and short TE to accentuate differences in longitudinal recovery. Conversely, a long TR/long TE sequence is a T2-weighted sequence, favoring differences in transverse decay. With prolonged TE sequences, as one waits longer to record signal from the excited protons, signal will be largely obtained from those tissues that maintain their phase coherence in the transverse plane. An example of such tissue is water, which is bright on a T2-weighted sequence. Cortical bone and structures made of type I collagen (tendons, ligaments) appear low signal or black on all pulse sequences in their normal state, because of their tightly organized cellular structure that restricts the motion of water molecules.

Additional sequences used in musculoskeletal imaging include gradient echo techniques, which exploit short excitation pulses for rapid acquisition of imaging data. Gradient echo techniques produce less correction for field inhomogeneities and therefore accentuate areas of hemorrhagic and calcification. This may be useful when attempting to distinguish loose bodies from hemorrhagic debris in the setting of an acute dislocation. Gradient echo techniques may be recognized by the coarse appearance of trabecular bone because of its inherent magnetic susceptibility and relatively small sequence numbers (TR/TE) despite an arthrogram effect, where fluid is of bright signal intensity.

More recently developed fast spin-echo techniques are ideally suited for the unstable shoulder, as they allow for superior spatial resolution, without requiring lengthy examination times. In addition, fast spin-echo techniques impart superior refocusing of signal in the face of orthopedic instrumentation (1), which is essential in the postoperative patient after tack stabilization. A more in-depth discussion of MRI physics is beyond the scope of this chapter; more comprehensive discussion is readily available in recent literature (2–4).

NORMAL MAGNETIC RESONANCE ANATOMY

MRI of the unstable shoulder requires a thorough study of each individual image obtained, as important tissue pathology may be evident on a single imaging section. Ideally, axial images should be obtained from the level of the quadrilateral space to the acromioclavicular joint. Pulse sequences should be acquired that allow for adequate contrast between fibrocartilage, articular cartilage, subchondral bone, and the capsular labral complex. By allowing a minimum amount of T2 decay, an arthrogram effect may be achieved, exploiting the inherent high signal intensity of normal joint fluid (Fig. 1). Trabecular bone appears high signal (white), because of the presence of marrow fat. Subchondral bone and cortex appear low signal (black), while articular cartilage is typically of intermediate signal intensity (gray). It is important not to misinterpret the normal invagination of articular cartilage into the fibrocartilage of the labrum as a flap tear. The capsule and labrum, because of their type I collagen content, are low signal on all pulse sequences in the normal state. The glenohumeral ligaments may be recognized as thickenings of the shoulder capsule, best visualized in the axial plane, and identified immediately posterior to the anterior capsule (Fig. 1). Ligamentous variability exists, however, as cadaveric studies have noted an absence of the middle glenohumeral ligament in 27% of specimens (5). Glenohumeral ligaments are noted on multiple contiguous axial images, and should not be misinterpreted as displaced labral fragments, which are typically seen on only one or two axial images.

The anterior labrum is usually triangular in appearance. In the older patient, degenerative blunting of the apex of the triangle may be seen, and does not necessarily imply a displaced fragment. The posterior labrum, in contrast, may be rounded in the normal young patient. The superior labrum is best evaluated using a combination of axial and oblique coronal images, as the 12:00 axis is best seen only in the oblique coronal plane. As increased signal intensity without detachment may be seen in asymptomatic patients and arthroscopically normal labra (6), the diagnosis of labral tear should be made in the presence of both abnormal labral morphology and intrasubstance signal intensity. In the older patient, increased intralabral signal may indicate degeneration of fibrocartilage, as recently reported in an MR evaluation of 10 cadaveric specimens, where signal hyperintensity correlated to fibrovascular tissue, mucoid, and eosinophilic degeneration (7).

Normal variants also exist in the asymptomatic patient. Awareness of the imaging findings associated with these variants is essential if one is to properly interpret the MRI of the symptomatic patient. In a sublabral foramen, the mid to superior anterior labrum may appear detached from the subchondral bone (Fig. 2), and then appears restored at the superior or 12:00 axis. This normal variant may be recognized by a detached but morphologically normal labrum, without intrasubstance signal or displaced flaps, as well as a uniform, hypointense adjacent capsule. In addition, the Buford complex (8), defined as a band-like middle glenohumeral ligament with a deficient anterosuperior labrum, may be recognized by a markedly thickened middle glenohumeral ligament noted just posterior to the anterior capsule, as well as a lack of an identifiable labrum on the corresponding image (Fig. 3). A recent study evaluating the Buford complex on MR arthrography (9) led to a misdiagnosis of labral avulsion in two of the ten reported patients, and possible superior labral tear was diagnosed in an additional four of these patients. An awareness of these pitfalls is essential for the orthopedic radiologist who interprets MR images, so as to prevent misinterpretation of normal variants as labral pathology.

PATHOLOGIC FINDINGS

In an acute dislocation, the value of MRI is controversial. However, prompt recognition and distinction of a labral detachment from a primary capsular injury may be made, which may have prognostic significance regarding recurrent dislocation (10), and allows for prompt operative stabilization of Bankart lesions (11). The MRIs should be of sufficient contrast and resolution to accurately and reliably assess the integrity of the fibrocartilage, articular cartilage, and capsular labral complex (Fig. 4).

Acutely, extracapsular soft-tissue edema adjacent to the axillary pouch typically reflects extravasation of joint fluid from a torn capsule. In MR evaluation of the capsule, it is important to note the location and extent of capsular injury, which may be present in the absence of labral tears. While

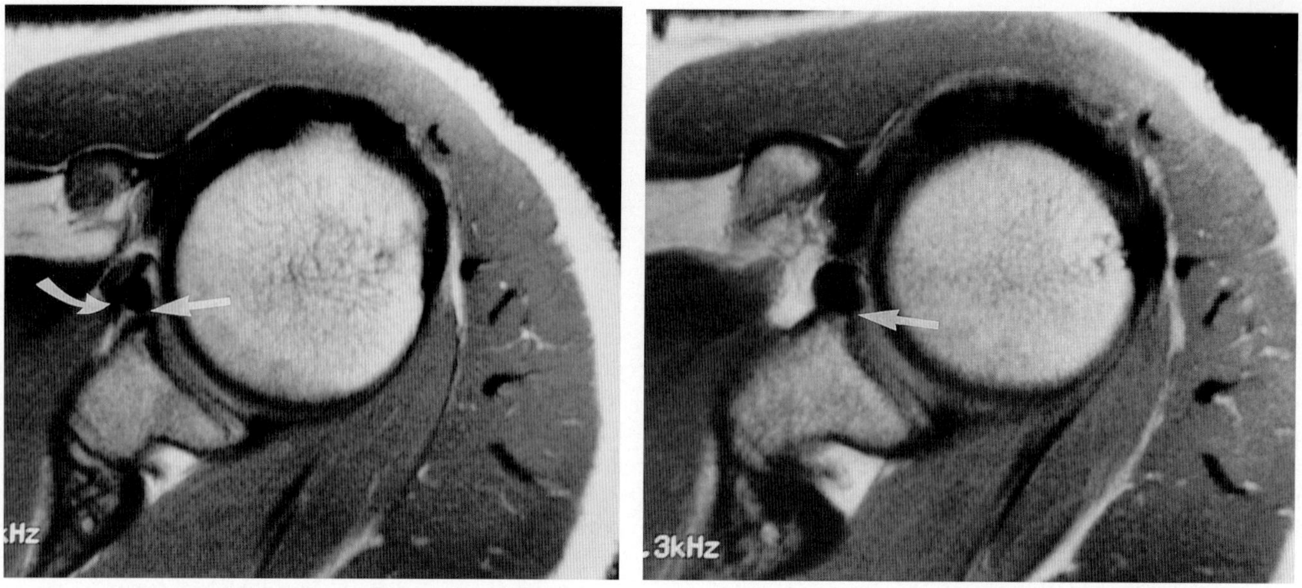

FIG. 2. Arthroscopically confirmed sublabral foramen. **A:** Axial fast spin-echo sequence demonstrating apparent detachment of the anterior labrum from the base of the glenoid *(straight arrow)*. Note the intact adjacent anterior capsule *(curved arrow)*. **B:** Axial fast spin-echo sequence at a more superior level now demonstrates a normal appearance of the anterosuperior labrum, which is situated at the base of the glenoid *(arrow)*.

capsular stripping at the glenoid is typically the rule (Fig. 4), lateral capsular detachment may also occur, and may be readily apparent on appropriately performed MRIs (Fig. 5).

Rotator interval defects in the capsule have recently come into increased attention in the orthopedic literature (13). The anatomic landmarks of the rotator interval are easily defined by MRI, specifically representing the space between the subscapularis and supraspinatus, reinforced by both the coracohumeral ligament and superior glenohumeral ligament. Joint fluid decompressing into this region may denote a rotator interval defect (Fig. 6). Preoperative knowledge of rotator interval defect may be helpful, as the surgeon may plan for concomitant rotator interval defect closure at arthroscopic or open stabilization.

In addition to labral and capsular injuries, preoperative recognition of chondral shear injuries may also be helpful;

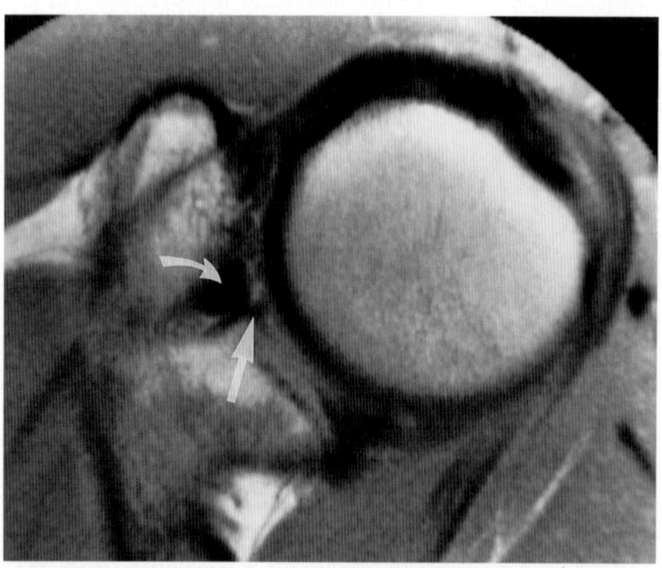

FIG. 3. Arthroscopically confirmed Buford complex. Axial fast spin-echo sequence demonstrates a deficient anterosuperior labrum *(long arrow)*, with a band-like thickened middle glenohumeral ligament *(curved arrow)*. The middle glenohumeral ligament should not be mistaken as a displaced glenohumeral fragment.

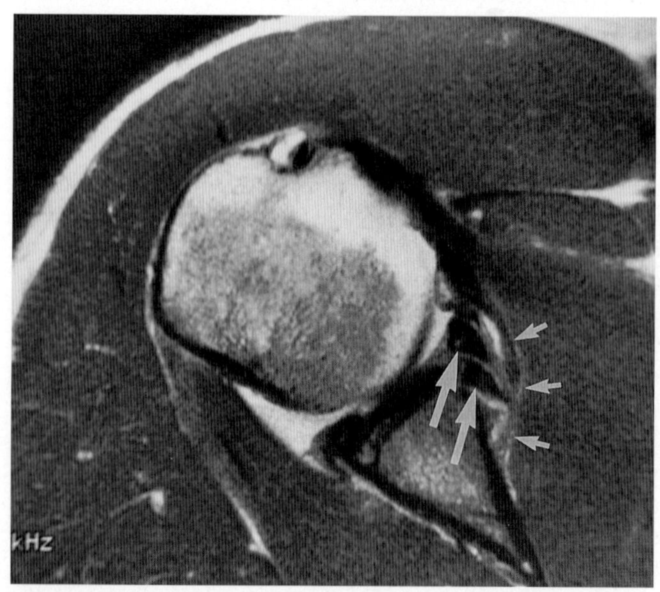

FIG. 4. Acute dislocation in a 26-year-old man. Axial fast spin-echo sequence through the anterior labrum demonstrates a fragmented anteroinferior labral tear. Note the fragmented anterior fibrocartilage *(long straight arrows)*, as well as the capsular stripping off the scapula *(short straight arrows)*.

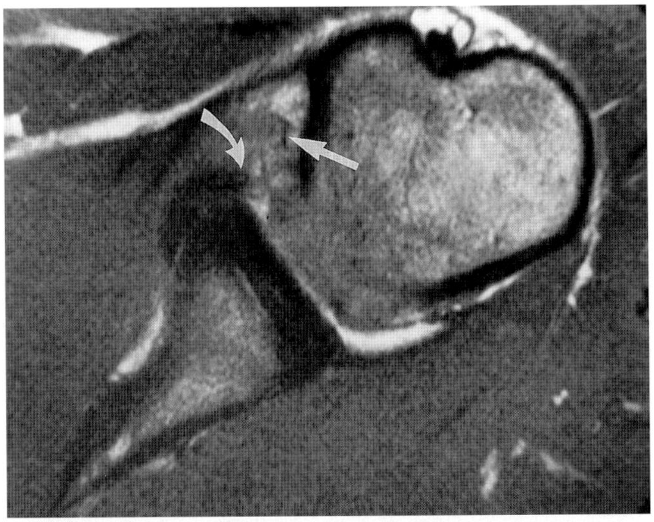

FIG. 5. Magnetic resonance imaging following anterior translational episode in a 16-year-old patient. Axial fast spin-echo sequence through the anteroinferior labrum demonstrates detachment of the anterior band *(curved arrow)* from its humeral insertion. The findings were confirmed at arthroscopy. Note the particulate debris and hemorrhage in the axillary pouch *(straight arrow).*

the surgeon may then provide the patient with a more realistic prediction of outcome, as severe cartilage shearing complicating a Bankart lesion may delay symptomatic improvement (12) (Fig. 7).

Massive dislocations, associated with osteochondral fractures, are best assessed by means of a combination of plain radiographs and MRI. When using appropriate pulse sequences, it is unnecessary to obtain concomitant CT in the setting of osseous trauma, as MRI may adequately assess the integrity and fragmentation of the glenoid or humeral

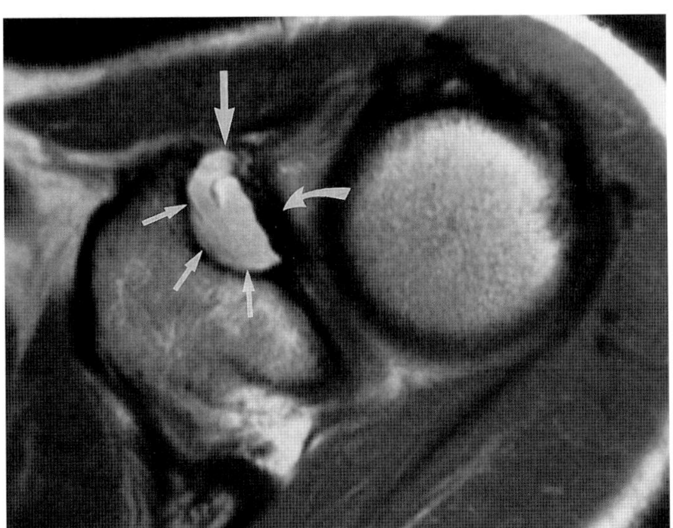

FIG. 6. Rotator interval defect. Axial fast spin-echo sequence demonstrates large fluid collection *(thin arrows)*, causing secondary deformity of the superior glenohumeral ligament *(curved arrow)*. Note the intact coracohumeral ligament *(straight arrow).*

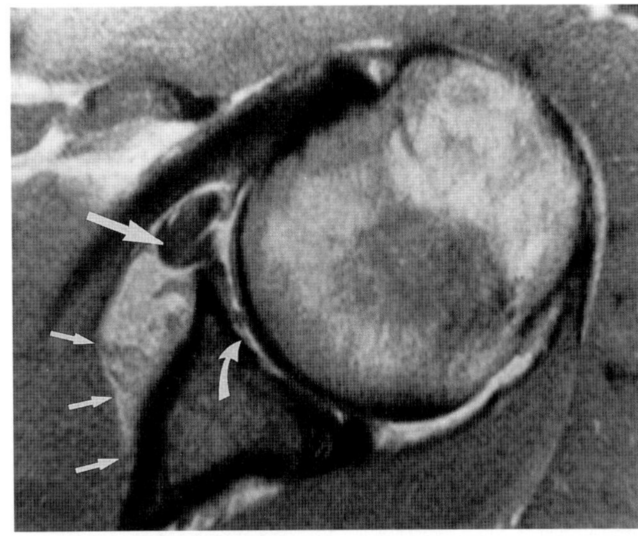

FIG. 7. Axial fast spin-echo sequence through the left shoulder in a 30-year-old patient following anterior dislocation. Stripping of the anterior capsule is noted *(small arrows)* as well as fraying of the middle glenohumeral ligament *(large arrow)*. Of greater note is the capsular shear injury, which was confirmed at arthroscopy, over the mid to anterior aspect of the glenoid *(curved arrow).*

surface (Fig. 8). Hill-Sachs lesions may be recognized on all three planes of imaging. On axial sequences, they are typically seen at and above the level of the coracoid (Fig. 9). In addition, MRI has the added advantage of depicting the degree of associated articular cartilage injury, without the use of contrast agent.

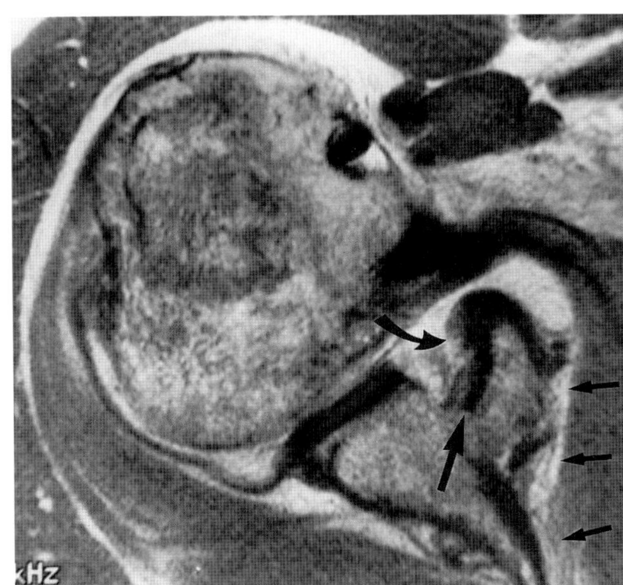

FIG. 8. Fracture dislocation in a 30-year-old patient following a severe ski injury. Axial fast spin-echo sequence demonstrates depressed central fragment of the glenoid *(large straight arrow)*, with intact overlying intermediate signal articular cartilage. Note the frayed appearance of the anterior glenoid cartilage *(curved arrow)*, as well as the capsular stripping off the scapula *(small arrows).*

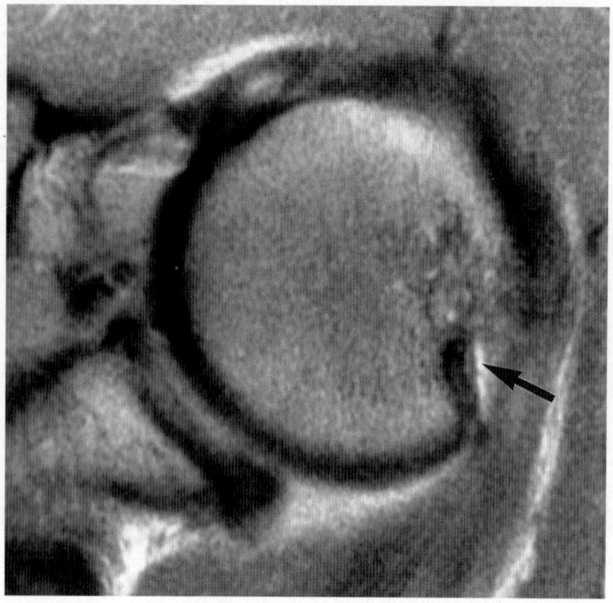

FIG. 9. Axial fast spin-echo sequence in a patient following an acute dislocation demonstrates a defect at the posterolateral aspect of the humerus *(arrow)*, indicating a Hill-Sachs lesion.

More subtle injury patterns may also be recognized, often with little fluid in the glenohumeral joint, provided that the images impart adequate resolution, and each individual image obtained is thoroughly studied (Fig. 10). Evaluation of the posterior and superior labrum is also important, as labral pathology may exist in the absence of clinically detected instability (Fig. 11).

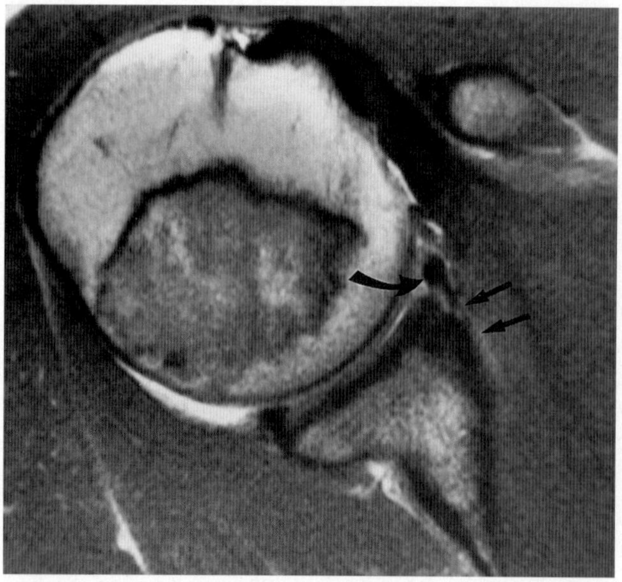

FIG. 10. Anterior labral tear with capsular tear off the scapula, in the absence of a large joint effusion. Axial fast spin-echo sequence demonstrates displaced anterior labral fragment *(curved arrow)*, as well as abnormal signal at the capsular insertion onto the scapula *(small arrows)*.

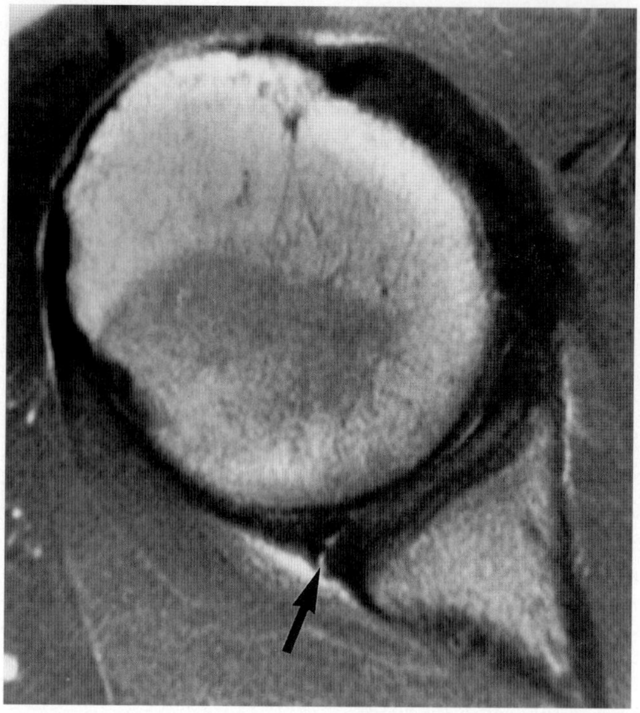

FIG. 11. Axial fast spin-echo sequence in a patient with no clinically detectable posterior instability. Arthroscopically confirmed posterior labral tear *(arrow)* is seen, with extracapsular soft-tissue edema adjacent to the posterior capsule.

The superior labrum anterior posterior (SLAP) lesions as described by Snyder et al. (14) may be difficult to diagnose consistently in a clinical examination. MR assessment of the superior labrum requires careful study of both axial and oblique coronal images, as well as a firm understanding of normal labral variants. Assessment of labrum, superior glenohumeral ligament, and the biceps anchor is important (Fig. 12). One of the benefits of higher-resolution imaging lies in its ability to detect displaced fragments (Fig. 13). Anterior glenolabral recesses that mimic superior labral tears have been described using MR arthrography (15), potentially creating a false-positive diagnosis of superior labral tear.

Superior labral tears may be associated with ganglion cysts (16). When enlarged, these cysts may decompress into either the suprascapular or spinoglenoid notches, causing compressive suprascapular neuropathy (Fig. 14). Acutely denervated muscle will appear hyperintense and edematous on T2-weighted sequences, particularly those obtained with fat suppression, a technique that increases the inherent tissue contrast of structures with increased water content. The muscle appears globally hyperintense, in distinction to the patchy edema that may be seen in contused muscle following exertional or direct injury. Chronically denervated muscle (usually > 12 months) demonstrates atrophy with increased signal intensity on the T1-weighted sequences attributable to fatty replacement (17). Although associated with superior labral

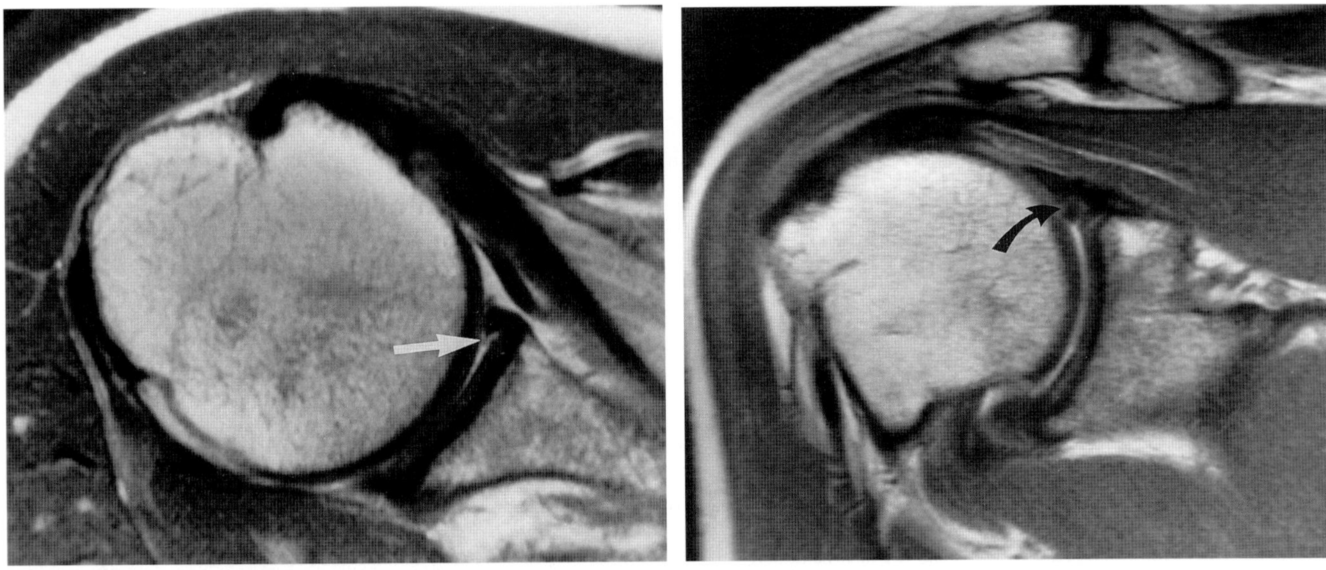

A B

FIG. 12. A: Axial fast spin-echo sequence demonstrates a flap tear of the anterosuperior labrum *(arrow).* **B:** Oblique coronal fast spin-echo sequence demonstrates abnormal signal intensity extending into the superior labrum *(curved arrow).* A type II SLAP tear was confirmed at arthroscopy.

tears, ganglion cysts may be seen in anterior, posterior, or superior labral tears; ganglia associated with inferior labral tears may preferentially decompress close to the neurovascular bundle at the quadrilateral space.

Chronic dislocation patterns may be more confusing, as the repetitive translational injury to fibrocartilage, capsule, and articular cartilage may lead to a rounded, denuded labrum, rather than to an acutely torn one. The differentiating MR features of chronic instability include a blunted, rounded appearance of the labrum, greater tendency for loose body formation, and post-traumatic osteoarthrosis. The capsule is chronically thickened, and the value of MRI in this setting is to distinguish acutely traumatized tissue from chronically injured tissue.

With regard to technique, the decision to convert the noninvasive MRI examination into an invasive MR arthrogram should be based on the individual preference of the radiologist and referring orthopedic surgeons. Some contro-

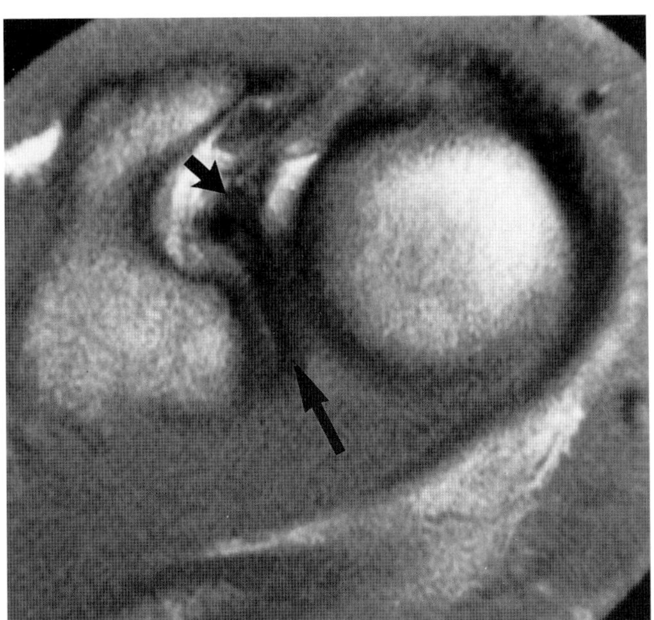

FIG. 13. Axial fast spin-echo sequence demonstrates bucket handle tear with anterior displacement of the superior labrum *(large arrow).* Note the frayed appearance of the superior glenohumeral ligament *(small arrow).*

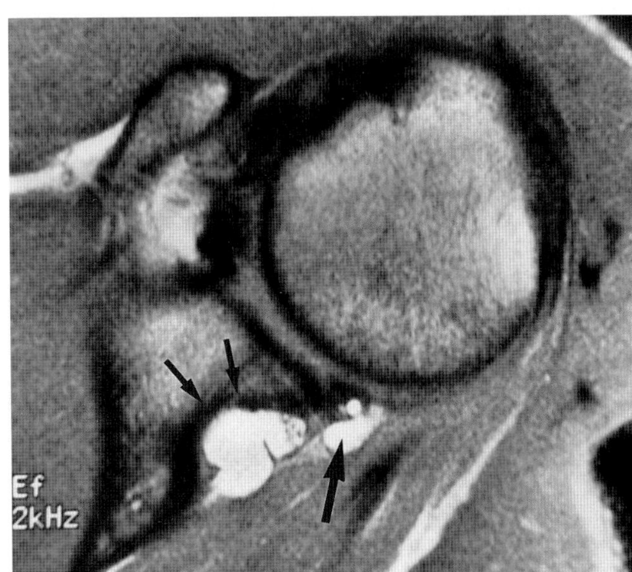

FIG. 14. Axial fast spin-echo sequence in a patient with a surgically confirmed posterosuperior labral tear, presenting with infraspinatus muscle weakness. A large soft-tissue ganglion *(large arrow)* arises from the posterosuperior labrum and decompresses preferentially into the spinoglenoid notch *(small arrows),* compressing the suprascapular nerve.

versy exists regarding the use of MR arthrography, as the intra-articular use of gadolinium MR contrast agents has not yet received Food and Drug Administration (FDA) approval. In addition, the increased cost of the gadolinium may not be reimbursed by third-party payers (18), and this additional cost may be absorbed by the patient. Previous investigators have maintained that MR arthrography is superior to noncontrast MRI in detecting labral (19) and capsular (20) injury. Chandnani et al. (21) reported 88% sensitivity and 100% specificity in detecting inferior glenohumeral ligament tears, with identification of the superior and middle glenohumeral ligaments in 85% of cases. Palmer et al. (22) reviewed 121 MR arthrograms prospectively, all surgically confirmed, and reported 76% sensitivity and 98% specificity in the detection of inferior labral ligamentous lesions. In the latter study, some false-positive diagnoses of capsular tears were attributed to extravasation of contrast into the periarticular soft tissues. All cases of capsular laxity noted at arthroscopy were interpreted as normal on the preoperative MR arthrogram. Of note, the location of the capsular insertion onto the glenoid did not correlate with clinically evident instability.

Using high-resolution noncontrast MRI, Gusmer et al. (23) prospectively evaluated 103 surgically confirmed patients. All 37 surgically noted anterior labral tears were seen and, in addition, 31 of the 36 superior labral tears of the study were correctly interpreted on the preoperative images. In this latter study, the sensitivity for detection of tears in the anterior labral was 100%, 86% in the superior labrum, and 74% in the posterior labrum, with specificity at 95%, 100% and 95%, respectively. Overall, high-resolution noncontrast MR technique in the latter study was 95% accurate in the detection of labral injuries. Because of these results, it may not be necessary to convert to MR arthrography in detecting labral pathology.

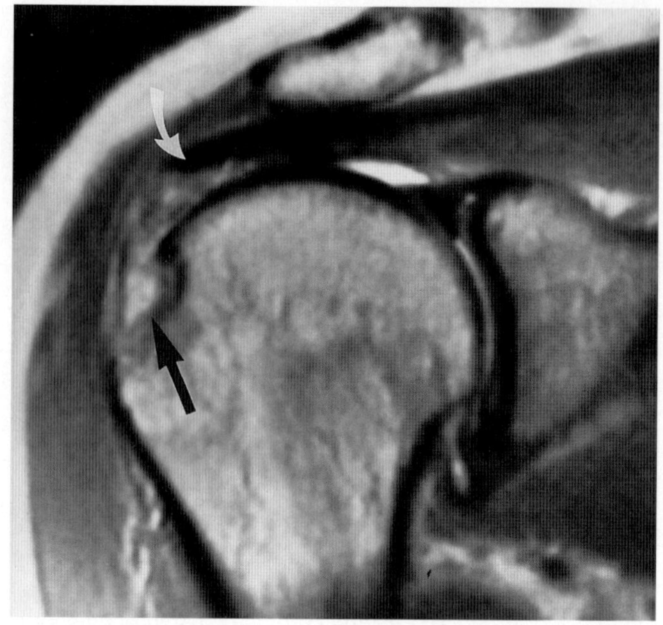

FIG. 16. Cuff avulsion in a patient who also sustained a labral tear. Oblique coronal fast spin-echo sequence demonstrates avulsion of the supraspinatus tendon *(curved white arrow)* from the greater tuberosity, with an associated bony defect *(straight black arrow).*

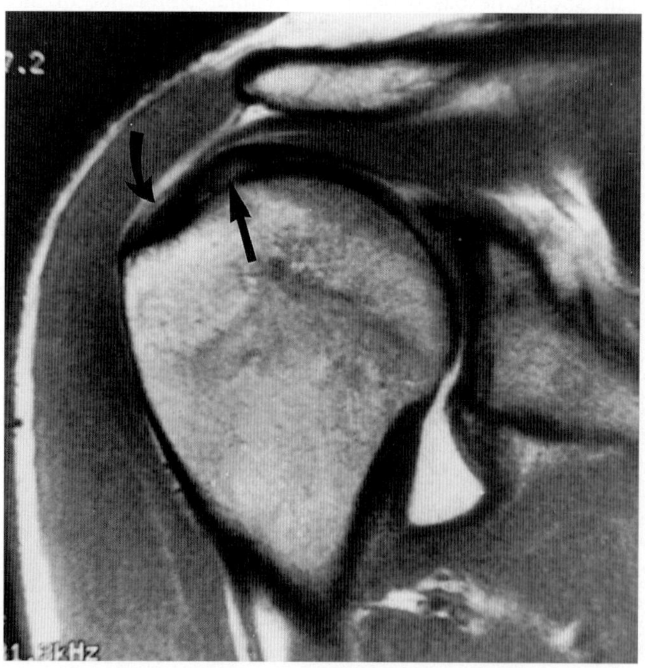

FIG. 15. Cuff contusion in a 26-year-old patient following acute dislocation. Oblique coronal fast spin-echo sequence demonstrates slight fraying at the bursal edge of the supraspinatus tendon *(curved arrow)*, as well as thickening and signal hyperintensity on the undersurface of the tendon *(straight arrow).* No discrete partial thickness defect is noted. The cuff was thought to be intact at arthroscopy.

ASSOCIATED ROTATOR CUFF PATHOLOGY IN SHOULDER INSTABILITY

MRI has been well recognized as an effective tool in evaluating the rotator cuff (24,25). This emphasizes the importance of providing a complete MR exam with all three planes of imaging, regardless of the respected diagnosis. In the unstable shoulder, the value of MR is distinguishing partial from complete tendon tears, and even more commonly, distinguishing a true partial-thickness tear, which can be either arthroscopically debrided or undergo formal repair, or both, from cuff contusions, which may appear as an arthroscopically normal tendon. The classic cuff contusion on MRI appears as a thickened hyperintense tendon with mild fraying, but no discrete partial thickness defect is seen on either the articular or bursal side (Fig. 15). Not uncommonly, the bursa adjacent to the tendon is thickened because of the direct blow and contusion of the tissue. A partial-thickness tear is denoted by abnormal tendon morphology, with a discrete defect seen in the tendon. In more severe shoulder trauma, a cuff avulsion may complicate a labral tear (Fig. 16); in this setting, complete tendon dis-

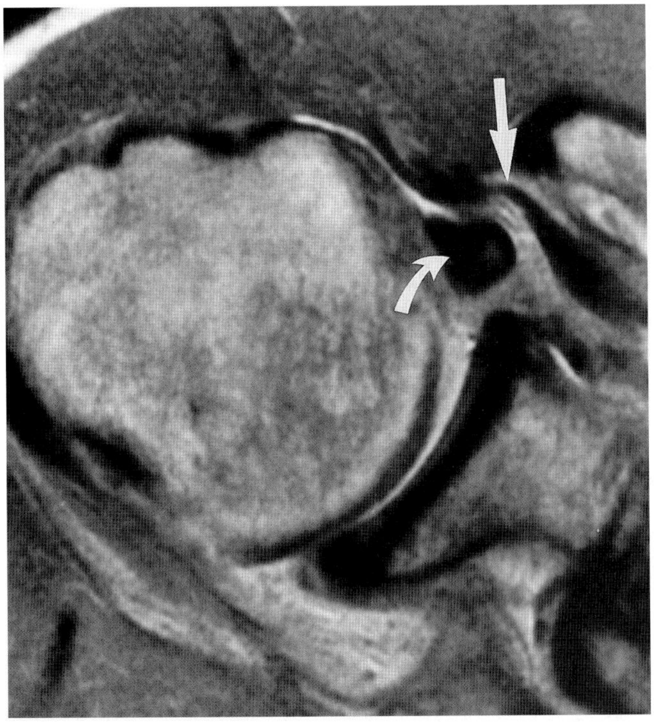

FIG. 17. Axial fast spin-echo magnetic resonance image demonstrates detachment of the subscapularis tendon *(straight arrow)* from the lesser tuberosity. Note the medially dislocated long head of the biceps tendon *(curved arrow)*, which lies posterior to the retracted subscapularis tendon. Intratendinous signal hyperintensity within the biceps indicates intrasubstance degeneration.

continuity is seen, sometimes with an associated bony fragment.

The role of the subscapularis tendon has been defined as a true dynamic stabilizer to anterior translation (26). Subscapularis tears may be difficult to assess despite a rigorous physical examination (27); axial MRIs are perhaps the most effective means of diagnosing a subscapularis tear (Fig. 17). As the subscapularis tendon fibers blend with the transverse humeral ligament, stabilizing the biceps tendon, tears of the subscapularis tendon will often lead to dislocation of the biceps tendon in a medial direction. On axial MRIs, if the biceps tendon is localized posterior to the subscapularis tendon, a full-thickness tear of the subscapularis must be present.

THE THROWING SHOULDER

The pathogenesis of instability in overhead athletes is complex, involving cuff pathology, capsular laxity and injury, labral trauma, and abnormal scapulothoracic motion. The extremes of motion consistently applied to the glenohumeral joint and surrounding soft-tissue stabilizers require a thorough MR evaluation of all structures. A painful shoulder in these athletes is evaluated in three planes of imaging, assessing for subtle undersurface posterior cuff injury, sustained by impingement of the cuff against the superior labrum in the abducted and externally rotated arm, as well as potential osteochondral impaction of the humeral head against the glenoid in a similar position (Fig. 18). Concom-

A

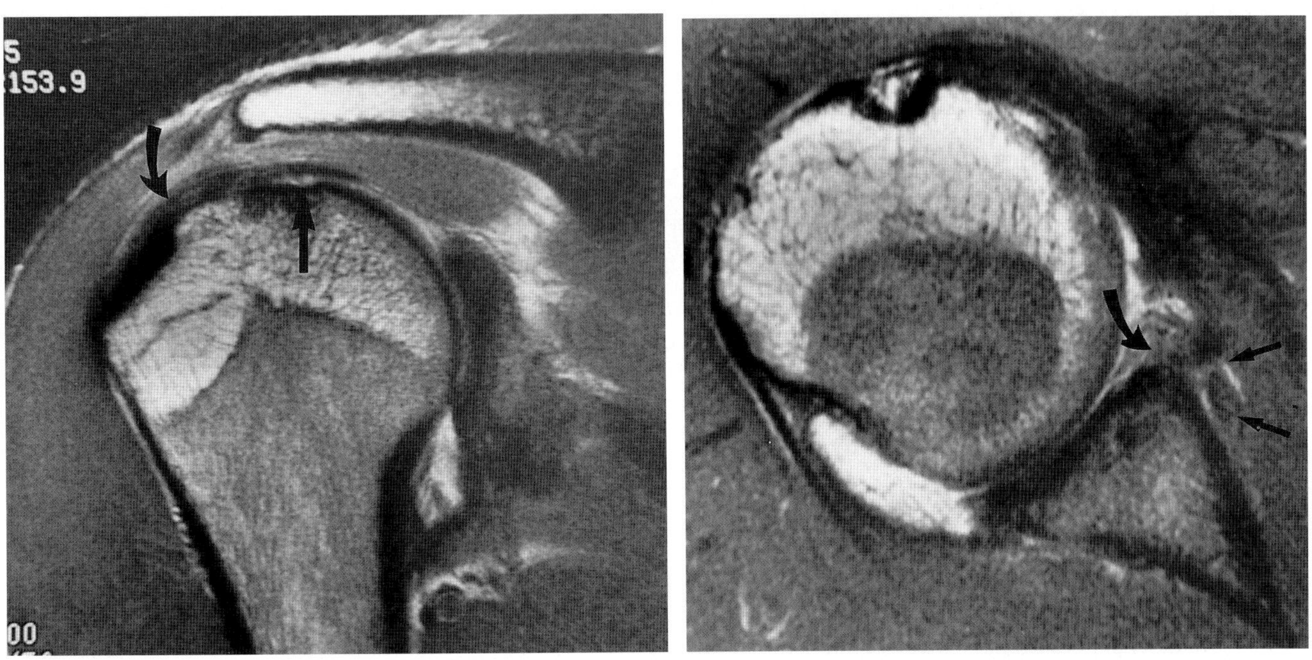

B

FIG. 18. A: Oblique coronal fast spin-echo sequence in a professional football player demonstrates fraying in the posterior margin of the supraspinatus tendon *(curved arrow)*, as well as an osteochondral injury over the superior portion of the humeral head *(straight arrow)* because of impaction against the superior glenoid rim. Note the full-thickness cartilage loss, manifested as the lack of overlying intermediate signal intensity articular cartilage. **B:** Axial fast spin-echo sequence in the same patient demonstrates a midanterior labral tear with fragmentation *(curved arrow)*, as well as associated capsular injury *(straight arrows)*.

itant capsular stretch may be seen, and recognition of a true capsular detachment from a primary capsular stretch, particularly in baseball pitchers, may be difficult. Correlation between the signal characteristics and morphology of the anterior capsule in these athletes on a preoperative MR evaluation, combined with a thorough examination under anesthesia, may provide the best diagnostic assessment of capsular–labral integrity in these patients.

POSTOPERATIVE EVALUATION

The value of fast spin-echo MR techniques has recently been established in the postoperative patient, in whom the use of traditional pulse sequences may obscure regional anatomy in the presence of orthopedic instrumentation. A recent trend toward the use of bioabsorbable tack fixation of the labrum has led to awareness of associated complications, including an ''inflammatory'' synovitis associated with these techniques. On MRI, this may appear as discrete filling defects with a distended capsule, simulating synovial chondromatosis or the ''rice body'' associated with inflammatory arthropathies (Fig. 19). Patients presenting with painful shoulders after tack stabilization may not require MRI in all cases. MRI is best reserved for those patients who have refractory pain despite the use of conservative measures, including nonsteroidal anti-inflammatory drugs (NSAIDs).

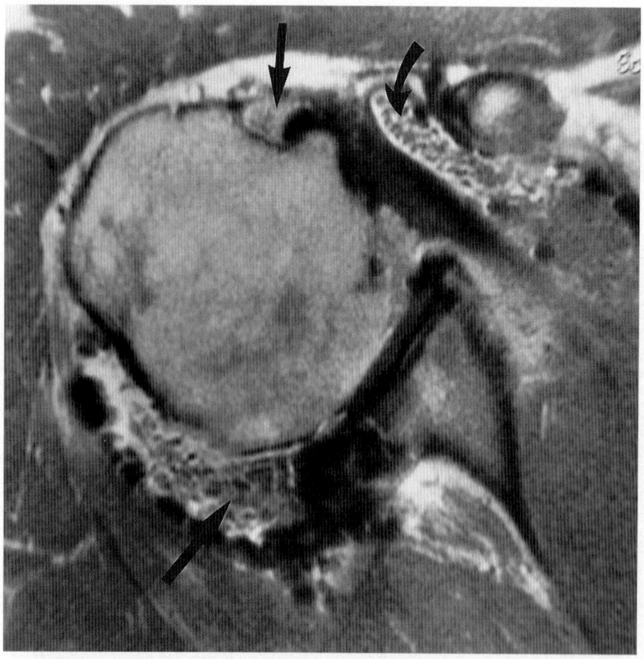

FIG. 19. Axial fast spin-echo sequence in a patient with clinical manifestations of synovitis. Patient had undergone a previous open posterior capsular repair, as well as tack stabilization of the labrum. Note the particulate debris in the posterior capsule *(large arrow)*, as well as decompressing into the biceps tendon sheath *(straight arrow)*, and subscapularis bursa *(curved arrow)*.

CONCLUSION

The utility of any diagnostic imaging technique is in combining the images with a thorough physical examination of the shoulder. MRI is only of use to the orthopedic surgeon if it will change the management of the patient. While routine MR assessment of the unstable shoulder is not necessary, appropriately performed, high-resolution noncontrast MRI may accurately and reliably assess the labrum, articular cartilage, and capsule of the shoulder, thus aiding in planning the operative or conservative management of the patient. Strict attention to imaging technique is essential, and simply obtaining T1- and T2-weighted images is not sufficient to accurately assess the supporting structures of the shoulder and is likely the cause for disappointing results reported by previous investigators (28), regarding the value of MRI in shoulder instability.

REFERENCES

1. Potter HG, Montgomery KD, Padgett DE, Salvati EA, Helfet DL. Magnetic resonance imaging of the pelvis: new orthopaedic applications. *Clin Orthop* 1995;319:223–231.
2. Plewes DB. The AAPM/RSNA physics tutorial for residents: contrast mechanisms in spin-echo MR imaging. *RadioGraphics* 1994;14:1389–1404.
3. Price RR. The AAPM/RSNA physics tutorial for residents: contrast mechanisms in gradient-echo imaging and an introduction to fast imaging. *RadioGraphics* 1995;15:165–178.
4. Hendrick RE. The AAPM/RSNA physics tutorial for residents: basic physics of MR imaging: an introduction. *RadioGraphics* 1994;14:829–846.
5. O'Brien SJ, Neves MC, Arnoczky SP, et al. The anatomy and histology of the inferior glenohumeral ligament complex of the shoulder. *Am J Sports Med* 1990;18:449–456.
6. McCauley TR, Pope CF, Jokl P. Normal and abnormal glenoid labrum: assessment with multiplanar gradient-echo MR imaging. *Radiology* 1992;183:35–37.
7. Loredo R, Longo C, Salonen D, et al. Glenoid labrum: MR imaging with histologic correlation. *Radiology* 1995;196:33–41.
8. Williams MM, Snyder SJ, Buford D. The Buford complex—the ''cord-like'' middle glenohumeral ligament and absent anterosuperior labrum complex: a normal anatomic capsulolabral variant. *Arthroscopy* 1994;10:241–247.
9. Tirman PFJ, Feller JF, Palmer WE, Carroll KW, Steinbach LS, Cox I. The Buford complex—a variation of normal shoulder anatomy: MR arthrographic imaging features. *AJR* 1996;166:869–873.
10. Baker CL, Uribe JW, Whitman C. Arthroscopic evaluation of acute initial anterior shoulder dislocations. *Am J Sports Med* 1990;18:25–28.
11. Arciero RA, Wheeler JH, Ryan JB, McBride JT. Arthroscopic Bankart repair versus nonoperative treatment for acute, initial anterior shoulder dislocations. *Am J Sports Med* 1994;22:589–594.
12. Potter HG, Schweitzer ME, Altchek DW. Advanced imaging in orthopaedics: current pitfalls and new applications. In: Springfield DS, ed. *Instructional course lectures,* vol. 46. Rosemont, IL: American Academy of Orthopaedic Surgeons, 1997:521–529.
13. Cole BJ, Rodeo SA, O'Brien SJ, et al. The developmental anatomy of the rotator interval capsule and the rotator interval defect: an anatomic and histologic analysis of fetal and adult cadaver specimens with clinical implications. *Transactions of the American Orthopaedic Society for Sports Medicine,* Specialty Day, American Academy of Orthopaedic Surgeons, San Francisco, CA, 1997.
14. Snyder SJ, Karzel RP, Del Pizzo W, Ferkel RD, Friedman MJ. SLAP lesions of the shoulder. *Arthroscopy* 1990;6:274–279.
15. Smith DK, Chopp TM, Aufdemorte TB, Witkowski EG, Jones RC. Sublabral recess of the superior glenoid labrum: study of cadavers

with conventional nonenhanced MR imaging, MR arthrography, anatomic dissection, and limited histologic examination. *Radiology* 1996;201:251–256.

16. Tirman PFJ, Feller JF, Janzen DL, Peterfy CG, Bergman AG. Association of glenoid labral cysts with labral tears and glenohumeral instability: radiologic findings and clinical significance. *Radiology* 1994;190:653–658.
17. Fleckenstein JL, Watumull D, Conner KE, et al. Denervated human skeletal muscle: MR imaging evaluation. *Radiology* 1993;187:213–218.
18. Quinn SF. Reply to ''Accuracy of fat-suppressed MR imaging of the shoulder for detection of partial-thickness rotator cuff tears'' (letter). *Radiology* 1996;198:293.
19. Palmer WE, Brown JH, Rosenthal DI. Labral–ligamentous complex of the shoulder: evaluation with MR arthrography. *Radiology* 1994;190:645–651.
20. Chandnani VP, Yeager TD, DeBerardino T, et al. Glenoid labral tears: prospective evaluation with MR imaging, MR arthrography, and CT arthrography. *AJR* 1993;161:1229–1235.
21. Chandnani VP, Gagliardi JA, Murnane TG, et al. Glenohumeral ligaments and shoulder capsular mechanism: evaluation with MR arthrography. *Radiology* 1995;196:27–32.
22. Palmer WE, Caslowitz PL. Anterior shoulder instability: diagnostic criteria determined from prospective analysis of 121 MR arthrograms. *Radiology* 1995;197:819–825.
23. Gusmer PB, Potter HG, Schatz JA, et al. Labral injuries: accuracy of detection with unenhanced MR imaging of the shoulder. *Radiology* 1996;200:519–524.
24. Iannotti JP, Zlatkin MB, Esterhai JL, Kressel HY, Dalinka MK, Spindler KP. Magnetic resonance imaging of the shoulder. *J Bone Joint Surg [Am]* 1991;73A:17–29.
25. Farley TE, Neumann CH, Steinbach LS, et al. Full-thickness tears of the rotator cuff of the shoulder: diagnosis with MR imaging. *AJR* 1992;158:347–351.
26. DePalma AF, Cooke AJ, Prabhakar M. The role of the subscapularis in recurrent anterior dislocations of the shoulder. *Clin Orthop* 1967;54:35–49.
27. Deutsch A, Altchek DW, Veltri DM, Potter HG, Warren RF. Traumatic tears of the subscapularis tendon: clinical diagnosis, magnetic resonance imaging findings, and operative treatment. *Am J Sports Med* 1997;25:13–22.
28. Green MR, Christensen KP. Magnetic resonance imaging of the glenoid labrum in anterior shoulder instability. *Am J Sports Med* 1994;22:493–498.

The Unstable Shoulder,
edited by R.F. Warren, E.V. Craig, and D.W. Altchek.
Lippincott–Raven Publishers, Philadelphia © 1999.

CHAPTER 8

Examination Under Anesthesia

Robert H. Cofield and Pierre Mansat

BACKGROUND

The shoulder has always been recognized as a complex joint. A number of studies have been undertaken throughout the 20th century to better describe shoulder mechanics. The modern era, though, appeared to be introduced to orthopedic surgeons during the mid-1970s, when materials such as the article by Poppen and Walker (1) were published describing the normal and abnormal motion of the shoulder. In normal shoulders, there was very little excursion of the humerus on the face of the glenoid through various arcs of motion; however, when significant previous injury had occurred, the mechanics of the shoulder were altered. Five years later, another publication from the same institution quite clearly identified that different structures were contributing to shoulder stability in different positions (2). Such studies and ideas served as a stimulus for the study of the various structures contributing to shoulder stability in various arcs of movement and in varying directions, as outlined in Chapter 3.

Clinically, during this period, clinicians focused their attention on directional testing, such as assessing humeral head translation in the inferior direction, as described in the article on inferior capsular shift for inferior and multidirectional instability of the shoulder (3). Drawer tests were also defined, assessing humeral translation in anterior and posterior directions (4,5).

During the mid-1980s, we became concerned, given the above background, that directional testing without more careful attention to arm position not only in flexion/extension or abduction/adduction, but also in rotation, would be necessary to evaluate more fully humeral head translation on the glenoid and identify pathologic (usually traumatic) changes in the shoulder supporting structures. As a result, in 1987 a system, seemingly quite complicated, for examination of the shoulder under anesthesia was proposed (6). Before this time, we could easily agree that the methods used for examining humeral translation clinically were not all that helpful, but we were also hopeful on the basis of developments in the understanding of shoulder biomechanics that a more refined examination would be found clinically useful.

Soon thereafter, the shoulder group from Seattle conducted very interesting *in vivo* assessments of the laxity of normal and unstable glenohumeral joints. In the first study of normal joints published in 1992, they defined that laxity of normal shoulders, represented by glenohumeral translation, varied substantially among subjects for the anterior drawer, posterior drawer and sulcus tests (7). These investigators recognized that the tests were being performed in the middle range of glenohumeral motion—in which capsular constraints would be expected to be lax. By contrast, when positioning the joint near the extreme of motion such as during the fulcrum test, tension was imparted to the shoulder capsule and while in this position, in normal subjects, no significant humeral translation occurred. This study was followed by the second *in vivo* evaluation of normal and unstable glenohumeral joints and, not surprisingly, they identified that there was significant overlap in the amount of humeral head translation in the anterior, posterior and inferior directions of patients who were normal, who had traumatic instability, or who had atraumatic instability—rendering these clinical laxity tests insufficient in specificity for diagnosis of glenohumeral instability (8).

During the period in which these laboratory tests were being performed, we were evaluating the diagnosis of shoulder instability using examination under anesthesia with the more complex assessment method, taking into consideration all three components of arm positioning (9). Fifty-five patients thought to have shoulder instability had been evaluated by the standard methods (history, physical

R. H. Cofield: Department of Orthopaedics, Mayo Medical School; and Department of Orthopaedics, Mayo Clinic and Mayo Foundation, Rochester, Minnesota 55905.

P. Mansat: Department of Orthopaedics, Mayo Graduate School of Medicine and Mayo Clinic, Rochester, Minnesota 55905.

examination, and plane radiographs with special views), examination under anesthesia, and either shoulder arthroscopy or operation. Twenty-five of those shoulders showed pathologic evidence of shoulder instability. All 25 had abnormal results on examination under anesthesia, whereas the 30 shoulders without demonstrable instability had normal examinations in 28 (two false-positive results). Thus, the accuracy of this testing method seem to be improving dramatically, warranting much more careful assessment of the test-examination under anesthesia—as a part of the armamentarium for the diagnosis of shoulder instability.

CONCEPTS

Based on this background, several concepts evolved:

1. Shoulder range of motion and classic drawer and sulcus testing allow appreciation of joint flexibility or laxity but are not sufficient for the diagnosis of shoulder instability.
2. The diagnosis of shoulder instability ideally includes the triad: appropriate signs and symptoms, abnormal translation of the humeral head on the glenoid, and identification of physical changes in the shoulder's supporting structures (usually by imaging studies or arthroscopy) that are associated with shoulder instability. However, some patients with shoulder instability have sustained a capsular injury and the physical structural changes are obscured by the repair process, reinforcing the importance of being able to distinguish normal from abnormal humeral head translation, if consistency in diagnosis is to be achieved.
3. Examination of humeral head translation under anesthesia should be designed to assess not only mid-range flexibility or laxity, but also end-range humeral head translation on the glenoid, in order to distinguish between normal and abnormal shoulders.

TECHNIQUE

Technique can be considered in four areas: patient and examiner position, arm positioning, testing sequence, and grading of humeral head translation.

The patient is placed in the supine position. Interscalene block anesthesia may be preferred if a subsequent procedure such as arthroscopy is to be performed. A short general anesthetic is desirable if both shoulders are to be examined, and if there is any evidence of remaining muscle tone, a paralyzing agent should be given. Both shoulders are exposed. The examiner stands by the side of the patient. For examination of the right shoulder, the right wrist of the patient is held by the right hand of the examiner while the left hand of the examiner is placed across the superolateral aspect of the shoulder. The palm of the left hand rests across the acromion and distal clavicle with the fourth and fifth fingertips resting near the coracoid process. The thumb is positioned on the posterior aspect of the humeral head, and the index and long fingers are placed on the anterior aspect of the humeral head. The right hand of the examiner positions the arm of the patient in varying degrees of abduction/adduction, flexion/extension, and rotation while the left hand of the examiner applies pressure to the head of the humerus during the translation maneuvers. The amount of pressure applied during this force-displacement evaluation is not large. I would estimate that it is 2 to 5 pounds. The positions of the hands of the examiner are then reversed for examination of the left shoulder. Before each translational maneuver the examiner must be certain the humeral head is centered on the glenoid. This is accomplished by performing minor translational maneuvers anteriorly and posteriorly before each test to ascertain with clarity that the humerus is centered in the glenoid fossa and by pressing the humeral head not directly anteriorly or posteriorly, but slightly anteromedially and posteromedially, to fully engage the humerus in the glenoid.

Humeral translation could be tested in an infinite number of arm positions. We have found it useful to define certain positions of testing for consistency and to add additional positions when they are thought to be clinically useful (Fig. 1). For translation of the humerus in the anterior direction, the arm is positioned in 20 to 30 degrees of abduction, 0 to 10 degrees of extension, and then in neutral rotation, 40 degrees of external rotation and 80 degrees of external rotation. For assessment of translation of the humeral head in the anteroinferior direction, the arm is positioned in 70 to 80 degrees of abduction, 0 to 10 degrees of extension, and 0, 40, and 80 degrees of

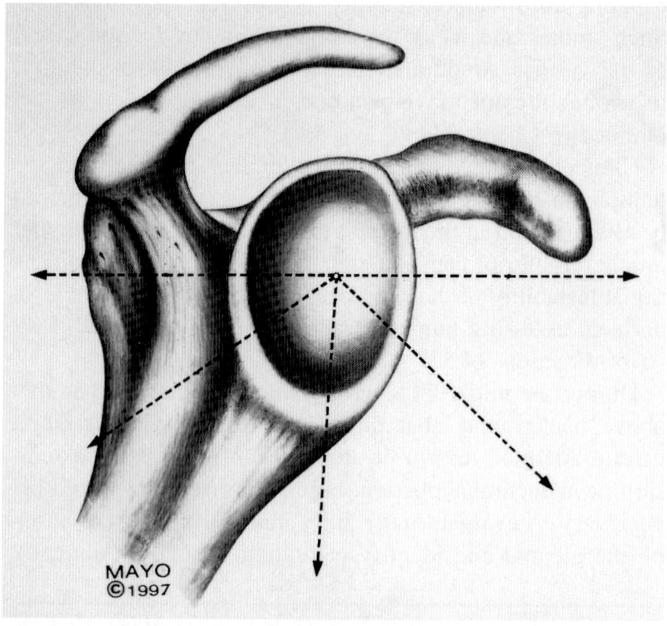

FIG. 1. Directions of humeral head translation on the glenoid that are assessed (measured) during examination under anesthesia: anterior, anteroinferior, inferior, posteroinferior, and posterior.

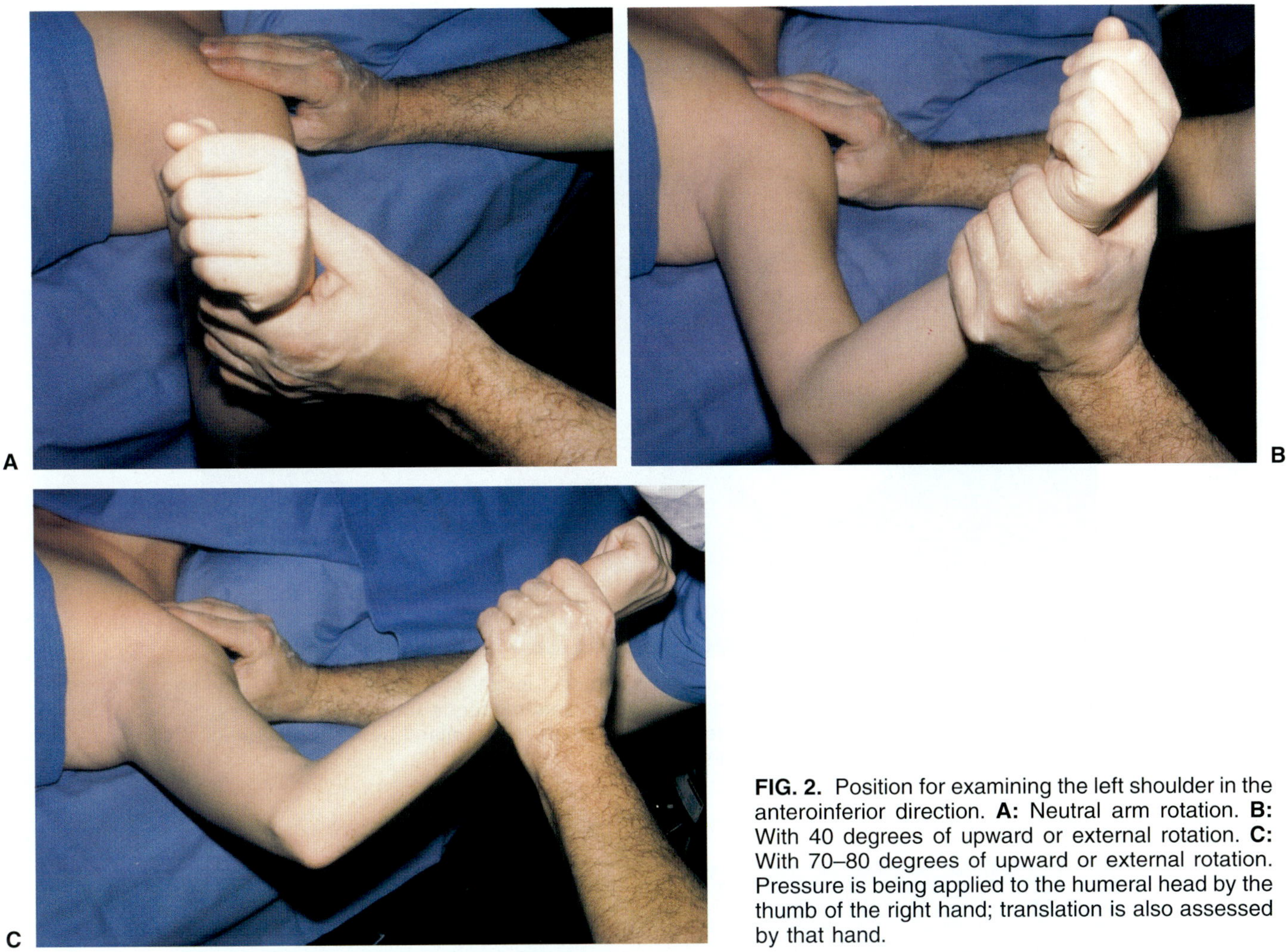

FIG. 2. Position for examining the left shoulder in the anteroinferior direction. **A:** Neutral arm rotation. **B:** With 40 degrees of upward or external rotation. **C:** With 70–80 degrees of upward or external rotation. Pressure is being applied to the humeral head by the thumb of the right hand; translation is also assessed by that hand.

external rotation (Fig. 2). For assessing translation of the humeral head in the posterior direction, the arm is positioned in 20 to 30 degrees of abduction, 0 to 10 degrees of flexion, and 0, 40 and 80 degrees of internal rotation. For assessing translation of the humeral head on the glenoid in the posteroinferior direction, the arm is positioned in 70 to 80 degrees of abduction, 0 to 10 degrees of flexion, and 0, 40, and 80 degrees of internal rotation. For assessing translation in the inferior direction, the arm is positioned in 20 degrees of abduction, 0 degrees of flexion/extension, and neutral rotation.

Typically, the involved shoulder is examined first. This is followed by examination of the opposite (often normal) shoulder, and then examination of the involved shoulder is repeated to confirm the accuracy and the reproducibility of the examination. Additional repeat examinations are done if there is any uncertainty about the amount of humeral head translation.

Translation of the humeral head could also be graded in a variety of ways. We have found it useful to establish some standards with introduction of other grading methods if they appear to be clinically useful (Fig. 3). When translation of the humeral head on the glenoid is absent or no translation is appreciated, the translation is graded as 1. When there is slight translation of the humeral head on the glenoid, but not enough to allow the head of the humerus to rise up on the rim of the glenoid cavity, the translation is considered mild, grade 2. When the head of the humerus is appreciated to move up on the rim of the glenoid cavity, translation is graded as moderate, grade 3. When the head of the humerus courses over the rim of the glenoid cavity and is dislocated, the translation is severe, grade 4. Inferior translation is graded differently; it seems most practical to assess it in terms of the distance of translation. It is graded as grade 1 when there is 0.5 cm of translation or less, as grade 2 when the translation is greater than 0.5 to 1.0 cm, as grade 3 when the translation is greater than 1 to 1.5 cm, and as grade 4 when the translation is greater than 1.5 cm. It is useful to have a grading sheet prepared so that these translations can be easily and consistently recorded as a part of the examination sequence. Such a sheet is illustrated in Figure 4.

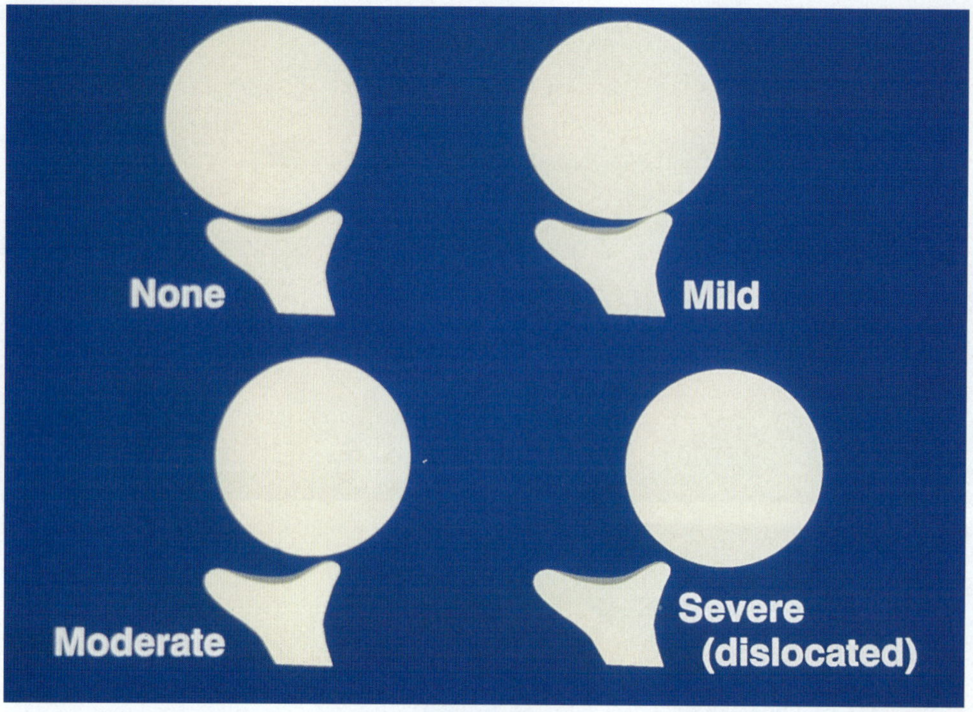

FIG. 3. Method for grading humeral head translation. Grade 1 is equivalent to no humeral head translation, grade 2 represents mild translation, grade 3 represents moderate translation with the humeral head perching on the glenoid rim, and grade 4 represents severe humeral head translation or dislocation of the humeral head over the glenoid rim.

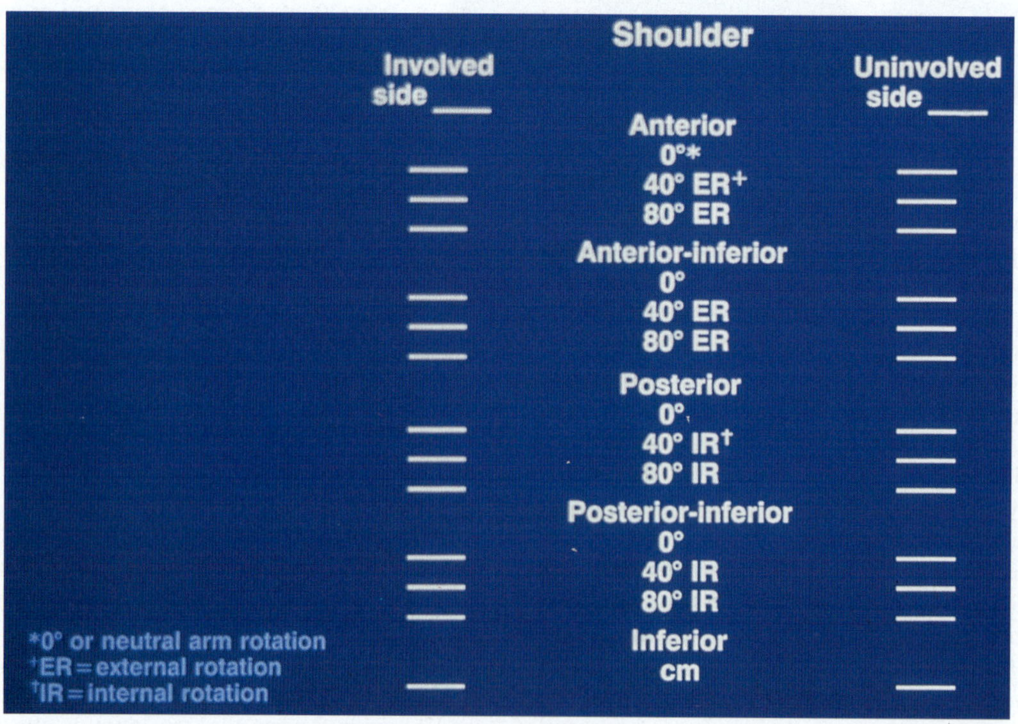

FIG. 4. Data sheet for recording humeral head translation during the examination under anesthesia.

INTERPRETATION OF HUMERAL HEAD TRANSLATION

When evaluating humeral head translations on the glenoid and indeed when assessing examination under anesthesia, one can evaluate various test groups, assess group mean values and standard deviations, and apply statistical testing to the differences between groups. This is a quite realistic method to evaluate differences between or among groups and has been applied both clinically and in the laboratory. For example, Warner et al. (10) assessed the patterns of laxity in normal and abnormal shoulders and showed statistically significant increases in humeral head translation in those patients with instability when compared with patients who were normal or who had impingement. This abnormal increase in translation occurred in anterior, posterior and inferior directions. Hawkins et al. (11) performed a similar assessment of translation but with the patients under anesthesia. Again, differences were identified in translation in the various directions between the control group, a group with anterior instability, and a group with multidirectional instability. They did note, though, that significant overlap in the translation was seen between the normal subjects and those with shoulder instability. In the laboratory, Itoi et al. (12) identified differences in translation between groups of tests related to the amount of load applied and to the amount of humeral rotation. Thus, in assessing humeral head translation in the laboratory, in the awake subject, or in the patient undergoing anesthesia, differences among groups evaluated can often be recognized and statistically assessed.

However, when assessing the validity of a test such as examination under anesthesia, one is more interested not in group differences but in various other parameters such as test sensitivity or the ability to detect true cases and test specificity, as well as the ability to detect disease-free individuals. One might also consider false-positive or false-negative rates and the predictive value or diagnostic value of the test. In addition, it must be recognized that the validity of any procedure can only be determined if a gold standard for absolute truth is available. Although group differences as outlined above certainly are informative, it seems more appropriate to apply this latter set of test measures to an assessment such as examination under anesthesia.

In an attempt to make headway in this regard, we have evaluated examination of the shoulder under anesthesia as a test in two study groups. The first group reported in 1993 was a mixed group of patients referred with a suspicion that they had shoulder instability but in whom the diagnosis could not be made with certainty (9). The gold standard was arthroscopically or surgically identifiable glenoid or capsular lesions. The test criterion for an abnormal examination was moderate or severe translation in a given arm position two grades greater than the translation seen in that position in the uninvolved opposite shoulder. Using this criterion, there were 27 positive examinations—25 true-positive and 2 false-positive. There were 28 negative examinations, all 28 being true-negative with no false-negative examinations. Thus, the sensitivity of the examination was 100%; the specificity was 93.5%; the false-positive rate was 7.4%; the false negative rate was 0; and the predictive value of the examination was 92.6%.

A second study was conducted in 30 patients with stereotypical, unilateral, involuntary traumatic anterior shoulder instability who underwent examination under anesthesia before a surgical procedure (13). The opposite shoulder was normal and without symptoms. In this homogeneous group, group analysis demonstrated statistically increased humeral head translation in the anteroinferior direction at 40 and 80 degrees of external rotation, as compared with the opposite normal side. The difference in translation at 80 degrees of external rotation was significantly greater than the difference in the anteroinferior direction with 40 degrees of external rotation. The sensitivity of the test, according to the above criteria, was 84% in this group with a specificity of 100%. The positive predictive value was 100%. Interestingly, if less strict examination criteria were used with a positive test being defined as moderate to severe humeral translation but only one grade more than the opposite normal side, the sensitivity would have increased to 97% without a detrimental decrease in specificity.

In summarizing conceptually the interpretations of this test (and others), analysis by testing groups supplies useful information, but it is better to apply the various measurements contributing to the assessment of test validity. It can be readily seen that the expanded examination of the shoulder under anesthesia is reasonably accurate as a test but, as with most other tests, cannot be perfect. It is most important when considering this test to recall that there is a continuum of humeral head translation from no translation (e.g., arthrodesis) to extreme instability (e.g., fixed dislocation), and that we are attempting to draw a line somewhere along this continuum that will separate all abnormals from all normals. Clearly, this will never be possible to achieve. It is remarkable, though, that advances in knowledge about shoulder biomechanics, improved anatomic understanding of the shoulder capsule, increasingly refined recognition of structural changes indicative of shoulder instability, and the development of refinements in examination under anesthesia testing have all come together to create a situation in which examination under anesthesia has become a great addition to the overall evaluation of patients with shoulder instability.

There are some points of caution. There are really no firm gold standards as to what constitutes clinically significant posterior instability or multidirectional instability, and even in classic traumatic anterior instability there are a number of people who have had capsule tearing that has healed in an elongated position but without visible pathologic alterations. With this absence of firm standards, it becomes very difficult to define test accuracy in these settings. Correspondingly, the accuracy of examination under anesthesia has not been measured for posterior or multidirectional instability. In addition, there are undoubtedly some patients who possess instability that manifests itself between mid-range and end-range but are very difficult to assess. This includes a small group of patients who have had previous surgery for shoulder instability who have had capsular tightening and possess no end-range instability but by virtue of a still existing Bankart lesion, catch a humeral head impression defect in the Bankart lesion and manifest clinically significant instability in a position short of end range. The evaluation of these latter conditions are yet to be fully resolved, and it is quite possible that examination under anesthesia will not be able to do so to the exclusion of other adjunctive evaluative methods.

FUTURE CONSIDERATIONS

There is no doubt that increased understanding of the anatomy and the biomechanics of the shoulder will further refine examination of the shoulder both in the office and under anesthesia. These improvements in understanding of the concepts behind shoulder instability will undoubtedly modify the role of examination under anesthesia and perhaps modify it significantly. For example, the relationship between office examination and examination using an anesthetic is still to be defined. It is our experience that the classic anterior apprehension test can be negative in the office, even in a patient with typical historic features and symptoms. Yet, examination with an anesthetic using the described system clearly defines an anteroinferior instability. Conversely, most patients without a history of injury who profess to have shoulder instability and who have had a negative office examination will have a negative examination under anesthesia—eliminating the need for further testing.

This test is really a force-displacement test. It is hard in this setting, if not impossible, to accurately measure the forces involved and to measure the displacement with precision. Improved imaging may assist us with assessing displacements and various testing devices such as those now available for the knee may become practically usable for the shoulder (14). However, I sense that, as with many other physical examination type tests, it will be difficult to improve on the accuracy of a skilled, experienced examiner.

It is also unclear whether additional information about joint laxity (or flexibility) should influence surgical treatment, but probably it does (3). In our practice, if examination under anesthesia defines a focal anteroinferior instability and little laxity in other directions, correction of the existing Bankart lesion is performed without adjunctive tightening of the shoulder capsule. By contrast, when the shoulder is quite lax, in addition to having anteroinferior instability in the presence of a Bankart lesion, the capsule is tightened somewhat in addition to doing the Bankart repair at the time of surgery.

SUMMARY

Examination under anesthesia is but one component in the overall armamentarium of diagnostic tools for shoulder instability. A careful history combined with physical examination that includes specific maneuvers and plain radiographs with special views, such as the West Point axillary and Stryker notch views, will continue to serve as the foundation for diagnosis in this arena. Adjunctive imaging tests may prove useful, such as computed tomography (CT) arthrography or magnetic resonance imaging (MRI) with gadolinium. Arthroscopy can quite nicely assess the visual changes that are seen in association with shoulder instability, and this is quite important. However, to be absolutely secure in our diagnosis in addition to appropriate signs and symptoms and visual evidence of structural changes associated with instability, it seems sound relative to basic orthopedic principles to also be able to measure the amount of shoulder instability (humeral head translation) that is present and to compare it with the standard that describes the difference between normal and abnormal. Examination under anesthesia is probably the best contemporary tool to fulfill this latter need (15–18).

Currently it seems reasonable if a patient has by history, physical examination, and plain radiographs, a rather firm diagnosis of shoulder instability to confirm the presence of instability under anesthesia before undertaking operative reconstruction. Alternatively, when the diagnosis is not as secure after the basic investigations, performing examination under anesthesia in conjunction with additional diagnostic testing such as MRI or arthroscopy would seem prudent.

REFERENCES

1. Poppen NK, Walker PS. Normal and abnormal motion of the shoulder. *J Bone Joint Surg* 1976;58A:195–201.
2. Turkel SJ, Panio MW, Marshall JL, Girgis FG. Stabilizing mechanisms preventing anterior dislocation of the glenohumeral joint. *J Bone Joint Surg* 1981;63A:1208–1217.
3. Neer CS II, Foster CR. Inferior capsular shift for involuntary inferior and multidirectional instability of the shoulder. *J Bone Joint Surg* 1980;62A:897–908.
4. Gerber C, Ganz R. Clinical assessment of instability of the shoulder. With special reference to anterior and posterior drawer tests. *J Bone Joint Surg* 1984;66B:551–556.
5. Lintner SA, Levy A, Kenter K, Speer KP. Glenohumeral translation in the asymptomatic athlete's shoulder and its relationship to other clinically measurable anthropometric variables. *Am J Sports Med* 1996;24:716–720.
6. Cofield RH, Irving JF. Evaluation and classification of shoulder instability. With special reference to examination under anesthesia. *Clin Orthop* 1987;223:32–43.
7. Harryman DT, Sidles JA, Harris SL, Matsen FA III. Laxity of the normal glenohumeral joint: a quantitative in vivo assessment. *J Shoulder Elbow Surg* 1992;1:66–76.
8. Lippitt SB, Harris SL, Harryman DT II, Sidles JA, Matsen FA III. In vivo quantification of the laxity of normal and unstable glenohumeral joints. *J Shoulder Elbow Surg* 1994;3:215–223.
9. Cofield RH, Nessler JP, Weinstabl R. Diagnosis of shoulder instability by examination under anesthesia. *Clin Orthop* 1993;291:45–53.
10. Warner JJP, Micheli LJ, Arslanian LE, Kennedy J, Kennedy R. Patterns of flexibility, laxity and strength in normal shoulders and shoulders with instability and impingement. *Am J Sports Med* 1990;18:366–375.

11. Hawkins RJ, Schutte JP, Janda DH, Huckell GH. Translation of the glenohumeral joint with the patient under anesthesia. *J Shoulder Elbow Surg* 1996;5:286–292.
12. Itoi E, Motzkin NE, Morrey BF, An KN. Contribution of axial arm rotation to humeral head translation. *Am J Sports Med* 1994;22:499–503.
13. Cofield RH, Oliashirazi A. Diagnosis of traumatic shoulder instability by examination under anesthesia. Presented at the Sixth International Congress on Surgery of the Shoulder, Helsinki, Finland and Stockholm, Sweden, June 27–July 4, 1995.
14. Jørgensen U, Bak K. Shoulder instability. Assessment of anterior-posterior translation with a knee laxity tester. *Acta Orthop Scand* 1995;66:398–400.
15. Bahr R, Craig EV, Engebretsen L. The clinical presentation of shoulder instability including on field management. *Clin Sports Med* 1995;14:761–776.
16. Morton KS. The unstable shoulder: recurring subluxation. *Injury* 1978;10:304–306.
17. Pappas AM, Goss TP, Kleinman PK: Symptomatic shoulder instability due to lesions of the glenoid labrum. *Am J Sports Med* 1983;11: 279–288.
18. Warren RF. Subluxation of the shoulder in athletes. *Clin Sports Med* 1983;2:339–354.

The Unstable Shoulder,
edited by R.F. Warren, E.V. Craig, and D.W. Altchek.
Lippincott–Raven Publishers, Philadelphia © 1999.

CHAPTER 9

Diagnostic Shoulder Arthroscopy

Pathologic Findings

Champ L. Baker, Jr., and George M. McCluskey III

NORMAL ARTHROSCOPIC ANATOMY

To make accurate diagnoses and to perform arthroscopic surgical procedures, the shoulder surgeon must have a thorough knowledge of normal intra-articular (glenohumeral) and extra-articular (subacromial) shoulder anatomy and its normal variations. A reproducible and systematic pattern of arthroscopic shoulder examination should be developed to ensure its completeness, accuracy, and reliability. Orientation of the anatomic structures varies depending on the patient's position (beach chair versus lateral decubitus position) during the procedure.

Superficial Landmarks

The bony structures are useful as landmarks and should be outlined with a marking pen after the patient has been anesthetized but before the surgical procedure is begun. First, the posterolateral angle of the acromion is palpated and marked. Next, the lateral edge of the acromion up to its anterolateral corner should be marked. The shaft of the clavicle is then palpated to determine the location of the acromioclavicular joint. The supraclavicular fossa, or ''soft spot,'' is located immediately posterior to the acromioclavicular joint. The coracoid process is the most easily identified anterior landmark; it serves to identify the danger zone inferior to the coracoid in which the brachial plexus and axillary vessels are located. The coracoacromial ligament should also be marked to complete the topographic outline of the anatomic landmarks used in shoulder arthroscopy. The humeral head can be grasped easily with the thumb and long finger in the front and back of the shoulder in thinner patients and does not need to be marked with a pen.

C. L. Baker, Jr.: Department of Orthopaedics, Tulane University School of Medicine, New Orleans, Louisiana 70112; and The Hughston Clinic, Columbus, Georgia 31908.

G. M. McClusky III: The Hughston Clinic, Columbus, Georgia 31908.

Glenohumeral Joint Anatomy

With the arthroscope in the posterior portal, the glenohumeral joint anatomy should be viewed in a systematic fashion.

Biceps Tendon

The long head of the biceps tendon should be the first structure seen when the shoulder joint is entered. The biceps has a firm attachment to the supraglenoid tubercle at the posterosuperior glenoid. The biceps tendon appears to be confluent with the superior glenoid labrum. The tendon is smooth and glistening with no attachments or structures superior to it. Followed laterally, the biceps tendon can be seen to exit the glenohumeral joint by passing through the bicipital groove, thus becoming extra-articular (Fig. 1). At this lateral location, the biceps tendon demarcates the interval between the supraspinatus and subscapularis tendons of the rotator cuff.

Glenoid Labrum

The glenoid labrum is a variable fibrous structure that forms a ring around the glenoid and provides stability to the glenohumeral joint (Fig. 2). The labrum attaches to the glenoid through a thin, fibrocartilaginous transitional zone and functions primarily as the attachment site on the glenoid for the capsuloligamentous structures (1). The glenoid labrum also acts to increase the overall surface area and load-bearing surface on which the humeral head articulates with the glenoid (2).

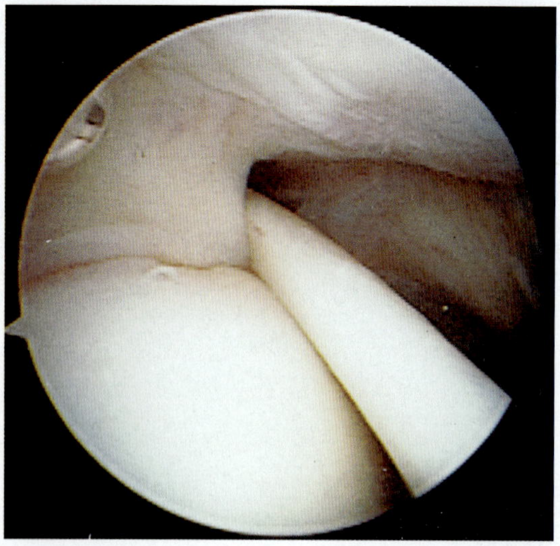

FIG. 1. Biceps tendon viewed from inside the glenohumeral joint as it runs between the supraspinatus and subscapularis tendons into the bicipital groove.

Significant anatomic variation of the labrum exists in the anterosuperior and posterosuperior quadrants of the glenoid and will be discussed in more detail later. Generally, the superior half of the labrum is loosely attached to the glenoid and resembles the knee meniscus in appearance. In this wedge-shaped portion of the labrum, the free-tapered edge of the labrum is directed toward the center of the glenoid. However, in the inferior quadrants below the equator of the glenoid, the labrum is normally attached firmly to the articular cartilage of the glenoid without much variation (1).

Articular Surfaces of the Humeral Head and Glenoid

The articular surface of the glenoid is approximately one-fourth the size of the surface of the humeral head. Thus, little inherent joint stability is derived from the bony architecture of this joint. The glenoid is shaped like an inverted comma with the superior portion narrower than the inferior portion. In any shoulder position, it is estimated that only 25% of the humeral head is covered by the glenoid socket (3).

The articular cartilage of the glenoid is thickest at the periphery (average, 3.81 mm) and thinnest at its center (average, 1.14 mm) (2). The "bare spot" as described by DePalma et al. (4) at the center of the glenoid is often misinterpreted as an area of chondromalacia. Although the articular cartilage is thinnest here, the subchondral bone density is increased in this central area.

The articular surface of the humeral head should appear smooth and regular, except for the inferior nonarticulating portion. At the bare area of the humeral head, adjacent to the posterolateral rotator cuff attachment, the articular cartilage is noticeably absent, and the area often has pits or indentations representing nutrient vascular channels into the bone (Fig. 3). This region should not be confused with the Hill-Sachs lesion associated with glenohumeral instability that is often seen in this area.

Glenohumeral Ligaments

The articular capsule has thickenings that collectively form the glenohumeral ligaments. There are no named ligaments in the posterior capsule above the posterior band of the inferior glenohumeral ligament. These ligaments are quite variable in structure (*vide infra*). The superior, middle, and inferior glenohumeral ligaments are named according to their location on the humeral head. They vary considerably in shape, insertion, and size.

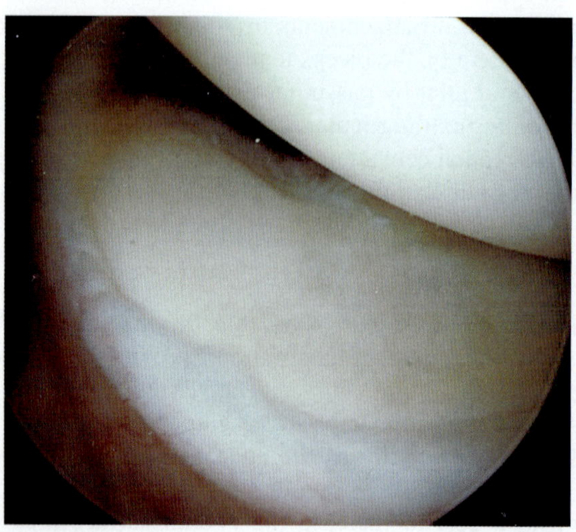

FIG. 2. Intra-articular view of the glenoid labrum as it encircles the glenoid.

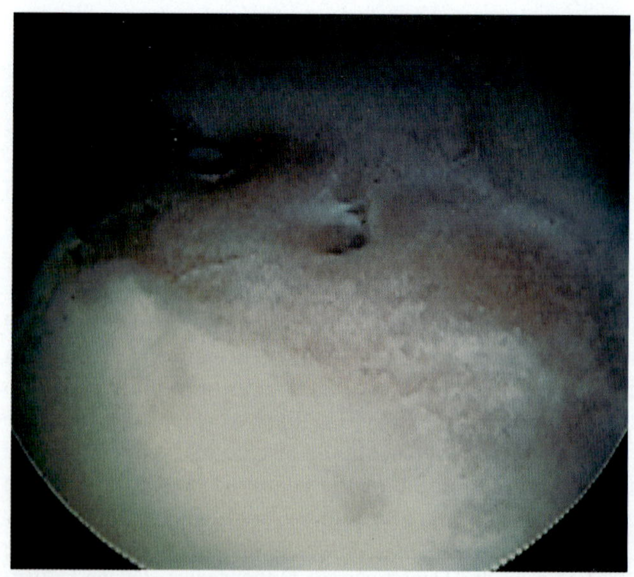

FIG. 3. Bare area located between the articular cartilage and the attachment site of the infraspinatus and teres minor tendons. Vascular pits are often present and can give the false impression of a pathologic Hill-Sachs lesion.

The superior glenohumeral ligament courses vertically to the joint. It arises from the supraglenoid tubercle from the base of the coracoid just anterior to the long head of the biceps tendon (5) (Fig. 4). It then attaches to the medial ridge of the bicipital groove and the anatomic humeral neck anteriorly. This superior ligament is often difficult to see behind the long head of the biceps tendon, especially from the standard posterior arthroscopic portal. It functions with other structures in the rotator interval to stabilize the adducted dependent arm and to prevent inferior translation of the joint. This ligament was invariably present in cadaveric specimens (5).

The middle glenohumeral ligament varies most in size and shape and is absent in 8% to 30% of shoulders (6,7). It arises from the superior glenoid just beneath the superior glenohumeral ligament along the anterosuperior glenoid neck, and it inserts just medial to the lesser tuberosity. As it courses at an oblique angle across the posterior aspect of the subscapularis tendon, the two common morphologic variations of the middle glenohumeral ligament can be seen. One is sheet-like and confluent with the anterior band of the inferior glenohumeral ligament, and the second is cord-like with a foramen, or recess, between it and the anterior band of the inferior glenohumeral ligament. This ligament stabilizes the joint when the arm is abducted to 45 degrees (5).

The inferior glenohumeral ligament is the primary ligamentous stabilizer of the shoulder joint, particularly at 90 degrees of abduction and is the easiest ligament to visualize arthroscopically (5). This inferior glenohumeral ligament complex, as described by O'Brien et al. (6), consists of thick anterior and posterior bands in the joint capsule with a thinner hammock-like area inferiorly between these two bands. This inferior capsular pouch is often quite patulous, allowing for considerable laxity in the joint. This complex arises from the anteroinferior glenoid labrum and glenoid neck and inserts into the surgical neck of the humerus. The reciprocal tightening and loosening of the glenohumeral ligaments during rotation is best demonstrated at 90 degrees of abduction by viewing the inferior glenohumeral ligament complex (7). At 90 degrees of abduction, the humeral head is supported during external rotation by the tightening and fanning out of the anterior band while the posterior band relaxes. During internal rotation, the posterior band fans out while the anterior band relaxes.

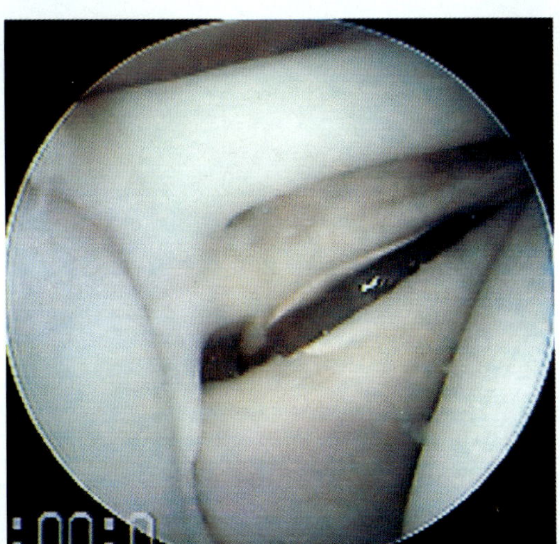

FIG. 4. The superior glenohumeral ligament is often difficult to visualize arthroscopically. When seen, it courses from the supraglenoid tubercle of the glenoid just behind the biceps tendon to the medial ridge of the bicipital groove.

It was disruption of this anteroinferior glenoid capsulolabral complex that was termed the ''essential lesion'' by Bankart, when dealing with acute or recurrent anterior shoulder dislocations (8).

Subscapularis Recess

The subscapularis recess is a foramen located between the subscapularis and the neck of the glenoid. It can originate either above or below the middle glenohumeral ligament, or both, and can be quite large when the middle glenohumeral ligament is absent. This recess becomes a bursa that extends to the coracoid base from the glenoid rim and is often a hiding place for loose bodies. The entire recess or bursa is difficult to see with the arthroscope.

Rotator Cuff

The rotator cuff comprises the supraspinatus, infraspinatus, teres minor, and subscapularis tendons. The posterosuperior portion of the subscapularis tendon is located behind the superior glenohumeral ligament and middle glenohumeral ligaments and can be seen arthroscopically.

Visualization of the undersurface of the remaining cuff tendons is done systematically. The biceps tendon is a useful landmark for localizing the anterior border of the supraspinatus tendon. Although the supraspinatus, infraspinatus, and teres minor tendons and associated capsule form the superior and posterior walls of the glenohumeral joint, the individual borders of the tendons cannot be distinguished from inside the joint. The lateral attachments of the infraspinatus and teres minor tendons are beyond the lateral extent of the articular surface, and the bare area is located in this interval. The articular surfaces must be inspected closely for signs of fraying or tearing, especially near their lateral humeral attachment sites.

Subacromial Space

After the intra-articular portion of the shoulder is examined, the subacromial space must be visualized (Fig. 5). The subacromial bursa, which is the largest bursa in the body, extends anteriorly to the glenohumeral joint and laterally beyond the greater tuberosity (9). The bursa may be large and thin walled with a very benign appearance or

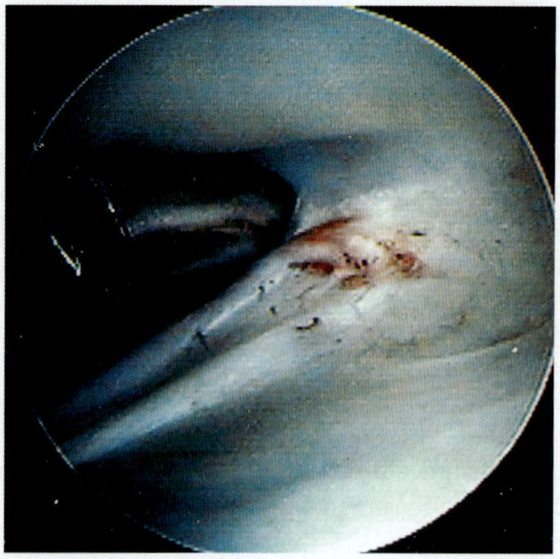

FIG. 5. Normal view of the subacromial bursa showing the smooth glistening structure in the subacromial space. The undersurface of the acromion can be seen with the coracoacromial ligament above and bursal surface of the cuff below.

thickened and loculated with multiple fibrous bands. It is usually necessary to debride this bursa for adequate visualization of the other structures in the subacromial space.

Other structures in the subacromial space are the acromion, acromioclavicular joint, coracoacromial ligament, and the bursal surfaces of the supraspinatus, infraspinatus, and teres minor tendons. A thick periosteum covers the undersurface of the acromion (10). The coracoacromial ligament is usually visible and prominent as it attaches to the anterior edge of the acromion and extends along the inferior surface of the anterior one-third of the acromion (Fig. 5). It often sends slips to the acromioclavicular joint capsule as well. The coracoacromial ligament is most prominent at the anterolateral portion of the acromion.

The distal clavicle and the acromioclavicular joint are usually covered by a thick, fibrous capsule. Its location is often marked preoperatively with a needle passed through the acromioclavicular joint. The bursal surfaces of the rotator cuff tendons are easily identified and form the floor of the subacromial space. The musculotendinous junctions are readily seen along with the tendinous insertions of the cuff into the greater tuberosity.

NORMAL VARIANTS

Variations of the intra-articular anatomy of the shoulder joint are common, and the surgeon must be familiar with the spectrum of what is normal. The glenoid labrum has a variable appearance with two primary patterns that have been described by Detrisac and Johnson (11). The superior portion of the labrum is detached centrally, but attached peripherally while the inferior, posterior, and anterior portions are attached centrally and peripherally in the first type. In the second type, all portions of the labrum are attached centrally and peripherally.

The anterosuperior labrum is attached to the glenoid rim in 88% of shoulders (12). In 11%, a sublabral hole or foramen was noted beneath the anterosuperior labral attachment (Fig. 6). This foramen varied in size from a few millimeters to inclusion of the entire anterosuperior quadrant. It should not be confused with a traumatic labral injury because it is a normal variant.

Another infrequent variant, the Buford complex, occurs in 1.5% of shoulders (12). This interesting complex has a thin, cord-like middle glenohumeral ligament that crosses the subscapularis tendon (Fig. 7). The ligament attaches to the superior labrum just anterior to the base of the long head of the biceps tendon. There is complete absence of the anterosuperior labrum at the glenoid rim.

Johnson and others (13,14) have shown that variations in the glenohumeral ligaments are the rule, rather than the exception. Rames and associates (14) reported that normal variations occurred in the glenohumeral ligaments in 34% of the cadaver specimens they examined. They found variations in size, shape, plane, and connection, as well as variation in the recesses between the ligaments. The most variable structure is the middle glenohumeral ligament. Normally, the ligament appears as a sheet-like thickening in the capsule that crosses the subscapularis obliquely with the subscapularis recess located above the superior edge of the ligament. In 19% of shoulders, the middle glenohumeral ligament is a cord-like structure with the subscapularis recess located either above or below the cord (12) (Fig. 8). In 5% of shoulders, the middle glenohumeral ligament ap-

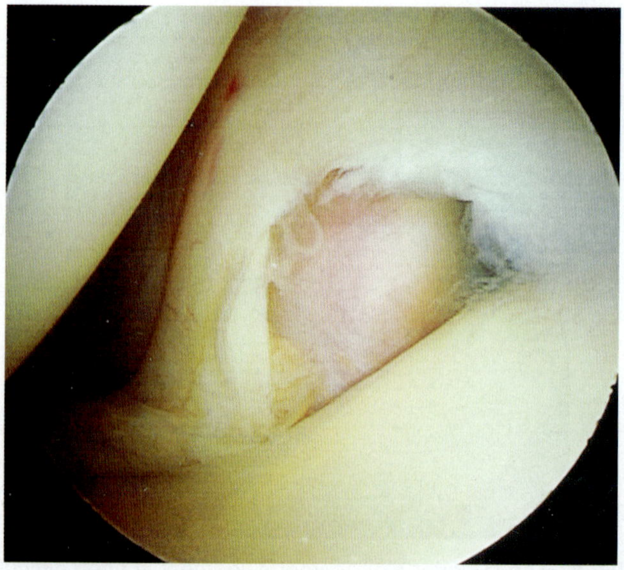

FIG. 6. A sublabral foramen is a normal variant seen arthroscopically in 11% of shoulders. It should not be confused with the glenoid labrum tear.

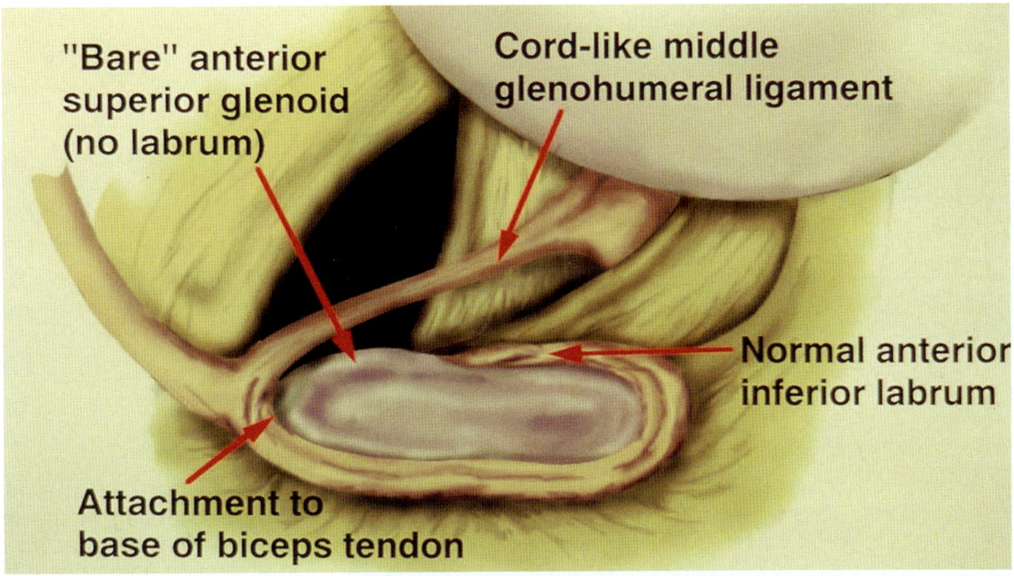

FIG. 7. The Buford complex consists of a thin, cord-like middle glenohumeral ligament that attaches to the superior labrum just anterior to the long head of the biceps tendon. The anterosuperior labrum is absent. This rare variant should not be confused with a labral tear.

pears as a thin transparent sheet with or without a few thin fibrous bands. The middle glenohumeral ligament is completely absent in 1% of shoulders, usually in conjunction with a congenital hyperlaxity syndrome.

In 3% of shoulders, an os acromiale—a failure of the acromial epiphysis to fuse by age 25—can be seen in the subacromial space (15) (Fig. 9). This lesion is often confused with a fracture or nonunion on the preoperative radiograph. The lesion has implications in the impingement syndrome and with rotator cuff lesions.

ARTHROSCOPIC TECHNIQUE

Lateral Decubitus Position

The lateral decubitus position is the most commonly used position for shoulder arthroscopy. Advantages of this patient position are easy access to the shoulder for the surgeon, visual orientation of shoulder structures on the video monitor that mimics the lateral decubitus orientation of the patient's shoulder to the surgeon, ease of repositioning the arm in forward elevation and abduction when viewing various parts of the shoulder, and ready access to the rotator cuff and acromioclavicular joint should an open procedure become necessary.

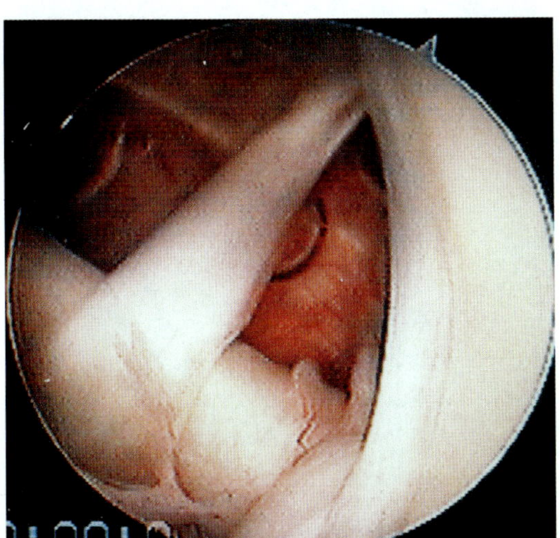

FIG. 8. In approximately 19% of patients, the middle glenohumeral ligament appears as a thin, cord-like structure instead of the more common sheet-like condensation that crosses obliquely over the subscapularis tendon.

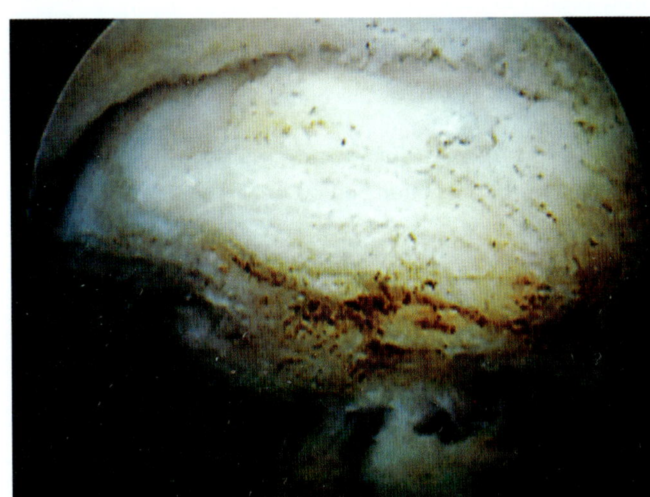

FIG. 9. Arthroscopic view of a mesoacromion (os acromiale), which is a persistent unfused acromial epiphysis.

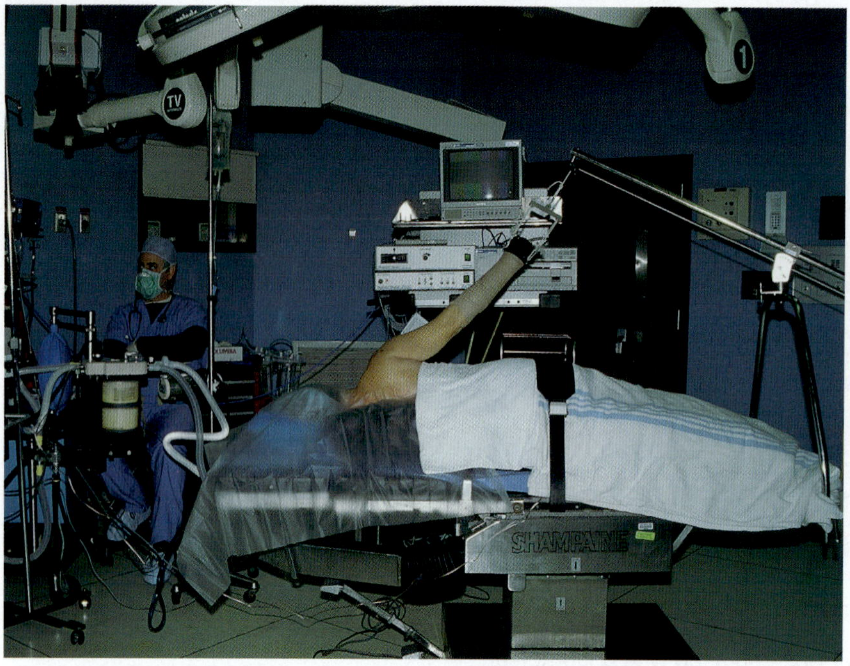

FIG. 10. The patient is placed on an inflatable beanbag in the lateral decubitus position with the affected arm suspended in abduction and forward flexion. Pressure areas, such as the head, knees, and feet, are properly padded and secured with a chest roll.

The patient is placed in the lateral decubitus position on an inflatable beanbag with the affected extremity up and the pelvis perpendicular to the table (Fig. 10). A chest roll is placed in the dependent axilla and the patient's head, neck, knees, and feet are properly padded and secured. The dependent arm is placed on a padded arm board. A safety strap is placed at waist level. The patient is then tilted posteriorly twenty degrees and the beanbag is inflated (Fig. 11). This position orients the glenohumeral joint horizontally. Kidney rests are placed to support the beanbag. Protective sterile plastic U-drapes are used to protect the patient's head and neck from the preoperative solution and irrigating fluid that can accumulate during the procedure. Wide access to the anterior, posterior, and lateral shoulder girdle region is necessary.

The arm and hand are then suspended from a shoulder traction device with 10 to 15 lb of weight applied. Various devices are available, but the one selected must allow for varying degrees of abduction (20 to 60 degrees). Our preferred position for procedures in the lateral position is 20 to 30 degrees of abduction and 10 to 15 degrees of forward flexion.

Nerve injuries have been reported with the arm in traction while in the lateral decubitus position. The minimum amount of weight needed to suspend the arm should be used, and no more than 15 lb should ever be used. Pitman et al. (16) reported that 10% of patients who had had arthroscopic shoulder surgery in the lateral position with the arm in traction showed the development of a clinically evident transient neuropraxia.

The lateral decubitus position is best for arthroscopic procedures, such as subacromial decompression, debridement, Bankart repairs, and acromioclavicular joint procedures. The mini-open deltoid-splitting approach for rotator cuff repair can be done with the patient in the lateral decubitus position and the arm released from the traction de-

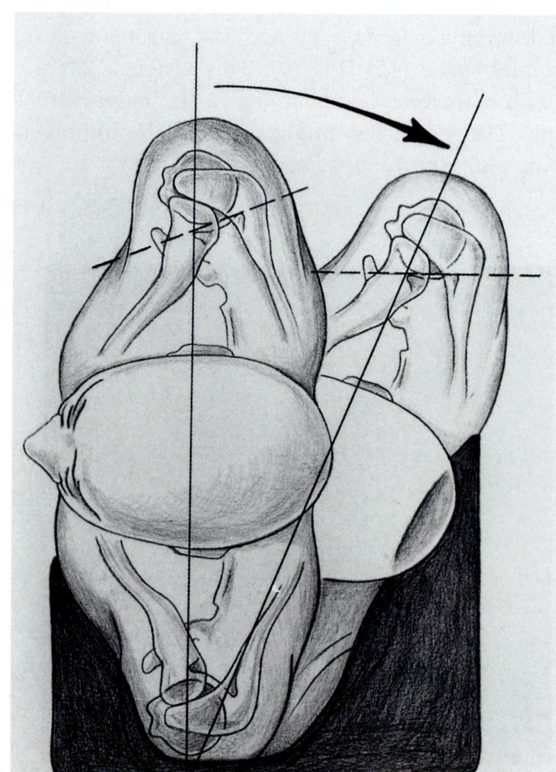

FIG. 11. While in the lateral decubitus position, the patient is tilted 20 degrees posterior to neutral *(arrow)* to orient the glenohumeral joint horizontally.

vice. Other open procedures (i.e., instability procedures), however, necessitate either changing the patient's position to the beach chair or supine position and reprepping and draping or using the beach chair position for the arthroscopic procedure initially.

Beach Chair Position

The beach chair position is the alternative to the lateral decubitus position for shoulder arthroscopy (17,18). The primary advantage of this position is the ease with which an arthroscopic procedure can be converted to an open one, such as when performing an open capsular technique for instability after diagnostic arthroscopy or debridement. Other advantages include the decreased time and effort needed to reposition the patient for improved joint visualization. The arm can be flexed, abducted, and rotated easily in this position. An interscalene block for anesthesia can be used independently with the beach chair position, whereas it is most often used in conjunction with general anesthesia and endotracheal intubation for patients in the lateral decubitus position. Also, the use of gravity for joint distraction decreases the risk of nerve injury.

The anesthetized patient is positioned supine on the operating table. First, the patient is placed in a 30-degree Trendelenburg position; the head is then slowly raised to a 60-degree beach chair position (Fig. 12). Pillows are placed under the knees to keep the patient from sliding down on the table during the procedure. The head is securely attached to a Mayfield-type neurosurgical head rest with the neck positioned to avoid hyperflexion or hyperextension. Protective pads are placed over the eyes. The hips must be located at the table break. The feet and ankles are strapped together to prevent external rotation of the lower extremities and pressure on the peroneal nerve at the fibular head region. The contralateral arm is tucked into the patient's side in a neutral position with a foam pad around the elbow to protect the ulnar nerve. A folded towel is placed under the medial scapular border to bring the shoulder girdle forward, and the patient is positioned so that the entire shoulder and scapular region is off the edge of the table. This allows free access to the anterior and posterior aspects of the shoulder. The entire arm and shoulder girdle are prepared and draped for the procedure.

Anesthesia

General anesthesia with endotracheal intubation is commonly used for shoulder arthroscopy. Many surgeons now augment the general anesthesia with an interscalene block, and some use the interscalene block alone (19). The block improves muscle relaxation and greatly reduces or eliminates postoperative pain for 12 to 16 hours. When a block is used in conjunction with general anesthesia, the need for narcotics and other agents during surgery is lessened, significantly decreasing postanesthesia sedation and nausea. An interscalene block alone is difficult for the patient in the lateral decubitus position. However, patient satisfaction has been high when it is used with the beach chair position. Obviously, the success of the block is improved with increased experience and interest on the part of the anesthesiologist. If operative procedures are performed without an interscalene block, we recommend injection of a local anesthetic into the skin edges, around the portal sites, and into the subacromial bursa and joint.

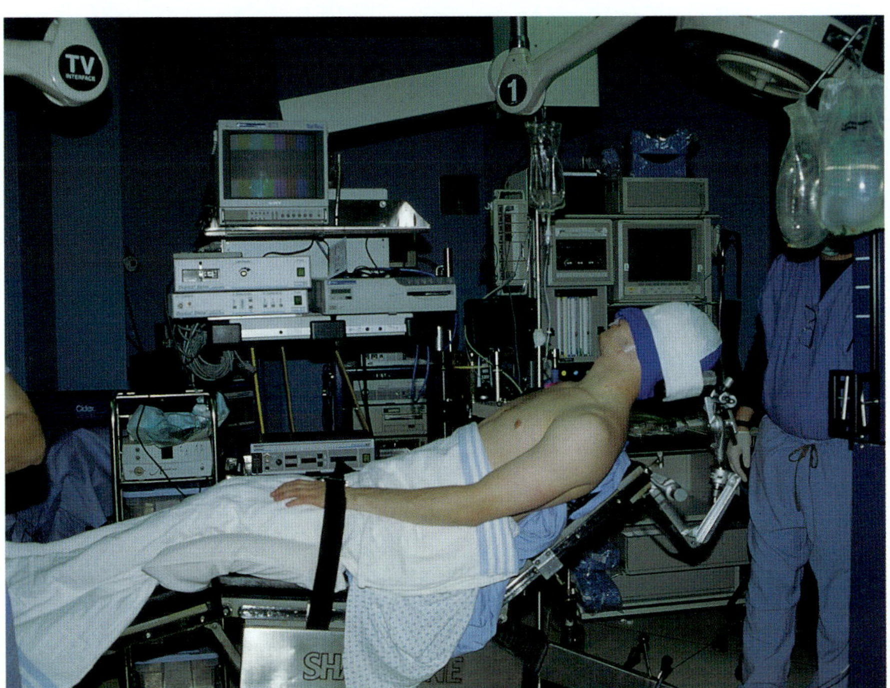

FIG. 12. The patient is placed in the 60-degree beach chair position with the head secured to a Mayfield head rest. The affected extremity is draped free so the arm can be placed in multiple positions.

Portal Placement

Various portals have been described for use during shoulder arthroscopy (13,20–30). Careful placement and orientation of the portals can only be accomplished if the surgeon is quite familiar with the superficial landmarks and the danger zones around neurovascular structures. Improper portal placement increases the risk of intra-articular injury and nerve injury and decreases the surgeon's ability to perform the technical procedure smoothly.

The five portals used for most arthroscopic procedures are the posterior, anterosuperior, anteroinferior, midlateral, and, occasionally, the supraclavicular (Fig. 13A, B). Before beginning either a diagnostic or an operative arthroscopic procedure, the superficial bony landmarks—the coracoid process, the acromion, and the acromioclavicular joint—and the course of the coracoacromial ligament must be marked on the skin. The portal incisions are then marked to enhance accuracy of placement.

Posterior Portal

The standard posterior portal for viewing is made in the "soft spot" located 1 cm medial and 2 cm inferior to the posterolateral corner of the acromion. This soft spot corresponds to the interval between the infraspinatus and teres minor just above the equator of the glenoid (Figs. 13 and 14). A blunt trochar is advanced through the skin portal, muscles, and capsule into the glenohumeral joint. Sharp trochars are not used, as they can damage the articular surfaces. The direction of the trochar is determined by placing the thumb in the soft spot and the index finger on the coracoid process. The trochar is then directed toward the coracoid tip. The axillary nerve is at risk if portal placement or trochar penetration is too inferior, and the suprascapular nerve and artery are at risk if the direction is too superior and medial.

Anterior Portals

Placement of the two anterior portals is next (Figs. 13 and 15). In diagnostic and operative arthroscopy, the anterosuperior portal is usually made along with the posterior portal. The other portals are used when the operative procedure requires them.

The anterosuperior portal is located 1 cm lateral and 1 cm superior to the coracoid process. A spinal needle is

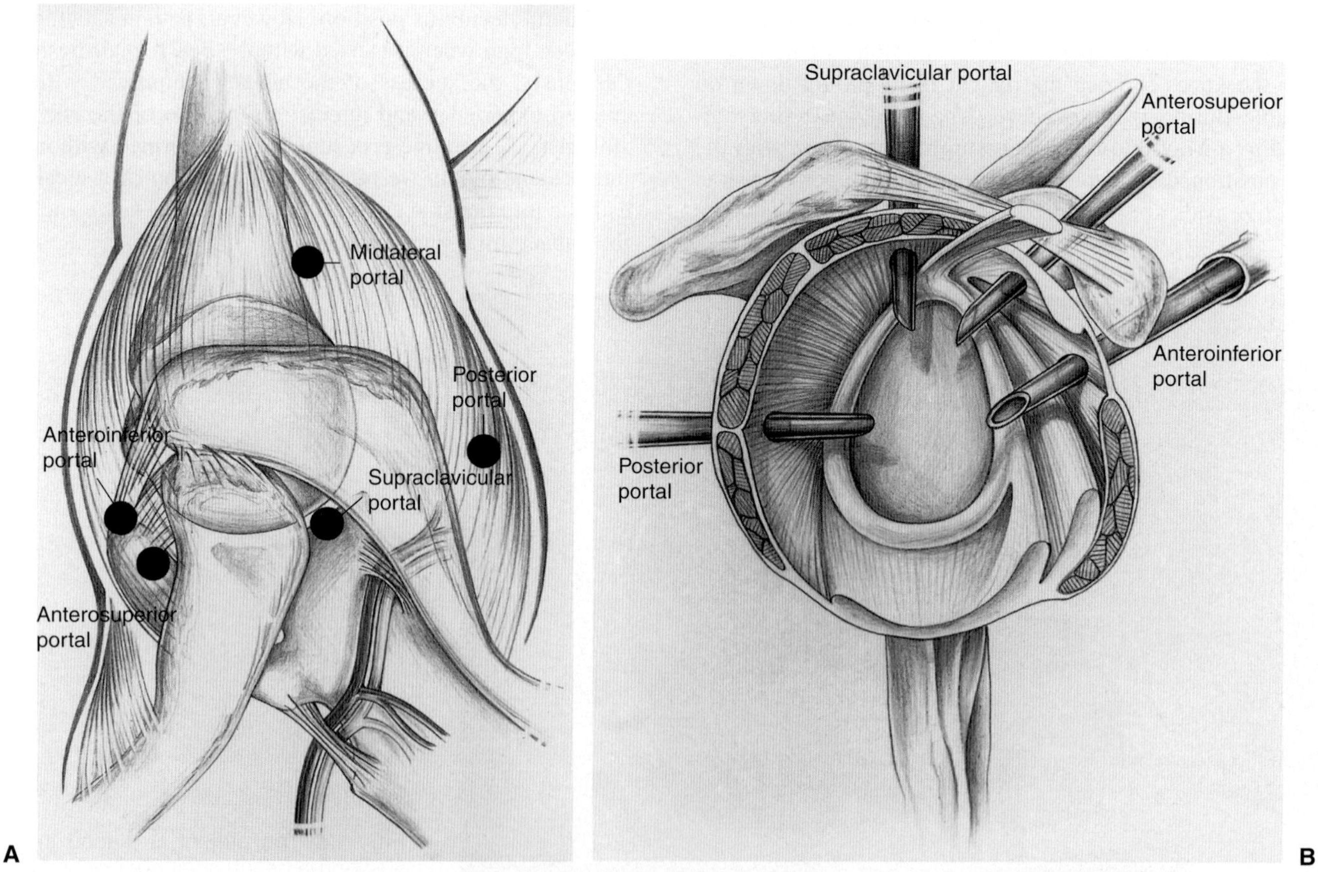

FIG. 13. A: Superior view of the shoulder showing the five portals commonly used in arthroscopy of the shoulder: the posterior, anterosuperior, anteroinferior, midlateral, and supraclavicular portals. **B:** Intra-articular view showing the entry points of the posterior, anterosuperior, anteroinferior, and supraclavicular portals. Relationships to other anatomic structures are illustrated.

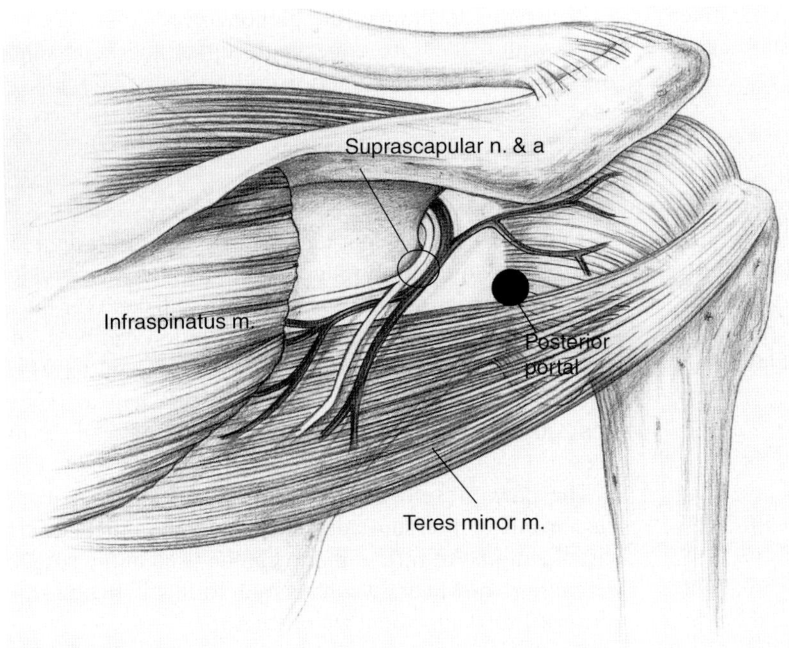

FIG. 14. The standard posterior portal is established between the infraspinatus and teres minor tendons in the soft spot located 1 cm medial and 2 cm inferior to the posterolateral corner of the acromion. The suprascapular nerve must be avoided medially.

placed from "outside in," just under the biceps tendon and under direct visualization with the arthroscope. This portal is versatile and can be used for gravity inflow or as a working or viewing portal. The anteroinferior portal is created with a Wissinger rod from "inside out." The arthroscope is used to visualize the area just above the subscapularis superior edge of the tendon, and the Wissinger rod is placed through the cannula in the posterior portal exiting through the capsule just inferior to the coracoid tip. A small incision is made over the prominent rod tip and a 4.5-mm cannula is slid over the rod and into the joint. There is usually an approximately 1-cm bridge of skin between the two anterior

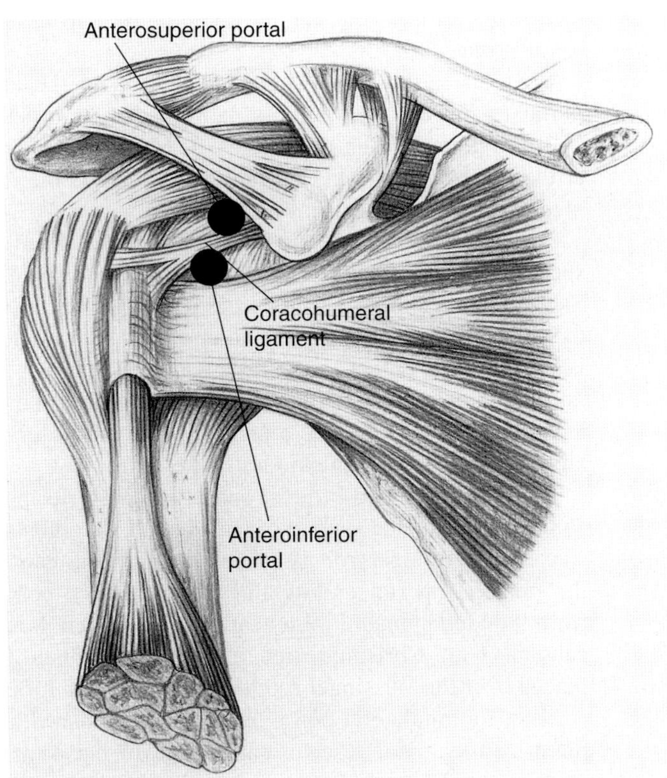

FIG. 15. Two anterior portals are commonly used in shoulder arthroscopy. The anterosuperior portal is located just lateral and superior to the tip of the coracoid process. The anteroinferior portal is located just inferior and lateral to the coracoid tip.

portals. We use these two portals together during operative procedures for debridement, removal of loose bodies, and labral repairs in the glenohumeral joint.

Midlateral Portal

The midlateral portal is used to introduce probes and motorized instruments when working in the subacromial space. The incision is made 2 cm distal to the midpoint on the lateral edge of the acromion. This portal gives excellent access to all structures in the subacromial space, including the anterior portion of the acromion, the acromioclavicular joint and all bursal surfaces of the rotator cuff.

Supraclavicular Portal

The supraclavicular portal can be used as an accessory inflow portal or for arthroscopic instrumentation (30). For safety, the patient's arm should be brought to a position of no more than 45 degrees of abduction and no forward flexion as the trochar is introduced. The trochar is directed laterally 30 degrees in the sagittal plane and neutral in the coronal plane. The entry point in the superior soft spot is then located, just posterior to the distal clavicle and acromioclavicular joint and just anterior to the spine of the scapula (Figs. 13 and 16). The acromion is lateral to the soft spot.

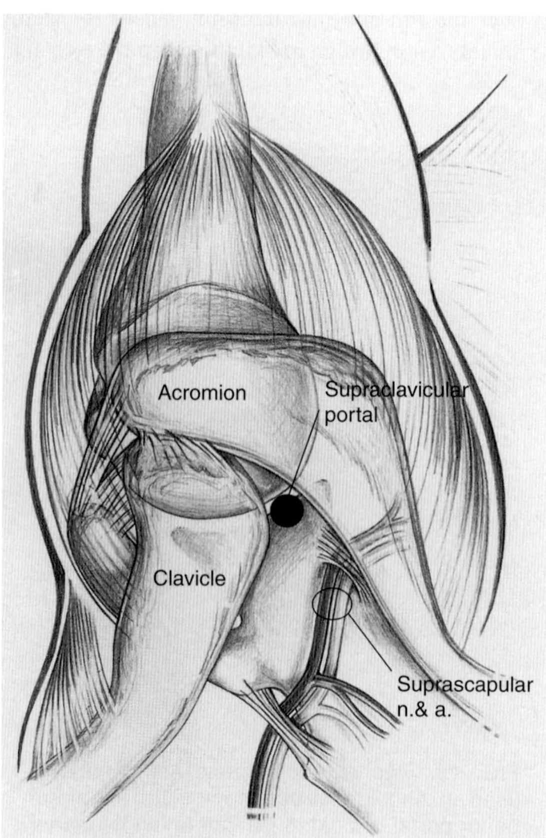

FIG. 16. The supraclavicular portal is located just posterior to the acromioclavicular joint in the superior soft spot.

Using this technique, the glenohumeral joint can be entered within the safe zone made up of the supraspinatus muscle belly and the superior portion of the shoulder capsule.

Diagnostic Arthroscopy

After the posterior portal is established, a 30-degree arthroscopic camera is introduced into the glenohumeral joint. The anterosuperior portal is then established for inflow. Normal saline or lactated Ringer's solution can be used for joint distention. Epinephrine, in a ratio of 1 ml to 100,000 ml of saline, is often added to each 3-L bag to facilitate hemostasis if there are no medical contraindications to its use.

The bags are elevated 7 to 8 feet above the patient to ensure inflow pressure adequate to maintain distention and visualization. An inflow pump can be used at the surgeon's discretion; however, we have not found it necessary for most arthroscopic shoulder procedures.

From the posterior portal, arthroscopic evaluation of the glenohumeral articulation begins by identifying the biceps tendon. The insertion of the tendon into the superior glenoid labral complex is identified and any fragmentation or injury to the tendon noted. If necessary, an anteroinferior portal can be established using an inside-out technique; a probe can be placed through the anterior triangular space to palpate the superior glenoid labral complex. Likewise, the subscapularis tendon should be palpated to look for evidence of attenuation, ruptures, or tears. The middle glenohumeral ligament variations, as well as the inferior glenohumeral ligament complex, can be seen from the posterior portal.

Next, the arthroscope should be placed in the anterior portal to inspect the posterior labrum and its articulation with the glenoid. The arthroscope is rotated down to look at the anteroinferior edge of the glenoid to see the inferior glenohumeral ligament inferiorly.

From the posterior approach, the humeral head is inspected for Hill-Sachs lesions and chondromalacia. Hill-Sachs lesions should be graded I, II, or III, depending on the degree of articular surface injury (31). A grade I lesion is defined as a defect in the articular surface down to, but not including, subchondral bone. A grade II lesion includes the subchondral bone, and a grade III lesion is reserved for large defects in the subchondral bone.

To look in the subacromial space, the posterior portal is again used and the cannula is placed in the subacromial space. A Wissinger rod is placed through the cannula in the posterior portal exiting the anterosuperior portal site from the glenohumeral joint examination earlier. A 4.5-mm cannula with Christmas tree and inflow tubing is then placed over the Wissinger rod; this portal is used for inflow.

Next, the midlateral portal should be established and the motorized synovial resector introduced to perform a bursectomy, if indicated. In some shoulders, the bursa is thickened; such cases necessitate a bursectomy to visualize the remaining subacromial structures. The anterolateral and anteromedial corners of the acromion can be marked at this point with spinal needles. The coracoacromial ligament insertion into the acromion is identified, along with the bursal surfaces of the rotator cuff. The acromioclavicular joint region must often be debrided as well, to expose the joint capsule. An electrocautery system should be employed to assist in controlling hemostasis in the more vascular areas.

If acromioclavicular joint debridement or distal clavicle resection is required, the inflow should be placed through the midlateral portal and the anterosuperior portal used to introduce the motorized instruments needed for the operative procedure.

PATHOLOGIC CHANGES IN ACUTE AND RECURRENT DISLOCATION

Acute Shoulder Dislocation

In 1990, Baker et al. (32) described the changes found at arthroscopy in acute initial dislocations of the shoulder. In a series of 42 patients with an average age of 21 years, arthroscopy was performed within an average of 3 days after the injury. The marked damage these investigators observed allowed them to describe and classify the lesions into three groups according to physical examination and arthroscopic findings. Their findings corresponded with earlier studies that associated surgical findings with those documented by arthrography in acutely dislocated shoulders.

In group I, six shoulders were stable during examination under anesthesia with hemarthrosis of less than 10 ml. From a posterior portal, hemorrhage was seen in the subscapularis tendon and in the inferior capsule between the middle and inferior glenohumeral ligaments. It appeared as either a hemorrhage or a frank rupture in the capsular surface. The glenoid labrum was preserved and no glenoid fractures or Hill-Sachs lesions were identified. In group II, 11 shoulders had subluxation during examination under anesthesia with a 10- to 15-ml hemarthrosis. The anterior labrum was mildly separated from the glenoid. Tearing began inferiorly and ran proximally to the biceps tendon with possible involvement of the biceps tendon. In group II, the glenoid labrum was not completely separated, although incomplete separation was found. Hill-Sachs lesions and chondral fractures were identified.

In group III, 28 shoulders showed gross instability during examination under anesthesia with moderate hemarthrosis. From the posterior portal, the humeral head was seen sitting anterior and inferior to the glenoid and was easily displaced. Complete disruption of the glenohumeral ligament and the glenoid labrum was also seen (Fig. 17). A fissure was identified inferiorly consistent with acute trauma to the soft tissues from the impact of the humeral head against the glenoid rim. The anterior portal provided the best means of viewing the separation of the glenoid labrum and the ligament from the rim of the glenoid. Glenoid rim fractures and full-thickness rotator cuff tears were seen in group III patients.

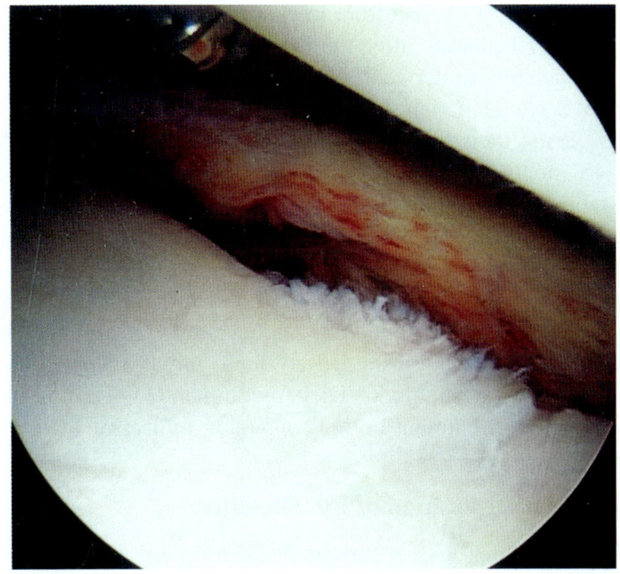

FIG. 17. Intra-articular arthroscopic view of an avulsion of the glenoid labrum complex from the superior to the inferior quadrant—the classic Bankart lesion.

In 1989, Wheeler et al. (33) described their arthroscopic findings in nine patients who had acute initial anterior shoulder dislocations. In each case, frank disruption of the labrum from the anteroinferior glenoid was found. No appreciable interstitial damage to the inferior or middle glenohumeral ligaments was identified; however, five of the nine patients had avulsion fractures of the glenoid contained within the substance of the detached labrum. All patients had Hill-Sachs lesions described as either a chondral fracture or an osteochondral defect.

Arciero et al. (34) recently updated their earlier series and reported their findings in 36 patients. From September 1988 to October 1991, these investigators followed 495 patients who were treated for instability of the shoulder. Thirty-six of these (7%) met the following inclusion criteria: (a) an acute anterior shoulder dislocation, (b) no history of impingement or subluxation, (c) a dislocation that required manual reduction by a physician or certified athletic trainer, and (d) no concomitant neurologic injury. They divided their patients into two groups based on whether they received nonoperative (group I) or operative (group II) treatment. The regimen for patients in group I consisted of shoulder immobilization for 1 month, supervised rehabilitation, and resumption of full activity at 4 months. The patients in group II underwent an arthroscopic transglenoid Bankart repair, followed by the same immobilization and rehabilitation program instituted for group I.

Group I, which was followed for up to 23 months, consisted of 15 patients whose average age was 19.5 years. In

12 patients (80%), recurrent instability developed at an average of 10 months after the initial dislocation, for which seven patients underwent subsequent open Bankart repair. There were 21 patients in group II with an average age of 20.5 years; their follow-up averaged 32 months (range, 15 to 45 months). Eighteen patients (80%) had no recurrent instability at follow-up examination. One patient had an open Bankart repair for recurrent instability, and three had postoperative complications.

Arciero and colleagues found arthroscopic Bankart repair to attain significant reduction in the rate of recurrence in young athletes who sustained an acute initial anterior dislocation of the shoulder. They recommended repair as a viable initial treatment option for young athletes.

Recurrent Dislocation of the Shoulder

The shoulder with recurrent dislocation has tissue damage that is strikingly similar to that seen with an acute dislocation. The most common arthroscopic findings in the shoulder with recurrent instability after a traumatic initial dislocation or subluxation are stretching or attenuation of the anteroinferior capsuloligamentous complex; fraying, tearing, or avulsion of the anteroinferior labrum; and the Hill-Sachs lesion.

The classic Bankart lesion is easily seen with the arthroscope and confirms the diagnosis of instability (35). Occasionally, this lesion has undergone a healing response and appears to be intact with scar tissue filling the defect. However, the inferior glenohumeral ligament is stretched and elongated, allowing continued instability of the glenohumeral joint. If the labrum is also torn posteriorly, some degree of instability in this direction is created.

Labral degeneration with capsular stripping from the glenoid neck, which was best described by Neviaser (36) in his report on the anterior labrum ligamentous periosteal sleeve avulsion lesion, can also be present. It is characterized by an avulsion of the labrum and the periosteum, which then drops down inferiorly on the glenoid and no longer provides an anteroinferior buttress to instability. When viewed from the anterior portal during arthroscopy, the absence of the inferior labrum is noted but, with palpation, the labrum can be identified inferiorly in the glenoid. It can usually be pried loose from the glenoid neck anteriorly and reattached to its normal position as a buttress on the anteroinferior glenoid.

Anterosuperior labrum tears are frequently seen in throwing athletes and may or may not be associated with recurrent instability. Some investigators have reported good results with simple debridement of these tears (37). Snyder et al. (38) classified superior labrum tears (SLAP) lesions into four types. Their cause is most often traumatic, and they are frequently encountered in athletes with recurrent instability. These lesions are discussed in more detail in Chapter 23.

The Hill-Sachs lesion is a compression defect in the posterolateral aspect of the humeral head (31). Arthroscopic visualization of this lesion differentiates this pathologic lesion from the normal bare area. Occasionally, an anterior Hill-Sachs lesion is seen in patients with recurrent posterior dislocations.

Chondral injury, especially along the anterior rim of the glenoid, may be seen in recurrent instability, especially when the instability is long-standing with multiple instability events. The labrum may detach from the glenoid and pull off a small portion of bone from the anterior glenoid rim. This bony Bankart lesion can be seen arthroscopically, as well as in preoperative radiographs. After an initial dislocation, the presence of this lesion on radiographs may convince the surgeon to treat the patient with surgical instability repair because it is usually refractory to nonoperative treatment.

Tearing or stretching of the anteroinferior glenohumeral ligament may occur in 50% of cases (35). This injury may occur in the ligament's midsubstance and, less frequently, at its humeral attachment. Experience with arthroscopic shoulder surgery is required to determine physiologic from pathologic attenuation of the glenohumeral ligaments.

Articular surface rotator cuff tears are frequently seen in athletes and older patients with recurrent instability of the shoulder joint. These are generally tensile failure lesions and are secondary to the instability lesion.

Multidirectional Instability

Often, a patient with global laxity of the shoulder has few obvious intra-articular changes. The humeral head can be found to displace anteriorly, posteriorly, or inferiorly within the capsule; however, impaction injuries or damage to the glenoid labrum are usually minimal. Capsular thinning and stretching can create a patulous capsule with increased capsular volume and no distinct abnormalities.

Acquired Instability in the Throwing Athlete

The throwing athlete who presents with shoulder pain and inability to perform is often a diagnostic dilemma for the surgeon. Athletes who participate in sporting activities that require repetitive overhead arm motions, such as volleyball, swimming, and tennis, may develop signs consistent with rotator cuff impingement. These patients are often thought to have impingement and secondary rotator cuff tendinitis.

Kvitne and Jobe (39) described four groups of throwing athletes with shoulder pain. Group I includes patients with pure impingement. These patients have a stable examination under anesthesia, but at arthroscopy, they may be found to have a tear of the rotator cuff on the glenohumeral articular side and subacromial bursitis. The labrum and glenohumeral ligaments are believed to be normal.

Group II includes patients with impingement findings and concurrent instability caused by labral and capsular trauma. These patients have an unstable examination under anesthesia, as well as a partial rotator cuff tear on the articular side. There may be labral damage, humeral head chondromalacia, and clinically demonstrable subluxation of the humeral head on arthroscopic testing. Group III includes patients who have impingement findings and associated instability caused by hyperelasticity of the joint. Arthroscopically, they have an unstable examination under anesthesia and have an incomplete tear of the rotator cuff. The labrum is attenuated but intact, and there is glenohumeral capsular laxity on examination with subluxation of the humeral head over the labrum. Group IV includes patients with true anterior instability. Arthroscopically, they have a normal rotator cuff examination, but they are unstable to testing under anesthesia. These patients may have a subluxating humeral head, as well as lateral head chondromalacia and labral damage or capsular laxity.

With the arthroscope in the standard posterior portal, inflow can be brought in either on the scope through a pump or through the anterior portal. A standard lateral portal is established as an operating portal. Findings in the subacromial space and unstable shoulder are dictated by the injury. Patients with pure impingement and minimal instability often develop subacromial bursitis and may or may not show evidence of a rupture of the bursal side of the rotator cuff with a button under the cuff against the coracoacromial ligament. Younger patients usually present with minimal changes in the subacromial space, although examination should be carried out to be complete. Surgical intervention other than minimal bursectomy or debridement of soft tissue is seldom needed in athletes with instability who are younger than thirty years old. Patients with a grade II or III impingement and pure rotator cuff damage may require further subacromial decompression or cuff debridement.

Arthroscopic findings in the unstable shoulder range from functional instability with loose labral fragments to occult findings of instability or labral tears and from Bankart and Hill-Sachs lesions to the marked trauma associated with acute dislocations of the shoulder. The advent of arthroscopy over the past 10 years has enabled the surgeon to better define the tissue damage seen with instability, and, therefore, to develop a better treatment plan for these patients (40).

Associated Findings of the Rotator Cuff and Biceps Tendon

Impingement and rotator cuff lesions are one of the most common shoulder conditions that require arthroscopic surgery. The spectrum of cuff pathology includes tendinitis, tendinosis, partial tendon tear, complete tendon tear, massive cuff avulsion with retraction, and cuff tear arthropathy. The arthroscope can be used as a diagnostic tool and as an operative tool to treat these lesions.

Neer (41) described the impingement lesion that we now refer to as mechanical or outlet impingement. With this lesion, mechanical attrition of the cuff tendon or tendons is caused by a prominent coracoacromial arch. The offending structures in this arch include type II and III morphologic acromions, distal clavicle spurring associated with acromioclavicular joint arthritis, anterior acromial spurs, and a thickened coracoacromial ligament. Neer classified the impingement and rotator cuff lesions into three stages. In stage I, edema and hemorrhage of the cuff is caused by repetitive use of the arm above shoulder level and usually occurs in patients younger than 25 years of age. Most often, this lesion can be treated nonoperatively and is reversible. Arthroscopic findings include inflammation of the bursa with little scarring and a normal cuff.

In shoulders with stage II lesions, fibrosis and thickening of the bursa are the result of repetitive motion and microinjuries. This condition is usually found in patients aged 25 to 40 years and results in chronic pain after activity. If nonoperative treatment is unsuccessful, arthroscopic subacromial decompression is indicated when an anteroinferior prominence is present under the acromion. Bursectomy is always indicated in the surgical treatment of a type II lesion. Typical arthroscopic findings in stage II impingement are a thickened, inflamed, fibrotic subacromial bursa with fraying and fibrillation of the periosteum and soft tissue on the undersurface of the acromion. The coracoacromial ligament is occasionally obscured by hypertrophic bursal tissue. A prominent anteroinferior acromion and an anterior acromial spur can be seen arthroscopically. The bursal cuff surface is often frayed, but without significant partial or complete fiber disruption. Distal clavicle spurring and acromioclavicular joint arthritis often cause impingement on the supraspinatus at the musculotendinous junction.

Subacromial bursal thickening, inflammation, and other pathologic findings characteristic of stage II lesions are seen in the stage III impingement lesion. Additionally, rotator cuff tearing is seen. Wear and erosion of the bursal surface of the cuff most often involves the supraspinatus tendon located just medial to its insertion onto the greater tuberosity. With the arm abducted and slightly internally rotated, impingement of the cuff against the coracoacromial arch can be reproduced and visualized arthroscopically.

Neer's outlet impingement, however, does not adequately account for all pathologic lesions of the cuff seen in younger patients. Other causes of injury and degeneration to the cuff have been described. Several investigators (39,41–44) have described an internal impingement lesion that occurs in overhead throwing athletes. The articular surface of the cuff impinges against the posterosuperior portion of the glenoid as the arm is placed in the cocking position of abduction and external rotation. Chronic fraying of the cuff can be seen in these shoulders along with partial tearing and wear of the involved labrum. Another common mechanism is found in younger patients with primary recurrent glenohumeral instability. As the static restraints fail from repetitive microtrauma, such as that caused by the throwing motion, the cuff and shoulder girdle muscles fatigue as they try to maintain joint stability and compensate for the failed static restraints. Secondary impingement of the cuff tendons against the coracoacromial arch due to superior migration of the overworked rotator cuff muscles causes inflammation and thickening of the subacromial bursa with fraying and tendinitis of the cuff. Treatment is directed at correcting the primary instability problem unless advanced secondary lesions of impingement such as significant cuff tearing and acromial spurring are profound.

Partial rotator cuff tears can occur on the bursal or articular surface, or they can be intratendinous. Ellmann (45) stated that 13% of partial tears occurred within the substance of the tendon and were not visible arthroscopically. The depth and area of partial tears of the articular and bursal surfaces should be measured accurately so a classification system can be used to determine proper treatment of the various sized tears. Contrary to Neer's outlet impingement, entailing wear and tear on the tendons from the bursal surface, a large percentage of partial rotator cuff tears occur on the articular surface (Fig. 18). Several mechanisms for this finding have been described as they relate to internal impingement and secondary impingement. In the area of the supraspinatus tendon's distal attachment to the tuberosity, the more proximal and medial cuff fibers that attach to the greater tuberosity undergo increased stress compared with the larger more distally attached superficial fibers. These articular surface tears result from repetitive tensile forces acting on the cuff.

Full-thickness rotator cuff tears are generally easy to diagnose clinically. However, arthroscopy allows the surgeon to scrutinize the integrity of the tissue, the size of the cuff tear, and associated injuries directly. The location of the tendon's ''critical zone'' is the area of the supraspinatus tendon just medial to its attachment site on the greater tuberosity. This is the most common starting point for all cuff tears (46).

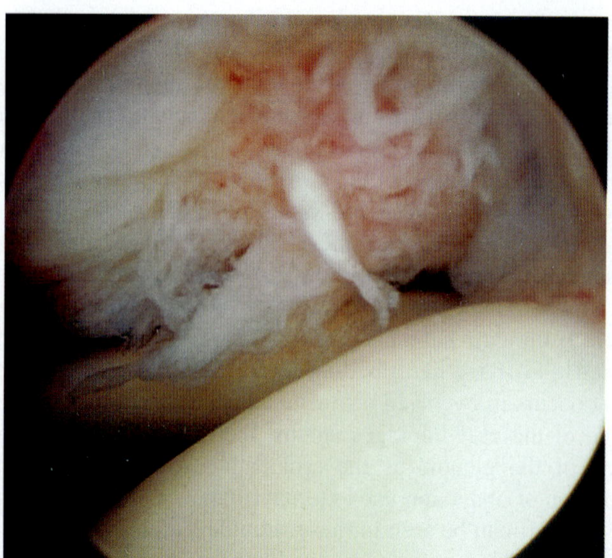

FIG. 18. Intra-articular arthroscopic view of a partial rotator cuff tear involving the articular surface of the supraspinatus tendon. Synovitis and inflammatory tissue is noted around the biceps–labral complex.

Massive avulsion of the cuff from the greater tuberosity is visualized initially from the glenohumeral joint. The supraspinatus tendon is retracted medially and the infraspinatus anterius minor tendons can be seen below the equator of the humeral head. In chronic tears, the edges of these tendons are usually thin, smooth, and rounded with scarring and prominent retraction. Articulation of the superior portion of the humeral head with the undersurface of the acromion is seen in chronic massive cuff tears, and eburnation of the lateral humeral articular surface and greater tuberosity area with sclerosis of the anterior acromial rim can be seen in these areas. It is often difficult to assess accurately the degree of mobilization that will be available to the surgeon for repair of the torn rotator cuff tendons and a massive cuff tear. In most shoulders, a full attempt should be made to repair these massive rotator cuff tears. The biceps tendon is often found to be diseased in these situations. Hypertrophy of the tendon can occur because the tendon assumes the role of the cuff in depressing the humeral head as the arm is elevated and abducted. The biceps tendon is often frayed and inflamed. In 14% of large to massive tears, the biceps ruptures at its intra-articular site or as it travels under the transverse bicipital ligament in the bicipital groove.

Codman (47) described calcium deposits occurring within the rotator cuff tendons, usually involving the supraspinatus tendon just medial to its insertion into the greater tuberosity. In the acute phase of calcific tendinitis, the subacromial bursa becomes acutely inflamed, hypertrophic, and exceedingly painful. Occasionally, impingement of an enlarged deposit occurs under the coracoacromial arch. If the patient's symptoms are not relieved with rotator cuff exercises, arthroscopic treatment is indicated. The calcium deposit is first localized with a needle then evacuated or debrided (Fig. 19).

The biceps tendon is usually the first landmark structure seen when introducing the arthroscope into the glenohumeral joint. Erythema and inflammation around the biceps tendon are commonly seen in inflammatory conditions involving the joint, adhesive capsulitis, and bicipital tendinitis. Occasionally, mild, moderate, or severe partial tearing of the tendon is seen. Debridement of the tendon with the motorized resector in conjunction with palpation with a nerve hook, needle, or cannula is often necessary to establish the true extent of the biceps tendon tear. Occasionally, traction on the biceps tendon will demonstrate injury at the entrance of the bicipital groove. Often, bone spurs can be seen at the groove site that cause narrowing and may contribute to the deterioration of the tendon. When the tendon has completely ruptured, an intra-articular stump of tendon attached to the superior glenoid remains and should be de-

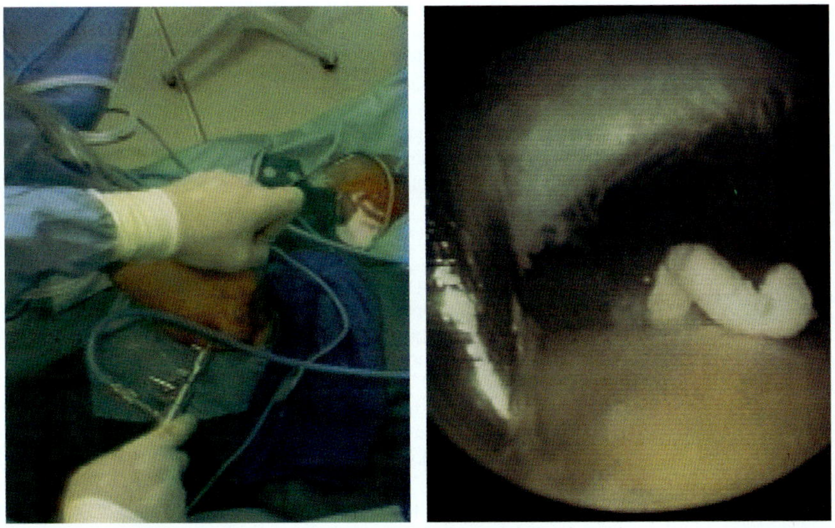

FIG. 19. A, B: Arthroscopic view of a calcium deposit in the supraspinatus tendon. The patient was treated with arthroscopic decompression.

brided. Injury to the biceps tendon in conjunction with labral tearing is discussed in Chapter 23.

In rare cases, dislocation of the biceps tendon medially occurs in conjunction with injury to the subscapularis tendon. Internal and external rotation of the humerus shows an abnormal relationship of the biceps tendon to the subscapularis in these shoulders.

CONCLUSION

The value of the arthroscope as a diagnostic tool has been established, and its usefulness to the shoulder surgeon has grown rapidly. However, its use in helping the surgeon make an accurate diagnosis depends on the throroughness and reproducibility of the arthroscopic shoulder examination. Knowledge of normal shoulder anatomy, as seen through the arthroscope, its normal variants, patient positioning, and portal placement allow the surgeon to examine the shoulder joint systematically and to recognize pathologic conditions.

REFERENCES

1. Cooper DE, Arnoczky SP, O'Brien SJ, Warren RF, DiCarlo E, Allen AA. Anatomy, histology, and vascularity of the glenoid labrum. *J Bone Joint Surg [Am]* 1992;74A:46–52.
2. Soslowsky LJ, Flatow EL, Bigliani LU, Mow VC. General orthopaedics. Articular geometry of the glenohumeral joint. *Clin Orthop* 1992;285:181–190.
3. Saha AK. *Theory of shoulder mechanism.* Springfield, IL: Charles C Thomas, 1961.
4. DePalma AF, Callery G, Bennett GA. Shoulder joint. Variational anatomy and degenerative lesions of the shoulder joint. *Instruct Course Lect* 1949;6:255–280.
5. Turkel SJ, Panio MW, Marshall JL, Girgis FG. Stabilizing mechanisms preventing anterior dislocation of the glenohumeral joint. *J Bone Joint Surg [Am]* 1981;63A:1208–1217.
6. O'Brien SJ, Neves MC, Arnoczky SP, et al. The anatomy and histology of the inferior glenohumeral ligament complex of the shoulder. *Am J Sports Med* 1990;18:449–456.
7. Warner JJP, Deng XH, Warren RF, Torzilli PA. Static capsuloligamentous restraints to superior-inferior translation of the glenohumeral joint. *Am J Sports Med* 1992;20:675–685.
8. Bankart ASB. The pathology and treatment of recurrent dislocation of the shoulder-joint. *Br J Surg* 1938;26:23–29.
9. Schobert WE. Shoulder arthroscopy: orientation and landmarks. *Techniques Orthop* 1988;3:15–21.
10. Matthews LS, Fadale PD. Subacromial anatomy for the arthroscopist. *Arthroscopy* 1989;5:36–40.
11. Detrisac DA, Johnson LL. *Arthroscopic shoulder anatomy. Pathological and surgical implications.* Thorofare, NJ: Slack, 1986.
12. Snyder SJ. *Shoulder Arthroscopy.* New York: McGraw-Hill, 1994:23–39.
13. Johnson LL. Shoulder arthroscopy. In: *Arthroscopic surgery: principles and practice.* St Louis: CV Mosby, 1986:1301–1445.
14. Morgan CD, Rames RD, Snyder SJ. Arthroscopic assessment of anatomic variations of the glenohumeral ligaments associated with recurrent anterior shoulder instability. *Orthop Trans* 1992;16:727–728.
15. Butler JBV, McCluskey GM. Os acromiale: incidence and preliminary results of surgical excision of the meso-acromion. *Orthop Trans* 1993;17:600.
16. Pitman MI, Nainzadeh N, Ergas E, Springer S. The use of somatosensory evoked potentials for detection of neuropraxia during shoulder arthroscopy. *Arthroscopy* 1988;4:250–255.
17. Rao JP, Tovey JE, Zoppi A, Mastromonaco E. Barber chair position for arthroscopy of the shoulder—a versatile approach. *Contemp Orthop* 1990;20:525–527.
18. Skyhar MJ, Altchek DW, Warren RF, Wickiewicz TL, O'Brien SJ. Shoulder arthroscopy with the patient in the beach-chair position. *Arthroscopy* 1988;4:256–259.
19. Arciero RA, Taylor DC, Harrison SA, Snyder RJ, Leahy KE, Uhorchak JM. Interscalene anesthesia for shoulder arthroscopy in a community-sized military hospital. *Arthroscopy* 1966;12:715–719.
20. Andrews JR, Carson WG Jr, Ortega K. Arthroscopy of the shoulder: technique and normal anatomy. *Am J Sports Med* 1984;12:1–7.
21. Wolf EM. Anterior portals in shoulder arthroscopy. *Arthroscopy* 1989;5:201–208.
22. Andrews JR, Angelo RL. Shoulder arthroscopy for the throwing athlete. *Techniques Orthop* 1988;3:75–81.
23. Esch JC. Shoulder arthroscopy: basic setup. *Techniques Orthop* 1988;1:9–14.
24. Richardson AB. Arthroscopic anatomy of the shoulder. *Techniques Orthop* 1988;3:1–7.
25. Nottage WM. Shoulder arthroscopy: portals and surgical techniques. *Techniques Orthop* 1988;3:23–26.
26. Carson WG Jr. Arthroscopy of the shoulder: anatomy and technique. *Orthop Rev* 1992;21:143–153.
27. Andrews JR, Heckman MM, Guerra JJ. Diagnostic arthroscopy of the shoulder. In: McGinty JB, ed. *Operative arthroscopy.* 2nd ed. Philadelphia: Lippincott–Raven, 1996:647–662.

28. Green A. Shoulder arthroscopy: techniques and indications. In: Pelmer CA, ed. *Surgery of the hand and upper extremity.* New York: McGraw-Hill, 1996:375–396.
29. Blachut PA, Day B. Arthroscopic anatomy of the shoulder. *Arthroscopy* 1989;5:1–10.
30. Souryal TO, Baker CL. Anatomy of the supraclavicular fossa portal in shoulder arthroscopy. *Arthroscopy* 1990;6:297–300.
31. Calandra JJ, Baker CL, Uribe J. Incidence of Hill-Sachs lesions in initial anterior shoulder dislocations. *Arthroscopy* 1989;5:254–257.
32. Baker CL, Uribe JW, Whitman C. Arthroscopic evaluation of acute initial anterior shoulder dislocations. *Am J Sports Med* 1990;18:25–28.
33. Wheeler JH, Ryan JB, Arciero RA, Molinari RN. Arthroscopic versus nonoperative treatment of acute shoulder dislocations in young athletes. *Arthroscopy* 1989;5:213–217.
34. Arciero RA, Wheeler JH, Ryan JB, McBride JT. Arthroscopic bankart repair versus nonoperative treatment for acute, initial anterior shoulder dislocations. *Am J Sports Med* 1994;22:589–594.
35. Caspari RB, Geissler WB. Arthroscopic manifestations of shoulder subluxation and dislocation. *Clin Orthop* 1993;291:54–66.
36. Neviaser TJ. The anterior labroligament periosteal sleeve avulsion lesion: a cause of anterior instability of the shoulder. *Arthroscopy* 1993;9:17–21.
37. Andrews JR, Carson WG. The arthroscopic treatment of glenoid labrum tears in the throwing athlete. *Orthop Trans* 1984;8:44.
38. Snyder SJ, Karzel RP, Del Pizzo W, Ferkel RD, Friedman MJ. SLAP lesions of the shoulder. *Arthroscopy* 1990;6:274–279.
39. Kvitne RS, Jobe FW. The diagnosis and treatment of anterior instability in the throwing athlete. *Clin Orthop* 1993;291:107–123.
40. Baker CL, Shalvoy RM. Arthroscopic evaluation of the unstable shoulder. *Operative Techniques Sports Med* 1993;1:268–275.
41. Neer CS II. Impingement lesions. *Clin Orthop* 1983;173:70–77.
42. Jobe FW. Unstable shoulders in the athlete. *Instruct Course Lect* 1985;34:228–231.
43. Jobe FW. Impingement problems in the athlete. *Instruct Course Lect* 1989;38:205–210.
44. Walch G, Boileau P, Noel E, Donell ST. Impingement of the deep surface of the supraspinatus tendon on the posterosuperior glenoid rim: an arthroscopic study. *J Shoulder Elbow Surg* 1992;1:238–245.
45. Ellmann H. Diagnosis and treatment of incomplete rotator cuff tears. *Clin Orthop* 1990;254:64–80.
46. Yamanaka K, Fakuda H. Pathologic studies of the supraspinatus tendon with reference to incomplete thickness tears. In: Takagishi N, ed. *The shoulder.* Tokyo: Professional Postgraduate Services, 1990:220–224.
47. Codman EA. The pathology of the subacromial bursa and the supraspinatus tendon. In: Codman EA, ed. *The shoulder: rupture of the supraspinatus tendon and other lesions in or about the subacromial bursa.* Boston: Thomas Todd, 1934;65–107.

Section 3

Treatment Considerations

The Unstable Shoulder,
edited by R.F. Warren, E.V. Craig, and D.W. Altchek.
Lippincott–Raven Publishers, Philadelphia © 1999.

CHAPTER 10

Acute Anterior Dislocations

Evaluation and Treatment

Robert A. Arciero

ACUTE DISLOCATIONS EVALUATION AND TREATMENT

Instability of the shoulder is an extremely common problem encountered in orthopedic practice. Several classification schemes have been developed to assist the orthopedist in appropriate clinical management (1–3). Thomas and Matsen (1,2) developed a classification distinguishing traumatic unidirectional instability from those with atraumatic multidirectional instability. They emphasized that the mechanism of injury, underlying pathology, and subsequent treatment is different for both groups. Bigliani et al. (3) expanded the understanding of shoulder instability and introduced the concept of instability as a clinical problem with wide variation and a spectrum of presentation. Within this scheme, the traumatic unidirectional patients form one end of the spectrum and the atraumatic, multidirectional, and hyperlax patients are at the other. Patients can present with considerable variation, and in any one patient clinical features may cross over between these two ends of the spectrum. This scheme would then take into account patients who present with a traumatic etiology but on physical exam may also have signs of ligamentous laxity. It also includes those patients, such as throwers or swimmers, in whom acquired instability develops from repetitive microtrauma.

With this as a basis for our understanding of the presentation of shoulder instability, acute traumatic anterior dislocation of the shoulder represents one of the most dramatic and frequently encountered shoulder instability problems. The history often includes a significant traumatic episode for the dislocation. Typically, a fall with the arm in the abducted and externally rotated position or arm tackling such as in football is an often cited mechanism. With the arm in this position, the anterior superior band of the inferior glenohumeral ligament complex is under tension and fails, leading to dislocation (4,5). The patient with an acute traumatic dislocation is in acute distress. The dislocated arm is held in a slightly abducted and internally rotated position and is frequently supported by the normal extremity. Visual inspection will demonstrate loss of the normal deltoid contour with a prominence of the acromion process. Many times the patient will relate that the shoulder "slipped" or "popped out" of joint. It is important to obtain an accurate description of the mechanism of injury and the position of the arm, as this will assist in the determination of direction. The patient will frequently resist attempts of motion of the arm and will indeed guard against abduction and external rotation.

A careful neurologic and vascular examination is essential in the initial evaluation of the acute anterior shoulder dislocation. The frequency of axillary nerve injuries increases with the age of the patient and has been reported to occur in 5% to 35% of patients with acute dislocations (6,7). Although the patient with the acutely dislocated shoulder usually has intense pain, it is possible to ascertain function of this nerve by simply having the patient contract the deltoid isometrically or minimally resist abduction of the arm. Although the sensory portion of the nerve innervates the lateral proximal arm region this clinical sign is an unreliable indicator of axillary nerve function (6,7). In addition, vascular injuries can occur as a complication of acute anterior dislocation of the shoulder (7). Most commonly this complication occurs in the elderly. Associated arthrosclerosis and vessel rigidity predispose this population group to axillary artery avulsions. A rapidly expanding

R. A. Arciero: Department of Orthopaedics, Keller Army Hospital, West Point, New York 10996.

hematoma or fullness in the axilla accompanied by marked pain may be indicative of this complication. A thorough evaluation of brachial, radial, and ulnar pulses is important in identifying these associated injuries. Swelling of the proximal humerus, ecchymosis, and crepitation is also indicative of associated greater tuberosity or glenoid rim fracture, which can occur with an anterior dislocation of the shoulder. It is important to also evaluate the entire shoulder girdle to include inspection and palpation of both the acromioclavicular and sternoclavicular joints.

Radiographic Evaluation

Three views of the glenohumeral joint are necessary to evaluate fully the acute traumatic dislocation of the shoulder. Not only is it paramount to determine the direction of dislocation, but these views are necessary to identify associated bony injuries. A standard anterior posterior view as the arm is held in slight internal rotation will assist in the identification of greater tuberosity fractures (7) (Fig. 1) Furthermore, this view usually permits the identification of an associated glenoid rim fracture. Displacement of the glenoid rim and glenoid fossa fractures associated with acute anterior dislocations are better appreciated on a true anteroposterior (AP) view of the shoulder (7) (Fig. 2) An axillary view or a modified axillary view, the so-called West Point radiograph, will confirm the direction of dislocation and will allow for the identification of rim fractures and small avulsion fractures associated with bony avulsion of the inferior glenohumeral ligament (8,9) (Fig. 3) The transcapular lateral view or Y view will also confirm the direction of dislocation (7) (Fig. 4) If there is severe pain or guarding, this radiograph requires no arm abduction and may be easier to obtain than the axillary radiographs.

Methods of Reduction

If the dislocation is evaluated acutely, occasionally reduction can be achieved without the use of analgesic medication. This treatment is frequently provided when a dislocation is witnessed on the playing field and evaluated during athletic events. Typically in these instances an injured player is evaluated within seconds of the dislocation and one can take advantage of the absence of spasm to perform the reduction. When an injured player is seen after a suspected anterior shoulder dislocation and before any closed reduction is attempted, inspection and palpation of the injured shoulder are necessary to observe for any crepitation that may indicate an associated proximal humerus fracture. In this instance, reduction should be delayed until sufficient radiographic documentation can be obtained. If no crepitus is appreciated and the loss of deltoid contour and prominence of the acromion appears to indicate an uncomplicated acute anterior dislocation, a traction countertraction method as described by Rockwood has been extremely effective in achieving a relatively painless reduction (7,9). Using this method, an assistant provides countertraction with a linen sheet or stockinette circled about the torso underneath the axilla of the involved side. With traction proximally, this effectively stabilizes the chest and

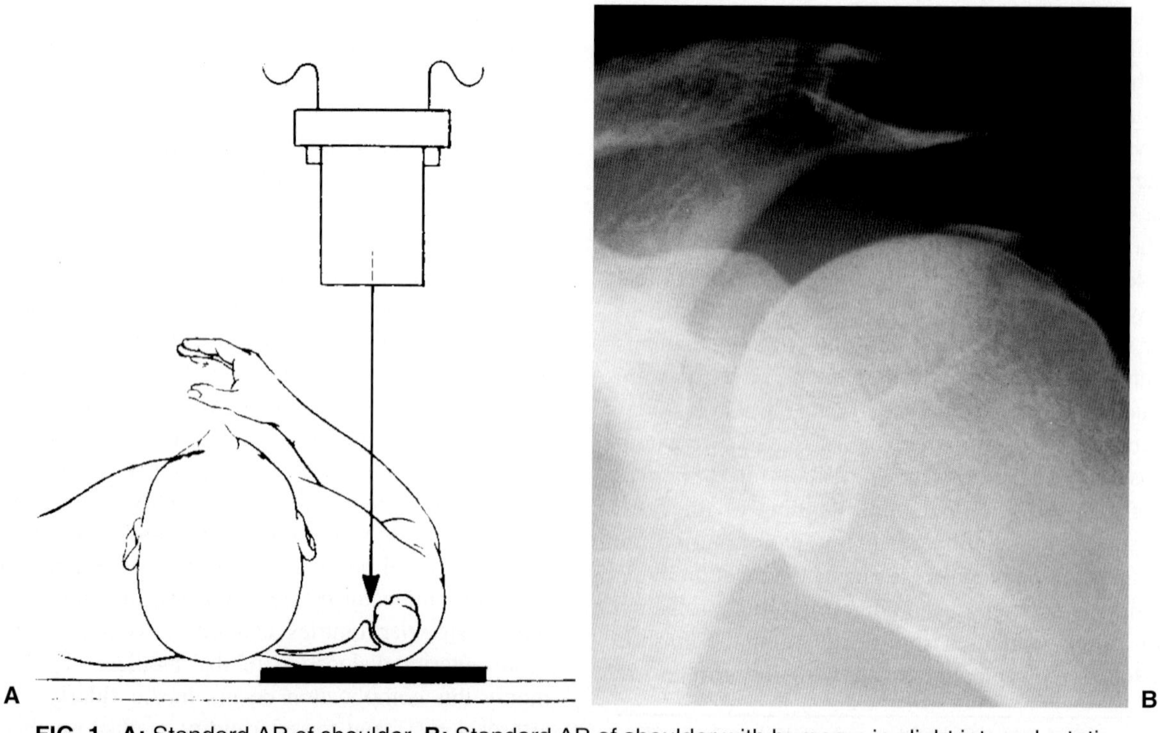

FIG. 1. A: Standard AP of shoulder. **B:** Standard AP of shoulder with humerus in slight internal rotation demonstrating associated greater tuberosity fracture.

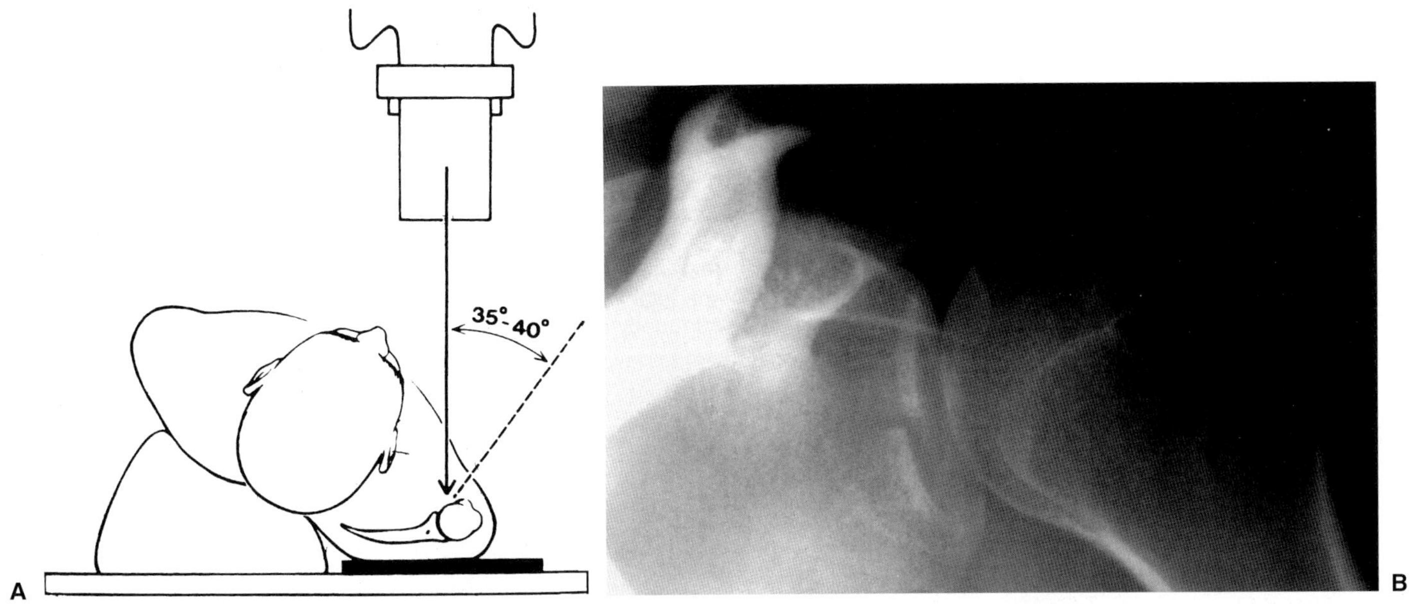

FIG. 2. A: True AP of shoulder requires 35 to 40 degrees of rotation. **B:** True AP of shoulder demonstrating displacement of associated glenoid fracture.

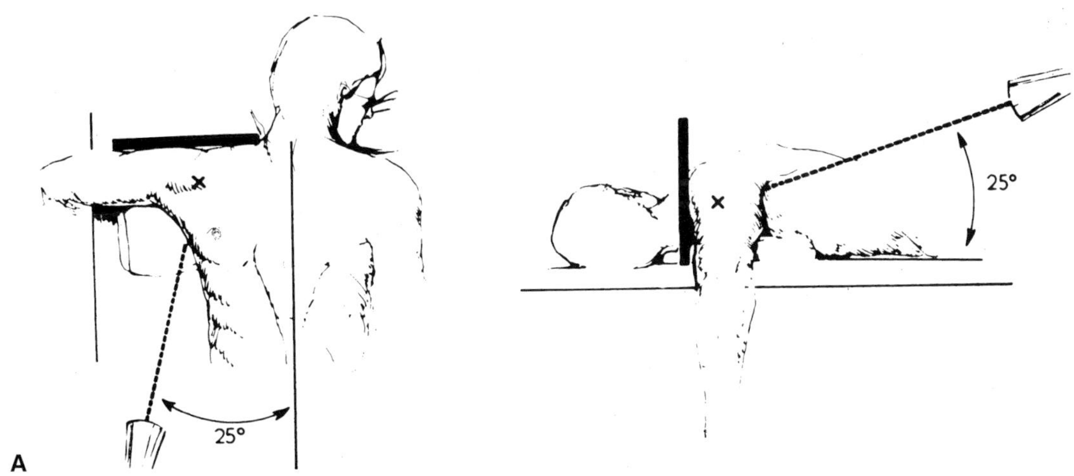

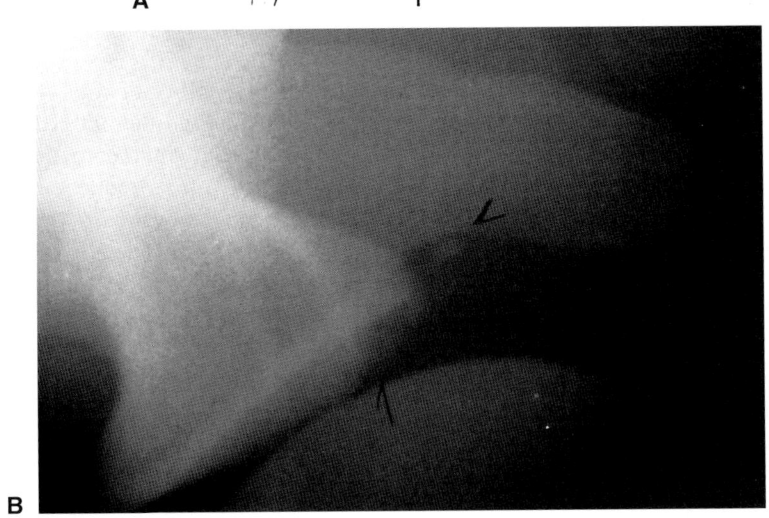

FIG. 3. A: Technique for West Point radiograph. **B:** West Point radiograph demonstrating subtle avulsion fracture of the inferior glenohumeral ligament.

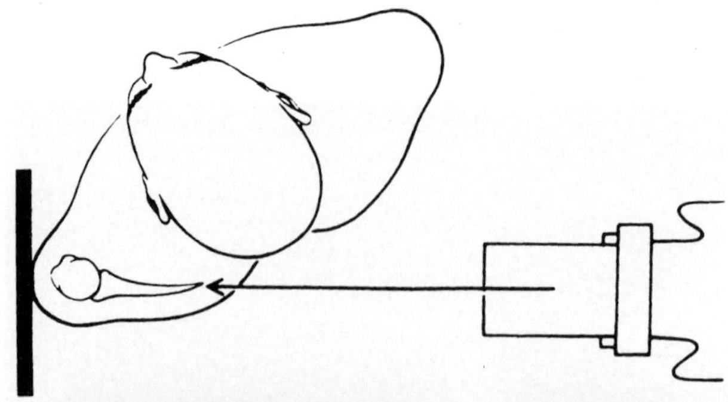

A

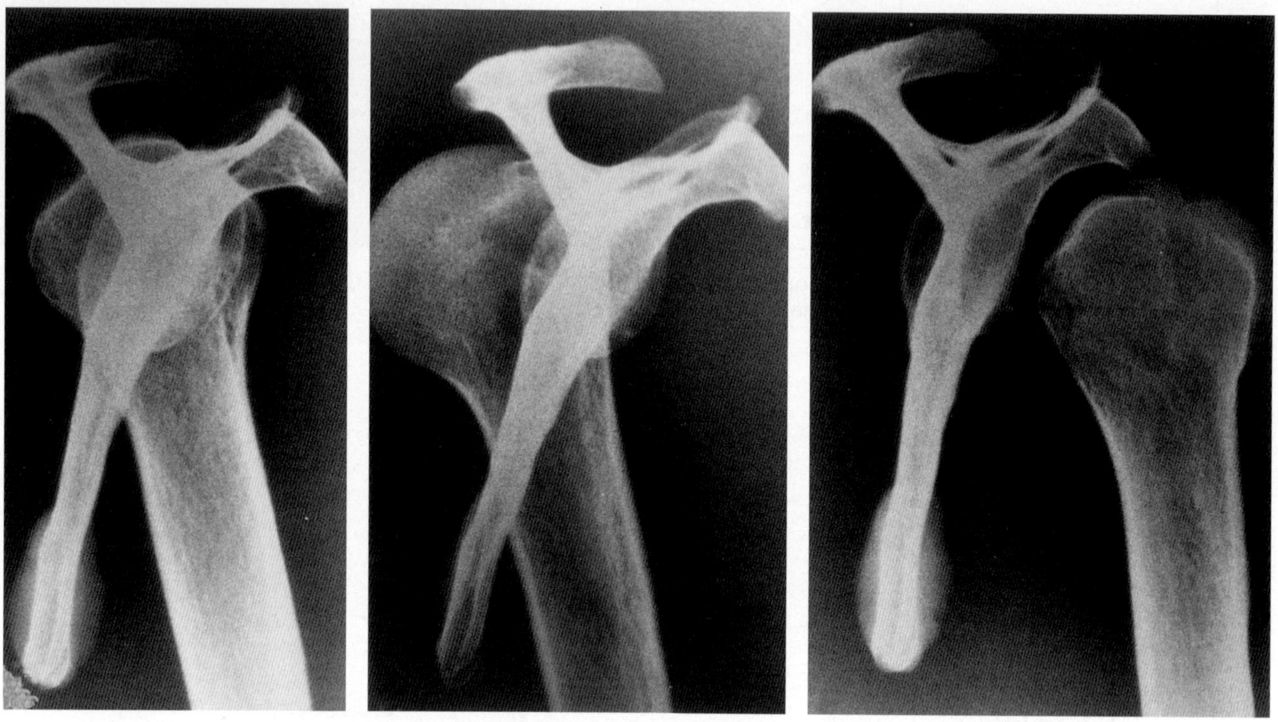

B

FIG. 4. **A:** Technique for transcapular "Y" radiograph. **B:** Transcapular radiograph demonstrating direction of dislocation and adequacy of reduction.

the scapula. The surgeon then provides counter-traction on the injured extremity distally to affect reduction (Fig. 5).

Many patients, however, will present to the emergency department several hours after their dislocation. In this instance, intravenous narcotics and muscle relaxant agents, such as benzodiazepines, will frequently be necessary to permit reduction. If this does become necessary, with the patient in a relaxed state, the traction countertraction method is highly effective. There are a number of other satisfactory reduction techniques. The reduction method of Stimpson places the patient in a prone position with the involved shoulder hanging over the edge of a table (2,7,9). The thorax and scapula are essentially supported by the table. A total of 5 to 10 lb of weight is hung from the wrist of the involved extremity and over a 15- to 20-minute period reduction will occur (Fig. 6). It is important to remember that this technique requires time to affect reduction.

Westin et al. (10) recently described a sitting technique employed in treating 118 anterior dislocations that occurred primarily at a ski resort. Here, a 3-foot loop of 4-inch-wide cast stockinette is placed around the proximal forearm of the involved extremity with the elbow flexed to 90 degrees. The patient must sit erect and upright as much as possible. An assistant stabilizes the chest and torso by clasping his or her hands around the chest in the axilla of the affected side. The physician simply places a foot in the stocking loop to provide firm downward traction (Fig. 7). This technique also affords the physician the capability of rotating the arm as needed for reduction. It was found that 93% of the patients treated with this technique required no narcotic, analgesia, or sedation. A total of 97% of these reductions were successful. There were no complications with this technique as well.

The scapula manipulation technique originally described by Bosley and Miles, and subsequently reported by Anderson et al. (11), is also employed by a number of orthopedists. With this technique, the patient is placed prone and the shoulder is slightly flexed with 5 to 15 lb of traction at the elbow. The scapula is rotated by pushing medially on the inferior tip and rotating the superior aspect of the scap-

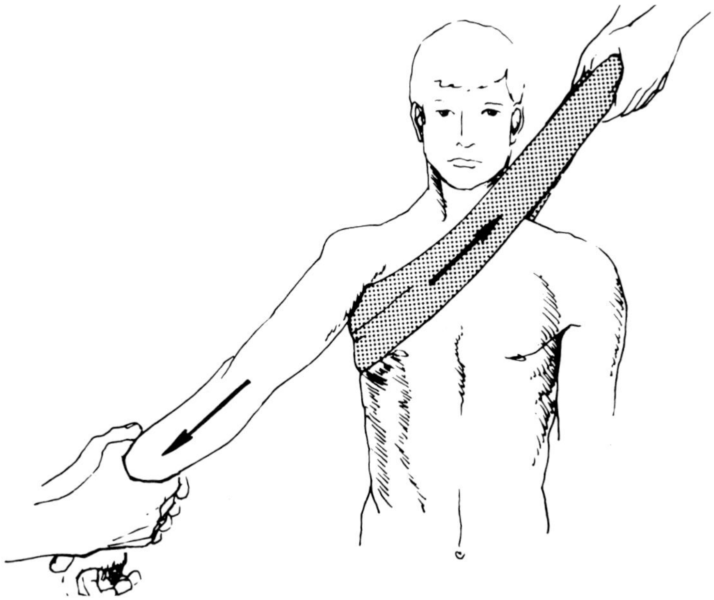

FIG. 5. Traction-counter traction reduction method.

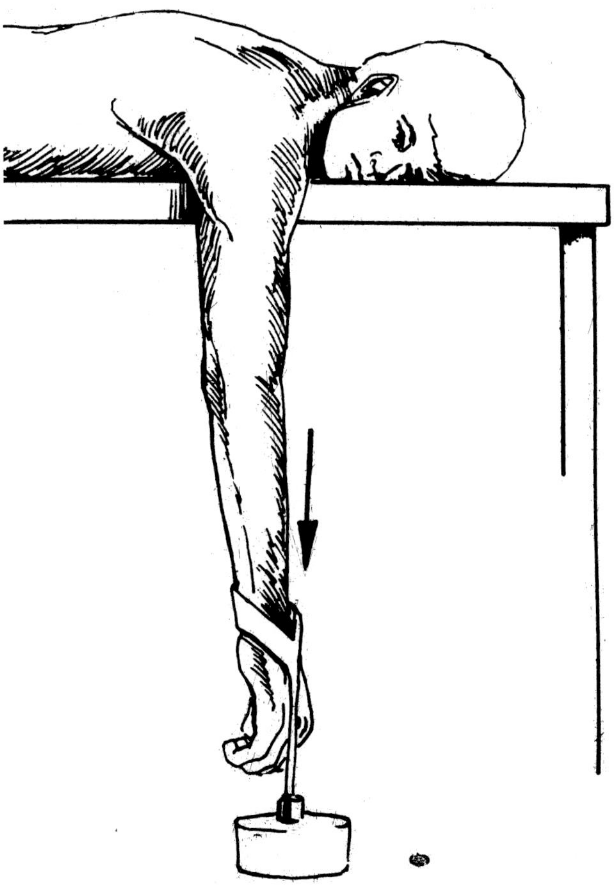

FIG. 6. Modified Stimpson reduction technique.

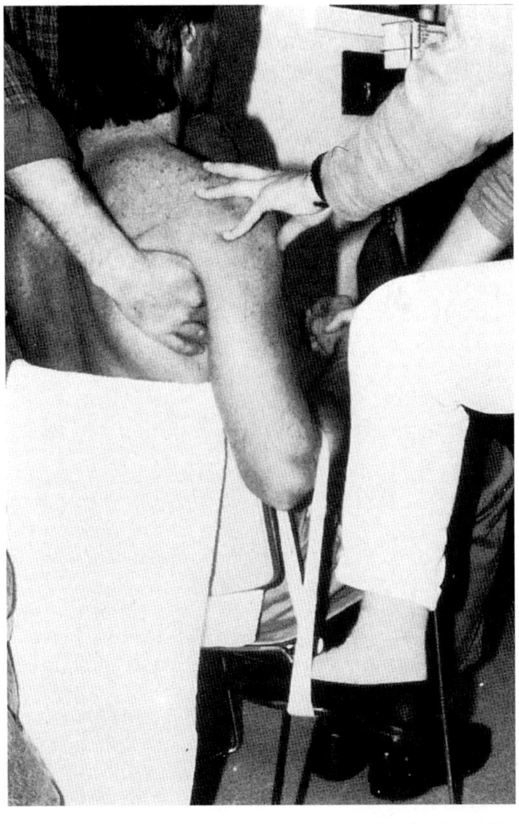

FIG. 7. Sitting-downward traction method described by Westin.

ula outward (Fig. 8A, B). Anderson et al. reported a 92% success rate in 51 patients with this technique.

With traction and patience, many reductions can be accomplished without the use of intravenous analgesics or sedation. Should analgesia be required a technique using a single intra-articular lidocaine injection has recently been reported for analgesia in the reduction of anterior shoulder reduction dislocations (12). In this report, Matthews and Roberts randomly compared a single intra-articular injection of 20 ml of 1% lidocaine with intravenous injections of morphine sulfate and midazolam. A 20-gauge needle was directed 2 cm inferior and lateral to the acromion in the lateral sulcus created by the absent humeral head. Two reduction techniques were used: the traction countertraction method and the scapula rotation method. The lidocaine injection technique was effective in 100% of the patients. They reported no complications with this technique and, when compared with intravenous analgesia and sedation, a statistically significant shorter emergency room visit was noted. On a practical note, many hospitals are requiring credentialing of competence for administering intravenous analgesia and sedation to include the ability to manage any side effects. In some instances, only anesthesiologists are credentialed to use intravenous sedation. The intra-articular lidocaine injection obviates the need for additional sub-specialty management and the expensive monitoring and documentation of the patient's vital status that is necessary with intravenous techniques.

The technique used by Milch (13), described in 1938 employs reduction by using external rotation. The patient is supine and the arm is forward and elevated slowly to 90 degrees. The arm is then abducted with slight traction. Finally, directed thumb pressure is used to gently push the head of the humerus gently back in place. Janecki and Shahcheragh (14) reported success in 50 consecutive cases. This technique is frequently a useful adjunct to the traction countertraction method, in which the treating surgeon can gently externally rotate the humerus while providing traction and then with the opposite hand gently use the thumb to assist reduction (Fig. 9A, B). Finally, the leverage technique of Kocher involves four steps for reduction (7). This method is being described for completeness, but the other methods previously described are recommended, as they are more gentle and are associated with a much lower complication rate. The Kocher maneuver positions the elbow flexed to 90 degrees, and traction is applied in the line of the humerus. The arm is slowly and smoothly brought into full external rotation and then adducted across the front of the chest approximately to the midline. The arm is then internally rotated until the hand is placed on the opposite shoulder. The humeral head is levered on the anterior glenoid and the shaft is essentially levered against the thorax. However, this technique has been associated with proximal humerus fractures, especially in the elderly.

After reduction, post-reduction radiographs are necessary to confirm the adequacy of reduction as well as to docu-

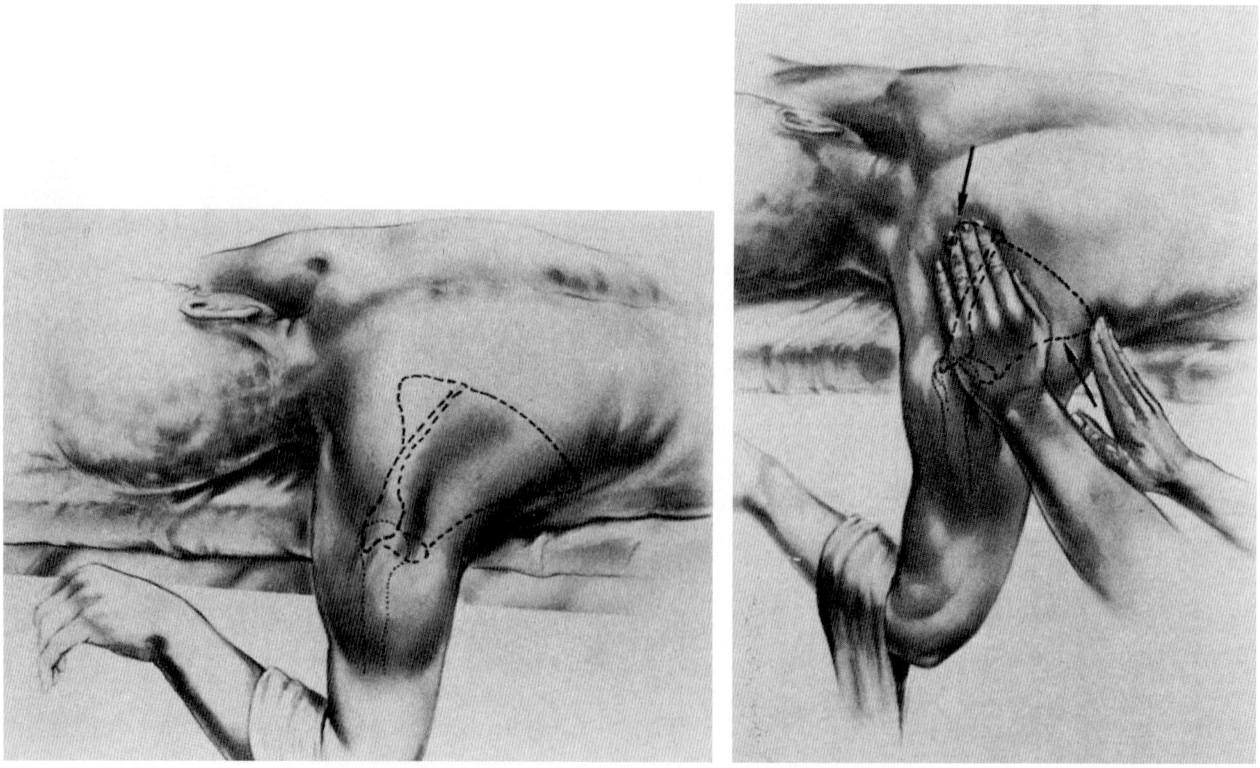

A B

FIG. 8. A, B: Scapular manipulation technique.

A 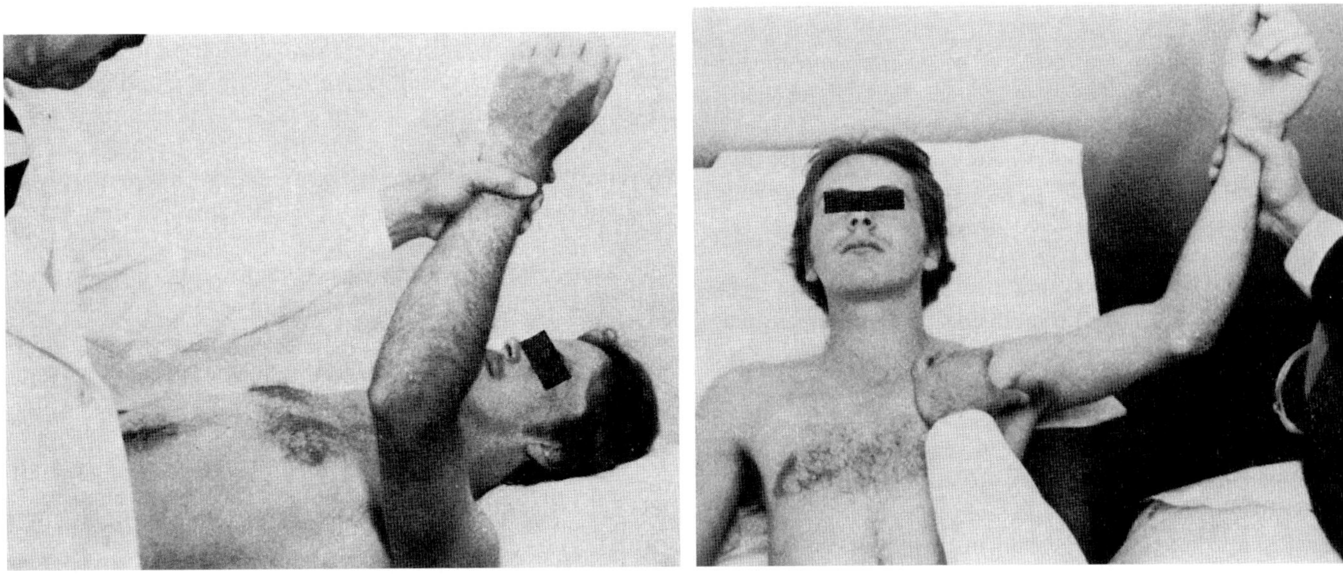 B

FIG. 9. A, B: Milch technique.

ment associated bony injuries. It is also important to document the neurologic and vascular status of the involved extremity at this time. Frequently, although the pain is improved by reduction, there will be sufficient guarding that causes a full neurologic examination to be difficult. However, it is usually possible to ascertain axillary, musculocutaneous, radial, median, and ulnar nerve function. Follow-up care should involve a re-evaluation within 10 to 14 days after reduction. At this point, pain and spasm have subsided and will permit better examination. An examination is also required to establish associated soft-tissue injuries. This becomes extremely important in patients over the age of 40. In this population group, injuries to the axillary nerve and rotator cuff occur with increasing frequency (15–18). In patients older than 40 years of age, tears at the rotator cuff can occur in 15% of those who sustain an anterior shoulder dislocation (15,17). The injury may, on occasion, be seen in younger patients. In one study, this rate increased to as high as 40% in patients older than 60 years of age (17). If, at 4 weeks post-reduction, there is no active abduction of the arm, magnetic resonance imaging (MRI) of the shoulder and/or EMG may be necessary to diagnose axillary nerve palsy and/or a tear of the rotator cuff.

Associated Injuries

Besides recurrence, injury to the axillary nerve is the most common complication of anterior dislocations of the shoulder. Blom and Dahlback (6) performed an EMG study in 73 patients who sustained either an anterior dislocation of the shoulder or a proximal humerus fracture. A total of 35% of 26 nerve injuries were documented, with 22 confined to the axillary nerve. There was EMG evidence of radial, musculocutaneous, and median nerve injury as well. The incidence of axillary nerve denervation is higher in older patient populations and has been estimated to be as high as 30% in elderly patients. Full functional and EMG recovery is typically documented within 3 to 6 months after this complication.

As mentioned, injuries to the rotator cuff can also occur after an anterior dislocation of the shoulder. Associated soft-tissue injury is known to increase over the age of 40. In the study by Ribbans et al., computerized arthrotomography, or arthro-CT, was performed in 33 patients after an acute primary anterior dislocation of the shoulder (16). Avulsion of the anterior glenoid labrum was seen in all younger patients and in 75% of patients who were older than 50. Associated fractures of the proximal humerus and a tear of the rotator cuff was demonstrated in 63% of the older patients, aged 50 or more. Tijmes reported a series of 14 patients with rotator cuff lesions and anterior dislocation of the shoulder; 11 of the patients were elderly (17). Neviaser et al. (15) reported on 31 patients with rotator cuff tears after anterior shoulder dislocations. All but one patient was older than 40, and the diagnosis was delayed an average of 8 months. Axillary nerve injuries also occurred in 7% of the patients. These findings underscore the importance of repeated examinations and the use of arthrography, MRI, and EMG in the patient older than 35 to 40 years of age who is unable to abduct the arm after an anterior shoulder dislocation. In this age group, treatment of the rotator cuff after adequate soft-tissue healing from the initial injury may take precedence in management to preserve shoulder function.

Associated fractures of the greater tuberosity have been observed in up to 40% of patients over the age of 50 who have sustained a primary shoulder dislocation. Displacement of greater than 1 cm may require surgical treatment, as this problem can lead to limited abduction and impingement syndrome with loss of rotator cuff function.

Natural History

The natural history and results of nonoperative treatment of acute, initital anterior shoulder dislocation have been studied by many investigators. McLaughlin and Cavallaro reported on 573 patients with primary anterior shoulder dislocation and observed a 95% recurrence rate in patients younger than 20 years of age, 60% in patients 20 to 40 years of age, and only 10% in patients older than 40 years of age (19,20). Later, McLaughlin and MacLellan (21) reported on 265 cases of recurrent dislocation and established similar findings. Ninety-six percent of those patients in whom recurrent dislocation developed were younger than 30 years of age at the time of the initial dislocation. Furthermore, recurrent dislocation occurred in only 10% of patients over the age of 40. In several classic studies, Rowe (22,23) documented similar findings with recurrence rates dependent on the age of the patient at the time of initial dislocation. In patients less than 20 years of age, a 94% recurrence rate was observed, 79% in patients 21 to 30 years of age, 50% in patients 31 to 40 years of age, and 14% in patients over the age of 40. These classic studies established age at the time of the initial dislocation as the primary predictor of recurrence. Furthermore, these investigators demonstrated that immobilization had little effect on prognosis.

Nonoperative treatment of the initial dislocation has been the subject of several major studies. Traditionally, nonoperative treatment after reduction consists of a period of immobilization, a rehabilitation and strengthening program of the rotator cuff and especially subscapularis muscle, and a delay in return to activity until pain and apprehension have disappeared. Despite these treatment efforts, nonoperative treatment has had inconsistent and unpredictable effects on the development of recurrent instability with contradictory results reported. As mentioned, Rowe found no evidence supporting immobilization for longer than 3 weeks. In a prospective study by Kiviluoto and colleagues of 226 patients with 1-year follow-up, 99 patients under the age of 50 were treated with either 1 or 3 weeks of immobilization (24). The remaining 127 patients were older than 50 years of age. The older patients were all treated with one week of immobilization and had a very low recurrence rate. A much higher frequency of recurrence in patients younger than 30 years of age was observed as compared with those aged 30 to 50. In those patients younger than 30 years old who were included in this study, a higher frequency of redislocation was established in 26 of those who were treated with only 1 week of immobilization as compared with those treated with 3 weeks of immobilization. Henry and Genung (25) found a 90% redislocation rate in 62 patients immobilized in a sling and swathe or shoulder immobilizer for varying amounts of time. An 85% redislocation rate was demonstrated in 59 patients who were treated without immobilization in this study. Many of the patients in this study were young athletes; this led the authors to conclude that immobilization had little effect on recurrence. In fact, in this particular study of 121 patients, all redislocations occurred within 18 months of the initial injury and 79 patients were operated on for recurrent dislocation. These investigators concluded that the high-demand young athlete has a high risk of recurrence and perhaps surgical repair of the primary dislocation should be considered.

By contrast, Watson-Jones (26) reported no episodes of recurrence in several hundred patients treated with strict immobilization for a minimum of 4 weeks. Yoneda et al. (27) reported the results of 104 patients treated with 5 weeks of immobilization in a sling and swathe followed by 6 weeks of graduated exercise. At an average 13-year follow-up, they reported a 17.3% recurrent dislocation rate. Aronen and Regan (28) reported on an aggressive rehabilitation program in 20 United States Naval Academy midshipmen with a marked restriction of activities for 3 months and observed a 25% redislocation rate. These three studies reported results of much greater success with nonoperative treatment.

Hovelius (29,30) has reported on 5- and 10-year follow-up of a series of 257 patients with primary anterior shoulder dislocation. These patients have been prospectively followed and treated with shoulder immobilization for 3 to 4 weeks versus a sling for 1 week. At 5 years, two or more recurrences had occurred in 55% of the shoulders in patients who were 22 years old or younger, in 37% of shoulders in patients who were 22 to 29 years old, and in 12% of shoulders in patients who were 30 to 40 years old (30). Hovelius most recently reported on the 10-year follow-up of this group. At the 10-year follow-up, 48% had sustained recurrent dislocation and 23% had required operative reconstruction; 20% of these patients had evidence of dislocation arthropathy on follow-up radiographs. On initial review of this study, it would appear that recurrence rates and the subsequent need for surgery is lower than previously reported. However, 37% of patients were between 30 to 40 years of age, an age group known to have lower recurrence rates. Furthermore, the study population is not well defined (e.g., job requirements, athletic activity). The functional level at the time of injury and at final follow-up is not described. Finally, there is no mention of an objective shoulder score to better understand the results in these patients. Although an excellent study, these limitations prevent it from being the definitive natural history paper.

Hovelius did, however, report in a separate study, the results of primary shoulder dislocation in young Swedish ice hockey players (32). He observed a 90% recurrence rate in hockey players under the age of 20 and a 65% recurrence rate in those aged 20 to 25 years. This particular report may represent a better cohort of high demand athletes rather than recreational or part-time participants who place a much lower demand on their shoulders.

Simonet and Cofield (33) likewise reviewed their results with nonoperative management of 116 patients. The recurrence rate in their patients was somewhat less than the previous classical studies by Rowe and McLaughlin. The overall recurrence rate in this study was 66%. They believed that 3 to 6 weeks of immobilization, restricting the return to full activity for at least 6 weeks, and extensive rehabilitation improved results. They noted, however, that despite these efforts, a much higher incidence of recurrence in athletes was demonstrated as compared with nonathletes. In fact, in athletes younger than 30 years old, the overall recurrence rate was 82%, compared with 30% in nonathletes of the same age. These investigators also noted continued symptomatic instability in the form of subluxation in another 22% of the patients in the group. Recurrent subluxation was observed in 11 of 14 patients who described recurrent dislocation and in 14 of 78 patients without recurrence of dislocation. These findings suggest that immobilization, rehabilitation, and delay in return to full activity have little predictable effect in decreasing recurrent dislocation in athletes. In addition, they demonstrate recurrent subluxation as a significant problem.

Wheeler et al. (34) reported our initial experience with nonoperative treatment for cadet-athletes at the United States Military Academy. In an attempt to reproduce the findings by Aronen and Regan, 38 cadets were treated with 3 weeks of shoulder immobilization, completion of a supervised therapy rehabilitation program and a restriction from contact activity and overhead sports for 3 months. Thirty-five of 38 cadet-athletes or 92% sustained recurrent instability. Strict adherence to a supervised nonoperative treatment program had no effect on the recurrence rate. All recurrences of instability occurred within 14 months of the initial injury.

Making firm recommendations regarding the management of the initial anterior shoulder dislocation is difficult after review of the literature presented. Many studies lack prospective design, randomization or proper cohort groups. Classically, the results of nonoperative treatment has been determined by the rates of recurrent dislocation after treatment. However, many studies lack detailed documentation of the functional or athletic activity level that the patient has returned to after such treatment. Also with the exception of one study, recurrent subluxation has not been evaluated which in athletes can compromise functional return and also require further treatment. The literature appears to suggest a high recurrent dislocation rate in patients younger than 25 years old who continue to participate in athletic activities, regardless of nonoperative treatment. Contact or collision athletes appear to be particularly susceptible to recurrent shoulder instability in the form of recurrent dislocation subluxation, or both. As mentioned previously, little attention has been paid to the functional assessment after treatment (particularly for athletes), activity modification as a result of the injury, or the incidence of recurrent subluxation that would have a significant effect on athletic activity.

It is the author's opinion that the development of recurrence after an initial traumatic anterior dislocation is based on age and activity level. Although patients under the age of 25 would be expected to be at risk of recurrence, a sedentary lifestyle may be protective. However, in young patients who are athletically active, the recurrence rates are high.

Rationale for Surgical Treatment of Acute Anterior Shoulder Dislocation

Natural History

Before proceeding with the discussion regarding surgical management of the acute initial anterior shoulder dislocation, it is important to outline the rationale for considering this more aggressive operative management. First, and perhaps foremost, nonoperative treatment leads to a high incidence of recurrent instability in young athletes. A critical review of the literature as described previously reports that recurrence rates in the young athletic population range from 65 to 95%. For a young athlete who desires to return to full activity that includes collision and contact sporting events, the results of nonoperative treatment to date are extremely disappointing and unpredictable.

Pathoanatomy (Cadaveric Studies)

Second, primary repair after an acute initial dislocation is attractive when the pathoanatomy is considered. Turkel and others demonstrated that the inferior glenohumeral ligament complex is the primary restraint for glenohumeral translation especially with the arm in the abducted position (5). O'Brien et al., in a histologic and arthroscopic evaluation, described the inferior glenohumeral ligament complex as an anterior band, a posterior band, and an interposed axillary pouch (4). Both Turkel and O'Brien determined that the anterior band of the inferior glenohumeral ligament was the primary restraint to anterior translation at 90 degrees of abduction. The detachment of the anterior band of the inferior glenohumeral ligament from the anterior glenoid is the Perthes or Bankart lesion and represents the major gross anatomic lesion in traumatic dislocation (35, 36). Currently, techniques are available that permit repair of this lesion. In a cadaveric study, Harryman et al. (37) detached the anterior inferior labrum and capsule from the glenoid. These specimens were then loaded and documented that anterior translation of the humerus on the glenoid was nearly doubled compared with the intact specimen. He then performed an arthroscopic Bankart repair that reduced translation to that of the intact specimens. Therefore, acute repair is supported by the concept that a detached capsulolabral complex of the anterior inferior glenohumeral ligament is observed frequently after an acute dislocation, and surgical repair of this lesion primarily should restore glenohumeral stability.

Bigliani and colleagues performed a cadaveric study in which the inferior glenohumeral ligament complex was loaded and tensioned to failure (38). They observed that strain before failure for all bone–ligament–bone preparations averaged 27%. They observed failure of the inferior glenohumeral ligament at the glenoid, in the ligament midsubstance and at the humeral insertion site. Furthermore, even when failure occurred at the glenoid, there was significant elongation of the capsule itself. These authors concluded that plastic deformation of the capsule is a fundamental component of anterior instability.

Speer et al., in contradiction to the study of Harryman, created a Bankart lesion in a cadaveric study and noted only small increases in translation when these specimens were loaded (39). The studies of Bigliani and Speer would perhaps underscore the importance of capsular laxity and deformation in contributing to an anterior dislocation. It must be stressed, however, that these studies were in elderly cadavers subjected to extremely low loads, and the specimens were loaded in tension. In the clinical setting, an anterior dislocation frequently occurs with abduction, external rotation and with significant shear forces in the glenohumeral joint. The cadaveric studies may not represent what happens in the young athlete who sustains this injury. To support this concept, studying failure mechanisms in the shoulders of young and old primates, Reeves observed that inferior glenohumeral ligament detachment occurred in young shoulders and that the capsular ligaments tended to tear in the older ones (40). In a study of CT arthrograms of primary anterior dislocation in humans, Ribbans (16) observed similar findings. One-half of the patients were under 50 years of age, with the other half older than 50 years of age. Avulsion of the anterior glenoid labrum (i.e., the Bankart lesion) was seen in 100% of the younger patients and in 75% of the older ones. Associated fractures, tears of the rotator cuff and capsular injuries were more common in those patients over 50. Their conclusions were that the pathoanatomy of a primary anterior shoulder dislocation is dependent on age and that this could explain the disparity in the cadaveric work mentioned previously.

Pathoanatomy (Arthroscopic Studies)

Arthroscopy was recently used in the evaluation of primary anterior dislocations of the shoulder. Baker et al. (41) performed arthroscopy on 45 patients with an acute primary anterior dislocation. These workers described three types of injury. The first group comprised six patients who had a capsular injury alone; interestingly, the examination under anesthesia demonstrated that these shoulders were stable. Eleven patients had a partial detachment of the anterior inferior labrum, and these shoulders were subluxable on examination under anesthesia.

The largest group, consisting of 28 patients, had a complete detachment of the anterior inferior glenoid labrum and these shoulders could be dislocated under anesthesia. In essence, 87% of the patients had either a partial or complete Bankart-type lesion after the initial dislocation. Norlin (42) reported on 24 cases of first-time anterior shoulder dislocation on which arthroscopy was performed within 72 hours of the dislocation. All patients in this study had an anterior capsulolabral detachment, and all 24 had a posterolateral humeral head defect. In none of the cases was gross capsular injury demonstrated. All shoulders were unstable to examination under anesthesia.

Finally, in our own experience at West Point with 75 consecutive cases, a capsulolabral avulsion has been observed arthroscopically 96% of the time (43,45). In summary, the pathoanatomy has been extremely consistent; that is, a Bankart lesion has been observed with high frequency and represents a very important structure with regard to stability of the shoulder. The special circumstances of an initial dislocation with hemarthrosis and excellent tissue quality make it attractive for intervention with acute stabilization. We support the concept of plastic deformation of the capsule prior to avulsion. However, as will be discussed, gross capsular disruption has been observed infrequently. As arthroscopic techniques continue to improve, the acute initial dislocation may be the optimum circumstance for success with this surgical option.

To summarize the rationale for acute stabilization of the initial anterior dislocation:

1. Recurrence rates are unacceptably high in the young high-demand patient.
2. A capsulolabral avulsion occurs with high frequency in this age group and is associated with anterior instability as an important pathologic entity.
3. After the initial dislocation, capsular injury and attenuation would be the least after the initial event.
4. Current arthroscopic techniques permit repair of the capsulolabral complex to the glenoid.

WEST POINT EXPERIENCE

Cadets at the United States Military Academy at West Point, New York, represent a young population of athletes with an age range of approximately 17 to 24 years. In addition to intercollegiate, intramural, and club sports participation, there are physical education requirements for graduation that include boxing, wrestling, rugby and military obstacle courses. Yearly, military training includes hand-to-hand combat, pugile sticks, and parachute training. Within this environment, acute shoulder instability presents as a frequent clinical problem. Wheeler and associates were the first investigators at West Point to evaluate the role of arthroscopic management after an acute initial shoulder dislocation (34). Despite immobilization for 3 weeks and supervised rehabilitation in restricting return to full activity for 3 months after injury, the recurrence rate was 92%. He reported an initial experience using arthroscopic treatment for 9 patients. Two patients (2%) developed recurrence. Although the follow-up was short, with a minimum follow-up of 14 months, these results suggested improved results after acute arthroscopic repair.

Subsequently, we designed a prospective study evaluating nonsurgical and arthroscopic treatment for the initial dislocation (44). The indication for surgical treatment was an initial anterior shoulder dislocation that required a manual reduction. There could be no prior history of shoulder instability or impingement-type pain possibly indicating occult subluxation. No greater tuberosity fractures or concomitant axillary nerve palsies were included in the group. In the nonsurgical group, patients were immobilized for 4 weeks, underwent supervised rehabilitation, and were allowed to return to full activity at 4 months. In the surgical group, arthroscopic Bankart repair using a transglenoid suture technique was performed within 10 days of injury. These patients were then immobilized for 4 weeks and followed a strengthening program and restriction of activity similar to that of the nonsurgical group. From 1988 to 1991, 36 patients met the inclusion criteria for study enrollment. During the same period, 495 cadets were evaluated for shoulder instability at the United States Military Academy. Therefore, only 7% satisfied the inclusion criteria. The average age of the patients was 19.6 years. In the nonsurgical group, 12 of 15 patients developed recurrent instability and 7 of these patients required open Bankart repair before completing their curriculum at the Academy. In the arthroscopic group, 3 of 21 patients developed recurrent instability and 1 patient subsequently required an open Bankart repair to treat residual instability. In essence, surgical treatment reduced recurrence rates to 14% compared with 80% in the nonoperative group. Furthermore, 1 patient in the arthroscopic group (5%) required subsequent open surgery to treat recurrent instability, whereas 50% of those treated nonoperatively required subsequent open Bankart repair.

Since December 1991, reflecting what we perceived as improvements in arthroscopic repair, our technique changed (45). We initiated the use of the sitting position as described by Skyhar (46–49). Our anesthetic technique employed interscalene regional anesthesia and our fixation method changed from a transglenoid suture technique to one using a bioabsorbable fixation device (Suretac, Smith-Nephew endoscopy, Andover, MA). The fixation device is a polymer of polyglycolic acid. In laboratory studies, the implant is absorbed over a period of 4 to 6 weeks. At 2 weeks, its initial pullout strength is reduced to nearly 50% at implantation. The pullout strength has been reported to be within the range of 100 to 120 N-m, or approximately 20 lb. An additional 45 patients have been treated with arthroscopic tack stabilization for the initial anterior shoulder dislocation. From our previous arthroscopic experience, the avulsed capsulolabral complex has been of excellent tissue quality and is an ideal situation for use in this fixation method.

Technique

Interscalene anesthesia is administered using a 50:50 mixture of 0.75% bubivacaine and 3% chloroprocaine. After satisfactory anesthesia, with the patient in the supine position, an examination under anesthesia is performed and recorded. Here, a modified load shift maneuver is performed with the arm in approximately 70 to 80 degrees of

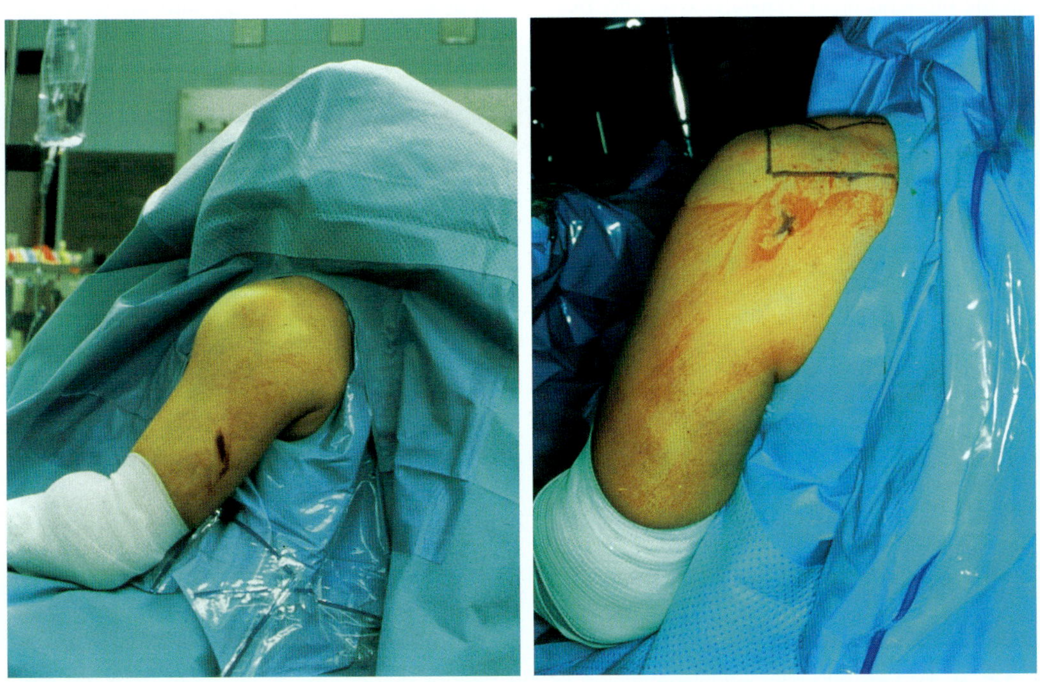

A B

FIG. 10. A, B: Left shoulder prepped and draped in sitting position for arthroscopy.

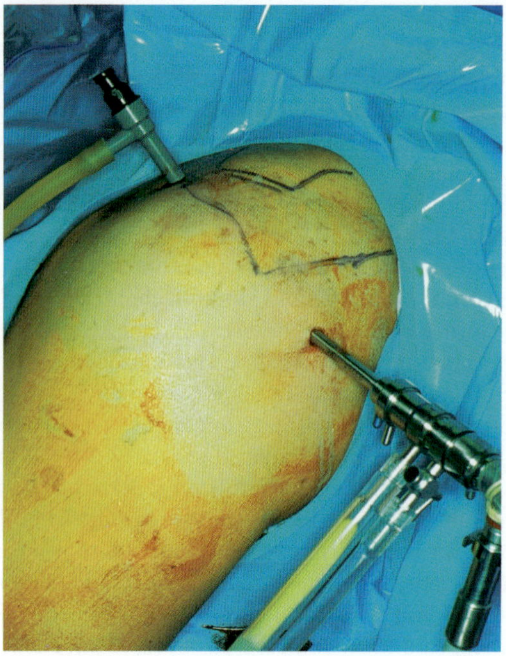

FIG. 11. Left shoulder. Arthroscope is posterior with anterosuperior portal adjacent to anterolateral corner of acromion.

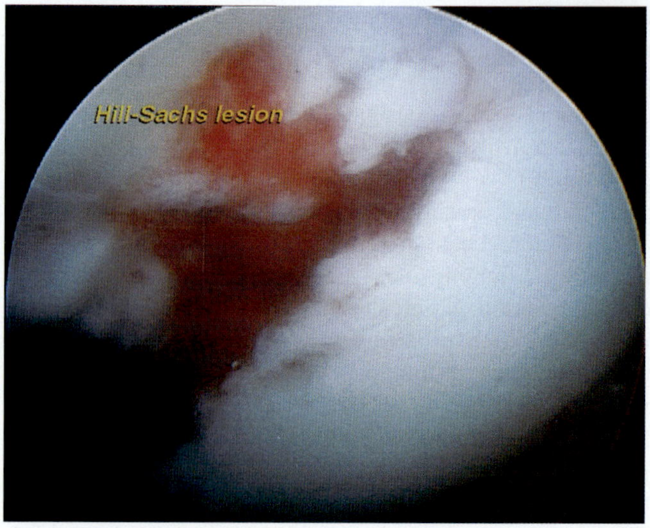

FIG. 13. Left shoulder. An acute posterolateral humeral head defect (Hill-Sachs lesion).

abduction and elevation in the plane of the scapula. With the humeral head compressed into the glenoid fossa, the proximal humerus is translated anteriorly, inferiorly or posteriorly. Trace or 1+ translation indicates that the humeral head could be translated to the glenoid rim only. A 2+ translation is when the humeral head jumps over the anterior glenoid rim but when the force is removed, the humeral head spontaneously reduces. The designation 3+ translation indicates that the humeral head translates over the glenoid rim and remains locked in this position when the force is removed. After the examination, the patient is placed in a sitting position by forward flexing the back of the table and flexing the end or foot of the table. A bean bag or commercially available positioner can be used to support the torso and allow exposure of the shoulder (Fig. 10).

The shoulder is prepped and draped in a sterile manner ensuring adequate exposure of pertinent anatomy. A surgical marker is used to outline the acromion, coracoid process and the sites for the potential posterior, anterosuperior, and anteroinferior portals. With the patient in the sitting position, one can easily palpate a soft spot in the region for appropriate level of entry into the posterior capsule. A he-

A

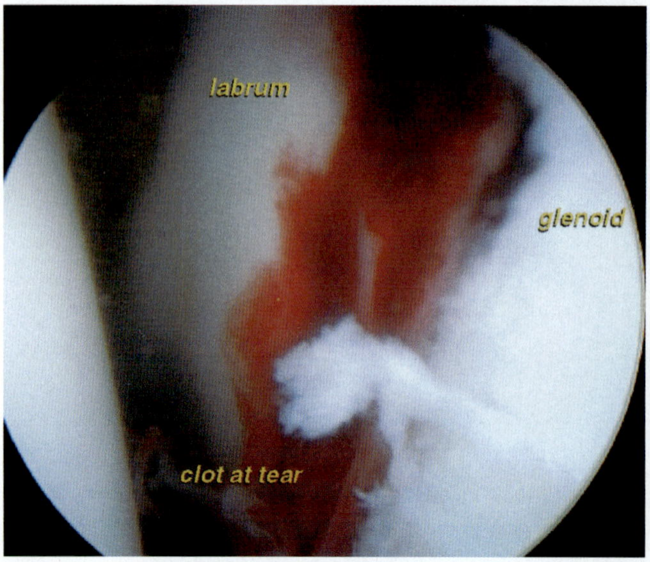

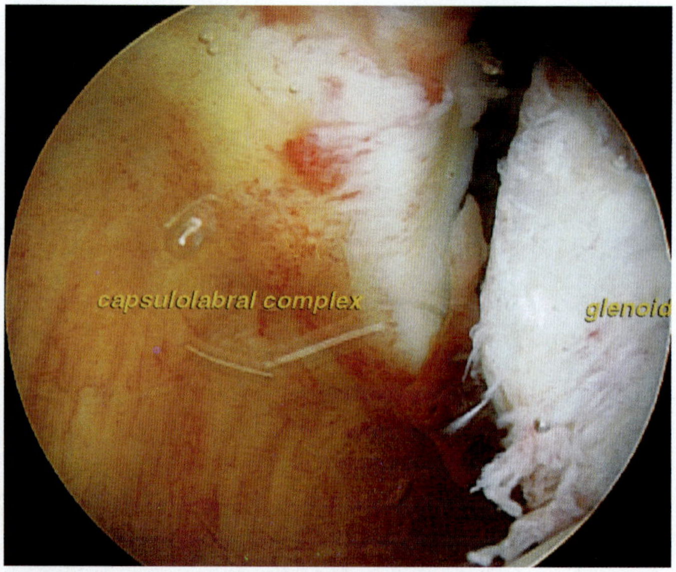

B

FIG. 12. A, B: Left shoulder—acute avulsion of the inferior glenohumeral ligament from the glenoid (Bankart lesion).

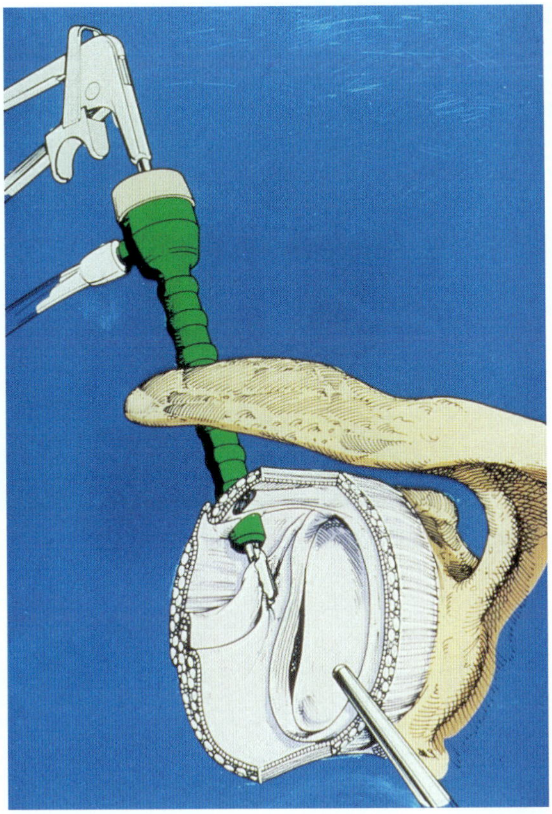

FIG. 14. Left shoulder. Soft-tissue grasper used to reduce Bankart lesion and reestablish tension of inferior glenohumeral ligament.

marthrosis after acute dislocation has been demonstrated in all of our cases and the use of a pump facilitates the evacuation of the hematoma. The anterior superior portal (ASP) is rapidly established with an 18-gauge spinal needle placed entering the joint just medial to the biceps tendon and as superior as possible (Fig. 11). The entry point outside the shoulder is at the anterolateral corner of the acromion. A 5.5 cannula is placed into the ASP. A probe can then be inserted through the ASP and thorough arthroscopic examination is performed. In 96% of our cases, a complete capsulolabral avulsion of the inferior glenohumeral ligament complex from the glenoid has been encountered (Fig. 12). The Hill-Sachs lesion is also frequently encountered but has not required treatment (Fig. 13). Next, abrasion and decortication of the scapula neck follows. To ensure better visualization, a 70-degree arthroscope can be placed from the posterior portal to allow the surgeon visualization of the anterior glenoid and scapular neck. Subsequently, a burr is used through the anterosuperior portal to perform the abrasion while viewing from posteriorly.

After abrasion a specifically designed soft-tissue grasper is placed through the anterosuperior portal and a trial reduction of the Bankart lesion is performed. This is to ensure that the capsulolabral complex can be brought to its anatomic position. It is important to grasp the capsulolabral complex and shift it superiorly over the rim of the glenoid and re-establish tension into the IGHL (Fig. 14).

The next step is to establish an anteroinferior portal. The anteroinferior portal should enter the shoulder just superior to the superior edge of the subscapularis tendon (Fig. 15). The surgeon should ensure that the angle of approach of the 18-gauge spinal needle is tangential to the glenoid fossa. This will minimize medial or inferior deflection of the drilling instruments that will be used later. The 18-gauge needle used to establish the AIP will start outside the shoulder just lateral to the coracoid process. The surgeon should attempt to maximize the distance between the anterior superior portal and the anteroinferior portal. This will facilitate triangulation. Once satisfied with the position of the needle, the

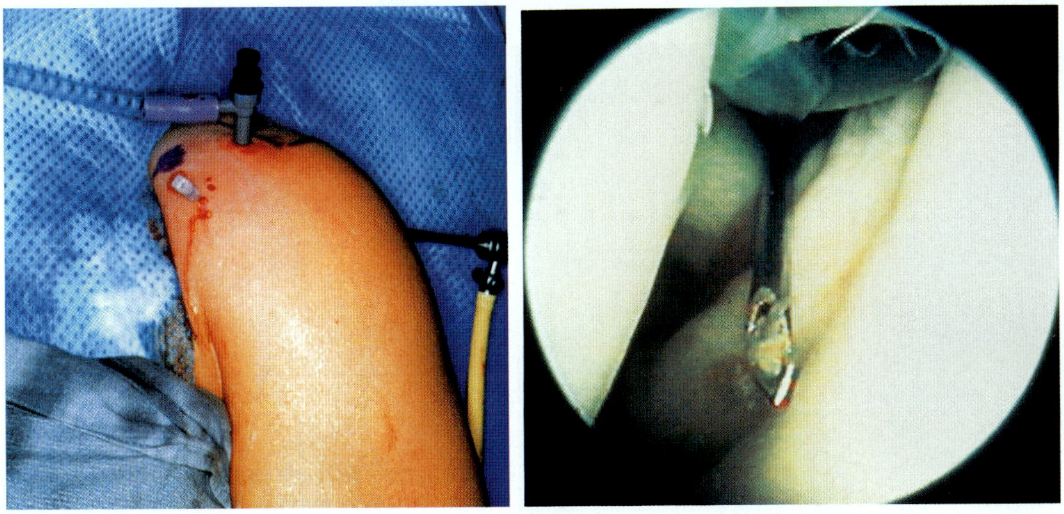

A B

FIG. 15. A: Left shoulder. Outside view with 18-gauge spinal needle used in outside-in fashion to establish anteroinferior portal. **B:** Left shoulder. Eighteen-gauge needle entering tangential to glenoid fossa just superior to subscapularis tendon.

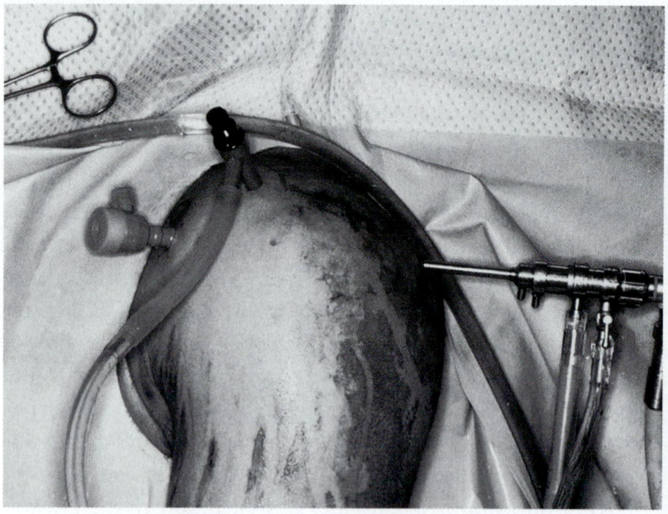

A

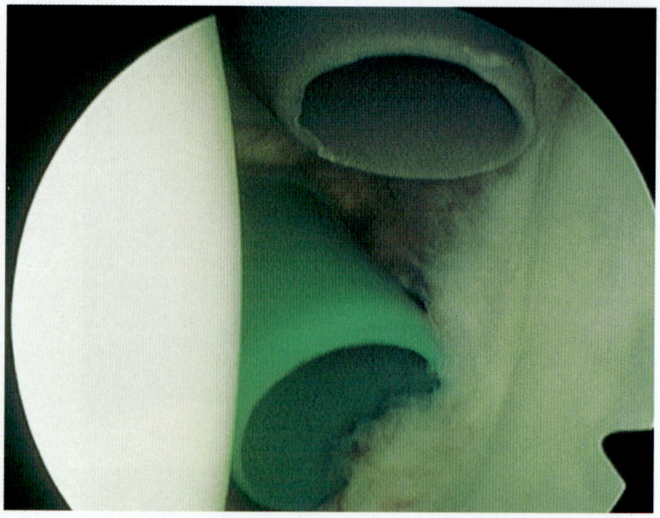

B

FIG. 16. A: Left shoulder. Outside view of anterosuperior and anteroinferior portals established. **B:** Left shoulder. Cannula for anterosuperior and anteroinferior portals in position.

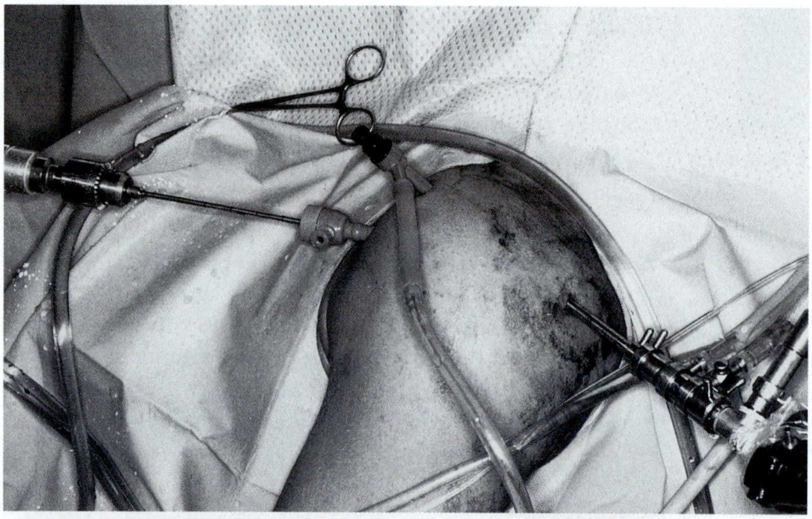

A

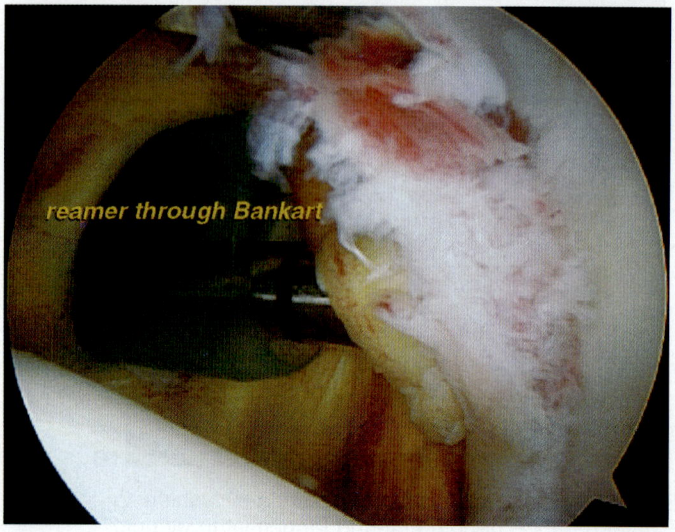

B

FIG. 17. A: Left shoulder. Outside view demonstrating drilling with reamer-guidewire. **B:** Left shoulder. Arthroscopic view of drilling with guidewire-reamer while maintaining reduction of Bankart lesion.

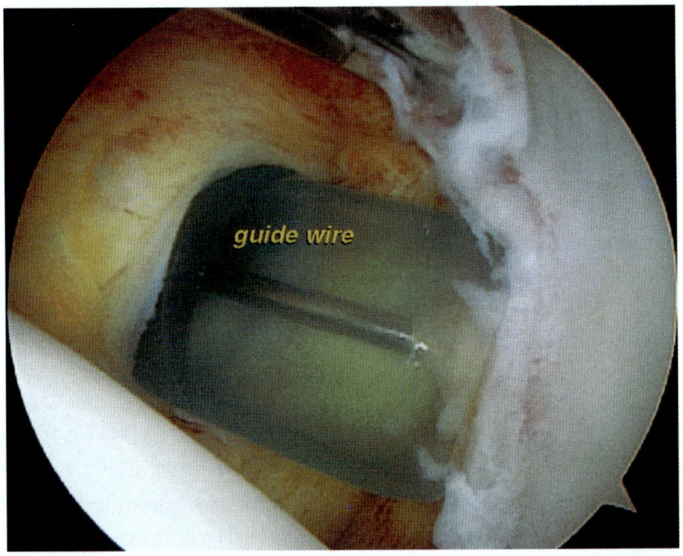

FIG. 18. Left shoulder. Reamer removed leaving guidewire in place inside cannula.

AIP is created with a No. 11 blade and a 7-ml cannula is positioned (Fig. 16).

The bioabsorbable fixation device requires initial drilling with a reamer and guide wire. To facilitate ease of piercing the capsulolabral tissue, it is recommended that the guidewire be locked to the reamer extending 3 to 4 mm beyond the tip of the reamer. A capable assistant provides visualization with the arthroscope and grasps the Bankart lesion with the grasper from the anterosuperior portal and reduces the lesion automatically. The surgeon can then pierce the avulsed capsulolabral tissue with the reamer guidewire in preparation for the first tack. Drilling commences at approximately the 8 o'clock position for a left shoulder (4 o'clock position for a right shoulder) to a depth of 1.5 cm (Fig. 17). Once the reamer has been drilled to the appropriate depth, the locking nut is loosened and a wire tamp is placed over the guidewire. Several light taps with a mallet will free the guidewire from the reamer. Using the specially designed hex-handled instrument, attached to the outside position of the reamer, the reamer is then backed out, leaving the guidewire in place (Fig. 18). Extreme attention to detail is necessary in this phase so as to not remove the guidewire inadvertently. After the reamer has been removed, an 8-mm cannulated tack is placed over the guidewire, and the impactor will allow full seating of the tack into its final position (Fig. 19). These steps are repeated for an additional tack placed at 2 o'clock for the right shoulder (10 o'clock for the left shoulder). The arthroscope is then placed through the ASP to review the repair from the front (Fig. 20). Postoperatively, the shoulder is immobilized for 4 weeks, followed by a rehabilitation program with full activity allowed at 4 months.

Since December 1991, 45 additional patients have been evaluated with arthroscopy after the acute initial anterior dislocation. The pathologic findings at surgery have been remarkably consistent. All patients have had a hemarthrosis and 42 patients had a capsulolabral disruption of the inferior glenohumeral ligament from the glenoid scapular neck. Two patients with Bankart lesions also had capsular tears extending into the inferior glenohumeral ligament as well. There have been two isolated capsular tears of the inferior glenohumeral ligament without evidence of a Bankart lesion and there has been one lateral detachment of the inferior glenohumeral ligament from the neck of the humerus (50). There have been four associated superior labral anterior to posterior lesions (''SLAP tears''), two of which were repaired with an additional 6-mm tack (51,52). The two patients with cap-

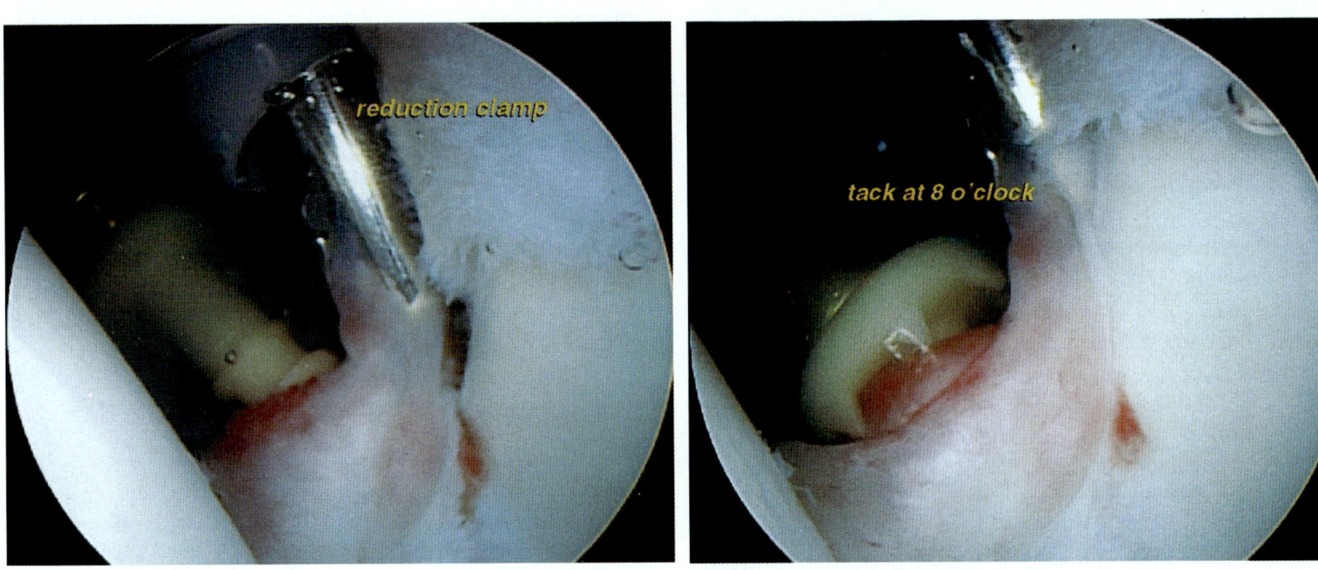

A B

FIG. 19. A, B: Left shoulder. Tack inserted at 8 o'clock. Note soft-tissue grasper maintaining reduction.

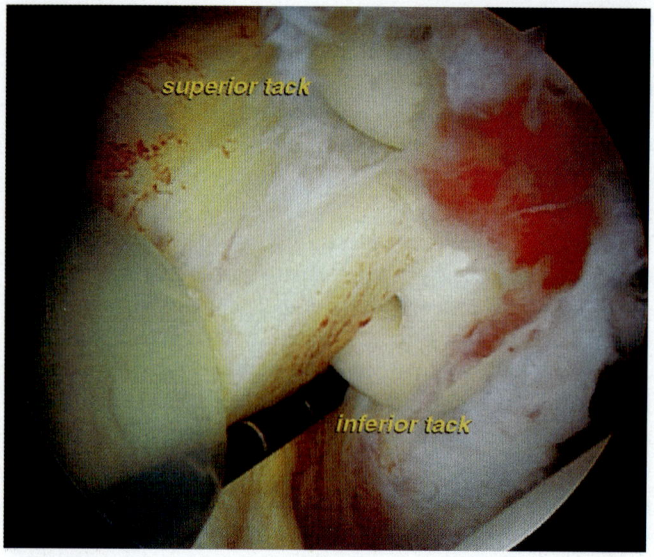

FIG. 20. Left shoulder. View from anterior portal of completed repair.

sular injuries and the one patient with a lateral detachment of the inferior glenohumeral ligament were treated with an open repair. Therefore, 42 patients have been treated with arthroscopic repair using the bioabsorbable tack. The average patient age has been 19.6 years and the average follow-up is now 24 months. An average of two tacks per case has been used. Of 32 patients with a minimum of 1-year follow-up, 29 have returned to full activity at the United States Military Academy without restriction or any incidence of recurrence, subluxation, or dislocation. There have been four cases of recurrent instability. Two patients had recurrent dislocation after reinjury in a collision sport and two developed recurrent subluxation after a fall. Two of these patients have required an open reconstruction to treat recurrent instability.

In summary, 130 patients at the United States Military Academy have been treated for an initial traumatic anterior shoulder dislocation since 1986. The average age has been 19.6 years and a manual reduction was required for initial treatment in all cases. Fifty-five patients were treated nonsurgically and 47 developed recurrent instability (85%) within the first 2 years after injury. Seventy-five patients have been treated with three different arthroscopic techniques reflecting perceived improvements in arthroscopic repair. Nine patients have developed recurrence (12%). The examination under anesthesia has demonstrated increased anterior translation in all patients. The arthroscopic examination has revealed a consistent, easily identifiable injury in 96% of the cases. An avulsion of the inferior glenohumeral ligament from the glenoid has been documented in 72 cases. Two of these cases also had gross evidence of capsular injury. The remainder of these 72 cases had no gross evidence of capsular disruption. Only three cases have deviated from this presentation.

More recently, Jakobsen and Sojbjerg reported their results of open primary surgical repair for acute initial dislocations. Preliminary results with early follow-up indicate a recurrent instability rate of 3% (53). In this study, 76 consecutive patients, with an average age of 22, were randomized to nonoperative or open Bankart repair treatment protocol. At an average follow-up of nearly 1 year, 27% of the nonoperative group had sustained recurrent instability and 62% had a positive apprehension sign. Only one patient, 3% in the operative repair group, sustained recurrent dislocation with only 8% having a positive apprehension test at 12 months after the injury.

SUMMARY

The management of the initial anterior shoulder dislocation is dependent on the age and activity demands of the patient. After a thorough examination and appropriate radiographs, a gentle closed reduction is the initial treatment. Many investigators have recommended a period of immobilization, followed by a rehabilitation program emphasizing rotator cuff strengthening. Restricting return to athletic activities to allow adequate soft-tissue healing also appears appropriate. This will effectively treat the vast majority of patients with this injury. In patients older than 25 years of age, one would expect a relatively low recurrence rate, especially those with low activity demands or those willing to modify activity.

However, in the young active patient desiring a return to strenuous athletic activity, nonoperative treatment has been unpredictable and often leads to high recurrence rates that require subsequent treatment. Acute operative treatment of an initial anterior shoulder dislocation is therefore considered in the young, active high-risk patient. In the author's experience, the examination under anesthesia and the arthroscopic examinations have confirmed an avulsion of the anterior inferior capsulolabral complex as the most commonly encountered pathoanatomic lesion. The special circumstances of an initial dislocation with a hemarthrosis and excellent tissue quality make it ideal for arthroscopic stabilization. With no labral degeneration or marked capsular attenuation, as is frequently observed in chronic instability, these unique circumstances may be optimal for an arthroscopic stabilization technique. Our early results have been encouraging and we believe this approach is a viable option in the management of this injury in young athletes (aged 17 to 24).

REFERENCES

1. Thomas SC, Matsen FA III. An approach to the repair of avulsion of the glenohumeral ligaments in the management of traumatic anterior glenohumeral instability. *J Bone Joint Surg* 1989;71A:506–513.
2. Matsen FA, Thomas SC, Rockwood CA Jr. Anterior glenohumeral instability. In: Rockwood CA Jr, Matsen FA, eds. *The shoulder*, vol 1. 1st ed. Philadelphia: JB Lippincott, 1990:526–622.

3. Bigliani LU, Kurzweil PR, Schwartzbach CC, et al. Inferior capsular shift procedure for anterior-inferior shoulder instability in athletes. *Am J Sports Med* 1994;22:578–584.
4. O'Brien SJ, Neves MC, Arnoczky SP, et al. The anatomy and histology of the inferior glenohumeral ligament complex of the shoulder. *Am J Sports Med* 1990;18:449–456.
5. Turkel SJ, Panie MW, Marshal JL, et al. Stabilizing mechanisms preventing anterior dislocation of the glenohumeral joint. *J Bone Joint Surg* 1981;63A:1208–1217.
6. Blom S, Dahlback LO. Nerve injuries in dislocations of the shoulder joint and fractures of the neck of the humerus: a clinical and electromyographical study. *Acta Chir Scand* 1970:136:461–466.
7. Neer CS II, Rockwood CA Jr. Fractures and dislocations of the shoulder. In: Rockwood CA Jr, Green DP, eds. *Fractures in adults*, vol. 1, 2nd ed. Philadelphia: JB Lippincott, 1984:675–985.
8. Rokous JR, Feagin JA, Abbott HG. Modified axillary roentgenogram: a useful adjunct in the diagnosis of recurrent instability of the shoulder. *Clin Orthop* 1972;82:84–86.
9. Arciero RA. Acute traumatic anterior dislocation of the shoulder. In: Bigliani LU, ed. *The unstable shoulder*, 1st ed. American Academy of Orthopaedic Surgeons, 1996:37–45.
10. Westin CD, Gill EA, Noyes ME, Hubbard M. Anterior shoulder dislocation. A simple and rapid method for reduction. *Am J Sports Med* 1995;23:369–371.
11. Anderson D, Zvirbulis, Ciullo J. Scapular manipulation for reduction of anterior shoulder dislocations. *Clin Orthop* 1982;164:181–183.
12. Matthews DE, Roberts T. Intraarticular lidocaine versus intravenous analgesic for reduction of acute anterior shoulder dislocations: a prospective randomized study. *Am J Sports Med* 1995;23:54–58.
13. Milch H. Treatment of dislocation of the shoulder. *Surgery* 1938;3: 732–740.
14. Janecki CJ, Shahcheragh GH. The forward elevation maneuver for reduction of anterior dislocations of the shoulder. *Clin Orthop* 1982;164:177–180.
15. Neviaser RJ, Neviaser TJ, Neviaser JS. Concurrent rupture of the rotator cuff and anterior dislocation of the shoulder in the older patient. *J Bone Joint Surg* 1988;70A:1308–1311.
16. Ribbans WJ, Mitchell R, Taylor GJ. Computerized arthrotomography of primary anterior dislocation of the shoulder. *J Bone Joint Surg* 1990;72B:181–185.
17. Tijmes J, Loyd HM, Tullos HS. Arthrography in acute shoulder dislocations. *South Med J* 1979;72:564–567.
18. Reeves B. Arthrography in acute dislocation of the shoulder. *J Bone Joint Surg* 1966;48B:182.
19. McLaughlin HL, Cavallaro WU. Primary anterior dislocation of the shoulder. *Am J Surg* 1950;80:615–621.
20. McLaughlin HL. Dislocation of the shoulder with tuberosity fracture. *Surg Clin North Am* 1963;43:1615–1620.
21. McLaughlin HL, MacLellan DI. Recurrent anterior dislocation of the shoulder. II. A comparative study. *J Trauma* 1967;7:191–201.
22. Rowe CR. Prognosis in dislocation of the shoulder. *J Bone Joint Surg* 1956;38A:957–977.
23. Rowe CR, Sakellarides HT. Factors related to recurrences of anterior dislocations of the shoulder. *Clin Orthop* 1961;20:40–48.
24. Kiviluoto O, Posila M, Jaronia H, et al. Immobilization after primary dislocation of the shoulder. *Acta Orthop Scand* 1980;51:915–919.
25. Henry JH, Genung JA. Natural history of glenohumeral dislocation revisited. *Am J Sports Med* 1982;10:135–137.
26. Watson-Jones R. Recurrent dislocation of the shoulder [editorial]. *J Bone Joint Surg* 1948;30B:6–8.
27. Yoneda B, Welsh RP, MacIntosh DL. Conservative treatment of shoulder dislocation in young males. *J Bone Joint Surg* 1982;64B: 254–255.
28. Aronen JG, Regan K. Decreasing the incidence of recurrence of first time anterior shoulder dislocations with rehabilitation. *Am J Sports Med* 1984;12:283–291.
29. Hovelius L, Eriksson K, Fredin H, et al. Recurrence after initial dislocation of the shoulder. *J Bone Joint Surg* 1983;65A:343–349.
30. Hovelius L. Anterior dislocation of the shoulder in teenagers and young adults. *J Bone Joint Surg* 1987;69A:393–399.
31. Hovelius L, Augustini BG, Fredin OH, et al. Primary anterior dislocation of the shoulder in young patients. *J Bone Joint Surg* 1996;78A: 1677–1684.
32. Hovelius L. Shoulder dislocation in Swedish ice hockey players. *Am J Sports Med* 1979;6:373–377.
33. Simonet WT, Cofield RH. Prognosis in anterior shoulder dislocation. *Am J Sports Med* 1984;12:19–24.
34. Wheeler JH, Ryan JB, Arciero RA, et al. Arthroscopic versus non-operative treatment of acute shoulder dislocations in young athletes. *Arthroscopy* 1989;5:213–217.
35. Bankart ASB. The pathology and treatment of recurrent dislocation of the shoulder-joint. *Br J Surg* 1938;26:23–29.
36. Perthes G. Uber operationen bei: Habitueller Schulterluxation. *Dtsch Ztschr Chir* 1906;85:199–227.
37. Harryman DT, Ballmer FP, Harris SL, Sidles JA. Arthroscopic labral repair to the glenoid rim. *Arthroscopy* 1994;10:20–30.
38. Bigliani LU, Pollack RG, Soslowsky LJ, et al. Tensile properties of the inferior glenohumeral ligament. *J Orthop Res* 1992;10:187–197.
39. Speer KP, Deng X, Borrero S, et al. Biomechanical evaluation of a stimulated Bankart lesion. *J Bone Joint Surg* 1994;76A:1819–1826.
40. Reeves B. Acute anterior dislocation of the shoulder: clinical and experimental studies. *Ann R Coll Surg Engl* 1969;44:255–273.
41. Baker CL, Uribe JW, Whitman C. Arthroscopic evaluation of acute initial anterior shoulder dislocations. *Am J Sports Med* 1990;18:25–28.
42. Norlin R. Intraarticular pathology in acute, first-time anterior shoulder dislocation. An arthroscopic study. *Arthroscopy* 1993;9:546–549.
43. Taylor DC, Arciero RA. Pathologic changes associated with shoulder dislocations. Arthroscopic and physical examination findings in first-time traumatic anterior dislocation. *Am J Sports Med* 1997;25:306–311.
44. Arciero RA, Wheeler JH, Ryan JB, et al. Arthroscopic Bankart repair vs. non-operative treatment for acute, initial, anterior shoulder dislocations. *Am J Sports Med* 1994;22:589–594.
45. Arciero RA, Taylor DC, Snyder RJ, et al. Arthroscopic bioabsorbable tack stabilization of initial anterior shoulder dislocations: a preliminary report. *Arthroscopy* 1995;11:410–417.
46. Skyhar MJ, Altchek DW, Warren RF, et al. Shoulder arthroscopy with the patient in the beach-chair position. *Arthroscopy* 1988;4:256–259.
47. Altchek DW. Arthroscopic shoulder stabilization using a bioabsorbable fixation device. *Sports Med Arthrosc Rev* 1993;1:266–271.
48. Warner JP, Warren RF. Arthroscopic Bankart repair using a cannulated, absorbable fixation device. *Op Tech Orthop* 1991;1:192–198.
49. Pagnani MJ, Warren RF. Arthroscopic shoulder stabilization. *Op Tech Sports Med* 1993;1:276–284.
50. Bach BR, Warren RF, Fronek J. Disruption of the lateral capsule of the shoulder: a cause of recurrent dislocation. *J Bone Joint Surg* 1988;70B:274–276.
51. Snyder SJ, Karzel RP, Del Pizzo W, et al. SLAP lesions of the shoulder. *Arthroscopy* 1990;6:274–279.
52. Warner JJ, Kann S, Marks P. Arthroscopic repair of combined Bankart and superior labral detachment anterior and posterior lesions: technique and preliminary results. *Arthroscopy* 1994;10:383–391.
53. Jakobsen BW, Sojbjerg JO. Primary repair after traumatic anterior dislocation of the shoulder joint. *Orthop Trans* 1995;19:459.

The Unstable Shoulder,
edited by R.F. Warren, E.V. Craig, and D.W. Altchek.
Lippincott–Raven Publishers, Philadelphia © 1999.

CHAPTER 11

Rehabilitation and Nonoperative Treatment

Joshua M. Zimmerman, John G. Skedros, Mark T. Dean, Peter O'Rourke, and Wayne Z. Burkhead, Jr.

The appropriate nonoperative treatment of the unstable shoulder has received considerable attention in the literature during the past 15 years. Until recently, the mainstay of nonoperative treatment of the unstable shoulder had consisted mainly of varying periods of immobilization. With the exception of an early report by Davis (1) in 1936, the concept of muscle rehabilitation as an adjunct to immobilization had been largely ignored. Refinements in our understanding of anterior shoulder instability now allow us to design patient-specific rehabilitation programs as well as to counsel patients on the likelihood of success of these programs (2–4).

Rehabilitation of the scapular stabilizing muscles, in addition to the dynamic glenohumeral stabilizers, is now recognized as an essential component in the management of the unstable shoulder (5,6). Electromyographic (EMG) studies have delineated which muscles and groups of muscles are activated during specific rehabilitative exercises (7–9). EMG analysis has also been instrumental in demonstrating muscle group imbalances in those patients with anterior instability (10). This information, in combination with a patient-specific diagnosis, can provide a rational basis for designing and implementing an effective rehabilitation program for shoulder instability.

The purpose of this chapter is to address the nonoperative management of anterior shoulder instability. The discussion focuses primarily on three entities: (a) first-time acute dislocators, (b) chronic anterior instability, and (c) anterior subluxation in the throwing athlete. Clinical evaluation and diagnostic imaging are discussed in Section 2 and are included in this chapter only as they pertain to rehabilitative recommendations.

J. M. Zimmerman, J. G. Skedros, M. T. Dean, P. O'Rourke: W. B. Carrell Memorial Clinic, Dallas, Texas 75204.

W. Z. Burkhead, Jr.: Department of Orthopaedics, University of Texas—Southwestern Medical School, and W. B. Carrell Memorial Clinic, Dallas, Texas 75204.

ACUTE FIRST-TIME DISLOCATORS

Immobilization

The appropriate length and value of immobilization after an initial episode of dislocation remain controversial. Most early studies recommend immobilization of 2 to 6 weeks duration, and little or no mention is made of a muscle strengthening program. In 1956, Rowe (2) reviewed 500 shoulder dislocations, 96% of which were traumatic in origin. Of those patients younger than 20 years of age at the time of dislocation, 83% experienced recurrent dislocations, compared with 63% of those aged 20 to 40 years and 16% of those older than 40 years of age. The nonoperative treatment of these patients consisted of varying periods of immobilization in a sling and swath. No correlation was noted between length of immobilization and recurrence. An earlier study conducted by McLaughlin and Cavallaro (11) noted recurrence rates of 90% in patients under 20 years using similar nonoperative methods. More recently, Henry and Genung (12) prospectively studied the recurrence rate in young athletes treated with immobilization for 2 to 6 weeks versus those treated with no immobilization. These investigators found an 85% to 90% recurrence rate in both groups. A 10-year prospective study by Hovelius et al. (13) noted somewhat lower redislocation rates in first time dislocators but also concluded that the type and duration of the initial treatment had no effect on the rate of recurrence. Simonet and Cofield (14) found a recurrence rate of 66% in patients less than 20 years of age, 40% in patients aged 20 to 40 years, and no recurrences in patients older than 40 years. The only treatment factor that significantly influenced recurrence in their study was a 6-week restriction on return to sports.

By contrast, two studies have demonstrated the efficacy of immobilization as a component of nonoperative treatment. In 1982, Yoneda et al. (15) reviewed the recurrence rate in young athletes treated with immobilization for 5 weeks, followed by a graduated exercise routine for 6 weeks. These investigators reported the recurrence rate with this program to be only 17%. Similarly, Aronen and Regan (16) reported a recurrence rate of 25% in Naval cadets treated with 3 weeks of immobilization followed by a specific rehabilitation program of isometric, isotonic, and isokinetic exercises.

Although the literature remains controversial, our preference is for a 6-week period of immobilization in those patients who elect nonoperative treatment. Our rationale for this decision is based on the fact that a significant degree of capsular injury typically occurs before the traumatic detachment of the inferior glenohumeral ligament from the labrum (17). Also, cadaveric studies have demonstrated that a Bankart lesion alone, in the absence of capsular stretching or rupture, is *unlikely* to allow significant anterior translation of the humeral head in the glenoid fossa (18). The repair and regenerative phase of tendon and ligament healing occur between 72 hours and 6 weeks (19). Basic science studies evaluating tensile strength demonstrate that in this phase of healing, ligaments are relatively weak at 3 weeks with gradually increasing strength thereafter (20,21). Therefore, although immobilization in internal rotation may not result in anatomic healing of the inferior glenohumeral ligament to the glenoid labrum, our hope is that 6 weeks of immobilization will allow for the best nonoperative chance for optimizing healing of the static stabilizers of the shoulder.

Rehabilitation Protocol for First-Time Dislocators

After reduction of an acute first-time dislocation, as much information about the pathoanatomy of the patient's dislocation should be obtained as is safely and comfortably possible. Appropriate radiographs of the affected shoulder should be obtained, and include a Stryker notch, axillary lateral, true anteroposterior (AP), West Point axillary lateral, and apical oblique views as described by Garth et al. (22). These radiographs will define most of the bony defects in the humeral head and the glenoid, which have been noted in approximately 80% of patients with anterior dislocations (3). Several studies have noted a poorer prognosis in those patients with humeral head impression defects (Hill-Sachs lesion) compared with patients without other defects (3,13). Conversely, dislocations associated with a greater tuberosity fracture have a significantly better prognosis (23). In young patients at high risk of recurrence, computed tomography (CT), arthrography, or diagnostic arthroscopy should be considered to rule out a repairable Bankart lesion as well to document a chondral Hill-Sachs defect. The role of magnetic resonance imaging (MRI) continues to evolve in the evaluation of the unstable shoulder. Several recent studies comparing MR arthrography with CT arthrography in the detection of Bankart lesions and labral pathology have concluded that MRI is the superior modality (24,25). Rehabilitation recommendations are guided by patient age, history, and radiographic studies in most cases. MRI scanning is not routinely performed. We continue to reserve MR arthrography for the older first-time dislocator who is suspected of having rotator cuff pathology in addition to labral pathology.

The results of the imaging evaluation along with the patient's age and the magnitude of trauma causing the dislocation can be used to counsel the patient on the probable success of a nonoperative treatment program. If the patient, after being given this information, chooses nonoperative treatment, we insist on 6 weeks of immobilization. The patient is instructed to avoid exacerbating activities including overhead use of the involved extremity, as well as the abducted externally rotated "at-risk" position. The patient should also be informed that the period of immobilization will be followed by a long-term strengthening program that must be sustained to increase the probability of a successful outcome. Cessation of the rehabilitation protocol even in the remote future may increase the risk of recurrent symptoms.

After discharge from the hospital, the patient should use ice, nonsteroidal anti-inflammatory drugs (NSAIDs), and other modalities to control pain and reduce inflammation. As the pain subsides over the first few days, the patient begins isometric exercises in the sling with resisted contractions of 8 to 10 seconds with a 2-second intervening rest period. This consists primarily of deltoid isometric contractions. At 3 to 4 weeks postinjury, the patient is given instruction on isotonic rehabilitation exercises. These exercises are performed with a pulley, surgical tubing, weights, or Therabands (Hygienic, Akron, OH, U.S.A.). We prefer to use Therabands, as they facilitate both eccentric and concentric strengthening, are easy to use at home without expensive equipment and are not cumbersome. Therabands are available in six different thicknesses, providing progressive resistance from 1 to 6 lb in 1-lb increments. The initial program emphasizes isotonics with internal rotation and adduction, limiting external rotation to the neutral position. During the 5th and 6th weeks, the patient may progress to a comprehensive strengthening program emphasizing the three parts of the deltoid, the rotator cuff, and the scapular stabilizers (26) (Fig. 1A,B). Theraband exercises are performed two to three times per day. The exercises should be short arc, avoiding the end ranges of motion. Exercises are performed at low intensity and low speeds with high repetitions. Initially, five repetitions are performed holding each repetition isometrically for a 5-second count. The patient is advanced to 12 repetitions, with an isometric 10-second count, before advancing to the next level. After completion of the last level of a Theraband program, the patient performs the same exercises with either a pulley and weight kit or free weights. The weights are usually begun at 8 to 10 lb for an average patient, and

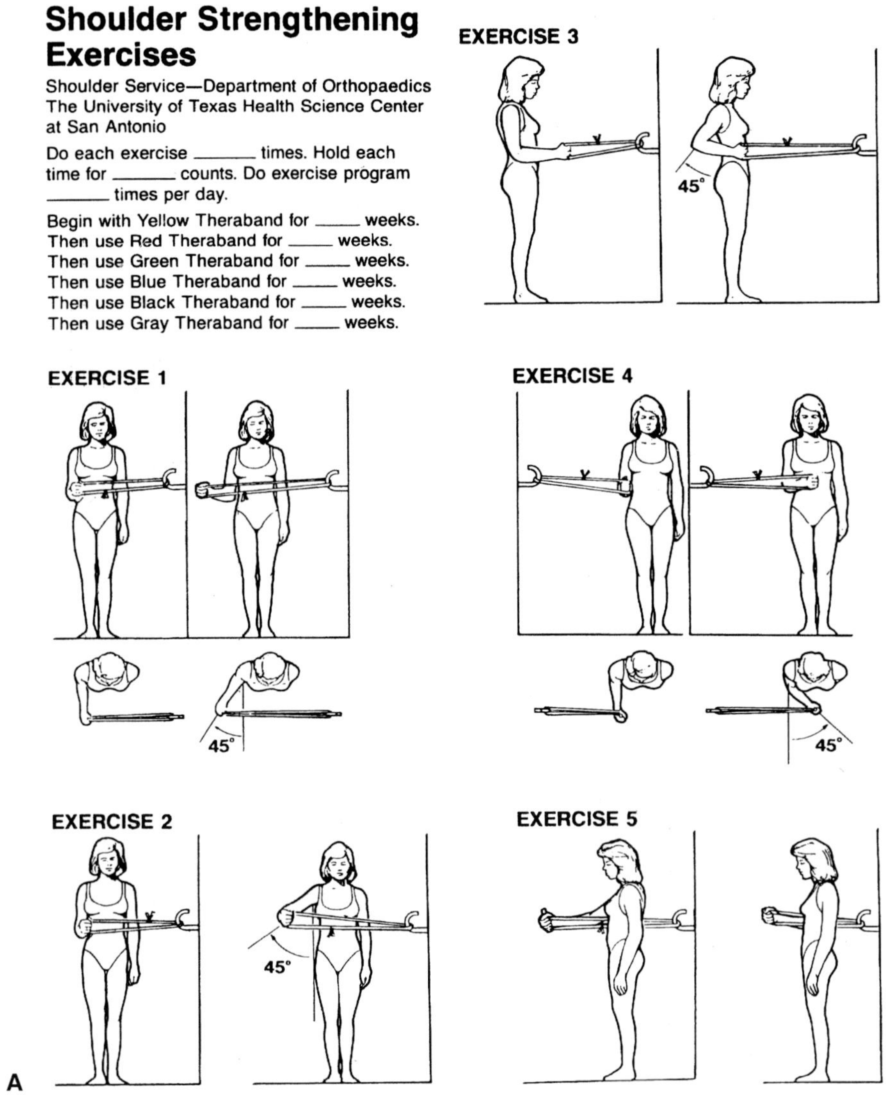

FIG. 1. Rehabilitation program to strengthen the deltoid, rotator cuff, and scapular stabilizer muscles. **A:** Initially, only internal rotation in adduction is performed. During the 5th or 6th week, the patient progresses to all five Theraband exercises. (*figure continues*)

then increased in 2-lb increments. The weights may be increased to as much as 20 to 25 lb for men and 15 lb for women. Patients are not progressed to the next level if they experience increasing exercise-related pain. When not performing exercises, the patient continues to wear the shoulder immobilizer. At 6 weeks, the immobilizer is discontinued, but the patient is restricted from returning to sports and is instructed to avoid at-risk positioning of the arm. A long-term rehabilitation program is instituted at this time. From a practical standpoint, rehabilitation is continued for 8 to 12 weeks after the immobilizer has been discontinued. Return to play is generally allowed at this point if full strength and range of motion are restored. Ideally, shoulder rehabilitation will be continued indefinitely, throughout the season and off-season.

When designing a program of specific exercises, it is extremely important to strengthen both the glenohumeral and scapular musculature. A broad rehabilitation protocol may include internal rotation, external rotation, flexion, extension, cross-body adduction, abduction, horizontal adduction, abduction in the plane of the scapula in both internal and external rotation, forward flexion, shoulder shrugs, press-ups, and rows. However, in acute first-time dislocators with no pre-existing muscle weakness, a simpler and more specific rehabilitation protocol may be designed.

Muscle-specific EMG studies have demonstrated core groups of exercises that effectively work the glenohumeral and the scapulothoracic musculature (10,27). For rehabilitation of the dynamic glenohumeral stabilizers, a set of four exercises has been shown to adequately address all of the involved muscles. These muscles include the four rotator cuff muscles, the three portions of the deltoid, the pectoralis major, and the latissimus dorsi. All nine of these muscles demonstrate adequate activity with a combination of scap-

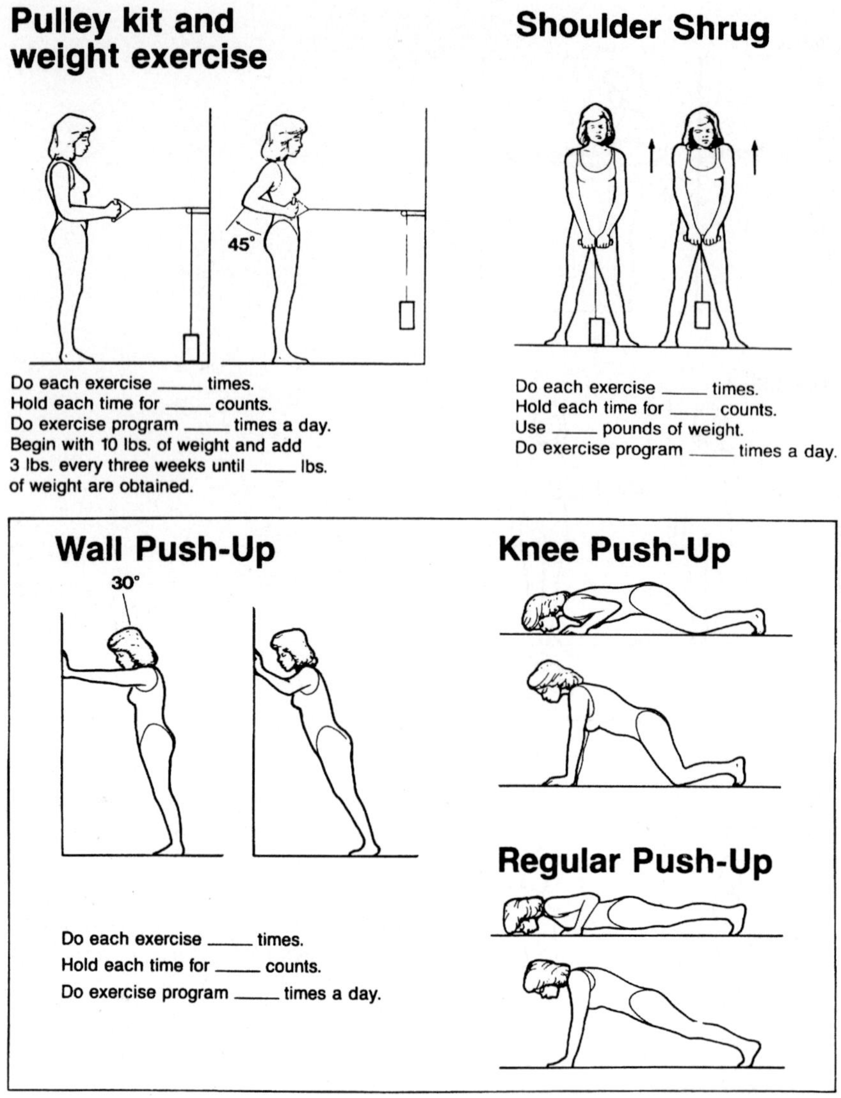
Pulley kit and weight exercise
45°
Do each exercise ____ times.
Hold each time for ____ counts.
Do exercise program ____ times a day.
Begin with 10 lbs. of weight and add
3 lbs. every three weeks until ____ lbs.
of weight are obtained.
Shoulder Shrug
Do each exercise ____ times.
Hold each time for ____ counts.
Use ____ pounds of weight.
Do exercise program ____ times a day.
Wall Push-Up
30°
Do each exercise ____ times.
Hold each time for ____ counts.
Do exercise program ____ times a day.
Knee Push-Up
Regular Push-Up

B

FIG. 1. *Continued.* **B:** Strengthening of the scapular stabilizers is begun at the same time as the shoulder shrugs, wall push-ups, and the five Theraband exercises. Wall push-ups are then advanced to knee push-ups, then to modified regular push-ups (see Figs. 6 and 9). When the 5th Theraband level has been completed, a rope and pulley system is utilized for all five exercises, beginning initially with 5 to 10 lb. (From Young DC, Rockwood CA Jr. Complications of failed Bristow procedures and their management. *J Bone Joint Surg [Am]* 1991;73A:972–973, with permission.)

tion in internal rotation (Fig. 2), external rotation (Fig. 3), horizontal abduction with the arm externally rotated (Fig. 4), and press-ups (Fig. 5). Scaption in internal rotation resulted in the highest amount of EMG activity in the anterior deltoid, middle deltoid, subscapularis, and supraspinatus (27). External rotation produced the highest activity in the teres minor, infraspinatus, and the posterior deltoid (27). Later in the rehabilitation protocol, when the patient is able to abduct the arm without danger of instability, horizontal abduction in the prone position with external rotation may be performed. This has been shown to produce the highest EMG activity for the posterior deltoid, infraspinatus, and teres minor (27). This exercise has also shown to have very high EMG activity for the middle trapezius, upper trapezius, lower trapezius, and levator scapulae (27). The press-up (Fig. 5) has been shown to have the highest amount of EMG activity for the pectoralis major, pectoralis minor, and the latissimus dorsi; however, this exercise may be difficult to perform initially in the rehabilitation program for the

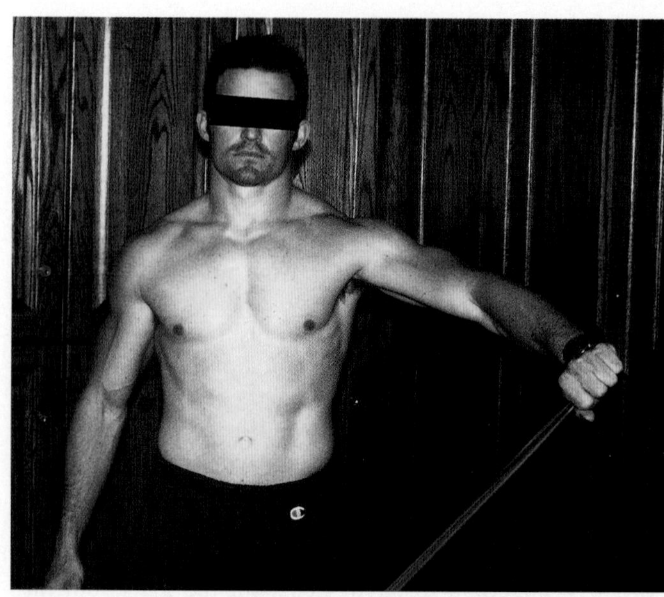

FIG. 2. Scaption in internal rotation.

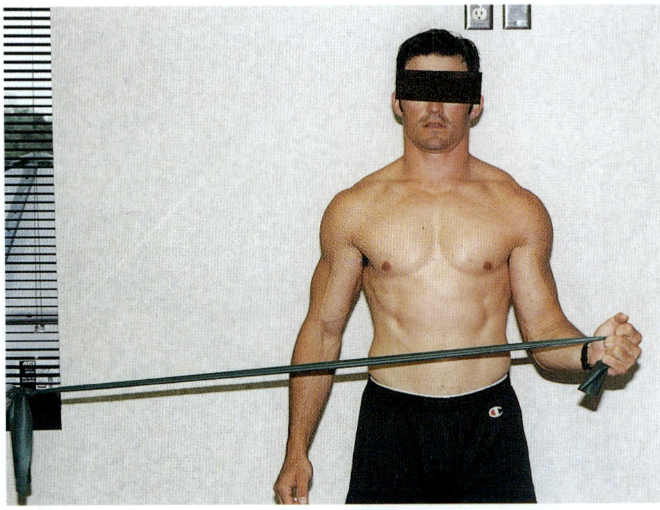

FIG. 3. External rotation.

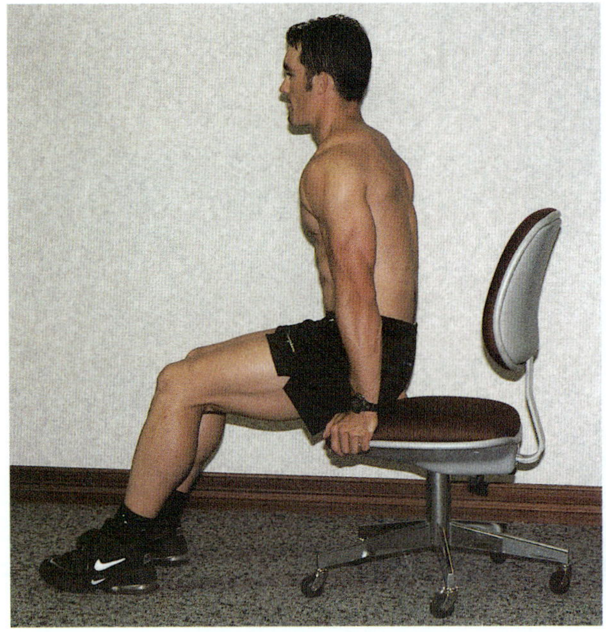

FIG. 5. The press-up.

acute dislocator. Push-ups against the wall followed by knee push-ups may be substituted initially for press-ups. The push-ups should be performed with the hands together to reduce the strain on the anterior capsule (Fig. 6). Interestingly, very limited subscapularis activity is produced with internal rotation of the shoulder with the arm in the adducted position, although this exercise has long been considered specific for maximally activating this muscle (9,27). High subscapularis activity is actually produced by internally rotating the arm in the 90-degree abducted position (9)(Fig. 7). Because of the degree of abduction required, this exercise should be instituted in the later stages of rehabilitation.

For rehabilitating the scapular stabilizers, EMG studies have demonstrated a core group of four exercises that effectively activate these muscles (10). These muscles include the upper, middle, and lower trapezius, the levator scapulae, the rhomboids, the pectoralis minor, and the middle and lower serratus anterior. All eight of these muscles demonstrate adequate EMG activity with a combination of scaption in external rotation (Fig. 8), rowing (Fig. 9A,B), press-ups, and push-ups with a plus (Fig. 10). We have included the first three of these exercises in our rehabilitation protocol. Scaption in external rotation has been shown to have the highest EMG activity for the lower serratus, as well as very high activity for the rhomboid and middle serratus (10). Rows exhibit high EMG

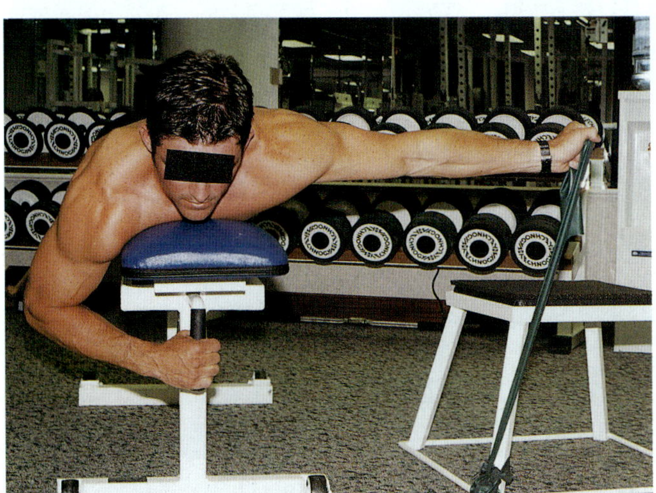

FIG. 4. Horizontal abduction with the arm externally rotated.

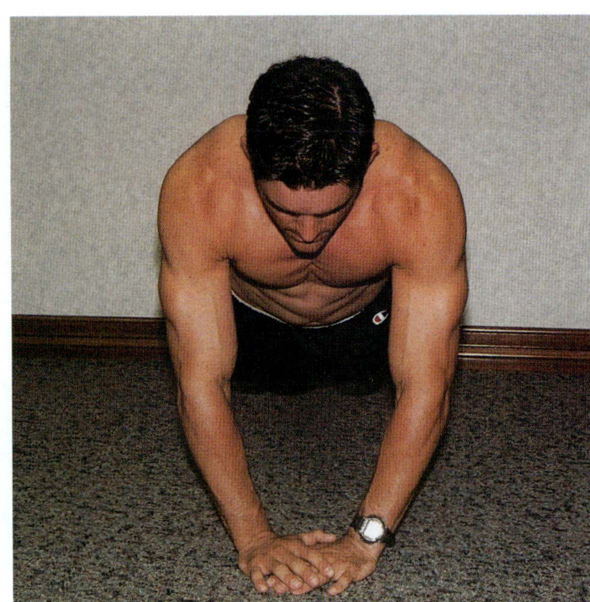

FIG. 6. Push-ups with hands together.

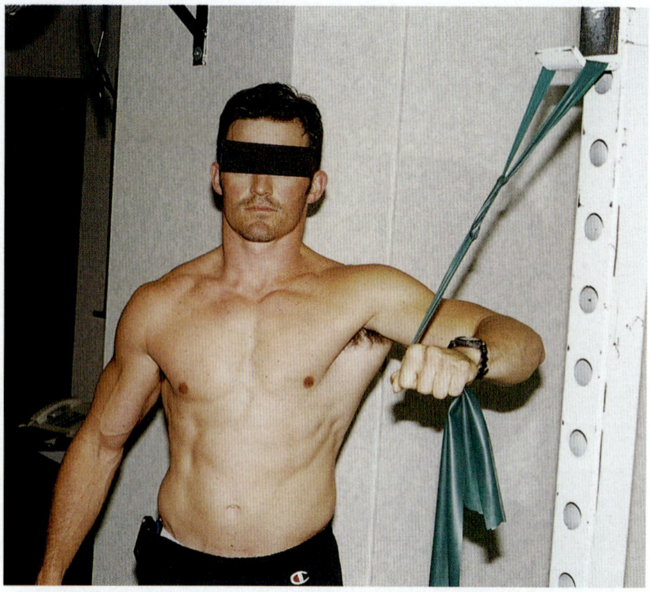

FIG. 7. Internal rotation with the arm in 90 degrees of abduction. This position is recommended in the later stages of rehabilitation for maximal subscapularis activity.

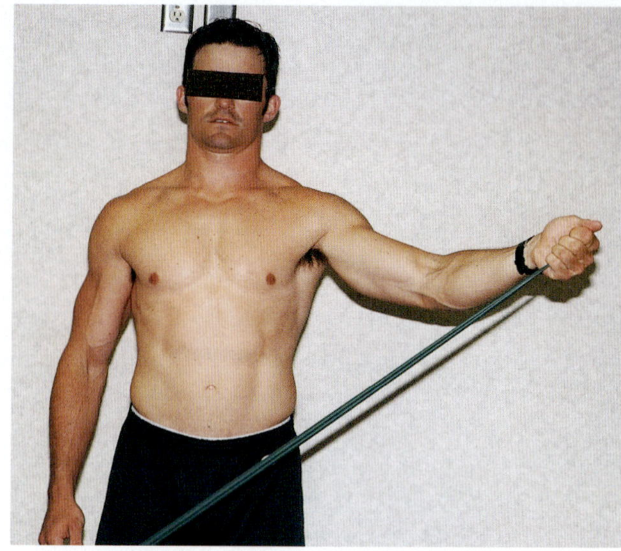

FIG. 8. Scaption in external rotation.

activity for the upper, middle, and lower trapezius, the rhomboids, and levator scapulae. Press-ups, as previously mentioned, demonstrate high activity in the pectoralis minor. Because of concerns that the push-up with a plus causes undue stress on the anterior capsule, we have excluded it from our rehabilitation protocol.

Isokinetic exercises (e.g., using Cybex or Biodex exercise machines), if available, may be added to the muscle-strengthening program. Initially, the isokinetic exercises should be performed with the elbow at the side. In the final stages of the rehabilitation program, these exercises may be performed with 90 degrees of shoulder flexion (Fig. 11).

The patient may return to full activity with no restrictions when there are no signs of apprehension and the upper extremity is approximately equal in strength to the opposite extremity. This generally does not occur before 3 months from the time of injury. Isokinetic strength testing is useful for assessing the strength of the extremity before return to full activities.

A

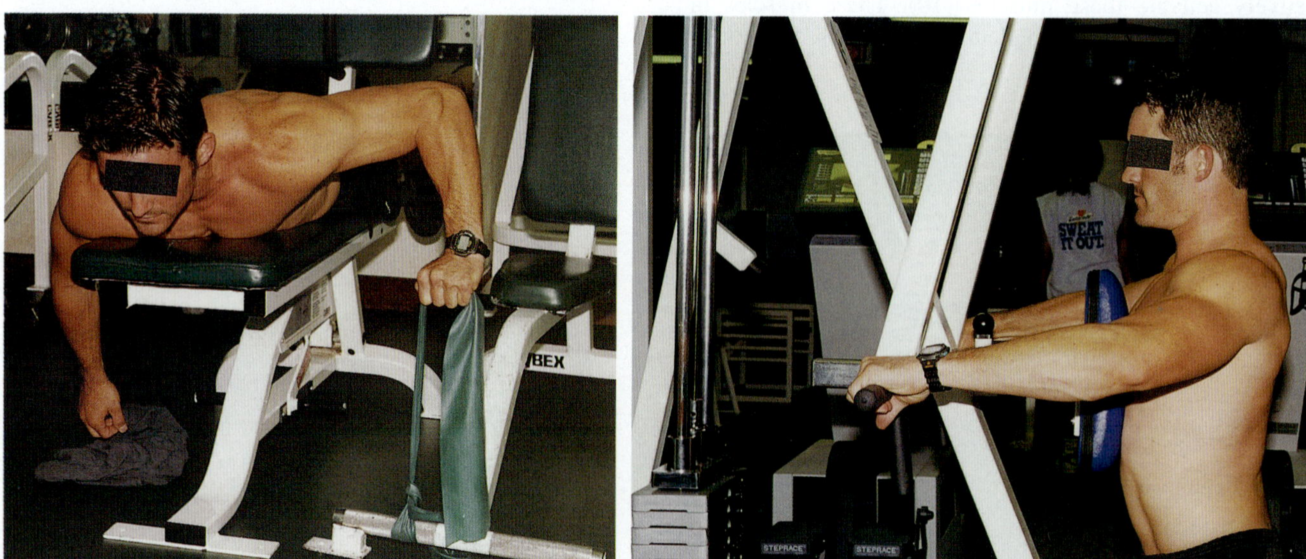

B

FIG. 9. **A:** Rowing using a Theraband. **B:** Rowing on a rowing machine.

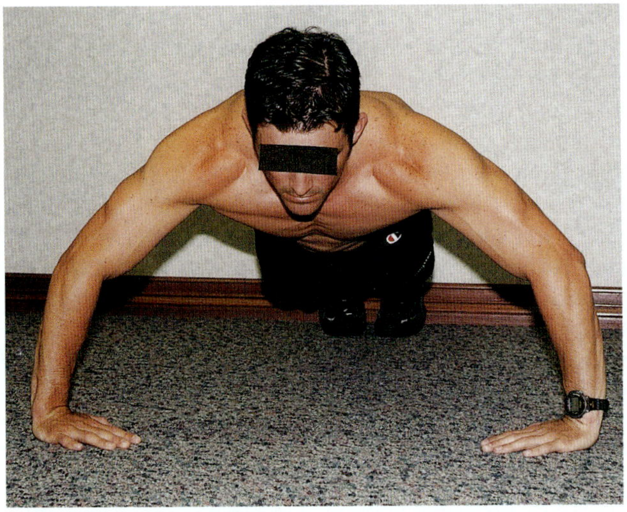

FIG. 10. Push-up with a plus.

Impact of Associated Injuries

As mentioned previously, fractures associated with acute dislocations have significant impact on prevalence of recurrent instability (13,23). Although no specific alterations in the rehabilitation protocol are recommended, this information is important to consider in counseling the patient on the probability of a nonoperative treatment program. A patient with a greater tuberosity fracture can be reassured of a low probability of redislocation. A patient with an associated Hill-Sachs defect, particularly in the young athlete, can be cautioned that nonoperative treatment will likely result in a high failure rate (3).

The frequency of an associated rotator cuff injury increases with age and may exceed 30% in patients older than 40 years of age (28). The diagnosis should be suspected in patients who are unable to abduct the arm after shoulder relocation (29). These patients are commonly misdiagnosed as having an axillary nerve injury, as an explanation for their continued weakness. We obtain an MRI with intra-articular contrast for those patients who exhibit continued abduction weakness at a 3-week follow-up. When a significant rotator cuff tear is confirmed by imaging studies, we recommend prompt surgical treatment. Hawkins and Koppert (30) noted that a low redislocation rate can be anticipated in these patients—only one redislocation occurred in 36 patients with this injury. Passive range-of-motion exercises, including pendulum, forward flexion with a pulley, and internal rotation, are permitted immediately after surgery. Passive external rotation is limited to neutral for 3 weeks. Depending on the strength of the rotator cuff and deltoid repairs, active range of motion is permitted at 4 to 6 weeks after surgery. Patients may begin Theraband exercises limited to internal and external rotation at 10 weeks. At 12 weeks, a full Theraband program may be instituted as described above. At the discretion of the surgeon, larger tears or tears with tenuous repairs, or both, may require a modified program.

Injuries to the axillary nerve are common after anterior shoulder dislocations and have been reported to occur in up to 25% of patients (31). Most of these are neuropraxic injuries, which typically recover spontaneously. Full recovery may take 3 to 5 months (32). We modify our rehabilitation protocol by the addition of an electrical muscle stimulating unit for rehabilitation of the deltoid. This is generally worn for 6 to 8 hours each day. These patients continue the regular rehabilitation protocol to the best of their abilities. If deltoid function fails to return by 3 months, surgical exploration of the nerve is recommended. Exploration is delayed if function is improving, but incomplete, at the 3-month mark.

Vascular injury after an anterior shoulder dislocation is relatively uncommon. Immediate surgical management is often necessary to restore circulation to the arm. The focus in these cases is on limb salvage, and we have no specific rehabilitation recommendations. When the vascular repair allows, a gradual rehabilitation program may be instituted.

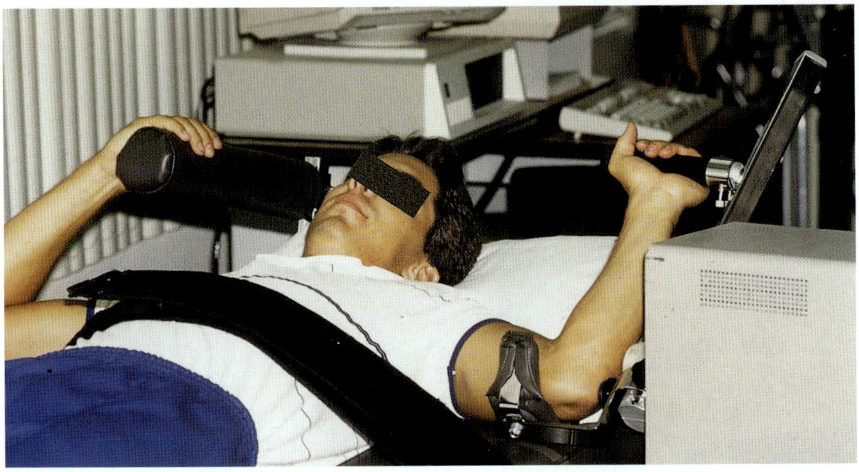

FIG. 11. Isokinetic exercises using a Biodex machine.

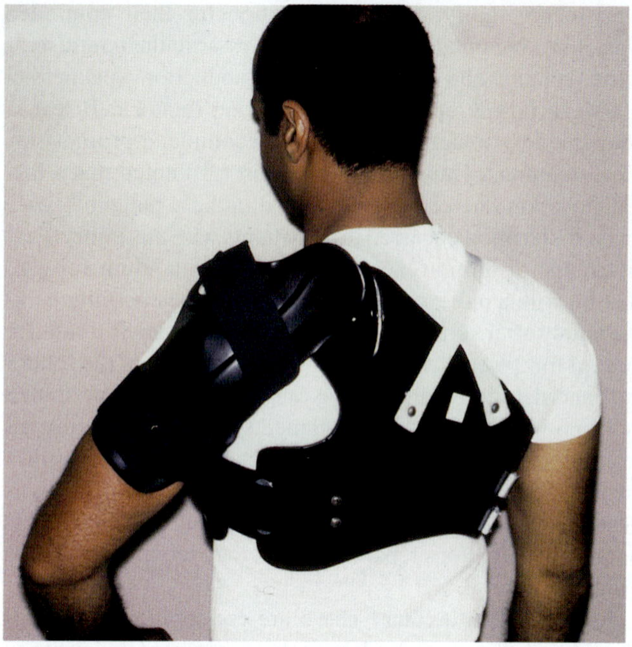

FIG. 12. SSI Shoulder Brace (Boston Brace International, Avon, MA, U.S.A.).

Bracing for Return to Sports

Shoulder braces are used to limit motion of the glenohumeral joint, specifically by limiting the "at-risk" position of abduction and external rotation. In selected patients, braces may be offered as a nonoperative alternative. This indication is typically for the athlete who wishes to complete the season after an anterior shoulder dislocation. Several commercially available braces are designed for this purpose. The SSI brace (Boston Brace International, Avon, MA, U.S.A.) (Fig. 12) limits motion and protects against direct blows. The Sawa Shoulder Orthosis (Brace International, Atlanta, GA, U.S.A.) (Fig. 13) also provides some anterior support and acts as a check rein. The Duke-Wire harness (not pictured) has a fairly cumbersome lace-up corset. In 1996, DeCarlo et al. (33) reported the results of a study that evaluated the ability of each of these braces to limit motion during isokinetic testing. Although test subjects considered the Sawa brace the most comfortable, the SSI brace was most effective in limiting motion likely to result in anterior instability.

In our practice, we have found that a simple and inexpensive shoulder strap can be made out of a football belt and is effective at limiting deleterious positions (Fig. 14). Of the commercially available braces, the Sawa Shoulder Orthosis is our preference for its ease of wear and effective check rein. Athletes involved in sports such as football, who sustain a shoulder dislocation during the season, may be offered a brace to wear during practice and games. The brace should be used in conjunction with ongoing shoulder rehabilitation. Brace wear is also recommended for contact athletes returning to sports after anterior shoulder reconstruction. Tackling athletes, in particular, are recommended to continue brace wear until they are 6 months postoperative and strength and confidence in the shoulder have been restored. A second group of patients who may be considered for bracing are recurrent dislocators who are nonoperative candidates for medical reasons. These patients generally must experience significant instability before a brace is recommended, as full-time brace wear is difficult.

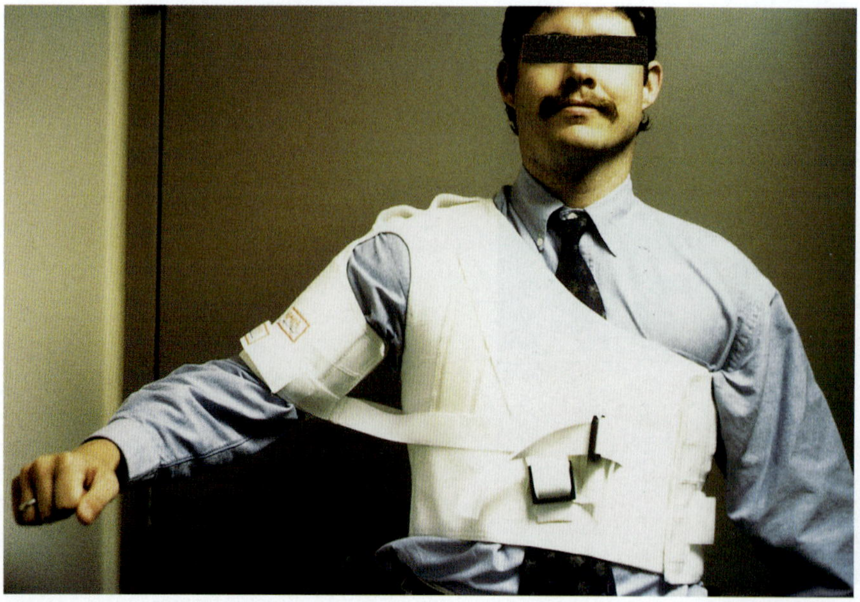

FIG. 13. Sawa Shoulder Brace (Brace International, Atlanta, GA, U.S.A.).

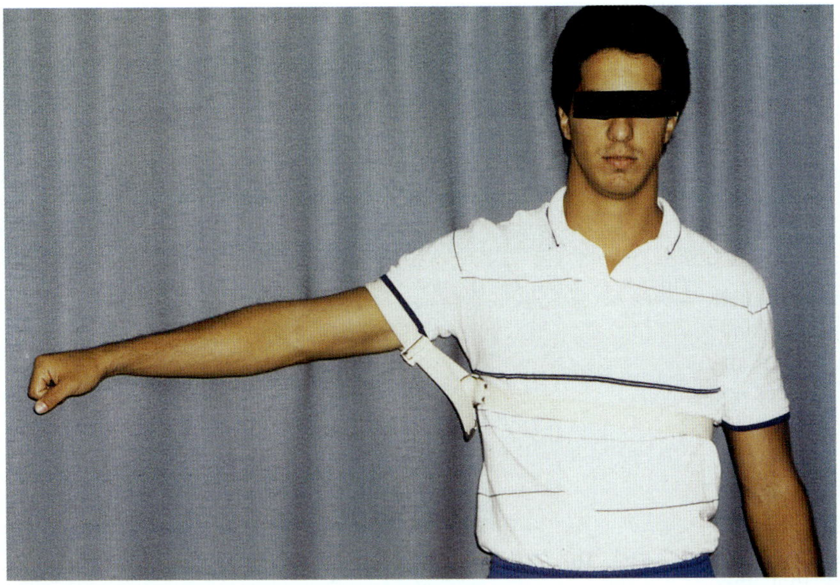

FIG. 14. Simple shoulder strap.

Rehabilitation for Atraumatic Recurrent Anterior Instability

The prognosis for successful rehabilitation in patients with recurrent atraumatic anterior subluxation, including those with multidirectional instability, appears to be much better as compared with that of patients with acute traumatic dislocations. A 1992 report by Burkhead and Rockwood (3) documented a 80% success rate in treatment of this group of patients when using a program of progressive resistance exercises. This represents a substantial improvement in comparison to the 16% success rate for those with traumatic subluxation.

In contrast to the patient with an acute traumatic dislocation, the patient with recurrent anterior instability may have developed chronic muscle imbalance. McMahon et al. (34) used EMG analysis to compare the rotator cuff and scapular muscles in normal shoulders *versus* shoulders of patients with anterior instability. The subscapularis, supraspinatus, infraspinatus, rhomboids, serratus anterior, and trapezius muscles were studied in three arcs of motion: scaption, flexion and abduction. Subjects with anterior shoulder instability consistently demonstrated relative deficiencies in the serratus anterior and the supraspinatus muscles. None of the other muscles tested demonstrated significant differences in activity between the two subject groups. This information suggests that additional emphasis should be spent on the rehabilitation of these muscles in a rehabilitation program designed for chronic anterior instability.

Careful manual muscle testing is performed on the initial evaluation of these patients. Particular attention is given to subtle winging of the scapula and asynchronous movements of the scapulothoracic and glenohumeral joints. Specific muscular imbalances are recorded and are addressed with a specific rehabilitation protocol.

Immobilization is avoided in these patients in order to avoid exacerbation of muscle weakness and imbalance. Physical examination often demonstrates significant tightness of the posterior capsule and deltoid, which can contribute to anterior subluxation (35). To address this problem, a stretching program emphasizing cross-body adduction and internal rotation is instituted early in the rehabilitation protocol.

A comprehensive Theraband program involving rehabilitation of the glenohumeral and scapulothoracic musculature (see also the section on acute dislocations) is instituted at the outset. Alterations in the basic rehabilitation protocol can be made if muscle imbalances are noted at the initial examination. This generally involves increased rehabilitative efforts directed toward the serratus anterior and supraspinatus by emphasizing scaption and push-ups with a plus (Fig. 12), which have been demonstrated to elicit high EMG activity in these muscles. Although scaption has traditionally been performed in an internally rotated (thumb-down) position (36), recent EMG analysis by Kelly et al. (9) suggests that optimal supraspinatus activity occurs with scaption in external rotation (palm up). In patients with a component of subacromial impingement, scaption in external rotation better avoids the position of impingement and is recommended in favor of scaption in internal rotation.

Rehabilitation of Throwing Athletes with Anterior Instability

The throwing athlete subjects the shoulder to repetitive high-energy forces. This may cause repetitive microtrauma that can lead to progressive damage to the anterior stabilizing structures of the shoulder (37). Kronberg et al. (38) demonstrated that coordinated muscle activity plays a significant role in stabilizing the shoulder. Initially, this coordinated muscular activity is able to compensate for the progressively attenuated anterior structures, allowing the shoulder to maintain stability. With continued throwing and continued damage, the muscular activity is unable to compensate and anterior translation of the humeral head in the glenoid occurs. With increased anterior translation, the humeral head can contact the coracoacromial arch or glenoid rim leading to an impingement syndrome and a painful throwing motion (37).

In the uninjured shoulder, the abducted externally rotated position of late cocking is accompanied by posterior translation of the humeral head in the glenoid fossa. When anterior instability develops, this posterior translation does not occur and anterior translation is observed. In EMG analyses of throwing shoulders in pitchers with anterior instability, Glousman et al. (37) demonstrated markedly diminished activity in the pectoralis major, subscapularis, serratus anterior, and the latissimus dorsi in the late cocking and acceleration phases. These investigators concluded that this imbalance contributes to, and propagates, the instability syndrome, whether this instability is a consequence of the primary pathology or a secondary effect.

The rehabilitation program for the throwing athlete begins with an initial period of rest. No throwing is allowed and inflammation is brought under control with an oral NSAID and physical therapy modalities. Most of these athletes demonstrate excessive external rotation on the dominant side with a reduction in internal rotation. This is usually accompanied by posterior capsular tightness, which can contribute to anterior subluxation (35,39) (Fig. 15). To manage this, a stretching program is instituted that includes cross-body adduction (Fig. 16) and abduction with internal rotation. Hancock and Hawkins have recommended a towel stretch with the athlete's hand behind her or his back to further address deficient internal rotation (7) (Fig. 17). A general rehabilitation program similar to that for anterior instability should be instituted along with the stretching exercises. Strengthening exercises for the entire upper extremity including the triceps, biceps, forearm, wrist, and hand are also instituted to improve overall fitness and endurance. The serratus anterior, pectoralis major, subscapularis, and latissimus dorsi are specifically emphasized, as they are important in the throwing motion. Scaption in external rotation and press-ups, or alternatively push-ups with a plus, are emphasized to strengthen these muscles. The forward

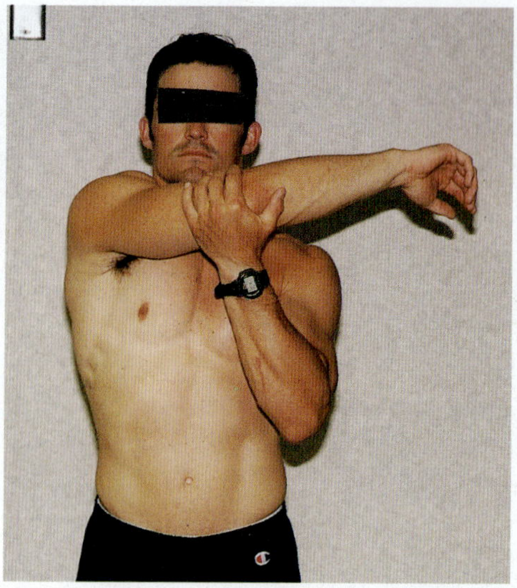

FIG. 16. Cross-body adduction to stretch the posterior capsule.

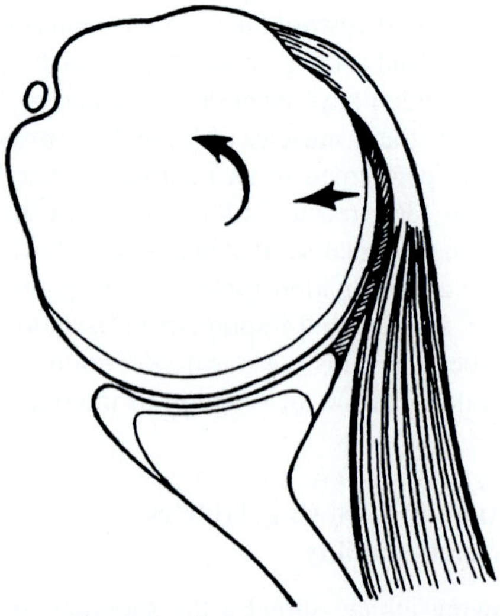

FIG. 15. Effect of asymmetric tightening of the capsule. Excessive posterior tightness contributes to translation of the humeral head in the opposite direction contributing to anterior subluxation. (From Harryman DT, Sidles JA, Clark JM, et al. Translation of the humeral head on the glenoid with passive motion. *J Bone Joint Surg [Am]* 1990;72A:1341, with permission.)

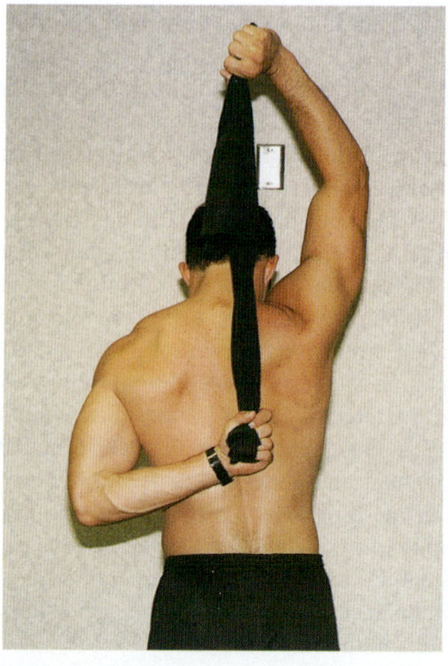

FIG. 17. Internal rotation stretching with a towel to address posterior capsular tightness.

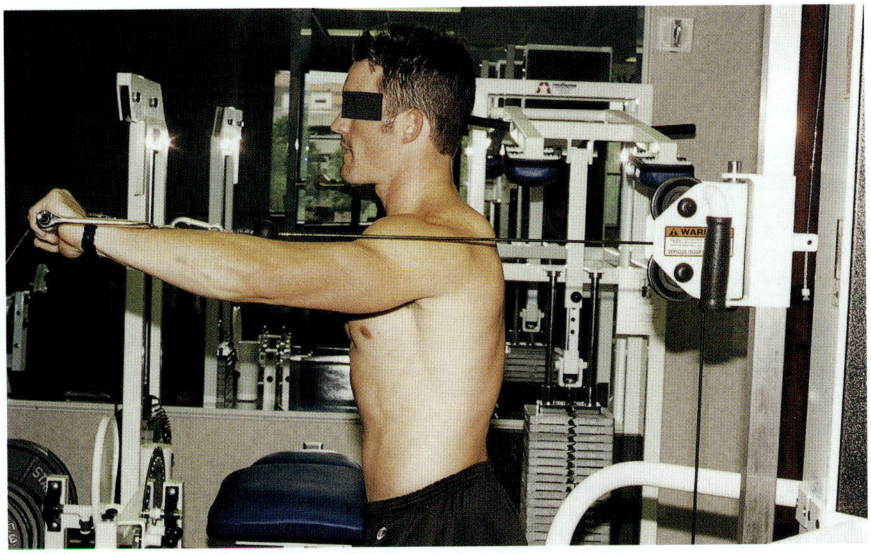

FIG. 18. Forward punch using a pulley to work the subscapularis further.

punch has been recommended by Hawkins et al. (7), which can also be added to work the subscapularis muscle further (Fig. 18). Eccentric contractions are emphasized in throwers to aid in strengthening for the deceleration phases of throwing. Isokinetic exercises can also be useful in improving the strength and endurance of the upper extremity. The athlete may return to throwing activities once there is full range of motion, no apprehension or impingement, and approximately equal strength to the contralateral extremity. Isokinetic testing is useful for determining when adequate strength has been achieved. The athlete is not immediately released to previous levels of throwing but, rather, is placed on a graduated throwing program. During the graduated program, the patient should continue strengthening exercises. When throwing activity is resumed, the strengthening program is performed later in the day, after the throwing program, to avoid reinjury secondary to fatigue.

FUTURE CONSIDERATIONS

Proprioception

A recent study conducted by Lephart et al. (40) demonstrated proprioceptive deficits in shoulders with anterior instability, as compared with stable shoulders. These investigators evaluated three groups of patients: a healthy group of normal volunteers, a group of patients with recurrent anterior instability at the completion of a rehabilitation program, and a group of patients who had a surgical reconstruction of the shoulder for anterior instability and had completed 6 months of postoperative rehabilitation. They were able to demonstrate significant proprioceptive deficits in the unstable shoulders, as compared with the healthy volunteers. No significant differences were demonstrated between the postsurgical group and the healthy volunteers. They concluded that reconstructive surgery appears to restore normal proprioceptive sensibility to the shoulder. In another study designed to evaluate proprioception, Wallace et al. (41) studied 12 subjects with anterior shoulder instability. The contralateral shoulder served as an internal control (41). A pneumatic cylinder was used to produce a sudden external rotation movement of the glenohumeral joint. The latency between the onset of movement and the detection of muscle contraction was used as an index of proprioception. These workers found no significant difference in muscular reflex activity between the stable and unstable shoulders and concluded that these results do not support the use of proprioception-enhancing physical therapy in the treatment of post-traumatic anterior shoulder instability.

Neural end organs in the form of Pacinian corpuscles and two types of Ruffini end organs are present in the ligamentous structures and connective tissues of the shoulder joint capsule (42). Disruption of these elements may interrupt the normal proprioceptive sensibility of the glenohumeral joint. Undoubtedly, normal proprioception is essential in providing the appropriate feedback to balance complex muscle-firing sequences as the joint position rapidly changes. Although it is clear that operative stabilization can improve proprioception, it has not been established whether a nonoperative rehabilitation protocol can have a significant impact on this parameter and thereby reduce the incidence of recurrent dislocation. For this reason, we do not currently include a specific proprioceptive program in our rehabilitation protocols.

Although the value of proprioceptive training remains to be verified in shoulder rehabilitation, several investigators have elected to include proprioceptive training in their rehabilitation protocol on an investigational basis (43). They recommend the following progression of activities to maximally restore proprioception and neuromuscular control: (a) joint position sense and kinesthesia, (b) dynamic joint stabilization, (c) reactive neuromuscular control, and (d) functionally specific activity. If these investigations and others are able to demonstrate improved stability with a proprioceptive program, this may prove to be an advance in our ability to understand and treat shoulder instability.

REFERENCES

1. Davis AG. The conservative treatment for habitual dislocations of the shoulder. *JAMA* 1936;107:1012–1015.
2. Rowe C. Prognosis in dislocations of the shoulder. *J Bone Joint Surg [Am]* 1956;38A:957–976.
3. Burkhead WZ, Rockwood CA. Treatment of instability of the shoulder with an exercise program. *J Bone Joint Surg [Am]* 1992;74A: 890–896.
4. Blazina ME, Satyman JS. Recurrent anterior subluxation of the shoulder in athletes—a distinct entity. Proceedings of the American Academy of Orthopaedic Surgeons. *J Bone Joint Surg [Am]* 1969;51A: 1037–1038.
5. Paine RM, Voight M. The role of the scapula. *J Orthop Sports Phys Ther* 1993;10:386–391.
6. Dines DM, Levinson M. The conservative management of the unstable shoulder including rehabilitation. *Clin Sports Med* 1995;14:797–816.
7. Hancock RF, Hawkins RJ. Applications of electromyography in the throwing shoulder. *Clin Orthop* 1996;1330:84–97.
8. McMahon PJ, Jobe FW, Pink MM, Brault JR, Perry J. Comparative electromyographic analysis of shoulder muscles during planar motions: anterior glenohumeral instability versus normal. *J Shoulder Elbow Surg* 1996;5(pt I):118–123.
9. Kelly BT, Kirkendall DT, Levy AS, Speer KP. Current research on muscle activity about the shoulder. *Instruct Course Lect* 1997;46:53–66.
10. Mosely JB, Jobe FW, Pink M, Perry J, Tibone J. EMG analysis of the scapular muscles during a shoulder rehabilitation program. *Am J Sports Med* 1991;19:264–272.
11. McLaughlin HL, Cavallaro WV. Primary anterior dislocation of the shoulder. *Am J Surg* 1950;80:615.
12. Henry J, Genung J. Natural history of glenohumeral dislocation—revisited. *Am J Sports Med* 1982;10:135–137.
13. Hovelius L, Augustine BG, Freoin H, Johasson O, Nurlen R, Thorling J. Primary anterior dislocation of the shoulder in young patients. *J Bone Joint Surg [Am]* 1996;78A:1677–1684.
14. Simonet W, Cofield R. Prognosis in anterior shoulder dislocation. *Am J Sports Med* 1984;12:19–24.
15. Yoneda B, Welsh RP, McIntosh DL. Conservative treatment of shoulder dislocation in young males. *J Bone Joint Surg [Br]* 1982;64B: 254–255.
16. Aronen J, Regan K. Decreasing the incidence of recurrence of first time anterior shoulder dislocations with rehabilitation. *Am J Sports Med* 1984;12:283–291.
17. Bigliani LU, Pollock RG, Suslowsky LJ, et al. Tensile properties of the inferior glenohumeral ligament. *J Orthop Res* 1992;10:187–197.
18. Speer KP, Deng X, Borrero S, et al. Biomechanical evaluation of a simulated Bankart lesion. *J Bone Joint Surg [Am]* 1994;76A:1819–1826.
19. Fu FH, Hundu CD, Johnson DL, Meuer MD, Woo SY. Biomechanics of knee ligaments: basic concepts and clinical applications. *J Bone Joint Surg [Am]* 1993;75A:1716–1727.
20. Mason ML, Allen HS. The role of healing of tendons. *Ann Surg* 1941;113:424–459.
21. Clayton ML, Weir GS. Experimental investigations of ligamentous healing. *Am J Surg* 1959;93:373–378.
22. Garth WP, Slappey CE, Ochs CW. Roentgenographic demonstration of instability of the shoulder: the apical oblique projection—a technical note. *J Bone Joint Surg [Am]* 1984;66A:1450–1453.
23. Rowe CR. Acute and recurrent anterior dislocations of the shoulder. *Orthop Clin North Am* 1980;2:253–270.
24. Sand H, Kato Y, Haga K, Irvin E, Tabata S. Magnetic resonance arthrography comparison with double-contrast computed tomography arthrography. *J Shoulder Elbow Surg* 1996;5:280–285.
25. Gusmer PB, Potter HG. Imaging of shoulder instability. *Clin Sports Med* 1995;1:777–795.
26. Young DC, Rockwood CA Jr. Complications of a failed Bristow procedure and their management. *J Bone Joint Surg [Am]* 1991;73A: 972–973.
27. Townsend H, Jobe F, Pink M, Perry J. Electromyographic analysis of the glenohumeral muscles during a baseball rehabilitation program. *Am J Sports Med* 1991;19:264–272.
28. Matsen FA, Thomas SC, Rockwood CA Jr. Anterior glenohumeral instability. In: Rockwood CA Jr, Matsen FA III, eds. *The shoulder*. Philadelphia: WB Saunders, 1990;961–990.
29. Neviaser RJ, Neviaser TJ, Neviaser JS. Concurrent ruptures of the rotator cuff and anterior dislocation of the shoulder joint in the older patient. *J Bone Joint Surg [Am]* 1988;70A:1308–1311.
30. Hawkins RJ, Koppert C. The natural history following anterior dislocation of the shoulder in the older patient. *J Bone Joint Surg [Br]* 1982;64B:225.
31. Brom JT. Nerve injuries complicating dislocation of the shoulder. *J Bone Joint Surg [Br]* 1952;34B:526.
32. Brom S, Dahlback LO. Nerve injuries in dislocations of the shoulder joint and fractures of the neck of the humerus. *Acta Chir Scand* 1970;136:461–466.
33. DeCarlo M, Malone K, Geric B, Hunker M. Evaluation of shoulder instability braces. *J Sports Rehabil* 1996;5:143–150.
34. McMahon PJ, Jobe FW, Pink MM, et al. Computive electromyographic analysis of shoulder muscles during planar motions: anterior glenohumeral instability versus normal. *J Shoulder Elbow Surg* 1996; 15:118–123.
35. Harryman DT, Sidles JA, Clark JM, et al. Translation of the humeral head in the glenoid with passive glenohumeral motion. *J Bone Joint Surg* 1990;72A:1334–1343.
36. Jobe FW, Monynes DR. Delineation of diagnostic criteria and a rehabilitation program for rotator cuff injuries. *Am J Sports Med* 1982; 10:336–339
37. Glousman RE, Jobe FW, Tibone JE, et al. Dynamic electromyographic analysis of the throwing shoulder with glenohumeral instability. *J Bone Joint Surg [Am]* 1988;70A:220–226.
38. Kronberg M, Nemeth G, Brusham LA. Muscle activity and coordination in the normal shoulder: an electromyographic study. *Clin Orthop* 1990;257:76–85.
39. Howell SM, Galinat BJ, Renzi AJ, Marone PJ. Normal and abnormal mechanics of the glenohumeral joint in the horizontal plane. *J Bone Joint Surg [Am]* 1988;70A:227–232.
40. Lephart SM, Warner JP, Borsa PA, Fu FH. Proprioception of the shoulder joint in healthy, unstable and surgically repaired shoulders. *J Shoulder Elbow Surg* 1994;3:371–380.
41. Wallace DA, Beard DJ, Gill RHS, Eng B, Carr AJ. Reflex muscle contraction in anterior shoulder instability. *J Shoulder Elbow Surg* 1997;6:150–155.
42. Vangsness CT, Ennes M, Taylor JG, Atkinson R. Neural anatomy of the glenohumeral ligaments, labrum and subacromial bursa. *Arthroscopy J Arthrosc Rel Surg* 1995;2:180–184.
43. Lephart SM, Pincovero DM, Giraldo JL, Fu FH. The role of proprioception in the management and rehabilitation of athletic injuries. *Am J Sports Med* 1996;25:130–137.

The Unstable Shoulder,
edited by R.F. Warren, E.V. Craig, and D.W. Altchek.
Lippincott–Raven Publishers, Philadelphia © 1999.

CHAPTER 12

Decision Making in Recurrent Shoulder Instability

Edward V. Craig, Russell F. Warren, and Edgar K. Ragsdale

The story is told of a taxicab ride in which two masters of shoulder surgery, Charles Neer and Richard Hawkins, were discussing various aspects of the problem shoulder. Somewhere into their cab ride, Neer turned to his partner, his face reflecting puzzlement, and inquired ''Don't you think that instability is confusing?'' Now here is a man who had made the study of the shoulder his passion for 40 years—whose lasting contributions had spanned all aspects of shoulder reconstruction, anterior acromioplasty and cuff disease, classification and treatment of fractures, multidirectional and unidirectional instability, and shoulder arthroplasty—giving voice to something that has an impact on most surgeons' practice, that is, that the evaluation and treatment of the unstable shoulder involves decision making that is multifaceted and complex. This decision-making process, by its very nature, has the following characteristics.

1. *Challenging.* As continued laboratory and clinical research has increased our understanding of the normal stabilizing mechanisms of the shoulder, long-term outcomes of standard instability treatments have become available, and our concepts of shoulder instability have changed as well. From the ''essential lesion'' of a Bankart avulsion and Hill-Sachs to such anatomic structures as capsular laxity, rotator interval defects, and cuff insufficiency, traditional approaches to the shoulder have been challenged. Patient expectations and demands have evolved, so few patients are willing to sacrifice motion and function for a stable shoulder. Technologic advances have demanded that surgeons become familiar with new technology and their applications, with the attendant struggle to fit emerging technology into the day-to-day management of patients.

The demographics of patients with instability add to the challenge; the very young child with voluntary instability or congenital hypoplasia of the glenoid, the elite athlete with more subtle instability, even the elderly patient with a locked anterior dislocation following trauma—each require different thought processes for successful management.

Adding to this challenge is the fact that even the diagnosis of instability can be problematic. Two patients may have equally ''lax'' shoulders, yet one will have symptomatic instability while the other is unaffected. Frequently, left and right shoulders in the same patient may have the same degree of laxity, yet only one is painful. An elite athlete may not have instability as the primary complaint, but may complain of ''pain,'' ''failure to get loose,'' ''dead arm,'' and ''catching.'' A ''loose'' shoulder may not necessarily be an ''unstable'' one.

Finally, the challenge is magnified by the fact that the final common pathway, a shoulder that ''comes out of joint and shifts,'' can be produced by such variable pathology as ligament tearing, capsular laxity, fractures of the glenoid or greater tuberosity, congenital hypoplasia, rotator cuff tearing, and systemic or distant problems such as Ehler-Danlos, birth palsy, or neuropathic shoulder. Truly, the more we know regarding the stabilizing and destabilizing factors around the shoulder, the more precise and better treatment we can give to the patient.

2. *Comprehensive.* All aspects of the patient evaluation produce relevant information that has an impact on the ability to treat the patient successfully. Decision making can

E. V. Craig: Department of Orthopaedics, Cornell University Medical College, New York, New York, 10021; and Department of Orthopaedics, New York Hospital, New York, New York 10021; and The Hospital for Special Surgery, New York, New York 10021.

R. F. Warren: Department of Orthopaedics, Cornell University Medical College, New York, New York 10021; and Department of Orthopaedics, The Hospital for Special Surgery, New York, New York 10021.

E. Ragsdale: Department of Orthopaedic Surgery, Southwest Washington Medical Center, Vancouver, Washington 98688; and Northwest Surgical Specialists, Vancouver, Washington 98664-6440.

be influenced by, and dependent on, accurate information from patient history, clinical examination, appropriate radiographic and imaging data, examination under anesthesia, arthroscopic findings, and intraoperative evaluation of pertinent anatomy.

3. *Personal.* From the standpoint of both the physician—patient relationship and one's personal assessment of one's own skill, the management of instability frequently depends on factors other than simply the pathomechanics and pathoanatomy. Knowing the patient is a tremendous help. What are the patient's needs, wants, and expectations? In a litigious society, are these wants and expectations practical, and can we live up to them?

Hand dominance, age, activity level, profession, recreational pursuits, and economic impact of lost time from work all significantly influence the way we manage the unstable shoulder.

Personal factors must be answered by each surgeon. "Can you deliver what the patient wants?" What can be reasonably certain about treatment and what is unpredictable? Do your skills in arthroscopic or open surgery make successful outcome predictable? If your track record in open repairs has been well established, should you be doing an arthroscopic repair? If your practice is arthroscopically focused, are you comfortable with the variability of anatomy with open reconstruction? What is an acceptable "learning curve" for new technology? These are the elements we all wrestle with in orthopaedics, but perhaps we wrestle harder and more frequently with these elements as they relate to the unstable shoulder.

4. *Ongoing.* The decision making does not end with the early management of the unstable shoulder, either nonoperatively or operatively. Length of immobilization, rapidity of return to school, work, recreational pursuits, noncontact, and contact sports all require an element of sophisticated decision making. What about treatment failure? A patient who has undergone a successful reconstruction suffers new trauma, and another instability episode. Should this be considered a surgical failure, treated as an initial dislocation, be treated with immobilization, or have early repeat surgery?

5. *Evolving.* Surgical treatment has taken major steps away from most procedures that had been practiced for years, and that were intentionally designed to restrict external rotation of the humerus, thereby preventing a Hill-Sachs lesion from engaging in the Bankart avulsion of the labrum.

Much like the evolution in knee reconstruction, we and our patients "want it all." We want to control the instability episode without sacrificing motion, strength, function or activity level. We have learned much from shoulder arthroscopy, including associated pathology, what seems to work and under what conditions it does work. As with replantation surgery of the hand, in the early stages of evaluation everything was replanted before the indications for applying this new technology became more clear, the ideal indications for arthroscopic treatment have continued to evolve as well. And now, the basic science dealing with thermal effects on collagen have brought us the capability of shrinking soft-tissue capsule of the shoulder, in theory giving us the opportunity to fine-tune our arthroscopic intra-articular repair. But what of the unintended effects or side effects and the long-term effects on joint mechanics? As knowledge is gained, decision making will evolve as well in these areas.

6. *Impact on Success.* The complexity of treating the unstable shoulder is magnified by the fact that critical decisions and understanding of the shoulder impact so directly on the success of treatment. The decision that a patient has unidirectional instability with a surgical approach geared to the anterior shoulder can prove disastrous if the problem is global or multidirectional instability. An extensive decompression for cuff impingement in a thrower with "subtle instability" can lead to treatment failure and an end to the elite athlete's career. A decision to bring a competitive football player back too early can convert a potential successful outcome to a unsuccessful one.

It seems that each step of the way, there are elements of decision making that impact on a successful outcome in treating this potentially complex problem. The following is intended to offer some guidelines related to decision making, which may shed some light on instability and how this instability can be approached and managed under a variety of circumstances.

IMPORTANT QUESTIONS THAT GUIDE DECISION MAKING

Decisions regarding the management of the unstable shoulder can be more effectively and easily made if the answers to a number of questions can be dealt with successfully:

1. *Is the problem shoulder instability or something else* (Fig. 1)? If the patient presents with the history that the shoulder dislocated with trauma, and presents with a radiograph showing the shoulder dislocated, the elements of decision making may include things that, while challenging therapeutically, may be fairly straightforward diagnostically. However, the presenting symptoms may be more subtle, and there are elements in the presentation of some unstable shoulders that are identical to cuff disease, impingement syndrome, symptomatic superior labral anterior and posterior (SLAP) lesions, or catching from a loose or sublaxing biceps tendon body. A patient may say that the shoulder "goes out," while what he means is he is having pain. A patient can give a history of shoulder dislocation in the distant past, when what really occurred was a previous acromioclavicular separation. A shoulder that is "loose" may have pain caused from a symptomatic AC joint, a suprascapular nerve lesion, or associated tendinitis. The first thing to determine is whether the presenting problem is one of pain secondary to instability or not.

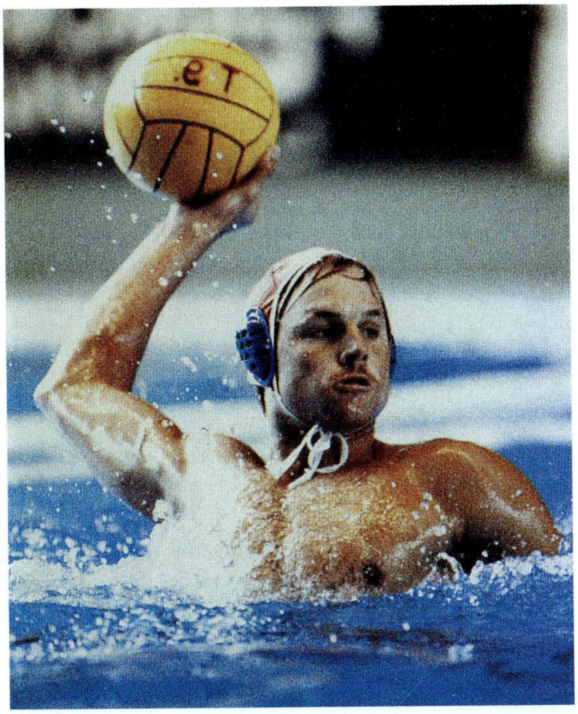

FIG. 1. Pain or an injury with the arm above shoulder level is frequently indicative of anterior instability.

2. *What is the direction of the instability* (Fig. 2)? Is the shoulder loose in one direction or in all directions? Is inferior laxity the main problem or only a component of the problem? The treatment for isolated posterior, isolated anterior, or isolated inferior instability is very different from that of multidirectional shoulder instability. A shoulder with anterosuperior instability after cuff repair has issues relative to the bone and soft-tissue constraints of the superior shoulder that may not even be solvable.

3. *What degree of trauma produced the instability* (Fig. 3A-C)? Was the instability essentially atraumatic, as might occur with congenital dysplasia or minimal trauma, such as when a young mother picks up a baby, or traumatic, as in the classic abduction external rotation injury of a high school quarterback suffering an anterior dislocation? Was it something such as a repetitive microtrauma that might be associated with "acquired laxity" over time, such as a swimmer, baseball pitcher, or tennis player.

The answer to the issue of degree of trauma is important, because it is usually directly related to the next question, which needs to be addressed.

4. *What is the pathology responsible* (Fig. 4)? What restraining structures have been altered to allow the dislocation? Have the static stabilizers, i.e., the capsule, the glenohumeral ligaments, the glenoid labrum, been altered? Is the instability more dynamic, as may occur with scapular winging and posterior subluxation? Is the rotator cuff, the main dynamic stabilizer of the shoulder, incompetent or torn? Has the lateral capsule been avulsed? Has the rotator interval been torn or enlarged? Is there a bony problem associated with instability such as a glenoid rim fracture, large Hill-Sachs defect, or greater tuberosity fracture? Or are there combinations of things involved?

Knowing the precise pathology involved in the destabilization of the shoulder gives us a better chance to gear our treatment in a more focused fashion. By repair of only that pathology responsible for the instability, we are less likely to have unintended consequences in the areas of the shoulder that remain normal, and thus get closer to solving the problem while not sacrificing motion, strength, or function.

5. *Who is the patient* (Fig. 5)? Age and gender have an impact on recurrence. Hovelius has shown in a large prospective study that below age 22, there is a 55–60% chance of recurrence, while in patients over 40 the recurrence rate drops to 10–12%. What is the lifestyle of the person? A sedentary person may be more inclined to favor activity modification or bracing. Will what the patient does or enjoys (lifestyle, work, or sports) pose a danger to him/her if recurrent dislocation should occur? A steelworker working

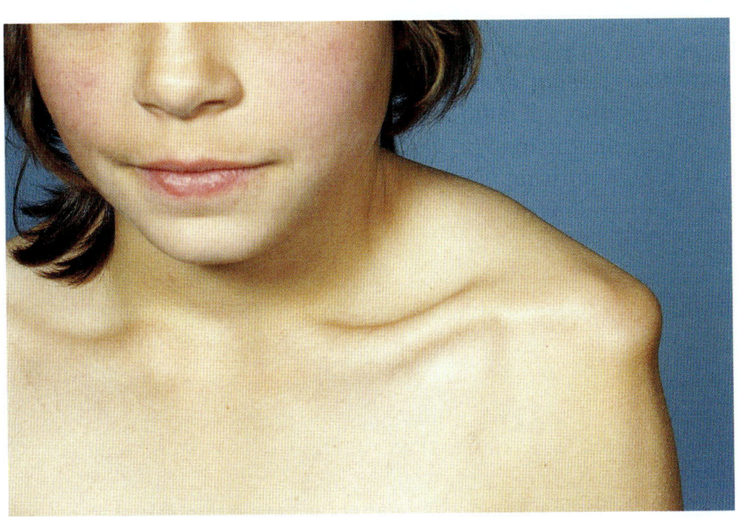

FIG. 2. Voluntary instability can be identified by history. Surgery on these patients is frequently not helpful.

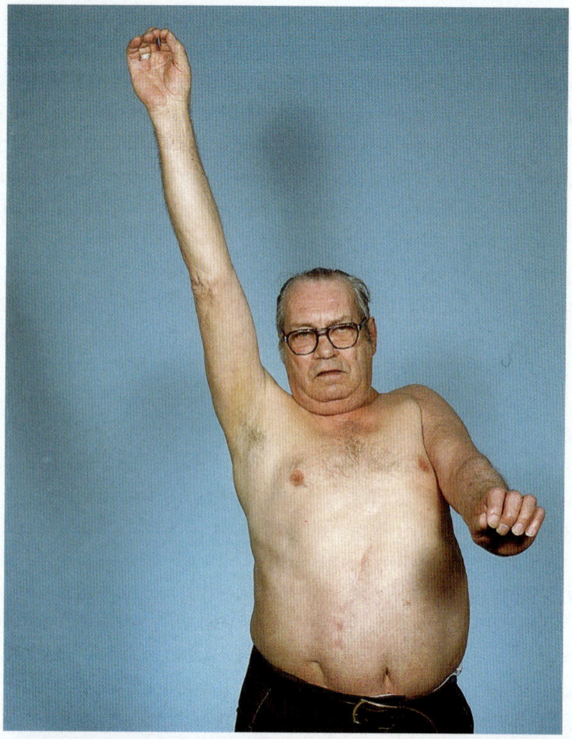

A

FIG. 3. **A:** A 67-year-old man with inability to raise arm after an acute dislocation. **B:** Radiograph showing his anterior dislocation. **C:** Radiograph following reduction. Note the cystic changes in the greater tuberosity. His weakness was caused by a massive rotator cuff tear.

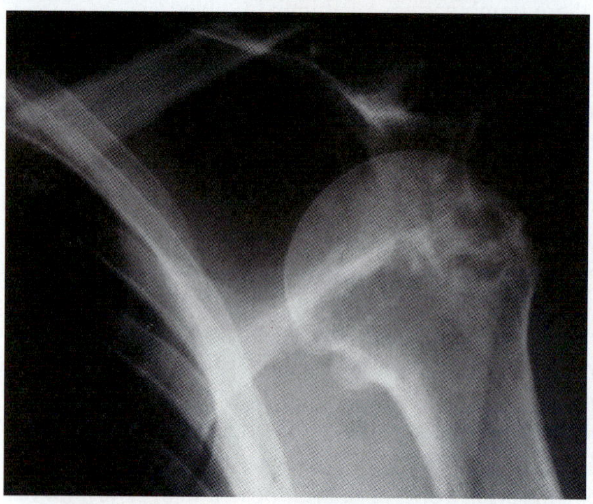

B

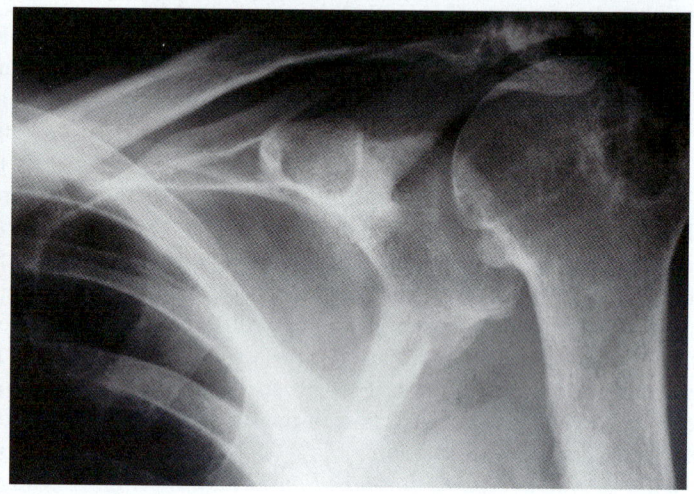

C

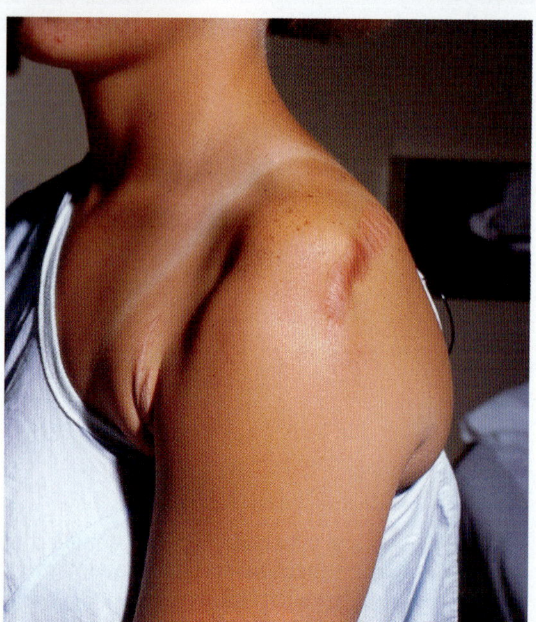

FIG. 4. A "sulcus" sign in a woman with multidirectional instability with failed anterior and posterior surgery.

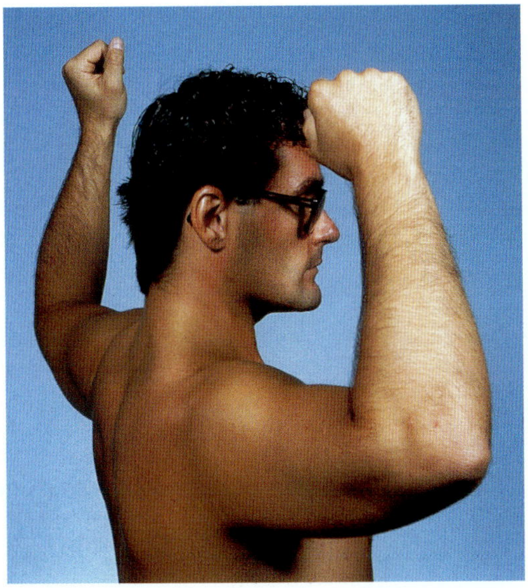

FIG. 5. A patient who is "apprehensive" about dislocation will guard against extension with the arm externally rotated.

at significant heights or a white-water kayaker in dangerous terrain may be in life-threatening situations if the recurrence occurs. Does the patient exist in an environment where emergency treatment is available if need be? Are there psychological or emotional factors that would adversely impact on treatment?

The same fundamental problem, with the same pathology, leading to the same direction of instability, with the same degree of trauma, may well be approached differently simply because individuals are different. Thus the importance of careful and complete history cannot be over emphasized.

6. *Is there "hidden pathology"* (Fig. 6)? Could this impact on treatment directly? For example, there is a high incidence of rotator cuff tear in a patient above age 40 who suffers a primary traumatic anterior dislocation. This may involve the subscapularis, or any and all of the external rotators. This has been called the "posterior mechanism" for acute anterior dislocations. In younger patients, a healthy cuff is not a weak link in the stabilizing system. Traumatic instability will usually tear the anterior glenohumeral ligaments or labrum, permitting the shoulder to dislocate. In the older patient, the rotator cuff, weakened by aging, degeneration, or impingement may be the weak link. Trauma to the shoulder can cause destruction of this weak link, permitting the shoulder to dislocate anteriorly, effectively having the humeral head hinge on intact glenohumeral joint ligaments and labrum. Different pathology and different mechanisms mean different approaches to the treatment. But postreduction weakness can be ascribed to pain, nerve injury, disuse, and the cuff injury essentially can be hidden, as the patient is put through rehabilitation of the "postdislocated shoulder." In addition, the surgical repair is aimed primarily at the anterior capsule, while the main pathology is a massive posterior cuff avulsion, the problem of anterior dislocation can be magnified. Thus, in an older patient who has an initial traumatic dislocation, if weakness persists after reduction of the shoulder, or if there is external rotation weakness on physical examination, a magnetic resonance imaging scan (MRI) or arthrogram should be part of the evaluation and work-up early after the closed reduction, since a considerable number of these patients will have an associated rotator cuff tear as the primary pathologic mechanism responsible for their dislocation.

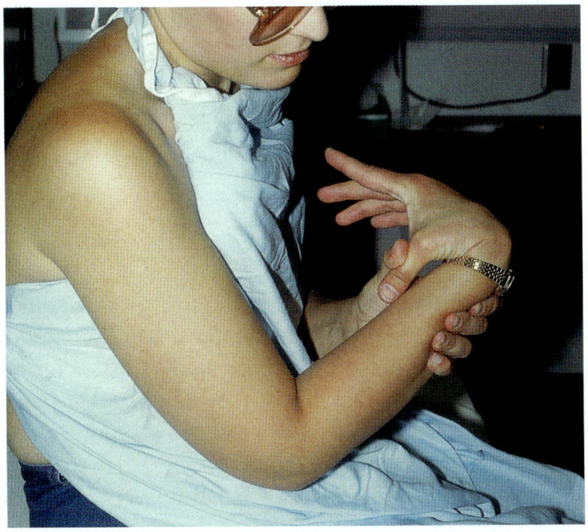

FIG. 6. General laxity may indicate multidirectional instability.

Likewise, anterior dislocations of the shoulder can be complicated by nerve injury, and the most frequent nerve involved is the axillary nerve. In the presence of an acute dislocation, the pain of the patient and the splinting of the arm may make a sensory examination of the shoulder unreliable. It is probably prudent to detect presence of axillary nerve injury before manipulating the shoulder for a closed reduction, and certainly if surgical repair is going to be undertaken.

Alternatively, weakness after relocation of a dislocating shoulder may be ascribed to cuff tear, splinting, or pain, while actually the deltoid is not functioning because of nerve injury. Therefore, palpation of the deltoid muscle for contraction, even if done isometrically, is an easy way to determine a functioning axillary nerve even in the presence of an acute dislocation of the shoulder.

7. *What is the impact of nonoperative treatment* (Fig. 7)? How successful will nonoperative treatment be in controlling symptoms? For example, frequently a rehabilitation program aimed at dynamic stabilizers can keep patients with multidirectional instability or isolated posterior instability comfortable. However, traumatic unidirectional instability is not likely to be successfully treated with rehabilitation, because of the associated damage to the labrum ligament complex.

Are there activity magnifications that can be done to affect solution to the problem? For a baseball pitcher, im-

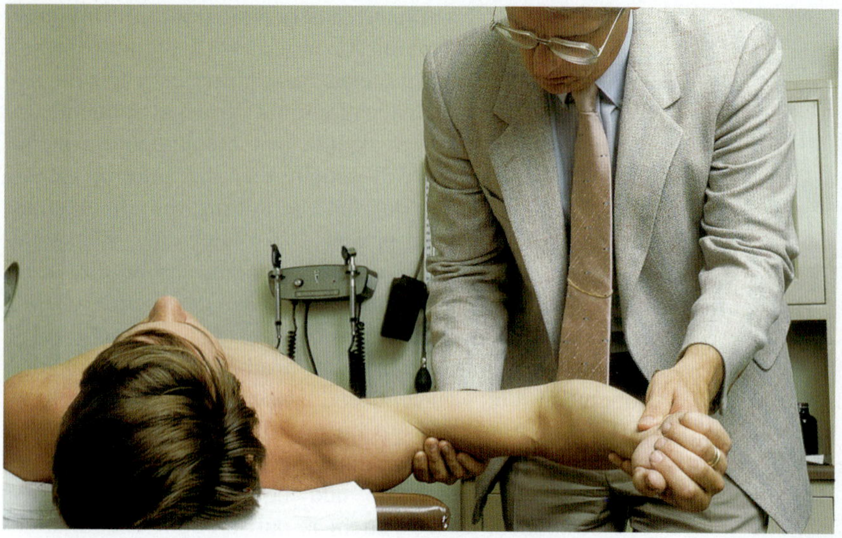

FIG. 7. Anterior apprehension in the abducted-external rotated position frequently accompanies anterior instability.

proving throwing mechanics or limiting the number of pitches may be an option. But, for a swimmer, it may mean altering the height of recovery of the stroke while eliminating some of the events performed. For a kayaker, it may mean avoiding high bracing. For many athletes, altering or changing style or sport is impractical or impossible.

Bracing externally can be used as an adjunct to treatment and may permit surgical timing to be planned for a more opportune moment relative to the athletic season.

8. *Impact and timing of operative procedure*. If nonoperative treatment is unlikely to help, how successful is surgical treatment likely to be? For example in the young, voluntary dislocator, surgical treatment is likely to be fraught with frustration and failure for all involved. In an elite athlete, the shoulder may be tight but at what cost in terms of effect on performance, time away from sport, and ultimate success?

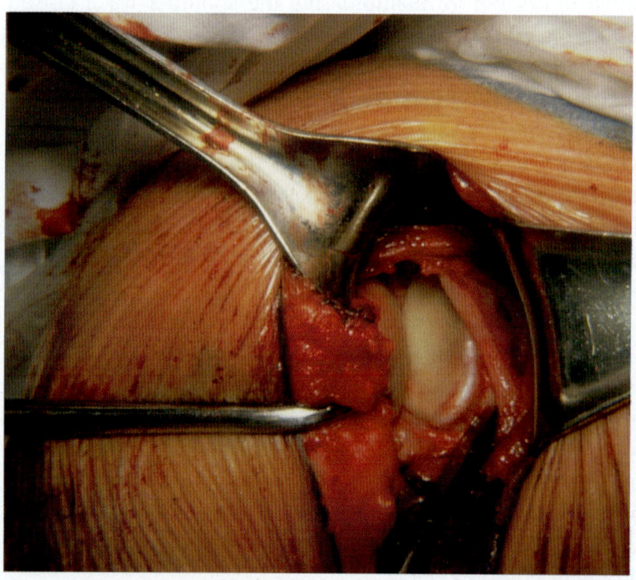

FIG. 8. Intraoperative photo of a Bankart lesion.

Is the repair likely to be one that is amenable to arthroscopic treatment? If it is, given that the arthroscopic success rate is generally thought to be lower than open surgery, can the person afford a failure in return for an attempt at an arthroscopic repair?

What about timing of surgical repair (Fig. 8)? Under what circumstances should a shoulder be repaired after the first dislocation independent of whether this is done arthroscopically or open?

THE DECISION-MAKING PROCESS

The answers to each of the questions above are important, as specific treatment is tailored to the patient, depending on these answers. The process of information gathering is a process geared toward answering the above questions. Each of the elements in information gathering—history, physical examination, radiographic studies, imaging studies, and examination under anesthesia play a role in the decision-making process. The following is an approach to each of these areas and how the information impacts on the decision regarding treatment. Is it the only way? No. Is it necessarily complete? No. But it is an approach that has helped us cope with some of the decisions that must be made in the treatment of the unstable shoulder.

HISTORY

There are important elements in the history that help answer the question as to whether the presenting problem is, in fact, instability. Matsen was once quoted as saying that if one required for the diagnosis of instability that the patient come into the office and state "my shoulder came out" or "my shoulder keeps coming out," that we would be diagnostically correct 99% of the time, and that if the shoulder does not "feel unstable" to the patient, it is "not unstable.'' Certainly there is an element of truth to this statement. In patients who have had a clear-cut dislocation, the diagnosis is not subtle. However, I think that two critical questions need to be answered when a patient presents after an initial dislocation episode: (a) ''what was the degree of trauma required to produce the instability,'' and (b) ''did someone need to put it back in'' or was it self-reduced? If the degree of trauma was minimal, or atraumatic, or if the dislocation was self reduced, then there should at least be the question of whether the surgeon is dealing with multidirectional or global instability. A young mother who lifts up the child and her shoulder ''pops out,'' the backstroker whose shoulder comes out while doing a flip turn, the tennis player whose shoulder slips out while serving, these may well be considered events with minimal trauma, and probably reflect pathology that is not a labrum or ligament tearing. Contrast this with the typical picture of the high school football player or cheerleader presenting in the emergency department after a fall on an outstretched arm, with the shoulder locked anteriorly, with the muscles in considerable spasm, for which significant anesthesia is required to manipulate the shoulder back into place. Therefore, if there is minimal or no trauma associated with the initial dislocation, one should suspect multidirectional instability. Alternatively, if there has been major trauma associated with the initial dislocation, it is unlikely to get better with rehabilitation, and consideration might be given for early surgical treatment, depending on the patient, because the damage is usually to the capsuloligamentous complex.

Second, the position of the arm at the time of instability is helpful in shedding light on the direction of the instability. Most anterior instability occurs with the position of the arm above the shoulder level, frequently in abduction external rotation—whether this is a hyper rotation injury above shoulder level or a fall on an outstretched arm. Isolated posterior instability frequently occurs with a direct posterior push or blow transmitted axially through a stiff arm, as might occur to a defensive lineman. Clearly, a history of seizures or an electrical shock event should alert the examiner to the possibility of a posterior dislocation.

Third, the frequency of the instability episodes or the length of time the problem has been going on is useful in deciding appropriate treatment. A shoulder that is coming out with less and less injury or trauma, or is coming out in the patient's sleep, is unlikely to be made better with nonoperative treatment. Likewise, a patient who has had many dislocations over a long period of time has usually altered the capsular restraints, even in the presence of a Bankart lesion, and is unlikely to be an ideal candidate for arthroscopic treatment.

The throwing athlete not infrequently presents as a diagnostic dilemma. Elements of the history can be helpful here as well. If there is a history of the arm ''going dead'' after a particularly hard throw, this may be a clue to anterior subluxation of the shoulder. A pitcher may be having a difficult time ''getting loose,'' may have trouble with diminishing speed or accuracy after a few innings, or may be fatiguing easily. The athlete may feel a click or a pop as the humeral head glides over the anterior labrum. And finally, in a thrower, if the pain onset has been gradual, over time, rather than with a specific inciting event, it is more likely to reflect subtle instability of the static stabilizers that have been stretched out over time.

Although these elements in the history seem to help with the diagnosis of instability, what to do about it and how quickly it should be done are more determined by factors that are related to the unique conditions of each patient.

Finally, an adequate history should investigate prior medical treatment, as this may impact on the successful outcome. Someone may have been labeled a ''rehabilitation failure'' in whom the actual rehabilitation consisted of ultrasound, heat, and stretching exercises, when the main problem that needed rehabilitation was the endurance and the strength of the rotator cuff and scapula stabilizers. Prior emergency department notes, prior radiology reports, and prior operative reports also may shed important light on the successful treatment, including elements of secondary gain or social factors likely to impact on success.

PHYSICAL EXAMINATION

One of the first things that can be determined is whether a patient's instability can be produced willfully, and whether these voluntary dislocations are painful. Voluntary instability can occur in an anterior or posterior direction (Fig. 6). Some patients can raise the arm up and the shoulder will subluxate posteriorly, while continued elevation relocates and recenters the shoulder in the glenoid. Other patients may wing the scapula and produce posterior subluxation of the shoulder. Stabilizing the scapula against the chest wall may prevent this posterior subluxation and offers a clue that scapula exercises and biofeedback techniques to control specific muscle groups may improve the situation. Nonpainful, voluntary instability need not be surgically treated, and there is a real question as to whether it need be treated at all. However, it is probably wise to begin a program of dynamic exercises to strengthen the glenohumeral joint and scapula in a voluntary dislocator, as a certain percentage of people who begin as voluntary dislocators will over time become involuntary and symptomatic. Voluntary anterior instability is less common and is usually associated with ''trick maneuvers'' to relax a series of muscles and contract others to selectively bring the shoulder out anteriorly. Treatment should probably be simply supportive with or without rehabilitation.

Inspection can provide valuable information. Atrophy of the deltoid can be a clue to a prior axillary nerve injury, which certainly would impact on the risk of reinjury with surgical treatment if atrophy exists. An electromyogram (EMG) should be considered. Atrophy of the infraspinatus in combination with the supraspinatus in a younger patient may suggest a suprascapular nerve lesion rather than shoulder instability in a young patient or a cuff tear that is chronic and difficult to treat in a patient who is older. Inspection may reveal scapula winging in a serratus anterior palsy, parascapula wasting in a brachial plexopathy, or distal atrophy in a non-plexus peripheral nerve lesion.

Before examining the involved shoulder, it is helpful to get a sense as to whether there is generalized joint laxity as might be reflected by recurvatum of the elbow, recurvatum of the proximal interphalangeal (PIP) joint, decreased thumb to wrist distance (Fig. 6), and patella hypermobility, all clues to the presence of multidirectional laxity of the shoulder. In addition, the contralateral shoulder should be examined for laxity, translatability, and subluxation. Frequently a relaxed, nonpainful, nonapprehensive examination of the contralateral shoulder can give a clue to the presence or absence of capsular laxity in a symptomatic shoulder.

Checking passive range of motion and comparing it with the contralateral shoulder is often helpful. A patient with painful recurrent subluxations of the shoulder may have apprehension limiting voluntary passive range of motion, especially in the abducted position. Some patients with multidirectional instability may have excessive external rotation compared with the contralateral shoulder, as may some patients who have a rupture of the subscapularis tendon. Alternatively, a stiff, solid end point in the direction tested, especially if there has not been prior surgery, essentially excludes the diagnosis of shoulder instability, as the shoulder cannot be stiff and loose at the same time. In the presence of prior surgery, however, if one side has been tightened up, a shoulder can exhibit elements of symptomatic instability in other directions. Finally, limitations of passing range of motion may give a subtle clue to the presence of early glenohumeral arthrosis.

Active motion is helpful in assessing the overall strength of the arm (Fig. 3A). A patient with limitation of active elevation may have this because of pain and apprehension. External rotation weakness with the arm at the side may be the first clue to a rotator cuff tear as the source of the problem in the patients who have a traumatic instability episode. A positive lift-off test may be a clue to subscapularis rupture. Subscapularis rupture may be either a component of a larger global rotator cuff tear or as an isolated subscapularis avulsion, in cases following prior instability surgery in which the subscapularis has been repaired.

Finally, provocative tests are often extremely helpful. With the arm in neutral position, inferior stress is applied, and, if there is an increased space between acromion and humeral head, a dimple or ''sulcus,'' this implies an element of inferior laxity (Figs. 2 and 4). Some investigators have suggested that the difference between the degree of sulcus and neutral and external rotation can pinpoint the cause and the location of the pathologic anatomy, whether this is inferiorly (inferior capsular laxity), or superiorly (an excessively large rotator interval or an incompetent coracohumeral ligament). If the sulcus decreases when the arm is externally rotated, as the coracohumeral ligament tightens, this suggests that the pathology is inferiorly, as the ligament responsible for checking external rotation seems to be functioning adequately. By contrast, if the sulcus is the same in any degree of rotation, this may be evidence that an abnormal rotator interval lesion, or a coracohumeral ligament that is not functioning well may be the prime component allowing inferior translation.

The load and shift, or ''draw'' test, centers the humeral head in the glenoid while translational stresses are applied. This not only gives a clue to the presence of laxity, that is excessive translation, but if this maneuver produces pain, apprehension, or a ''that's it'' response from the patient, it can help with the diagnosis of the degree and a direction on the instability. In addition, a grinding or grating as the humeral head is moved over the anterior or posterior glenoid rim may give a clue to associated labral pathology or cartilage wear in the affected glenoid region.

The ability to translate anteriorly, posteriorly, or inferiorly is gaged in the positions in which the normal restraining ligaments would be affected. This has also been called an apprehension (Fig. 7). Most patients with anterior symptomatic instability will not let the examiner stress the arm in abduction external rotation enough to subluxate the shoulder, but if the patient feels uncomfortable or does not like the arm being placed in that position, that is usually enough to call it a positive apprehension test. As the patient guards against this maneuver or this position, the muscles tighten and the examiner is given a clue to the diagnosis.

When a posterior apprehension test is performed, it frequently is not positive in patients despite posterior subluxation, as they usually will not experience discomfort or pain apprehension.''

And, finally, the relocation test is performed. If the relocation test is truly positive, apprehension is diminished as pressure is placed on the humeral head, effectively maintaining it within the joint, and this is strongly suggestive of anterior instability. If, however, it is pain rather than apprehension that is eliminated, this may reflect not a positive response for instability, but rather other causes of pain eliminated by preventing forward movement of the humeral head in the glenoid, such as might occur with deep surface rotator cuff tear, (the so-called internal impingement as the undersurface of the cuff abuts against the glenoid labrum).

RADIOGRAPHY STUDIES

Radiography studies (Figs. 9 and 10) are used to help determine the presence of, the direction of, and the degree of instability. Toward that end, they are intended to identify the presence of glenoid rim lesions or fractures, Hill-Sachs lesions of the humeral head, fractures of the greater tuberosity, or the presence of glenohumeral arthrosis.

The most useful radiographs for obtaining this information are the anterior posterior in neutral and internal rotation, the Stryker Notch view, (which identifies Hill-Sachs

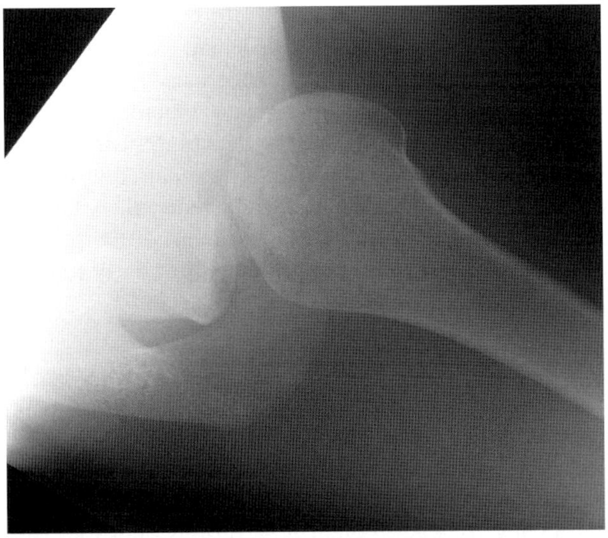

FIG. 9. Axillary radiograph of an anterior dislocation. Note the Hill-Sachs lesion.

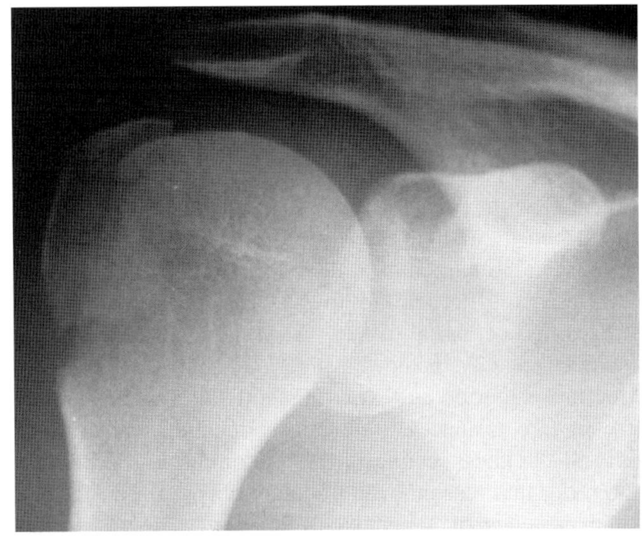

FIG. 10. A radiograph following reduction of an anterior dislocation. The greater tuberosity fractured permitting the dislocation via a "posterior mechanism."

lesions, and shoulder arthrosis), or the West Point axillary view that usually shows the anterior posterior glenoid rim away from overlapping bone (may also show glenoid rim fracture, reaction from repetitive trauma, or the extent of glenoid wear or bone deficiency). Plain radiology is not helpful for determining abnormal degrees of version of the humeral head or glenoid, but may indicate the presence or absence of a hypoplastic glenoid.

Although some have advocated stress or weighted radiographs, muscle guarding usually limits their effectiveness, and, indeed, it is only useful if compared to the contralateral shoulder. Overall, not much information is usually gained from stress or weighted radiograph views.

Computed tomography (CT) scans may give information if a fracture is suspected or present, and if accompanied by arthrographic may give information as to the presence or absence of labral detachment. However, a well-performed MRI scan with or without gadolinium, probably is much more useful in supplying the same degree of information.

Use of MRI scans (Fig. 11) is particularly useful if one is trying to decide about repairing a shoulder acutely after the first dislocation, or if trying to decide whether an arthroscopic approach is likely to be effective or successful. If the MRI scan demonstrates a clear-cut Bankart lesion, well-defined glenohumeral ligaments, with a competent capsule, arthroscopic repair is something that should certainly be considered, especially if the patient gives a history of recent instability, with few dislocations. Use of the MRI scan is not routine, but is useful for finding out if the presence or absence of a Bankart lesion will impact directly on the treatment approach, or if a rotator cuff tear is sus-

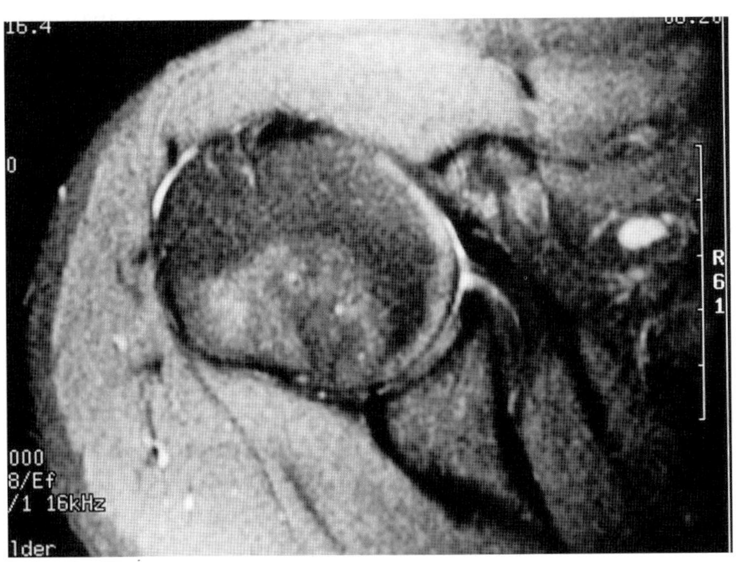

FIG. 11. Magnetic resonance image showing subscapularis rupture.

pected as a primary pathologic mechanism causing the dislocation. The MRI scan in the presence of a rotator cuff tear will give specific information about the posterior cuff, subscapularis, the location of the biceps tendon, and the quality or the repairability of the cuff tissue. If the MRI scan shows a full thickness rotator cuff tear, and this is associated with a demonstrable cuff weakness after dislocation, then the patient is offered a surgical repair acutely. The surgical treatment should be geared toward decompression and cuff repair, not toward stabilizing the shoulder by capsular or labral tissue. Adequate exposure to the shoulder probably includes a superior approach as the posterior and superior cuff are frequently the areas that are torn. In rare instances, traumatic dislocation can produce both full-thickness tearing of the rotator cuff and a Bankart lesion. For that reason, even if planning a rotator cuff repair in the presence of a positive MRI scan, a diagnostic arthroscopy to look at the labrum is useful. If there is a Bankart lesion, this can be repaired either at the time of the arthroscopy or the time of the cuff repair, usually through an extensive rotator interval exposure.

If the radiograph reveals the presence of a significant glenoid rim fracture, particularly if the humeral head remains subluxated on the anterior glenoid rim, plans are made for open reduction internal fixation of the glenoid fracture. Ordinarily, if the main surgical treatment will be repair of the glenoid fracture, additional capsular repair need not be contemplated. If a glenoid rim fracture is displaced and involves more than 25% of the anterior glenoid, this is usually the criteria for direct surgical repair of the glenoid fracture.

If following the relocation of the shoulder the radiograph reveals a greater tuberosity fracture (Fig. 10), what is done with the tuberosity depends on the resting position of the greater tuberosity relative to the humeral head and its normal anatomic location once the humeral head has been manipulated into place. For a two-part greater tuberosity anterior fracture dislocation, Neer suggested that once the shoulder was relocated, if more than one centimeter displacement of the greater tuberosity posteriorly or superiorily existed, the shoulder should be considered for surgical repair. However, the greater tuberosity fracture is probably the one fracture in which the one centimeter rule should be re-examined, as small degrees of superior displacement of the greater tuberosity fragment, if permitted to heal on the superior malunited position, can have dramatic effects on the subacromial space in the cuff mechanics, leading to significant tuberosity and rotator cuff impingement. With malunited greater tuberosity segments, anterior acromioplasty alone is usually not adequate surgical treatment, and an osteotomy and repositioning of the tuberosity are more likely to be necessary. Therefore, in the presence of an acute fracture, if the top of the greater tuberosity in the final position of the shoulder is above the top of the humeral head, it is wisest to anatomically repair the greater tuberosity through a deltoid split via an anterior superior approach. A low tolerance for superior greater tuberosity displacement has become more widespread as surgeons have had to deal with late sequelae of tuberosity malunion. It is also important to recognize that greater tuberosity displacement is associated with rotator cuff tearing, usually along the rotator interval, and this should be repaired at the time the greater tuberosity is anatomically reduced. A CT scan or MRI to evaluate posterior displacement of the fragment may be helpful in determining the need for early repair.

EXAMINATION UNDER ANESTHESIA

The issue of examination under anesthesia is frequently spoken about as part of the decision-making process. Certainly, if the humeral head cannot be made to subluxate or dislocate under anesthesia, the history of shoulder instability as a cause of the problem is in serious question. However, the contrary is not necessarily true. Many patients have laxity under anesthesia and this may not be reflected in abnormal intra-articular pathology. The examination under anesthesia is most helpful if it can be directly compared in all positions of stress with the contralateral shoulder. Adding to this difficulty of interpreting the examination under anesthesia is the fact that at many institutions, shoulder surgery is performed under regional anesthesia, so that the contralateral shoulder is not helpful as a direct control. While the examination under anesthesia may have some value in suspected instability, it is only helpful if the obtained increased translation can be explained by observed intra-articular pathology, usually at the time of arthroscopy.

Examination under anesthesia alone, without a diagnostic arthroscopic evaluation, has little practical value.

The examination under anesthesia, however, can be a valuable means of determining whether the shoulder has laxity in one or more directions. For instance, if the examination under anesthesia shows predominantly anteroinferior laxity, but there is also straight inferior and posterior subluxation this should give the surgeon to pause, and the other directions of instability and translation may need to be addressed at the time of surgery.

DECISION MAKING

Nonoperative Treatment

Treating the unstable shoulder by nonoperative means involves issues of length of immobilization (following acute dislocation), whether or not to implement rehabilitation exercises, and if so, which kind, and whether the rehabilitation may be playing a role in the treatment or producing further problems.

In the first place, a patient with multidirectional instability or isolated posterior subluxation is the patient most likely to respond to a rehabilitation program. Matsen coined the pneumonic AMBRII (Atraumatic, Multidirectional, Bilateral, Rehabilitation, Inferior capsular shift, Interval) to distinguish the patient with severe laxity from the more common traumatic patient, which he called TUBS (Traumatic, Unidirectional, Bankart, Surgery). Many patients without major trauma have multidirectional instability and global laxity, and can be treated with exercises. On the other hand, unidirectional patients often have had a significant traumatic event that has produced a Bankart lesion, with a concomitant Hill-Sachs lesion, and there is a high degree of recurrence if the same level of activity is kept up. These patients should be considered for repair. Certainly, if a patient has already demonstrated that the problem has become recurrent, if there are repeat dislocations and particularly if they are anterior, there is little role for rehabilitation in managing this patient.

Another important issue is the specific rehabilitation to order for the unstable shoulder. For anterior instability, it makes sense to strengthen and increase the endurance of the scapula and cuff muscles, especially the anterior subscapularis. If the problem is posterior subluxation, concentrating on the external rotators and the scapula is probably more fruitful, while global shoulder exercises are added at a later date.

Global laxity and multidirectional instability is often more of a problem. This condition frequently is accompanied by associated rotator cuff tendonitis and pain, so early abduction, resistance, or strengthening exercisers are frequently painful. In addition, the position of the shoulder at the extremes of internal and external rotation can reproduce subluxation in a globally lax shoulder. Therefore, it is probably best to begin in these patients with isometric exercises in the neutral position, followed by resistive exercises with the arm in the neutral position to keep the head centered without stressing it at the extremes of motion. When these exercises are no longer painful, end range of motion resistance exercises are added.

Using Arthroscopic Findings

The usefulness of arthroscopy in decision making lies with the information it gives about pathoanatomic structures by direct visualization and direct instrument palpation. In addition, the presence of arthroscopic findings can confirm the diagnosis of instability. For instance, frayed, torn, fragmented, or split anterior inferior labrum, with cartilage wear in the anterior inferior quadrant, essentially confirms the presence of repeated anterior inferior trauma and excess translation in that direction, as does the presence of a Hill-Sachs lesion. Specific localized labral pathology can be identified as well as pathologic changes in the undersurface of the rotator cuff. Less helpful is the fact that increased translation is frequently directly observed under arthroscopy. Much has been discussed about the so-called ''drive-through sign,'' that is, the ease with which the arthroscope can be passed from back to front, implying increased volume and laxity of the capsule. However, it must be remembered that laboratory experiments by multiple investigators have shown that simply venting the joint, a process that is done with the first capsular puncture at the time of arthroscopy, significantly increases the translation of the humeral head on the glenoid. However, the drive-through may be most utilized in decision making not by its presence or absence but by its ability to be directly compared before and after the instability repair.

Two areas can be directly identified at arthroscopy that can be helpful in the identification of an instability presence and in direction. First, the superior labrum, the presence of a SLAP lesion, can have an impact on stability of the shoulder through its biceps anchor. If instability and an unstable SLAP lesion are present, it is much easier to correct this arthroscopically than open, whether either excision or direct repair of the superior labrum is contemplated. Second, capsular inspection of the capsular may reveal either capsular tearing or plastic deformation. A capsular repair seen anteriorly and inferiorly confirms anterior inferior instability. A stress line in the capsule may be seen between the middle and the superior glenohumeral ligament, essentially confirming rotator interval enlargement, which should be addressed at the time of repair.

Circumferential capsular inspections enable one to see the lateral capsular attachment on the humerus, which may be an occasional site of tearing and may be one source of anterior instability. The lateral capsular rupture and failure are difficult to see at open surgery, and can be overlooked in an open instability repair, unless they are looked for or the subscapularis is opened.

Finally, if inspection of the capsular reveals that the predominant pathology is laxity and a loose capsule, the surgeon needs to be ready to reduce the capsular volume, decrease the inferior pouch, and tighten the capsule in a direction in which the laxity occurs.

If the degree of instability is minor, if no Bankart or capsular repair is done, and the primary pathology is increased capsular volume, consideration may be given to shrinking the capsular tissue by a thermal means. Heat has been shown to denature collagen, and, secondarily, to create scarring, and thus shrink capsular tissue. It is this thermal effect on collagen that has been responsible for capsular shrinkage observed with laser energy. More recently, radiofrequency probes to deliver heat to the capsule have been thought to be a safe and effective way to deliver thermal energy to the capsule without necessarily the associated distant effect on bone or cartilage that has been observed using laser within the glenohumeral joint.

The entire attachment of the labrum is easily visually inspected and probed, first to confirm the pathologic anatomy, and second to identify the degree or extent of labral detachment.

If a relatively small step-off exists in the anterior inferior labrum, and the shoulder has clear-cut anterior inferior dislocations, it is difficult to imagine a small area of step-off as the sole pathologic process, and the capsular procedure is usually added at this time.

Furthermore, in the setting of dislocations, with a relatively short instability history, if the probed labrum tissue reveals thick, good quality, easily identifiable tissue, which is nonfragmented, if preliminary fixation of the labrum to the anterior glenoid rim decreases the degree of instability to the shoulder, then consideration can be given to any one of a number of direct arthroscopic repairs of the Bankart lesion. The decision to repair the shoulder arthroscopically is a difficult one, given the fact that open instability repairs have a long history, with more predictable results are usually technically less difficult. In addition, many surgeons are more familiar with open techniques in practice and training. The recurrence rate with open instability repair, has been traditionally quite acceptable. Contrast this with published reports of arthroscopic repairs. Though many good series have been reported, even series in the hands of experienced arthroscopists have shown recurrences in as high as 40%.

The reason for variability of recurrence rate in published arthroscopic repairs is commonly multifactorial. First, arthroscopic instability repairs are technically difficult, with a steep learning curve. Second, they have a mixed pathology, with only one element of the pathology traditionally able to be addressed at arthroscopy—the reattachment and the approximation of the labrum (Bankart lesion)—leaving the capsular unaddressed at the time. Newer techniques such as heat shrinkage of the capsule gives some "backup" if the Bankart direct repair is inadequate and now probably will expand indications for arthroscopic repairs. Third, different criteria are used to measure surgical success; most of the series in the literature of failed open surgeries is based on redislocation rates, and this may significantly underestimate the failure attributable to resubluxation or remaining apprehension.

It seems reasonable that direct arthroscopic repairs have an important place in the surgical treatment of instability of the shoulder if: (a) the pathology is clearly a large Bankart lesion; (b) the labrum tissue is of good quality and can be manipulated easily; (c) the history is of short duration with few dislocations (or one dislocation), and (d) the patient is willing to accept the fact that failure rate is higher in the published literature for arthroscopic repairs than open repairs.

By contrast, it is probably not wise to do a purely arthroscopic repair if (a) there is poor quality (i.e., frayed and thin) labral tissue, (b) the patient is an elite or contact athlete and may not be able to afford a surgical failure, or (c) the patient has multidirectional instability, unless some global capsular tightening procedure is added arthroscopically.

With this in mind, thermal shrinkage of the capsule brings a new tool to the armament in the arthroscopic treatment of shoulder instability. The ability to precisely place heat-delivering probes on the capsule at carefully controlled temperature (65°C), directly visualizing the shrunken tissue, and eliminating the component of capsular laxity, has given surgeons another option (Fig. 12). What must be recognized is that what information we have on this procedure reveals that collagen is denatured, under direct visualization can be seen to shrink and to contract, and that scarring of the capsule is seen in the joint. What we don't know yet is whether structures in an area other than the capsule are affected by the heat, such as the subscapularis muscle, axillary nerve, and so forth, and whether these can be injured at the time. We don't know the mechanical properties of the heat-altered capsule and whether over the long term the contracture of the capsule directly seen at arthroscopy will hold up.

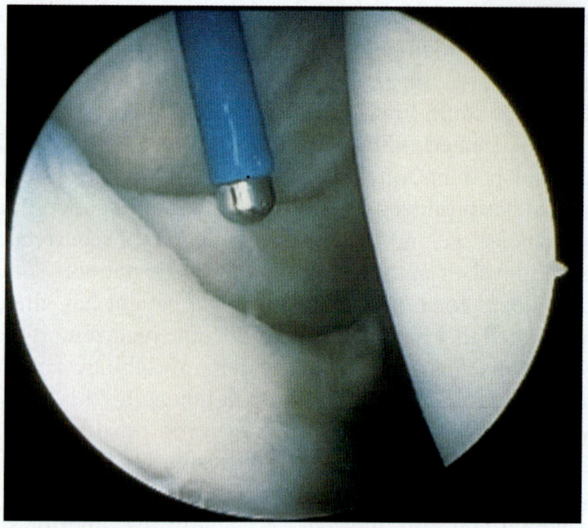

FIG. 12. For a thermal shrinkage of the capsule a precisely controlled "heat" probe is used to shrink the capsule.

However, this technique is considered if it is recognized by the patient that it is still investigational and (a) if the pathology is global laxity and the capsule can be shrunk in all three directions; (b) the degree of instability is not great—subtle instability or subluxation in conjunction with cuff irritation; (c) as an adjunct to arthroscopic direct repair of the Bankart lesion, in which, after repair of the Bankart lesion (the arthroscopic tack technique is preferred), the capsular tissue is then shrunk with the probe.

At arthroscopy, the presence and degree of degeneration of the joint is noted. Early osteoarthritis is frequently associated with loose bodies and these should be searched for if significant degenerative joint disease is present. In addition, peripheral osteophytes can be trimmed, and a synevectomy can be performed within the joint. If degenerative joint disease is present, even if mild, early postoperative passive range of motion is mandatory, as immobilization in the presence of osteoarthritis after surgery leads to considerable degree of stiffness in the shoulder.

Intraoperative Treatment—Open Surgery

The timing of surgical repair is clearly dependent upon the type of instability present, the needs of each patient, and how disabling, dangerous, or inconvenient a recurrent dislocation would be to each individual patient.

For example, a patient with isolated atraumatic posterior instability or a patient with global laxity and multidirectional instability, has a much better chance of solving his/her instability problems with rehabilitation than a patient with unidirectional, traumatic, anterior instability. In addition, the pain and morbidity of recurrence is less with this type of instability, and relocation is often self-manipulated or not difficult to perform. Thus, it seems reasonable to wait a longer period of time before recommending shoulder reconstruction in atraumatic, global, or isolated posterior instability. If, after a period of 3 to 4 months in a well-organized rehabilitation program, subluxation continues or apprehension is still present, reconstruction is usually recommended.

With traumatic unidirectional instability, the classic teaching has been to wait for recurrence before proceeding with surgery, given the information that the recurrence rate is probably 50% to 70% (that is, 30% to 50% will not recur, particularly with activity modification). A major step in our rethinking of this tenet problem was the experience at West Point, a patient group whose activity level requires continued shoulder stress.

In West Point cadets, with traumatic unidirectional instability, virtually 100% of the cadets with nonoperative treatment had recurrence. Given this experience, Arciero and colleagues went to immediate surgical repair following the initial event, with near elimination of recurrence and without significant untoward effects. While this is a unique population, their rationale can probably be applied to any very active group, including the athletic group, in whom recurrence is likely, who are unable to or unwilling to modify activity, in which the disability can be lengthy and extensive, career-threatening, if one waits for a second dislocation event. Similarly, in athletes who throw, subluxation or traumatic labral injury is usually poorly-tolerated, resulting in loss of control and velocity. In these patients, early repair is frequently suggested.

Therefore, in patients who have an anterior traumatic dislocation, in whom the MRI or arthroscopy has shown a clear-cut Bankart avulsion of the labrum by the glenohumeral ligaments, which is amenable to direct repair, and whose lifestyle would be severely impacted if a second dislocation should appear, surgery is offered after the first dislocation. An example of this is the white-water kayaker, who suffers a dislocation. A recurrence while kayaking in this patient could be life threatening. Another example is a highschool athlete in his sophomore year, wanting to play ball or dependent on a scholarship for college, who dislocates during the season. If rehabilitation alone is performed, if he is permitted to return to sports, and a second dislocation occurs, the athlete will probably miss most of the two seasons rather than only one. Surgery would be offered to this type of patient. This logic has been extended to offer acute surgical treatment after the first dislocation depending on who does not want the down time from activities, or the inconvenience of waiting until a second dislocation occurs for surgery to be performed. In the case of an elite athlete who can play with restricted arm motion in season, bracing is useful and surgery performed after the season is concluded.

It is recognized that with this approach to acute stabilization, surgery may be done on someone who might otherwise have stabilized without repair. However, if patients understand the risk, their choice, given the high likelihood of recurrence in traumatic instability, will often be for early surgical repair.

There are a number of technical decision-making issues that surgeons face. While the standard approach is a long deltopectoral incision, as the long skin incision makes exposure easy, burying the incision in the axillary area with a more limited skin incision, will certainly be more cosmetic. In patients in whom cosmesis is very important, this skin incision can be made. But in the patient who has a large, muscular shoulder, a long deltopectoral incision is preferred.

The coracoid muscles can be taken down when additional exposure is needed, but the risk with detachment of the coracoid process is traction on the brachial plexus, particularly with significant forceful retraction. Our preference is to leave the conjoined tendon attached to the coracoid process without coracoid osteotomy.

The subscapularis can be split, or taken down in part or entirely. The argument for subscapularis split is that in the dominant arm of a thrower, this approach may interfere less with propriception and motion and is a safer approach with less interference with the interaction of the important cuff muscles. Yet, exposure is more difficult when the subscapularis is simply split; it is less easy to separate the capsule entirely from the subscapularis muscle, and there is less flexibility to precisely tension the capsule in different directions. In addition, the rotator interval is not identified. The subscapularis split is not done if a significant capsular shifting is contemplated. In most cases, for the most control of the capsule, the subscapularis is divided formally, vertically and superior laterally, and separated from the anterior capsule before the anterior repair is to be done.

Much has been written about capsular division (Figs. 13–15), and whether to divide the capsule laterally (at the humeral head), medially (at the glenoid), or in the middle. It clearly does not matter significantly, as the capsular tightening can be accomplished no matter where the capsule is divided.

Selective capsular repair has been described by Warren et al. as when a horizontal capsulotomy is initially made toward the glenoid and the glenoid is inspected, a decision then is made whether to do a formal Bankart repair. If work needs to be done on the glenoid, a vertical capsular incision is made adjacent to the glenoid. If there is not going to be a direct labral repair, the vertical limb is made laterally for a capsular shift.

However, as an alternative in all circumstances, Craig has advocated capsular division laterally. The rationale is since the lateral capsular attachment to the humeral head is

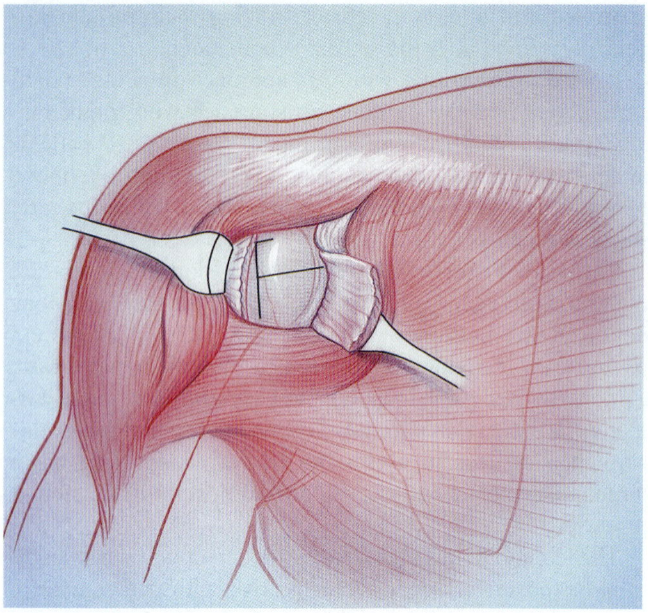

FIG. 13. One method of capsular repair. Superior and inferior flaps are developed for later transposition.

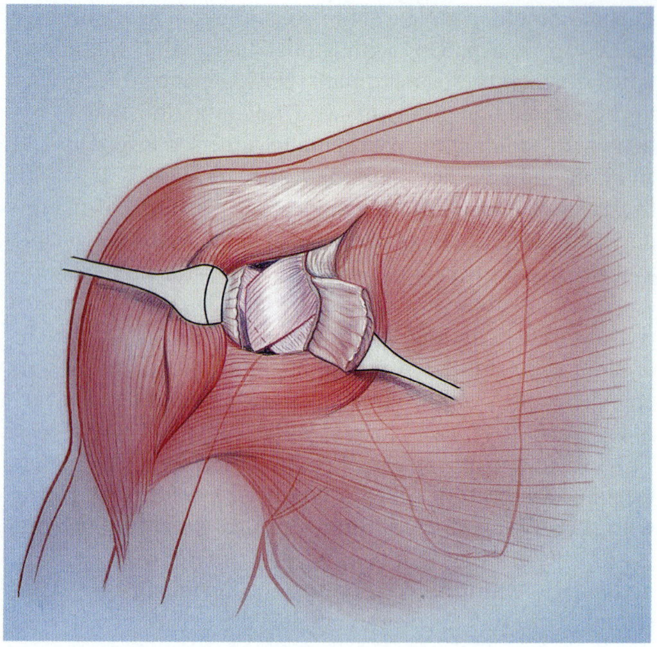

FIG. 14. Transposing two flaps permits capsular tightening.

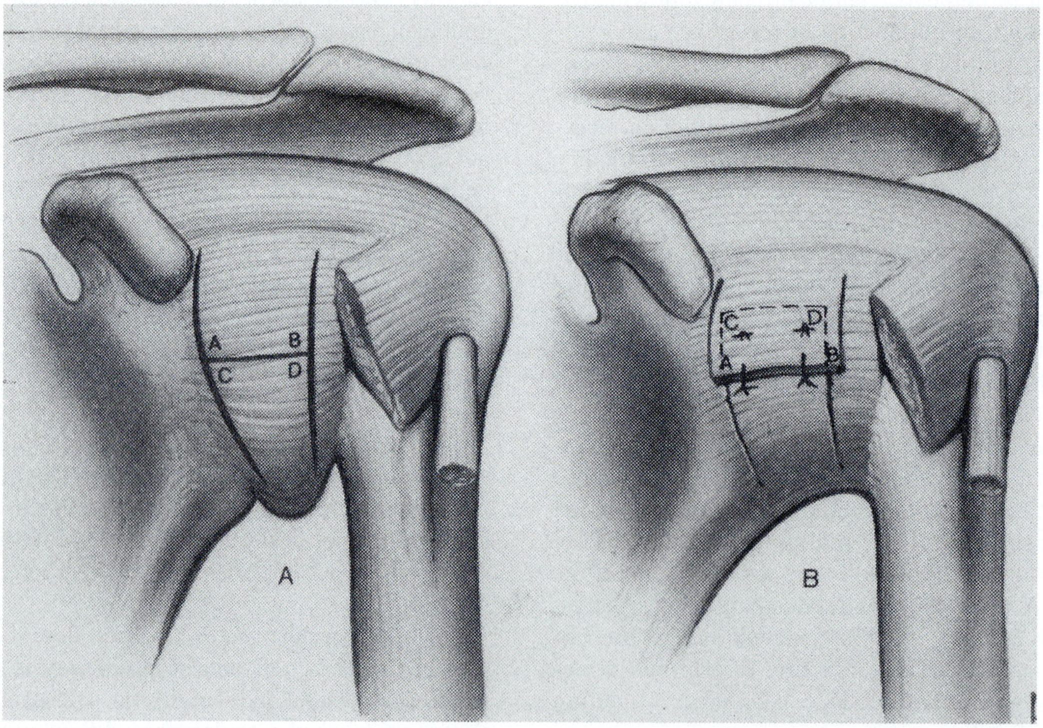

FIG. 15. A, B: Capsule can be divided in a number of ways, depending on what part of the capsule is to be tightened. Here, a horizontal incision is made. Two vertical capsular incisions from an H-shape, permitting inferior laxity to be eliminated.

more extensive than that to the glenoid, the capsule is actually a funnel with a wider base around the humerus, resulting in more flexibility to fine-tune the capsular tightening laterally, the capsular may even be released ''around the corner'' for multidirectional instability if more control of the capsule is desired. In addition, cutting through the capsule at the glenoid divides the capsule at the thickest and most clearly developed aspect of the glenohumeral ligaments, while a lateral division of the capsule divides the soft tissue before the ligaments become so clearly defined.

For repair of the Bankart lesion (Fig. 8), the decision is usually between drill holes from the glenoid neck to the articular surface, while passing the suture through an intact ridge of bone, or use of any one of a number of soft tissue anchors to the bone. Suture anchoring is frequently done incorrectly, with the anchor hole along the glenoid neck, so that the labrum and capsule are not reattached directly to the edge of the glenoid rim. However, if the anchoring hole is precisely at the rim, the suture anchor technique has served attractive features, and this is our preference.

After repair of the Bankart lesion, the decision is made whether to tighten the capsule and how much tension to apply. We advocate capsulorrhaphy if the Bankart lesion is small (unlikely to explain the entire pathomechanics of instability) or if the instability is multidirectional (based on large inferior pouch, a large rotator interval) and recommend revision surgery where the tissue is often less satisfactory.

How much to tension the capsule depends on the needs and wants of each individual. If you make the capsule too tight, this can dramatically restrict range of motion, and contracture postoperatively can be a serious problem. Indeed, secondary osteoarthritis can develop if one over tightens the capsule. It is difficult to give precise guidelines for how much to tighten the capsule. For instance, a baseball pitcher or a football quarterback needs every bit of their shoulder motion, and range of motion should not be restricted at all. On the table, we like to be able to achieve 90 degrees of external rotation with the arm elevated 90 degrees. Capsular tightening should therefore be minimized. On the other hand, an interior lineman will often sacrifice small degrees of range of motion for additional security of the shoulder, and the capsule can be tightened somewhat without worry of small degrees of restricted motion. In general, if the capsule is tensioned with the arm at 45 degrees of abduction and 50 to 60 degrees of external rotation, overtightening is avoided. Following capsular repair, in the operating room (OR), 75 degrees of external rotation is able to be achieved easily without undue tension on the capsule, it is unlikely that significant postoperative stiffness will be problematic, particularly if early motion is begun.

One word about bone grafting a worn, a rounded, or deficient glenoid: if the capsular and labrum complex is directly repaired to the remaining edge of the glenoid rim, one need not bone graft any deficiency of the glenoid. The Hill-Sachs lesion will not engage on the area of the glenoid if the capsule is directly reapproximated to it, and stability will be maintained. In the patient with multidirectional instability, the issues are a little different. The pathology is usually a patulous capsule, a large inferior pouch, or a large rotator interval, and each of these areas needs to be dealt with as well. Some have advocated rotator interval closure alone in some patients with multidirectional instability. While this may be reasonable, particularly if the patient does not have a large inferior pouch, the best control of the entire capsule (anteriorly, inferiorly, posteriorly) is found with a capsulotomy and an inferior capsular shift, with closure of the rotator interval at the time of the capsular shift.

Revision Surgery

In patients who have had failed surgery, what needs to be done at the time of revision depends upon the problem and the reason for failure. If the problem is one of over tightening and surgical contracture with restricted motion, the capsule can be released either arthroscopically (with or without laser) or openly, effectively lengthening the capsule and subscapularis and restoring external rotation (the most frequent motion lost with overtightening). If internal rotation is too tight, the posterior capsule might be released, and this is usually done more easily arthroscopically than with an open procedure.

If the reasons for a failed surgery are attributable to recurrence, the reason for the recurrence dictates the decision making at the time of surgery. The most common reasons for failed surgical treatments of instability are failure to repair a Bankart lesion, failure to recognize multidirectional instability, failure to recognize subscapularis or lateral capsular rupture, or too early return to activities with new trauma. These are usually readily addressed with open revision surgery.

In the case of a shoulder that has been multiply operated on and has had multiple failed procedures, the subscapularis may be thin, retracted, and may not provide satisfactory tissue for surgical repair during revision reconstruction. In this case, an Achilles tendon allograft can be used to augment the subscapularis repair and suture the Achilles either to the remaining edge of the subscapularis, or as a reinforcement to the subscapularis, or directly anchored to the glenoid and humeral lesser tuberosity. In addition, some have suggested a pectoralis tendon for substitution for subscapularis muscle, although the power and the vector of this muscle may not be ideal for use as a subscapularis substitute. Alternatively, the hamstring tendon may be considered to rebuild specific glenohumeral ligaments, if the ligaments themselves are deficient.

In the case of a failed Bristow operation, usually the coracoid process causes a tremendous degree of scarring in the subscapularis as this is the muscle that has been violated. The coracoid process is often ununited, and hardware is frequently prominent. Our approach has been to remove the hardware, leave the bone graft (if united) alone, repair the Bankart lesion, and re-repair the subscapularis.

Postoperative

Decision making in the postoperative period centers on the length of immobilization, the timing of the initiation of rehabilitation, and the timing of return to activities. This also depends on the type of pathology (capsular laxity vs. Bankart lesion.) If the Bankart repair is secure, early range of motion can be begun safely with active range of motion permitted when there is subscapularis healing (6 weeks). In patients whose pathology is predominantly capsular laxity or a large inferior pouch, it is usually not difficult to regain a range of motion, and the patients can safely be immobilized for 6 weeks or longer before initiating range of motion. If a thermal capsular shrinkage has been undertaken, the collagen should be allowed to scar before beginning range of motion, and motion exercises are not begun for two to three weeks.

Returning to sports is permitted when range of motion returns to normal or plateaus, and the strength of the deltoid and cuff combination (enough to protect the repair) in 90% of the contralateral side. It is unusual to permit contact athletes to return to contact sports before 5 months. Precise guidelines for return are different, because they are sport-, position-, and patient-specific.

In general, a graduated program of increasing the muscles that are sports-specific can be trained once the range of motion has been obtained, and once the overall endurance and muscle strength of the shoulder approaches normal.

The Unstable Shoulder,
edited by R.F. Warren, E.V. Craig, and D.W. Altchek.
Lippincott–Raven Publishers, Philadelphia © 1999.

CHAPTER 13

Recurrent Anterior Glenohumeral Instability

Open Surgical Treatment

Robert F. LaPrade and Gregory A. Brown

It is essential to properly evaluate the patient with recurrent anterior glenohumeral instability to determine the frequency of recurrent dislocations, how the dislocations occur, and whether it is a true dislocation or a subluxation event. Overall, the decision to proceed with an open surgical-stabilization procedure will depend on the amount of pain and loss of function of the patient. In some cases, pain, such as that which occurs with an impingement syndrome resulting from anterior glenohumeral instability, may be the only presenting complaint of the patient, and a careful physical examination must be performed to supplement the patient's history to arrive at a correct diagnosis. Plain radiographs, and occasionally magnetic resonance imaging or computed tomography (CT) arthrograms, are also an essential portion of the evaluation of these patients to evaluate the possible presence of a Hill-Sachs or bony Bankart lesion.

The purpose of this chapter is to review the indications, techniques, complications, and the history behind open anterior glenohumeral–instability surgery. In addition, we present a comparison of and summary of the published results for open anterior-instability surgery.

INDICATIONS FOR OPEN INSTABILITY REPAIR

The indications for open anterior glenohumeral–instability repair are for those patients who have functional limitations of their glenohumeral joints primarily for the following reasons:

1. Recurrent anterior/anteroinferior glenohumeral dislocations/subluxations.
2. Failed arthroscopic stabilization procedures with recurrence of instability.
3. Anterior glenohumeral microinstability and secondary impingement nonresponsive to rehabilitation modalities.

In most instances, patients who sustain a traumatic anterior glenohumeral dislocation can initially be treated nonoperatively. A brief period of treatment in a sling should be performed until the patient is comfortable. An attempt to return to normal activity should be performed only after an appropriate period of rehabilitation for the intrinsic rotator-cuff muscles, the three parts of the deltoid, and the scapular stabilizers. However, patients who have symptomatic recurrent anterior glenohumeral dislocations and are unable to participate in overhead activities, or who have an impingement syndrome resulting from anterior instability that does not respond to a period of rehabilitation, should be offered the opportunity to have an open anterior capsulolabral reconstruction to improve their overall glenohumeral function. Although it is recognized that younger patients have a higher incidence of recurrent anterior glenohumeral instability, age should not be the sole determining factor in making a recommendation for an open anterior-shoulder reconstruction. It is important also to assess the time interval between the dislocations and the functioning level achieved between the episodes of anterior dislocations. The decision to proceed with an open anterior reconstruction should be individualized, depending on both the functional demands and the limitations of the patient.

The role of arthroscopic stabilization procedures to treat anterior glenohumeral instability is still in the process of

R. F. LaPrade and G. A. Brown: Department of Orthopaedic Surgery, Sports Medicine Division, University of Minnesota, Minneapolis, Minnesota 55455.

evolving. As longer follow-up has been obtained on arthroscopic anterior glenohumeral–stabilization procedures, it has become apparent that the rates of recurrent instability after arthroscopic procedures are much higher than those after open procedures (see Published Results section). Koss et al. (1) reported a 30% recurrence rate with an arthroscopic suture anchor technique in 27 patients with an average follow-up of 40 months. They found that patients with five or fewer dislocations before surgery and patients who did not participate in contact sports were better candidates for arthroscopic stabilization. Green et al. (2) found an overall failure rate of 42% in 47 patients with 2 to 5 years of follow-up by using the transglenoid suture repair technique. They found that patients with simple detachment of the glenoid labrum had a 4.5% failure rate, whereas those with significant degeneration of the glenoid labrum–inferior glenohumeral ligament complex had an 87% failure rate. Mologne et al. (3) reported that 41% of 41 patients with an arthroscopic transglenoid suture repair technique had recurrent instability at a mean follow-up of 30 months. In their study, it was reported that the recurrence rate was lower in patients with 6 weeks of postoperative immobilization and that the transglenoid pin technique jeopardized the suprascapular nerve. Mologne et al. (3) also analyzed the results of failure of arthroscopic stabilization procedures in a series of 20 patients and found that 40% had recurrent Bankart lesions and 75% had redundant anterior capsules. The patients with capsular laxity were noted to have more problems with recurrent postoperative subluxation events rather than with frank dislocations. It is apparent from reviewing the results of these series that proper patient selection is important preoperatively in making the decision to proceed with an open anterior glenohumeral–instability procedure as opposed to an arthroscopic stabilization procedure in most patients. It is generally recommended that open stabilization procedures be considered as the primary surgery for patients who participate in contact sports, have a history of recurrent anterior glenohumeral instability, or appear to have capsular redundancy clinically.

Athletes with recurrent symptomatic anterior glenohumeral subluxation (4) that has proven to be nonresponsive to an extensive rehabilitation program may be candidates for an open anterior-stabilization procedure. It should be emphasized that the vast majority of patients with this clinical problem will respond to a well-managed rehabilitation program. However, for those overhead-throwing athletes who did not respond to this program over a period of 6 to 9 months or more, an open anterior glenohumeral stabilization procedure may be indicated. Whereas the role of lasers and other means of capsular shrinkage procedures have been promoted recently, we believe that further basic-science and clinical-outcome studies are necessary to determine whether this form of treatment provides acceptable long-term functional results.

CONTRAINDICATIONS

Contraindications and relative contraindications to open anterior glenohumeral reconstruction are as follows:

Absolute Contraindications:

1. Psychiatric voluntary dislocators
2. Advanced glenohumeral arthritis
3. Paralysis of extremity

Relative Contraindications:

1. Multidirectional instability
2. Large Hill-Sachs lesions

Fortunately, most of the contraindications to an open glenohumeral reconstruction can be recognized by an appropriate history, clinical examination, and plain radiographic work-up. Patients with voluntary shoulder instability should be carefully evaluated to determine whether they have any associated psychological or emotional problems. Patients who are voluntary dislocators with psychiatric disorders should not be considered to be surgical candidates. Another contraindication to an open anterior glenohumeral reconstruction is advanced glenohumeral arthritis. Patients with this condition should be recognized by decreased internal rotation on their physical examination and the presence of degenerative changes on their plain radiographs. Patients with shoulder instability due to paralysis are also not candidates for an open anterior reconstruction. These patients need a careful work-up of the cause of their paralysis, if necessary, to determine whether it is a reversible or permanent condition (syrinx). Patients with instability of their shoulder due to permanent paralysis should be evaluated for a possible glenohumeral arthrodesis, rather than an open instability procedure, to improve their function. Patients with evidence of multidirectional instability can be recognized by a careful assessment of their posterior apprehension test, sulcus sign, and the amount of posterior translation on the load-and-shift test. Multidirectional instability should be considered to be a relative contraindication to an anterior-stabilization procedure. These patients should first be enrolled in an extensive shoulder-rehabilitation program and monitored over a long period to make sure that their symptoms remain consistent and they have no evidence of voluntary dislocations related to a psychiatric condition. Only after failure of an extensive trial of physical therapy over 9 to 12 months should these patients be considered to be surgical candidates. Patients with a large Hill-Sachs lesion contributing to anterior instability may need either a bone-grafting procedure in addition to their anterior capsulolabral reconstruction or may be candidates for a glenohumeral arthroplasty procedure. Patients with this condition can be properly evaluated preoperatively with plain radiographs [an anteroposterior (AP) view in internal rotation and an axillary view] or a CT scan (if necessary) to supplement their clinical examination.

TECHNIQUES OF OPEN ANTERIOR GLENOHUMERAL–INSTABILITY RECONSTRUCTION

Anterior/Capsular Exposure and Arthrotomy Techniques

A common anterior approach to the glenohumeral joint can be followed in the majority of anterior shoulder-stabilization procedures. In our description of techniques for an open anterior reconstruction, our positions are in reference to a right shoulder and should be reversed for left shoulder anterior reconstructions. A vertical skin incision is made extending over the anterior midaxillary crease in line with the coracoid (Fig. 1). The length of the incision depends somewhat on the size of the patient. Larger patients may require a slightly longer incision to allow adequate soft-tissue retraction to gain access to the anterior capsule and capsulolabral complex. The incision will be more cosmetic the lower it is placed along the anterior midaxillary crease. Sharp dissection should be performed down to the delto-pectoral fascia to develop the relatively avascular skin flaps in this area. The deltopectoral interval is developed, and the cephalic vein is retracted laterally with the deltoid muscle fibers. The clavipectoral fascia is then incised along the lateral border of the conjoined tendon and the coracobrachialis muscle fibers. The conjoined tendon and associated coracobrachialis muscle fibers are then retracted medially, and the arm is externally rotated to expose the subscapularis tendon. The inferior edge of the subscapularis tendon is readily identified, as it is well defined anatomically by a series of three to four relatively horizontal small blood vessels.

Our preferred method of dividing the subscapularis tendon to gain exposure to the anterior glenohumeral capsule is to dissect the superior 80% of the tendon from the capsule with a vertical incision 1 cm from the bicipital groove and to leave the inferior portion of the tendon with its vessels intact (Fig. 2A). Excellent exposure can be obtained with this method, and leaving the inferior portion of the subscapularis tendon intact allows extra protection of the axillary nerve. The superior portion of the subscapularis tendon is dissected free with a needle-tipped electrocautery, and stay sutures are placed at the medial edges of the incised tendon to aid in retraction and dissection of the tendon from the capsule. Attempts are made to dissect the majority of the subscapularis tendon off the capsule. In the majority of patients, it is usually easier to gain access to the correct tissue plane by finding the tendon–capsular interval off the medial extent of the inferior horizontal extension of the subscapularis takedown incision near the musculotendinous junction. A small blunt, curved periosteal elevator is an excellent tool to develop this tissue plane and can be used to retract the more lateral aspect of the subscapularis tendon away from the capsule during dissection with the fine-tipped electrocautery. Once the subscapularis tendon has been dissected free of the capsule, a careful examination of the anterior capsule can be performed.

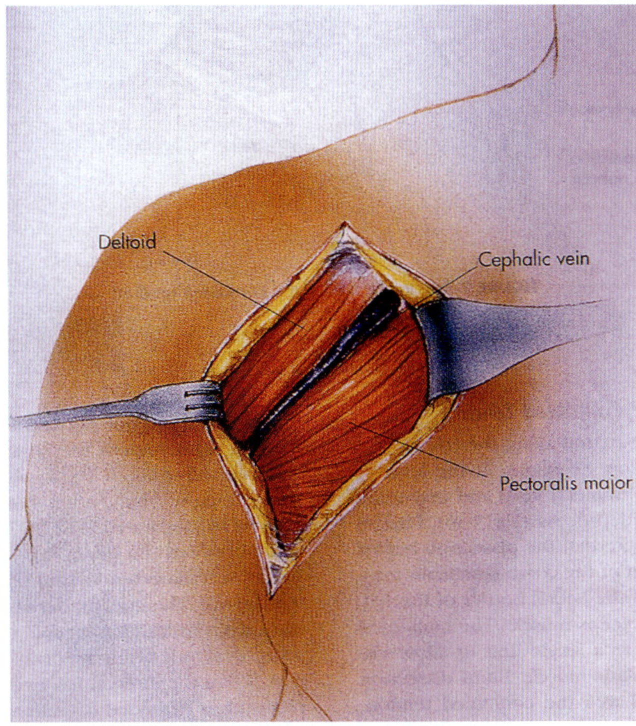

FIG. 1. Skin incision for an open anterior shoulder reconstruction. (From Jobe FW. *Operative techniques in upper extremity sports injuries.* St. Louis: Mosby, 1996, with permission.)

Jobe et al. (5) described a technique for a longitudinal split of the subscapularis tendon at the interval of the lower third and upper two thirds of the tendon (Fig. 2B). Dissection of the capsule from the subscapularis tendon is initiated medially within the muscular portion of the subscapularis and then extended laterally. Special modified Gelpi retractors are necessary to provide adequate retraction of the subscapularis with this technique. The technique of Jobe et al. is especially useful in throwing athletes, as it allows a more rapid early rehabilitation protocol for the subscapularis muscle.

Once the subscapularis tendon has been dissected from the anterior capsule, the rotator interval is then assessed. The rotator interval is the normal interval between the supraspinatus tendon and the subscapularis tendon, which occurs because the coracoid process of the scapula is located between these two structures. As Plancher et al. (6) showed from their anatomic studies, the anterior glenohumeral capsule in the region of the rotator interval is very thin (but always present). A capsular defect can be easily created in the rotator interval during the course of attempting to develop the tissue plane between the subscapularis tendon and the anterior capsule. If the capsule of the rotator interval has been violated and the capsule is noted

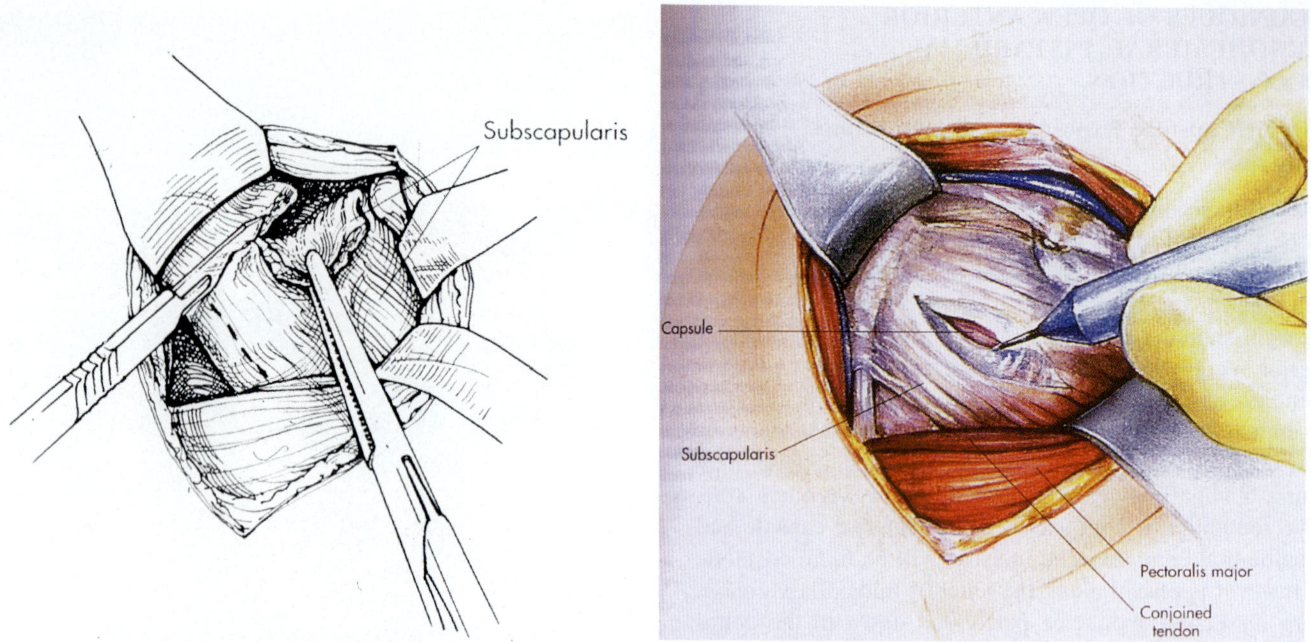

A B

FIG. 2. Retraction of subscapularis tendon. **A:** Dissection of superior 80% from capsule. **B:** Subscapularis-splitting incision. (From Jobe FW. *Operative techniques in upper extremity sports injuries.* St. Louis: Mosby, 1996, with permission.)

to be very redundant, either the rotator-interval defect can be repaired side-to-side or an inverted humerus-based L-capsular incision can be performed at this point, extending medially to the glenoid rim (Fig. 3). An assessment of the glenoid labrum and glenohumeral ligaments can then be performed.

After exposure of the anterior glenohumeral capsule, it is important to make certain that the capsule has been exposed adequately in its inferior aspect so that an accurate assessment of the amount of capsular redundancy can be performed. The axillary nerve is identified either grossly or by direct palpation. With care being taken to protect the axillary nerve, a small, curved periosteal elevator can be used bluntly to dissect the capsule away from the remaining subscapularis tendon and the axillary pouch tissues. The anterior capsule should be dissected down to at least the 6 o'clock position to allow proper evaluation of the laxity of the anterior glenohumeral capsule. In those cases in which

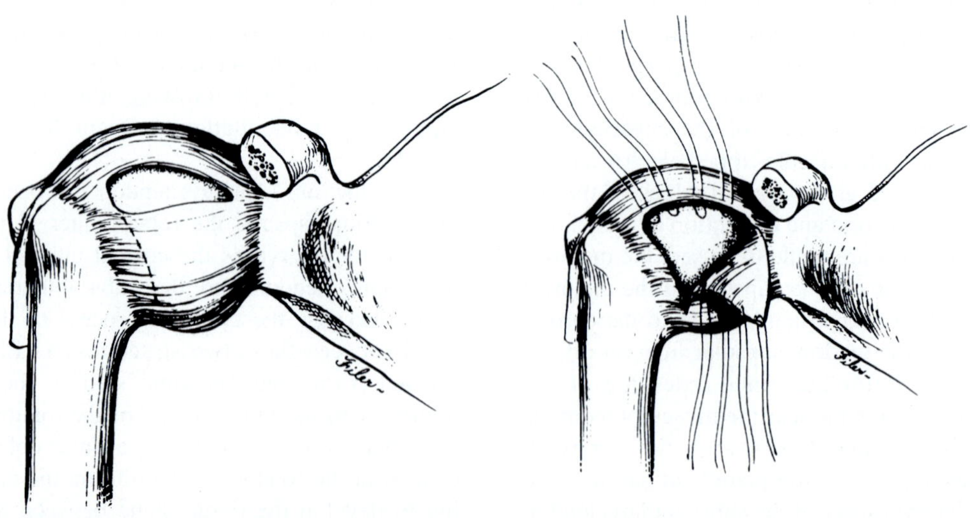

FIG. 3. Method of anterior capsular approach in a patient with a rotator-interval defect. (From Warner JP, Johnson D, Miller M, Caborn DN. Technique for selecting capsular tightness in repair of anterior-inferior shoulder instability. *J Shoulder Elbow Surg* 1995;4:352–364, with permission.)

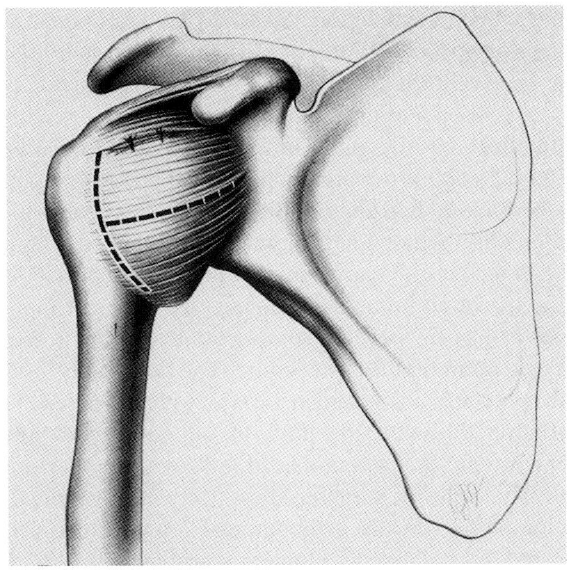

FIG. 4. Method of anterior capsular approach for a humerus-based T-capsular incision. (From Neer CS. *Shoulder reconstruction.* Philadelphia: WB Saunders, 1990, with permission.)

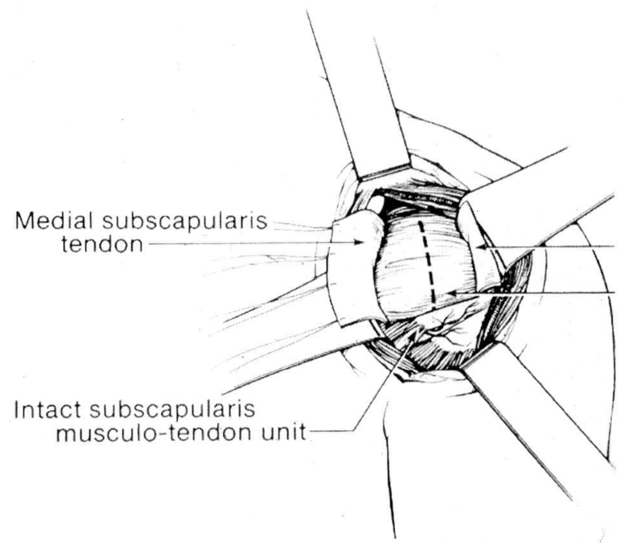

FIG. 6. Method of anterior capsular approach for a vertical midcapsular-splitting incision. (From Rockwood CA, Matsen FA. *The shoulder.* Philadelphia: WB Saunders, 1990, with permission.)

the surgeon chooses to take down the entire subscapularis tendon from the anterior capsule, it is essential to identify the axillary nerve to protect it from injury during exposure of the inferior capsule.

Once the anterior capsule has been adequately exposed, it can be incised in one of four ways. Our preferred method is a humerus-based T-capsular incision with the horizontal portion of the incision ending at the midportion of the anterior glenoid rim (Fig. 4). The vertical portion of the incision is located just medial to the lateral attachment of the capsule on the humerus and is extended distally to approximately the 6 or 7 o'clock position on the neck of the humerus. A glenoid-based T-capsular incision also can be used, with the vertical portion of the incision based 5 mm lateral to the anterior glenoid rim (Fig. 5). The horizontal limb of the incision extends to the lateral attachment of the anterior capsule on the humerus. Wirth et al. (7) also described making a midcapsular vertical incision to gain access to the glenohumeral joint (Fig. 6). Jobe et al. (5) also described a horizontal capsular incision completed along the midanterior glenoid rim at about the 4 o'clock position in line with their subscapularis tendon–splitting incision (Fig. 2B). In this approach, it is important not to incise the anterior labrum as part of the horizontal capsular incision and to extend the incision only to the lateral edge of the anterior glenoid labrum. Jobe et al. (5) noted that it is es-

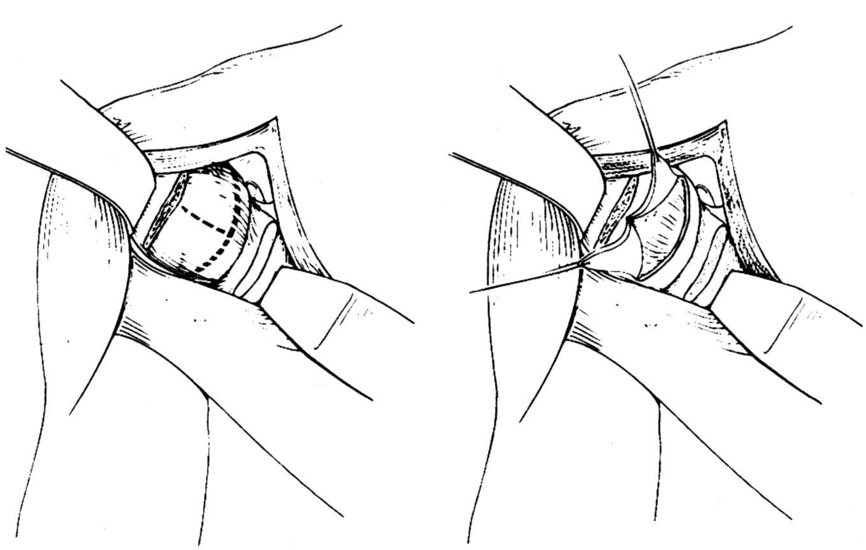

A B

FIG. 5. A, B: Method of anterior capsular approach for a glenoid-based T-capsular incision. (From Crenshaw AH. *Campbell's operative orthopaedics.* 8th ed. St. Louis: Mosby, 1992, with permission.)

pecially important in patients with a redundant anterior capsule not to drift superior or inferior along the glenoid when making this incision.

After the anterior capsulotomy incision has been made, a humeral-head retractor is inserted, and the humeral head is gently retracted laterally. A glenoid-rim pitchfork retractor can then be placed to evaluate the integrity of the anterior glenoid rim and glenoid labrum.

Bankart Lesion Repairs

The majority of patients with an initial traumatic or recurrent anterior glenohumeral dislocation have either a soft-tissue or bony Bankart lesion (8). Although it is not the sole cause of recurrent instability (9), it is an essential anatomic lesion to repair in patients to prevent a recurrence of instability.

The diagnosis of a Bankart lesion is made either preoperatively with a magnetic resonance imaging (MRI) scan with gadolinium (Fig. 7), during the diagnostic arthroscopy, or at the time of open stabilization. We do not routinely obtain MRI scans in everyone with anterior glenohumeral instability and tend to reserve it for our athletic or overhead-throwing population. In our institutions, we have found MRI scans without gadolinium to be inaccurate in the diagnosis of Bankart or other labral tears. We routinely perform a diagnostic arthroscopy before an open anterior-stabilization procedure to assess the entire glenohumeral joint. The arthroscopy is performed in the beach-chair position with the patient stabilized with the use of an inflatable beanbag. We have not found it necessary to use a special operating table to perform the arthroscopic portion of this procedure. The beanbag is inflated after the patient is positioned in the beach-chair position. During inflation, the anesthetist holds the superior portion of the beanbag around the patient's head to provide support intraoperatively, while the surgeon adjusts the beanbag around the posterior portion of the glenohumeral joint so that arthroscopic access is allowed without any problems. In addition, if the patient must be positioned more laterally after the beanbag has been inflated, the whole beanbag can be shifted laterally with the patient remaining securely fixed in position.

A

B

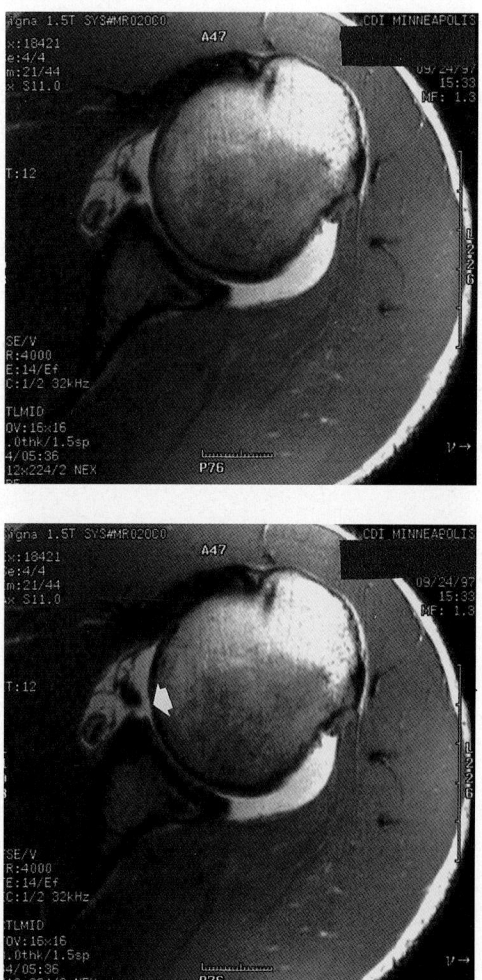

FIG. 7. A, B: Magnetic resonance imaging scan of a left glenohumeral joint demonstrating a soft-tissue Bankart lesion (gadolinium enhanced).

The key to the technique of Bankart lesion repairs is to recreate the anterior buffer of the native anterior capsulolabral complex on the glenoid. The most important factor in this portion of the reconstruction is to make sure that the repair is performed as far laterally on the glenoid neck as possible, preferably at the junction of the articular surface of the glenoid with the glenoid neck. Repairs that are placed medial to this junction with the articular surface are at an increased risk of failure because of an inability to prevent anterior humeral subluxation on the glenoid.

The surgical approach for the Bankart repair is the same as described previously for the anterior approach. After the capsular incision has been performed, a humeral-head retractor is carefully placed intra-articularly to allow easier exposure of the anterior capsulolabral complex. Once the anterior capsulolabral complex has been exposed, and it is verified that a Bankart lesion is present, a small, sharp, hand-held osteotome is used to elevate the remaining tissue medially off the anterior glenoid rim to create a bleeding bony surface. Three-pronged glenoid retractors are then inserted to expose the anterior glenoid rim. Further decortication of the anterior glenoid rim may then be performed with an osteotome or a curette if necessary.

Once the capsulolabral complex has been stripped medially off the anterior glenoid rim, and visualization of the anterior glenoid rim is adequate, two methods of repair of the Bankart lesion may be used. Our preferred method is to use Mitek suture anchors (Mitek Products, Westwood, MA, U.S.A.) loaded with a No. 2 Ethibond suture (Ethicon, Inc., Somerville, NJ, U.S.A.) and placed at the articular margin of the anterior glenoid rim. Usually between three and four suture anchors can be used to perform this portion of the repair from approximately the 2 o'clock to the 6 o'clock position on the anterior glenoid rim (Fig. 8). An alternate method to perform the repair of the Bankart lesion

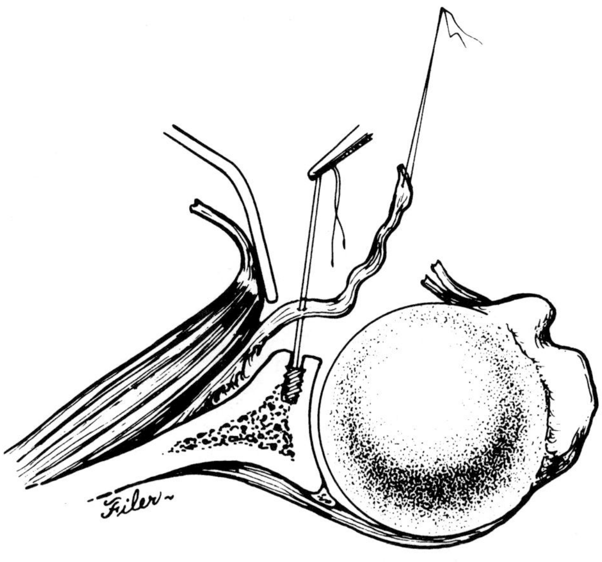

FIG. 8. Method of repair of Bankart lesion with suture anchors to the anterior rim. (From Warner JP, Johnson D, Miller M, Caborn DN. Technique for selecting capsular tightness in repair of anterior-inferior shoulder instability. *J Shoulder Elbow Surg* 1995;4:352–364, with permission.)

is to repair it back to the anterior glenoid rim through drill holes (Fig. 9). This technique is more tedious because of the difficulty in developing the drill holes, especially in larger patients. In either technique, the most important factor is to restore the normal anterior buffer of the capsulolabral complex by placing the repaired Bankart lesion as far laterally on the anterior glenoid rim as possible.

Once the suture anchors have been placed, the sutures are brought out anteriorly through the capsule from inside to outside and tied over the capsule. It is important in this step to make sure that the sutures come out medially when they pass through the anterior capsule. No attempt should be made to shift the capsule at this time. If the sutures pass from the inside to outside along the lateral aspect of the capsule, a loss of external rotation could occur, or the capsular repair may be too tight as the capsule is tightened too much in a medial to lateral direction. After the Bankart lesion has been repaired, an assessment of the amount of anterior capsular tightening can then be performed.

Adjusting Tension of the Capsule

Addressing the issue of the proper amount of capsular tightness is very important. Patients who do not have enough of the redundant capsule tightened may have recurrent glenohumeral subluxation or dislocation, whereas patients who have too much capsular tightness can have a loss of external rotation or posterior subluxation of the humeral head. Preservation of external rotation is especially important in the throwing athlete, in whom preservation of normal external rotation may mean the difference between a successful result and failure. Addressing the amount of capsular tightening will follow the surgical repair of the Bankart lesion or may be the essential step in those patients without a Bankart lesion at the time of exploration of the anterior glenoid labrum. In these latter patients, it is especially important to assess the amount of capsular redundancy and whether they may have a humerus-based capsular-avulsion lesion that also may require repair.

Arm position at the time of capsular closure is very important in determining the amount of tension on the capsule. Jobe et al. (5) emphasized the importance of not making the capsular repair too tight and of checking capsular repair by putting the shoulder through 90 degrees of abduction, 45 degrees of external rotation, and 30 degrees of forward flexion intraoperatively. Altchek et al. (10) reported that they performed their capsular repair with the shoulder in 45 degrees of abduction and external rotation. They verified that their repair was not too tight by making sure that they could achieve at least 30 to 40 degrees of external rotation with the arm at the patient's side intraoperatively.

Warner et al. (11) conducted a survey in which 80% of the members of the American Shoulder and Elbow Surgeons responded about their technique of capsular closure and arm position. The most common responses for arm position were flexion, 0 degrees; abduction, 30 degrees; and external rotation, 30 degrees. In addition to this survey, Warner et al. (11) also reported on a technique of selective capsular repair that they thought was useful in attempting to gauge the amount of capsular tightening necessary for patients with capsular injury or laxity. With a humerus-based T-capsular incision, they repaired the inferior leaf of the capsule first with the shoulder in 10 degrees of forward flexion, 60 to 80 degrees of abduction, and 45 to 60 degrees

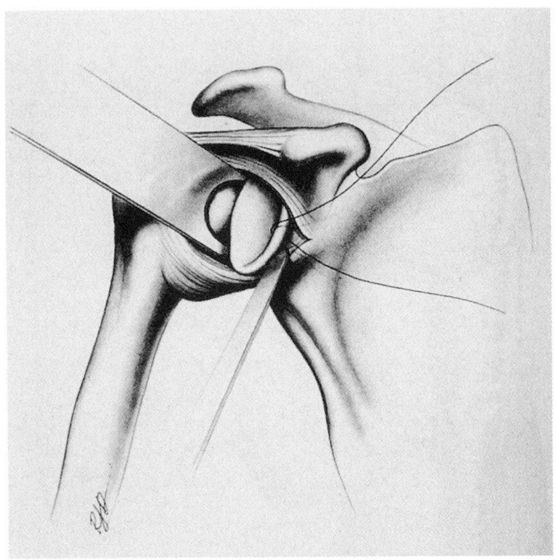

FIG. 9. Method of repair of Bankart lesion through drill holes in the anterior glenoid rim. (From Neer CS. *Shoulder reconstruction.* Philadelphia: WB Saunders, 1990, with permission.)

of external rotation (Fig. 10A). The superior capsular flap was then repaired to the inferior flap in a pants-over-vest technique with the shoulder in 0 degrees of abduction and 45 degrees of external rotation (Fig. 10B). They then checked the tightness of their repair by verifying that they could intraoperatively achieve 90 degrees of abduction of the shoulder in the scapular plane and 60 degrees of external rotation before the capsular repair became tight. They reported that the 18 patients repaired by using this technique had minimal loss of external rotation with no recurrences of instability after an average follow-up of 27 months.

It is recommended that each patient be assessed for capsular laxity after repair of an intra-articular Bankart lesion, especially in those patients with multiple recurrent episodes of anterior glenohumeral instability. Our preferred arm position at the time of a humerus-based T-capsular closure is 0 to 10 degrees of forward flexion, 20 to 30 degrees of abduction, and 45 degrees of external rotation. The inferior capsular leaf is repaired first by suturing it to the humerus-based stump of the remaining capsular edge. All attempts are made at this point to reduce capsular laxity. The superior capsular leaf is then advanced over the inferior leaf in a pants-over-vest manner and imbricated to the inferior leaf and remaining edge of the capsule on the humerus (Fig. 11). We then verify the security of our suture repair by

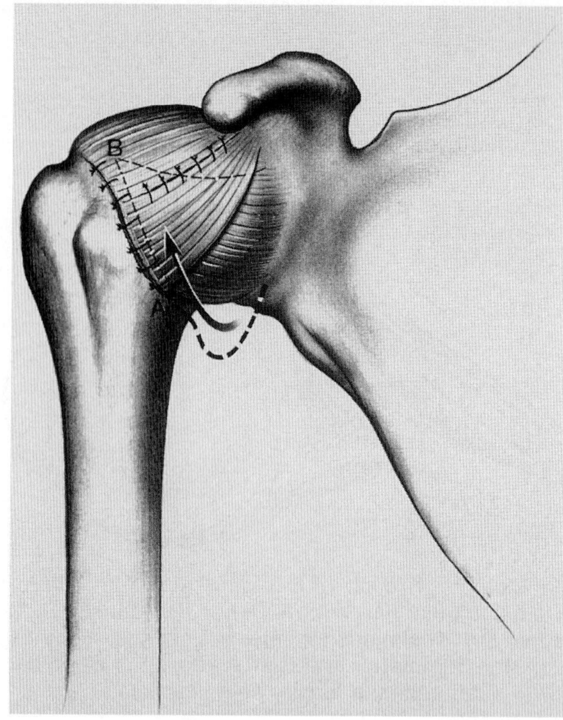

FIG. 11. Method of modified capsular shift after Bankart repair or for an anteroinferior capsular shift. (From Neer CS. *Shoulder reconstruction.* Philadelphia: WB Saunders, 1990, with permission.)

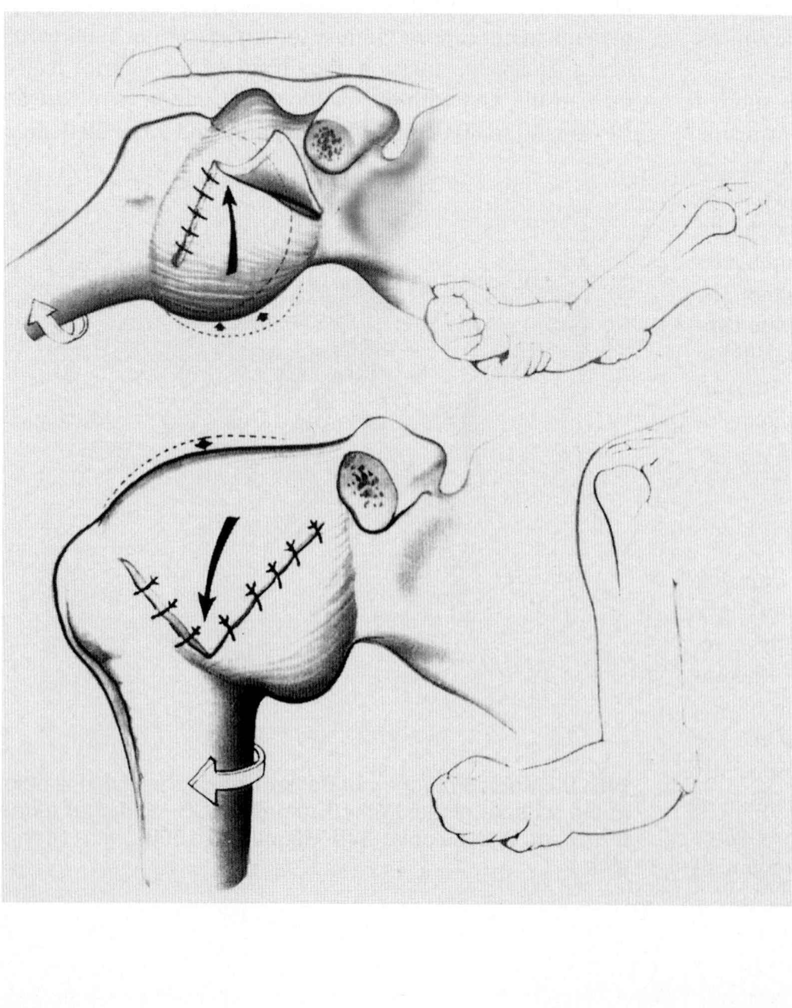

A

B

FIG. 10. Method of selective capsular repair. **A:** Repair of inferior leaf. **B:** Repair of superior capsular flap. (From Warner JP, Johnson D, Miller M, Caborn DN. Technique for selecting capsular tightness in repair of anterior-inferior shoulder instability. *J Shoulder Elbow Surg* 1995;4:352–364, with permission.)

verifying that full forward elevation of the glenohumeral joint can be achieved intraoperatively after each leaf of the capsular repair on the humerus has been secured. If there is any doubt about whether the repair is too tight or too loose, the sutures are removed and replaced to attempt to achieve the desired amount of capsular plication within the desired amounts of glenohumeral motion. If there is a concern about whether the sutures will hold the repair adequately in the initial postoperative period, soft-tissue suture anchors are placed in the humerus to supplement the soft-tissue repair.

Indications for a Bone Block

Patients with a previous anterior glenoid rim fracture or chronic erosion of the anterior glenoid rim due to recurrent anterior glenohumeral dislocations may need an anterior bone-block procedure to prevent recurrent anterior instability. In these patients, strong consideration should be given to performing a modified Bristow procedure (12), in which the transferred coracoid process will provide a bone-block effect to prevent anterior subluxation of the humerus on the glenoid.

The surgical approach to the anterior aspect of the glenohumeral joint is the same initially as for the previously mentioned procedures until the clavipectoral fascia has been exposed. The coracoid process is then exposed and may be predrilled with a 3.2-mm AO drill bit. The coracoid is then osteotomized with the conjoined tendons of the coracobrachialis and the short head of the biceps brachii and a 1- to 2-cm wedge of bone. It is important at this point to protect the musculocutaneous nerve where it penetrates the coracobrachialis muscle just distal to the coracoid tip during mobilization of the conjoined tendons. The arm is externally rotated to expose the subscapularis tendon, and a horizontal splitting incision is made through the subscapularis tendon and anterior glenohumeral capsule at approximately the 4 o'clock position (at the junction of the mid to lower third of the subscapularis tendon). The anterior glenoid neck is then exposed subperiosteally, and a 3.2-mm drill is used to drill a bicortical hole at the anteroinferior portion of the glenoid neck. A 4.5-mm cortical or malleolar screw can then be used to fix the coracoid tip with its tendinous attachments to the anterior glenoid (Fig. 12). The capsular incision is closed side-to-side at this point. It is important to check that there is no bony overhang of the transferred coracoid tip into the glenohumeral joint, or impingement could occur.

The Bristow procedure does not address the issue of capsular laxity and does not restore normal anatomy. However, for those patients with a deficient anterior glenoid rim, it may be a useful procedure to prevent recurrent anterior glenohumeral instability.

COMPLICATIONS OF OPEN ANTERIOR GLENOHUMERAL RECONSTRUCTIONS

Recurrent dislocation, neurovascular injury, restricted motion, osteoarthritis, and hardware problems are the principal complications of the surgical treatment of anterior-shoulder instability. The reported rates of recurrent instability and loss of motion are included in Tables 1 and 2. The neurovascular injuries and hardware complications are combined with complications of infection, hematoma, coracoid fractures/nonunion, deep vein thrombosis/pulmonary embolus, and adhesive capsulitis to form Table 3. All series that included complications are tabulated here. Table 3 is subdivided into Bankart/capsular-shift procedures and bone-block procedures.

After coracoid fractures and nonunions, hardware complications are the second most common complication for bone-block procedures. There are multiple case reports and series describing screw complications related to the shoulder (64–67). The complications related to screws include screw fracture, screw migration, secondary arthrosis, and

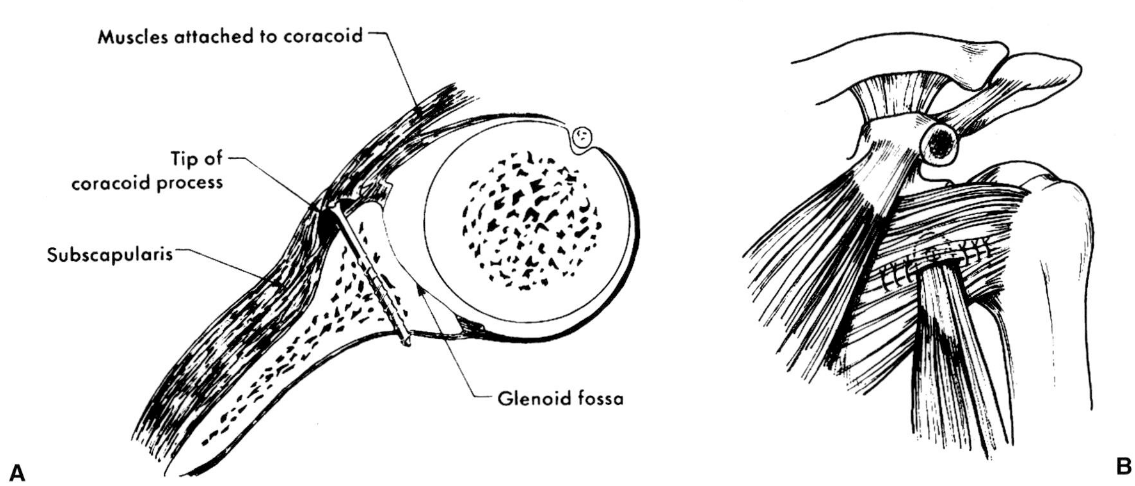

FIG. 12. A,B: Method of fixation of bone block to the anterior glenoid rim in the Bristow procedure. (From Crenshaw AH. *Campbell's operative orthopaedics.* 8th ed. St. Louis: Mosby, 1992, with permission.)

neurovascular injury. Given similar rates of instability recurrence after Bankart/capsular-shift procedures and bone-block procedures, the Bankart/capsular-shift procedures are recommended over the bone-block procedures because of a lower rate of hardware complications. Hawkins and Hawkins (68) concluded that screws and staples should be avoided near the shoulder joint in their review of failed anterior-shoulder instability reconstructions.

Glenohumeral arthrosis has been identified as a possible long-term result of Bankart and bone-block procedures for anterior-shoulder stabilization. Hindmarsh and Lindberg (39) examined the radiographic findings of 106 shoulders after an Eden–Hybbinette bone-block procedure with a mean follow-up of 102 months. They found 76 of 106 operative shoulders had moderate or severe radiographic changes of arthrosis compared with 10 of 104 control shoulders. They also noted that the radiographic findings did not correlate with subjective symptoms, and 19 of 22 shoulders with severe arthrosis had no or slight subjective symptoms. Rosenberg et al. (34) evaluated 33 shoulders for glenohumeral arthrosis after a Bankart reconstruction with a mean follow-up of 180 months. The radiographic changes were three moderate and one severe for 31 operative shoulders and two moderate for 27 nonsurgical shoulders. They found a statistically significant correlation between degenerative radiographic changes and restricted abduction/external rotation ($p = 0.004$) and length of follow-up ($p = 0.03$).

The prevalence of glenohumeral arthrosis after anterior-shoulder stabilization appears to be related to two other factors. First, untreated shoulder instability can result in glenohumeral arthrosis. Samilson and Prieto (69) described shoulder-dislocation arthropathy. In their series, 10 of 15 shoulders with severe glenohumeral arthrosis and six of 14 shoulders with moderate glenohumeral arthrosis were never treated surgically for the dislocations. Almost half the patients in the Hindmarsh and Lindberg series (39) had a 5-year interval from the first dislocation to surgery, and this may have resulted in dislocation arthropathy with degenerative changes. This would suggest that the surgical procedures are not necessarily the cause of the arthrosis. Second, loss of external rotation can result in glenohumeral arthrosis. Lusardi et al. (70) reviewed 20 shoulders with an average loss of external rotation of 11 degrees after anterior capsulorrhaphy for recurrent anterior instability. They concluded that severe loss of external rotation could result in posterior subluxation and glenohumeral arthrosis. They recommended an anterior-shoulder release if external rotation is limited to 0 degrees six months after surgery. In addition, it is recommended that a subscapularis-lengthening procedure be considered for all patients with a symptomatic loss of external rotation.

PUBLISHED RESULTS OF ANTERIOR GLENOHUMERAL RECONSTRUCTIONS

The compiled results from Bankart/modified Bankart procedures and capsular-shift procedures are tabulated in Table 1. The compiled results from Eden–Hybbinette and Bristow–Helfet–Laterjet bone-block procedures are tabulated in Table 2. The procedures are principally for recurrent anterior instability, but Neer and Foster (24), Loomer and Fraser (27), Altchek et al. (10), Cooper and Brems (32), Bigliani et al. (33), and Rosenberg et al. (34) included multidirectional instability (MDI) or anteroinferior instability or both in their series.

TABLE 1. *Published results of anterior*

Author (ref.)	Year	Procedure	Instability	Initial		Follow-up		Previous surgeries	Mean follow-up (mo)	Follow-up range (mo)
				Patients	Shoulders	Patients	Shoulders			
Bankart (13)	1938	Bankart	Ant	27	27	27	27	—	—	—
Bost and Inman (14)	1942	Modified Bankart	Ant	10	10	9	9	—	23	7–39
Robertson and Stark (15)	1947	Bankart	Ant	12	12	12	12	—	—	7–18
Adams (16)	1948	Bankart	Ant	—	—	—	18	—	—	>24
Eyre-Brook (17)	1948	Bankart	Ant	12	12	7	7	2	25	15–30
Dickson and Devas (18)	1957	Bankart	Ant	88	—	50	53	—	—	—
Rowe (19)	1963	Bankart	Ant	—	—	—	90	—	>120	—

The mean follow-up ranged from 22 to 180 months (15 years). Morrey and Janes (21) suggested that recurrence rates increase with time. They found that seven of the 20 dislocations occurred more than 24 months postoperatively, and longer follow-up times are needed to assess adequately the success of stabilization procedures.

The results were graded excellent, good, fair, or poor in many of the series. Most authors used the Bankart rating system developed by Rowe and Patel (22) for grading results. The Rowe rating system combines stability (50 points), motion (20 points), and function (30 points). The results are graded excellent (90 to 100 points), good (75 to 89 points), fair (51 to 74 points), or poor (50 or fewer points).

The recurrence rates varied from 0.0 to 13.3% for the Bankart and capsular-shift procedures and 0.0 to 20.0% for the bone-block procedures. The recurrences were subdivided as anterior dislocations, posterior dislocations, and subluxations. The recurrence rate was determined by calculating the total number of shoulders with anterior dislocations, posterior dislocations, and subluxations and dividing the total by the number of follow-up shoulders. This may result in a higher recurrence rate than that stated in the original article because posterior dislocations and subluxations were not included in the recurrence totals, or the total was divided by the initial number of patients or shoulders.

Hovelius et al. (63) performed a follow-up analysis of the Bristow–Laterjet bone-block procedure to determine which technical aspects of the procedure resulted in optimal results regarding recurrent dislocations. They had no redislocations in 40 patients with a fibrous or osseous coracoid union below the glenoid equator and within 1 cm of the glenoid rim. To ensure adequate union, they recommended avoiding coracoid-tip fracture and fixing the coracoid tip with a bicortical screw engaging the posterior cortex of the scapula.

Rowe et al. (71) reported a series of 39 patients with redislocation after unsuccessful anterior-shoulder stabilization surgical treatment. Thirty-two of the patients were treated with reoperation (25 Bankart, four Putti-Platt, and three modified capsular shifts); and 24 (92%) patients were graded excellent or good, and two (8%) patients had recurrent instability (dislocation and subluxation). They recommended revision stabilization in patients with recurrent anterior dislocation after surgical repair and attempts at rehabilitation had failed.

Loss of range of motion (ROM) has been reported in different manners in these series. The most common loss reported was external rotation (ER), but authors also included abduction (Abd), external rotation in 90 degrees of abduction (Abd/ER), forward elevation (FE), internal rotation (IR), and internal rotation in 90 degrees of abduction (Abd/IR). The results were reported as a range for all patients, percentage of patients within a range of lost motion, mean loss of motion (represented as ''mean'' in Tables 1 and 2), mean arc of motion (not loss of motion, represented as ''mean absolute'' in Tables 1 and 2), or median loss of motion.

Postoperative-strength changes are difficult to report. Wirth et al. (7) reported that 98% of traumatic recurrent instabilities treated with a capsular imbrication had normal (strength grade, five/five) or good (strength grade, four/five) strength compared with only 88% normal and good strength from the article on atraumatic recurrent instabilities treated with capsular imbrication. The strength was graded

glenohumeral reconstruction

Rating																				
Excellent		Good		Fair		Poor		Recurrence					ROM loss				Return to activities			
n	(%)	*n*	(%)	*n*	(%)	*n*	(%)	Ant	Post	Sublux	Total	(%)	Motion	(deg)	*n*	(%)	Activity	*n*	(%)	Total
—	—	—	—	—	—	—	—	0	0	0	0	0.0						—		
—	—	—	—	—	—	—	—	1	0	0	1	11.1								
—	—	—	—	—	—	—	—	0	0	0	0	0.0	ER	10–15						
													Abd	10–15						
—	—	—	—	—	—	—	—	1	0	0	1	5.6	ER	51	Mean absolute					
													Abd	166	Mean absolute					
—	—	—	—	—	—	—	—	0	0	0	0	0.0								
—	—	—	—	—	—	—	—	2	0	0	2	3.8	ER	<10	25	52.1				
													ER	20	9	18.8				
													ER	40	7	14.6				
													ER	60	6	12.5				
													ER	>60	1	2.1				
—	—	—	—	—	—	—	—	3	0	0	3	3.3								

TABLE 1.

Author (ref.)	Year	Procedure	Instability	Initial		Follow-up		Previous surgeries	Mean follow-up (mo)	Follow-up range (mo)
				Patients	Shoulders	Patients	Shoulders			
Werner and Reimers (20)	1972	Modified Bankart	Ant	—	93	—	77	—	94	—
Morrey and Janes (21)	1976	Bankart	Ant	—	—	11	12	—	—	—
Rowe et al. (22)	1978	Bankart	Ant	161	162	145	146	8	72	12–360
Hovelius et al. (23)	1979	Bankart	Ant	51	51	46	46	—	—	18–120
Neer and Foster (24)	1980	Inferior capsular shift	Inf/MDI	—	—	36	40	11	26	<12–72
Protzman (25)	1980	Lateral T capsulorrhaphy	Ant	—	97	89	89	—	37	12–69
Rowe and Zarins (26)	1981	Bankart	Ant	—	32	—	32	—	—	—
		Modified Bankart	Ant	—	18	—	18	—	—	—
				48	50	48	50	7	49	24–192
Loomer and Fraser (27)	1989	Modified Bankart/ capsular shift	Ant/Inf	—	—	30	30	—	38	34–58
Thomas and Matsen (28)	1989	Modified Bankart	Ant	61	63	37	39	—	66	26–136
Varmarken and Jensen (29)	1989	Bankart	Ant	31	31	23	23	—	48	12–180
Berg and Ellison (30)	1990	Modified Bankart	Ant	63	69	63	69	—	72	24–141
Altchek et al. (10)	1991	T-plasty modified Bankart	MDI	45	48	40	42	4	36	24–84
Jobe et al. (5)	1991	Anterior capsulolabral reconstruction	Ant	25	25	25	25	—	40	27–53
Richmond et al. (31)	1991	Modified Bankart with suture anchors	Ant	32	32	17	17	—	15	12–24
Cooper and Brems (32)	1992	Inferior capsular shift	MDI	43	48	38	43	25	39	24–71
Bigliani et al. (33)	1994	Inferior capsular shift	Ant/Inf	63	68	63	68	25	48	12–108
Rosenberg et al. (34)	1995	Modified Bankart	Ant/Inf	52	56	31	33	3	180	120–264
Wirth et al. (7)	1996	Capsular imbrication	Ant (traumatic)	—	—	106	108	65	—	—
			Ant (atraumatic)	—	—	32	34	45	—	—
			Ant (total)	178	182	138	142	110	60	24–244
Gill et al. (35)	1997	Modified Bankart	Ant	71	—	56	60	0	143	96–192

MDI, multidirectional instability; ROM, range of motion; ER, external rotation; IR, internal rotation; Abd, abduction; FE, forward elevation.

Continued

Rating								Recurrence					ROM loss				Return to activities			
Excellent		Good		Fair		Poor														
n	(%)	*n*	(%)	*n*	(%)	*n*	(%)	Ant	Post	Sublux	Total	(%)	Motion	(deg)	*n*	(%)	Activity	*n*	(%)	Total
—	—	—	—	—	—	—	—	5	0	0	5	6.5	ER	15–20	Mean					
—	—	—	—	—	—	—	—	0	0	0	0	0.0								
108	74	33	23	0	0	4	3	5	0	0	5	3.4	ER	0%	86	69.4	Throwing	10	33.3	30
													ER	<25%	30	24.2	Sports	75	97.4	77
													ER	>50%	8	6.5				
													FE	0%	86	69.4				
—	—	—	—	—	—	—	—	1	0	0	1	2.2	ER	0–5	2	9.5	Throwing	13	86.7	15
													ER	10–15	12	57.1				
													ER	20–25	3	14.3				
													ER	30–35	4	19.0				
													ER	16	Mean					
—	—	—	—	—	—	—	—	0	0	1	1	2.5								
—	—	—	—	—	—	—	—	1	0	7	8	9.0	ER	9	Mean					
													Abd/ER	12	Mean					
													Abd	7	Mean					
25	78	6	19	1	3	0	0	0	0	1	1	3.1								
10	56	6	33	2	11	0	0	0	0	0	0	0.0								
35	70	12	24	3	6	0	0	0	0	1	1	2.0					Throwing	21	63.6	33
																	Sports	41	85.4	48
13	43	12	40	1	3	4	13	4	0	0	4	13.3	ER	4	Mean		Sports	21	70.0	30
													Abd/ER	7	Mean					
													Abd	1	Mean					
													FE	2	Mean					
													IR	2 seg	Mean					
34	87	4	10	0	0	1	3	1	0	0	1	2.6	ER	68	Mean absolute		Work	35	89.7	39
													Abd/ER	84	Mean absolute					
													FE	171	Mean absolute					
—	—	—	—	—	—	—	—	3	0	0	3	13.0	ER	20	Median					
58	84	4	6	4	6	3	4	1	0	5	6	8.7	ER	5	Mean					
													Abd/ER	4	Mean					
—	—	—	—	—	—	—	—	0	1	3	4	9.5	ER	10	Mean		Throwing	0	0.0	3
													Abd/ER	10	Mean		Sports	33	82.5	40
17	68	6	24	1	4	1	4	0	0	0	0	0.0	ER	0	17	68.0	Throwing	18	72.0	25
14	82	2	12	0	0	1	6	1	0	0	1	5.9	ER	0						
—	—	—	—	—	—	—	—	3	1	0	4	9.3	ER	8	Mean		Sports	16	48.5	33
													FE	2	Mean		Work	29	67.4	43
													IR	2 seg	Mean					
42	67	17	27	2	3	2	3	2	0	0	2	2.9	ER	7	Mean		Throwing	5	50.0	10
													FE	175	Mean absolute		Sports	47	74.6	63
21	64	3	9	7	21	2	6	0	0	3	3	9.1	ER	18	Mean		Sports	26	83.9	31
													Abd/ER	15	Mean					
													FE	3	Mean					
													IR	1 seg	Mean					
103	95			4	4	1	1	0	0	1	1	0.9	ER	7	Mean		Sports	42	76.4	55
													FE	5	Mean		Work	98	90.7	108
													IR	2 seg	Mean					
29	85			3	9	2	6	1	0	1	2	5.9	ER	5	Mean		Sports	9	60.0	15
													FE	7	Mean		Work	29	85.3	34
													IR	1 seg	Mean					
132	93			7	5	3	2	1	0	2	3	2.1								
43	77	9	16	3	5	1	2	3	0	0	3	5.0	ER	12	Mean		Work	55	98.2	56
													Abd/ER	10	Mean					
													Abd	5	Mean					
													FE	5	Mean					
													IR	1 seg	Mean					

TABLE 2. *Compiled results*

Author (ref.)	Year	Procedure	Instability	Initial		Follow-up		Previous surgeries	Mean follow-up (mo)	Follow-up range (mo)
				Patients	Shoulders	Patients	Shoulders			
Speed (36)	1927	Speed	Ant	3	3	2	2	0	6	4–7
		Eden	Ant	4	5	4	5	0	45	22–60
Palmer and Widen (37)	1948	Hybbinette–Eden	Ant	—	90	60	60	—	—	18–144
Helfet (12)	1958	Bristow	Ant	—	—	30	30	—	—	—
Lavik (38)	1961	Eden–Hybbinette	Ant	21	22	21	22	2	—	20–120
Hindmarsh and Lindberg (39)	1967	Eden–Hybbinette	Ant	119	120	113	114	7	102	24–210
Bonnin (40)	1969	Bristow	Ant	—	16	—	16	—	—	—
May (41)	1970	Modified Bristow	Ant	22	22	16	16	—	>13	—
Solonen and Rokkanen (42)	1972	Eden–Hybbinette	Ant	—	51	—	40	—	90	—
		Eden–Hybbinette–Lange	Ant	—	33	—	25	—	84	—
Werner and Reimers (20)	1972	Hybbinette	Ant	—	22	—	15	—	131	—
Lindholm (43)	1974	Eden–Hybbinette	Ant	118	124	118	124	8	—	—
Halley and Olix (44)	1975	Bristow	Ant	27	31	21	24	—	—	—
Lombardo et al. (45)	1976	Modified Bristow	Ant	66	66	51	51	—	17	7–46
MacKenzie (46)	1980	Modified Bristow	Ant	21	21	16	16	6	22	9–38
Hill et al. (47)	1981	Modified Bristow	Ant	—	224	100	107	4	58	37–105
Nielsen and Nielsen (48)	1982	Modified Bristow	Ant	18	18	17	17	—	52	7–120
Bodey and Denham (49)	1983	Eden–Hybbinette	Ant	—	18	15	16	—	92	4–180
Hovelius et al. (50)	1983	Bristow–Latarjet	Ant	112	113	111	112	12	30	24–60
MacKenzie (51)	1984	Bristow	Ant	31	31	25	25	3	38	12–66
Paavolainen et al. (52)	1984	Eden–Hybbinette	Ant	—	48	—	41	—	—	—
Shively and Johnson (53)	1984	Modified Bristow	Ant	23	23	23	23	—	25	5–36
Shroder and Fristed (54)	1985	Modified Eden–Hybbinette	Ant	33	33	31	31	—	60	24–168
Carol et al. (55)	1985	Modified Bristow	Ant	49	52	44	47	0	44	8–113
Barry et al. (56)	1985	Modified Bristow	Ant	47	—	34	36	0	70	28–120
Braly and Tullos (57)	1985	Modified Bristow	Ant	28	—	20	20	1	43	12–74
Torg et al. (58)	1987	Modified Bristow	Ant	207	212	131	131	—	47	24–132
Gerber et al. (59)	1988	Trillat	Ant	52	57	48	52	—	69	36–120
Schauder and Tullos (60)	1992	Modified Bristow	Ant	33	—	19	20	1	55	38–83
Banas et al. (61)	1993	Modified Bristow	Ant	78	86	71	79	0	103	24–164
Singer et al. (62)	1995	Modified Bristow–Latarjet	Ant	17	17	14	14	—	246	240–270

Abd, abduction; ant, anterior; ER, external rotation; FE, forward elevation; IR, internal rotation; ROM, range of motion.

of reconstructions

Rating: Excellent n	(%)	Good n	(%)	Fair n	(%)	Poor n	(%)	Recurrence: Ant	Post	Sublux	Total	(%)	ROM loss: Motion	(deg)	n	(%)	Return to activities: Activity	n	(%)	Total
—	—	—	—	—	—	—	—	0	0	0	0	0.0								
—	—	—	—	—	—	—	—	0	0	1	1	20.0								
—	—	—	—	—	—	—	—	4	0	0	4	6.7								
—	—	—	—	—	—	—	—	2	1	0	3	10.0								
—	—	—	—	—	—	—	—	1	0	0	1	4.5								
57	50	41	36	13	11	3	3	2	0	0	2	1.8					Work	112	98.2	114
—	—	—	—	—	—	—	—	0	0	0	0	0.0								
—	—	—	—	—	—	—	—	0	0	0	0	0.0	ER	<15	16	100.0				
—	—	—	—	—	—	—	—	5	0	0	5	12.5	ER	0	13	43.3	Work	32	80.0	40
													Abd/ER	0	12	40.0				
													Abd	0	24	80.0				
													FE	0	25	83.3				
—	—	—	—	—	—	—	—	1	0	0	1	4.0	ER	0	9	40.9	Work	24	96.0	25
													Abd/ER	0	6	27.3				
													Abd	0	18	81.8				
													FE	0	16	72.7				
—	—	—	—	—	—	—	—	3	0	0	3	20.0	ER	5–10	Mean					
—	—	—	—	—	—	—	—	5	0	0	5	4.0								
—	—	—	—	—	—	—	—	1	0	0	1	4.2	ER	0	18	75.0	Throwing	4	44.4	9
													ER	<10	6	25.0	Sports	17	70.8	24
—	—	—	—	—	—	—	—	1	0	0	1	2.0	Abd/ER	11	Mean		Throwing	0	0.0	18
													Abd/IR	4	Mean					
—	—	—	—	—	—	—	—	0	0	1	1	6.3								
—	—	—	—	—	—	—	—	2	0	7	9	8.4	Abd/ER	13	Mean		Throwing	6	14.6	41
													Abd/IR	2	Mean		Tennis	10	33.3	30
—	—	—	—	—	—	—	—	0	0	0	0	0.0								
—	—	—	—	—	—	—	—	0	0	0	0	0.0	ER	0%	2	14.3				
													ER	25%	6	42.9				
													ER	50%	5	35.7				
													ER	60%	1	7.1				
70	63	31	28	8	7	3	3	7	0	8	15	13.4	ER	19	Mean					
													Abd/ER	21	Mean					
													IR	13	Mean					
													Abd/IR	2 seg	Mean					
—	—	—	—	—	—	—	—	0	0	1	1	4.0	ER	15–30						
30	73	7	17	3	7	1	2	3	0	0	3	7.3	ER	<10	21	51.2	Work	40	97.6	41
													ER	10–30	19	46.3				
													ER	31–50	1	2.4				
—	—	—	—	—	—	—	—	0	0	0	0	0.0	ER	13	Mean					
													IR	12	Mean					
—	—	—	—	—	—	—	—	3	0	2	5	16.1	ER	10	Median					
													Abd	3	Median					
													IR	0	Median					
29	62	12	26	5	11	1	2	0	0	1	1	2.1	ER	15	Mean		Work	42	95.5	44
													Abd/ER	12	Mean					
25	69	5	14	4	11	2	6	0	0	2	2	5.6	Abd/ER	10	Mean					
7	35	12	60	1	5	0	0	0	0	0	0	0.0	Abd/ER	10	Mean		Throwing	14	87.5	16
—	—	—	—	—	—	—	—	8	0	10	18	13.7	Abd/ER	15	Mean static D		Throwing	3	15.8	19
													Abd/ER	20	Mean static ND					
													Abd/ER	18	Mean dynamic D					
													Abd/ER	23	Mean dynamic ND					
—	72	—	9	—	10	—	9	2	0	0	2	3.8	Abd/ER	>30	31	62.0				
													ER	>30	23	46.0				
11	55	6	30	2	10	1	5	1	0	0	1	5.0	Abd/ER	5	Mean		Throwing	10	83.3	12
35	74	5	11	4	9	3	6	3	0	9	12	15.2	Abd/ER	9	Mean		Sports	42	67.7	62
													Abd/IR	5	Mean					
5	36	8	57	1	7	0	0	0	0	1	1	7.1	ER	52	Mean absolute					

TABLE 3. *Injuries*

Authors (ref.)	Year	Procedure	Number of procedures	Superficial infection	Deep infection	Hematoma	Thrombophlebitis
Bankart/capsular-shift procedures							
Werner and Reimers (20)	1972	Modified Bankart	93	1	—	—	—
Rowe et al. (22)	1978	Bankart	162	1	—	5	1
Neer and Foster (24)	1980	Inferior capsular shift	40	—	—	—	—
Rowe and Zarins (26)	1981	Bankart	50	0	0	1	1
Thomas and Matsen (28)	1989	Modified Bankart	63	1	—	—	—
Berg and Ellison (30)	1990	Modified Bankart	69	1	3	—	—
Altchek et al. (10)	1991	T-plasty modified Bankart	48	—	—	1	—
Cooper and Brems (32)	1992	Inferior capsular shift	48	0	0	—	—
Bigliani et al. (33)	1994	Inferior capsular shift	68	2	—	1	—
Bone-block procedures							
Helfet (12)	1958	Bristow	30	—	—	—	—
Hindmarsh and Lindberg (39)	1967	Eden–Hybbinette	120	1	—	—	—
May (41)	1970	Modified Bristow	22	0	0	—	—
Solonen and Rokkanen (42)	1972	Eden–Hybbinette	86	1	—	—	—
Halley and Olix (44)	1975	Bristow	31	1	—	—	—
Lombardo et al. (45)	1976	Modified Bristow	66	—	—	1	—
Hill et al. (47)	1981	Modified Bristow	224	1	1	1	—
Nielsen and Nielsen (48)	1982	Modified Bristow	18	—	—	—	—
Bodey and Denham (49)	1983	Eden–Hybbinette	18	—	0	—	—
Hovelius et al. (50)	1983	Bristow–Latarjet	113	3	0	—	—
Paavolainen et al. (52)	1984	Eden–Hybbinette	48	1	—	—	—
Shively and Johnson (53)	1984	Modified Bristow	23	1	—	—	—
Shroder and Fristed (54)	1985	Modified Eden–Hybbinette	33	1	—	—	—
Carol et al. (55)	1985	Modified Bristow	52	0	0	—	—
Barry et al. (56)	1985	Modified Bristow	47	—	—	—	—
Braly and Tullos (57)	1985	Modified Bristow	28	—	—	—	—
Torg et al. (58)	1987	Modified Bristow	212	—	1	—	—
Gerber et al. (59)	1988	Trillat	57	—	—	—	—
Schauder and Tullos (60)	1992	Modified Bristow	33	—	—	—	—
Banas et al. (61)	1993	Modified Bristow	86	—	—	1	—
Singer et al. (62)	1995	Modified Bristow–Latarjet	17	—	—	—	—

DVT, deep vein thrombosis.
[a] Subcoracoid impingement.

according to the American Shoulder and Elbow Surgeons (ASES) grading system (72). Regarding the Bristow–Helfet–Laterjet bone-block procedures, Hovelius et al. (50) found 10% to 13% strength reduction in the operated-on shoulder relative to the contralateral shoulder by using a dynamometer for abduction, abduction/external rotation, and abduction/internal rotation. Torg et al. (58) found a decrease in strength in abduction and extreme rotation (cocking) and the initiation of internal rotation (early acceleration) after a Bristow procedure by using Cybex testing compared with the contralateral shoulder. This partially explains the difficulty in returning to throwing, particularly after a Bristow procedure.

Because the Bristow procedure transposes the origin of the biceps short head from the coracoid tip to the anterior glenoid, Chen et al. (73) used dynamic electromyography (EMG) and Cybex testing to determine whether the Bristow procedure affected elbow-flexion strength. They found that there is a reduced dynamic response in the short head of the biceps brachii, but that there was increased activity in the long head of the biceps brachii and brachialis. This compensation for the short head of the biceps resulted in normal elbow function.

The functional outcomes of the procedures are represented by the patients' return to activities in Tables 1 and 2. The return to activities was divided into throwing, sports not restricted to throwing, and work. Whenever possible, successful return to activity was defined as returning to the preinjury level of activity. This definition is more restrictive than that used by some of the authors. For example, an athlete whose preinjury level was collegiate sports and postsurgical level of activity was recreational sports was not included as a successful return to sports, for purposes of this review, but may have been classified as a successful return to sports in some of the reviewed series. Not all articles provided sufficient information to determine the preinjury and postsurgical levels of activity, so those results are tabulated as reported in the articles.

Gartland (74) expressed concern that orthopedic clinical research focused too much attention on the procedures and technology and not on the functional outcome of the patient. The return-to-activity data provide the functional outcomes necessary to evaluate the procedures. The Bankart/capsular-shift procedures allowed 85.3% to 98.2% of the patients to return to work (excluding series with MDI;

and complications

Musculocutaneous injury	Axillary injury	Median injury	Ulnar injury	Radial injury	Total nerve injuries	Coracoid fracture/ nonunions	Screw problems	DVT or pulmonary embolism	Adhesive capsulitis
1	—	—	—	1	2	–	—	—	—
—	1	—	—	—	1	–/0	—	—	—
—	3	—	—	—	3	—	—	—	—
—	—	—	—	—	—	–/0	—	—	—
—	—	—	—	—	0	—	—	—	—
—	—	—	—	—	—	—	—	1	1
1	—	1	—	—	2	—	—	—	—
—	0	—	—	—	0	—	—	—	—
1	—	—	—	—	1	—	—	—	—
1	—	—	—	—	1	—	—	—	—
—	—	—	—	—	—	—	—	—	—
—	—	—	—	—	—	—	—	—	—
—	—	—	—	—	—	—	—	—	—
—	—	—	—	—	—	—	—	—	—
—	—	—	—	—	—	1/6	4	1	—
—	—	—	—	—	—	7/2	3	1	—
—	—	—	—	—	—	–/8	4	—	—
—	—	—	—	—	0	—	—	0	—
1	—	—	—	—	1	16/17	5	—	—
—	—	—	—	—	—	–/5	—	—	—
—	—	—	1	—	1	—	0	—	—
—	—	—	—	—	—	—	—	—	—
—	—	—	2	—	2	—	—	—	—
—	—	—	—	—	—	–/4	1	—	—
—	—	—	—	—	—	2/–	3	—	—
—	—	—	—	—	—	—	10	—	—
—	—	—	—	—	8[a]	—	—	—	—
—	—	—	—	—	—	–/0	0	—	—
2	—	—	—	—	2	–/1	8	—	—
—	—	—	—	—	—	—	0	—	—

32). The bone-block procedures allowed 80.0% to 96.0% of the patients to return to work. Future prospective studies will need to provide further analysis of patient satisfaction and functional outcome to provide sufficient data to determine the overall effectiveness of the different treatment options for open anterior glenohumeral stabilization procedures.

REFERENCES

1. Koss S, Richmond JC, Woodward JS. Two-to-five year follow-up of arthroscopic Bankart reconstruction using a suture anchor technique. *Am J Sports Med* 1997;25:809–812.
2. Green MR, Christensen KP. Arthroscopic Bankart procedure: two-to-five year followup with clinical correlation to severity of glenoid labral lesion. *Am J Sports Med* 1995;23:276–281.
3. Mologne TS, Lapoint JM, Morin WD, Zilberfarb J, O'Brien TJ. Arthroscopic anterior labral reconstruction using a transglenoid suture technique. *Am J Sports Med* 1996;24:268–274.
4. Garth WP, Allman FL, Armstrong WS. Occult anterior subluxation of the shoulder in noncontact sports. *Am J Sports Med* 1987;15:579–585.
5. Jobe FW, Giangarra CE, Kvitne RS, Glousman RE. Anterior capsulolabral reconstruction of the shoulder in athletes in overhead sports. *Am J Sports Med* 1991;19:428–434.
6. Plancher KD, Johnston J, Peterson R. Quantitative and qualitative dimensions of the rotator interval. *J Shoulder Elbow Surg* (in press).
7. Wirth MA, Blatter G, Rockwood CA Jr. The capsular imbrication procedure for recurrent anterior instability of the shoulder. *J Bone Joint Surg [Am]* 1996;78:246–259.
8. Baker CL, Uribe JW, Whitman C. Arthroscopic evaluation of acute initial anterior shoulder dislocations. *Am J Sports Med* 1990;18:25–28.
9. Speer KP, Deng X, Borrer S, Torzilli PA, Altchek DA, Warren RF. Biomechanical evaluation of a simulated Bankart lesion. *J Bone Joint Surg [Am]* 1994;76:1819–1826.
10. Altchek DW, Warren RF, Skyhar MJ, Ortiz G. T-Plasty modification of the Bankart procedure for multidirectional instability of the anterior and inferior types. *J Bone Joint Surg [Am]* 1991;73:105–112.
11. Warner JP, Johnson D, Miller M, Caborn DN. Technique for selecting capsular tightness in repair of anterior-inferior shoulder instability. *J Shoulder Elbow Surg* 1995;4:352–364.
12. Helfet AJ. Coracoid transplantation for recurring dislocation of the shoulder. *J Bone Joint Surg [Br]* 1958;40:198–202.
13. Bankart ASB. The pathology and treatment of recurrent dislocation of the shoulder-joint. *Br J Surg* 1938;26:23–29.
14. Bost FC, Inman VT. The pathological changes in recurrent dislocation of the shoulder: a report of Bankart's operative procedure. *J Bone Joint Surg* 1942;24:595–613.
15. Robertson R, Stark WJ. Diagnosis and treatment of recurrent dislocation of the shoulder. *J Bone Joint Surg* 1947;29:797–800.
16. Adams JC. Recurrent dislocation of the shoulder. *J Bone Joint Surg [Br]* 1948;30:26–38.
17. Eyre-Brook AL. Recurrent dislocation of the shoulder: lesions discovered in seventeen cases, surgery employed, and intermediate report on results. *J Bone Joint Surg [Br]* 1948;30:39–48.

18. Dickson JW, Devas MB. Bankart's operation for recurrent dislocation of the shoulder. *J Bone Joint Surg [Br]* 1957;39:114–119.
19. Rowe CR. The results of operative treatment of recurrent dislocations of the shoulder. *Surg Clin North Am* 1963;43:1667–1670.
20. Werner HH, Reimers J. The operative treatment of recurrent, anterior dislocation of the shoulder: a review of 151 operations. *Acta Orthop Scand* 1972;43:375–383.
21. Morrey BF, Janes JM. Recurrent anterior dislocation of the shoulder: long-term follow-up of the Putti-Platt and Bankart procedures. *J Bone Joint Surg [Am]* 1976;58:252–256.
22. Rowe CR, Patel D. The Bankart procedure: a long-term end-result study. *J Bone Joint Surg [Am]* 1978;60:1–16.
23. Hovelius L, Thorling J, Fredin H. Recurrent anterior dislocation of the shoulder: results after the Bankart and Putti-Platt operations. *J Bone Joint Surg [Am]* 1979;61:566–569.
24. Neer CS, Foster CR. Inferior capsular shift for involuntary inferior and multidirectional instability of the shoulder: a preliminary report. *J Bone Joint Surg [Am]* 1980;62:897–908.
25. Protzman RR. Anterior instability of the shoulder. *J Bone Joint Surg [Am]* 1980;62:909–918.
26. Rowe CR, Zarins B. Recurrent transient subluxation of the shoulder. *J Bone Joint Surg [Am]* 1981;63:863–872.
27. Loomer R, Fraser J. A modified Bankart procedure for recurrent anterior/inferior shoulder instability: a preliminary report. *Am J Sports Med* 1989;17:374–379.
28. Thomas SC, Matsen FA. An approach to the repair of avulsion of the glenohumeral ligaments in the management of traumatic anterior glenohumeral instability. *J Bone Joint Surg [Am]* 1989;71:506–513.
29. Varmarken J-E, Jensen CH. Recurrent anterior dislocation of the shoulder: a comparison of the results after the Bankart and the Putti-Platt procedures. *Orthopedics* 1989;12:453–455.
30. Berg EE, Ellison AE. The inside-out Bankart procedure. *Am J Sports Med* 1990;18:129–133.
31. Richmond JC, Donaldson WR, Fu F, Harner CD. Modification of the Bankart reconstruction with a suture anchor: report of a new technique. *Am J Sports Med* 1991;19:343–346.
32. Cooper RA, Brems JJ. The inferior capsular-shift procedure for multidirectional instability of the shoulder. *J Bone Joint Surg [Am]* 1992;74:1516–1521.
33. Bigliani LU, Kurzweil PR, Schwartzbach CC, Wolfe IN, Flatow EL. Inferior capsular shift procedure for anterior-inferior shoulder instability in athletes. *Am J Sports Med* 1994;22:578–584.
34. Rosenberg BN, Richmond JC, Levine WN. Long-term followup of Bankart reconstruction: incidence of late degenerative glenohumeral arthrosis. *Am J Sports Med* 1995;23:538–544.
35. Gill TJ, Micheli LJ, Gebhard F, Binder C. Bankart repair for anterior instability of the shoulder. *J Bone Joint Surg [Am]* 1997;79:850–857.
36. Speed K. Recurrent anterior dislocation at the shoulder: operative cure by bone graft. *Surg Gynecol Obstet* 1927;44:468–477.
37. Palmer I, Widen A. The bone block method for recurrent dislocation of the shoulder joint. *J Bone Joint Surg [Br]* 1948;30:53–58.
38. Lavik K. Habitual shoulder luxation. *Acta Orthop Scand* 1961;30: 251–264.
39. Hindmarsh J, Lindberg A. Eden-Hybbinette's operation for recurrent dislocation of the humero-scapular joint. *Acta Orthop Scand* 1967;38: 459–478.
40. Bonnin JG. Transplantation of the tip of the coracoid process for recurrent anterior dislocation of the shoulder. *J Bone Joint Surg [Br]* 1969;51:579.
41. May VR. A modified Bristow operation for anterior recurrent dislocation of the shoulder. *J Bone Joint Surg [Am]* 1970;52:1010–1016.
42. Solonen KA, Rokkanen P. The results of operative treatment for recurrent dislocation of the gleno-humeral joint. *Acta Orthop Scand* 1972;43:101–108.
43. Lindholm TS. Results of treatment for anterior recurrent dislocation of the shoulder joint with the Eden-Hybbinette operation. *Acta Orthop Scand* 1974;45:508–517.
44. Halley DK, Olix ML. A review of the bristow operation for recurrent anterior shoulder dislocation in athletes. *Clin Orthop* 1975;106:175–179.
45. Lombardo SJ, Kerlan RK, Jobe FW, Carter VS, Blazina ME, Shields CL. The modified Bristow procedure for recurrent dislocation of the shoulder. *J Bone Joint Surg [Am]* 1976;58:256–261.
46. MacKenzie DB. The Bristow-Helfet operation for recurrent anterior dislocation of the shoulder. *J Bone Joint Surg [Br]* 1980;62:273–274.
47. Hill JA, Lombardo SJ, Kerlan RK, et al. The modified Bristow-Helfet procedure for recurrent anterior shoulder subluxations and dislocations. *Am J Sports Med* 1981;9:283–287.
48. Nielsen AB, Nielsen K. The modified Bristow procedure for recurrent anterior dislocation of the shoulder: results and complications. *Acta Orthop Scand* 1982;53:229–232.
49. Bodey WN, Denham RA. A free bone block operation for recurrent anterior dislocation of the shoulder joint. *Injury* 1983;15:184–188.
50. Hovelius L, Akermark C, Albertsson B, et al. Bristow-Latarjet procedure for recurrent anterior dislocation of the shoulder: a 2-5 year follow-up study on the results of 112 cases. *Acta Orthop Scand* 1983;54:284–290.
51. MacKenzie DB. The treatment of recurrent anterior shoulder dislocation by the modified Bristow-Helfet procedure. *South Am Med J* 1984;65:325–330.
52. Paavolainen P, Bjorkenheim J-M, Ahovuo J, Slatis P. Recurrent anterior dislocation of the shoulder: results of Eden-Hybbinette and Putti-Platt operations. *Acta Orthop Scand* 1984;55:556–560.
53. Shively J, Johnson J. Results of modified Bristow procedure. *Clin Orthop* 1984;187:150–153.
54. Schroder HA, Fristed PB. Recurrent dislocation of the shoulder: the Alvik modification of the Eden-Hybbinette operation. *Acta Orthop Scand* 1985;56:396–399.
55. Carol EJ, Falke LM, Kortmann JOJPM, Roeffen JFW, Van Acker PAM. Bristow-Latarjet repair for recurrent anterior shoulder instability; an eight-year study. *Neth J Surg* 1985;37 (4):109–113.
56. Barry TP, Lombardo SJ, Kerlan RK, et al. The coracoid transfer for recurrent anterior instability of the shoulder in adolescents. *J Bone Joint Surg [Am]* 1985;67:383–387.
57. Braly WG, Tullos HS. A modification of the Bristow procedure for recurrent anterior shoulder dislocation and subluxation. *Am J Sports Med* 1985;13:81–86.
58. Torg JS, Balduini FC, Bonci C, et al. A modified Bristow-Helfet-May procedure for recurrent dislocation and subluxation of the shoulder: report of two hundred and twelve cases. *J Bone Joint Surg [Am]* 1987;69:904–913.
59. Gerber C, Terrier F, Ganz R. The Trillat procedure for recurrent anterior instability of the shoulder. *J Bone Joint Surg [Br]* 1988;70: 130–134.
60. Schauder KS, Tullos HS. Role of the coracoid bone block in the modified Bristow procedure. *Am J Sports Med* 1992;20:31–34.
61. Banas MP, Dalldorf PG, Sebastianelli WJ, DeHaven KE. Long-term follow-up of the modified Bristow procedure. *Am J Sports Med* 1993;21:666–671.
62. Singer GC, Kirkland PM, Emery RJH. Coracoid transposition for recurrent anterior instability of the shoulder: a 20-year follow-up study. *J Bone Joint Surg [Br]* 1995;77:73–76.
63. Hovelius L, Korner GL, Lundberg B, et al. The coracoid transfer for recurrent dislocation of the shoulder. *J Bone Joint Surg [Am]* 1983;65: 926–934.
64. Artz T, Huffer JM. A major complication of the modified Bristow procedure for recurrent dislocation of the shoulder: a case report. *J Bone Joint Surg [Am]* 1972;54:1293–1296.
65. Zuckerman JD, Matsen FA III. Complications about the glenohumeral joint related to the use of screws and staples. *J Bone Joint Surg [Am]* 1984;66:175–180.
66. Lower RF, McNiesh LM, Callaghan JJ. Computed tomographic documentation of intra-articular penetration of a screw after operations on the shoulder. *J Bone Joint Surg [Am]* 1985;67:1120–1122.
67. Stromqvist B, Wingstrand H, Egund N. Recurrent shoulder dislocation and screw failure after the Bristow-Latarjet procedure: a case report. *Arch Orthop Trauma Surg* 1987;106:260–262.
68. Hawkins RH, Hawkins RJ. Failed anterior reconstruction for shoulder instability. *J Bone Joint Surg [Br]* 1985;67:709–714.
69. Samilson RL, Prieto V. Dislocation arthropathy of the shoulder. *J Bone Joint Surg [Am]* 1983;65:456–460.
70. Lusardi DA, Wirth MA, Wurtz D, Rockwood CA Jr. Loss of external

rotation following anterior capsulorrhaphy of the shoulder. *J Bone Joint Surg [Am]* 1993;75:1185–1192.

71. Rowe CR, Zarins B, Ciullo JV. Recurrent anterior dislocation of the shoulder after surgical repair: apparent causes of failure and treatment. *J Bone Joint Surg [Am]* 1984;66:159–168.
72. Barrett WP, Franklin JL, Jackins SE, Wyss CR, Matsen FA III. Total shoulder arthroplasty. *J Bone Joint Surg [Am]* 1987;69:865–872.
73. Chen S-K, Perry J, Jobe FW, Healy BS, Radovich Moynes D. Elbow flexion analysis in Bristow patients: a preliminary report. *Am J Sports Med* 1984;12:347–350.
74. Gartland JJ. Orthopaedic clinical research: deficiencies in experimental design and determination of outcome. *J Bone Joint Surg* 1988; 70A:1357–1364.

The Unstable Shoulder,
edited by R.F. Warren, E.V. Craig, and D.W. Altchek.
Lippincott–Raven Publishers, Philadelphia © 1999.

CHAPTER 14

Special Considerations in the Treatment of Shoulder Instability in the Throwing Athlete

David W. Altchek and Peter T. Simonian

The art of pitching a baseball at a competitive level places extreme demands on the soft-tissue structures of the shoulder joint. These structures—the labrum, capsule, and tendons of the rotator cuff—all act in concert to stabilize the humeral head into the glenoid fossa. Injuries to any of these structures can lead to a loss of stability and resultant symptoms.

To understand shoulder injuries of this sort, one must accept a broad definition of instability, whereby instability is defined as a pathologic increase in glenohumeral translation that results in symptoms. In nonthrowing activities in which less rotational torque is placed across the shoulder joint, symptoms are produced only if a severe capsulolabral injury is present, as with patients with recurrent anterior subluxation dislocation. Throwers, however, place such high loads across the shoulder joint that even moderate injuries to any of the structures (rotator cuff tendons, capsule, or labrum) will often produce symptoms. The clinician must remember that the symptoms of instability in the thrower are usually more subtle than those in the nonthrower, consisting primarily of pain, occasionally dead-arm syndrome, and only rarely, actual episodes of subluxation.

This chapter reviews the pertinent biomechanics, as well as issues of the diagnosis and treatment of the unstable shoulder in the throwing athlete.

THE BIOMECHANICS OF THROWING

The art of throwing is a transfer of kinetic energy from the legs, through the hips, spine, shoulder, elbow, and wrist. Throughout the throw, the arm is maintained at approximately 100 degrees of abduction. In the horizontal plane, the arm moves from 30 degrees of abduction at maximal cocking to 10 degrees adduction at follow-through. The act of accelerating the ball occurs at astonishing speed as the arm goes from a maximum of 175 degrees of external rotation to completion of the throw at 105 degrees of internal rotation. Andrews and Dillman (1–3) estimated this speed at 7,000 degrees/second, with the torque estimated at 52 Nm. When analyzed further, it appears that during the cocking phase, the humeral head experiences a force of anterior translation measured to be 40% of body weight, whereas the follow-through phase creates a distraction force of 80% of body weight. These translation forces about the glenohumeral joint are resisted by the labrum, capsular ligaments, and rotator cuff muscle–tendon units.

To better understand how the rotator-cuff musculature acts on the glenohumeral joint, several electromyogram (EMG) studies have been performed (4). It appears from these studies that the rotator-cuff musculature and biceps are relatively inactive during the acceleration phase of throwing, whereas the larger torso muscles, the pectoralis major, serratus anterior, subscapularis, and latissimus dorsi are most active. During deceleration, when the muscle must act eccentrically, the rotator cuff primarily is active (4).

The rotator cuff acts in concert with the glenoid labrum and capsular ligaments to restrain abnormal motion. Presumably the labrum allows the muscular tension within the rotator cuff to center the humeral head on the glenoid socket. The capsular-ligament anatomy and function are described in detail elsewhere in this book. The role of the ligaments in restraining motion during the throw has not been well documented. Many authors hypothesize, as do we, that these ligaments function primarily as end-range stabilizers at the extremes of motion (5–7). In these positions, the ligaments are under maximal tension, and the

D. W. Altchek: The Hospital for Special Surgery, New York, New York 10021; and Department of Surgery (Orthopaedics), Cornell University Medical College, New York, New York 10021.
P. T. Simonian: Department of Orthopaedic Surgery, University of Washington, Seattle, Washington 98195.

musculature is at a mechanical disadvantage, in a position that is too short (cocking) or too long (follow-through) for its fibers to be well aligned.

There is obviously a complex interaction between the static restraint structures and the dynamic restraint structures that requires further in-depth study for better comprehension.

DIAGNOSIS OF SHOULDER INSTABILITY IN THE THROWING ATHLETE

History

The majority of injuries to the thrower's shoulder occur insidiously from repetitive microtrauma. By far the most common complaint is pain. But in competitive athletes, what often motivates them to seek medical attention is pain associated with a decreased performance level. Other symptoms that can be specifically associated with instability are clicking, a sense of the shoulder coming apart, dead-arm syndrome, and rarely, actual subluxation of the joint. The pain can be localized to different portions of the shoulder, often related to the injured portion of the stabilizing system.

Pain in the anterolateral deltoid is common and is usually referred from injury to the supraspinatus tendon. Pain posteriorly at the joint line is often due to injury to the posterior labrum and infraspinatus tendon. This combination injury has been termed internal impingement and is discussed in a subsequent portion of this chapter (8). Pain at the anterior joint line at the coracoid is often associated with labral injury, most often the superior labrum—a superior labral anterior and posterior (SLAP) lesion (9).

If the athlete can isolate the pain to a portion of the throw, that also can be helpful in detecting the site of injury. Most injuries will cause pain during the high-load phase of the throw—the acceleration phase. Internal impingement, however, will classically result in pain at cocking, when the shoulder is minimally horizontally adducted and externally rotated (8,10–12). At this point, it appears that the posterior rotator-cuff attachment can abut the posterior labrum. The cause of internal impingement is not always known, but in some throwers, it is related to excessive anterior capsular stretch, causing anterior subluxation of the humeral head on the glenoid (8,10–12).

Pain in the follow-through phase, when the arm is internally rotated and relatively adducted, can be a symptom of instability of the shoulder. In this phase of the throw, the rotator cuff is contracting maximally, and the capsular ligaments are under maximal tension. If these stabilizing mechanisms are injured, the athlete will often experience pain severe enough to create a sense that the shoulder is actually coming apart.

Physical Examination

It is essential that the examiner have an understanding of the ''normal'' variants that exist in the throwing athlete's shoulder, in particular, laxity and loss of internal rotation.

Laxity is a measure of the translation of the humeral head on the glenoid. It is clear from several prior studies, as well as our experience, that the dominant shoulder of the throwing athlete has increased laxity compared with the nondominant shoulder and with the those of the nonthrowing population. This laxity is manifested by an increased sulcus sign (a measure of inferior translation of the humeral head on the glenoid) and increased anterior and posterior translation. In such a setting, it is difficult to differentiate this ''normal'' laxity from instability.

Physical examination tests for instability in the throwing athlete must do more than simply measure laxity. Such tests, more importantly, must attempt to determine whether translation of the humeral head on the glenoid produces symptoms.

Several physical examination tests have been developed to address this issue. The first, and arguably the most popular, is the relocation test, as described by Jobe (10–12). To perform this examination, the athlete is placed supine; the examiner kneels behind and maximally externally rotates the abducted arm 90 degrees. At the end point of external rotation, an anteriorly directed force on the humeral head is applied. The athlete's symptoms are then gauged. From the same position, the examiner then releases the anterior pressure and applies a posterior pressure to the humeral head. In theory, if abduction/external rotation is causing subluxation, this posterior force should reduce the humeral head, and the symptoms should be relieved. Although it was initially believed that this test was an accurate test for anterior instability, subsequent studies have shown that the specificity of the relocation test is mediocre for anterior instability (13). Jobe now admits that this test, although useful for anterior instability, may be a better test for internal impingement (F.W. Jobe, personal communication, 1996). Internal impingement, a term coined by Walch and Jobe (8,10–12), is the abnormal contact between the posterosuperior labrum and the posterior rotator-cuff insertion. This injury occurs at the maximal cocking phase of throwing. The result is injury to the labrum and cuff in these areas, which manifests in the athlete as posterior joint-line pain in the cocking phase of the throw.

Of the many other instability tests described, we prefer the supine stress test. With the scapula stabilized on the examining table, the examiner kneels behind the athlete. With one hand, he or she stabilizes the humerus in the plane of the scapula by applying an axial load from the elbow along the axis of the humerus, trying to center the humeral head on the glenoid. The other hand is placed on the mid-humerus, and, with the humerus maintained in neutral rotation, the humerus is then driven anteriorly, posteriorly, and inferiorly. The examiner analyzes three data points for each direction:

1. Amount of translation (usually compared with the contralateral side)

2. Degree of subluxation: 0, 1+, being able to place the humeral head onto the glenoid rim; 2+, being able barely to sublux the humeral head over the rim, but on release of the examiner's pressure, the humeral head spontaneously reduces; 3+, instability, implying that the humeral head is easily and completely subluxed over the glenoid rim and requires manipulation to reduce
3. The examiner should carefully assess the presence of clicking/crunching and whether translation in a single direction reproduces symptoms

All are possible signs of labral pathology.

The examiner should expect a normal throwing athlete to have a moderately loose posterior capsule, to at least 2+, and that anterior laxity be typically 1 to 2+, with a 2+ sulcus sign. We have regarded 3+ anterior laxity in the thrower usually as a sign of anterior instability. An exception would be a loose-jointed individual in whom the examination is identical on the opposite side. This is similarly true in the posterior direction, where 2+ laxity is common but 3+ is suggestive of instability.

Labral Signs

Labral injury, such as a detached inferior labrum, can be the cause of shoulder instability. In the throwing athlete, labral tearing, particularly of the superior labrum, is often an associated finding in the unstable shoulder.

Detection of labral injury by physical examination can be challenging. The previous tests described for instability include tests for the inferior portion of the labrum. Four tests have been popularized for the physical examination of superior labral tears, also known as SLAP lesions: the crank test, scapular slide, clunk test, and O'Brien sign. The common denominator of these tests is to rotate and adduct the humerus internally. We have the most experience with the O'Brien sign, whereby the arm is maximally adducted and internally rotated; the athlete is then asked to maintain the arm in that position against a downward force (14). The test is positive if pain is produced at either the anterior or posterior joint line. False positives will occur with a painful acromioclavicular (AC) joint.

Impingement and Rotator Cuff

Impingement is abnormal contact between the superior surface of the rotator cuff and overlying coracoacromial arch. This can occur in conjunction with instability. Rotator-cuff injury without impingement can occur as well. The mechanisms by which these injuries occur in the throwing athlete are not well understood. Most authors hypothesize that an injury occurs to a portion of the stabilizing system, either labrum, capsule, or rotator cuff. With continued use, this leads to gradual malfunction of all systems, and abnormal translation or instability of the shoulder occurs. This abnormal translation is not limited to the anterior and posterior directions but can occur as well superiorly, as a weakened rotator cuff allows abnormal superior translation of the humeral head. This abnormal superior translation can result in subacromial impingement (15).

The rotator-cuff tendon can be directly injured by the extreme tensile forces that are produced during the follow-through phase of the throw. This is particularly true if a labral or capsular injury is already present, and the rotator cuff must work harder to compensate for the excess laxity already present.

The physical examination for rotator-cuff injury and impingement is performed as follows: the shoulders are inspected for atrophy. In the throwing athlete, hypertrophy of the shoulder-girdle musculature is to be expected. Relative atrophy can be an important sign of malfunction. Profound atrophy of the infraspinatus fossa is usually a sign of suprascapular neuropathy. Range of motion of the shoulder is next assessed. The examiner should expect a percentage decrease of adduction and internal rotation compared with the contralateral shoulder. This loss of motion is due to contracture of either the posterior cuff or posterior capsule and has been noted by many authors to be common in asymptomatic, elite throwers. It remains to be seen what degrees of contracture are truly pathologic. Further study is needed in that area.

Routine examination for impingement is carried out by assessing the presence or absence of impingement signs and subacromial bursitis, as well as the integrity of the AC joint.

Rotator-cuff strength is assessed in abduction in the scapular plane and internal rotation both in positions of abduction and adduction. The parameters of these tests are used to measure absolute strength as well as the production of symptoms during the testing. Extreme weakness of the rotator cuff, out of proportion to pain, is a sign of suprascapular neuropathy. Typical rotator-cuff pathology, such as tendinitis or partial-thickness tears, will generally result in minimal demonstrable weakness and moderate pain reproduced by these resistance tests.

The AC joint is directly palpated and compressed with crossed-arm adduction. If the athlete has a symptomatic AC joint, these maneuvers will reproduce pain at the AC joint.

The stability examination includes an evaluation of the capsular and labral integrity. At all times during this portion of the examination, the examiner must remember that there are important differences between laxity and instability. Laxity represents the amount of translation normally present in the glenohumeral joint. This "normal" amount of laxity can vary tremendously from individual to individual. Of course, in elite throwing athletes, experience has shown us that the normal pitcher's dominant shoulder is considerably more lax than the nondominant shoulder (16).

Translation tests are carried out in the straight "inferior" direction by using the well-known sulcus sign to assess the integrity of the superior capsular ligaments. The size of the sulcus produced is proportional to the amount of laxity present. The range is typically 1 to 3 cm. The sulcus sign is usually performed with the athlete seated.

Anterior–posterior stability is tested with the athlete supine and with the scapula stabilized on the examining table. The examiner kneels behind the athlete, grasping the elbow and humeral shaft. With his ''elbow'' hand, the examiner applies an axial load, centering the humeral head, and maintains the humerus in neutral rotation. By using the opposite hand, the examiner translates the humerus directly anterior, anteroinferior, and posterior. Translation is graded as 1+, 2+, or 3+. A 1+ implies that the humeral head cannot be brought as far as the glenoid rim; 2+, the humeral head can be subluxed over the glenoid rim; and 3+, the humeral head can be locked over the glenoid rim. A typical laxity pattern for a thrower's shoulder is 1+ anterior, 2+ posterior. Laxity in excess of this is often pathologic, caused by capsular stretch, capsular tear, or labral detachment. Rarely do throwing athletes experience frank instability. For that reason, typical apprehension tests are rarely helpful in this type of athlete.

The relocation test popularized by Jobe (10–12) was originally thought to be an excellent test for subtle instability. Over time, Jobe's own experience and studies such as those by Speer et al. (13) showed that the relocation test, although highly sensitive, is not highly specific for instability. Instead this test, in which the arm is placed in a position of maximal abduction and external rotation, has evolved into a test for internal impingement. As described by Walch (8), internal impingement is an abnormal collision between the posterosuperior labrum and posterior rotator cuff during the cocking/acceleration phase of throwing. The cause of this injury is unknown, but it is postulated to be due to abnormal anterior translation of the humeral head on the glenoid. To test for internal impingement, the examiner places the humerus to 90 degrees of abduction and maximal external rotation. In patients with internal impingement, this position will reproduce the symptoms of posterior pain at the level of the joint line. Relief by creating posterior pressure on the humeral head with the examiner's hand is confirmatory of either articular side-cuff injury or labral injury.

SLAP lesions, or tears of the superior labrum, will produce symptoms of clicking and pain (9). The pain typically occurs at the joint line anteriorly or posteriorly during activity. Detection of a SLAP lesion on physical examination is difficult. Many physical examination maneuvers have been described to detect SLAP lesions, and all have in common placing the humerus in adduction/internal rotation. Of these tests, we use the adduction compression sign described by O'Brien (14). In this test, the humerus is abducted 90 degrees to the body and horizontally adducted across the midline of the body. With the humerus internally rotated (thumb toward the floor), the examiner places a downward force on the arm while the patient resists. Pain will be produced at the AC joint in cases of abnormalities of the AC joint and at the joint line, either anteriorly or posteriorly, in cases in which a SLAP lesion is present.

IMAGING

When ordering imaging studies of throwing athletes, the clinician must remember that these tests provide further insights, but that this information must be used in conjunction with the history and physical examination data.

Plain radiographs are always necessary. A series includes anteroposterior (AP) in neutral rotation and a West Point axillary view. From the AP, we can assess the overall alignment of the glenohumeral joint, the presence of lateral sloping of the acromion, and the status of the AC joint. The West Point axillary view allows assessment of the AP alignment of the glenohumeral joint, the presence of a posterior Bennett lesion, the presence of an anterior or posterior bony Bankart lesion, and the thickness of the glenohumeral articular cartilage. Unusual variants, such as os acrominale, can also be identified in the axillary view. If a posterior glenoid calcification or Bennett lesion is suspected, a Stryker notch view is ordered.

In general, most shoulder injuries in throwing athletes are to the soft-tissue structures rather than to the bone, making the magnetic resonance imaging (MRI) more valuable than plain radiographs.

MRI must be performed by using only the highest-quality imaging equipment and software. The injuries are often subtle and will be overlooked on mediocre studies. With an appropriate study, the radiologist and clinician can evaluate the following structures:

- rotator cuff
- labrum
- subacromial bursa
- capsule

The rotator-cuff assessment can usually be performed with a high degree of accuracy. The typical injuries will range from a tendinosis-type of degeneration, partial-thickness articular tears, and rarely, full-thickness tears.

The labrum is more difficult to assess. The examiner must understand the many variations of the labrum to avoid the confusion of normal variants with injury. Labral injuries that are commonly seen are:

- SLAP lesions with or without detachment
- anteroinferior labral tears or detachment
- posterosuperior labral injury typical of internal impingement

An impingement-like syndrome can occur in throwing athletes because of either rotator-cuff weakness or glenohumeral instability. This will often result in a thickening of the subacromial bursa, which should be recognizable on MRI.

The capsular ligaments are the most difficult structures to evaluate. Two types of injuries will occur, capsular stretch or capsular tears. Capsular tears are severe injuries, but fortunately, they are rare. Our experience has demonstrated that this injury should be visible on proper imaging studies (see Chapters 6 and 7).

In contrast, capsular stretch is not now identifiable on MRI scanning. Unfortunately this is the most common capsular injury. Detection of this lesion must be performed by other means.

REHABILITATION

The cornerstone of treatment of shoulder instability is rehabilitation. The essence of the rehabilitation program is to develop the proprioceptive and muscular systems to compensate for the injuries present. This approach is based on the concept that injury to the stabilizing structures (the rotator cuff, the labrum, and the capsular ligaments) will result in a pathologic increase in glenohumeral translation (i.e., shoulder instability). The goal of the rehabilitation is to develop the athlete's shoulder-girdle musculature to allow him or her to compensate. The parameters are that this process will take time and will require a skilled and knowledgeable therapist. Please refer to Chapter 11 for details.

SURGICAL TREATMENT

Surgical treatment is reserved for throwing athletes for whom conservative treatment has failed. The surgeon must identify the following factors in choosing the proper candidates for surgery:

- the athlete's symptoms have not been reduced by conservative treatment to the degree that he or she can compete at the necessary level
- the surgeon can identify by perioperative testing that a lesion or lesions are present that the surgeon believes are repairable
- the surgeon is confident that the athlete can attempt a painful, lengthy, and intermittently discouraging recovery process
- the surgeon is confident that the surgical trauma required to ''fix'' the problem can be minimized to a degree such that the chances of recovery are maximized

Surgical Procedure

Anesthesia is generally by intrascalene block. The first step in the surgical procedure is a thorough examination under anesthesia. This is performed in the same position as in the preoperative stability examination. The data from this are a crucial step in deciding what the surgical procedure will be.

The goal of surgery in the throwing athlete is to effect repair of the labrum, capsule, and rotator cuff such that, with extensive strengthening, the athlete can return to sports at the preinjury level. This represents a true challenge for the surgeon and the athlete.

In the case of the throwing athlete, the final surgical plan is made after the examination under anesthesia and the diagnostic arthroscopy. This information is combined with the data from the history and the awake physical examination. Factors weighted particularly are (a) Does the athlete complain of a distinct sense of subluxation? If this is present, the surgical procedure will usually require labral repair, capsular tightening, or both; and (b) Does the athlete have distinct, persistent rotator-cuff weakness on examination, with MRI evidence of a significant (50% thickness) rotator-cuff tear? This situation will usually require direct repair of the rotator cuff.

The surgical procedure is begun after a complete examination under anesthesia. The glenohumeral stability is assessed in inferior, anterior, and posterior directions replicating the awake stability examination. Normal stability for a throwing athlete will demonstrate a 2+ posterior laxity and 1+ anterior laxity with a 1 to 2+ sulcus. Laxity of 3+ in the posterior direction or 2+ or greater in the anterior direction should raise suspicion that capsulolabral repair will be required.

Diagnostic arthroscopy is then performed. We prefer the beach-chair position (17). Beginning with the arthroscope in the posterior portal, the surgeon visualizes the biceps and biceps anchor. This area of the labrum is often meniscoid in shape and can have a recessed attachment at the supraglenoid tubercle.

Differentiation of a normal recessed superior labrum and a type II SLAP lesion (a detached biceps anchor) requires that the surgeon clearly visualize the *undersurface* of the labrum in this region. Detachment due to injury will be accompanied by evidence of tearing or fraying of the labral undersurface. In contrast, a normal but ''mobile'' superior labrum will have a ''clean'' undersurface with no evidence of detachment injury. Warren pointed out that the normal recessed superior labrum will exhibit articular cartilage contiguous to the attachment site (R.F. Warren, personal communication, 1996).

Next the anterosuperior labrum is visualized. This area is important to stability because it represents the attachment site of the superior and middle glenohumeral ligaments. Confusion can arise because of the variations of ligament attachment and labral structure in this region. Two important variations exist. The first is a ''band-like'' middle glenohumeral ligament, which is usually accompanied by a complete absence of anterosuperior labral tissue. The second is a ''sublabral hole,'' a defect in the anterosuperior labrum occurring below the attachment site of the middle glenohumeral ligament. In both of these, it is important to recognize the difference between these normal variants and injury. As in the prior case, labral detachment usually has accompanying distinct evidence of injury, such as fraying or tearing of the labrum. If "repair" is performed without actual injury (i.e., in normal variants), this will result in overtightening of the middle glenohumeral ligament, and the athlete will lose glenohumeral external rotation.

After completion of the evaluation of the anterosuperior labrum, the arthroscopic view is shifted inferiorly. The anteroinferior labrum has minimal variability. This portion of the labrum is normally attached securely to the glenoid margin. Any detachments in this region are pathologic.

Evaluation of the integrity of the anterior portion of the inferior glenohumeral ligament is complex and somewhat subjective. Ideally the anterior band of this ligament, as described by O'Brien et al. (7), is a distinct, robust structure that takes up tension quickly as the arm is externally rotated. As stretch injury occurs, the anterior band loses a robust appearance, and the ligament fails to tighten with external rotation. Warren (18,19) described the drive-through sign as a tool to evaluate the degree of ligament stretch.

The term "drive-through" refers to the ability of the surgeon to pass the arthroscope into the anterior capsular pouch. As that pouch gets larger, the "drive-through" becomes easier. In the normal shoulder, external rotation of the humerus quickly eliminates any drive-through. When anterior instability is present, the ability to drive through remains despite humeral external rotation (18,19).

The inferior glenohumeral ligament also must be evaluated for the presence of tears, which are rare but do occur, particularly as Wolf (20) described, on the humeral end of the ligament.

After completion of evaluation of the anterior labrum and capsule, attention is directed to the rotator cuff. During evaluation of the anterior capsule, the superior tendon of the subscapularis is clearly evident. Injury to the subscapularis has rarely been reported in a young throwing athlete. Most injuries to the subscapularis that we have seen have been muscular "sprains" rather than tendon tears.

The supraspinatus attachment to the tuberosity is visualized by placing the humerus in the plane of the scapula with distal traction. Undersurface tears are commonly seen, and all frayed tissue must be thoroughly debrided to allow visualization of the remaining tendon. Conflicting data have been reported about the results of debridement. Andrews (21) generally reported good results with debridement alone. Payne (22), from our institution, found that debridement in the overhead athlete has been unpredictable. Currently, we believe that tears greater than 50% of the thickness of the tendon should undergo repair to maximize the potential for symptom relief and return to function. Quantification of the degree of tearing can be difficult. Gerber (23) pointed out that one clue is the amount of exposed tuberosity. Normally, the tendon attaches directly at the edge of the articular cartilage. When tearing occurs, progressive recession of the remaining tendon from the articular edge develops. Gerber (23) stated that a space greater than 5 mm is associated with a tear of approximately 50% of the tendon thickness. Snyder (24) described placing a suture from the subacromial space through the conjoined tendon, allowing the surgeon to visualize precisely the superior surface (from a subacromial view) of the injured area of the tendon. None of these techniques is precise. The surgeon must use his or her judgment based on the visualized appearance, the MRI appearance, and as mentioned, the degree of tendon-type pain and weakness present in the physical examination.

Once the supraspinatus has been evaluated, the arthroscope is switched to an anterior portal, and the infraspinatus tendon and posterior labrum are evaluated. A not-infrequent injury encountered in this region is that of internal impingement. This is evidenced by partial tearing of the infraspinatus and fraying without detachment of the posterosuperior labrum. Again, debridement is performed to remove all frayed tissue to evaluate the integrity of the remaining tendon and labrum. In cases of internal impingement in which posterior joint-line pain is reproduced with the position of humeral abduction and external rotation, simple debridement is often adequate treatment, unless coexistent anterior instability is present.

Posterior labral detachment is less common but can occur in conjunction with posterior instability. These lesions are present in the inferior half of the posterior labrum and are evident after probing.

The final step of the diagnostic arthroscopy is to evaluate the subacromial space. The bursa is predistended with epinephrine solution from a lateral position, ensuring that the needle is anterior enough to penetrate the subacromial bursa. The arthroscopic trocar is then placed from the posterior portal and should be felt to "pop" through the posterior bursal wall. The status of the bursa is evaluated first. A normal bursa will be a large open space, and the coracoacromial ligament will be clearly visible. If the bursa is abnormal, crisscrossing adhesions will be present, the tissue will be thickened, and the coracoacromial ligament will usually not be visible. All abnormal bursal tissue is debrided with a full-radius resector until the coracoacromial ligament and superior surface of the rotator cuff are clearly evident, which will demonstrate fraying and degeneration if impingement is present. In the young athlete, bony spurs on the acromion are rare. If the bursa is abnormal, indicating the presence of subacromial impingement, the coracoacromial ligament should be carefully evaluated. In some athletes, the ligament will hypertrophy and may contribute to impingement. In these cases, partial, if not complete, debridement of the ligament is indicated (25).

Surgical Procedure for Instability in the Throwing Athlete

The following algorithm should guide the choice of surgical procedures.

Type I

Athlete complains of pain with no discernible symptoms of true instability.

1-A: Minor Rotator-Cuff Injury, Subacromial Bursitis With or Without a Thickened Coracoacromial Ligament

In this case, minor dynamic instability is occurring because of chronic rotator-cuff dysfunction.

Surgical Treatment. Debridement of undersurface cuff tear. This is performed with the shaver in the anterior portal.

Arthroscopic subacromial decompression. With shaver in the lateral portal, all abnormal subacromial bursa is debrided. If the coracoacromial ligament is thickened, it is debrided.

I-B: Rotator-Cuff Injury Is Severe (More Than 50% of the Tendon Thickness)

The anterior capsule and labrum are intact.

Surgical Treatment. A mini-open repair is performed on the torn portion of the rotator cuff. Most of these tears are not full thickness, requiring the surgeon to complete the tear. This is generally performed with the arthroscope in the joint. A blunt instrument is used through a lateral subacromial portal to locate the area of the torn tendon. Next, by using a knife, the tear is completed under direct vision. A shaver is then passed through the subacromial space and through the tendon defect. The shaver is then used further to debride any nonviable tendon and to abrade the tuberosity to bleeding bone. The arthroscope is then inserted into the subacromial space as described earlier.

After performing the subacromial decompression, the rotator-cuff repair is performed. By using a mini-open exposure (deltoid split incorporating the portal), the rotator cuff is repaired to the previously prepared tuberosity bed. The technique of repair is to maximize the length of tendon attached to the tuberosity. To do this, fixation is performed at the articular margin by using suture anchors and laterally by using traditional tuberosity drill holes.

I-C: Internal Impingement

Athletes with posterior pain that is reproduced by the position of abduction and external rotation. Arthroscopy reveals the typical lesion of internal impingement.

Surgical Treatment. Surgical treatment includes debridement of the frayed posterior labrum and cuff. Careful inspection of the subacromial space is performed, and subacromial decompression is performed as necessary. Again, remember that acromial bone removal is rarely indicated in this population.

I-D: SLAP Lesion

Athletes with joint-line pain (at the coracoid or posterior joint line) in association with an MRI confirms a SLAP lesion.

Surgical Treatment. Surgical treatment involves debridement and/or repair of the labrum, depending on whether the labrum is torn or detached. Labral repair is performed with an absorbable Suretac (Acufex Microsurgical Inc., Norwood, MA, U.S.A.). The debridement of the glenoid neck and the tack placement are usually performed through a superolateral portal, placed in the lateral aspect of the rotator interval. SLAP lesions typically occur in conjunction with partial-thickness undersurface rotator-cuff tears and bursitis of the subacromial space. When treating a SLAP lesion, the surgeon must carefully evaluate the rotator cuff and subacromial space. Usually, it is necessary only to debride the rotator-cuff tear and perform a bursectomy in conjunction with a SLAP repair.

Type II

This group of athletes is thought to have anterior instability. Symptomatically, they complain primarily of pain, but may, if questioned, admit that the shoulder feels excessively loose, and that the shoulder "comes apart" during throwing. Examination under anesthesia reveals 2 to 3+ anterior laxity, and arthroscopy reveals a loose anterior capsule with a large drive-through.

II-A: Capsular Laxity Without Rotator-Cuff Tear

Surgical Treatment. The surgeon's goal in this type of patient is to tighten the anterior capsule such that the humeral head remains centered on the glenoid during the act of throwing. The difficulty facing the surgeon is that errors in capsular tensioning, even slight, lead to restriction of motion and can cause significant disability in the throwing athlete. There is no exact formula for how to tension a capsule in this situation. The principles typically used to perform capsular surgery for recurrent instability will usually lead to overtightening and loss of motion. In these athletes, the surgeon must remember that slight excessive laxity can be compensated for by dynamic (muscular) stabilization. Two methods are used to reduce excessive laxity. The most traditional is open capsular shift. Jobe (12) popularized the technique of capsulolabral reconstruction

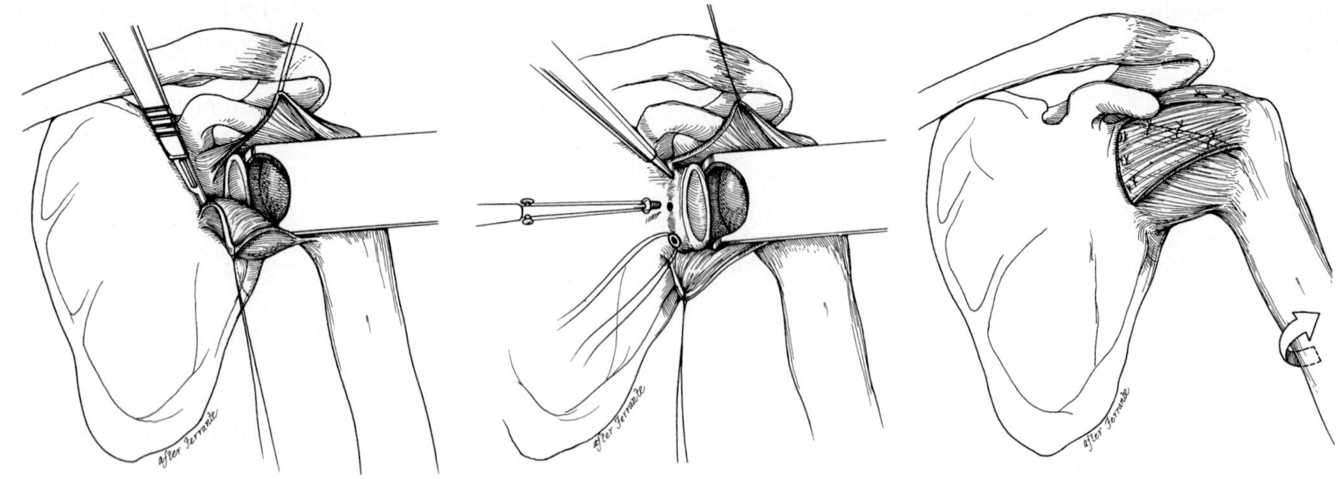

A,B C

FIG. 1. A–C: Technique for capsulolabral reconstruction, particularly when marked anterior capsular laxity is present. The capsule is incised horizontally and then T-plasty performed along the vertical margin of the glenoid. Labral repair can be performed where necessary, and a large capsular shift can be performed along the glenoid neck.

performed through a subscapularis split. In this procedure, the capsule is divided horizontally and T-plasty performed from the glenoid neck, leaving the labrum intact. Anchors are then placed medial to the intact labrum, and the capsular flaps are tensioned superiorly and inferiorly, eliminating excess capsular redundancy (Fig. 1). This procedure has been used in a large series of competitive pitchers with results of 69% returning to the prior level of play (26).

We developed a modification of this procedure, whereby the capsule is divided horizontally and no T-plasty performed. This approach simplifies capsular shift and limits the degree to which the capsule can be tightened (12; Fig. 2).

The alternative to these open capsular-shift procedures is thermal capsular shrinkage. The principles for this procedure are outlined in Chapter 22. The advantages of this procedure over open capsular surgery in this athletic population are obvious. First, the surgical trauma is minimized, making recovery easier. Second, the chance of overtightening is minimized, making recovery easier. Of course, this procedure is in its preliminary stages, and further study will be needed before it can be clearly recommended.

In most cases, we perform the modified capsular tightening by using only a horizontal capsular incision. This is performed through a subscapularis split. The capsule is exposed superiorly and inferiorly. A horizontal capsular incision is made just above the inferior glenohumeral ligament, and care is taken not to transect the middle glenohumeral ligament. The incision is made from the humeral insertion to the capsular reflection on the glenoid neck. The inferior capsule is then shifted superiorly, overlapping the superior and inferior capsule, by using nonabsorbable mattress sutures. The sutures are tensioned without tying, and the shoulder is reexamined. Motion should allow 90 degrees of abduction with 90 degrees of external rota-

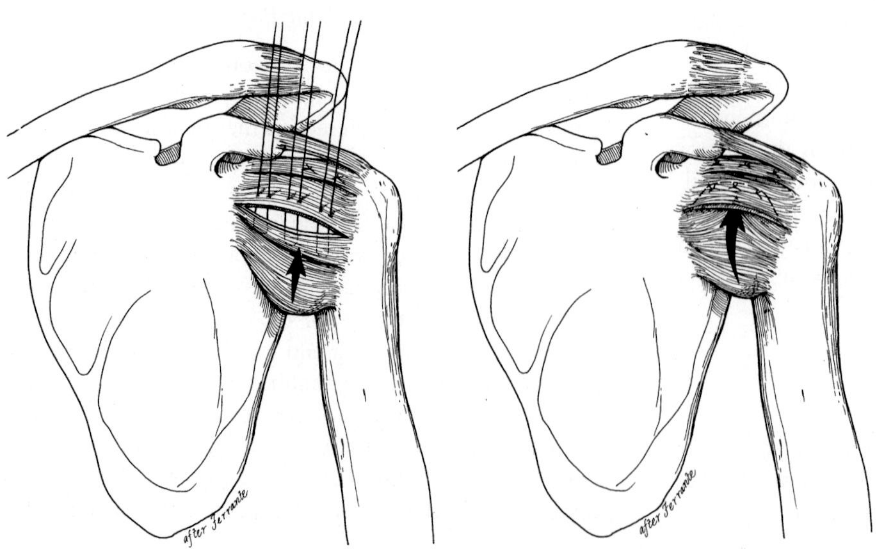

A,B

FIG. 2. A,B: A modification of the capsulolabral reconstruction, which uses only a horizontal incision. The labrum may be repaired at the medial aspect of the incision when necessary. The capsule is shifted in a north–south fashion, but the degree of capsular shift is more limited than in the previous procedure.

tion. Anterior subluxation should be reduced. The sutures are then tied, and the subscapularis is closed anteromedially by using absorbable sutures.

II-B: Capsular Laxity with Rotator-Cuff Tear

If the athlete demonstrates anterior instability on the basis of capsular laxity and a rotator-cuff tear, both issues must be addressed surgically. The rotator cuff is assessed as described previously. If the tear is believed to extend greater than 50% of the tendon thickness, repair is performed as previously outlined by using a mini-open approach. Concomitant subacromial decompression is performed only if distinct arthroscopic evidence of subacromial impingement is present, as previously described in this chapter. We have found that subacromial decompression is rarely necessary in the group of patients who have distinct instability.

II-C: Capsular Tear With or Without Rotator-Cuff Tear

As described by Wolf (20) and Bach (27), capsular tears can occur in throwing athletes. Such injuries usually involve the anterior portion of the inferior glenohumeral ligament. In our limited experience with this injury, conservative treatment does not ameliorate the symptoms, and surgical repair is indicated for definitive treatment of this injury. Operative repair can be difficult, particularly if the injury is chronic. Arthroscopy is used to confirm the injury. Open capsular repair is performed through a subscapularis split. The surgeon should be aware that these capsular tears often appear larger than anticipated by the arthroscopic view. Repair is performed by using nonabsorbable sutures and a mattress closure, doubling the capsular layer at the repair junction. Postoperative management is handled in the same fashion as the typical capsular repair for instability.

POSTOPERATIVE MANAGEMENT

The first principle of postoperative management of the throwing athlete is restoration of motion. Although a sling may be used for protection, motion exercises must begin on postoperative day 1 and progress in a steady fashion. The exact details of each program depend on the procedure performed. In general, basic motion (full forward flexion with 90 degrees of external rotation) should be restored no later than 8 weeks postoperatively.

Strengthening begins with the scapular musculature and progresses to the rotator-cuff muscles. Trunk, buttock, and leg muscle groups are trained simultaneously.

Throwing, in the form of tossing, is begun when motion is full and muscle strength around the shoulder is at approximately 80% of normal. The throwing program progresses gradually over a period of months until the athlete is prepared to return to competitive throwing. The time frame for postoperative rehabilitation of a throwing athlete to full return is lengthy. We have found that 6 months of rehabilitation is needed for minor shoulder procedures and 12 months or more for major surgery, such as stabilization or rotator-cuff repair (Table 1).

SUMMARY

The throwing athlete with shoulder instability presents a diagnostic and treatment challenge to the orthopedic surgeon. The physician must understand the role of the system of static and dynamic restraints that function to keep the shoulder stable during the complex throwing motion. Treatment is directed toward restoring the equilibrium between shoulder laxity and dynamic stabilization of the rotator cuff and scapular musculature, such that the athlete can return to sports at his or her prior, competitive level.

TABLE 1. *Interval throwing program*

Phase I: Long-toss program			
45-ft Stage			
Step 1	a. Warm-up throwing b. 45 ft (25 throws) c. Rest 15 min d. Warm-up throwing e.45 ft (25 throws)	Step 2	a. Warm-up throwing b. 45 ft (25 throws) c. Rest 10 min d. Warm-up throwing e. 45 ft (25 throws) f. Rest 10 min g. Warm-up throwing h. 45 ft (25 throws)
60-ft Stage			
Step 3	a. Warm-up throwing b. 60 ft (25 throws) c. Rest 15 min d. Warm-up throwing e. 60 ft (25 throws)	Step 4	a. Warm-up throwing b. 60 ft (25 throws) c. Rest 10 min d. Warm-up throwing e. 60 ft (25 throws) f. Rest 10 min g. Warm-up throwing h. 60 ft (25 throws)

(continued)

TABLE 1. *Continued.*

90-ft Stage			
Step 5	a. Warm-up throwing b. 90 ft (25 throws) c. Rest 15 min d. Warm-up throwing e. 90 ft (25 throws)	Step 6	a. Warm-up throwing b. 90 ft (25 throws) c. Rest 10 min d. Warm-up throwing e. 90 ft (25 throws) f. Rest 10 min g. Warm-up throwing h. 90 ft (25 throws)
120-ft Stage			
Step 7	a. Warm-up throwing b. 120 ft (25 throws) c. Rest 15 min d. Warm-up throwing e. 120 ft (25 throws)	Step 8	a. Warm-up throwing b. 120 ft (25 throws) c. Rest 10 min d. Warm-up throwing e. 120 ft (25 throws) f. Rest 10 min g. Warm-up throwing h. 120 ft (25 throws)
150-ft Stage			
Step 9	a. Warm-up throwing b. 150 ft (25 throws) c. Rest 15 min d. Warm-up throwing e. 150 ft (25 throws)	Step 10	a. Warm-up throwing b. 150 ft (25 throws) c. Rest 10 min d. Warm-up throwing e. 150 ft (25 throws) f. Rest 10 min g. Warm-up throwing h. 150 ft (25 throws)
180-ft Stage			
Step 11	a. Warm-up throwing b. 180 ft (25 throws) c. Rest 15 min d. Warm-up throwing e. 180 ft (25 throws)	Step 12	a. Warm-up throwing b. 180 ft (25 throws) c. Rest 10 min d. Warm-up throwing e. 180 ft (25 throws) f. Rest 10 min g. Warm-up throwing h. 180 ft (25 throws)
Step 13	a. Warm-up throwing b. 180 ft (25 throws) c. Rest 10 min d. Warm-up throwing e. 180 ft (25 throws) f. Rest 10 min g. 180 ft (25 throws)	Step 14	Begin throwing from mound or return to respective position.
Phase II: Starting off the mound			
Stage I: Fastball only			
Step 1	a. Interval throwing b. 15 throws from mound, 50%		
Step 2	a. Interval throwing b. 30 throws from mound, 50%		
Step 3	a. Interval throwing b. 45 throws from mound, 50%		
Step 4	a. Interval throwing b. 60 throws from mound, 50%		
Step 5	a. Interval throwing b. 30 throws from mound, 75%		
Step 6	a. 30 throws from mound, 75% b. 45 throws from mound, 50%		
Step 7	a. 45 throws from mound, 75% b. 15 throws from mound, 50%		
Step 8	a. 60 throws from mound, 75%		

(continued)

TABLE 1. *Continued.*

Stage II: Fastball only	
Step 9	a. 45 throws from mound, 75%
	b. 15 throws in batting practice
Step 10	a. 45 throws from mound, 75%
	b. 30 throws in batting practice
Step 11	a. 45 throws from mound, 75%
	b. 45 throws in batting practice
Stage III	
Step 12	a. 30 throws from mound, 75% warm-up
	b. 15 throws from mound, 50% breaking balls
	c. 45–60 throws in batting practice, throws from mound, 50% (fastball only)
Step 13	a. 30 throws from mound, 75%
	b. 30 breaking balls, 75%
	c. 30 throws in batting practice
Step 14	a. 30 throws from mound, 75%
	b. 60–90 throws in batting practice, 25% breaking balls
Step 15	Simulated game progressing by 15 throws per workout. Use interval throwing to 120-ft. phase as warm-up. All throwing from the mound should be done in the presence of the pitching coach to stress proper throwing mechanics. A speed gun should be used to aid in effort control.

Throwing is performed every other day, Prethrowing and postthrowing exercises must be performed.
Each Step should be 2 weeks. If pain occurs during any step, back up to previous step.

(From Andrews JA, Wilk KE, eds. *The athlete's shoulder.* New York: Churchill Livingstone, 1994:672–674.)

REFERENCES

1. Dillman CJ, Fleisig GS, Andrews JR. Biomechanics of pitching with emphasis upon shoulder kinematics. *J Orthop Sports Phys Ther* 1993;18 (2):402–408.
2. Pappas AM, Zawacki RM, Sullivan TJ. Biomechanics of baseball pitching: a preliminary report. *Am J Sports Med* 1985;13:216–222.
3. Altchek DW, Dines DM. Shoulder injuries in the throwing athlete. *J Am Acad Orthop Surg* 1995;3:159–165.
4. Jobe FW, Moynes DR, Tibone JE, et al. An EMG analysis of the shoulder in pitching: a second report. *Am J Sports Med* 1984;12:218–220.
5. Matsen FA III, Harryman DT II, Sidles JA. Mechanics of glenohumeral instability. *Clin Sport Med* 1991;10:783–788.
6. Warner JJP, Deng XH, Warren RF, et al. Static capsuloligamentous restraints to superior-inferior translation of the glenohumeral joint. *Am J Sports Med* 1992;20:675–685.
7. O'Brien SJ, Neves MC, Arnoczky SP, et al. The anatomy and histology of the inferior glenohumeral ligament complex of the shoulder. *Am J Sports Med* 1990;18:449–456.
8. Walch G, Bioleau P, Noel E, Donnell ST. Impingement of the deep surface of the supraspinatus tendon on the posterosuperior glenoid rim: an arthroscopic study. *J Shoulder Elbow Surg* 1992;1:238–245.
9. Snyder SJ, Karzel RP, Del Pizzo W, et al. SLAP lesions of the shoulder. *Arthroscopy* 1990;6:274–279.
10. Kvitne RS, Jobe RW, Jobe CM. Shoulder instability in the overhand or throwing athlete. *Clin Sports Med* 1995;14:917–935.
11. Kvitne RS, Jobe FW. The diagnosis and treatment of anterior instability in the throwing athlete. *Clin Orthop* 1993;291:107–123.
12. Jobe FW, Kvitne RS, Giangarra CE. Shoulder pain in the overhand or throwing athlete: the relationship of anterior instability and rotator cuff impingement. *Orthop Rev* 1989;18:963–975.
13. Speer KP, Hannafin JA, Altchek DW, et al. An evaluation of the shoulder relocation test. *Am J Sports Med* 1994;22:177–183.
14. O'Brien SJ, Pagnani MJ, McGlynn SR, Fealy S, Wilson JB. The active compression test: a new and effective test for diagnosing labral tears and acromioclavicular joint pathology. *Am J Sports Med* (in press).
15. Paletta GA, Warner JJP, Warren RF, Deutsch A, Altchek DW. Shoulder kinematics with two-plane x-ray evaluation in patient with anterior instability or rotator cuff tearing. *J Shoulder Elbow Surg* 1997;6 (6): 516–527.
16. Bigliani LU, Codd TP, Connor PM, Levine WN, Littlefield MA, Hershon SJ. Shoulder motion and laxity in the professional baseball player. *Am J Sports Med* 1997;25 (5):609–613.
17. Skyhar MJ, Altchek DW, Warren RF, et al. Shoulder arthroscopy with the patient in the beach-chair position. *Arthroscopy* 1988;4:256–259.
18. Pagnani M, Warren R. Arthroscopic shoulder stabilization. *Oper Tech Sports Med* 1993;1:276–284.
19. Warner JJP, Warren RF. Arthroscopic Bankart repair using a cannulated absorbable fixation device. *Oper Tech Orthop Surg* 1991;1:192–198.
20. Wolf E. Arthroscopic management of shoulder instability. Arthroscopy Association of North America Annual Meeting, Instructional Course No. 201, Boston, MA, April 23–26, 1992.
21. Andrews JR. Rotator cuff repairs in the throwing athlete. AAOS Shoulder and Knee Course: the athletic perspective to treatment, controversies and problem solving. Steamboat Springs, CO, March 18–22, 1997.
22. Payne LZ, Altchek DW, Craig EV, Warren RF. Arthroscopic treatment of partial rotator cuff tears in young athletes: a preliminary report. *Am J Sports Med* 1997;25:299–305.
23. Gerber C. L'epaule operee du joueur de tennis. 2eme Conference Internationale Medicine et Tennis, Paris, France, May 31, 1997.
24. Snyder SJ, Banas MP, Belzer JP. Arthroscopic treatment of anterior shoulder instability using threaded suture anchors and nonabsorbable suture. *Instr Course Lect* 1996;45:71–81.
25. Bigliani LU, Rodsky MW, Newton PD, et al. Arthroscopic coracoacromial ligament resection for impingement in the overhead athlete. *J Shoulder Elbow Surg* 1995;4 (1):S54.
26. Montgomery WH III, Jobe FW. Functional outcomes in athletes after modified anterior capsulolabral reconstruction. *Am J Sports Med* 1994;22:352-358.
27. Bach BR, Warren RF, Fronek J. Disruption of the lateral capsule of the shoulder. A cause of recurrent dislocation. *J Bone Joint Surg* 1998;70B:274–276.

The Unstable Shoulder,
edited by R.F. Warren, E.V. Craig, and D.W. Altchek.
Lippincott–Raven Publishers, Philadelphia © 1999.

CHAPTER 15

Recurrent Posterior Subluxation

Open Surgical Treatment

Mark K. Bowen and Russell F. Warren

The diagnosis and treatment of posterior instability of the glenohumeral joint continues to present a significant challenge to orthopedic surgeons. Published case reports and small series of patients have brought attention to its frequent misdiagnosis and have caused some confusion by using the terms posterior subluxation and dislocation interchangeably (1–14). The increased discussion and awareness of posterior instability has led to clearer definitions and terminology. This clinical entity has been focused by advances in our understanding and treatment of sports-related injuries of the shoulder (9,15–19). Thus, recurrent posterior subluxation has been recognized and diagnosed as a cause of shoulder pain and instability with increasing frequency. In our experience, recurrent posterior instability of the glenohumeral joint most commonly manifests itself as recurrent subluxation rather than dislocation. Important to the therapeutic decision-making process is an understanding of the etiologies of instability and the natural history of the rehabilitated and surgically stabilized shoulder.

DIAGNOSTIC CONSIDERATIONS

Etiology

The onset of symptoms has been attributed to a traumatic event (macrotrauma) by approximately 50% of our patients (16,20). Others have described precipitation of symptoms related to major repetitive indirect trauma to the adducted, flexed, and internally rotated upper extremity. This is most frequently seen in athletes who perform heavy incline and flat bench-press weightlifting, as well as football linemen who use locked, straight-arm, pass-blocking techniques.

Repetitive vigorous stress to the upper extremity (microtrauma) that occurs in many different overhead sports can also lead to symptoms from posterior subluxation of the humeral head on the glenoid. The most common sports that we associate with this group of patients include baseball, tennis, and swimming. High stresses on the posterior capsule are generated in these activities during the follow-through phase as the humerus is flexed, adducted, and internally rotated. In swimming, the stresses occur during the pull-through phase in the free-style stroke.

Some patients ultimately diagnosed as having recurrent posterior subluxation are unable to attribute the onset of their symptoms to any particular activity or trauma (atraumatic). Many of these patients have an association of other physical characteristics consistent with generalized ligamentous laxity.

Voluntary Subluxation

Approximately 50% of the patients we have diagnosed with recurrent posterior subluxation were able to demonstrate their instability on a voluntary basis (16,20). Two patterns of voluntary posterior subluxation have been observed. The most common voluntary subluxation (positional type) is demonstrated when the patient forward flexes, adducts, and internally rotates the arm. This subluxed position becomes apparent when the arm is moved horizontally from a flexed to an extended position, and the humeral head dramatically reduces. A second type of voluntary subluxation (muscular

M. K. Bowen: Department of Orthopaedic Surgery, Northwestern University, Chicago, Illinois 60611; and Department of Orthopaedic Surgery, Northwestern Memorial Hospital, Chicago, Illinois 60611-2950.

R. F. Warren: Department of Orthopaedics, Cornell University Medical College, New York, New York 10021; and Department of Orthopaedics, The Hospital for Special Surgery, New York, New York 10021.

type) is demonstrated by patients who are able to selectively suppress or activate muscles (or both) to displace the humeral head posteriorly on the glenoid. This subluxation typically occurs with the arm positioned at the side. In both types of voluntary subluxation, patients appear to develop a sensitivity to the subluxation and the arm position or muscular maneuver necessary to achieve the mechanically apparent extreme of joint position.

In most patients who are ultimately diagnosed with posterior subluxation, the instability occurs involuntarily. These same patients may also be able to demonstrate the subluxation on a voluntary basis. We believe that it is important to differentiate between patients who are able to sublux their shoulders by position or muscular activation and those who use this as a trick to attract attention, create an apparent disability, or otherwise manipulate their environment. The majority of patients, in our experience, are not manipulative and should not be excluded from consideration of surgery because of their ability to sublux their shoulders voluntarily. However, those who are the voluntary muscular type should generally be treated with exercises, avoiding surgery. In the past, Rowe (12) advised against surgical treatment of patients with voluntary posterior instability because of the high frequency of emotional disorders he observed in these patients. He warned of the high failure rate of surgery in these patients, perhaps because of secondary gain issues in continuing the disability. Awareness of this potential problem, careful patient selection, and appropriate psychiatric evaluation will minimize this issue as a complicating factor of the surgical management of recurrent posterior subluxation.

Presentation

The symptoms of recurrent posterior subluxation are similar to those of other shoulder problems, and therefore, making a definitive diagnosis is frequently quite difficult. The most common presenting complaint, like that of many other shoulder conditions, is pain. Location of pain is variable and not particularly helpful or specific to this condition. The pain may be related to edge loading of the humeral head on the glenoid or due to excessive stress on the rotator cuff as it acts to contain the humeral head on the glenoid. Similar to the "impingement syndrome" recognized with anterior instability, patients with posterior instability can develop secondary rotator-cuff injury. Symptoms and findings referable to the rotator cuff may cause some confusion in establishing the diagnosis of posterior subluxation.

Patients with posterior subluxation will often describe a sensation of clicking or crepitation of the shoulder when it is placed in certain positions. Excessive motion may not be appreciated initially by the patient, or it may be a secondary issue compared with pain. In many patients, the sensation of the shoulder moving out of joint develops over time, and it is common for patients to experience an increase in the frequency of instability episodes over time as well. The history of a voluntary ability to "shift" the shoulder in and out of the socket is also often very helpful in building suspicion for the diagnosis of recurrent posterior subluxation.

A careful history will help clarify the etiology of the instability. As discussed, the patient may recall a specific initial traumatic episode or describe a history of recurrent stress to the shoulder. There may also be no recollection of any prior event or activity. Patients may relate that the shoulder is symptomatic only in certain positions or with specific activities. The position of the arm at the time of injury and when symptoms occur are among the most important diagnostic considerations. Shoulder pain experienced primarily during follow-through, or with the arm in an adducted, flexed, and internally rotated position, is often a significant clue that posterior subluxation may be occurring.

Evaluation

Along with important data from the patient's description of the shoulder problem, the physical examination helps confirm the diagnosis of posterior subluxation. Routine examination of shoulder range of motion and muscle testing is often unrevealing. In some patients, a loss of internal rotation, particularly with the arm at 90 degrees of abduction, may be detected. Instability testing of the shoulder in the office may be difficult to interpret because of variables of patient relaxation and guarding. Posterior stress testing is performed with the patient supine and the arm at 90 degrees of abduction and neutral rotation. Translation of the humeral head on the glenoid is carefully tested on both shoulders and is graded as described in Chapter 5. Although studies have demonstrated equal anterior and posterior translation in cadaveric specimens and normal volunteers (21,22), routine stress testing often appears to show posterior translation greater than anterior. Most commonly, the apparent increased posterior translation is due to the favorable orientation of the glenoid and the leverage and feedback possible when translating the head posteriorly on the glenoid. This impression on physical examination must be interpreted carefully and related to the history of arm position and symptoms.

In contrast to anterior instability, apprehension with examination in the provocative position is an uncommon finding. If posterior translation does produce symptoms, it can be quite helpful in confirming the diagnosis of posterior subluxation. When present, it is usually seen in patients after an acute indirect trauma to the shoulder. Stress testing also should be carefully performed in the anterior and inferior directions to assess the shoulder for multidirectional instability.

Typically, the diagnostic features distinguishing between posterior subluxation and multidirectional instability are the position of the arm when symptoms are generated, the degree of inferior translation on stress testing, and whether the patient is able to demonstrate the posterior instability voluntarily. This distinction is particularly critical when surgery is being considered, as the impression of the direction of abnormal translation that causes symptoms will determine the surgical approach.

When the history and examination are consistent with recurrent posterior subluxation, we have typically approached the shoulder from posterior to restore tension to the posterior band of the inferior glenohumeral ligament and capsule. The degree of inferior translation as a second direction of instability has not particularly changed this approach, except when the sulcus sign is excessive (3+). In these patients, the choice between performing a capsular shift from an anterior approach and performing a shift from a posterior approach can be difficult. As stated earlier, if the symptoms are clearly related to the arm in an adducted, flexed position, we approach the shoulder from the posterior direction. Recently, there has been interest in a surgical approach from the front to close the rotator interval (decreasing inferior translation), followed by a traditional posterior capsular repair. It is not yet clear whether this is necessary or adds significantly to joint stability to warrant approaching the shoulder from two directions.

Radiographic evaluation of patients with posterior subluxation should include a typical instability series: anterior–posterior view in internal rotation, West Point axillary view, and Stryker notch view. Findings suggestive of posterior instability may be present; however, radiographs frequently show little unless the shoulder is posteriorly subluxed with positioning of the axillary view. In the past, we noted a 20% incidence of calcification along the posterior aspect of the glenoid rim and capsule (20). A computed tomography (CT) scan of the shoulder can be useful in assessing the version of the glenoid and humeral head. Arthrography and CT arthrography have been advocated by some as useful in visualizing labral and capsular pathology. We have not found these techniques to be particularly helpful in making the diagnosis and have found arthroscopic evaluation to be more revealing when and if it becomes indicated.

NONOPERATIVE MANAGEMENT

Indications and Results

Many patients with shoulder symptoms due to recurrent posterior subluxation will respond to conservative treatment. Burkhead (23) found that among a group of patients with instability, those with posterior subluxation responded better to nonoperative management than did those with anterior subluxation. One recent study presented a comparatively good success rate of conservative versus operative treatments in assessing satisfaction and return to sports (24). We found that patients without a history of shoulder trauma or with a history of microtrauma respond best to strengthening exercises (16,20). Patients who have a macrotraumatic etiology are less likely to be aided by an exercise program. In a group of 16 patients treated with a rehabilitation program, 10 (63%) reported improvement in pain, stability, or both. The program best controlled pain and instability in patients in whom the instability was of an atraumatic or microtraumatic origin. All seven patients who had an episode of major trauma had some degree of persistent instability after strengthening. Four (25%) patients went on to surgical stabilization. Without surgery, only 37% of patients were able to return to sports and strenuous activities. Return was associated with a decrease in level of competition in all patients (16).

Techniques

Nonoperative management is directed toward decreasing pain by rest, antiinflammatory medications, and avoidance of provocative arm positions and activities, particularly voluntary subluxations. Physical therapy is structured to develop a stable scapular platform by closed- and open-chain exercises. In addition, exercises to strengthen the rotator cuff are used, with some particular attention to the external rotators. Development of the rotator cuff will enhance its joint-compressive effects and therefore dynamic stabilization of the glenohumeral joint.

Indications for Surgery

Surgical stabilization of the glenohumeral joint is an option in those patients for whom an extensive rehabilitation program has failed because of continued pain, instability, or both. Persons who have symptoms during desired activities or who are unable to participate in their sports may also elect a surgical approach to treat their instability. Surgery is also appropriate for patients who, despite aggressive strengthening, experience persistent episodes of voluntary, positional subluxation.

SURGICAL TECHNIQUE

The following description of our surgical technique for recurrent posterior subluxation involves use of a glenoid-based, posterior capsular shift or capsulorrhaphy. We have found it to be reliable, reproducible, and successful (16,20). A lateral-based capsular shift was also described as an approach to this problem (15). In our opinion, the advantages of a medial-based capsulorrhaphy include ease of exposure through a muscle-splitting approach with low morbidity, direct treatment of abnormal capsular pathology, and repair of the capsulolabral complex if detached (reverse Bankart lesion).

In most instances, techniques to augment the capsular repair are not necessary. However, in primary surgeries or revisions when the capsule is deemed inadequate, augmentation may be desired. Options and techniques for augmentation are reviewed after the description of our capsulorrhaphy.

Position

Our initial experience with this procedure was to perform the surgery with the patient in the lateral decubitus position (Fig. 1A). The patient's chest is actually rolled semiprone to enhance retraction and visualization. More recently, we frequently have the patient seated upright in a ''beach-chair'' position (Fig. 1B). This position is considered when we first perform an arthroscopy, which we routinely do in the beach-chair position. If the beach-chair position is used, the approach is facilitated by having nearly all the scapula exposed and the operating table height adjusted so the shoulder is at eye level. Regardless of patient position, the skin incision and subsequent approach are identical.

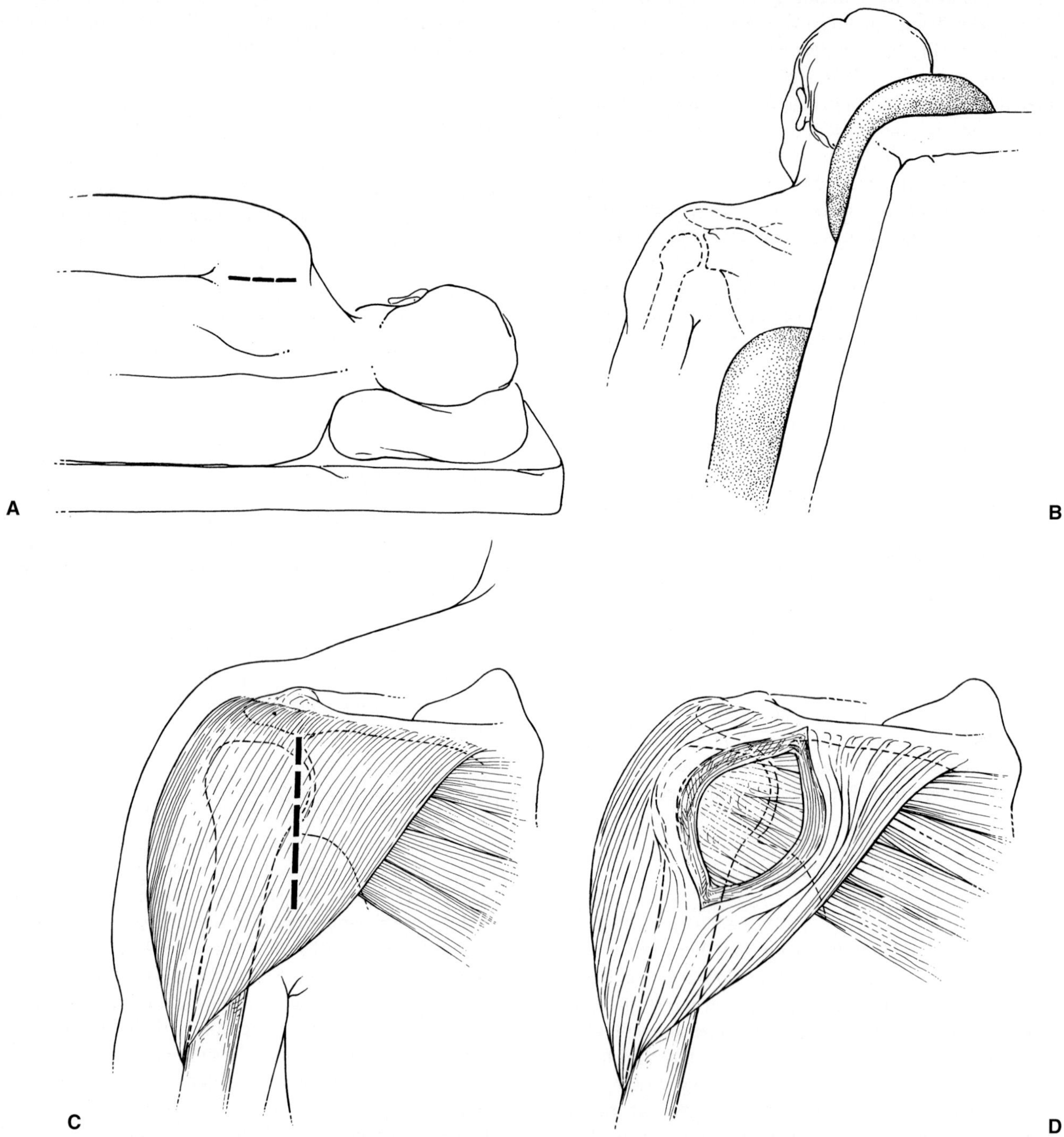

FIG. 1. A: Lateral decubitus position for a posterior approach to the glenohumeral joint. Thorax is rolled semiprone to facilitate retraction and visualization. **B:** Beach-chair position for a posterior approach to the glenohumeral joint may be used after diagnostic arthroscopy. **C:** Skin incision for a posterior approach is vertical and centered over the glenohumeral joint. **D:** Initial approach is by deltoid split located by palpating center of the glenohumeral joint. The posterior rotator-cuff musculature is then fully exposed. The capsule is visualized by splitting and developing an avascular interval between the infraspinatus and teres minor muscles.

Approach

Our preferred skin incision is oriented vertically and is centered over the glenohumeral joint (Fig. 1C). The incision extends from the axillary crease superiorly to the acromion, approximately 2 cm medial to its posterolateral corner. It may be helpful to consider the approach as a ''large'' extension of the posterior portal used for glenohumeral arthroscopy.

Subcutaneous dissection in the prefascial plane helps to define the orientation of the deltoid muscle fibers. The deltoid fascia is incised, and the muscle is next split in a plane that centers the deeper approach over the glenohumeral joint (Fig. 1D). The deltoid split is limited superiorly by the spine of the scapula and inferiorly by concerns over injury to the axillary nerve. If greater exposure is necessary, the deltoid can be released laterally from the scapular spine. This is rarely necessary if the full extent of the deltoid split is used and effective retraction is available.

The fascia overlying the infraspinatus and teres minor muscles and tendons should be exposed beneath the deltoid. Deeper exposure is accomplished by splitting the posterior rotator-cuff musculature or by incising the infraspinatus. Our preference is to develop a horizontal plane between the infraspinatus and teres minor or through the infraspinatus itself (see Fig. 4A). The location of the split is again determined by estimating the center of the glenohumeral joint by palpation. Additionally, there is frequently a fatty yellow stripe in the muscle that defines an avascular plane. It is very important to determine this interval carefully to avoid being inferior where there is risk of injury to the axillary nerve and posterior humeral circumflex vessels (Fig. 2). The infraspinatus may be incised either for exposure or to later reinforce the capsular repair. The vertical incision is usually placed at or just lateral to the glenoid rim with the arm in neutral rotation (Fig. 3).

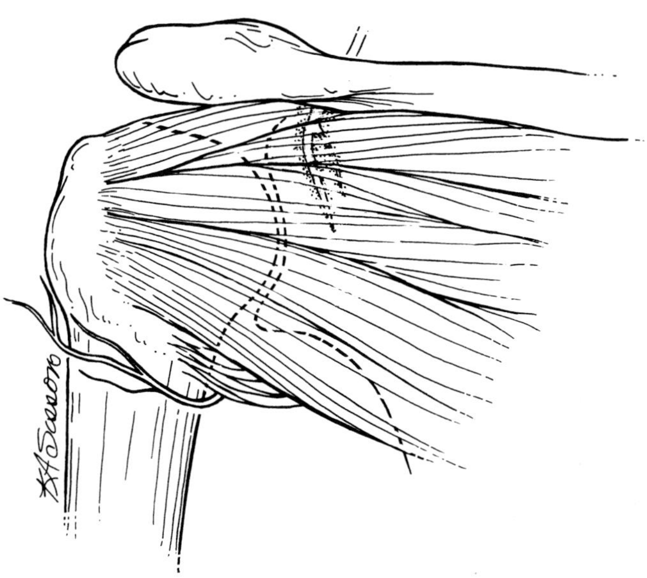

FIG. 2. Anatomy of the posterior rotator-cuff musculature with location of axillary nerve.

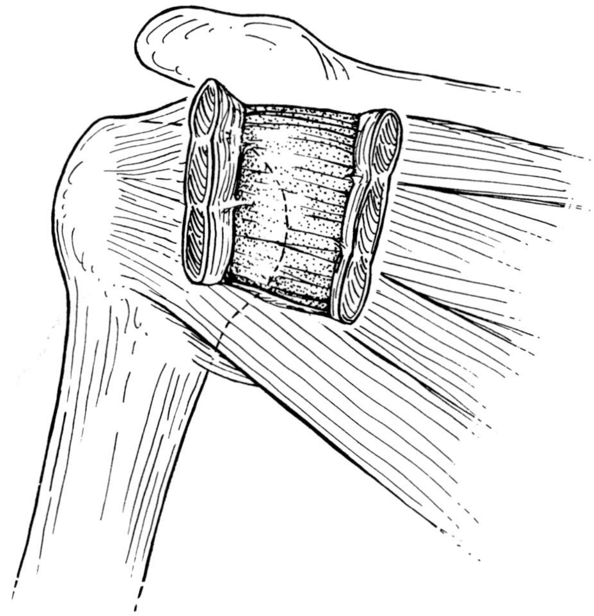

FIG. 3. Incision in infraspinatus at level of glenoid to obtain exposure of the capsule and for later use for reinforcement of the capsulorrhaphy.

It is important to expose completely the posterior capsule before performing a capsulotomy. This is facilitated by using deep right-angled retractors to retract the rotator-cuff muscle inferiorly and superiorly. Two areas of the dissection are tedious but critical to visualize fully the capsule (Fig. 4A). Laterally, where the tendon and capsule blend together and insert, the tendon must be sharply freed from the capsule to retract it inferiorly and superiorly. Inferiorly, the rotator-cuff musculature is adherent to the capsule; careful dissection of the fibers from the capsule allows an assessment of capsule laxity and accurate mobilization for the capsulorrhaphy. Dissection more than 1 cm medial to the glenoid is avoided because of the risk of injury to the suprascapular nerve (Fig. 4A).

Capsulorrhaphy

Once the posterior capsule is well defined, we perform a horizontal capsulotomy beginning at the glenoid and extending laterally (Fig. 4B). Next, we typically carry the horizontal incision medially through the capsulolabral attachment on to the glenoid. The attachment is stripped from the glenoid superiorly and inferiorly, exposing the entire posterior glenoid rim. A T-shaped incision, medial to the glenoid rim, can then be made, creating two mobile flaps of capsule. The intra-articular aspect of the posterior glenohumeral joint is then examined for abnormalities of the bony or cartilaginous glenoid rim. We have not seen ''reverse Bankart'' lesions of the posterior labrum as frequently as we have with anterior instability.

The medial (glenoid)-based capsular shift is performed

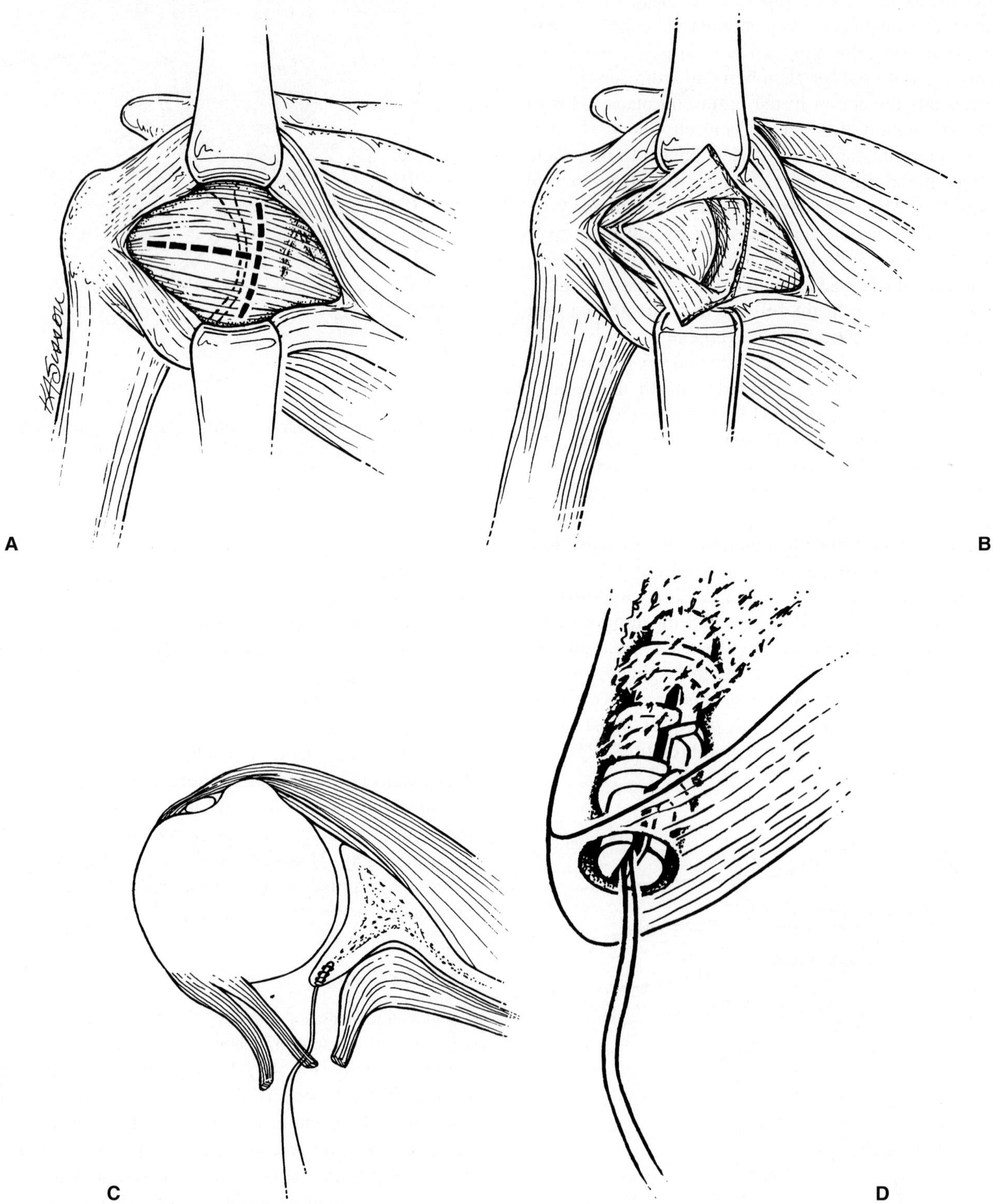

FIG. 4. A: Complete exposure of the posterior capsule is critical before performing a capsulotomy. Care is taken medially to avoid injury to the suprascapular nerve. **B:** The horizontal capsulotomy is performed from midglenoid and extends laterally. The capsulolateral attachment is stripped off the glenoid inferiorly and superiorly, forming a T-shaped release and exposing the entire posterior rim of the glenoid. **C:** Capsular repair to the glenoid is typically performed by using suture anchors. **D:** After roughening the glenoid surface, suture anchors are placed as close to the rim as possible.

by repairing the capsule to the glenoid (Fig. 4C). If the labrum is intact and secure, sutures can be placed in the labrum, and the capsule secured to it. Typically, however, we strip the labrum and capsule from the glenoid together and then reattach them as a flap to the bony glenoid. Suture anchors are placed along the glenoid rim to facilitate the capsular repair. After roughening the posterior glenoid with a burr, we usually place three spaced suture anchors as close to the rim as possible (Fig. 4D).

The capsulorrhaphy is performed by adjusting the capsular tension with the arm in approximately 20 degrees of abduction and neutral humeral rotation. With the arm in this position, the inferior capsule is advanced superiorly and slightly medially along the glenoid (Fig. 5A and B). Sutures

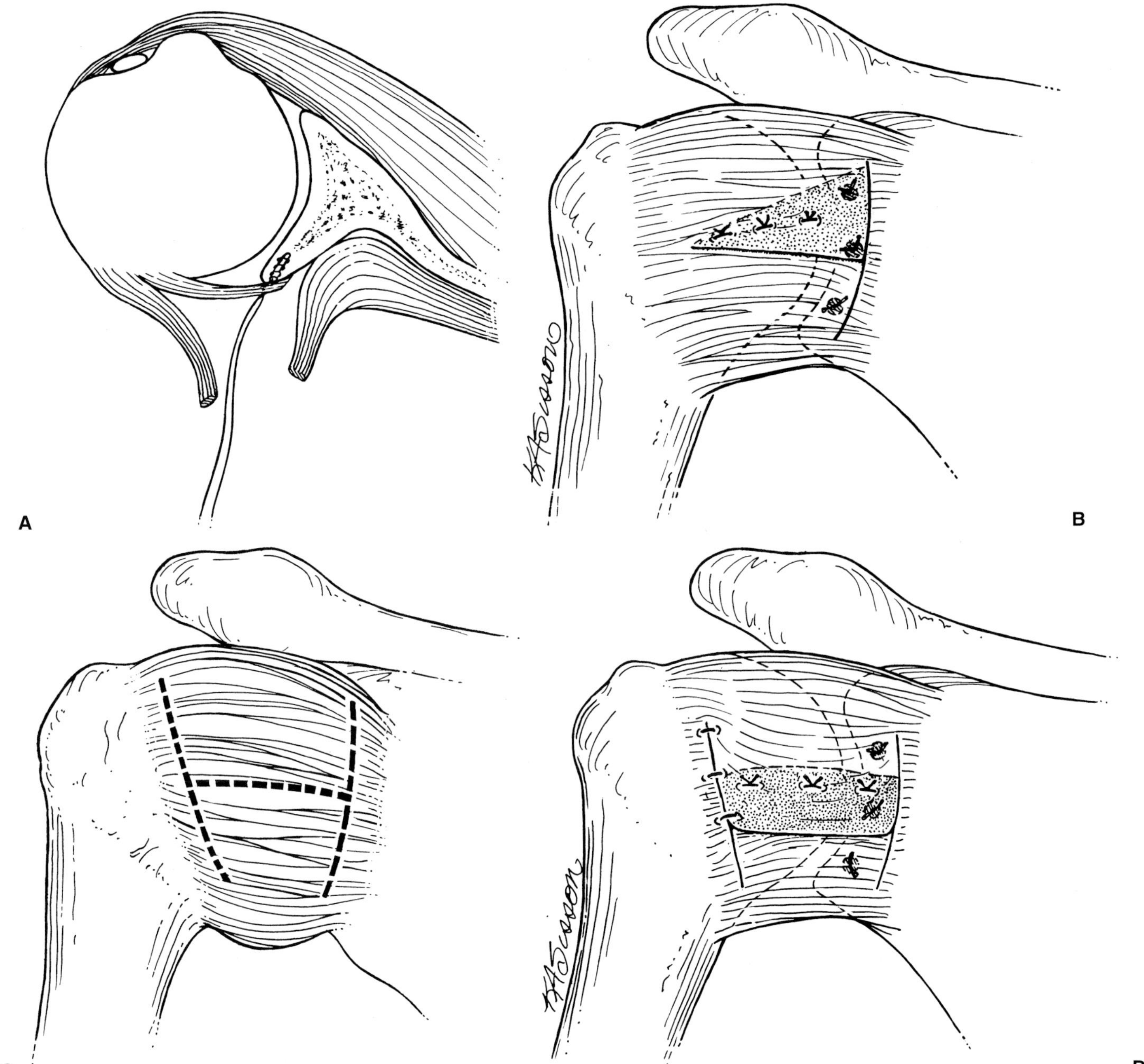

FIG. 5. A: Posterior capsulorrhaphy is performed by using the sutures from the anchors. **B:** The repair involves tensioning the capsule as the inferior capsule is advanced superiorly and the superior flap is advanced inferiorly. The posterior capsule may be tensioned further by overlapping the capsule as the horizontal interval is closed. **C:** If capsular laxity persists after the medial repair, a vertical incision may be made laterally. **D:** A lateral-based tensioning of the capsule should eliminate any remaining laxity in the posterior capsule.

from the anchors are placed through the capsule, starting with the most inferior anchor. After being tied, these sutures are also used to secure the superior capsule as it is advanced inferiorly. Capsular laxity should be eliminated by this medial-based shift. If inferior laxity persists, tension can be increased by overlapping the capsule when closing the horizontal opening. If necessary, the capsule can also be tensioned laterally, by using a vertical lateral incision and an H-type repair (Fig. 5C and D). Once the capsulorrhaphy is completed, we usually check the repair by testing translation in all three directions.

Augmentation

In primary or revision cases when there is inadequate capsular tissue, it may be necessary to augment the capsulorrhaphy. Augmentation by using the infraspinatus has been necessary in about 10% of our cases in the last 3 years. It is not used in throwers because of subsequent muscle defects. To use the infraspinatus for augmentation, it is incised vertically at the level of the glenoid, while the tendon is left attached to the humerus laterally (Fig. 6A). The medial portion is secured to the glenoid by using the previously placed capsular sutures (Fig. 6B). Humeral rotation is usually maintained at neutral to very slight internal rotation. To complete the repair, the remaining infraspinatus muscle is advanced laterally and secured over the lateral portion of the tendon (Fig. 6C).

An extracapsular posterior bone block may be added to reinforce the security of the capsular repair. Its use is reserved for cases with deficiency of the glenoid rim or revisions in which the posterior tissues are attenuated and inadequate. This technique has not been necessary in our surgeries in the past 8 years. The bone graft is obtained from the spine of the scapula because it is convenient and avoids the morbidity of iliac crest bone-graft harvest. The ideal bone graft is tricortical and measures 4 × 2.5 cm.

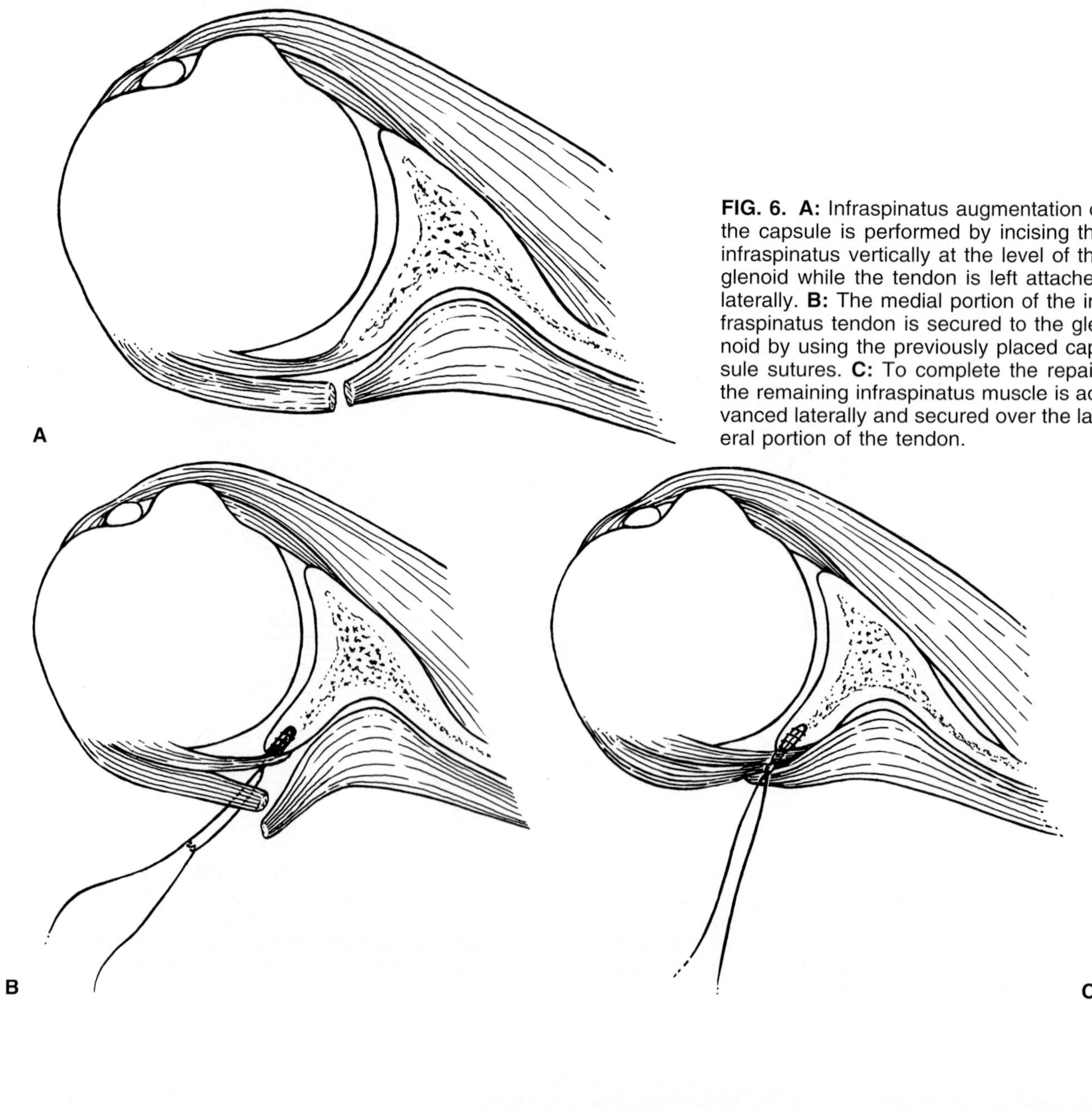

FIG. 6. A: Infraspinatus augmentation of the capsule is performed by incising the infraspinatus vertically at the level of the glenoid while the tendon is left attached laterally. **B:** The medial portion of the infraspinatus tendon is secured to the glenoid by using the previously placed capsule sutures. **C:** To complete the repair, the remaining infraspinatus muscle is advanced laterally and secured over the lateral portion of the tendon.

Before capsular repair, accurate placement is determined, and the graft and posterior scapular neck are predrilled. This minimizes the risk of intra-articular penetration of the glenoid. The graft is placed to increase the depth of the glenoid without contacting the humeral head. It is positioned along the posteroinferior quadrant of the glenoid, contiguous with the normal glenoid curvature (Fig. 7A and B). The capsule itself is repaired before securing the graft to the glenoid. Postoperative care is not altered when this technique is used.

Alternative Surgical Procedures

Numerous reconstructive procedures have been performed for recurrent posterior instability (1–4,7,9,15,16,19, 20,24–39). Several surgical procedures attempted to address posterior instability by altering the bony anatomy. These include glenoid osteotomy (2,9,25,26,31,32,34,36,39), proximal humeral rotation osteotomy (28,37), and posterior bone block (3,4,16,25,26,29). Soft-tissue stabilization procedures include biceps tendon transfer with and without capsular plication (1), reverse Putti–Platt procedure (24,30, 31), reverse Bankart procedure (16,19), staple capsulorrhaphy (19,38), infraspinatus tendon reinforcement (16,18,31), and posterior capsular shift (35,37). Reported results of the various procedures described demonstrated inconsistent success in terms of eliminating recurrent instability. Taken together, there is a higher incidence of recurrent subluxation and complications with these procedures compared with the various stabilization procedures performed for recurrent anterior instability. The relative infrequency of posterior subluxation has made it difficult for most surgeons to develop significant experience treating this problem. Limited individual clinical experience and the reported results of surgeries have contributed to the generally pessimistic view of surgery for posterior subluxation.

Several potential pitfalls are encountered in reviewing the reported studies of surgical treatments for posterior subluxation. Confusion exists with regard to the definition of subluxation and dislocation. These diagnostic definitions have been used imprecisely and interchangeably in the literature and make comparing patient populations difficult. In some patients, coincident inferior, anterior, or multidirectional instability is missed, and inappropriate treatment may result. It is difficult to be certain that patients in the same study are a homogeneous group with the identical diagnosis and underlying pathology.

The initial popularity of glenoid osteotomy was based on the theory that these patients have abnormally increased glenoid retroversion (2,24,27,36,39). Abnormal glenoid retroversion is probably an uncommon finding or cause of posterior subluxation, and thus we have not used this procedure (25,40,41). Glenoid osteotomy also adds an unnecessary degree of complexity and risk of complications. Penetration of the glenohumeral joint has been reported to lead to accelerated joint destruction (31).

Role of Arthroscopy

Arthroscopy of the glenohumeral joint in patients with subluxation may be indicated for several reasons. Examination of the posterior glenoid, labrum, and capsule may

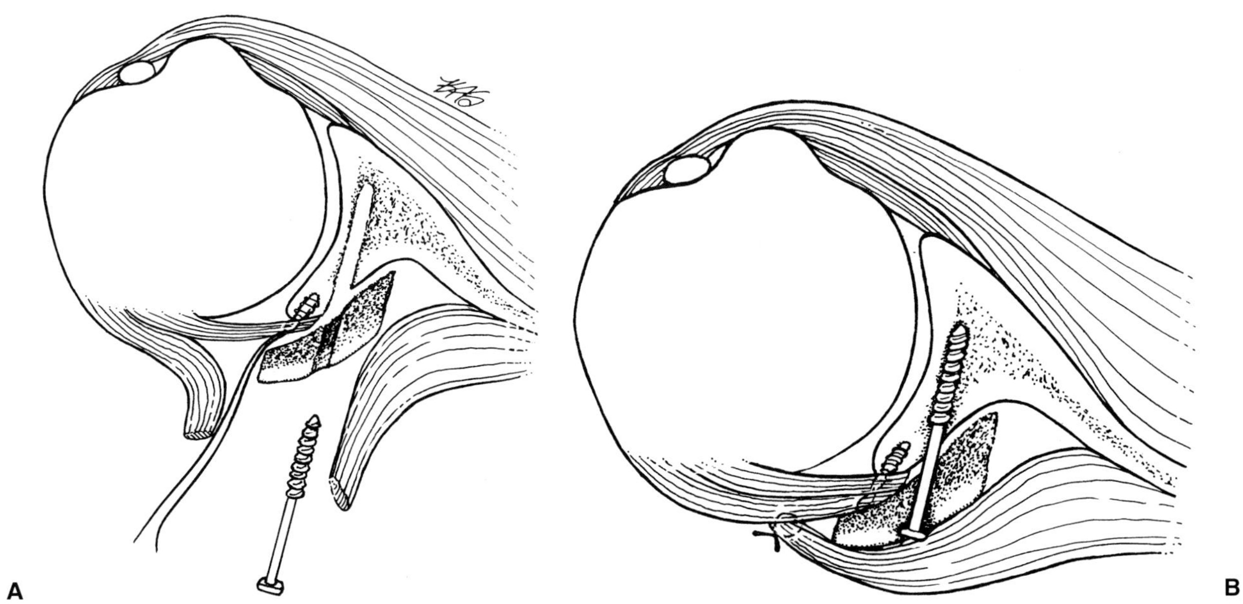

FIG. 7. A: Extracapsular bone-block augmentation may be added to reinforce the repair when the glenoid is deficient or for revisions. Correct placement is determined before capsular repair to minimize risk of glenoid penetration. **B:** The capsule repair and infraspinatus augmentation are completed before final graft placement.

demonstrate lesions consistent with posterior subluxation. Arthroscopy also allows the surgeon to make an intra-articular assessment of the capsuloligamentous anatomy to rule out findings suggestive of excessive anterior translation. This is useful in confirming the diagnosis made on the basis of history, office examination, and examination under anesthesia. We have at times only debrided the labrum when a significant, detached lesion exists. This may provide temporary relief; however, the symptoms frequently will return if the instability is not addressed. When a posterior capsulolabral detachment is identified, arthroscopic repair may be attempted. We have used a cannulated absorbable Suretac (Acufex Microsurgical, Mansfield, MA, U.S.A.) to fix the tissue to the posterior glenoid. Alternatively, suture-fixation techniques may be used. The role of laser or thermal treatment of the capsule to shorten the collagen and reduce capsular volume is of interest, but its effectiveness has yet to be determined.

POSTOPERATIVE CARE

Postoperatively, patients wear a splint for 4 to 6 weeks, immobilizing the arm in neutral rotation and slight abduction. The splint can be made preoperatively out of orthoplast or plaster; adjustable splints are also commercially available. After the period of immobilization, the splint is removed, and the patient begins a program that includes range-of-motion and muscle-strengthening exercises. We are quite concerned about restoring full range of motion in throwing and overhead athletes and so begin these patients on an early motion program. While the shoulder is otherwise protected in the brace, passive external rotation is not limited and internal rotation is allowed to neutral rotation. Passive elevation is instructed in the plane of the scapula. As with nonoperative management of shoulder instability, postoperative rehabilitation emphasizes the scapular stabilizers. Patients also focus on the rotator-cuff musculature, especially the external rotators. Rubber tubing internal and external rotation resisted exercises are begun during week 7 postoperatively. Light free weightlifting is started during week 12 and progresses to heavy weights at week 20. Noncontact and nonthrowing sports are resumed at 5 months. Contact sports are allowed between 6 and 9 months, whereas full return to throwing or repetitive overhead sports is delayed until approximately 9 months. Sports or other strenuous activities requiring the shoulder to be placed in the adducted and flexed position are avoided for the first 6 months after surgery. In general, when the patient demonstrates asymptomatic full range of motion and near-normal strength, sports-related activities are allowed to resume.

COMPLICATIONS

Unsuccessful surgery and complications are more frequent with surgery for recurrent posterior subluxation than with anterior instability procedures. The most likely factors that influence this general experience include failure to make an accurate diagnosis and unfamiliarity with the surgical techniques. Common surgical errors include failure to address the pathology directly and insufficient tensioning of the posterior capsule. Historically, the posterior capsule has often been described as insufficient and thin. This has not typically been our experience, particularly if the inferior capsule is carefully dissected, visualized, and advanced superiorly. Nonanatomic soft-tissue procedures do not directly address capsular laxity, may overtighten the joint, and increase the possibility for anterior subluxation. In addition, it is clear that anterior surgical procedures that overtighten the joint may lead to the development of glenohumeral arthrosis (42,43). This is certainly also a possible complication of similar surgery performed on the posterior side of the glenohumeral joint.

Complications of bony stabilization procedures for recurrent posterior subluxation appear to be more probable than for soft-tissue procedures. Glenoid osteotomy and bone-block augmentation carry the risk of intra-articular fracture, nonunion, and loss of graft fixation or position. Glenoid osteotomy may also lead to osteonecrosis of the glenoid and degenerative arthritis or cause anterior displacement of the humeral head, leading to contact, or impinge on the coracoid process.

Neurovascular injuries can occur during surgery for recurrent posterior subluxation. The axillary nerve and posterior humeral circumflex vessels are at risk in the approach to the posterior aspect of the glenohumeral joint if the dissection strays inferior to the teres minor (Fig. 2). Maintaining the deep dissection through the posterior rotator-cuff musculature and centered over the middle of the glenohumeral joint will minimize this problem. The axillary nerve is also at risk during deeper dissection and exposure of the capsule. The suprascapular nerve and vessels are medial to the rim of the posterior glenoid after they pass around the spinoglenoid notch (Fig. 4A). Palpation of the rim of the glenoid and the spinoglenoid notch will keep the surgeon from dissecting dangerously and unnecessarily medially.

RESULTS OF SURGERY

Patients treated surgically with posterior capsulorrhaphy have generally benefited in terms of pain relief and stability. In an initial review of 11 patients treated with surgical stabilization, nine (82%) had a decreased level of pain after surgery (16). Six patients were completely free of pain, and the other five reported pain only when involved in stressful activities or in competitive sports. Ten (91%) of 11 patients had no further episodes of instability. One patient developed recurrent instability 4 years postoperatively. He was mildly symptomatic but continued to be an active swimmer and believed he had significant improvement compared with his preoperative status.

We recently reviewed the surgical results of these original 11 patients and 15 subsequent patients at longer follow-up. All 26 patients had either severely disabling symptoms or insufficient success with an intensive rehabilitation program. The posterior stabilization procedure consisted of a capsulorrhaphy in all patients. Based on the quality of the repair, an infraspinatus augmentation was used in 17 patients, and a bone block was added in seven. At an average follow-up of 5 years, only three (12%) patients reported any episodes of instability postoperatively. None of the 21 patients who had a history of significant trauma to the shoulder reported postoperative instability. Postoperative pain was improved in all patients: 54% of patients were completely free of pain, 31% noted mild discomfort only with stressful activities or with competitive sports, and 15% described occasional discomfort with daily activities. Based on an overall shoulder evaluation, significant improvement was reported by 92% of patients at the follow-up.

After surgical stabilization, 38% of patients were able to return to sports without a change in level of competition. Half of these were involved in professional or collegiate contact sports; 62% returned to some level of athletic involvement, but with reduction in the level of participation. This was described as voluntary in 39%. Thus, only 23% thought they were unable to return to their previous level of athletic competition. This group included three nationally ranked swimmers. The average length of time after surgery to return to effective sports participation was 11 months.

In our experience, posterior stabilization with capsulorrhaphy and augmentation as necessary has proven to be an effective surgical procedure for patients with symptomatic and disabling recurrent posterior subluxation.

REFERENCES

1. Boyd HB, Sisk TD. Recurrent posterior dislocation of the shoulder. *J Bone Joint Surg [Am]* 1982;54:779–786.
2. English E, Macnab I. Recurrent posterior dislocation of the shoulder. *Can J Surg* 1974;17:147–151.
3. Hindenach JCR. Recurrent posterior dislocation of the shoulder. *J Bone Joint Surg* 1947;29:582–586.
4. Jones V. Recurrent posterior dislocation of the shoulder: report of a case treated by posterior bone block. *J Bone Joint Surg [Br]* 1958;40:203–207.
5. Kretzler HH Jr. Scapular osteotomy for posterior shoulder dislocation. *J Bone Joint Surg [Am]* 1974;56:197.
6. May VR Jr. Posterior dislocation of the shoulder: habitual, traumatic, and obstetrical. *Orthop Clin North Am* 1980;11:271–285.
7. McLaughlin HL. Posterior dislocation of the shoulder. *J Bone Joint Surg [Am]* 1952;34:584–590.
8. Nobel W. Posterior traumatic dislocation of the shoulder. *J Bone Joint Surg* 1962;44:523–537.
9. Norwood LA, Terry GC. Shoulder posterior subluxation. *Am J Sports Med* 1984;12:25–30.
10. Rockwood CA Jr. Subluxations and dislocations about the shoulder. In: Rockwood CA Jr, Green DP, eds. *Fractures in adults.* Philadelphia: Lippincott, 1984:722–860.
11. Rowe CR. Prognosis in dislocations of the shoulder. *J Bone Joint Surg [Am]* 1956;38:957–977.
12. Rowe CR, Pierce DS, Clark JG. Voluntary dislocation of the shoulder: a preliminary report on a clinical electromyographic and psychiatric study of twenty-six patients. *J Bone Joint Surg* 1973;55:445–460.
13. Rowe CR, Zarins B. Chronic unreduced dislocations of the shoulder. *J Bone Joint Surg [Am]* 1982;64:S494–S505.
14. Samilson RL. Posterior dislocation of the shoulder in athletes. *Clin Orthop* 1983;2:369–378.
15. Bigliani LU, Pollock RG, McIlveen SJ, et al. Shift of the posteroinferior aspect of the capsule for recurrent posterior glenohumeral instability. *J Bone Joint Surg* 1995;77:1101–1120.
16. Fronek J, Warren RF, Bowen M. Posterior subluxation of the glenohumeral joint. *J Bone Joint Surg [Am]* 1989;71:205–216.
17. Goss TP, Costello G. Recurrent symptomatic posterior glenohumeral subluxation. *Orthop Rev* 1988;17:1024–1032.
18. Hawkins RJ, Janda DH. Posterior instability of the glenohumeral joint: a technique of repair. *Am J Sports Med* 1996;24:275–278.
19. Tibone JE, Prietto C, Jobe FW, et al. Staple capsulorrhaphy for recurrent posterior shoulder dislocation. *Am J Sports Med* 1981;9:135–139.
20. Bowen MK, Warren RF, O'Brien SJ, Altchek DW. Posterior subluxation of the glenohumeral joint treated by posterior stabilization. *Orthop Trans* 1991;15:764–765.
21. O'Brien SJ, Schwartz RS. Capsular restraints to anterior-posterior motion of the abducted shoulder: a biomechanical study. *J Shoulder Elbow Surg* 1995;4:298–308.
22. Harryman DT II, Sidles JA, Clark JM. Translation of the humeral head on the glenoid with passive glenohumeral motion. *J Bone Joint Surg* 1990;72:1334–1343.
23. Burkhead WZ Jr, Rockwood CA Jr. Treatment of instability of the shoulder with an exercise program. *J Bone Joint Surg [Am]* 1992;74:890–896.
24. Hurley JA, Anderson TE, Dear W, et al. Posterior shoulder instability: surgical versus conservative results with evaluation of glenoid version. *Am J Sports Med* 1992;20:396–400.
25. Mowery CA, Garfin SR, Booth RE, et al. Recurrent posterior dislocation of the shoulder: treatment using a bone block. *J Bone Joint Surg [Am]* 1985;67:777–781.
26. Ahlgren SA, Hedlund T, Nistor L. Idiopathic posterior instability of the shoulder joint: results of operation with posterior bone graft. *Acta Orthop Scand* 1978;49:600–603.
27. Brewer BJ, Wubben RC, Carrera GF. Excessive retroversion of the glenoid cavity: a cause of non-traumatic posterior instability of the shoulder. *J Bone Joint Surg [Am]* 1986;68:724–731.
28. Chaudhuri GK, Sengupta A, Saha AK. Rotation osteotomy of the shaft of the humerus for recurrent dislocation of the shoulder: anterior and posterior. *Acta Orthop Scand* 1974;45:193–198.
29. Fried A. Habitual posterior dislocation of the shoulder joint: a report of 15 operated cases. *Acta Orthop Scand* 1949;18:329–345.
30. Greenhill BJ. Persistent posterior shoulder dislocation: its diagnosis and its treatment by posterior Putti-Platt repair. *J Bone Joint Surg [Br]* 1972;54:763.
31. Hawkins RJ, Koppert G, Johnston G. Recurrent posterior instability (subluxation) of the shoulder. *J Bone Joint Surg [Am]* 1984;66:169–174.
32. Hernandez A, Drez D. Operative treatment of posterior shoulder dislocations by posterior glenoidplasty, capsulorrhaphy, and infraspinatus advancement. *Am J Sports Med* 1986;14:187–191.
33. Neer CS II, Foster CR. Inferior capsular shift for involuntary inferior and multidirectional instability of the shoulder: a preliminary report. *J Bone Joint Surg [Am]* 1980;62:897–908.
34. Pouget G. Recurrent posterior dislocation of the shoulder treated by glenoid osteotomy. *J Bone Joint Surg [Br]* 1984;66:140.
35. Santini A, Nevaiser R. Long term results of posterior inferior capsular shift. *J Shoulder Elbow Surg* 1995;4(suppl):S65.
36. Scott DJ Jr. Treatment of recurrent posterior dislocations of the shoulder by glenoplasty: report of three cases. *J Bone Joint Surg [Am]* 1967;49:471–476.
37. Surin V, Blader S, Markhede G, et al. Rotational osteotomy of the humerus for posterior instability of the shoulder. *J Bone Joint Surg [Am]* 1990;72:181–186.
38. Tibone J, Ting A. Capsulorrhaphy with a staple for recurrent posterior subluxation of the shoulder. *J Bone Joint Surg [Am]* 1990;72:999–1002.
39. Wilkinson JA, Thomas WG. Glenoid osteotomy for recurrent posterior dislocation of the shoulder. *J Bone Joint Surg [Br]* 1985;67:496.
40. Gerber C, Ganz R, Vinh TS. Glenoplasty for recurrent posterior shoulder instability: an anatomic reappraisal. *Clin Orthop* 1987;216:70–79.
41. Randelli M, Gambrioli PL. Glenohumeral osteotomy by computed tomography in normal and unstable shoulders. *Clin Orthop* 1986;208:151–156.
42. Hawkins RJ, Angelo RL. Glenohumeral osteoarthrosis: a late complication of the Putti-Platt repair. *J Bone Joint Surg [Am]* 1990;72:1193–1197.
43. Bigliani LU, Weinstein DM, Glasgow M, et al. Glenohumeral arthroplasty for arthritis after instability surgery. *J Shoulder Elbow Surg* 1995;4:87–94.

The Unstable Shoulder,
edited by R.F. Warren, E.V. Craig, and D.W. Altchek.
Lippincott–Raven Publishers, Philadelphia © 1999.

CHAPTER 16

Multidirectional Shoulder Instability

Open Surgical Treatment

Frank A. Cordasco and Louis U. Bigliani

DIAGNOSTIC CONSIDERATIONS

Patients with multidirectional instability have symptomatic glenohumeral subluxation or dislocation in more than one direction: anterior, inferior, and posterior. The primary pathology is a loose redundant capsule (1–4). This problem is more common than previously recognized (2,3,5). There is a common misconception that multidirectional instability is limited to young sedentary patients with generalized ligamentous laxity, bilateral symptoms, and an atraumatic history (Fig. 1). Although there is a group of such patients, shoulders with multidirectional instability are often seen in athletic patients, many of whom have had injuries (2). Repetitive microtrauma, from gymnastics or butterfly swimming for example, may have selectively stretched out their shoulders so that their other joints may not be lax on examination (Fig. 2). Furthermore, shoulders with multidirectional instability may have Bankart lesions and humeral head impression defects, although less commonly than unidirectional cases resulting from hard trauma (2,6).

Patients with shoulder instability do not always easily separate into clear categories (unidirectional vs. multidirectional). This is especially true of athletes, often lax to begin with, who subject their shoulders to repetitive microtrauma on a daily basis but who also may have a superimposed injury. We have found athletes with anterior instability to constitute a spectrum from unidirectional anterior instability to frank multidirectional instability with pronounced inferior capsular laxity, rather than simple discrete groups (1, 7). For this reason, we have used an inferior capsular shift approach in all cases, modifying the repair so that only as much inferior capsule was shifted as was necessary to reduce the degree of inferior laxity found in each instance (1, 3,7,8).

In 1980, Neer and Foster (3) introduced the inferior capsular shift for the treatment of involuntary and multidirectional instability of the shoulder. They noted that few articles had been published regarding the treatment of inferior and multidirectional instability of the glenohumeral joint. Not only was there a relative dearth of information regarding the management of this problem, but also there was little consensus concerning the operative treatment of choice. Before 1980, several authors (9–13) recognized the importance of distinguishing this disorder from the more common unidirectional form of instability and recommended a comprehensive trial of strengthening exercises before considering surgical intervention. Neer (2,14–16) emphasized the problems encountered when standard procedures used to correct unidirectional anterior or posterior instability are performed in patients with multidirectional instability. These procedures may fail because they do not reduce the excessive inferior capsular redundancy. Furthermore, excessive tightness created on one side of a hypermobile joint may result in a fixed subluxation or dislocation in the opposite direction, possibly leading to severe glenohumeral arthritis (1,16–34).

Material property studies of the inferior glenohumeral ligament have disclosed two principal modes of failure: at the glenoid insertion (analogous to a Bankart lesion) and in midsubstance (analogous to capsular stretching or laxity; 35). Significant midsubstance ligament strain before failure

F. A. Cordasco: Department of Orthopaedic Surgery, Columbia University College of Physicians and Surgeons, New York, New York 10032; and Department of Orthopaedic Surgery, St. Luke's—Roosevelt Hospital Center, New York, New York 10019.

L. U. Bigliani: Department of Orthopaedic Surgery, Columbia University College of Physicians and Surgeons, New York, New York 10032; and The Shoulder Service, Columbia—Presbyterian Medical Center, New York, New York 10032.

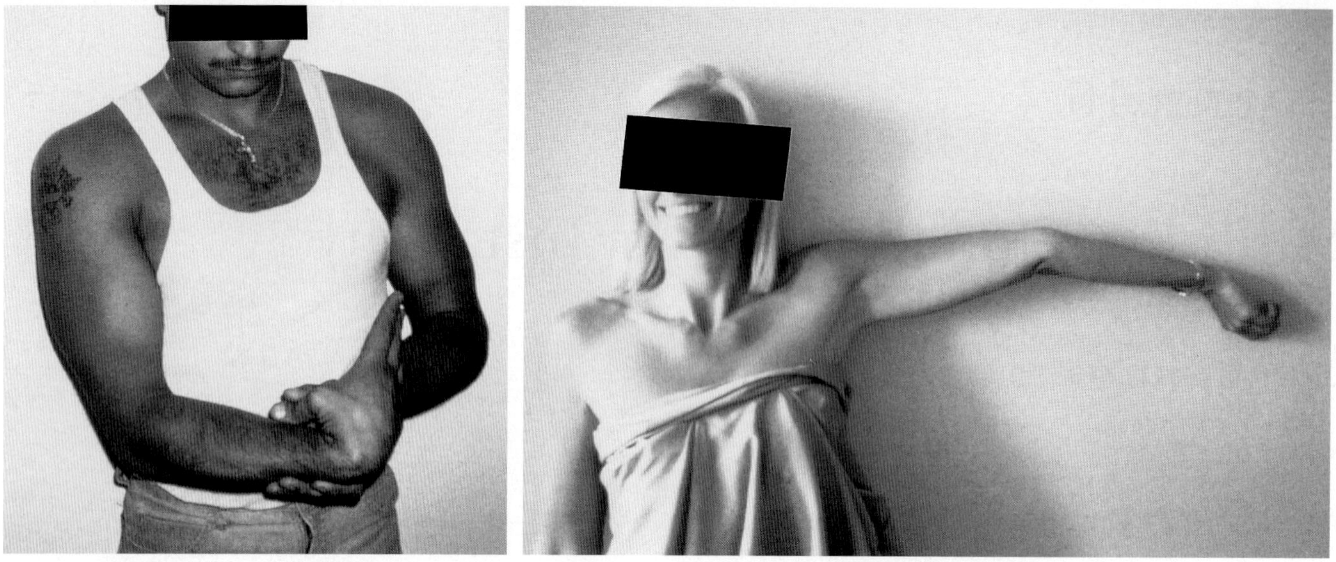

FIG. 1. Generalized ligamentous laxity. A: Laxity of the thumb is demonstrated in this patient with approximation of thumb to forearm. B: Laxity of the elbow is demonstrated in this patient with hyperextension of the elbow.

was noted even in the specimens that ultimately failed at the glenoid insertion. These findings are consistent with the results of another biomechanical study (36) that demonstrated that a Bankart lesion alone does not increase instability enough to allow anterior dislocation. These studies suggest that reconstructive procedures for shoulder instability must correct capsular laxity as well as the avulsion of the glenohumeral ligaments.

A methodical approach to the evaluation and treatment of patients with multidirectional instability, addressing the primary pathology within the glenohumeral ligament complex, has led to satisfactory results in a high proportion of cases (1–3,6,19,25,37–45).

INDICATIONS AND CONTRAINDICATIONS FOR OPEN REPAIR

Patients with multidirectional instability may be seen in a variety of ways. The patient is often athletic, and swimmers, weight lifters, and gymnasts may be particularly predisposed. The instability episode may have occurred without significant injury and spontaneously reduced or self-reduced. Extremely hypermobile shoulders can become symptomatic without unusual trauma and possibly even from the activities of daily living. A typical presentation is an individual with a relatively loose shoulder who stresses it repetitively in athletic activities or work-related events.

A subgroup of patients has a family history of hypermobility. Although investigations into the association between connective tissue disorders such as Ehlers–Danlos syndrome, biochemical abnormalities, and ligamentous laxity syndromes have been performed, no definitive relations have been demonstrated (11,46–50).

The direction of instability may occasionally be determined from the patient's symptom complex. Inferior instability may be seen with the patient's description of pain associated with carrying heavy suitcases or shopping bags. Occasionally, these symptoms are accompanied by traction paresthesias. Pain associated with pushing open heavy or revolving doors, or use of the arm in a forward flexed and internally rotated position, usually suggests a component of posterior instability, while discomfort in the overhead, abducted, and externally rotated position might generally suggest anterior instability. However, symptoms can be complex, vague, and difficult to sort out.

The physical examination may demonstrate evidence of generalized ligamentous laxity such as hyperextension at the elbows (Fig. 1), the ability to approximate the thumbs to the forearms (Fig. 1), hyperextension of the metacarpophalangeal joints, or patellofemoral subluxation. In some of these patients, we have noted hypermobile acromioclavicular and sternoclavicular joints, which can be sources of symptoms. Therefore, it is important to examine these joints for tenderness. A significant finding is the sulcus sign (Fig. 3), documenting inferior laxity. Additionally, close inspection of the scapulothoracic articulation should be performed because concomitant scapulothoracic instability may occasionally be present (2,51). There may be multiple positive findings by using the following maneuvers: anterior and posterior load-and-shift tests, anterior and posterior apprehension tests, fulcrum test, relocation test, Fukuda test, and push–pull or supine stress test (1–3,51,52). The aim is to produce humeral translations anteriorly, posteriorly, or inferiorly (relative to the glenoid) and to document that these translations are reliably accompanied by the patient's report of the usual pain and discomfort.

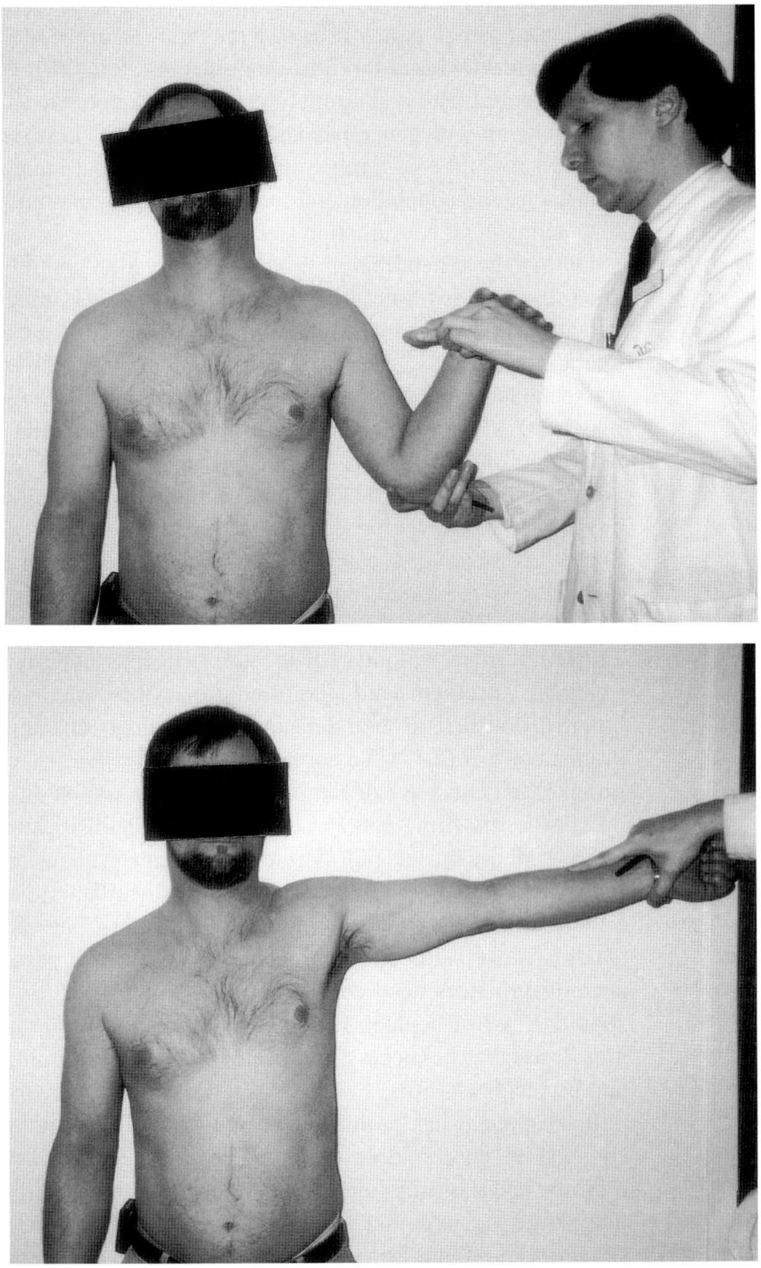

A

B

FIG. 2. Acquired shoulder laxity. **A:** This patient had multidirectional shoulder instability. He has a history of extensive gymnastics during youth, including the rings. Although his shoulders were stretched out over years of repetitive microtrauma, he does not have thumb laxity. **B:** He does not have elbow laxity.

At times, it can be difficult to determine the primary direction of instability on physical examination. Determining whether the shoulder is moving from a dislocated to a reduced position or from a reduced to a dislocated position can be challenging. Maintaining the fingers of one hand on the coracoid anteriorly and the posterolateral acromion can aid in this determination. For this reason, multiple physical examinations are helpful in assessing these patients.

It is important that symptoms be reproduced with such maneuvers, because laxity in and of itself is not an indication for surgical-stabilization procedures (2,53). Biomechanical studies have demonstrated that normal asymptomatic shoulders may show substantial translation on clinical testing (54). In addition, joint laxity may be remarkable enough to distract the examiner from the primary source of pain, such as a painful acromioclavicular joint or a cervical radiculopathy. Conversely, laxity may be hard to demonstrate, even in a shoulder with multidirectional instability, if pain, muscle spasm, and guarding prevent subluxation. It is helpful to examine the contralateral, asymptomatic shoulder for laxity. If it is extremely loose, it may be a clue to the multidirectional nature of the affected side (2,55).

Plain radiographs are generally normal but should be evaluated for the presence of humeral head defects or glenoid lesions or both, such as osseous Bankart fragments, reactive bone, or wear. Double-contrast computed tomography (CT) arthrograms may demonstrate an increased capsular volume. Recently, we have been using magnetic res-

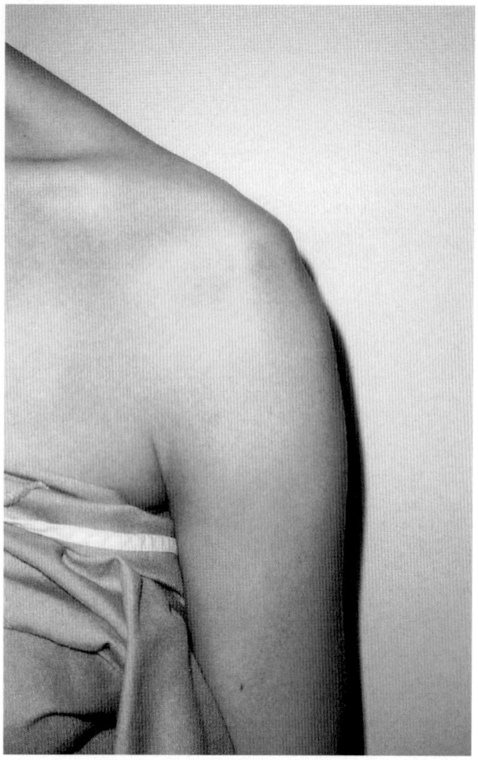

FIG. 3. This 22-year-old woman has a 3+ sulcus sign.

onance imaging (MRI) enhanced with an intra-articular mixture of saline and gadolinium. This has provided the joint distention necessary to evaluate the capsular volume and the uncommon labral or capsular detachments. Inferior subluxation can be demonstrated by stress radiographs; however, this technique is generally not needed (56). Cine MRI is currently under investigation, but has the potential to demonstrate dynamically capsular and labral defects in varying positions (57).

Once the diagnosis of multidirectional instability has been established, a prolonged course of rehabilitation is instituted with emphasis on strengthening the deltoid and rotator-cuff muscles with the arm below the horizontal (44, 58,59). The scapulothoracic stabilizing muscles are strengthened as well. Patients with multidirectional instability may have an associated synovitis and will occasionally develop a secondary impingement syndrome. Nonsteroidal anti-inflammatory drugs will be helpful in these instances. At times, a subacromial injection of a steroid preparation will provide relief sufficient for the patient to resume his or her exercise regimen.

The role of proprioception in shoulder stability has been supported by a study demonstrating that athletic individuals with chronic shoulder instability have significant deficits in proprioception, and surgical stabilization normalizes proprioceptive sensibility. Because mechanoreceptors must be deformed or loaded to function, they may not be sufficiently stimulated in a lax or injured capsule (60). Alteration of the normal state of negative intra-articular pressure also has been implicated as potentially affecting the function of the mechanoreceptors and contributing to shoulder instability (61–63). Muscle-coordination abnormalities have been noted in studies of patients with generalized laxity as well (64). These studies are supportive of a rehabilitation program that includes neuromuscular adaptation and focuses on improving muscle tone and general coordination (59,65).

During the rehabilitation program, motivation should be carefully assessed both to be sure that the patient is mature enough to cooperate in the rehabilitation effort required postoperatively and to screen out those manipulating their disease for secondary gain (2,12). Patients with acquired instability may have developed the ability to dislocate the shoulder at will or on command. This is especially true if certain positions will reliably result in a dislocation (the humeral head falls out posteriorly whenever the arm is raised in the forward plane). Such ''positional dislocators'' may demonstrate this for the examiner, if requested, but otherwise will do their best to avoid such positions. However, these patients must be differentiated from true voluntary dislocators, who have underlying psychiatric problems and who often use asymmetric muscle pull to dislocate their shoulders, or even to hold it out, to great dramatic effect (2,12). To complicate things further, a small group of patients have developed a habitual initiation of improper muscle-firing patterns that also produce dislocations by asymmetric muscle pull. These patients can be unaware of this pattern and may be without psychiatric disturbance. Nevertheless, both groups of ''muscular dislocators'' are poor candidates for stabilization procedures. Those with psychiatric disturbances need counseling and, with respect to the shoulder, skillful neglect. The group with habitually improper muscle use may be successfully treated with muscle retraining and biofeedback (66).

If the patient has prolonged symptoms that have not responded to conservative treatment, including an exercise regimen and the occasional use of anti-inflammatory drugs, then surgery is recommended. Surgery may be considered sooner if additional factors are noted, such as a documented glenohumeral ligament avulsion on double contrast CT arthrogram or MRI.

TECHNIQUES

The primary pathology in multidirectional instability is the presence of a loose, redundant capsule. This pathologic capsular laxity is directly addressed by the inferior capsular-shift procedure, which reduces the volume of the glenohumeral joint anteriorly, inferiorly, and posteriorly. The inferior capsular shift is designed to reduce capsular volume on all sides by thickening and overlapping the capsule on the side of greatest instability and tensioning the capsule on the inferior and opposite sides. For example, in a shoulder that dislocates anteriorly and inferiorly and subluxes posteriorly, an inferior capsular shift would be performed from an anterior approach. The anterior "T" capsulorrhaphy thickens and tightens the anterior capsule. The inferior capsular pouch is obliterated. Finally, shifting the inferior capsule anteriorly, around the humeral neck, tensions the posterior capsule. In addition, the rotator interval is often widened, and closing this interval (and the associated "cleft" between the superior and middle glenohumeral ligaments as described by Neer) from an anterior approach, as well as drawing the superior flap of the T capsular incision down, tensions the anterosuperior capsule and ligaments.

Neer (3) believed that the rotator interval between the supraspinatus and subscapularis and the deeper cleft between the superior and middle glenohumeral ligaments was widened in patients with multidirectional instability. He described closing it before shifting the superior flap inferiorly "to act as a sling against inferior subluxation." Recent studies of the rotator interval confirm its important role in instability and substantiate the importance of addressing this area at the time of reconstructive surgery, as described by Neer (45,67–69). The inferior capsular shift corrects the redundant inferior pouch associated with inferior instability in the abducted arm and the widened rotator interval responsible for inferior instability in the adducted arm. This concept was supported by subsequent biomechanical and clinical studies (7,35–37,43,45,54,61–63,67–74). Thus, the soft tissues are balanced in a systematic way to meet the pathology actually present.

The capsular attenuation or redundancy may be addressed in three ways. The capsular approach to the joint may be lateral (humeral) as described by Neer (3), intermediate (middle) as advocated by Wirth et al. (75), or medial (glenoid) as described by Altchek et al. (6). We prefer the lateral capsular incision, as it offers several advantages. The capsule is shaped like a cone or funnel with a broader insertion and surface area on the humeral side. For this reason, more capsule can be shifted, as the tissue can be shifted a greater distance and reattached to a broader insertion. This is particularly consequential in patients whose shoulders have significant inferior redundancy or a patulous capsule. The lateral capsular incision also affords relative protection to the axillary nerve if the shoulder is maintained in a position of external rotation and adduction during the dissection (Fig. 4), as the nerve is more medial in this situation (1,2,8). Additionally, in the unusual instance of capsular tears at the humeral insertion, a lateral approach facilitates diagnosis and repair. The intermediate (middle) incision in the capsule has been recommended because it is thought to be technically easier than a medial approach, improves medial visualization of the glenoid rim, and allows double-breasting of the glenohumeral ligaments (75). A primary disadvantage is that inferior dissection must be done with great care, as injury to the axillary nerve is quite possible. The medial (glenoid) approach to the capsule (Fig. 5) has the advantage of facilitating repair of the capsule and labrum to bone when a concomitant Bankart lesion is present (6).

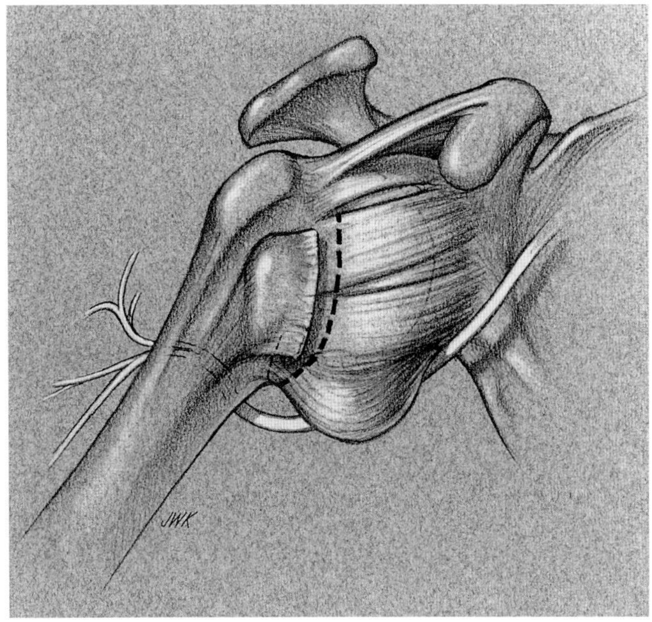

FIG. 4. The capsular incision is performed 5 mm medial to the lateral cuff of subscapularis tendon as the arm is maintained in external rotation and adduction to avoid injury to the axillary nerve.

An interscalene regional block is the anesthesia of choice when possible. Some infiltration of the skin and subcutaneous tissues of the axilla aid in comfort because of overlap with thoracic segmental nerves. The patient is placed in the beach-chair position, and all bony prominences are carefully padded to avoid skin and neurovascular compromise. Head and neck positioning is greatly simplified in an awake patient under regional anesthetic. However, if the patient is asleep, hyperextension or hyperflexion, or both, of the cervical spine are avoided by securing the head and neck in a stable position. The upper extremity is prepared and draped from the sternum, base of neck, and medial border of the scapula, with the upper extremity free. Prophylactic antibiotics are administered intravenously.

The examination under anesthesia is then performed. Biomechanical studies have contributed to the fund of knowledge regarding the static stabilizers of the glenohumeral joint, and this has aided in the performance of the examination under anesthesia (35,36,53,54,61–63,68,70–74,76,77). Because different portions of the capsule and ligament system are brought into play in different arm positions, the glenohumeral joint is stressed anteriorly, posteriorly, and inferiorly in adduction, 45 degrees of abduction, 90 degrees of abduction, and internal and external rotation. Usually, the direction of greatest instability has been determined preoperatively after the assessment of the history, multiple repeated examinations, plain radiographs, and any additional imaging studies, such as a double-contrast CT arthrogram or MRI or both. It is rare to change the approach intraoperatively on the basis of the examination under anesthesia.

A

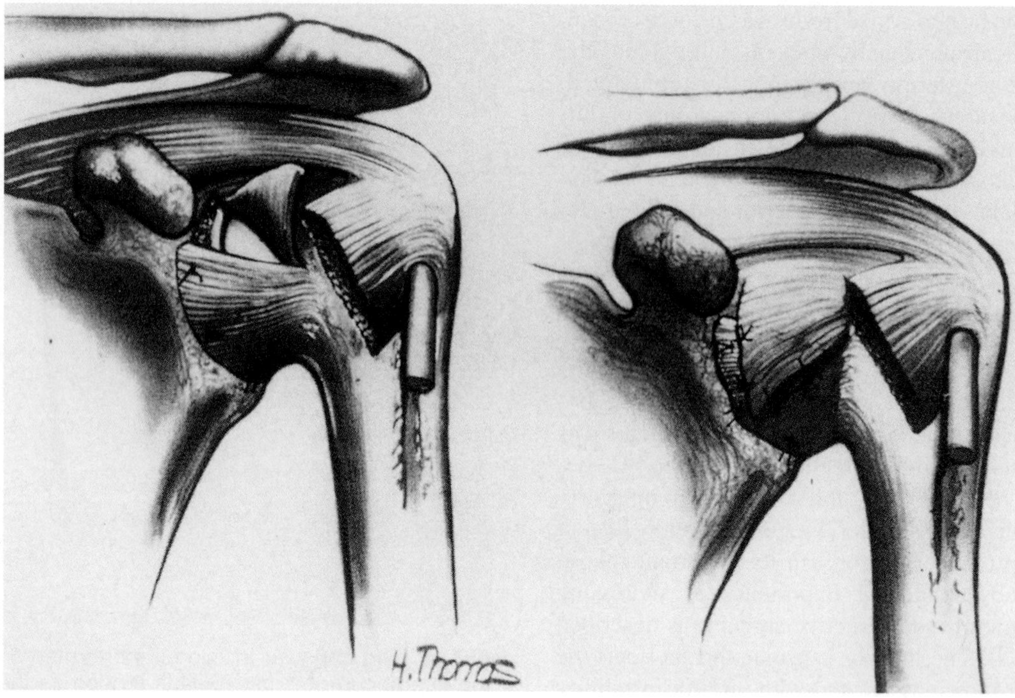

B

FIG. 5. T-Plasty modification of the Bankart procedure. **A:** A superior shift of the inferior flap and suture to the glenoid margin. **B:** The superior flap is to be advanced anteriorly to make a better layered closure. (From Altchek DW, Warren RF, Skyhar MJ, et al. T-plasty modification of the Bankart procedure for multidirectional instability of the anterior and inferior types. *J Bone Joint Surg [Am]* 1991;73:105–112, with permission.)

This technique is usually performed from one surgical approach, anterior or posterior. Over the years, we have found that the majority of our inferior capsular shifts have been approached from the anterior side. The capsulorrhaphy is reinforced on the side of the direction of greatest instability, which is also the side chosen for the approach (1,2, 8,37). Sometimes, it is difficult to decide on the best side for the approach; our method for this determination is outlined in Table 1. Essentially, the side that dislocates takes precedence over lesser degrees of instability. Shoulders that dislocate both anteriorly and posteriorly should be approached from the anterior side. Cooper and Brems (38) preferred to approach all cases from the anterior aspect of the shoulder.

An axillary skin incision is made as described by Leslie and Ryan (78). A concealed incision within the axillary-crease skin folds, it begins at a point midway between the tip of the coracoid and the inferior border of the pectoralis major and extends to the inferior border of the pectoralis major (Fig. 6). The incision is taken through the

TABLE 1. *Indications for approach (anterior vs. posterior)*

Anterior approach	Anterior: subluxation + posterior: stable or subluxation
	Anterior: dislocation + posterior: stable or subluxation or dislocation
Posterior approach	Anterior: stable + posterior: subluxation or dislocation
	Anterior: subluxation + posterior: dislocation

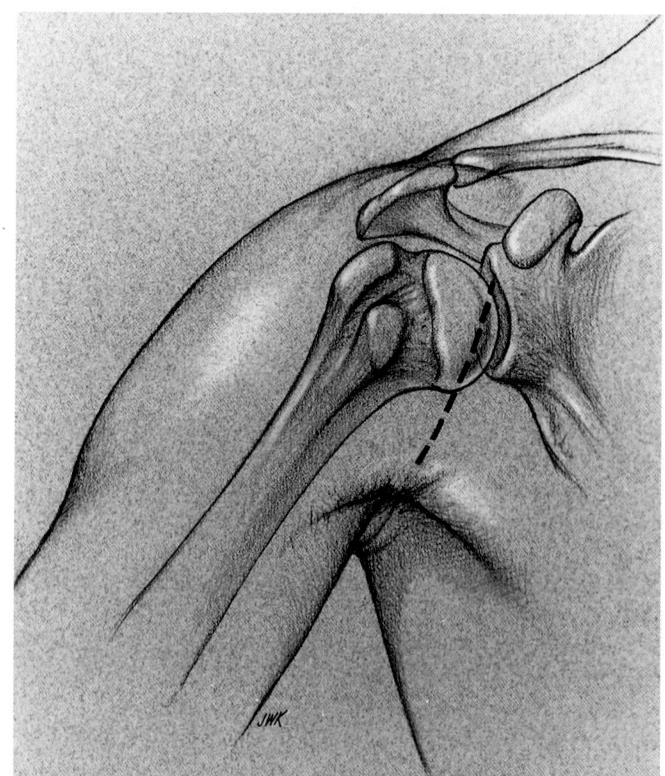

FIG. 6. The skin incision begins at a point midway between the tip of the coracoid and the inferior border of the pectoralis major and extends to the inferior border of the pectoralis major, concealed within the anterior axillary skin crease.

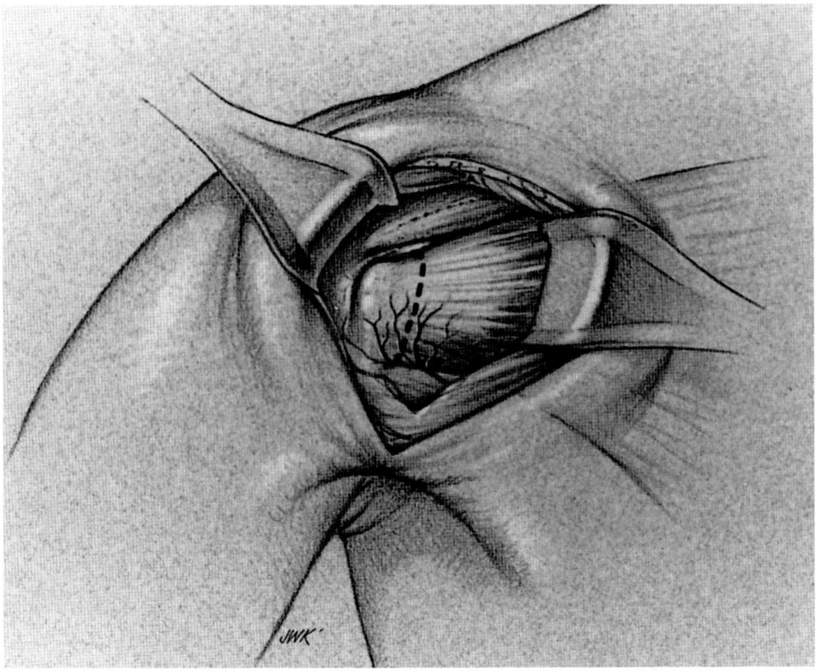

FIG. 7. Subscapularis tendon identification begins superiorly at the level of the rotator interval and inferiorly in the region of the anterior humeral circumflex vessels. The incision begins 1 cm medial to the lesser tuberosity.

subcutaneous tissues to the level of the deltopectoral interval. Careful hemostasis is obtained with the use of the needle-tip electrocautery. The subcutaneous tissues are mobilized superiorly to the inferior aspect of the clavicle and anteroinferior acromion. The cephalic vein is mobilized with the deltoid laterally, and retractors are placed beneath both the pectoralis major for medial retraction and the deltoid for lateral retraction. The superior third of the pectoralis major insertion may be taken down if needed and tagged for later repair. The long head of the biceps tendon is carefully protected during this maneuver.

Next, the clavipectoral fascia is incised lateral to the strap muscles, which are gently retracted. Osteotomizing the coracoid or incising the strap muscles may place the musculocutaneous nerve at risk and is not necessary for exposure. The arm is then placed in a slight degree of external rotation to facilitate identification of the superior and inferior borders of the subscapularis. After excising any overlying subdeltoid bursa, the lesser tuberosity is identified. A small wedge of the anterior portion of the coracoacromial ligament may be excised to facilitate visualization of the superior border of the subscapularis tendon.

The importance of the subscapularis muscle cannot be overemphasized, and meticulous care throughout the approach and repair is imperative (79,80). The subscapularis tendon is generally incised approximately 1 cm medial to its insertion on the lesser tuberosity. The incision is oriented from superior to inferior, perpendicular to the tendon fibers, and extends from the rotator interval superiorly to the lower border of the subscapularis inferiorly (Fig. 7). The anterior humeral circumflex vessels are cauterized to prevent bleeding. The subscapularis tendon is elevated from the under-

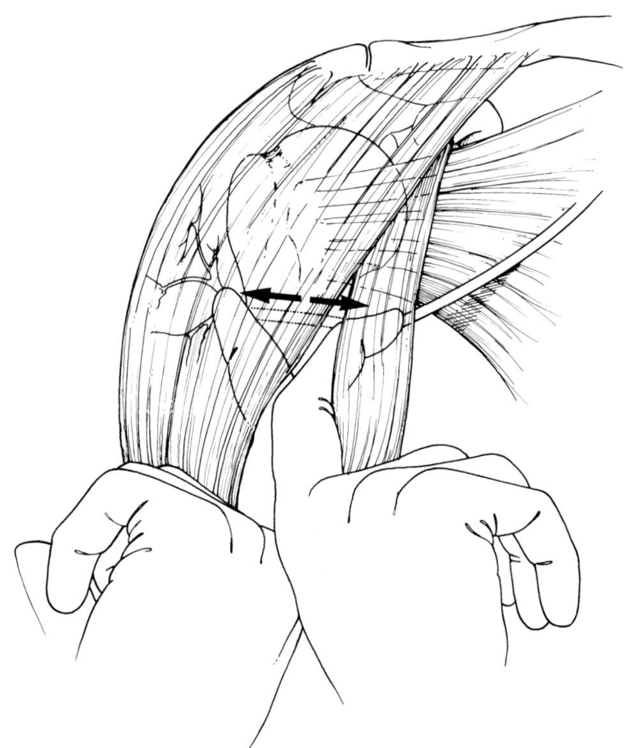

FIG. 8. The "tug test." One finger is placed on the axillary nerve at the front of the subscapularis, and the other finger under the deltoid on the anterior branch. A gentle tug applied by either finger will be transmitted to the other finger and is usually easily palpable.

lying capsule. Stay sutures are placed in the subscapularis tendon, which is retracted medially. A stay suture is placed in the rotator interval for later repair. The remaining lateral insertion of the subscapularis is elevated (undercut) from the underlying capsule. This facilitates differentiating the capsular and subscapularis flaps so that they may be later individually repaired. The surgeon must be cognizant of the position of the axillary nerve, because it courses quite close to the inferior portion of the capsule (Fig. 4). We have found the ''tug test'' (Fig. 8) to be quite helpful in locating the anterior aspect of the axillary nerve (81). If the vertical incision is too far medial, muscle fibers may be damaged, thereby compromising the subscapularis repair. Wirth and Rockwood (75) recommended preservation of the inferior portion of the subscapularis in an effort to protect the axillary nerve and anterior humeral circumflex vessels. An anatomic study (79) demonstrated that 40% of the subscapularis tendon insertion into the proximal humerus is inferior to the anterior humeral circumflex vessels. Neglecting to release the inferior subscapularis will severely compromise the inferior capsular dissection and may limit the ability to shift the inferior capsule superiorly. Whereas the possibility of compromise to humeral head vascularity was suggested, Steinmann et al. (82) found no significant reduction after ligation of the anterior humeral circumflex artery.

The lateral (humeral) approach to the capsule begins 5 mm medial to its humeral insertion. The incision starts at the level of the rotator interval. As the inferior aspect is approached, the arm is maintained in external rotation to avoid injury to the axillary nerve. Stay sutures are placed in the capsule as it is mobilized (Fig. 9). As the humerus is externally rotated and flexed, the capsule is incised around the neck of the humerus, extending as far posteriorly as necessary, depending on the degree of instability. A finger may be placed in the inferior pouch to assess how large it is and how much redundant capsule needs to be released from the humerus before repair. In a shoulder with classic multidirectional instability, the capsule is taken down all the way to the posterior capsule, which can then be tensioned as the detached inferior capsule is shifted anteriorly.

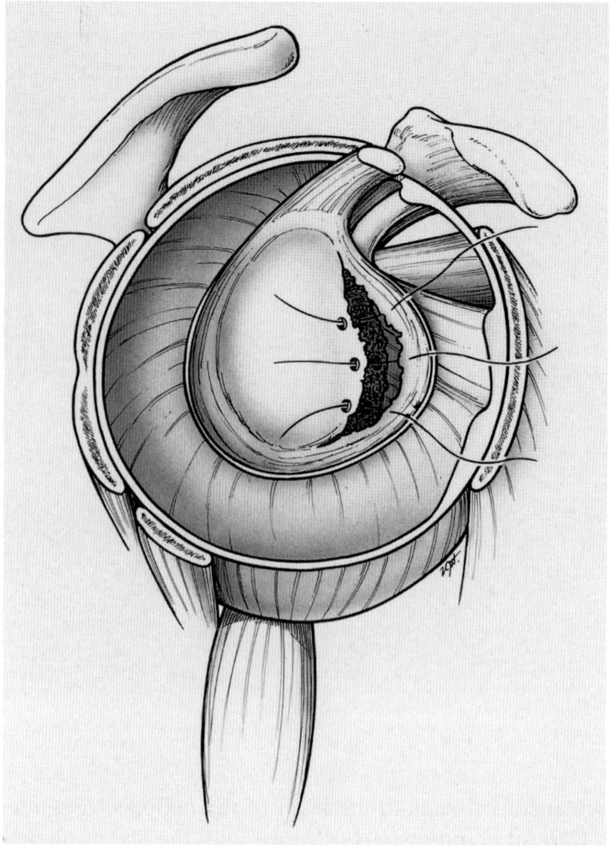

FIG. 10. A capsulolabral avulsion from the bony neck of the glenoid should be repaired before any attempt at capsulorrhaphy or shifting of the anterior capsule. Bone sutures or suture anchors can be used.

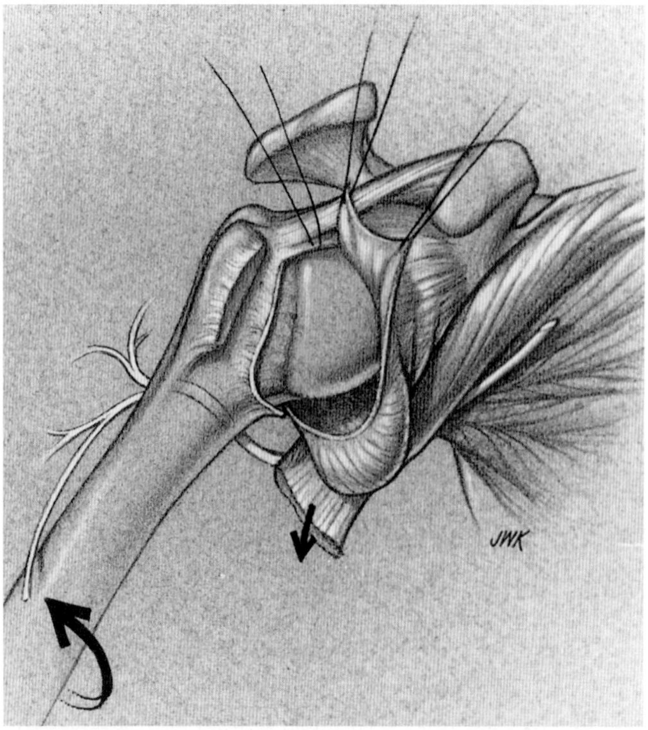

FIG. 9. Stay sutures are placed in the capsule as it is incised, and progressive external rotation facilitates inferior dissection.

A Fukuda ring retractor (Tiemann Co., Hauppage, NY, U.S.A.) is placed, and the joint is inspected carefully. Intra-articular pathology, loose bodies, and articular cartilage defects are noted. At this stage, special steps are added as the pathology indicates. If there is detachment of the glenohumeral ligament complex (Broca–Perthes–Bankart lesion), it is repaired. Although less frequently observed, glenohumeral ligament detachments do occur in patients with multidirectional instability (1,2,6). Sutures through drill holes in the bone and or suture anchors may be used for fixation. Both ends of the suture are passed through the medial capsule and tied down to secure the capsule, labrum, and ligaments to the roughened anterior glenoid neck (Fig. 10). Bone grafting is

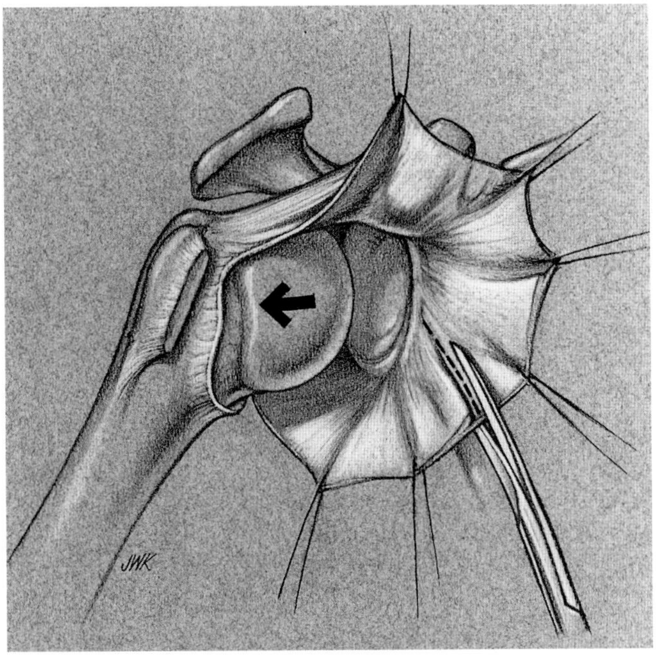

FIG. 11. The capsule is incised horizontally in a "T" fashion between the middle and inferior glenohumeral ligaments.

rarely required for patients with multidirectional shoulder instability (2). If there is anterior glenoid bone deficiency involving more than 25% of the glenoid articular surface (resulting from erosion from multiple previous dislocations or from prior fracture), a bone graft may be performed.

After the joint is carefully evaluated, the capsule is incised horizontally in a "T" fashion. This is generally performed between the middle and inferior glenohumeral ligaments (Fig. 11). The superior flap thus has the superior and middle glenohumeral ligaments, whereas the inferior flap consists of the three portions of the inferior glenohumeral ligament. At this time, the inferior capsular flap should be mobilized superiorly. The pouch should be obliterated, and this can be evaluated by placing a finger inferiorly and placing traction on the sutures in a superior direction. If there is any remaining subscapularis muscle on the inferior part of the capsule, there may be difficulty mobilizing this flap superiorly. Shifting the inferior capsular flap should effectively eliminate the redundant inferior pouch and tension the posterior capsule. The bone of the humerus just lateral to the articular margin is freshened to facilitate healing. The "T" incision allows adjustment of medial–lateral and superior–inferior tension independently, which can be especially helpful in athletes in whom restriction of motion must be avoided.

The capsule is repaired in general with the arm in approximately 25 degrees of external rotation and 20 degrees of abduction. This is modified for the individual patient. We repair the dominant shoulders in throwers in relatively more external rotation and abduction. The repair is performed beginning with the inferior flap, which is shifted superiorly (Fig. 12). The sutures are placed in a simple interrupted manner progressing superiorly, repairing the inferior flap to the lateral stump of capsular insertion. Occasionally, when the quality of the capsular tissue remaining on the humerus is poor, sutures through humeral bone or suture anchors, or both, are used. Next, the superior cleft is repaired in a simple interrupted manner, closing the enlarged rotator interval. The superior capsular flap is then shifted inferiorly and repaired (Fig. 12).

The subscapularis muscle is reattached to its insertion in an anatomic manner. It is not transferred laterally. If release of the pectoralis major insertion was necessary, it is repaired by using nonabsorbable sutures. The deltopectoral interval is closed with absorbable sutures in a simple interrupted manner, and the skin is closed in a running subcuticular fashion.

As noted, in recent years we have found that the majority of our inferior capsular shifts for the treatment of multidirectional instability have been performed from an anterior approach. Because posterior instability is discussed elsewhere in this volume, we refer the interested reader to previously published work for details regarding the posterior approach (2,3,8).

Several investigational techniques are being evaluated (26,83–85). Arthroscopy has been advocated as a diagnostic aid (86), and a preliminary report of an arthroscopic medial-based capsular shift has demonstrated satisfactory results (83). The effect of thermal heating on the glenohumeral joint capsule is being investigated, and arthroscopic laser contraction of the capsule has been described (84,85). The indications for these procedures have yet to be established, and long-term follow-up is unavailable.

REHABILITATION

For those patients with classic multidirectional instability and a significant degree of posterior instability, a special brace that holds the arm in a slightly abducted position with neutral rotation is used. The arm is immobilized in this brace for 6 weeks; only gentle isometric exercises and supervised elbow range of motion are allowed during that time. At 6 weeks, the brace is discontinued, and range-of-motion exercises are gradually introduced. At 12 weeks postoperatively, progressive strengthening is instituted on an individualized basis.

Those patients with "bidirectional" (anterior and inferior) instability without a significant posterior component are protected in a sling for 6 weeks, but after 10 days, the arm is removed from the sling for exercises, including isometrics and external rotation to 10 degrees and forward elevation to 90 degrees. From 2 to 4 weeks, external rotation is increased to 30 degrees and forward elevation to 140 degrees, and isometric strengthening is added. From 4 to 6 weeks, external rotation is increased to 40 degrees and forward elevation to approximately 160 degrees, and resistive exercises are begun. After 6 weeks, external rotation is increased to 60 degrees and forward elevation to 180 degrees. After 3 months, external rotation may be progressed.

A

B

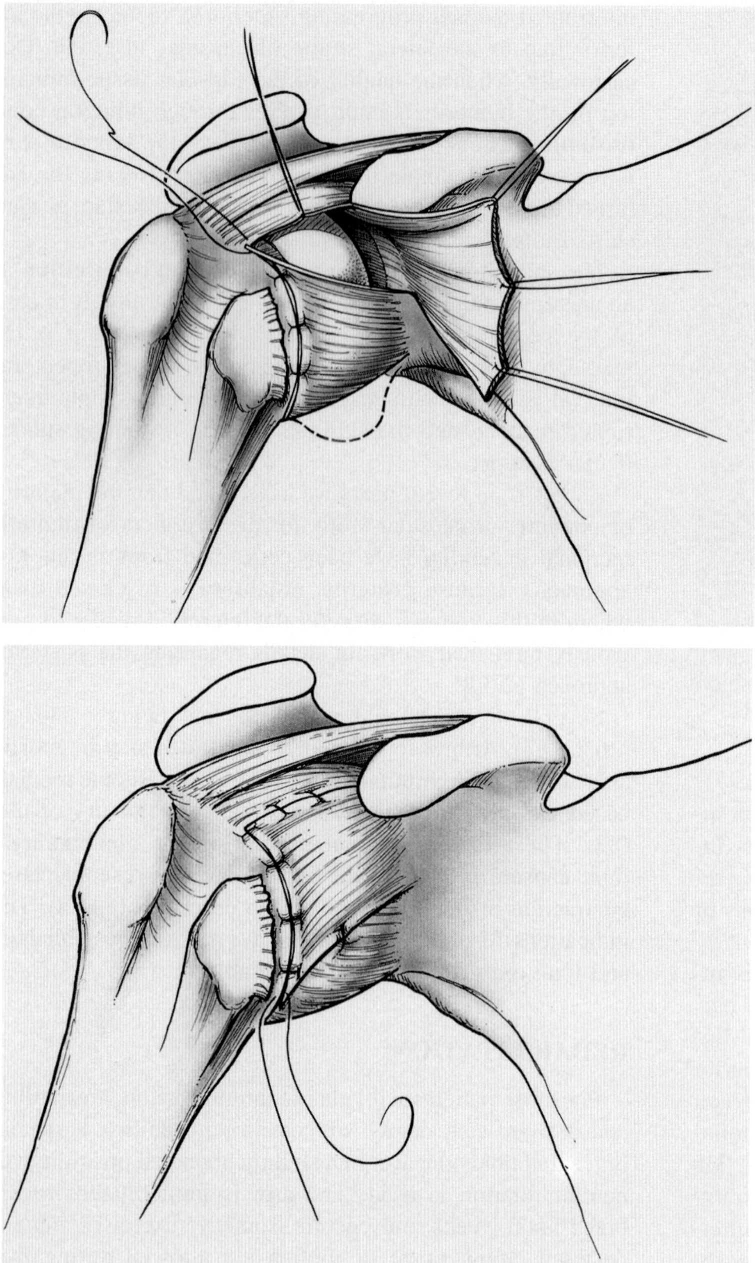

FIG. 12. A, B: The capsular shift begins as the inferior flap of the capsule is shifted superiorly and repaired to the lateral cuff of the capsule. After repair of the superior cleft, the superior capsular flap is then shifted inferiorly and repaired.

Strengthening begins with the arm in neutral below 90 degrees. As the rehabilitation progresses, more dynamic-strengthening exercises are introduced. These exercises include the use of medicine balls in various sizes and weights, as well as plyometric exercises (59,65).

These are general protocols and are modified on an individual basis as indicated. For example, the dominant shoulder of throwers would be progressed more quickly, particularly with reference to external rotation. The objective is to regain motion over several months, because progression that is too quick may lead to recurrent instability. This is especially true in patients with some degree of generalized ligamentous laxity and in younger patients in late adolescence. Careful and frequent postoperative follow-up is necessary, because patients who are not progressing quickly enough may need an accelerated program, whereas those who are regaining motion too quickly may need to be slowed down. Return to contact sports is generally restricted until 9 to 12 months have elapsed.

RESULTS

Since 1980, several investigators have reported on the treatment of patients with multidirectional instability (2,5, 20,37,38,40,42). Operative management by using the inferior capsular shift has been quite successful. Neer's initial report (3) in a series of 32 patients noted only one unsatisfactory result. One decade later, he reported ''more than

100 additional inferior capsular shifts have been done with similar satisfactory results'' (2). Cooper and Brems (38) reviewed their series of 43 shoulders in 38 patients with a minimum 2-year follow-up after inferior capsular shift. Thirty-nine (91%) of 43 shoulders were rated by the patient as satisfactory with no recurrent instability. Postoperatively, recurrent symptomatic instability developed in four (11%) patients. Two of these patients required subsequent revision inferior capsular shifts, and one of those later required a humeral head replacement for arthritis. The latter patient had had a prior Bristow procedure. They concluded that the inferior capsular shift procedure provided satisfactory objective and subjective results. Failures and recurrences of symptomatic instability generally occurred in the early postoperative period less than 2 years after surgery. Their findings did not demonstrate a deterioration of the results with follow-up to 6 years. Our service reported the results after inferior capsular shift for classic multidirectional instability in 52 shoulders. Average follow-up of 5 years was present, and all patients were immobilized in a brace for 6 weeks. Satisfactory results were noted in 94% of patients (37). Hawkins et al. (87) reported less favorable results in a series of 31 patients followed up for 2 to 5 years. Just fewer than 40% of the patients (12) went on to failure.

Altchek and Warren (6) reported their results after a T-plasty modification of the Bankart procedure for multidirectional instability in 42 shoulders. The patient population differed somewhat in that 38 of the 42 cases had a Bankart lesion or detachment of the labrum and glenohumeral ligament complex. Patient satisfaction was rated excellent for 40 (95%) of the shoulders. The average loss of external rotation was 5 degrees. They noted that throwing athletes had found they were unable to throw a ball with as much speed as before the operation. Additionally, 7 (16%) of 42 shoulders demonstrated 2+ or greater posterior instability postoperatively. There were four cases of symptomatic recurrent instability, one anterior and three posterior, and one patient required a posterior stabilization 2 years postoperatively.

The results after capsular-shift procedures for patients with anteroinferior instability demonstrated satisfactory results as well (7,43). Our service published preliminary results after 75 inferior capsular shifts performed in young athletes. Eighty-nine percent were able to return to their major sports, whereas 73% maintained the same level of competitiveness. Seven (9.3%) patients reported a single episode of probable subluxation that was not followed by recurrent instability and did not affect the result, whereas two (2.7%) patients had dislocations postoperatively, and both cases were associated with a traumatic episode. The average loss of external rotation was 7 degrees (7). Our experience with the inferior capsular shift in 171 anterior repairs was reported (43). The cause was primarily traumatic in 122 (71%) shoulders, repetitive microtrauma in 22 (13%), and atraumatic in 27 (16%). The direction of instability was unidirectional (anterior) in 50 (29%), bidirectional (anterior and inferior) in 87 (51%), and multidirectional (anterior, inferior, and posterior) in 34 (20%). At follow-up averaging 5 years (range, 2 to 13 years), 97 (57%) were rated excellent, 61 (36%) good, four (2%) fair, and eight (5%) poor. Seven (4%) shoulders had recurrent instability. The cause (traumatic, atraumatic, or acquired) and direction (anterior vs. anterior–inferior vs. multidirectional) of the instability were not found to influence the rate of success (43).

CONCLUSIONS

The operative treatment of choice for patients with multidirectional instability has become the inferior capsular shift since the landmark article by Neer and Foster in 1980 (3). Anatomy-deforming procedures, bony procedures, muscle transfers, and procedures designed for unidirectional instability have fallen into disfavor (1,2,19,21,22,25, 27–29,31–34,37,38,40,43,45).

Turkel et al. (72) demonstrated that anterior glenohumeral stability is provided by varying regions of the capsule, depending on arm position. Similarly, Warner et al. (45,74) demonstrated that inferior humeral translation is restrained by the anterosuperior capsule and ligaments with the arm at the side, and by the inferior capsule and ligaments with the arm in abduction. This is consistent with the clinical findings of Neer and Foster (3), who described inferior humeral translation with the arm at the side and with the arm in abduction in patients with multidirectional instability and emphasized reducing redundant capsular volume on all sides at the time of surgical reconstruction. Isolated tensioning of the anterosuperior capsular structures and rotator interval were proposed to treat the inferior component of instability (67,69). Although preliminary results are favorable, the role for these variations in technique has not yet been established.

The capsular-shift procedure eliminates laxity in the rotator interval, anterosuperior capsule, and anteroinferior capsule, and can be continued around the humeral neck to reduce as much laxity in the posteroinferior and posterior capsule as is actually found. Thus, it is a highly versatile procedure, allowing precise soft-tissue balancing on several sides of the joint. Because of the shifting of load between different capsular regions, as shown by Turkel et al. (72), the capsular shift affords stability in varying functional positions while preserving motion and is especially useful in the reconstruction of the unstable athletic shoulder.

The advantage of a versatile surgical approach to shoulder instability is that the surgeon is not committed to any one technique at the start. Varying degrees of instability can be dealt with precisely by using a utility approach. We have found that overlap syndromes are especially common in overhead athletes, given their associated repetitive stress and injury. Thus, rather than there being two discrete groups, unidirectional and multidirectional, there is a spectrum of varying amounts of inferior and posterior laxity on which, for example, a traumatic anterior stress may be superimposed. We have found the inferior capsular shift approach very valuable, allowing precise takedown of as much inferior capsule as is actually needed on an individual basis to eliminate a redundant pouch. Thus, we can perform only a modified shift, essentially an anterior capsulorrhaphy, if anterior instability is found (7,8,43,88), or a full inferior capsular shift for classic multidirectional instability (3,37). Additionally, when a labral or ligamentous detachment is encountered, it can be repaired to the medial glenoid rim to anchor the capsule before shifting the capsular flaps. In this way, both elements of capsular damage may be addressed. The inferior capsular-shift procedure is a versatile and reliable treatment for patients with multidirectional shoulder instability.

REFERENCES

1. Cordasco FA, Pollock RG, Flatow EL, Bigliani LU. Management of multidirectional instability. *Oper Tech Sports Med* 1993;1:293–300.
2. Neer CS II. *Shoulder reconstruction.* Philadelphia: WB Saunders, 1990:273–341.
3. Neer CS II, Foster CR. Inferior capsular shift for inferior and multidirectional instability of the shoulder: a preliminary report. *J Bone Joint Surg [Am]* 1980;62:897–908.
4. Ozaki J. Glenohumeral movements of the involuntary inferior and multidirectional instability. *Clin Orthop* 1989;238:107–111.
5. Welsh RP, Trimmings N. Multidirectional instability of the shoulder. *Orthop Trans* 1987;11:231.
6. Altchek DW, Warren RF, Skyhar MJ, Ortiz G. T-Plasty modification of the Bankart procedure for multidirectional instability of the anterior and inferior types. *J Bone Joint Surg [Am]* 1991;73:105–112.
7. Bigliani LU, Kurzweil PR, Schwartzbach CC, et al. Inferior capsular shift procedure for anterior inferior shoulder instability in athletes. *Am J Sports Med* 1994;22:578–584.
8. Bigliani LU. Anterior and posterior capsular shift for multidirectional instability. *Tech Orthop* 1989;3:36–45.
9. Bateman JE, ed. *The shoulder and neck.* 2nd ed. Philadelphia: JB Lippincott, 1978:475–564.
10. Depalma AF, ed. *Surgery of the shoulder.* 2nd ed. Philadelphia: JB Lippincott, 1973:403–432.
11. Endo H, Takigawa T, Takata K, et al. A method of diagnosis and treatment for loose shoulder. *Cent Jpn J Orthop Surg Traumatol* 1971;14:630–632.
12. Rowe CR, Pierce DS, Clark JG. Voluntary dislocation of the shoulder: a preliminary report on a clinical electromyographic and psychiatric study of twenty-six patients. *J Bone Joint Surg [Am]* 1973;55:445–460.
13. Thompson FR, Moga JJ, Fielding JW. Unusual habitual shoulder dislocations: combined operative repair. Audiovisual presentation at the Annual Meeting of the American Academy of Orthopaedic Surgeons, New York, 1965.
14. Neer CS II. Involuntary inferior and multidirectional instability of the shoulder: etiology, recognition, and treatment. In: Stauffer ES, ed. *American Academy of Orthopaedic Surgeons Instructional Course Lectures XXXIV.* St. Louis: CV Mosby, 1985:232–238.
15. Neer CS II. Recent concepts in dislocation and subluxation, In: Takagishi N, ed. *The shoulder: proceedings of the third International Conference on Surgery of the Shoulder.* Tokyo: Professional Postgraduate Services, 1987:7–12.
16. Neer CS II, Perez-Sanz JR, Ogawa K. Causes of failure in repairs for recurrent anterior dislocations. Presented at New York Orthopaedic Hospital Alumni Annual Meeting. In: Neer CS II, ed. *Shoulder reconstruction.* Philadelphia: WB Saunders, 1990:279.
17. Arendt EA. Multidirectional shoulder instability. *Orthopedics* 1988;11:113–120.
18. Bigliani LU, Weinstein DM, Glasgow MT, Pollock RG, Flatow E. Glenohumeral arthroplasty for arthritis after instability surgery. *J Shoulder Elbow Surg* 1995;4:87–94.
19. Flatow EL. Multidirectional instability. In: Bigliani LU, ed. *The unstable shoulder.* Park Ridge, IL: American Academy of Orthopaedic Surgeons, 1996:79–90.
20. Hawkins RJ, Abrams JS, Schutte J. Multidirectional instability of the shoulder: an approach to diagnosis. *Orthop Trans* 1987;11:246.
21. Hawkins RJ, Angelo RL. Glenohumeral osteoarthrosis. *J Bone Joint Surg [Am]* 1990;72:1193–1197.
22. Hawkins RH, Hawkins RJ. Failed anterior reconstruction for shoulder instability. *J Bone Joint Surg [Br]* 1985;67:709–714.
23. Lusardi DA, Wirth MA, Wurtz D, Rockwood CA. Loss of external rotation following anterior capsulorrhaphy of the shoulder. *J Bone Joint Surg [Am]* 1993;75:1185–1192.
24. MacDonald PB, Hawkins RJ, Fowler PJ, Miniaci A. Release of the subscapularis for internal rotation contracture and pain after anterior repair for recurrent anterior dislocation of the shoulder. *J Bone Joint Surg [Am]* 1992;74:734–737.
25. Mallon WJ, Speer KP. Multidirectional instability: current concepts. *J Shoulder Elbow Surg* 1995;4:54–64.
26. Nobuhara K, Ikeda H. Glenoid osteotomy for loose shoulder. In: Bateman JE, Welsh RP, eds. *Surgery of the shoulder.* Philadelphia: BC Decker, 1984:100–103.
27. Norris TR, Bigliani LU. Analysis of failed repair for shoulder instability: a preliminary report. In: Bateman JE, Welsh RP, eds. *Surgery of the shoulder.* Philadelphia: Decker, 1984:111–116.
28. O'Driscoll SW, Evans DC. Long term results of staple capsulorrhaphy for anterior instability of the shoulder. *J Bone Joint Surg [Am]* 1993;75:249–258.
29. Rockwood CA, Gerber C. Analysis of failed surgical procedures for anterior shoulder instability. *Orthop Trans* 1985;9:48.
30. Rowe CR, Zarins B, Ciullo JV. Recurrent anterior dislocation of the shoulder after surgical repair: apparent causes of failure and treatment. *J Bone Joint Surg [Am]* 1984;66:159–168.
31. Samilson RL, Prieto V. Dislocation arthropathy of the shoulder. *J Bone Joint Surg [Am]* 1983;65:456–460.
32. Steinmann SR, Flatow EL, Pollock RG, et al. Evaluation and surgical treatment of failed shoulder instability repairs. *Orthop Trans* 1992;16: 727.
33. Young DC, Rockwood CA. Complications of a failed Bristow procedure and their management. *J Bone Joint Surg [Am]* 1991;73:969–981.
34. Zuckerman JD, Matsen FA III. Complications about the glenohumeral joint related to the use of screws and staples. *J Bone Joint Surg [Am]* 1984;66:175–180.
35. Bigliani LU, Pollock RG, Soslowsky LJ, Flatow EL. The tensile properties of the inferior glenohumeral ligament. *J Orthop Res* 1992;10: 187–197.
36. Speer KP, Deng X, Borrero S, et al. Biomechanical evaluation of a simulated Bankart lesion. *J Bone Joint Surg [Am]* 1994;76:1819–1826.
37. Bigliani LU, Pollock RG, Owens JM, et al. The inferior capsular shift procedure for multidirectional instability of the shoulder. *Orthop Trans* 1994;17:576.
38. Cooper RA, Brems JJ. The inferior capsular shift procedure for multidirectional instability of the shoulder. *J Bone Joint Surg [Am]* 1992;74:1516–1521.
39. Foster CR. Multidirectional instability of the shoulder in the athlete. *Clin Sports Med* 1983;2:355–368.
40. Lebar RD, Alexander AH. Multidirectional shoulder instability: clinical results of inferior capsular shift in an active-duty population. *Am J Sports Med* 1992;20:193–198.
41. Marberry TA. Experience with the Neer inferior capsular shift for multidirectional shoulder instability. *Orthop Trans* 1988;12:747.
42. Mizuno K, Itakura Y, Muratsu H. Inferior capsular shift for inferior and multidirectional instability of the shoulder in young children: report of two cases. *J Shoulder Elbow Surg* 1992;1:200–206.
43. Pollock RG, Owens JM, Nicholson GP, et al. Anterior inferior capsular shift procedure for anterior glenohumeral instability: long term results. *Orthop Trans* 1993–1994;17:1109.
44. Rockwood CA. Management of patients with multidirectional instability of the shoulder. *Orthop Trans* 1994;18:328.
45. Warner JJP, Johnson D, Miller M, Caborn DNM. Technique for selecting capsular tightness in repair of anterior-inferior shoulder instability. *J Shoulder Elbow Surg* 1995;4:352–364.
46. Belle RM. Collagen typing in multidirectional instability of the shoulder. *Orthop Trans* 1989;13:680–681.

47. Carter C, Sweetnam R. Recurrent dislocation of the patella and of the shoulder: their association with familial joint laxity. *J Bone Joint Surg [Br]* 1960;42:721–727.
48. Emery RJ, Mullaji AB. Glenohumeral joint instability in normal adolescents: incidence and significance. *J Bone Joint Surg [Br]* 1991;73:406–408.
49. Finsterbush A, Pogrund H. The hypermobility syndrome: musculoskeletal complaints in 100 consecutive cases of joint hypermobility. *Clin Orthop* 1982;168:124–127.
50. Jerosch J, Castro WH. Shoulder instability in Ehlers-Danlos syndrome: an indication for surgical treatment? *Acta Orthop Belg* 1990;56:451–453.
51. Hawkins RJ, Bokor DJ. Clinical evaluation of shoulder problems. In: Rockwood CA, Matsen FA, eds. *The shoulder.* 1st ed. Philadelphia: Saunders, 1990:167–171.
52. Silliman JF, Hawkins RJ. Classification and physical diagnosis of instability of the shoulder. *Clin Orthop* 1993;291:7–19.
53. Hawkins RJ, Schutte JP, Janda DH, Huckell GH. Translation of the glenohumeral joint with the patient under anesthesia. *J Shoulder Elbow Surg* 1996;5:286–292.
54. Harryman DT, Sidles JA, Harris SL, Matsen FA. Laxity of the normal glenohumeral joint: a quantitative in vivo assessment. *J Shoulder Elbow Surg* 1992;1:66–76.
55. O'Driscoll SW, Evans DC. The incidence of contralateral shoulder instability in patients treated for recurrent anterior instability: an epidemiological investigation. *Orthop Trans* 1991;15:762.
56. Jalovaara P, Myllyla V, Paivansalo M. Autotraction stress roentgenography for demonstrating anterior and inferior instability of the shoulder joint. *Clin Orthop* 1992;284:136–143.
57. Friedman RJ, Bonutti PM, Genez B, et al. Cine magnetic resonance imaging of the glenohumeral joint. Presented at the American Academy of Orthopaedic Surgeons, Sixtieth Annual Meeting, San Francisco, California, February 18–23, 1993.
58. Burkhead WZ, Rockwood CA. Treatment of instability of the shoulder with an exercise program. *J Bone Joint Surg [Am]* 1992:74:890–896.
59. Kennedy K. Rehabilitation of the unstable shoulder. *Oper Tech Sports Med* 1993;1:311–324.
60. Lephart SM, Warner JJP, Borsa PA, Fu FH. Proprioception of the shoulder joint in healthy, unstable, and surgically repaired shoulders. *J Shoulder Elbow Surg* 1994;3:371–380.
61. Gibb TD, Sidles JA, Harryman DT II, McQuade KJ, Matsen FA III. The effect of capsular venting on glenohumeral laxity. *Clin Orthop* 1991;268:120–127.
62. Habermeyer P, Schuller U, Wiedemann E. The intra-articular pressure of the shoulder: an experimental study on the role of the glenoid labrum in stabilizing the joint. *Arthroscopy* 1992;8:166–172.
63. Warner JJP, Deng X, Warren RF, Torzilli PA, O'Brien SJ. Superior-inferior translation in the intact and vented glenohumeral joint. *J Shoulder Elbow Surg* 1993;2:99–125.
64. Kronberg M, Brostrom L-A, Nemeth G. Differences in shoulder muscle activity between patients with generalized joint laxity and normal controls. *Clin Orthop* 1991;269:181–192.
65. Cordasco FA, Wolfe IN, Wootten ME, Bigliani LU. An electromyographic analysis of the shoulder during a medicine ball rehabilitation program. *Am J Sports Med* 1996;24:386–392.
66. Beall MS Jr, Diefenbach G, Allen A. Electromyographic biofeedback in the treatment of voluntary posterior instability of the shoulder. *Am J Sports Med* 1987;15:175–178.
67. Field LD, Warren RF, O'Brien SJ, Altchek DW, Wickiewicz TL. Isolated closure of rotator interval defects for shoulder instability. *Am J Sports Med* 1995;23:557–563.
68. Harryman DT, Sidles JA, Harris SL, Matsen FA. The role of the rotator interval capsule in passive motion and stability of the shoulder. *J Bone Joint Surg [Am]* 1992:74:53–66.
69. Nobuhara K, Ikeda H. Rotator interval lesion. *Clin Orthop* 1987;223:44–50.
70. O'Brien SJ, Neves MC, Arnockzky SP, Warren RF. The anatomy and histology of the inferior glenohumeral ligament complex of the shoulder. *Am J Sports Med* 1990;18:449–456.
71. Speer KP, Deng X, Torzilli PA, Altchek DA, Warren RF. Strategies for an anterior capsular shift of the shoulder: a biomechanical comparison. *Am J Sports Med* 1995;23:264–269.
72. Turkel SJ, Panio MW, Marshall JL, et al. Stabilizing mechanisms preventing anterior dislocation of the glenohumeral joint. *J Bone Joint Surg [Am]* 1981;63:1208–1217.
73. Warner JJP, Caborn DNM, Berger R, Fu FH, See M. Dynamic capsuloligamentous anatomy of the glenohumeral joint. *J Shoulder Elbow Surg* 1993;2:115–133.
74. Warner JJP, Deng X, Warren RF, Torzilli PA. Static capsuloligamentous restraints to superior-inferior translation of the glenohumeral joint. *Am J Sports Med* 1992;20:675–685.
75. Wirth MA, Blatter G, Rockwood CA. The capsular imbrication procedure for recurrent anterior instability of the shoulder. *J Bone Joint Surg [Am]* 1996;78:246–259.
76. Cofield RH, Nessler JP, Weinstabl R. Diagnosis of shoulder instability by examination under anesthesia. *Clin Orthop* 1993;291:45–53.
77. Pagnani MJ, Warren RF. Stabilizers of the glenohumeral joint. *J Shoulder Elbow Surg* 1994:3:173–190.
78. Leslie JT Jr, Ryan TJ. The anterior axillary incision to approach the shoulder joint. *J Bone Joint Surg [Am]* 1962;44:1193–1196.
79. Hinton MA, Parker AW, Drez D, Altchek D. An anatomic study of the subscapularis tendon and myotendinous junction. *J Shoulder Elbow Surg* 1994;3:224–229.
80. McCann PD, Cordasco FA, Ticker JB, et al. An anatomic study of the subscapular nerves: a guide for the electromyographic analysis of the subscapularis muscle. *J Shoulder Elbow Surg* 1994;3:94–99.
81. Flatow EL, Bigliani LU. Locating and protecting the axillary nerve in shoulder surgery: the tug test. *Orthop Rev* 1952;21:503–505.
82. Steinmann SR, Gaccione DR, McGee TH, et al. Effect of anterior shoulder reconstruction on humeral head vascularity. *Orthop Trans* 1994–1995;18:1066.
83. Duncan R, Savoie FH III. Arthroscopic inferior capsular shift for multidirectional instability of the shoulder: a preliminary report. *Arthroscopy* 1993;9:24–27.
84. Hayashi K, Thabit G III, Massa KL, et al. The effect of thermal heating on the length and histologic properties of the glenohumeral joint capsule. *Am J Sports Med* 1997;25:107–112.
85. Thabit G III. Laser-assisted capsular shift for the treatment of glenohumeral instability. *Orthopaedics* 1994;3:10–12.
86. Mok DW, Fogg AJ, Hokan R, et al. The diagnostic value of arthroscopy in glenohumeral instability. *J Bone Joint Surg [Br]* 1990;72:698–700.
87. Hawkins RJ, Kunkel SS, Nayak NK. Inferior capsular shift for multidirectional instability of the shoulder: 2-5 year follow-up. *Orthop Trans* 1991;15:765.
88. Neer CS II, Fithian TF, Hansen PE, et al. Reinforced cruciate repair for anterior dislocations of the shoulder. *Orthop Trans* 1985;9:44.

The Unstable Shoulder,
edited by R.F. Warren, E.V. Craig, and D.W. Altchek.
Lippincott–Raven Publishers, Philadelphia © 1999.

CHAPTER 17

Fixed and Chronic Shoulder Dislocations

William C. Standeffer, Jr., Michael J. Pagnani, and Allen F. Anderson

Chronic shoulder dislocations present a difficult and challenging problem for the shoulder surgeon. Patients with chronic dislocations often are first seen with significant morbidity. Chronic dislocations are uncommon and are usually the result of a missed diagnosis on initial evaluation. Once the diagnosis is made, however, appropriate treatment frequently produces acceptable results (1). Chronic dislocations are usually seen in elderly and debilitated patients. Schultz et al. (2) reported on 58 patients with chronic shoulder dislocations in which 44 were in their sixth decade of life or older. Chronic dislocations may also be seen in patients with seizure disorders, alcohol and drug abuse, or multitrauma (3). In these patients, the diagnosis of the acute dislocation may be overlooked because of the patient's inability or unwillingness to cooperate or because of other injuries that divert attention away from the appropriate shoulder examination.

Chronic dislocations of the shoulder have been referred to by many terms including ''old,'' ''locked,'' and ''fixed,'' but the time interval distinguishing acute from chronic is poorly defined. Furthermore, the term locked or fixed dislocation has been used to describe irreducible acute dislocations associated with impaction of the humeral head on the glenoid (4). In practice, any dislocation that is not treated in the first few hours after injury or is irreducible by closed methods can be managed according to the principles outlined in this chapter.

CHRONIC POSTERIOR DISLOCATION

Acute posterior dislocations of the shoulder are uncommon, making up approximately 2% to 4% of all shoulder dislocations. There may be only subtle changes on standard radiographs, and a high index of suspicion as well as a good physical examination is essential in making the diagnosis. Reportedly up to 80% of all acute posterior dislocations go undiagnosed at the time of initial presentation (1). Hawkins et al. (5) noted that the average time to diagnosis was approximately 1 year in their series of 41 chronic posterior dislocations. Because of the frequent delay in diagnosis of the acute posterior dislocation, the majority of chronic dislocations are of the posterior type.

In reported series, the most common misdiagnoses are frozen shoulder, massive rotator-cuff tear, strain, bursitis, and malingering. The patients frequently will either receive no treatment or conservative treatment such as physical therapy initially. The most common presenting complaint is loss of range of motion of the involved shoulder, especially the inability to carry out daily activities. Loss of rotation results in difficulty with daily activities such as combing the hair, washing the face, and eating. Forward elevation is usually limited to approximately 90 degrees. Interestingly, only 20 of 41 patients in the series by Hawkins and McCormack (3) complained of moderate or severe pain. There is a correlation between pain and the duration of the dislocation such that the discomfort diminishes with time.

On physical examination, the patient typically holds the arm in an internally rotated, adducted position (6). Inspection of the shoulder may reveal a prominent coracoid process, a prominent humeral head posteriorly, and a ''squared off'' appearance of the anterior and lateral aspects of the acromion (7). Range of motion is limited, especially in external rotation, as most patients cannot even reach neutral rotation. Rowe and Zarins (1) described a test that demonstrates this fixed deformity in which the patient is asked to extend the arms and turn up the palm of the hand. Despite full forearm supination, the palm remains in an apparently pronated position because of the internal-rotation deformity of the shoulder (Fig. 1). The degree of limited motion appears to be directly related to the size of the humeral head defect that accompanies this injury (3).

W. C. Standeffer, Jr., M. J. Pagnani and A.F. Anderson: Tennessee Orthopaedic Alliance/The Lipscomb Clinic, Nashville, Tennessee 37205; and Departments of Orthopaedics and Rehabilitation, Vanderbilt University Medical Center, Nashville, Tennessee 37232.

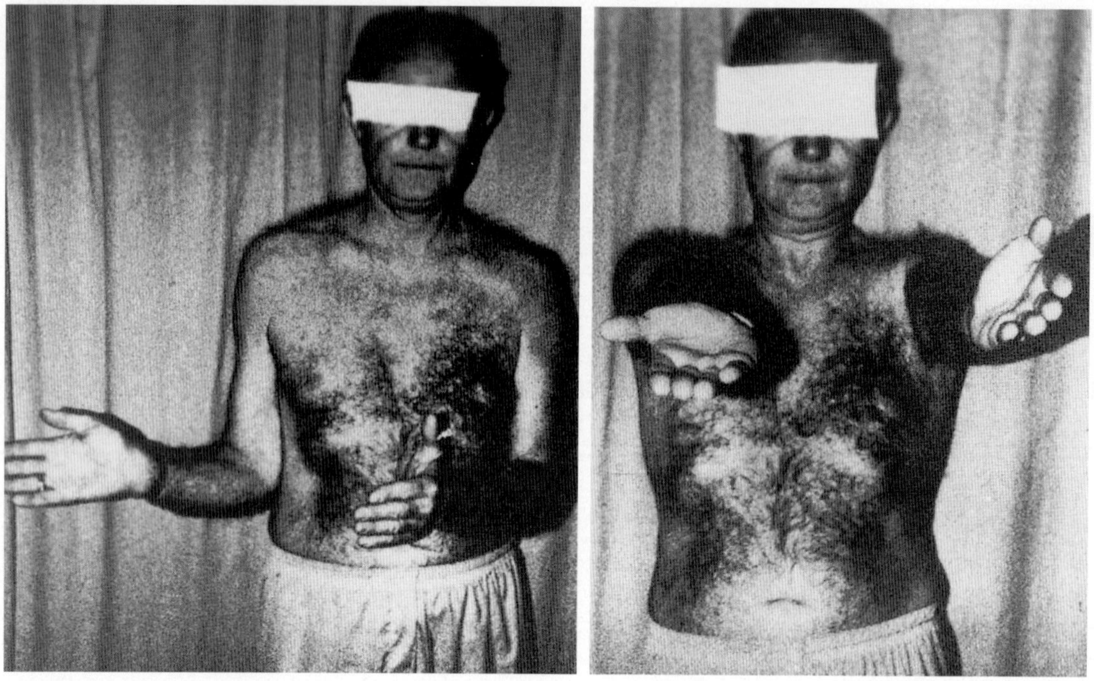

FIG. 1. A, B: The Rowe sign. The patient with a chronic posterior dislocation has limited external rotation and inability to supinate fully the flexed arm because of the internal-rotation deformity of the shoulder. (From Schwartz E, Warren RF, O'Brien SJ, et al. Posterior shoulder instability. *Orthop Clin North Am* 1987;18 [3]:409–419, with permission.)

Standard radiographic evaluation can give the treating physician a false sense of security, as posterior dislocations can appear normal or reveal only subtle abnormalities on standard anteroposterior views. Radiographic signs of posterior dislocation include the vacant glenoid sign (Fig. 2), the ''light bulb'' appearance of the humeral articular surface when seen in maximal internal rotation, and the ''rim sign,'' in which there are more than 6 mm between the anterior as glenoid rim and the humeral head (8). These serve only as diagnostic clues at best and are not direct evidence of posterior dislocation (9). A trauma series including an axillary view is essential in the work-up of a patient thought to have a posterior dislocation. An appropriately performed axillary view should confirm a posteriorly dislocated shoulder in all cases. This projection can be obtained with as little as 20 degrees of abduction. In patients in which limited abduction is not possible, a Velpeau view can be obtained with similar diagnostic accuracy (10). As mentioned previously, an impression fracture frequently accompanies chronic posterior dislocations, and an attempt to estimate the percentage of the humeral head involved is important in determining appropriate treatment. In addition, the glenoid should be inspected to rule out fracture or erosion. Associated tuberosity fractures or shaft fractures are usually nondisplaced. A computed tomography (CT) scan may be more accurate in evaluating the humeral head and glenoid (Fig. 3).

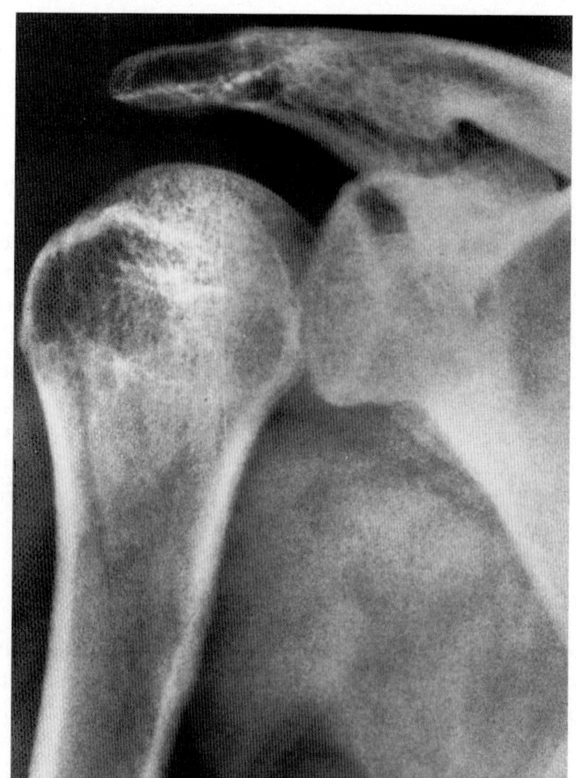

FIG. 2. The vacant glenoid sign in a patient with posterior dislocation. (From Schwartz E, Warren RF, O'Brien SJ, et al. Posterior shoulder instability. *Orthop Clin North Am* 1987;18 [3]:409–419, with permission.)

The chronic nature of the dislocation leads to specific pathoanatomy. Significant erosion of the glenoid can occur

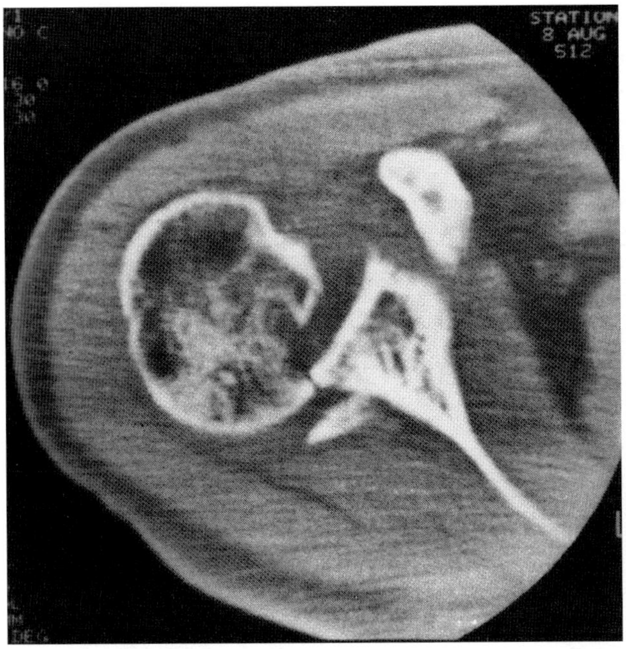

FIG. 3. Computed tomography (CT) scan of fixed posterior dislocation. Note the presence of the impression fracture of the humeral head. (From Schwartz E, Warren RF, O'Brien SJ, et al. Posterior shoulder instability. *Orthop Clin North Am* 1987;18 [3]:409–419, with permission.)

over time where it is in contact with the humeral head and can progress to a pseudoarticulation (11). The posterior capsule, infraspinatus, and teres minor become contracted and fibrotic. The glenoid fossa can become filled with granulation tissue, and the subscapularis and anterior capsule are tethered over the anterior glenoid rim. The articular surface undergoes degenerative changes over time. Samilson and Piieto (12) noted that "dislocation arthropathy" commonly develops in posterior dislocations in which the diagnosis is delayed. They observed moderate to severe arthrosis in 10 of 11 shoulders with chronic dislocations. Progressive wear of the posterior glenoid can be seen and may correlate with a decrease in patient pain as pressure on the humeral head decreases (13).

TREATMENT

Nonoperative Treatment

Careful consideration of treatment options and the individual patient are critical to obtain acceptable results. Some patients are best treated by observation. In patients with small impression fractures, reasonably functional range of motion may be present, and the patient may prefer to avoid surgery. These patients are generally elderly and less active (9,14). Patients who are not surgical candidates or are unable or unwilling to follow the postoperative rehabilitation can also be treated in this manner. Again, we can expect to see a diminution in pain as time progresses.

Most patients, however, fare much better with a more aggressive treatment protocol. Closed reduction of the dislocation may be attempted in selected patients. A careful evaluation of the radiographs should be undertaken to rule out a minimally displaced fracture before reduction. In these patients, an open reduction should be performed. In general, closed reduction may be considered within 6 weeks of the original injury in patients with less than a 20% defect in the humeral head. However, we must be wary of forceful manipulation in the patient with osteoporotic bone, as a fracture can easily be produced (Fig. 4). In these patients, closed reduction may best be avoided. Preparation should also be made to proceed surgically should the reduction fail or be unstable. Hawkins et al. (3) reported on 12 patients who fit these criteria and in whom a stable closed reduction was successful in only three. Closed reduction can be accomplished by placing the shoulder in flexion and adduction, applying longitudinal traction, and pushing the humeral head in an anterior direction (7).

Once a closed reduction is obtained, the joint should be assessed for stability in internal rotation. If there is no instability, the patient can be immobilized in a brace in approximately 10 to 20 degrees of external rotation for 3 to 4 weeks. When there is more than a 20% impression fracture of the humeral head, the reduction is usually unstable. Although there have been successful reports of pinning unstable joints temporarily (1,15), surgical reconstruction has been the general recommendation.

Operative Treatment

Historic

Among early recommendations for the surgical treatment of irreducible posterior dislocations were those made by Souchon (16) in 1897, in which he reported on resection of the humeral head as the treatment of choice. Neviaser (17) and Wilson and McKeever (18) preferred open reduction and temporary glenohumeral transfixation by using a screw or pin. In 1952, McLaughlin (13) described open reduction and transfer of the subscapularis tendon into the humeral head defect. Neer (3) modified this procedure by transferring the entire lesser tuberosity including the subscapularis into the defect by using screw fixation.

Open Reduction with Posterior Capsulorrhaphy

In patients who have an irreducible dislocation and less than a 20% impression fracture, an open reduction by using a posterior approach can often be accomplished with good results. Care must be taken not to damage the articular surface of the humeral head as the impression fracture is disengaged from the glenoid. The capsule is generally stretched or torn away from the glenoid. The capsule should be repaired at the time of reduction as a standard posterior capsular shift or reverse Bankart repair. The capsule can be

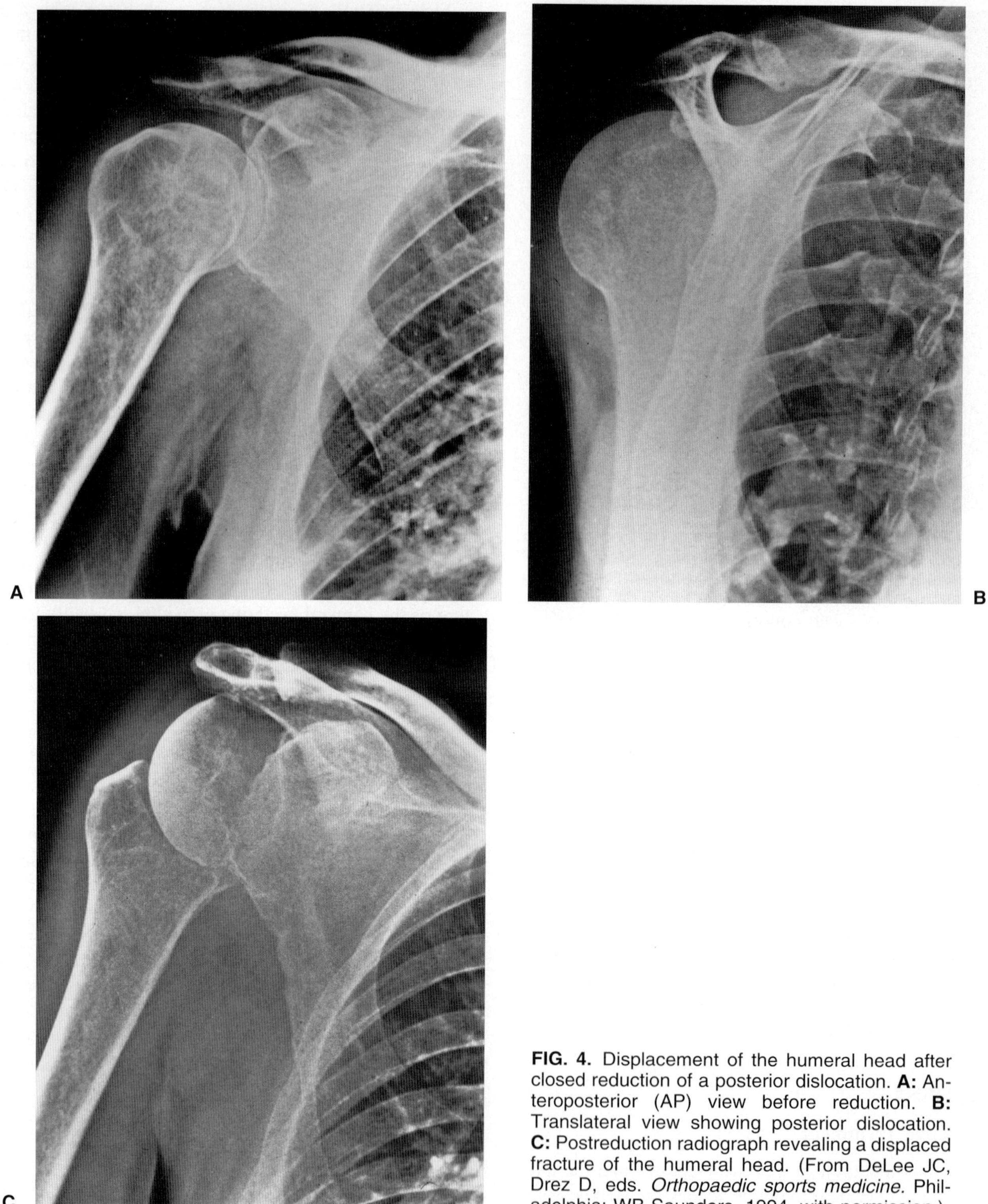

FIG. 4. Displacement of the humeral head after closed reduction of a posterior dislocation. **A:** Anteroposterior (AP) view before reduction. **B:** Translateral view showing posterior dislocation. **C:** Postreduction radiograph revealing a displaced fracture of the humeral head. (From DeLee JC, Drez D, eds. *Orthopaedic sports medicine.* Philadelphia: WB Saunders, 1994, with permission.)

very thin and weak after a chronic dislocation, and reinforcement with part of the infraspinatus tendon will significantly increase the strength of the repair. The patient is immobilized in 10 to 20 degrees of external rotation for 3 to 4 weeks, followed by aggressive physical therapy.

Open Reduction with Lesser Tuberosity Transfer

In cases in which the impression fracture is between 20% and 45%, an open reduction and lesser tuberosity transfer are recommended. We must make sure that the articular surfaces are fairly well preserved before proceeding with the transfer. Previous reports by Connolly (6), Oyston (19), and Hawkins (14) confirmed satisfactory results with this procedure. Although some authors (7) have suggested that the dislocation should be no more than 6 months from injury, we performed this procedure in chronic dislocations of up to 10 months with acceptable results. The limiting factor is the condition of the articular surfaces.

The shoulder is approached through an anterior deltopectoral incision. Usually, a significant internal-rotation deformity distorts the anatomy. The biceps tendon can be used as a reference point to find the lesser tuberosity, which is osteotomized with the subscapularis tendon attached. The capsule is opened to examine the joint and to perform the reduction under direct vision. The reduction can usually be accomplished by internal rotation to unlock the humeral head defect, followed by direct lateral distraction and external rotation. Once the reduction is completed, the articular surfaces should be examined. If they are well preserved, the lesser tuberosity can be fixed into the defect by using a screw or sutures (Fig. 5). If the articular cartilage is degenerated, a hemiarthroplasty or total shoulder should be performed. Assessment of posterior translation should be made, and if excessive, posterior capsulorrhaphy should be considered. The capsule can sometimes be plicated from an anterior approach, or a second, posterior incision may be required.

Postoperatively, the shoulder is immobilized in 20 degrees of external rotation for approximately 4 weeks, at which time, passive motion is begun. After 6 weeks, active motion is started, and progression to resistance exercises is allowed when active motion is regained.

Hawkins et al. (5) reported on nine patients who had undergone a transfer. Of the four operated on by the authors, forward elevation averaged 165 degrees, external rotation averaged 45 degrees, and internal rotation to vertebra 12 was possible. The remaining patients had been referred for failed lesser tuberosity transfers and complained of continued pain. Of these five, two had humeral head defects of greater than 45%, and three were dislocations of more than 1 year duration (3).

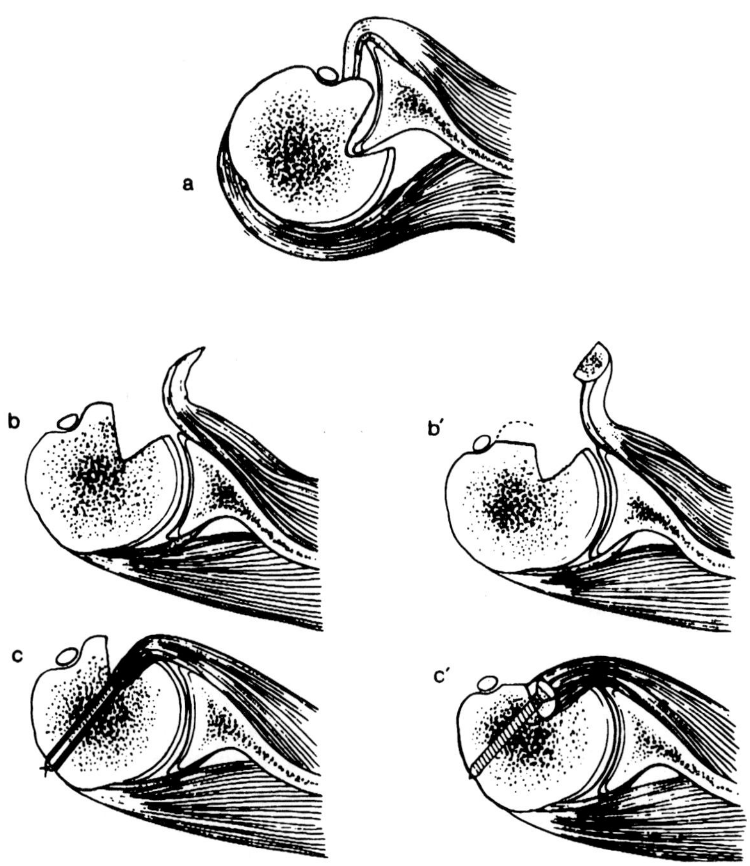

FIG. 5. Transfer of subscapularis tendon insertion into anteromedial defect. **a:** Posterior dislocation with anteromedial defect. **b, c:** McLaughlin procedure advances tendon into defect. **b', c':** Neer modification transfers lesser tuberosity to fill defect.

Hemiarthroplasty or Total Shoulder Replacement

A hemiarthroplasty is indicated in patients with an impression fracture involving more than 45% of the humeral head, and a total shoulder replacement with resurfacing of the glenoid may be necessary if there is significant erosion of the glenoid or glenoid articular degeneration. A large impression fracture can lead to difficulty in accessing the posterior humeral head from an anterior approach. An additional, posterior incision was advocated by Cheng et al. (20) to assist in removing the humeral head; however, we have not found this to be necessary in our experience. In general, retroversion of the humeral component should be decreased, as compared with standard procedures. Hawkins and McCormack (3) reported on nine patients who had a hemiarthroplasty and 10 who had a total shoulder for chronic posterior dislocation. In each group, redislocation occurred in one of four shoulders placed in 20 degrees of retroversion or greater. None of the shoulders placed in neutral version redislocated. An intraoperative assessment of stability by using trials can help in adjusting the version. If stability is difficult to obtain despite decreasing retroversion, the posterior capsule can be plicated to prevent subluxation or dislocation. Postoperative immobilization is unnecessary if good stability is obtained in the operating room. The patients can immediately begin passive range-of-motion exercises and progress to active and strengthening exercises.

Prosthetic replacement consistently provides the patient with alleviation of pain and some improvement in range of motion (3,21). Hawkins et al. (5) reported on three of nine patients with hemiarthroplasties that failed because of progressive glenoid erosions, but all did well after total revision shoulder procedures. Pritchett and Clark (21) reported on three patients who had undergone prosthetic replacement for a chronic dislocation. In two of these, a hemiarthroplasty was done, and in one, a total shoulder. All three had good results.

Other Procedures

Vukov (22) reported a case of rotational osteotomy of the proximal humerus for the treatment of chronic posterior dislocation, and Porteus and Miller (15) reported on two such patients in whom they used a modification of the procedure described by Vukov. The osteotomy is designed such that adequate range of motion can be obtained at the expense of external rotation, which usually will not improve past neutral. Indications for this procedure are not clear, but it may be considered in a young patient in whom the only other option is prosthetic replacement because of the size of the impression fracture. We have no experience with these procedures.

CHRONIC ANTERIOR DISLOCATIONS

Chronic anterior dislocations are uncommon although most acute dislocations are anterior. The diagnosis of anterior dislocation is usually evident on physical examination and radiographs and, therefore, is rarely missed. Patients with chronic anterior dislocations commonly do not immediately seek care, and, therefore, the dislocation goes undiagnosed. Many of these patients are elderly, debilitated, or mentally ill. The average age of the patients in the series by Flatow et al. (23) was 67 years. The signs and symptoms of anterior dislocation become less obvious with time. In particular, pain tends to decrease. However, the patient's arm typically rests in external rotation, and internal rotation is impossible. Abduction is usually significantly limited. A fullness can be appreciated in the anterior aspect of the shoulder, and the coracoid is difficult to see or feel. Although some patients have severe pain, the majority of patients seek medical care because of the functional deficit present (7,23,24). They are often unable to reach their faces or heads, and daily activities are severely limited.

The diagnosis is usually obvious on routine radiographic examination of the shoulder. A fracture of the posterolateral humeral head (Hill-Sachs lesion) is common and can involve a large area of the articular surface. The anterior glenoid commonly is eroded, too, but neither the humeral head defect nor the glenoid erosion can be completely appreciated by plain films. A CT scan is much more accurate in the assessment of bony pathology and can be helpful in planning management (11). Injuries to the rotator cuff are common, and evaluation with magnetic resonance imaging (MRI) may be helpful. This would also give added information about the articular surfaces, which can play a role in management decisions.

The pathoanatomy typically consists of a stretched and attenuated anterior capsule, while the inferior capsule is scarred to the humeral neck (23). A Hill-Sachs lesion is usually present and can vary in size. The size may correlate to the period of time the humeral head is dislocated as well as with the amount of motion attained through this pseudoarticulation (25,26). Again, associated rotator-cuff tears are common. Articular degeneration will occur with longstanding dislocations, although the period for this to occur is not known. Flatow et al. (23) reported that in their series all anterior dislocations present for more than 6 months had irreversible articular degeneration requiring prosthetic replacements.

TREATMENT

Nonoperative Treatment

As with chronic posterior dislocations, some patients with chronic anterior dislocations should be treated nonoperatively. This group includes patients who are poor anesthetic risks, those willing to accept their limitations, and those unable or unwilling to comply with postoperative therapy (Fig. 6). Although functional deficits vary between patients, chronic anterior dislocations seem to be more de-

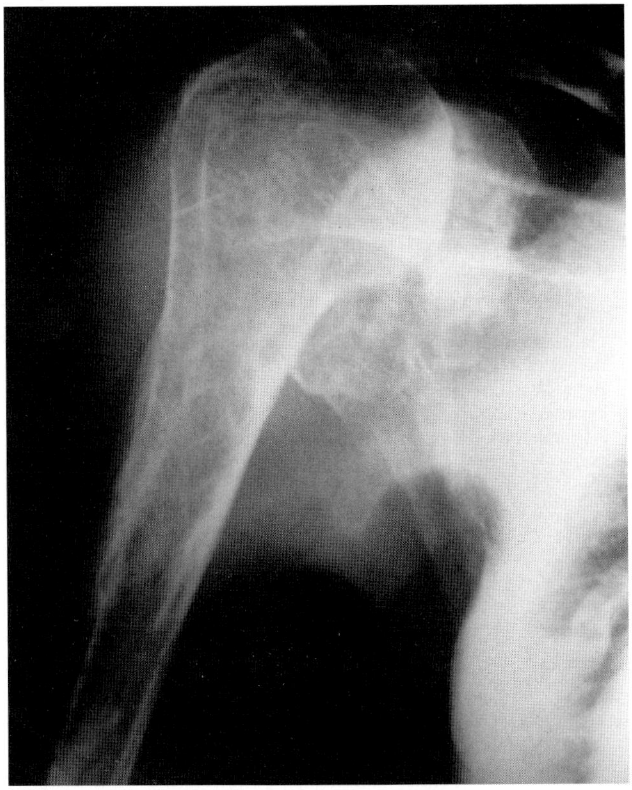

FIG. 6. Chronic anterior dislocation. This elderly woman was treated nonoperatively and functioned quite well despite an external-rotation deformity.

bilitating than their posterior counterpart (9). This is largely a result of the external-rotation deformity and the restriction of activities that accompany it.

Closed reduction is possible in chronic anterior dislocations, but the success is inversely proportional to the period of time it has been dislocated. Most authors have reported that closed reduction can be attempted up to 6 weeks after dislocation (14,24). Care must be taken to prevent an iatrogenic fracture or neurovascular injury; therefore, closed reduction may be best avoided in the elderly and osteoporotic patient. Once a reduction has been obtained, we must test for stability. Usually, there is instability in external rotation, and the patient requires immobilization in internal rotation for approximately 3 weeks (6). If gross instability is present, progression to open stabilization is advisable. Should the reduction be stable without an open procedure, we must be cognizant of the possibility of rotator-cuff injury and be prepared to evaluate it.

Operative Treatment

Open Reduction

Open reduction of a chronic anterior dislocation is appropriate in patients for whom attempts at closed reduction fail, for those who remain unstable after successful closed reduction, for those who have dislocations more than 6 weeks old, and for those who demonstrate poor bone quality and, therefore, are poor candidates for closed reduction. Preservation of the humeral head requires fairly well preserved articular cartilage as well as an impression fracture of no more than 20%. These parameters are not always accurately definable preoperatively, and preparations to modify the operative plan to hemiarthroplasty or total shoulder should be undertaken.

A standard deltopectoral approach is made. There is usually significant scarring of the anterior structures, and an extensive release of the subscapularis and the anterior capsule is necessary to accomplish the reduction. Great care must be taken, as the humeral head may be in close proximity to the brachial plexus. In addition, release of the pectoralis insertion is sometimes required. The glenoid must be examined for erosions and articular cartilage degeneration, and all scar tissue must be removed to allow a congruent reduction. The humeral head must be examined to ensure that the articular cartilage has not degenerated. Cartilage that appears relatively well preserved can actually be soft and will collapse with pressure and would not be functional after an open reduction (23). In cases in which erosion of the glenoid anteriorly renders the joint unstable (i.e., more than 30% of the glenoid surface), bone grafting the anterior glenoid rim is an option to confer stability. Flatow et al. (23) reported on such a case in which stability was obtained by performing a transfer of the coracoid into the glenoid erosion. The anterior capsule is tightened in the standard fashion to increase stability. After open reduction, the patient should be immobilized in internal rotation for approximately 3 weeks.

For patients with a Hill-Sachs lesion involving more than 20% but less than 40% of the humeral head, the Connolly procedure may be indicated (6). Through a posterior approach, the infraspinatus is transferred into the posterolateral humeral head defect. Usually, an anterior capsulolabral repair is also necessary to restore stability (Connelly, JF personal communication, 1997).

Hemiarthroplasty or Total Shoulder Replacement

Prosthetic replacement is necessary when the impression fracture involves more than 40% of the humeral head or when the articular cartilage of the humeral head or glenoid preclude their salvage. As a general rule, any chronic dislocation of longer than 1 year almost certainly will have significant articular cartilage damage and will require a prosthesis.

As with the approach for open reduction, an extensive release is necessary. The glenoid is cleared of all scar tissue, and an assessment of the glenoid articular surface is made to determine whether a hemiarthroplasty or a total shoulder replacement would be appropriate. Stability must be provided by an increase in the retroversion of the humeral component. The appropriate retroversion commonly is about 60 to 80 degrees for maximal stability. The version can vary depending on the wear of the glenoid and is best estimated intraoperatively (21). Excessive glenoid wear can necessitate bone grafting. It is important that the rotator cuff be intact or reparable if a glenoid resurfacing is to be performed. The postoperative protocol is similar to that for open reduction.

Pritchett and Clark (21) reported on their experience with prosthetic replacement. They had one good and one fair result in their patients who underwent hemiarthroplasty and one good and one fair result in their patients who underwent total shoulder replacement. Flatow et al. (23) reported on eight patients who had prosthetic replacement for chronic anterior dislocation, of whom four had an excellent result and four had a good result.

REFERENCES

1. Rowe CR, Zarins B. Chronic unreduced dislocations of the shoulder. *J Bone Joint Surg [Am]* 1982;64:494–505.
2. Schultz TJ, Jacobs B, Patterson RL. Unrecognized dislocations of the shoulder. *J Trauma* 1969;9:1009–1021.
3. Hawkins RJ, McCormack RG. Posterior shoulder instability. *Orthopaedics* 1988;11:101.
4. Matsen FA, Thomas SC, Rockwood CA. Glenohumeral instability. In: Rockwood C, Matsen F, eds. *The shoulder.* Philadelphia: Saunders, 1990:541.
5. Hawkins RJ, Neer CS II, Pianta RM, Mendoza FX. Locked posterior dislocation of the shoulder. *J Bone Joint Surg [Am]* 1987;69:9–18.
6. Connolly JF. Humeral head defects associated with shoulder dislocations: their diagnostic and surgical significance. *Instr Course Lect* 1972;xx:42–54.
7. Bennett GE. Old dislocations of the shoulder. *J Bone Joint Surg* 1936;18:594–606.
8. Arndt JH, Sears AD. Posterior dislocations of the shoulder. *Am J Radiol* 1965;94:639–645.
9. Bowen MK, Warren RY. Surgical approaches to posterior instability of the shoulder. *Op Tech Sports Med* 1993;1:301–310.
10. Bloom MH, Obata WG. Diagnosis of posterior dislocation of the shoulder with use of Velpeau and angle-up roentgenographic views. *J Bone Joint Surg [Am]* 1967;49:943–949.
11. Kirtland S, Resnick D, Sartorius DJ, Pate D, Greenway G. Chronic unreduced dislocations of the glenohumeral joint: imaging strategy and pathologic correlation. *J Trauma* 1988;28:1622–1631.
12. Samilson RL, Prieto V. Dislocation arthropathy of the shoulder. *J Bone Joint Surg [Am]* 1983;65:456–460.
13. McLaughlin HL. Posterior dislocations of the shoulder. *J Bone Joint Surg [Am]* 1952;34:584–590.
14. Hawkins RJ. Unrecognized dislocations of the shoulder. Instr Course Lect 1985;34:258–263.
15. Porteus MJLEF, Miller AJ. Humeral rotation osteotomy for chronic posterior dislocation of the shoulder. *J Bone Joint Surg [Br]* 1990;72:468–469.
16. Souchon E. Operative treatment of irreducible dislocations of the shoulder-joint, recent or old, simple or complicated. *Trans Am Surg Assoc* 1897.
17. Neviaser TJ. Old unreduced dislocations of the shoulder. *Orthop Clin North Am* 1980;11:287–294.
18. Wilson JC, McKeever FM. Traumatic posterior dislocation of the shoulder. *J Bone Joint Surg [Am]* 1949;31:160–172.
19. Oyston JK. Unreduced posterior dislocation of the shoulder treated by open reduction and transposition of the subscapularis tendon. *J Bone Joint Surg [Br]* 1964;46:256–259.
20. Cheng SL, Mackay MB, Richards R. Treatment of locked posterior fracture-disocations of the shoulder by total shoulder arthroplasty. *J Shoulder Elbow Surg* 1997;6:11–17.
21. Pritchett JW, Clark JM. Prosthetic replacement for chronic unreduced dislocations of the shoulder. *Clin Orthop* 1987;216:89–93.
22. Vukov V. Posterior dislocation of the shoulder with a large anteromedial defect of the humerus: a case report. *Int Orthop* 1985;9:37–40.
23. Flatow EL, Miller SR, Neer CS. Chronic anterior dislocation of the shoulder. *J Shoulder Elbow Surg* 1993;2:2–10.
24. Hejna WF, Fossier CH, Goldstein TB, Ray RD. Ancient anterior dislocation of the shoulder. *J Bone Joint Surg [Am]* 1969;51:1030–1031.
25. Hermodsson L. *Roentgenological studies of traumatic and recurrent anterior and inferior dislocations of the shoulder joint.* (Mosely HF, Overgaard BML, translators.) Montreal: McGill University Press, 1963.
26. Hill HA, Sachs MD. The grooved defect of the humeral head. *Radiology* 1940;35:690–700.

ADDITIONAL READINGS

Allard JC, Bancroft J. Irreducible posterior dislocation of the shoulder: MR and CT findings. *J Comput Assist Tomogr* 1991;15:694–696.

Boyd HB, Sisk TD. Recurrent posterior dislocation of the shoulder. *J Bone Joint Surg [Am]* 1972;54:779–786.

Craig EV. The posterior mechanism of acute dislocation. *Clin Orthop* 1984;190:212–216.

Cubbins WR, Callahan JJ, Scuderi CS. The reduction of old or irreducible dislocations of the shoulder joint. *Surg Gynecol Obstet* 1934;58:129–135.

Galinat BJ, Warren RF. Shoulder: trauma and related instability. In: Poss R, ed. *Orthopaedic knowledge update 3.* Park Ridge, IL: AAOS, 1990: 303–312.

Hill NA, McLaughlin HL. Locked posterior dislocation simulating a "frozen shoulder." *J Trauma* 1963;3:225–234.

Kuhnen W, Groves RJ. Irreducible acute anterior dislocation of the shoulder: case report. *Clin Orthop* 1979;139:167–168.

Lam SJS. Irreducible anterior dislocation of the shoulder. *J Bone Joint Surg [Br]* 1966;48:132–133.

Meadows T, Wallace WA. Missed posterior dislocations of the shoulder. *J Bone Joint Surg [Br]* 1987;69:152.

Neer CS. Dislocations. In: Neer C, ed. *Shoulder reconstruction.* Philadelphia: WB Saunders, 1990:273–362.

Neer CS, Miller SR, Flatow EL. Chronic unreduced anterior dislocation of the shoulder. *Orthop Trans* 1990;14 (3):596.

Neviaser JS. An operation for old dislocation of the shoulder. *J Bone Joint Surg [Am]* 1948;30:997–1000.

Neviaser JS. The treatment of old unrecognized dislocations of the shoulder. *Surg Clin North Am* 1963;43:1671–1678.

Rockwood CA. Subluxations and dislocations about the shoulder. In: Rockwood C, Green D, eds. *Fractures in adults.* Philadelphia: JB Lippincott, 1984:722–860.

Stableforth PG, Sarangi PP. Posterior fracture dislocation of the shoulder. *J Bone Joint Surg [Br]* 1992;74:579–584.

Section 4

Arthroscopic Techniques

The Unstable Shoulder,
edited by R.F. Warren, E.V. Craig, and D.W. Altchek.
Lippincott–Raven Publishers, Philadelphia © 1999.

CHAPTER 18

Arthroscopic Stabilization

An Overview

Daniel D. Buss, John R. Green III, and Raymond J. Meyer

INDICATIONS

The indications for arthroscopic reconstruction are similar to indications for open reconstruction. The ideal candidate for arthroscopic reconstruction is an overhead athlete, who participates in a noncontact sport, with traumatic unidirectional anterior instability with a well-defined Bankart lesion. Because these arthroscopic procedures are still relatively new, the indications and contraindications continue to evolve.

Contact sports, atraumatic lesions, multidirectional or voluntary instability, and intrasubstance damage to capsular and ligamentous tissue associated with shoulder dislocations are associated with higher rates of recurrent instability. Preoperative assessment should include examination for stigmata of ligamentous laxity (hyperextension of the knee, elbow, and fingers; ability to touch the volar aspect of the forearm with the thumb) as well as for multidirectional shoulder instability.

A careful diagnostic arthroscopy should be completed before the stabilization procedure to assess the extent of injury, associated injuries, and the quality of the tissue present for repair. Attention should be directed specifically to identify a significant bony Bankart defect, poor labral or capsular integrity, an enlarged rotator interval, intrasubstance tearing of the anterior inferior glenohumeral ligament or the axillary recess, a lateral capsular defect, or a significant Hill-Sachs lesion. All of these are relative contraindications to arthroscopic stabilization.

D. D. Buss: Department of Orthopaedics, University of Minnesota Medical School, Minneapolis, Minnesota 55454; and Minneapolis Sports Medicine Center, Minnepolis, Minnesota 55454.

J. R. Green III: Department of Orthopaedic Surgery, Louisiana State University Medical Center, Shreveport, Louisiana 71130-3932.

R. J. Meyer: Minneapolis Sports Medicine Center, Minnepolis, Minnesota 55454.

PUBLISHED RESULTS

Arthroscopic stabilization procedures represent recent advances in science and technology. As with any new procedure, the early results demonstrate wide variations between different techniques and different authors (see Table 1) and may be skewed by both the learning curve of the technique and the evolving indications for the procedure.

Metal-Staple Capsulorrhaphy

Arthroscopic staple capsulorrhaphy was first described in an instructional film by Johnson (1) in 1983, by using a metal staple designed for Bankart lesion repair. Detrisac and Johnson (2) reported on 148 patients with 4-year average follow-up. They had 16 (11%) recurrent dislocations. All of the shoulders obtained full elevation; however, external rotation was restricted an average of 10 degrees compared with the unoperated shoulder. In analyzing the 16 recurrent dislocations, 11 of the 31 shoulders were immobilized less than 3 weeks. In the group immobilized 3 or more weeks, redislocations occurred in five (4%) of 117, leading the authors to recommend 4 weeks of immobilization after surgery. Matthews et al. (3) reviewed their experience in 25 shoulders with 36-month average follow-up. These patients were evaluated with a Rowe score (4). By using this scale, 67% of patients achieved good or excellent results. They reported an average loss of 9 degrees of external rotation and 13 degrees of abduction. Six (24%) patients received a poor rating, five of whom required reoperation, four for instability and one for arthroscopic staple removal. Hawkins (5) reviewed his results of arthroscopic staple stabilization by using Johnson's surgical technique in 50 patients who were followed up an average of 39.4 months after surgery. Seven (16%) of the 50 shoulders had subsequent shoulder instability with additional trauma. Six of these seven patients had been asymptomatic from 1 to 2 years after the index procedure. Four patients had symptoms of recurrent instability severe enough to warrant a second stabilization procedure. Gross (6) reported 44.8-month follow-up on 12 patients, and by using the Rowe classification (4), six results were excellent, two good, two fair, and two poor. The two failures in this series were the first two cases, underscoring the relatively steep learning curve for arthroscopic stabilization.

Coughlin et al. (7) reviewed 47 patients with a 4-year follow-up. Twelve patients developed recurrent instability, eight of whom dislocated, and four complained of subluxation. Seven of the 13 with a preoperative diagnosis of subluxation continued with instability, whereas only five of the 34 shoulders with a history of dislocation developed recurrent instability. By using the Rowe scale (4), 21 (44%) patients had an excellent result, whereas five (11%) patients had a good result, eight (17%) patients had a fair result, and 13 (28%) patients had a poor result. Sixteen patients required reoperation; 12 were for instability, three for postoperative pain that required staple removal, and one patient for impingement-type symptoms.

In summary, the literature suggests that arthroscopic capsulorrhaphy with metal staples is associated with a high rate of recurrent instability, which may lead to further damage to the humeral head during subluxation or dislocation episodes resulting from poorly positioned staples. Metallic fixation devices used about the shoulders have had a high rate of complications including loosening, migration, and breakage (8). These problems with metal implants provided the impetus to develop bioabsorbable materials.

TABLE 1. *Arthroscopic techniques: summary of literature*

Technique	Reference	Year	Number of patients	Follow-up (mo)	Recurrence	Loss of external rotation	Complications
Transglenoid-suture capsulorrhaphy	Morgan and Bodenstab (13)	1987	25	17	None	None	None
	Caspari and Savoie (18)	1991	49	24–72	8%		
	Benedetto and Glotzer (14)	1992	22	29	None	>10 deg in five cases	None
	Landsiedl (15)	1992	65	35	14%	4 deg	5%: various minor
	Grana et al. (16)	1993	27	36	44%	6 deg	
	Goldberg et al. (17)	1993	38	36	11%	12 deg	13%: neurapraxia, other minor
	Youssef et al. (41)	1995	30	38	27%		None
	Walch et al. (40)	1995	59	49	49%	>10 deg in three cases	
	Torchia et al. (19)	1996	150	49	18%		5%: adhesions, neurapraxia, fistula, nerve injury
Metal-staple capsulorrhaphy	Mathews et al. (3)	1988	25	36	16%	9 deg	8%: loose staples, malpositioned staples
	Hawkins (5)	1989	50	39	16%		8%: neurapraxia, loose staples, broken staples
	Gross (6)	1989	12	45	17%	10 deg in two cases	17%: malpositioned staples
	Coughlin et al. (7)	1992	47	48	26%	15 deg	6%: painful staples
	Detrisac and Johnson (2)	1993	148	48	11%	10 deg	14%: infection, pain, loose staples, malpositioned staples
Biodegradable-staple capsulorrhaphy	Altcheck (10)	1993	150		20% of initial 50; 7% of next 100		
	Speer et al. (11)	1996	52	42	21%		
	Arciero et al. (12)	1995	26	19	4%	3 deg	None
Metal suture anchoring	Snyder et al. (20)	1996	37	22	11%	5 deg	3%: adhesive capsulitis

Biodegradable-Staple Capsulorrhaphy

Ideally, a bioabsorbable implant would maintain soft-tissue fixation until stable healing occurs and would absorb as the healing tissues become stronger. There have been several reports in the literature about a polyglyconate synthetic copolymer (Suretac; Acufex Microsurgical, Mansfield, MA, U.S.A.). The tack is cannulated for ease of insertion, has a ribbed shaft for fixation, and a broad, flat head with serrations to capture soft tissue. The implant loses most of its fixation strength by 4 weeks. The histologic evaluation demonstrated a very benign response within the bone without a foreign-body response (9).

Altchek (10) reported a large series with this tack. In his initial group of 50 patients, there was a 20% recurrent instability rate. By limiting the indications (excluding those patients with generalized ligamentous laxity and multidirectional instability) in the next 100 patients, the recurrent dislocation rate diminished to 7%. Patients with posttraumatic anterior glenohumeral instability were also evaluated arthroscopically to determine whether they were candidates for arthroscopic stabilization. A more recent study (11) of long-term outcomes (42 months) of 52 shoulders treated with this technique found that 41 (79%) of the patients were asymptomatic and able to participate in sports without restriction. Recurrent instability was present in 11 (21%) patients, and eight of these required further operation.

Arciero et al. (12) noted that inferior or middle glenohumeral ligament injury may involve plastic deformation or stretch, as well as detachment, in his series of first-time dislocators. For successful stabilization, restoration of the glenoid attachment and elimination of excessive laxity within the ligament itself must be obtained.

Arciero's (12) initial report with the Suretac in 19 West Point cadets who had sustained acute first-time anterior shoulder dislocation was encouraging. He performed arthroscopic stabilization within 10 days of the dislocation. At an average of 19-month follow-up, there were no recurrent dislocations and one episode of subluxation with an average loss of external rotation of 3 degrees. By using the Rowe score (4), 16 patients had an excellent result, two good, and one fair. All patients returned to preinjury athletic activities.

Transglenoid-Suture Capsulorrhaphy

Morgan and Bodenstab (13) reported their 17-month follow-up on 25 patients with recurrent anterior dislocations and a Bankart lesion. They performed an arthroscopic suture repair and had excellent results in all 25 patients by using Rowe's shoulder-rating system (4). They reported no loss of motion or recurrent instability during their follow-up. Benedetto and Glotzer (14) reported on 22 patients with a minimum of 2 years' follow-up. Two patients had limited abduction of 15 degrees, and five patients had limited external rotation of 10 to 20 degrees. No patients had recurrent instability within the follow-up period. Landsiedl (15) described 65 patients evaluated an average of 35 months postoperatively. Nine redislocations occurred, and one additional patient complained of instability symptoms. The average loss of external rotation was 3.6 degrees.

Grana et al. (16) reported on 27 patients followed up for an average of 36 months after arthroscopic suture stabilization of anterior shoulder instability. Functional grading, as described by Rowe (4), yielded 10 (37%) patients rated as excellent, five (19%) good, and 12 (44%) poor. Fourteen (52%) returned to their previous level of activity. The average loss of external rotation was 6.3 degrees with no loss of abduction or elevation. Recurrent instability occurred in 12 patients.

Goldberg et al. (17) performed a retrospective analysis on 38 shoulders with average follow-up of 36 months. Four (10%) shoulders had recurrent symptoms of instability. Fifteen (39%) had less than 10 degrees loss of external rotation, and two (5%) had more than 25 degrees loss of external rotation. Twenty-six of 35 athletes returned to the same level of athletic activity. Caspari and Savoie (18) reported on 49 consecutive patients who underwent arthroscopic reconstruction for traumatic anterior instability with 2- to 6-year follow-up. Satisfactory results were reported in 96% of the patients.

A more recent study by Caspari's group (19) reported on 150 patients with an average follow-up of 4.1 years. By using Kaplan–Meier survival analysis, they concluded that the probability of a recurrent instability event increased over time and was 18% at 5 years of follow-up. The group most at risk for recurrent instability were young patients with Bankart lesions. They concluded that their technique was most effective in patients older than 25 years and who did not have a Bankart lesion. They emphasized that their technique allows correction of both capsular laxity and labral detachment.

In summary, transglenoid suture capsulorrhaphy has a higher success rate than other reported techniques; however, it is a technically demanding procedure requiring multiple drill passes through the shoulder, which places the suprascapular nerve at risk.

Capsulorrhaphy By Using Metallic Suture Anchors

There is little in the literature on the results of capsulorrhaphy by using metallic suture anchors. Snyder et al. (20) reported on the Southern California Orthopedic Institute experience in 37 patients with average follow-up of 22 months after arthroscopic repair of anterior shoulder instability by using a threaded suture anchor. There were 27 excellent results by using the Rowe scoring system (4), five good results, one fair result, and four poor results. The average loss of external rotation was 5 degrees. The four poor results were all caused by recurrent instability. Two patients required revision surgery.

In well-positioned metallic suture anchors, the metal is completely enclosed in the bone, decreasing the likelihood of humeral head damage from the fixation device with recurrent instability. However, these devices may not stay intraosseous and may cause damage as a loose body in the joint. Use of these fixation devices requires intra-articular knot tying, which is technically demanding.

Arthroscopic Versus Open Bankart Procedures

Higher rates of recurrent instability have been reported in most articles for arthroscopic stabilization procedures compared with open surgery. Guanche et al. (21) compared a series of 15 arthroscopic and 12 open reconstructions of isolated Bankart lesions, in which the patient chose the surgical procedure. The arthroscopic group had significantly more recurrent instability (33% vs. 8%) compared with the open reconstructions. However, early reports included patients operated on during the learning curve, which is substantial with these technically demanding arthroscopic procedures. As more proficiency is achieved, improved range of motion and decreased postoperative pain can be expected for arthroscopic reconstructions compared with open surgery (22). Perhaps more important, the indications for arthroscopic stabilization have evolved to exclude patients who sustain significant intrasubstance damage to capsule and ligamentous structures, because current procedures have been unable to shift the capsule enough to stabilize this group of patients reliably.

Superior Labrum Anterior and Posterior Lesions

Isolated injuries of the superior labrum were classified by Snyder et al. (23) into four types, the most common being a type II superior labrum anterior and posterior (SLAP) lesion, a pathologic detachment of the labrum and biceps anchor from the superior glenoid. They favored repair with a titanium suture anchor and Ethibond suture (24). Several other methods of arthroscopic reattachment have been described. Field and Savoie (25) described a suture punch repair with polydioxanone suture (PDS). By using this technique in 20 patients, pain and function [with the American Shoulder and Elbow Society scoring system (26)] were significantly improved, and there were 16 excellent and four good results [with the Rowe scale (4)] at 21-month average follow-up. Yoneda et al. (27) reported on 10 athletes treated with arthroscopic stapling with average follow-up of 37 months, including second-look arthroscopies at 3 to 6 months at the time of staple removal. At the repeated arthroscopy, a stable biceps labral anchor had been reestablished in all 10 patients. The clinical results were excellent in five cases, good in three, fair in one, and poor in one patient, who had significant multidirectional instability.

Pagnani et al. (28) reported the result of arthroscopic stabilization of type II or IV SLAP lesions by using the Suretac biodegradable implant. At an average follow-up of 2 years, 19 of 22 patients were classified as having satisfactory results. Twelve of 13 overhead athletes were able to return to their preinjury levels of competition.

COMPLICATIONS

Successful surgery begins with appropriate patient selection. The first step to avoiding complications is making an accurate diagnosis, particularly distinguishing between unidirectional and multidirectional instability. The majority of articles reported a higher incidence of recurrent instability after arthroscopic compared with open stabilizations. Patients need preoperative counseling so their expectations of the treatment plan and outcome are realistic.

Avoiding intraoperative complications begins with patient positioning on the operating table. Extremes of head position, more than 15 pounds of traction, as well as excessive shoulder abduction and extension may lead to neurapraxia (29). Neurovascular structures may be injured during portal placement. To avoid injury to the musculocutaneous nerve, anterior portals must be superior and lateral to the coracoid and inserted with blunt tissue dissection (30). To decrease the chances of rotator-cuff tearing, the anterior superior (Neviaser) portal should be made with the arm at the side, and the posterior portal made with the arm in internal rotation to avoid puncturing the tendinous portion of the rotator cuff (31).

Intraoperative complications also include bleeding, particularly when working around the anterior glenoid. Bleeding can be controlled in most cases by increased hydrostatic pressure. Fluid extravasation is not typically a problem unless conversion to an open procedure is necessary. Articular-surface injury can occur during multiple portions of the procedure. Blunt technique during arthroscopic insertion, accurate portal placement, and direct visualization during instrument insertion, particularly drilling, can minimize articular injury.

Infection and synovial cyst formation at the portal sites are rare (32). Synovial cyst formation has been associated with the transglenoid suture technique (33). Arthroscopic techniques for shoulder stabilization are technically demanding, with difficult learning curves. Many authors have pointed out higher success rates with fewer complications at the end of their series compared with the beginning.

Capsulorrhaphies performed with metal staples were found by Small (34) to have the highest complication rate of any shoulder arthroscopic procedure. If the staple is driven in too far, tissue amputation causes loss of fixation. If the staple is too proud, humeral head impingement or subscapularis tendon injury may occur (2,35). Additional surgery may also be required for loose or malpositioned staples. As with any intra-articular fixation device, loss of fixation, breakage, and migration can produce a free fragment in the joint, which may necessitate reoperation. Zuckerman and Matsen (8) found articular damage in 40% of patients reoperated on for implant-related problems.

Wiley (36) developed a metal rivet, easily removed under local anesthesia, to minimize these complications. Biodegradable implants were also developed to address these same problems. Although the same mechanical problems that affect metal implants can theoretically occur, the polymers are relatively rapidly removed by hydrolysis, making reoperation for hardware problems unlikely. Tack hydrolysis may cause inflammation and clinical signs of joint irritation. It occurs at 6 to 8 weeks after surgery, generally has a 4-week, self-limited course, and can be treated with nonsteroidal anti-inflammatory drugs.

Transglenoid suture–type repairs place the suprascapular nerve at risk, from both pin passage in proximity to the nerve and tying the suture over the nerve. Newer suture anchors reduce the risk to the suprascapular nerve by eliminating the need for transglenoid drilling. Although most are designed to reside completely intraosseously, if placed improperly, they still have the potential problems of intra-articular metal staples. These anchors are used in conjunction with suture, which requires tying technically demanding intra-articular knots.

SUMMARY OF TECHNIQUES AND OVERVIEW OF REPAIR TYPES

Transglenoid Suture Techniques

Current arthroscopic techniques represent modifications of previously described open reconstructions. As an acceptable alternative to open reconstruction, the arthroscopic procedure should provide the same or improved results as the open techniques, minimal complications, and reduced postoperative discomfort. Johnson (1) is credited with the first successful arthroscopic procedure for anterior instability by using a metal staple. Subsequently, a multitude of procedures have been described for the unstable shoulder (2,11,13,18,37). Two arthroscopic stabilization procedures using the suture technique resulted in reports of excellent outcomes. The multiple suture technique of Caspari and Savoie (18) and the horizontal suture technique of Morgan and Bodenstab (13) are described later.

All reconstructions are performed under general anesthesia, interscalene block, or both. After appropriate anesthesia is obtained, the patient is positioned in either the lateral decubitus or beach-chair position. A thorough examination of the shoulder is performed to assess the instability pattern and extremes of range of motion. The examination should consist of anterior, posterior, and inferior translation maneuvers with quantification of instability. Range of motion should be determined in forward flexion, abduction, and external and internal rotation. This should always be compared with the contralateral normal side preoperatively. The following suture techniques were originally described with the patient in the lateral decubitus position but can also be completed in the beach-chair position.

To obtain the lateral position, the patient is placed in the lateral decubitus position with the uninvolved shoulder down. The patient is rolled back 30 degrees to provide adequate access to the anterior shoulder. A standard surgical preparation and draping is used. It is important that adequate exposure to both the anterior and posterior shoulder be obtained. Typically, draping free the medial boarder of the posterior scapula and to 3 cm medial to the coracoid process anterior is necessary. The arm is suspended sterilely to the traction apparatus so that it can be removed and replaced into traction without compromising the sterile field. The arm is positioned in approximately 45 degrees of abduction and 15 degrees of forward flexion. Ten to 15 pounds of weight are used to maintain distraction during the procedure.

A standard posterior visualization portal is established. It is important that the arthroscope enter the joint parallel to the face of the glenoid if the joint is to be adequately visualized. If necessary for joint distention, an anterosuperior inflow portal can be established. An anterior instrument portal is then established. Precise placement of the anterior portal is critical to the success of the procedure and should be established with an outside-in technique by localizing with a spinal needle. The location of the portal is at the lower edge of the rotator-cuff interval. The exterior location of the portal will typically be lateral and slightly superior to the coracoid process. The location of the anterior portal is dependent on the intra-articular pathology and the angle necessary to establish a working relation with the pathology on the anterior and inferior glenoid neck (Fig. 1).

Once adequate portals have been established, an arthroscopic examination of the shoulder is performed (18). Findings in the unstable shoulder will include the detached labrum–anterior inferior glenohumeral ligament (AIGHL) complex or avulsion of the AIGHL with an intact labrum. Secondary changes may be noted, including laxity of the anterior capsule and subscapularis tendon, flattening of the anterior glenoid margin, fraying or tearing of the anterior labrum, and an impaction fracture of the posterior humeral head adjacent to the normal bare-area lesion (Hill-Sachs lesion). The AIGHL–labrum complex is evaluated for the presence of a Bankart lesion. If the AIGHL–labrum complex is intact and the anterior capsule is incompetent, the anterior labrum and ligaments are detached from the anterior neck of the glenoid. A small portion of the capsule is resected to allow an anterior and superior shift of the capsule. If no capsule is present or if the capsule is markedly thin and atrophic, the patient is not a candidate for this type of repair, and an alternative form of reconstruction is selected.

The anterior glenoid neck is then abraded to a bleeding surface to facilitate a reactive response. The amount of anterior glenoid neck abrasion necessary is documented by visualization with the arthroscope from the anterior portal.

With the suture-punch cannula, five to eight sutures are placed into the detached labrum–AIGHL complex. Either 2-0 or zero monofilament absorbable suture may be used, and all sutures are retrieved from the anterior portal.

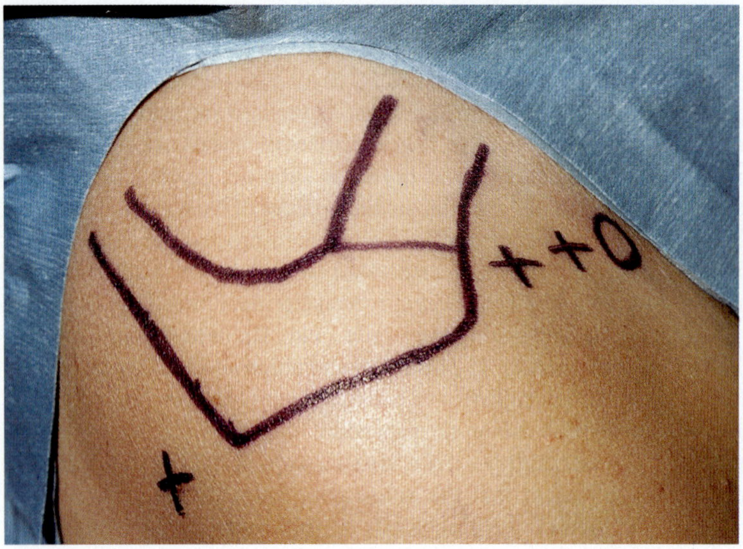

FIG. 1. Posterior and two anterior portal positions (marked X), in relation to palpable bony landmarks.

The transglenoid guide (Fig. 2) is then placed into the cannula and is used to direct a 3/16-inch long drill/suture passer through the glenoid neck from anterior to posterior and out into the infraspinatus fossa. A small incision is made posteriorly to allow the pin to exit the skin. The pin and sutures are pulled posteriorly through the glenoid neck and out the posterior incision. The shoulder is removed from traction, and the sutures are pulled tightly to approximate the repaired ligament to the glenoid neck. As traction is applied to the sutures, the capsule is shifted superiorly. Stability of the glenohumeral joint is confirmed, maintaining the arm in adduction and internal rotation. The AIGHL–labrum complex is reconstituted superiorly and medially against the abraded glenoid neck. The sutures are divided into two bundles and passed through the infraspinatus fascia by using a blunt needle. Keeping appropriate tension, the sutures are tied together. At the conclusion of the procedure, a shoulder immobilizer is applied, and the patient is placed on an outpatient-surgery protocol.

A shoulder immobilizer or sling is maintained for a total of 6 weeks. Pendulum exercises are begun at 3 weeks, and active/passive motion are initiated at 6 weeks. Full range of motion should be achieved by 12 weeks, including external rotation. Functional rehabilitation for athletes is started 3 to 4 months postoperatively. Regular sporting activities that require overhead activities (such as throwing) are allowed at 6 months; however, contact sports are withheld for the first year.

The Morgan transglenoid suture technique follows a similar set-up, portal placement, and diagnostic arthroscopy (13). The arthroscopic suture repair of the Bankart lesion is accomplished through the anterior operative cannula. Suture material is delivered through the soft tissue of the Bankart lesion and glenoid bone from anterior to posterior in a transglenoid fashion by using a modified Beath pin, which will be referred to as a suture pin. These suture pins measure 30 cm in length and 2 mm in diameter. The sharp tip allows accurate soft-tissue penetration and placement to the abraded bone surface.

Two separate anterior-to-posterior passes of the suture pin through the Bankart lesion and glenoid bone (one superior and one inferior) are required to create a single large anterior horizontal mattress suture. The inferior suture-pin passage is always done first, because it is important to bring up the inferior glenohumeral ligament to its anatomic attachment to the midportion of the glenoid rim with the inferior suture. The sharp tip of the suture pin is then used to shift the Bankart lesion 3 to 5 mm superiorly. The pin is then driven into the anterior abraded surface of the scapular neck 3 mm medial to the edge of the glenoid rim. The

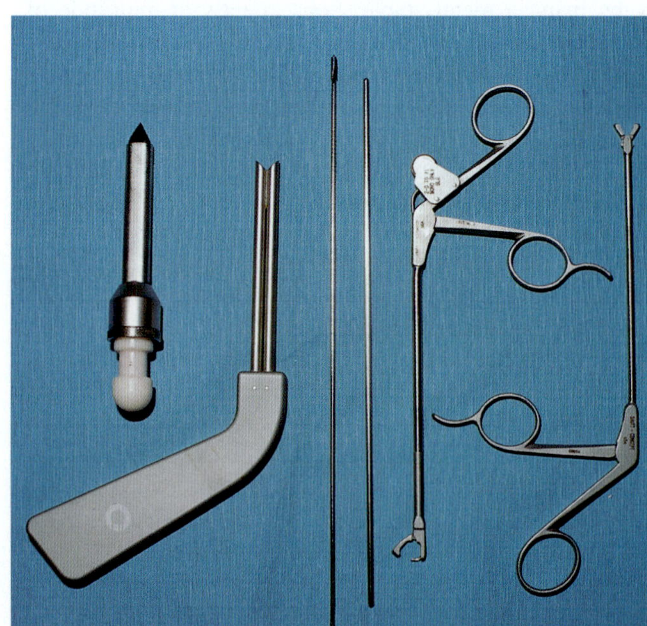

FIG. 2. Caspari transglenoid suture instrument set.

angle of the pin should be 30 degrees inferior to a perpendicular line, referenced to the long axis of the glenoid articular surface and parallel to the glenoid articular surface in an anterior-to-posterior direction. Cadaveric dissections of this procedure have shown that these pins will exit the scapular neck posteriorly more than 1 cm lateral to and more than 1.5 to 2 cm inferior to the suprascapular nerve. Placing the pins from anterior to posterior at an angle more than 45 degrees medially will place their exit close to the suprascapular nerve. It is important to place the pin parallel to the articular surface of the glenoid. Once the proper angle of the inferior pin is assessed, it is drilled through the glenoid bone until the pin exits the skin posteriorly. The exit point of this inferior pin (first pin passage) usually resides between 7 and 10 cm inferior from the midpoint of the scapular spine. A single strand of no. 1 PDS absorbable suture material is then placed through the eye of the suture pin anteriorly. The pin is delivered out through the shoulder posteriorly, doubling the suture material through the Bankart lesion and the transglenoid hole. The suture is tagged anteriorly and posteriorly outside the skin. A second suture pin is placed down the anterior cannula and positioned for passage through the Bankart lesion and glenoid bone. A similar technique as previously described for the first pin passage is used. The sharp end of the pin spears the anterior capsular attachments to the labrum in the upper third of the Bankart lesion. The location of the second passage usually resides 1.5 cm superior to the first pin passage anteriorly on the glenoid. The pin and captured soft tissue are brought to the abraded glenoid rim area. The pin is drilled in a transglenoid fashion from anterior to posterior by using the same angular orientation as described for the first passage, such that the second pin penetrates the scapular neck parallel to the first pin passage. The second pin will exit the skin posteriorly 2.5 cm superior to the portal created for the first pin passage. Again, suture is placed through the eye, and the pin is delivered posteriorly, bringing the second two strands of suture out through a separate posterior inferior portal. The second set of sutures is tagged both posteriorly and anteriorly outside the skin. Next, the first set of sutures is tied to the second set of sutures anteriorly outside of the anterior cannula with a double square knot. The suture tails posteriorly are pulled, delivering the knot down the cannula into the shoulder anteriorly under direct arthroscopic visualization. With further tension on the suture tails posteriorly, the horizontal mattress suture reduces the Bankart lesion to the abraded scapular neck and glenoid rim. In addition, this advances and tightens the inferior glenohumeral ligament complex. By maintaining tension on the posterior suture tails, the repair is assessed with a probe. The superior sutures are brought through the subcutaneous tissue into the inferior suture portal with a hemostat. Thus, both sutures exit through the inferior posterior portal. The sutures are then tied over the thick fascia of the posterior one third of the deltoid. After wound closure, the patient is placed in a shoulder immobilizer with the arm in internal rotation and is transferred to the recovery room and discharged as an outpatient.

To avoid tying the sutures over muscle and fascia, which may affect the muscle's ability to function and cause some loosening of the fixation, Morgan recently adopted the modified technique described by Maki (38). This involves tying interference knots in the sutures posteriorly and then pulling these knots down against the posterior glenoid neck. The sutures are then tensioned anteriorly and tied intra-articularly in a mattress fashion.

Arthroscopic transglenoid suture capsulorrhaphy is an effective alternative for correcting the pathology of anterior and anteroinferior shoulder instability. The procedure avoids the morbidity associated with open repairs as a result of anterior soft-tissue dissection and division of the subscapularis. The procedure, however, is technically demanding. To achieve predictable and reproducible results comparable to open Bankart stabilization, recognition and repair of the responsible pathology is essential. Equally important is appropriate patient selection. A minority of patients who require operative treatment should be considered for an arthroscopic procedure. Arthroscopic transglenoid suture capsulorrhaphy is best indicated for traumatic anterior instability with a Bankart lesion and good-quality glenohumeral ligaments. Arthroscopic suture capsulorrhaphy is not recommended for patients who do not have a Bankart lesion, those with a large glenoid rim defect, those with poorly defined capsular structures, those who do not report a specific traumatic or microtraumatic incident that initiated their instability complaints, and patients younger than 18 years (39). In addition, surgeons with limited arthroscopic experience should be cognizant of the steep learning curve in performing these stabilization techniques.

Goldberg et al. (17) stressed the importance of patient selection and cautioned against the use of arthroscopic techniques in the patient who has poorly defined capsular ligaments and other evidence of congenital laxity. Reasons for conversion to an open technique were described by multiple authors (17,40,41). Walch et al. (40) listed three: inferior hyperlaxity, confirmation of a bony Bankart lesion by preoperative radiography, and the presence of extended ligamentous lesions. Youssef et al. (41) stopped performing arthroscopic stabilizations in patients who are younger than 30 years and who participate in collision or competitive athletics.

Metal Implants

There are many variations on the suture anchor (Fig. 3). Two categories of anchors are currently used: metal and the bioabsorbable devices. Current techniques and implants have gained interest partly because they avoid the potential complications of injury to the suprascapular nerve and developing a posterior ganglion, which can occur with transglenoid drilling. The suture-anchor design must fulfill two criteria. First, the anchor should attach firmly to bone and

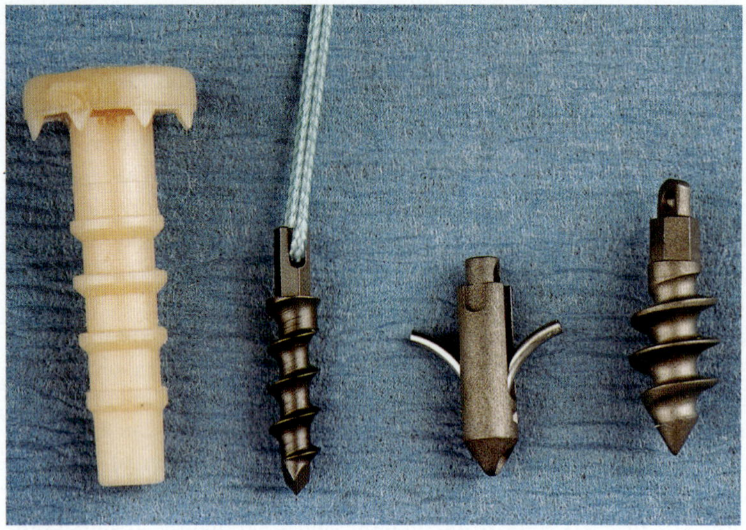

FIG. 3. Implants **(left to right)**: Suretac, Statac, GII Mitek, and Mini Revo screw.

should have a pull-out strength that approaches or surpasses the tensile strength of the suture being used. Second, the suture anchor must have an eyelet that permits sliding of the selected sutures to facilitate knot tying. In addition, a low-profile head or complete intraosseous location is preferred, to avoid injury to the articular cartilage on the humeral head if instability recurs. Two types of metal suture anchors are commonly used, the Mini Revo (Linvatec Inc., Largo, FL, U.S.A.) and the Mitek GII (Norwood, MA, U.S.A.; Fig. 3). Snyder (20,24) developed and reported a specific technique with the Mini Revo screw.

Patient positioning, examination under anesthesia, portal placement, and a diagnostic arthroscopy are performed as discussed earlier. Once the diagnostic portion of the arthroscopy is completed and a soft-tissue Bankart lesion has been documented, the surgeon may proceed with the anterior stabilization. The glenoid rim is prepared with the arthroscope in the anterosuperior (AS) portal, and a shaver is introduced through the anterior midglenoid portal (AMG) and used to debride scar tissue and labral and cartilage debris.

The thin cortical bone on the anterior scapular neck is abraded up to the anterior glenoid rim by using a motorized burr. The remaining loose articular cartilage and soft tissue are removed from the glenoid edge. This step allows direct visualization of the subchondral bone of the anterior glenoid rim for accurate placement of the suture anchors.

Care must be used with the motorized equipment in the anterior shoulder, because damage to the anterior soft tissue can limit the surgeon's ability to repair the ligaments adequately to bone. Similarly, excessive bone excision from the anterior glenoid decreases the anteroposterior (AP) dimension of the glenoid, which may exacerbate the possibility for redislocation. Thus, limited bone abrasion is recommended.

Pilot drill holes are made at the edge of the glenoid, slightly on the articular surface. If the holes are placed too far medially, they will fail to reconstitute the normal height of the labrum. Medial placement of the holes can also result in residual laxity of the ligamentous structures and possible recurrent instability. Two or three drill holes are made between the midglenoid region and the 5:30 o'clock position. Usually, two to three anchors are adequate to reapproximate the labrum to the glenoid. Once the anterior edge of the glenoid has been adequately prepared, it is necessary to exchange the AMG operating cannula for a larger screw-in operating cannula. This larger cannula is required for the use of the capsulorrhaphy-suturing instruments. Necessary equipment is pictured in Figure 4.

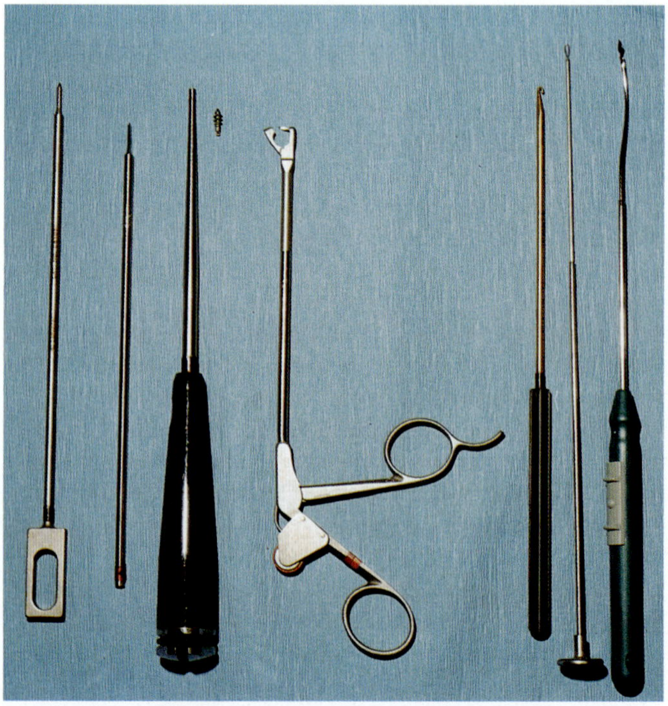

FIG. 4. Snyder Mini Revo screw instrument set.

While the surgeon is viewing through the AS portal, the first Mini Revo anchor is placed through the AMG cannula and is inserted into the inferiormost drill hole. The anchor is then fully seated by screwing in the implant. The inserter is then removed carefully to avoid pulling the sliding suture through the eyelet of the anchor. Once it is adequately seated, tension is placed firmly on the suture to confirm adequate fixation of the anchor in glenoid bone.

The arthroscope is then changed to the posterior portal for viewing. One strand of the suture is retrieved through the AS portal by using a crochet hook. Either a suture hook or a modified slotted-jaw suture punch is introduced through the AMG cannula and is passed through the inferior glenohumeral ligament and under the labrum. The instrument tip should exit near the anchor. A shuttle relay is passed through these structures into the joint. The number of anterior capsulolabral structures imbricated is dependent on the laxity of these structures.

The shuttle relay is grasped with an arthroscopic clamp and pulled out through the AS cannula until the eyelet is exposed. The shuttle is then loaded with Ethibond sutures outside the AS portal. By pulling on the limb of the shuttle outside the AMG cannula, the surgeon passes the suture retrograde through the appropriate anterior capsulolabral structures and delivers it out the AMG cannula. This step results in a simple stitch for securing the anterior structures to bone. The simple suture bolsters the labrum against the anterior glenoid, increasing the effective depth of the glenoid, thus increasing stability. A horizontal mattress stitch may be created by repeating these steps with the second strand of suture.

The sutures are then positioned for knot tying. Knot tying presents one of the more demanding aspects of this procedure. It is important to do it correctly with whatever knot-tying system is used. The surgeon has only one attempt to perform this task correctly. Knot integrity must be carefully checked; a loose stitch is functionless and must be replaced.

This procedure is repeated for a second and, if required, a third anchor. Once all sutures have been tied, the final repair is visualized and probed to assure firm fixation of the anterior capsulolabral structures to bone.

Wolf et al. (42) reported their experience by using Mitek GII suture anchors. These double-arched anchors have a holding strength comparable to a no. 2 polyester suture placed by a traditional open transosseous suture method. The technique involves arthroscopic placement of three to four suture anchors in the anterior glenoid rim after simple, PDS absorbable sutures are placed in the detached capsulolabral complex by using a suture hook. The sutures are then individually tied to their respective anchors by using an arthroscopic knot pusher. The suture hook enables the surgeon to place the sutures anywhere in the anterior capsulolabral complex. Thus, the anterior capsule can be plicated at the time the Bankart lesion is repaired.

Postoperative care and rehabilitation follows a similar protocol as previously described. The author advocated a slightly more conservative program (20).

Conversion to an open technique is based on similar guidelines as with the transglenoid suturing method. Arthroscopic stabilization is not attempted in patients who do not have a Bankart lesion, have poorly defined capsular structures, do not report a specific traumatic or microtraumatic incident, and are contact athletes. Incorrect anchor placement and position can require conversion to an open technique.

Degradable Implants

One technique for arthroscopic Bankart repair uses a cannulated, absorbable fixation device (Figs. 3 and 5). This

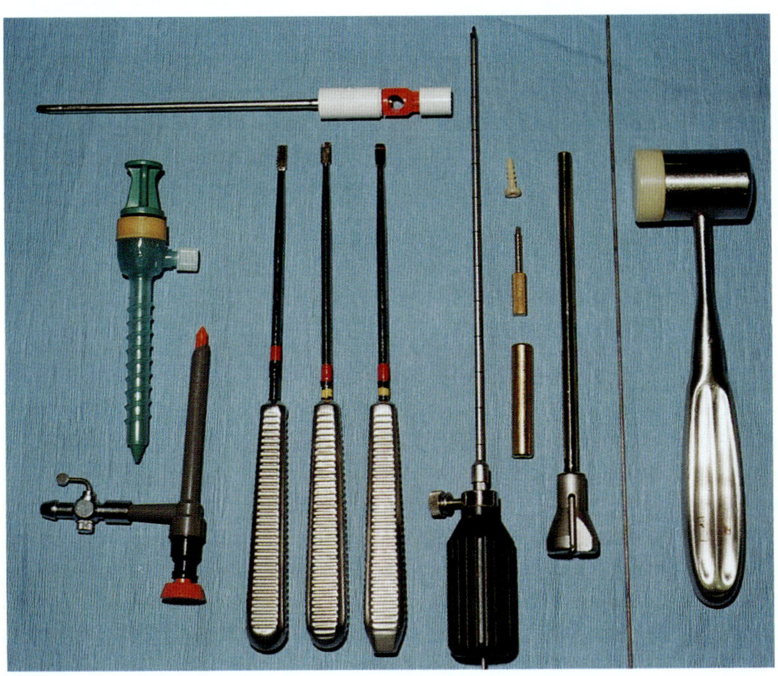

FIG. 5. Suretac cannulated instrument set.

device (Suretac) was designed to avoid the problems associated with metallic devices and suture-fixation techniques and to avoid having to tie knots intra-articularly. Proper patient selection is crucial for achieving a good result. The ideal candidate for an arthroscopic stabilization procedure is an individual with a history of traumatic anterior instability who is found to have a discrete Bankart lesion, robust and discrete capsuloligamentous structures, and neither arthritis nor rotator-cuff pathology (43). The technique also may be applied to patients with superior labral pathology, such as SLAP lesions (28,44).

The diagnostic arthroscopy and stabilization technique has been described in both the seated beach-chair and the lateral decubitus positions. Use of the beach-chair position allows unrestricted access to the entire shoulder and permits free movement of the arm in all planes. Conversion to an open procedure is easily accomplished without the need for repositioning.

After thorough examination under anesthesia, as previously described, a diagnostic arthroscopy is undertaken, and all intra-articular pathology is defined. Criteria that make an arthroscopic repair inappropriate include capsular injury, capsular laxity, a large bony Bankart lesion, glenohumeral arthritis, or a rotator-cuff tear (43). Absent or poorly defined glenohumeral ligaments indicate a poor prognosis for a successful outcome with an arthroscopic Bankart repair. Individuals noted to have tissue of this nature are best treated with open capsulorrhaphy.

The Bankart lesion is prepared by a series of steps designed to mobilize the tissue along the anterior glenoid neck so that it may be shifted superiorly and medially at the time of repair. Hand and motorized instruments are used to create a bleeding bony bed, to which the tissue will be approximated. If the labrum is incompletely detached, the Bankart lesion is extended to the 6 o'clock position by using an electrocautery device or small periosteal elevator. A rasp is placed through the anterior portal and used to detach soft tissue from the glenoid rim in both medial and inferior directions. After tissue mobilization, abrasion of the scapular neck with an arthroscopic rasp and motorized burr to create a bleeding surface will promote soft-tissue healing. In addition, the bony bed is shaped so that it is more perpendicular to the approach of the cannulated drill to prevent the drill from slipping during its advancement. An arthroscopic grasping instrument introduced through the AS portal is used to shift the capsulolabral tissue superiorly and medially while holding it reduced to the glenoid neck. A guide wire is locked in place within the cannulated drill with its tip protruding 3 mm beyond the tip of the drill. The cannulated drill with accompanying guide wire is introduced through the large cannula in the anterior–inferior portal, capturing the advanced tissue, and is drilled to a predetermined depth at about the 4 to 5 o'clock position (for a right glenoid). Drill holes should be positioned at the articular margin of the glenoid, with great care to direct the drill to avoid penetration of the articular cartilage. The drill is removed from over the guide wire, leaving the guide wire in place, transfixing the tissue. A Suretac device is placed over the guide wire and impacted into the prepared channel by using a cannulated pusher and mallet. The glenohumeral ligaments are captured by the head of the tack and held securely against the prepared bone surface. At least two Suretac devices are placed, the first as low as possible (typically the 4 to 5 o'clock position), and the second near the 2 o'clock position. Again, each tack should be placed immediately adjacent to the articular margin of the glenoid. The interface between the Suretacs and the capsulolabral complex should be probed to demonstrate sufficient compression against the bone. The arthroscope is now placed in one of the anterior portals to visualize the repair and to confirm further adequate placement and ligament tension (Fig. 6).

Postoperatively, the extremity is placed in a shoulder immobilizer for 4 weeks. Isometric exercises are performed during this period of immobilization. A graduated program of active and active-assisted motion, along with progressive strengthening, begins at 1 month. Swimming and light throwing are permitted at 4 months after surgery, whereas heavy labor, forceful overhead sports, and contact sports are restricted until 6 months postoperatively.

The importance of patient selection for arthroscopic shoulder stabilization cannot be overemphasized. A significant learning curve involving both proper patient selection and correct surgical technique exists for arthroscopic Bankart repair by using the Suretac device.

In addition to the previously described complications associated with arthroscopic techniques, postoperative tack lysis can occur. This causes glenohumeral joint inflammation, beginning 6 to 8 weeks postoperatively. It is self-limited and resolves in approximately 4 weeks with a course of nonsteroidal anti-inflammatory agents. Symptoms include pain and loss of motion.

The degree of capsular laxity is central to the success or failure of arthroscopic tack stabilization and perhaps to all arthroscopic techniques for anterior instability. Arthroscopic stabilization with a tack is best suited for repair of traumatic detachment of the anterior aspect of the labrum. The procedure is not a substitute for open capsulorrhaphy in all individuals with anterior instability.

ADVANTAGES COMMON TO ALL ARTHROSCOPIC TECHNIQUES

Open Bankart reconstructions have had good clinical results; however, limitations in range of motion, especially external rotation, have been reported (3). Arthroscopic stabilizations require smaller surgical incisions and less soft-tissue dissection than open procedures, which benefits the patient with less postoperative pain and scarring. Decreased soft-tissue scar enables patients stabilized arthroscopically to achieve better range of motion (21). Less-invasive surgery, after the learning curve, requires less time to perform than do open stabilizations.

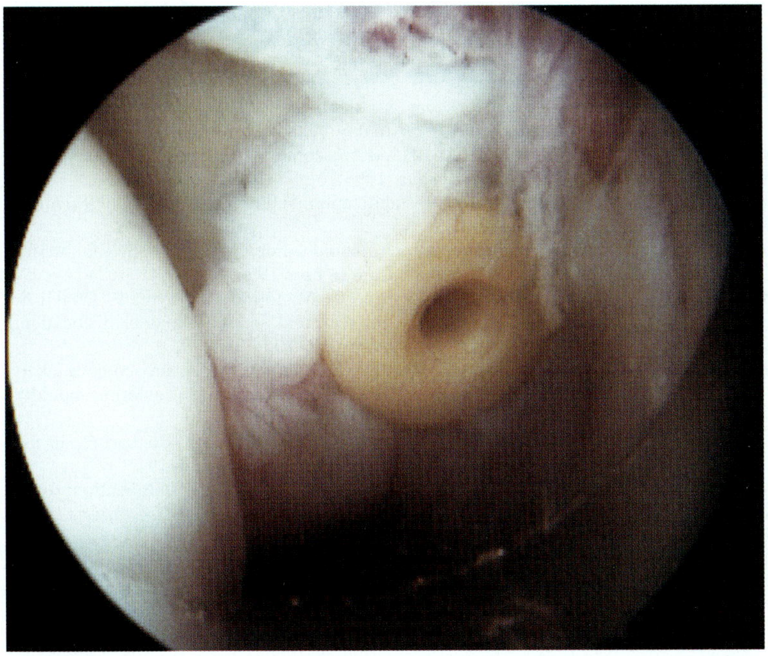

FIG. 6. Suretac placement in anterior capsulolabral structures, viewed from the anterior portal.

DISADVANTAGES COMMON TO ALL ARTHROSCOPIC TECHNIQUES

All arthroscopic stabilization procedures are technically demanding and have a difficult learning curve. The biggest disadvantage of these procedures is their high failure rate. This may be related to technique because many authors have pointed out the improvement in later results, as compared with earlier parts of their series.

As indications and contraindications have evolved, diagnostic arthroscopy has played an important role in identifying associated injuries, particularly intrasubstance injuries to the glenohumeral ligament and capsule, which may compromise the results of arthroscopic reconstruction. Diagnostic arthroscopy has not reliably been able to assess the rotator-interval size, another potential source of postoperative instability.

REFERENCES

1. Johnson LL. Instructional video: arthroscopic staple capsulorrhaphy. East Lansing, MI: Instrument Makar, 1983.
2. Detrisac DA, Johnson LL. Arthroscopic shoulder capsulorrhaphy using metal staples. *Orthop Clin North Am* 1993;24 (1):71–78.
3. Matthews LS, Vetter WL, Oweida SJ, Spearman J, Helfet DL. Arthroscopic staple capsulorrhaphy for recurrent anterior shoulder instability. *Arthroscopy* 1988;4:106–111.
4. Rowe CR, Patel D, Southmayd WW. The Bankart procedure: a long term end-result study. *J Bone Joint Surg [Am]* 1978;60:1–16.
5. Hawkins RB. Arthroscopic stapling repair for shoulder instability: a retrospective study of 50 cases. *Arthroscopy* 1989;5:122–128.
6. Gross RM. Arthroscopic shoulder capsulorrhaphy: does it work? *Am J Sports Med* 1989;17:495–500.
7. Coughlin L, Rubinovich M, Johansson J, White B, Greenspoon J. Arthroscopic staple capsulorrhaphy for anterior shoulder instability. *Am J Sports Med* 1992;20:253–256.
8. Zuckerman JD, Matsen FA. Complications about the glenohumeral joint related to the use of screws and staples. *J Bone Joint Surg [Am]* 1984;66:175–180.
9. Speer KP, Warren RF. Arthroscopic shoulder stabilization: a role for biodegradable materials. *Clin Orthop* 1993;291:67–74.
10. Altchek DW. Arthroscopic shoulder stabilization using a bioabsorbable fixation device. *Sports Med Arthosc Rev* 1993;1:266–271.
11. Speer KP, Warren RF, Pagnani M, Warner JJP. An arthroscopic technique for anterior stabilization of the shoulder with a bioabsorbable tack. *J Bone Joint Surg [Am]* 1996:78:1801–1807.
12. Arciero RA, Taylor DC, Snyder RJ, Uhorchak JM. Arthroscopic bioabsorbable tack stabilization of initial anterior shoulder dislocations: a preliminary report. *Arthroscopy* 1995;11:410–417.
13. Morgan CD, Bodenstab AB. Arthroscopic Bankart suture repair: technique and early results. *Arthroscopy* 1987;3:111–122.
14. Benedetto KP, Glotzer W. Arthroscopic Bankart procedure by suture technique: indications, technique, and results. *Arthroscopy* 1992;8: 111–115.
15. Landsiedl F. Arthroscopic therapy of recurrent anterior luxation of the shoulder by capsular repair. *Arthroscopy* 1992;8:296–304.
16. Grana WA, Buckley PD, Yates CK. Arthroscopic Bankart suture repair. *Am J Sports Med* 1993;21:348–353.
17. Goldberg BJ, Nirschl RP, McConnell JP, Pettrone FA. Arthroscopic transglenoid suture capsulolabral repairs: preliminary results. *Am J Sports Med* 1993:21:656–665.
18. Caspari RB, Savoie FH. Arthroscopic reconstruction of the shoulder: the Bankart repair. In: McGinty JB, Caspari RB, Jackson RW, Poehling GG, eds. *Operative arthroscopy.* New York: Raven Press, 1991:507–515.
19. Torchia ME, Caspari RB, Asselmeier MA, Beach WR. Arthroscopically assisted transglenoid suture repair for anterior shoulder instability: 2-8 year results in 150 shoulders [Abstract]. *Orthop Trans* 1996;20:79.
20. Snyder SJ, Banas MP, Belzer JP. Arthroscopic treatment of anterior shoulder instability using threaded suture anchors and nonabsorbable sutures. *Instr Course Lect* 1996;45:71–81.
21. Guanche CA, Quick DC, Sodergren KM, Buss DD. Arthroscopic versus open reconstruction of the shoulder in patients with isolated Bankart lesions. *Am J Sports Med* 1996;24:144–148.
22. Green MR, Christensen KP. Arthroscopic versus open Bankart procedures: a comparison of early morbidity and complications. *Arthroscopy* 1993:9:371–374.
23. Snyder S, Karzel R, Del Pizzo W, Ferkel R, Friedman M. S.L.A.P. lesions of the shoulder (lesions of the superior labrum both anterior and posterior). *Orthop Trans* 1990;14:257–258.

24. Snyder SJ, Banas MP, Belzer JP. Arthroscopic evaluation and treatment of injuries to the superior glenoid labrum. *Instr Course Lect* 1996;45:65–70.
25. Field LD, Savoie FH. Arthroscopic suture repair of superior labral detachment lesions of the shoulder. *Am J Sports Med* 1993;21:783–790.
26. Richards RR, An K-N, Bigliani LU, et al. A standardized method for the assessment of shoulder function. *J Shoulder Elbow Surg* 1994;3:347–352.
27. Yoneda M, Hirooka A, Saito S, Yamamoto T, Ochi T, Shino K. Arthroscopic stapling for detached superior glenoid labrum. *J Bone Joint Surg [Br]* 1991;73:746–750.
28. Pagnani MJ, Speer KP, Altchek DW, Warren RF, Dines DM. Arthroscopic fixation of superior labral lesions using a biodegradable implant: a preliminary report. *Arthroscopy* 1995;11:194–198.
29. Bigliani LU, Flatow EL, Deliz ED. Complications of shoulder arthroscopy. *Orthop Rev* 1991;20:743–751.
30. Matthews LS, Zarins B, Michael RH, Helfet DL. Anterior portal selection for shoulder arthroscopy. *Arthroscopy* 1985;1:33–39.
31. Norwood LA, Fowler HL. Rotator cuff tears: a shoulder arthroscopy complication. *Am J Sports Med* 1989;17:837–841.
32. Moran MC, Warren RF. Development of a synovial cyst after arthroscopy of the shoulder. *J Bone Joint Surg [Am]* 1989;71:127–129.
33. Pagnani MJ, Warren RF, Altchek DW, Wickiewicz TL, Anderson AF. Arthroscopic shoulder stabilization using transglenoid sutures. *Am J Sports Med* 1996;24:459–467.
34. Small NC. Complications in arthroscopic surgery of the knee and shoulder. *Orthopaedics* 1993;16:985–988.
35. Small NC. Complications in arthroscopic surgery performed by experienced arthroscopists. *Arthroscopy* 1988;4:215–221.
36. Wiley AM. Arthroscopy for shoulder instability and a technique for arthroscopic repair. *Arthroscopy* 1988;4:25–30.
37. Snyder SJ, Strafford BB. Arthroscopic management of instability of the shoulder. *Orthopedics* 1993;16:993–1002.
38. Maki NJ. Arthroscopic stabilization: suture technique. *Oper Tech Orthop* 1991;1:180–183.
39. Rose DJ. Arthroscopic transglenoid suture capsulorrhaphy for anterior shoulder instability. *Instr Course Lect* 1996;45:57–64.
40. Walch G, Boileau P, Levigne C, Mandrino A, Neyret P, Donell S. Arthroscopic stabilization for recurrent anterior shoulder dislocation: results of 59 cases. *Arthroscopy* 1995;11:173–179.
41. Youssef JA, Carr CF, Walther CE, Murphy JM. Arthroscopic Bankart suture repair for recurrent traumatic unidirectional anterior shoulder dislocations. *Arthroscopy* 1995;11:561–563.
42. Wolf EM, Wilik RM, Richmond JC. Arthroscopic Bankart repair using suture anchors. *Oper Tech Orthop* 1991;1:184–191.
43. Swenson TM, Warner JJP. Arthroscopic shoulder stabilization: overview of indications, technique, and efficacy. *Clin Sports Med* 1995;14:841–862.
44. Warner JJP, Kann S, Marks P. Arthroscopic repair of combined Bankart and superior labral detachment anterior and posterior lesions: technique and preliminary results. *Arthroscopy* 1994;10:383–391.

The Unstable Shoulder,
edited by R.F. Warren, E.V. Craig, and D.W. Altchek.
Lippincott–Raven Publishers, Philadelphia © 1999.

CHAPTER 19

Arthroscopic Labral Repair with the Suretac Device

Mark C. Deibert and Kevin P. Speer

DESIGN RATIONALE

The proposed benefits of arthroscopic labral-fixation techniques include a more anatomic repair, decreased surgical time, and less perioperative pain and surgical morbidity compared with open repairs/reconstructions (1–3). Despite these intended advantages, arthroscopic shoulder-stabilization procedures have traditionally been limited by complications associated with the fixation device used and by higher rates of recurrent instability compared with open reconstructive procedures with bone holes or suture anchors.

Arthroscopic stabilization of the shoulder by using metallic-staple fixation was initially described by Johnson in 1986 (4). In that study, an arthroscopically placed metallic staple was used to reattach the displaced labrum back to the glenoid rim. Follow-up studies found that arthroscopic staple capsulorrhaphy of the glenohumeral joint has the highest complications rate of any arthroscopic procedure (5). Complications related to the use of metallic staples include implant loosening and migration, pain, fracture of the implant, articular cartilage injury, and impingement (6–12).

Morgan and Bodenstab (13–15) designed an arthroscopic transglenoid suture technique for Bankart repair based on the open transosseous suture-repair technique of Reider and Inglis (7). In this procedure, a single large horizontal mattress stitch of no. 1 polydioxanone suture (PDS) is used to reduce the inferior glenohumeral ligament anatomically to the prepared midportion of the anterior glenoid rim. The suture is placed through the scapular neck with suture pins and exits posteriorly through two separate posterior–inferior skin incisions. The procedure is completed by tying the suture tails over the fascia of the posterior third of the deltoid (15). This procedure avoids the use of metallic fixation but requires separate posterior incisions and tying of the sutures over posterior muscular fascia. The posterior aspect of this suture construct lies over compressible soft tissue (muscular fascia), which may allow the capsulolabral repair to gap and compromise healing of the Bankart lesion (16). The long suture pins used in this technique have been associated with errant passage of the pin medial to the scapula (17).

Evolution of arthroscopic shoulder-stabilization techniques has led to the recent development of bioabsorbable tacks (18), which have less potential for articular injury while providing adequate tissue apposition. The Suretac (Acufex Microsurgical, Mansfield, MA, U.S.A.) is a cannulated bioabsorbable fixation device that provides tissue fixation without the risk of hardware-related complications associated with the placement of metallic fixation adjacent to joint surfaces. This bioabsorbable fixation tack eliminates the need for transglenoid drilling procedures and avoids the tying of suture over posterior deltoid or infraspinatus fascia in proximity to the suprascapular nerve. Arthroscopic labral repair with the Suretac device is in essence a labral-repair procedure. The technique allows a capsulorrhaphy but is limited by the repair design and is certainly less able to shift the capsule than are transglenoid techniques or open procedures.

DEVELOPMENT OF THE BIOABSORBABLE IMPLANT

The Suretac is a cannulated bioabsorbable tack that is molded from a polyglycolic acid polymer (polyglyconate) that is identical to the material used in Maxon sutures (Davis & Geck, Danbury, CT, U.S.A.). The head of the tack

M. C. Deibert: Alpine Orhtopedic and Sports Medicine, Bozeman, Montana 59715.
K. P. Speer: Duke Division of Orthopaedic Surgery, Duke University Medical Center, Durham, North Carolina 27710.

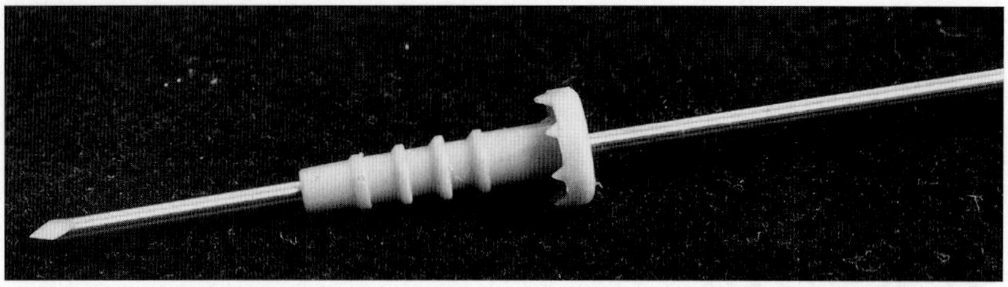

FIG. 1. Suretac II on a guide wire. Note the spiked surface of the head of the implant.

is 8 mm in diameter, and the shaft 1.5 cm in length and 3 mm in diameter. Ribs on the shaft of the tack increase its pull-out strength, and a broad, spiked head allows the tack to capture soft tissue and hold it to bone, as shown in Figure 1. The mechanical strength of the bioabsorbable tack falls to zero at 4 weeks after implantation (18).

The Suretac is designed to provide temporary mechanical fixation between soft tissue and bone. The bioabsorption profile of the Suretac occurs predictably as the healing tissues gain integrity and resistance to stress. If bioabsorption occurs too rapidly, the operative construct is likely to fail. If bioabsorption occurs too slowly, the implant might display a complication pattern similar to those of metallic implants: breakage, loosening, and migration, possibly leading to articular cartilage injury. The relatively longer bioabsorption profile of polyacetate polymers foils attempts to create bioabsorbable tacks from this material.

The bioabsorbable material, polyglyconate, is manufactured by reacting trimethylene carbonate and glycolytic acid with diethylene glycol as initiator and stannous chloride dihydrate as catalyst. The structure of the copolymer is represented, where the ratio is approximately 67.5x and 32.5y:

Glycolide moiety, -$(CH_2COOCH_2COO)x$
Trimethylene carbonate moiety, -$(CH_2CH_2CH_2OCOO)y$-

The Suretac is primarily degraded by hydrolysis. Therefore, an important criterion for packaging and delivery is that it be maintained absolutely dry. Prolonged exposure to hydrated air will initiate the degradative process.

INDICATIONS FOR ARTHROSCOPIC LABRAL REPAIR WITH THE SURETAC DEVICE

Arthroscopic anterior stabilization is primarily indicated for cases of instability caused by trauma, which require manual reduction. The patient should be at high risk for recurrent instability and is usually young and athletic. In addition, there should be few if any repeated dislocations after the initial traumatic episode to limit the magnitude of plastic deformation that may result from repeated instability episodes. Essentially, the instability should be entirely anterior in direction.

The results of a prospective study by Arciero et al. (19) suggest that the best candidate for this procedure may be a young athletic individual with an acute anterior dislocation. Arciero et al. (19) reported treating young athletic patients with initial traumatic dislocations with either acute arthroscopic stabilization or with immobilization followed by rehabilitation. These authors demonstrated a significant reduction in recurrent instability with acute arthroscopic repair of the Bankart lesion. Specifically, at an average of 32 months' follow-up, there was an 80% rate of recurrent instability in patients treated nonoperatively, whereas 14% of those treated with an acute repair developed recurrent instability.

Patients may also have a history consistent with primary mechanical labral pathology (tear) and not gross instability, as in the case of a superior (SLAP [superior labral anterior and posterior]; 20), inferior, or posterior labral (21) injury. Several findings on physical examination and imaging studies may diagnose these injuries; however, none is 100% accurate. We have found that history, with respect to the age of the patient, is most helpful in making these diagnoses. When patients with suspected labral injury have symptoms that are refractory to activity modification and rehabilitation, they may then be candidates for diagnostic arthroscopy and labral repair.

Patients with a (moderate) degree of inferior laxity (greater than 1+ sulcus sign) or posterior instability greater than 1+ are not candidates for the tack procedure. Patients demonstrating a sulcus sign of 2+ or greater, or 2+ posterior translation, who are surgical candidates, should be treated with an open reconstruction/repair as shown in Figure 2. In summary, anterior or posterior labral repair may be indicated for patients who require fixation of the labrum to the glenoid rim and a limited capsulorrhaphy and are not in need of a shift of the capsule.

OPERATIVE TECHNIQUE

An interscalene anesthetic is administered, and the patient is placed in the beach-chair position (22,37). A careful physical examination is then performed to confirm the severity and direction of the instability pattern. A comparison with the opposite shoulder should be made to establish baseline ligamentous laxity, and a careful assessment made for asymmetry. We assume that normal shoulders have symmetric shoulder laxity; however, this may not be the case (23).

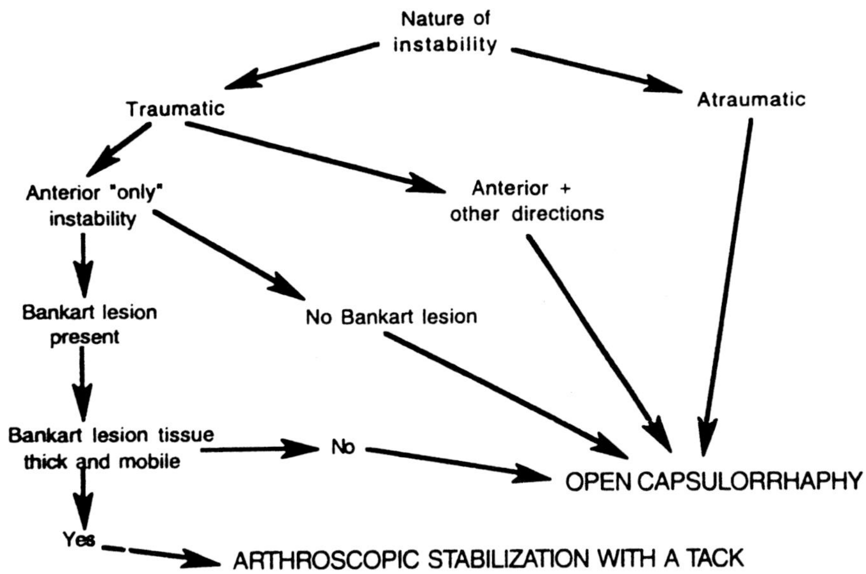

FIG. 2. Diagram showing variables that should be considered when selecting patients for arthroscopic stabilization with a bioabsorbable tack. (From Speer KP, Warren RF, Pagnani M, Warner JJP. An arthroscopic technique for anterior stabilization with a bioabsorbable tack. *J Bone Joint Surg [Am]* 1996;78:1801–1807, with permission.)

Technique for Repair of Anterior–Inferior Labral Detachment (Bankart Lesions)

A standard posterior portal is established, and a diagnostic arthroscopy is performed to document the mechanical basis for the instability pattern. A spinal needle placed in the anterior–superior portal position may be used as a probe until actual portal placement is established. Identification of a discrete Bankart lesion with an avulsed intact labrum, minimal capsular deformation, and robust inferior glenohumeral ligament (IGHL) would indicate ideal pathoanatomy for Suretac fixation. The magnitude and location of capsuloligamentous injury should be assessed, as well as the development of the inferior and middle glenohumeral ligaments (24,25). Despite direct arthroscopic visualization, assessment of the magnitude of plastic capsular deformity is very difficult. The presence of articular cartilage flaps, cartilage degeneration, labral detachment/fraying, and partial-thickness rotator-cuff tears is documented, and they are treated accordingly.

A second low anterior portal is next established by repositioning the spinal needle to the anterior glenohumeral joint line at the superior border of the subscapularis tendon. The position of the spinal needle is assessed for the ability to (a) instrument the anterior scapular neck from the 6 o'clock position upward, and (b) place a Suretac at the articular margin and angle obliquely away from the articular surface. The angle of insertion for the Suretac is approximately 20 degrees from the face of the glenoid. A large transparent cannula and trochar are inserted in the location determined by the spinal needle. We prefer a cannulated insertion-assembly system for insertion of the large cannula to reproduce the angle and placement of the spinal needle.

The labral and capsular tissue are detached with electrocautery from the anterior glenoid both medially and inferiorly to allow proper mobilization. The next step is preparation of the scapular neck with an angled sharp rasp, as shown in Figure 3, and an arthroscopic shaver. This critical step creates a bleeding bone surface that is necessary for healing of the capsulolabral complex to the glenoid rim and anterior inferior scapular neck. During the preparation of the glenoid, great care should be taken to avoid excessive removal of bone or injury to the substance of the labrum. The upper extremity is maintained at the side and in neutral

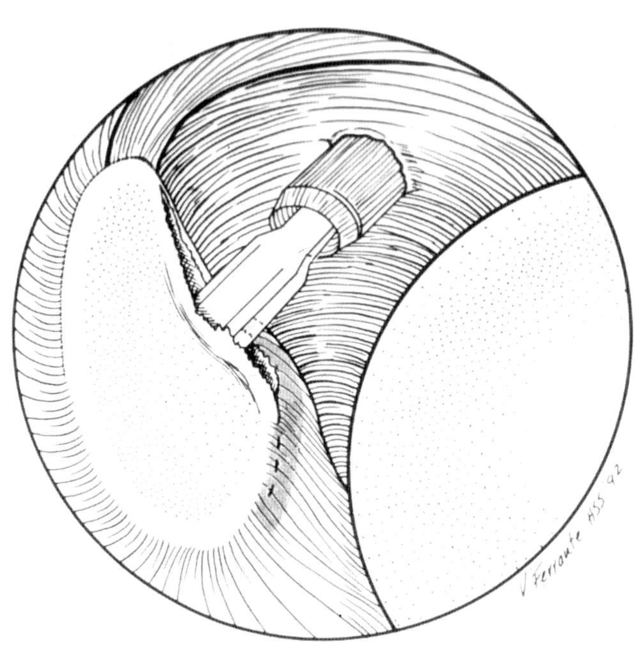

FIG. 3. Abrasion of the anterior and inferior glenoid rim to prepare site for soft-tissue attachment. Rasp enters joint through anterior portal. Bone preparation generally extends from 1 o'clock to 6 o'clock. (From Speer KP, Warren RF. Arthroscopic shoulder stabilization: a role for biodegradable materials. *Clin Orthop* 1993;291:67–74, with permission.)

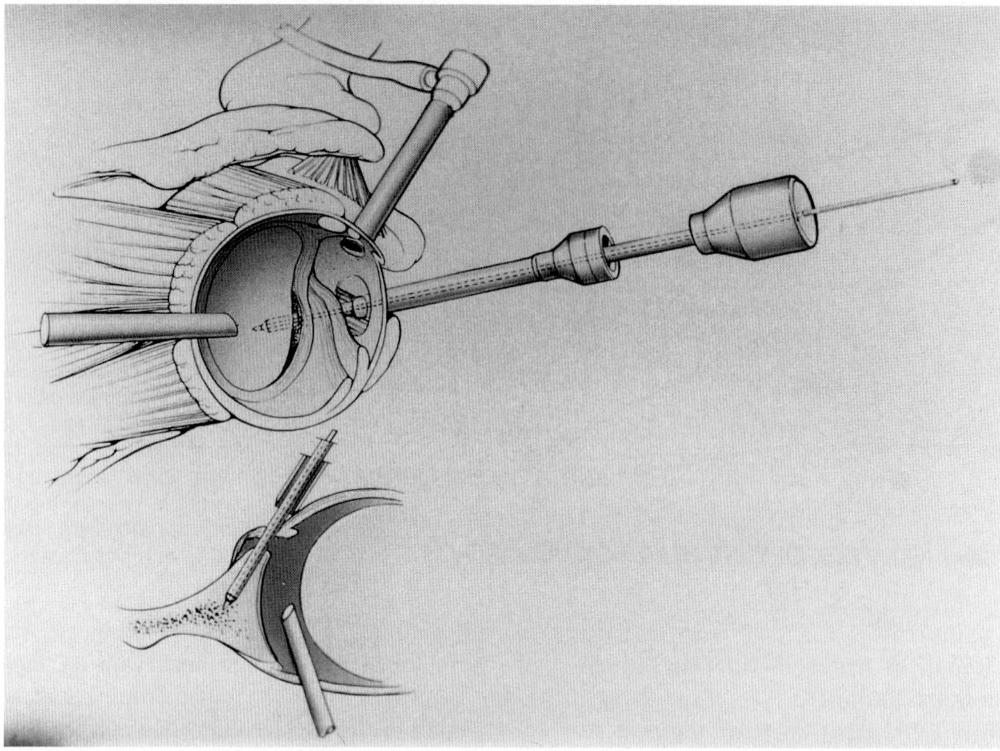

A

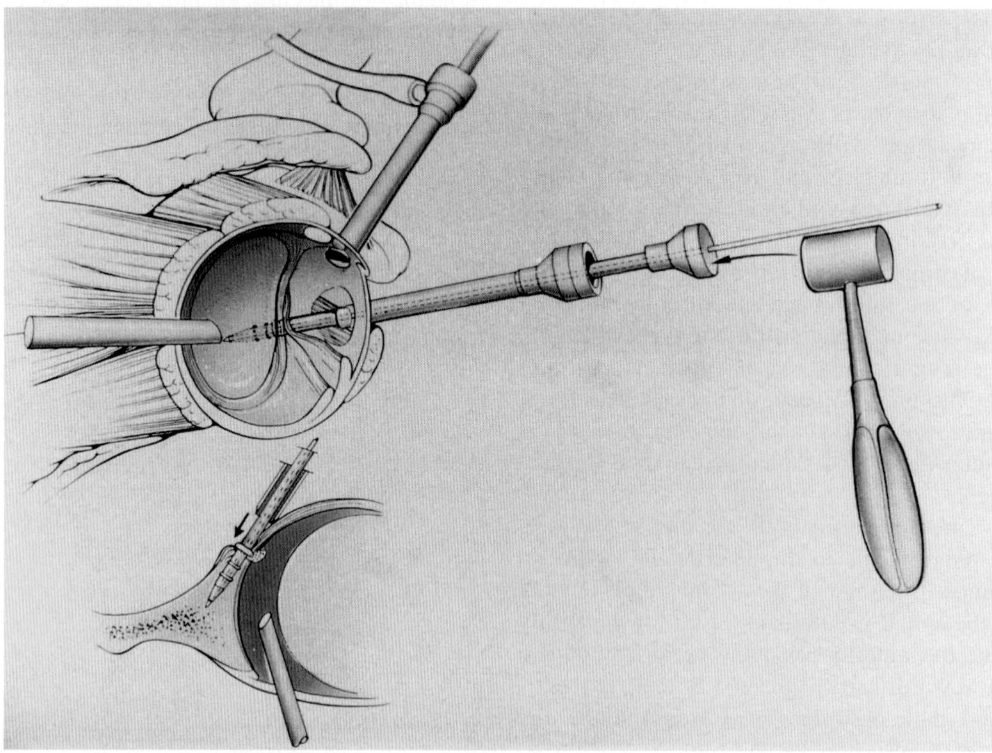

B

FIG. 4. Arthroscopic procedure for anterior stabilization with a bioabsorbable tack. **A:** All instrumentation for the insertion of the bioabsorbable tack comes through a cannula in an anterior portal. A cannulated drill creates the bone tunnel that is drilled both at the glenoid margin and obliquely away from the articular surface. A fine wire remains in the bone after removal of the drill to guide the tack into proper position. **B:** Cannulated tack is driven over the wire. Adequate apposition of the soft tissues to bone is confirmed by arthroscopic visualization. The arm is generally in neutral rotation and full adduction during the insertion of the implant.

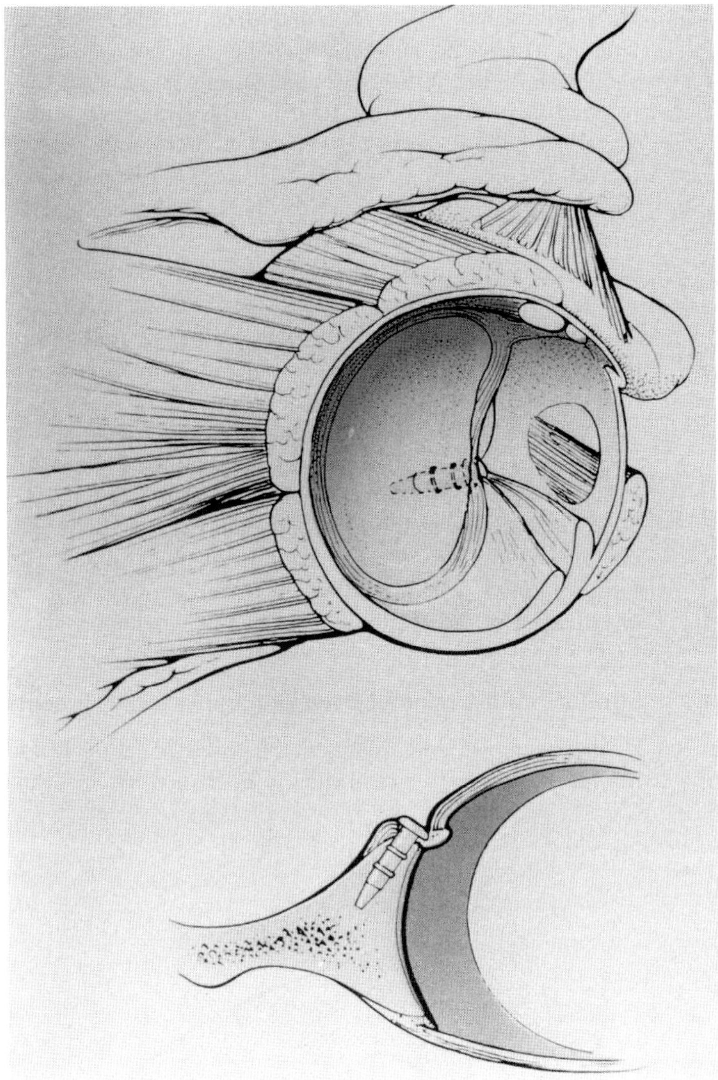

C

FIG. 4. *Continued.* **C:** Final construct must adequately reestablish the anterior–inferior glenohumeral ligament. (From Speer KP, Warren RF. Arthroscopic shoulder stabilization: a role for biodegradable materials. *Clin Orthop* 1993;291:67–74, with permission.)

rotation during placement of the Suretac. The cannulated drill with locked guide pin is then placed through the cannula and used to capture the capsulolabral complex. The detached labrum and capsuloligamentous tissue are shifted superiorly 1 cm, or as much as possible, on the scapular neck to the 4 o'clock position for the right shoulder, and to the 8 o'clock position for the left shoulder.

Alternatively, an anterior–superior portal may be established, and a grasping instrument may be used to advance the capsulolabral complex superiorly before placement of the drill and guide wire through the soft tissue. The drill and guide wire are then advanced into the glenoid neck at the articular margin, angling medially to prevent injury to the articular cartilage, as shown in Figure 4. The drill is then unlocked from the guide wire and carefully removed. The guide wire remains in the bone after removal of the drill to guide the tack into proper position. Care should be taken to avoid drilling completely through the scapular neck to avoid possible injury to the suprascapular nerve. A Suretac is then placed over the wire and driven into the scapular neck with a cannulated impactor and mallet. Clear arthroscopic visualization of the Suretac and impactor should be maintained to ensure accurate placement. A second Suretac may be placed at the 2 o'clock position. Normal anatomy of the IGHL should be restored and the drive-through sign eliminated. The repair is then examined with the arthroscope placed in the anterior working portal to confirm that the IGHL–labral complex is compressed against the glenoid rim (26).

Suretac Stabilization of Superior Labral/Biceps Anchor Lesions

Fixation of superior labral anterior to posterior (type II SLAP) lesions (20), illustrated in Figure 5, is carried out with a similar anesthetic, positioning, physical assessment of range of motion, laxity, and instability, and arthroscopic examination through a standard posterior portal. Localizing of the ideal position for the accessory anterolateral portal to instrument the SLAP lesion is again performed with a

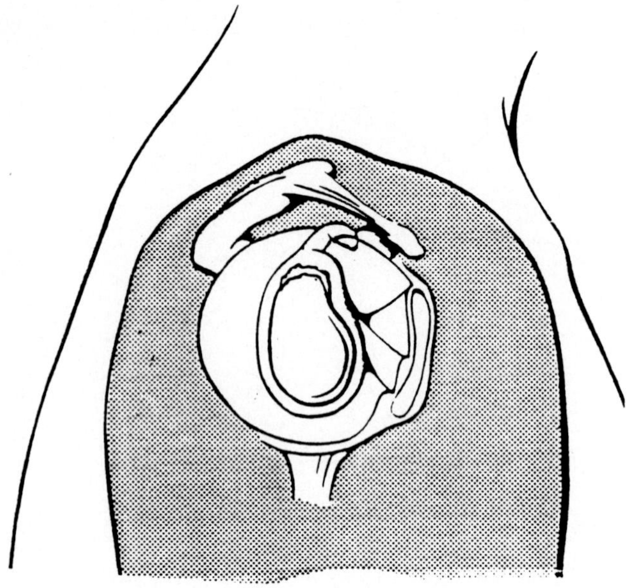

FIG. 5. Type II superior labrum anterior and posterior (SLAP) lesion according to Snyder (30). (From Resch H, Golser K, Thoni H, Sperner G. Arthroscopic repair of superior glenoid labral detachment [the SLAP lesion]. *J Shoulder Elbow Surg* 1993; May/June:149–151, with permission.)

spinal needle. Many times a SLAP lesion is found in overhead athletes who have impingement symptoms. An arthroscopic subacromial bursectomy and debridement is recommended in these patients. Acromioplasty is rarely indicated in overhead athletes and is performed only in the presence of a large anterior acromial spur.

Identification of the ideal location for the accessory anterolateral portal is important for completing the superior labral separation and preparation of the bleeding bone surface. The resulting angle of the cannula relative to the superior scapular neck must be appropriate for drilling and subsequent placement of the absorbable fixation tack. In general, the accessory anterolateral portal (Fig. 6) should be placed within 1 cm of the anterior lateral corner of the acromion, superior to the biceps tendon, and anterior to the leading edge of the supraspinatus tendon within the rotator interval. Figure 6 illustrates portal-placement options for instrumentation of a SLAP (20) lesion. Most arthroscopic shoulder surgeons in North America would not use the transacromial portal because of risk of acute or delayed acromial fracture, and we do not recommend it. The superior medial and anterior portals may be associated with excessive hemorrhage resulting from injury to the suprascapular artery or acromial branch of the thoracoacromial trunk, respectively.

Once the appropriate location and angle of approach are identified, the process of placement of the cannula and preparation of the bone and soft tissue are similar to that of repair of the Bankart lesion, as described earlier. After preparation of the bone and soft tissue, the 1-mm guide wire/drill assembly is used to pierce the origin of the biceps tendon within the substance of the superior labrum, as shown in Figure 7. The superior labrum is reduced to its original position, the pilot hole is drilled, and the Suretac placed. As illustrated in Figure 8, a second Suretac may be placed, if necessary, from an anterosuperior portal to secure the anterior superior labrum. Rarely, supplementary biceps anchor fixation may be required from a second tack brought in from an accessory high posterior portal.

The arthroscopic shoulder surgeon should be able readily to identify normal anatomic variants of the glenoid labrum, including an anterior–superior sublabral hole (27), a meniscoid, and medially based attachment of the superior labrum/biceps anchor. Recognition of these normal anatomic variations will assist the arthroscopic shoulder surgeon in avoiding inappropriate treatment. For example, Snyder et al. (27) reported consulting on a patient who had undergone inappropriate arthroscopic fixation of a sublabral hole (Buford complex), which resulted in frozen shoulder because of tethering of the middle glenohumeral ligament.

Suretac Stabilization of Posterior Labral Detachments

The diagnosis and treatment of posterior labral lesions in contact athletes were originally described by Speer and

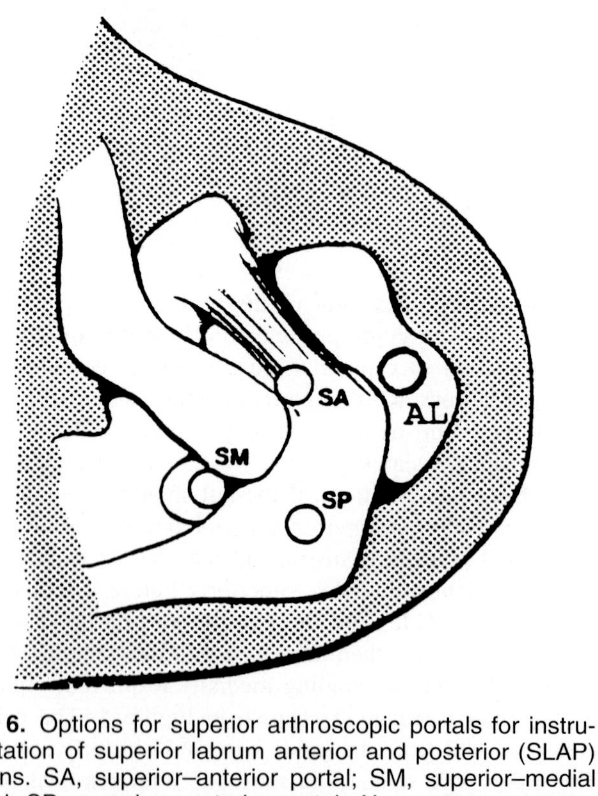

FIG. 6. Options for superior arthroscopic portals for instrumentation of superior labrum anterior and posterior (SLAP) lesions. SA, superior–anterior portal; SM, superior–medial portal; SP, superior–posterior portal; AL, accessory anterolateral portal. (Modified from Resch H, Golser K, Thoni H, Sperner G. Arthroscopic repair of superior glenoid labral detachment [the SLAP lesion]. *J Shoulder Elbow Surg* 1993; May/June:149–151, with permission.)

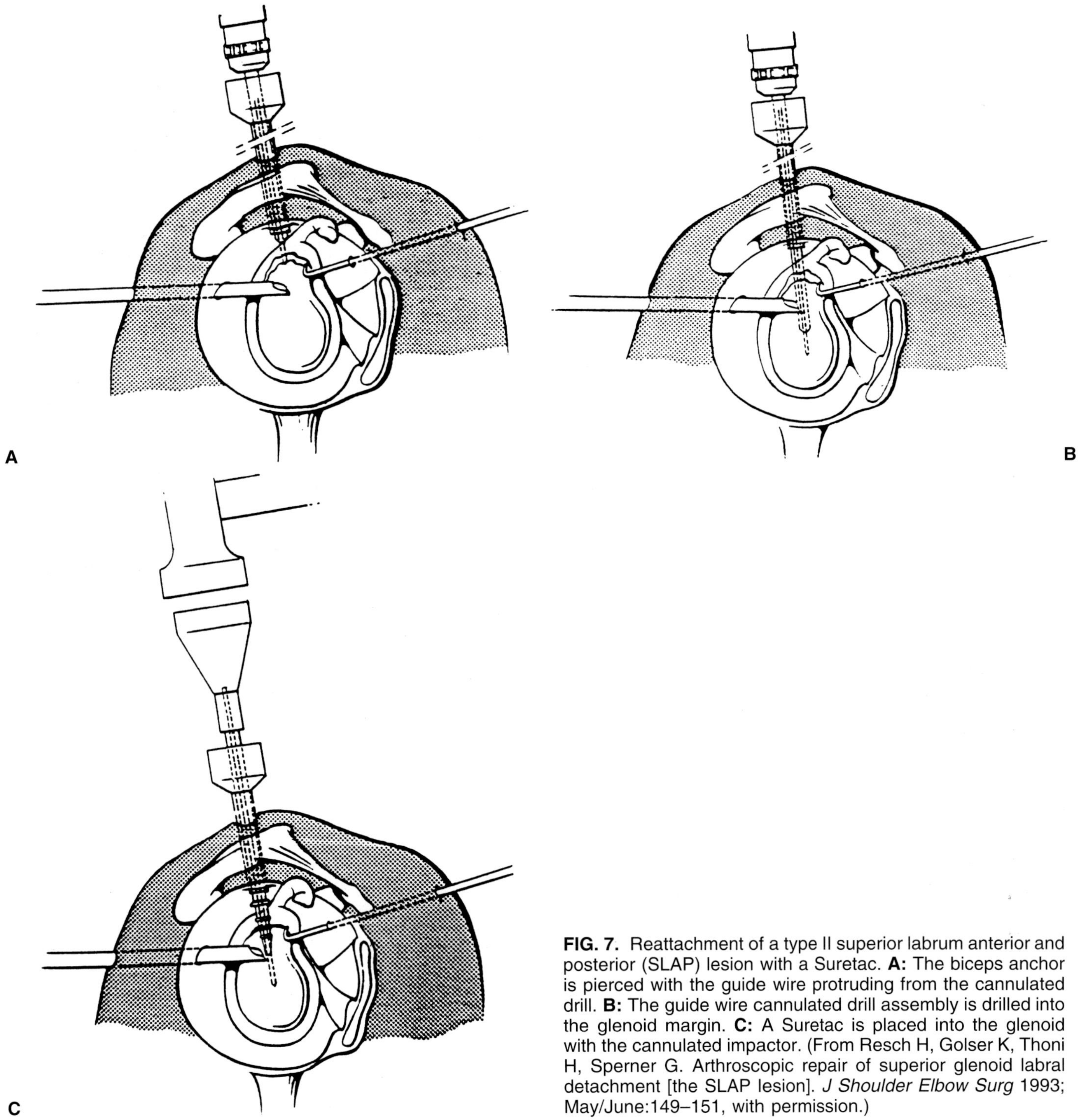

FIG. 7. Reattachment of a type II superior labrum anterior and posterior (SLAP) lesion with a Suretac. **A:** The biceps anchor is pierced with the guide wire protruding from the cannulated drill. **B:** The guide wire cannulated drill assembly is drilled into the glenoid margin. **C:** A Suretac is placed into the glenoid with the cannulated impactor. (From Resch H, Golser K, Thoni H, Sperner G. Arthroscopic repair of superior glenoid labral detachment [the SLAP lesion]. *J Shoulder Elbow Surg* 1993; May/June:149–151, with permission.)

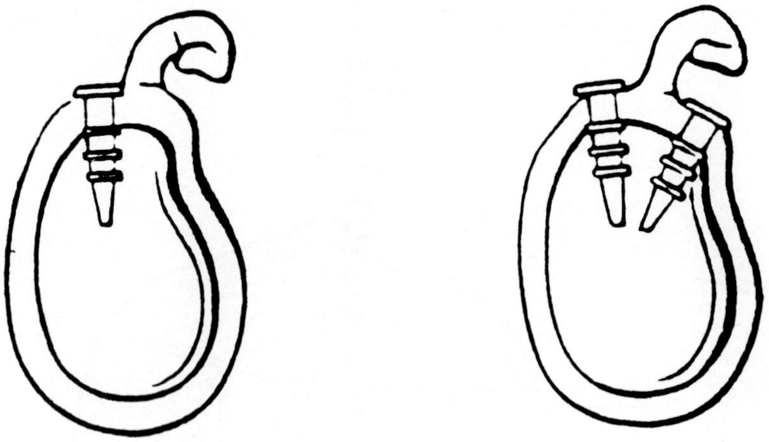

FIG. 8. One or two Suretacs may be used to repair the biceps anchor, if needed. (From Resch H, Golser K, Thoni H, Sperner G. Arthroscopic repair of superior glenoid labral detachment [the SLAP lesion]. *J Shoulder Elbow Surg* 1993; May/June: 149–151, with permission.)

Mair (21). The treatment of symptomatic posterior labral tears refractory to conservative management may include debridement at the site of the tear and labral fixation with the Suretac device. Preoperative evaluation may include a computed tomography (CT) arthrogram, which clearly demonstrates the posterior labral tear, as seen in Figure 9. The technique of posterior labral fixation begins with a thorough diagnostic arthroscopy. Assessment of the posterior labrum is greatly facilitated with visualization through an anterior portal, as seen in Figure 10. The actual process of preparation of the bone and insertion of the Suretac device is similar to that described in previous sections on labral repair. Figure 11 illustrates arthroscopic posterior labral repair of the lesion in Figure 10, with the Suretac device. The importance of establishing the proper angle of inclination for insertion of the Suretac relative to the face of the glenoid cannot be overemphasized. For example, if the posterior portal is placed too medially, it will be difficult to achieve the desired 20-degree angle between the line of insertion of the Suretac with respect to the face of the glenoid to avoid injury to the articular surface and achieve adequate fixation of the tack in bone.

Patients with symptoms of posterior shoulder instability refractory to rehabilitation, and a physical examination demonstrating a positive posterior apprehension test and an asymmetric posterior load-and-shift test, with a history, imaging study, or arthroscopic examination suggestive of posterior labral tear, should be treated with an open reconstruction rather than an arthroscopic labral-repair procedure. This is analogous to the surgical management of recurrent anterior shoulder instability in the setting of a capacious anterior capsule and Bankart lesion, which is appropriately treated with an open reconstruction rather than a Suretac labral repair, because of the inability of this procedure to sufficiently shift the plastically deformed capsule.

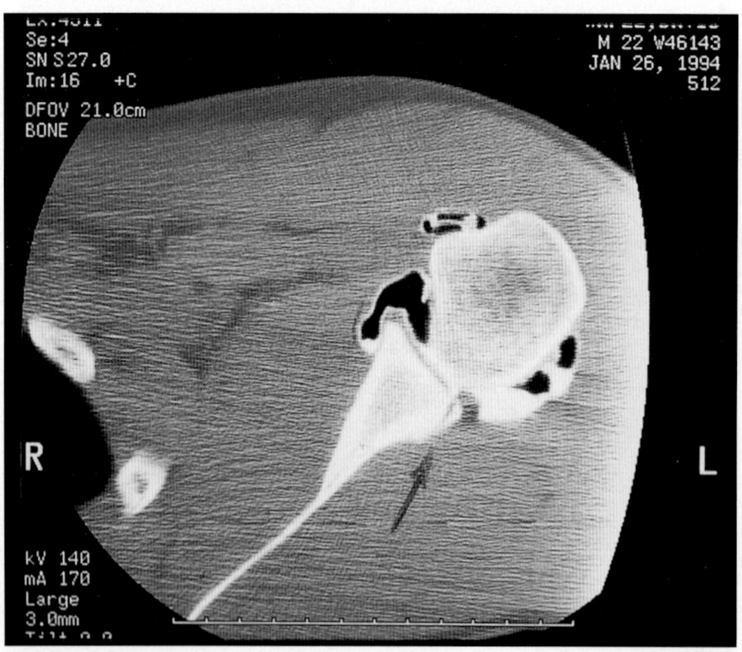

FIG. 9. Computed tomographic (CT) arthrogram of a left shoulder demonstrating a posterior labral tear.

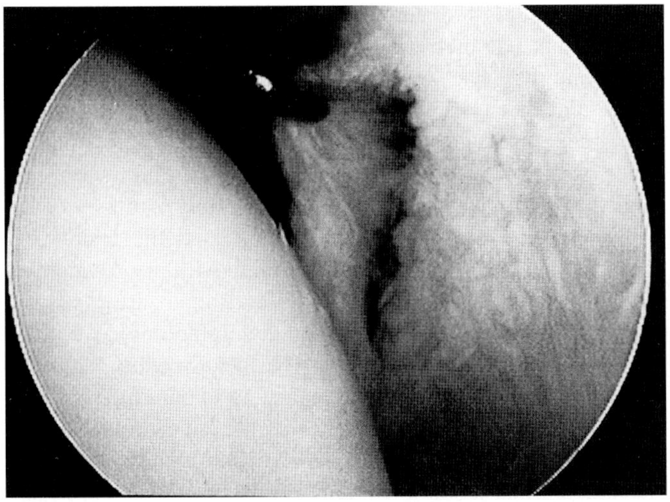

FIG. 10. Intraoperative photograph of a posterior labral detachment in a contact athlete.

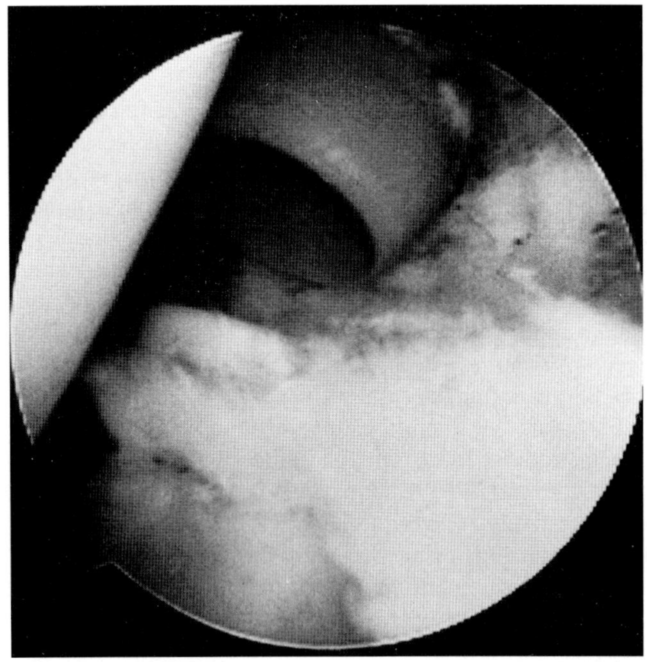

FIG. 11. Intraoperative photograph of an arthroscopic posterior labral repair with a Suretac.

TECHNICAL PITFALLS OF LABRAL FIXATION

Technical pitfalls of arthroscopic labral fixation with the Suretac include failure to establish a surface of bleeding bone on the glenoid rim, improper portal placement, inadequate restoration of tension to the IGHL, and failure to capture sufficient soft tissue with the head of the Suretac (38). Determination of the appropriate angle of approach to the glenoid for the Suretac instrumentation with a spinal needle and subsequent reproduction of this angle with the cannula will ensure that the Suretac will correctly engage the soft tissue and glenoid. Proper patient selection and adherence to strict technical standards, including arthroscopic assessment of plastic capsular deformation, may reduce the rate of recurrent instability after the Suretac labral-repair procedure.

The great uncertainty is arthroscopic assessment of plastic capsular deformity, which is exceedingly difficult at best. Currently, the side-to-side examination under anesthesia that assesses the magnitude of asymmetry is the standard for laxity comparison. Traction applied to the involved extremity, as is used in the lateral decubitus position, and distention of the glenohumeral capsule with a pressurized irrigation system may give the false impression that there is minimal plastic deformation of the anterior inferior capsule. Use of the "drive-through" sign (1) may be helpful by predicting the degree of plastic capsular deformation. The drive-through sign is present if the arthroscope can easily be placed from the posterior to anterior aspect of the joint and displaced in superior to inferior direction after the labrum has been reapproximated to the anterior glenoid margin. While assessing a shoulder for the presence of a drive-through sign, care should be taken not to injure the chondral surfaces of the humeral head or glenoid. A persistent drive-through sign indicates that arthroscopic stabilization should be aborted in favor of an open anterior reconstruction.

The key to avoiding recurrent instability after arthroscopic anterior inferior labral repair is identification of plastic anterior capsular deformation that cannot currently be treated with this procedure. In a redundant anterior capsule, an open capsular shift or transosseous technique of Caspari (28) should be performed in favor of arthroscopic labral repair with the Suretac. Baker et al. (29) identified primary capsular injury without a Bankart lesion in six of 45 patients who were assessed arthroscopically 10 days after an anterior shoulder dislocation. Anterior dislocations occurring without a Bankart lesion, as identified by Baker et al. (29), cannot be appropriately treated with a Suretac labral repair.

POSTOPERATIVE REHABILITATION

Our postoperative rehabilitation program begins with sling immobilization. Elbow range of motion, forearm and hand isometrics, axillary hygiene, and pendulum exercises are allowed during this time. Passive forward elevation to 90 degrees is encouraged from 4 to 6 postoperative weeks. External rotation to 0 degrees with the arm at the side is permitted, as well as deltoid isometrics and periscapular exercises.

At 6 weeks postoperatively, progression to full range of motion is encouraged. Resistive strength training is initiated at postoperative week 12 with isotonic and isokinetic training exercises. Participation in contact sports is not permitted until 5 months, and initiation of forceful overhead throwing is not permitted until 6 months after surgical repair.

CLINICAL RESULTS

Bankart Lesions

Speer et al. (18) presented the results of a retrospective study of 49 patients who underwent arthroscopic anterior stabilization of the glenohumeral joint by using a bioabsorbable tack. The injury mechanism was a traumatic dislocation in 36 patients and traumatic subluxation in 13 patients. One patient had prior surgical treatment, which consisted of arthroscopic excision of a labral tear. Postoperative follow-up was a minimum of 24 months and averaged 42 months. The average age at the time of surgery was 28 years (range, 16 to 50 years).

Forty-one (79%) of 49 patients returned to their preinjury athletic activity levels without evidence of recurrent instability. Eleven (21%) of 49 patients had recurrent instability postoperatively. Seven failures occurred from minimal trauma, and four resulted from a single traumatic reinjury during contact sports. Eight of these 11 patients were treated with open anterior reconstruction. At the time of surgery, the anterior inferior labrum was found to have healed to the anterior glenoid neck in seven of eight patients. In addition, a patulous anterior and inferior capsule was noted in all patients, and an open rotator interval in five. Assessment of range of motion at the most recent follow-up revealed an average loss of elevation of 3 degrees, an average loss of 3 degrees of external rotation with the arm at the side, and an average loss of 6 degrees of external rotation with the arm elevated 90 degrees. The results of this study modified the authors' indications for arthroscopic stabilization with a bioabsorbable tack. The ideal candidate should have anterior instability of traumatic origin, a robust detached anterior–inferior labrum, and minimal capsular laxity.

In an effort to identify the causes of clinical failures in seven of 96 patients with recurrent instability subsequent to an arthroscopic Suretac repair of a Bankart lesion, repeated arthroscopy was performed at an average of 9 months after arthroscopic stabilization by Warner et al. (26). The 96 patients in this study were treated for traumatic, recurrent unidirectional anterior shoulder instability. The authors made several observations: images obtained at the time of the index procedure revealed that five of seven patients had poorly developed glenohumeral ligaments; the head of the Suretac captured too little soft tissue or was noted to have torn through the capsular tissue in four cases; and a capacious anterior capsular tissue was noted in six of seven. The Bankart lesion was healed in three, partially healed in one, and detached in three. Four of the seven patients with recurrent instability returned to contact sports earlier than advised. All seven patients were revised with an open capsulorrhaphy and Bankart repair if necessary. The authors noted that the revision stabilization procedure was not complicated by scarring of overlying tissue planes.

In a prospective study, Arciero et al. (30) performed acute arthroscopic repairs of Bankart lesions with the Suretac device in 19 West Point cadets within 10 days of a first-time anterior dislocation that required manual reduction. At an average of 19 months of follow-up (range, 12 to 24 months), one patient had a single episode of subluxation, and there were no dislocations. All of the cadets in this study returned to their preinjury athletic performance level. Assessment of results with the Rowe point score revealed 16 excellent, two good, and one fair result.

Deberardino et al. (31) recently updated the results of their prospective study at the West Point Military Academy. In their study, 39 military cadets had acute arthroscopic repairs of Bankart lesions with the Suretac device within 10 days of a first-time anterior dislocation that required manual reduction. The average age of their patients was 19.5 years (range, 17 to 23 years). At an average of 22 months of follow-up (range, 4 to 24 months), 35 (90%) of 39 patients had a stable shoulder and returned to preinjury athletic performance. Four patients experienced recurrent instability. One of two patients with subluxation and one of two with traumatic redislocation were subsequently treated with an open Bankart repair.

In 1991, Warner and Warren (1) reported the results of 26 patients who underwent arthroscopic repair of Bankart lesions with the Suretac device with minimum 2-year follow-up. They noted recurrent instability in 8% of these patients. Five of eight throwing and racquet sports athletes and all four swimming athletes were able to return to full preinjury level of athletic activity. The authors noted that the average loss of external rotation with the shoulder abducted 90 degrees was 7 degrees. They described the ideal patient for arthroscopic Bankart repair as one with traumatic unidirectional instability.

Superior or Anteroinferior Labral Lesions or Both

Pagnani et al. (32) reported the results of treating 22 patients with superior labral lesions [16 type II, six type IV SLAP lesions (20)] by using the Suretac device. The patients ranged in age from 18 to 40 years. In 13 patients, the mechanism of injury related to overhead athletic activity, in five to contact sports, and in one to a distraction injury. The two remaining patients did not recall a specific inciting injury. The superior labrum was stabilized with one or two Suretacs, and two patients with significant anterior instability underwent a similar repair of a Bankart lesion. Four patients were treated with arthroscopic subacromial decompression. In addition, one of the four patients who underwent arthroscopic subacromial decompression was treated with a mini-open rotator-cuff repair. At 2-year follow-up, 12 of 13 overhead athletes were able to return to full preinjury function. Nineteen (86%) of 22 patients were satisfied with their outcomes. There was a statistically significant improvement in pain, instability, and function when pre- and postoperative American Shoulder and Elbow Surgeons scores were compared. The authors reported no complications related to the use of the Suretac device.

Warner et al. (33) identified SLAP (20) lesions in 10% of 72 individuals undergoing arthroscopic Bankart repair.

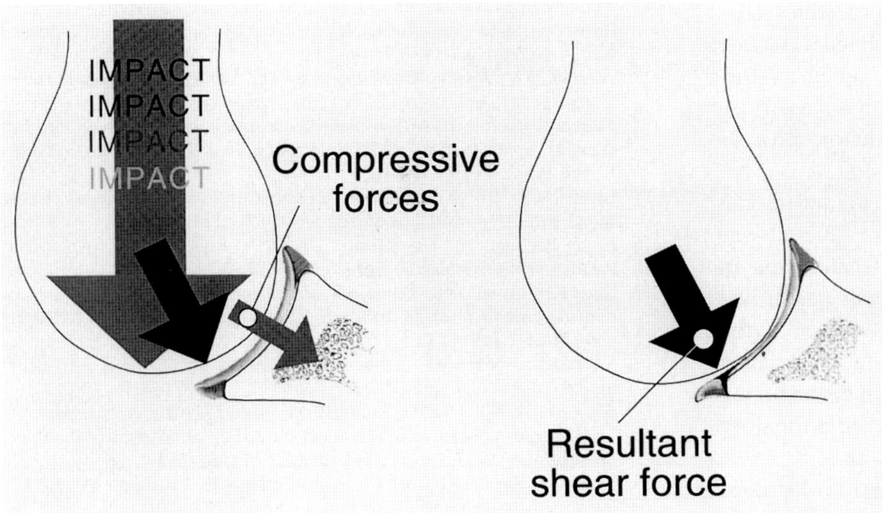

FIG. 12. Posterior shear forces.

Their study consisted of seven patients with recurrent shoulder instability who were treated with arthroscopic repairs of combined type II SLAP and Bankart lesions by using three to four Suretacs. Follow-up at 19 months (range, 15 to 22 months) revealed that five of the seven had returned to full preinjury activity levels, had no pain, and demonstrated full range of motion. One patient had recurrent dislocations 4 months after the arthroscopic Bankart repair and was treated with an open anterior reconstruction. One patient developed postoperative stiffness, which was successfully treated with arthroscopic capsular release and manipulation.

Resch et al. (2) treated 28 patients with superior, anterosuperior, or anteroinferior labral detachment by using the Suretac device. The presenting symptoms in these 28 patients included recurrent anterior instability in 18 with anteroinferior labral detachments, symptoms of impingement in five with anterosuperior labral detachments, and nonspecific in five with type II SLAP (20) lesions. At an average of 11 months (range, 4 to 18 months) of follow-up, one patient with anterior instability had recurrent instability after the arthroscopic labral-repair procedure. Four of five patients with repaired anterosuperior labral detachments had significant relief of impingement-type symptoms. Three of five patients with type II SLAP lesions obtained complete relief of painful symptoms, two returned to overhead sporting activity, one patient had only minimal pain relief, and one was continuing to improve at the most recent follow-up. The authors related that the singular complication that occurred in this series was that a guide wire failed during removal.

Posterior Labral Lesions

Mair and Speer (21) recently reported the results of treating nine contact athletes with posterior labral tears by using the Suretac device. None of the athletes, with an average age of 18.8 years (range, 16 to 21 years), complained of a history of instability or demonstrated evidence of instability or asymmetry when examined under anesthesia. The patient population in this study consisted of eight football linemen and one lacrosse player. All the patients were treated for a minimum of 6 weeks with physical therapy, anti-inflammatory medications, and cryotherapy. The average follow-up was 30 months (range, 24 to 42 months). All nine of the athletes returned to unrestricted contact athletics and bench pressing and completed a full season of their respective sports after the labral-repair procedure. The authors proposed that posterior labral detachments observed in this group of contact athletes were the result of repeated posterior shear forces, as depicted in Figure 12.

COMPLICATIONS

Edwards et al. (35) reported treating more than 100 patients with superior labral detachments with the Suretac device during the early 1990s. Five patients (six shoulders) noted increasing pain and loss of motion after the labral-repair procedure. Each patient was treated with arthroscopic lavage, debridement, and administration of local corticosteriods. At the time of repeated arthroscopy, the authors noted a dense synovial reaction within the glenohumeral joint. In each case, the superior labrum was noted to be healed. In one case, the head of a Suretac device was identified adjacent to the anterior wall 8 weeks after the index procedure. Histologic evaluation revealed a nonspecific granulomatous reaction in each case. All cultures were negative. All five patients had resolution of pain and stiffness within 4 to 8 weeks after repeated arthroscopy. Because of the time course and proximity of the histologic reaction to the implanted device, the authors suggested that these cases represented a reaction to the bioabsorbable implant.

In the study by Warner et al. (26), patients with recurrent anterior instability after arthroscopic Bankart repair underwent repeated arthroscopy. The authors noted the appearance a granuloma and "yellowish material" in the region of

Suretac fixation 6 to 8 months after the index procedure. Histologic evaluation of the labral-repair site revealed a chronic histiocytic infiltrate and polyglyconate surrounded by foreign-body giant cells. The authors suggested that these findings may indicate that this prolonged inflammatory process may lead to a weaker repair of the Bankart lesion.

The Suretac was initially evaluated in an animal model by M. Walton (unpublished data, 1989). The Suretac was used to reattach the distal patellar tendon to the tibia in sheep. Histologic analysis of the repair site was performed at 2, 6, and 12 weeks after implantation. At 6 weeks, the Suretac was noted to have a gelatinous consistency. At each time interval, there was progressive maturation of the bone–tendon site, and no adverse tissue reaction or inflammatory response was noted.

In our clinical experience, we have not had an instance of Suretac synovitis. Criteria for the diagnosis of Suretac synovitis are (a) excessive or increasing inflammatory type of pain at 6 to 8 weeks after labral repair, and (b) refractory stiffness after removal of the sling. Treatment of Suretac synovitis would include the use of nonsteroidal anti-inflammatory medications to treat inflammatory pain. Stiffness unresponsive to physical therapy would be addressed with an arthroscopic capsular release.

SUMMARY

In properly selected patients, arthroscopic labral repair with the Suretac device can predictably treat the detached posterior, superior, anterosuperior, and anteroinferior labrum. In addition to patient selection, several important technical guidelines deserve reiteration. Cannula placement and the resulting angle to the glenoid face are fundamental to accurate drilling and placement of the Suretac. Furthermore, preparation of the glenoid without causing injury to the substance of the labrum is essential.

REFERENCES

1. Warner JJP, Warren RF. Arthroscopic Bankart repair using a cannulated, absorbable fixation device. *Oper Tech Orthop* 1991;1:192–198.
2. Griffen LY, ed. *OKU: sports medicine.* Rosemont, IL: American Academy of Orthopaedic Surgeons, 1994:165–177.
3. Green MR, Christiansen KP. Arthroscopic versus open Bankart procedures: a comparison of early morbidity and complications. *Arthroscopy* 1993;9:371–374.
4. Johnson L. Shoulder arthroscopy. In: Johnson L, ed. *Arthroscopic surgery: principle and practice*. Vol. 1. St. Louis: Mosby, 1986:180.
5. Small N. Complications of arthroscopy: the knee and other joints. *Arthroscopy* 1936;2:253.
6. Zuckerman J, Matsen F. Complications about the glenohumeral joint related to the use of screws and staples. *J Bone Joint Surg* 1984;66:175.
7. Detrisac D. Arthroscopic staple capsulorrhaphy for traumatic anterior instability. In: McGinty J, ed. *Operative arthroscopy*. New York: Raven Press, 1991:517–528.
8. Hawkins RB. Arthroscopic stapling repair for shoulder instability: a retrospective study of 50 cases. *Arthroscopy* 1989;5:122–128.
9. Lane JG, Sachs RA, Riehl B. Arthroscopic staple capsulorrhaphy: a long-term follow-up. *Arthroscopy* 1993;9:190–194.
10. Burger RS, Shengel D, Bonatus T, Lewis J.Arthroscopic staple capsulorrhaphy for recurrent shoulder instability. *Orthop Trans* 1990;14: 596–597.
11. Coughlin L, Rubinovich M, Johansson J, White B, Greenspoon J. Arthroscopic staple capsulorrhaphy for anterior shoulder instability. *Am J Sports Med* 1992;20:253–256.
12. Mathews LS, Vetter WL, Oweida SJ, Spearman J, Helfet DL. Arthroscopic staple capsulorrhaphy for recurrent anterior shoulder instability. *Arthroscopy* 1988;2:106–111.
13. Altchek DW, Warren RF, Wickiewicz TL. Arthroscopic capsular shift: a retrospective analysis of 21 patients. *Arthroscopy* 1992;8:411–412.
14. Caperi R, Savoie F. Arthroscopic reconstruction of the shoulder: the Bankart repair. In: McGinty J, ed. *Operative arthroscopy*. New York: Raven Press, 1991:507–516.
15. Morgan CD, Bodenstab AB. Arthroscopic Bankart suture repair: technique and early results. *Arthroscopy* 1987;3:111–122.
16. Louis Bigliani, ed. *The unstable shoulder.* Rosemont, IL: American Academy of Orthopaedic Surgeons, 1996:47–58.
17. Shea KP, Lovallo JL. Scapulothoracic penetration of a Beath pin: an unusual complication of arthroscopic Bankart suture repair. *Arthroscopy* 1991;7:115–117.
18. Speer KP, Warren RF. Arthroscopic shoulder stabilization: a role for biodegradable materials. *Clin Orthop* 1993;291:67–74.
19. Arciero RA, Wheeler JH, Ryan JB, McBride JT. Arthroscopic Bankart repair versus nonoperative treatment for acute, initial anterior shoulder dislocations. *Am J Sports Med* 1994;22 (5):589–594.
20. Syder SJ, Karzel RP, Del Pizzo W, Ferkel RD, Friedman MJ. SLAP lesions of the shoulder. *Arthroscopy* 1990;6:274–279.
21. Mair SD, Speer KP. Posterior labral injury in contact athletes. *Am J Sports Med* (in press).
22. Skykar MJ, Altchek DW, Warren R, et al. Shoulder arthroscopy with the patient in the beach-chair position. *Arthroscopy* 1988;4: 256–259.
23. Lintner SA, Levy A, Kenter K, Speer KP. Glenohumeral translation in the asymptomatic athlete's shoulder and its relationship to other clinically measurable anthropometric variables. *Am J Sports Med* 1996;24 (6):716–720.
24. Warner JJP, Deng X, Warren RF, Torzelli PA. Static capsuloligamentous restraints to superior-inferior translation of the glenohumeral joint. *Am J Sports Med* 1992;20:675–685.
25. Warner JJP, Caborn DNM, Burger R, Fu FH, Seel M. Dynamic capsuloligamentous anatomy of the glenohumeral joint. *J Shoulder Elbow Surg* 1993;2:115–133.
26. Warner JJP, Miller M, Mark P, Fu F. Arthroscopic Bankart repair with the suretac device. Part I: clinical observations. *Arthroscopy* 1995;11 (1):2–13.
27. Williams MM, Snyder SJ, Buford D. The Buford complex: the cord like middle glenohumeral ligament and absent anterior superior labrum complex: a normal anatomic capsulolabral variant. *Arthroscopy* 1994;10:241–247.
28. Mcintyre LF, Caspari RB. The rationale and technique for arthroscopic reconstruction of anterior shoulder instability using multiple sutures. *Orthop Clin North Am* 1993;24 (1):55–58.
29. Baker CL, Uribe JW, Whitman C. Arthroscopic evaluation of acute initial anterior dislocations. *Am J Sports Med* 1990;18:25–28.
30. Arciero RA, Taylor DC, Snyder RJ, Uhorchak JM. Arthroscopic bioabsorbable tack stabilization of initial anterior shoulder dislocations: a preliminary report. *Arthroscopy* 1995;11 (4):410–417.
31. Deberardino TM, Arciero RA, Taylor DC. Arthroscopic stabilization of acute initial anterior shoulder dislocation: the West Point experience. *J South Orthop Assoc* 1996;5 (4):263–271.
32. Pagnani MJ, Speer KP, Altchek DW, Warren RF, Dines DM. Arthroscopic fixation of superior labral lesions using a biodegradable implant: a preliminary report. *Arthroscopy* 1995;11 (2):195–198.
33. Warner JJP, Kann S, Marks P. Arthroscopic repair of combined Bankart and superior labral detachment anterior and posterior lesions: technique and preliminary results. *J Arthrosc Rel Surg* 1994;10 (4): 383–391.
34. Resch H, Golser K, Sperner G, Thoni H. Die arthroskopische Labrumrefixation mit reorbierbaren Staples. *Arthroscopie* 1992;5:89–95.
35. Speer KP, Warren RF, Pagnani M, Warner JJP. An arthroscopic technique for anterior stabilization with a bioabsorbable tack. *J Bone Joint Surg [Am]* 1996;78 (12):1801–1807.
36. Edwards DJ, Hoy G, Saies AD, Hayes MG. Adverse reactions to an absorbable shoulder fixation device. *J Shoulder Elbow Surg* 1994;3: 230–233.
37. Pagnani MJ, Warren RF. Arthroscopic shoulder stabilization. *Oper Tech Sports Med* 1993;1:280.
38. Warner JJP, Miller M, Mark P. Arthroscopic Bankart repair with the Suretac device. Part II: Experimental observations. *Arthroscopy* 1995;11 (1):14–20.

The Unstable Shoulder,
edited by R.F. Warren, E.V. Craig, and D.W. Altchek.
Lippincott–Raven Publishers, Philadelphia © 1999.

CHAPTER 20

Arthroscopic Transglenoid Multiple-Suture Repair

Michael E. Torchia and Richard B. Caspari

In recent years, widespread interest has developed in the arthroscopic assessment and treatment of glenohumeral instability (1–23). It is now clear that a spectrum of instability exists, and the so-called Bankart lesion is only one of several anatomic lesions that may allow pathologic translation of the humeral head (7,13,16,19–21,24–34). Much like open capsulolabral repair, a variety of arthroscopic techniques is available, each technique with its own set of evolving indications, advantages, and disadvantages. Some are well suited for anatomic repair of a labral avulsion; other methods can be used to perform a capsulorrhaphy in the absence of a labral detachment. Even within the specific category of transglenoid suture techniques (3,9,12,35), significant differences exist in the methods. For the purposes of discussion, the technique devised and popularized by the senior author will be referred to as the arthroscopic transglenoid multiple-suture repair, and the technique popularized by Dr. Craig Morgan will be referred to as the arthroscopic transglenoid mattress-suture repair. The fundamental difference lies in the method of suture placement in the capsule. In the multiple-suture technique, a suture punch (3,36; Linvatec, Largo, FL, and Arthrotek, Warsaw, IN, U.S.A.) is used, whereas in the mattress-suture technique, a suture pin with an eyelet is used (11). In cases in which the pathology encountered is other than a simple Bankart lesion, these technical differences may affect the outcome (16,19, 37). This concept is developed later in the Results and Advantages/Disadvantages sections. The purpose of this chapter is to review the indications, surgical technique, results, complications, advantages, and disadvantages of the transglenoid multiple-suture method of capsular/labral repair.

M. E. Torchia: Mayo Clinic and Mayo Foundation, Rochester, Minnesota 55905.

R. B. Caspari: Department of Orthopaedics, Medical College of Virginia, Richmond, Virginia 23298; and Orthopaedic Research of Virginia, Glen Allen, Virginia 23060.

INDICATIONS AND CONTRAINDICATIONS

Recent studies have suggested that the indications for arthroscopic capsulolabral repair are variable, depending on the specific technique (see Chapters 10, 18, 19, 21). For example, the bioabsorbable tack has performed well for the treatment of first-time traumatic anterior dislocations that required a manual reduction (38). This technique can also be effective in shoulders with recurrent instability when a simple Bankart lesion is present, the tissue is robust, and there is minimal capsular laxity (24,32). Transglenoid suture repairs have been used effectively not only in this setting (7,12,16,19,20), but also in the absence of a Bankart lesion (19). The indications and contraindications for use of the multiple-suture technique with respect to the multiple variables that affect decision making are reviewed in detail later.

Origin of Instability

The multiple-suture technique has been used effectively when the cause is major trauma or repetitive microtrauma from long-standing overhead use of the arm. Atraumatic instability not responsive to an exercise program can also be treated effectively when the direction is primarily anterior or anteroinferior (19).Voluntary instability due to selective muscle contractions cannot be controlled effectively with this or any other capsular procedure.

Direction of Instability

As in open repairs, acceptable results have been obtained in anterior or anteroinferior instability (19,27). The multiple-suture technique has been used to treat symptomatic acquired multidirectional instability, but modifications of the technique are required to address the inferior and posterior capsule (27,39).

Chronicity

The indications for treatment of first-time traumatic dislocations are evolving (see Chapter 10). The multiple-suture technique can be used effectively in this setting (1, 14,20,38), provided the anterior capsule is not detached from its humeral insertion (8,22,24). Chronic recurrent instability likewise can be addressed, except in the rare case of anterior capsular deficiency (29). The pathologic changes that accompany chronic instability (capsular laxity, minor anterior glenoid erosion, and bony Hill-Sachs lesions; 3) were not associated with failure in our series; therefore, we do not exclude patients from consideration based on the number of previous dislocations or the duration of symptoms.

Athletic Participation

In our series, contact athletes had a higher rate of recurrent instability than did the remainder of the group (see Results section). This finding is not unique to the transglenoid method or the arthroscopic approach (12,13,29,40). The high recurrence rate in contact athletes seems to be related more to the risk activity than to the method of repair; therefore, we do not exclude contact athletes from consideration if the indications are otherwise sound. This technique has performed well in overhand athletes (18,19, 41), perhaps because it tends not to restrict motion of the shoulder.

Patient Age

More than any other variable, patient age seems to affect the rate of recurrent instability with this method. In two separate large series (18,19), youth was shown to have a significant effect on outcome. The reasons are not known with certainty. Younger patients seem to be less compliant with the necessary postoperative protection. In our series, several young patients failed early in the postoperative period because of gross noncompliance with the immobilization protocol. However, the effect of noncompliance alone was not enough to explain the strong association of youth with recurrent instability. More frequent high-risk activity, such as participation in collision sports, is a logical but unproven explanation for the higher recurrence rates in young patients regardless of treatment (nonoperative, open capsular repair or arthroscopic capsular repair; 18,19,42,43). It has also been suggested that the tissue characteristics of younger patients may be responsible for the less predictable outcomes (18,44).

Previous Surgery

This technique can be used effectively with prior surgery (43). Of the 150 shoulders in that series, 34 had had previous surgery ranging from open capsular repair to suprascapular nerve decompressions. In general, an arthroscopic approach may be preferred after failed open repairs that significantly alter the local extracapsular anatomy, such as the Bristow procedure.

SURGICAL PATHOLOGY

The multiple-suture technique can be used to address both labral detachment and capsular laxity. Contrary to some other methods of arthroscopic repair (16,32–34,45), results with the multiple-suture technique in cases of chronic instability have been more reliable in the absence of a Bankart lesion (19). This effect may be caused by the preservation of the glenoid labrum in patients with capsular laxity (28,46,47). This technique will not correct the instability in cases in which the capsule or subscapularis tendon has been avulsed from the humerus (24,27,48), or in cases of severe capsular deficiency (7,21,29).

Surgeon Experience and Training

As with any procedure, surgeon experience and training affects results. It is not surprising that the best results have been reported by those who developed these techniques or by those who have performed surgery in a very large number of cases (12,13,18,19). The frequency of complications may also be affected by experience and training. Prerequisites for effective and safe execution of this procedure include not only experience with arthroscopic surgery of the shoulder, but also a detailed knowledge of the anatomy of the shoulder girdle.

SURGICAL TECHNIQUE (3,18,19,36)

Room Set-Up, Anesthesia, and Positioning

General hypotensive anesthesia is administered. Both shoulders are examined for motion and stability. The patient is rolled to the lateral decubitus position and supported with a bean-bag device. The trunk is allowed to tilt posteriorly approximately 30 degrees. This position places the glenoid parallel to the floor and assists with orientation and portal placement. The operating table is then turned 90 degrees relative to the anesthetist. The essential feature in this set-up is surgeon access to the entire shoulder (anterior, superior, and posterior). Much of the procedure is done with the surgeon standing at the head of the table viewing from the posterior portal and working through the anterior portal; therefore, isolation drapes are best placed parallel to the long axis of the operating table rather than perpendicular to the head, as in most open procedures (Fig. 1). The

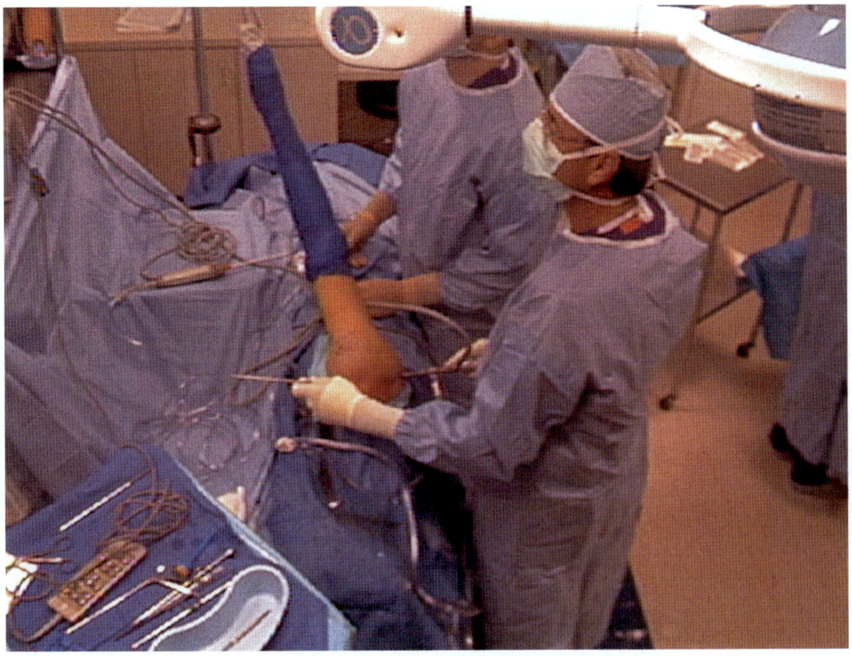

FIG. 1. The room set-up and positioning allows access to the posterior, superior, and anterior regions of the shoulder girdle.

monitor is ideally positioned directly opposite the surgeon. Standard prepping and draping are carried out, taking care to include the entire scapula in the field. The arm is suspended with 10 to 15 pounds of traction, and the superficial bony landmarks are palpated or marked to facilitate accurate placement of the portals.

Portal Placement

The standard posterior portal is established. The ideal position and trajectory allow the posterior capsule to be pierced with the trocar at the junction of the posterior labrum and humeral head, parallel to the articular surface of the glenoid. The anterior portal may be established in the rotator interval capsule by either the "inside-out" or "outside-in" technique. The anterior portal is made in such a way as to allow working access to the inferior aspect of the glenoid neck and capsule. Generally, this orientation is facilitated by placement of the portal somewhat superior and lateral in the interval capsule adjacent to the biceps tendon. A superolateral anterior portal also facilitates establishing the preferred inferomedial trajectory of the transglenoid pin (see Complications section). Appropriate position of both portals allows visualization of and working access to the entire labrum and capsule.

Diagnostic Arthroscopy

Examination of the articular surfaces, rotator cuff, biceps tendon, labrum, capsule, and ligaments is carried out by viewing from both the posterior and anterior portals. Classic pathologic lesions that confirm the diagnosis of anterior instability include the Bankart lesion (Fig. 2) or variation thereof (14; Fig. 3), and a Hill-Sachs lesion (superficial or deep; 26). The findings of a poorly developed anterior labrum, indistinct anterior ligaments, and a voluminous capsule (Fig. 4) should be interpreted along with the remainder of the arthroscopic examination (posterior labrum and capsule), clinical history, and examination under anesthesia (EUA) to arrive at the correct diagnosis (anterior vs. multidirectional instability) and degree of laxity.

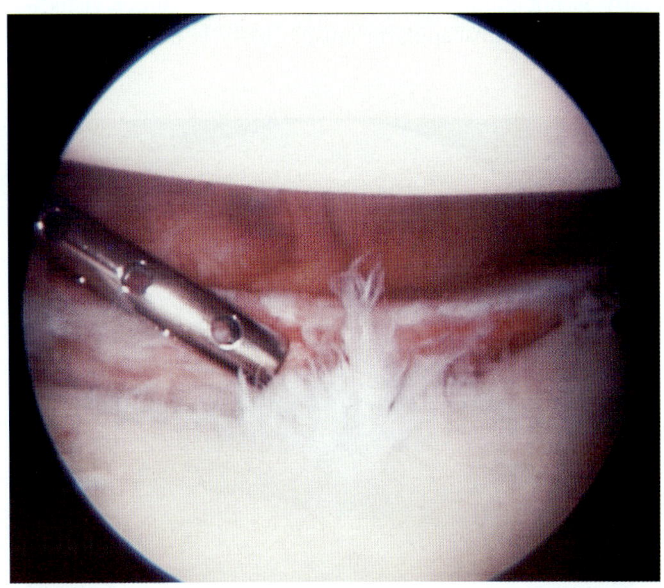

FIG. 2. A simple chronic Bankart lesion with minimal displacement of the labrum and minor chondromalacia of the anterior glenoid margin, as viewed from the posterior portal in a right shoulder. A Verres needle has been placed through the anterior portal and is used as a probe.

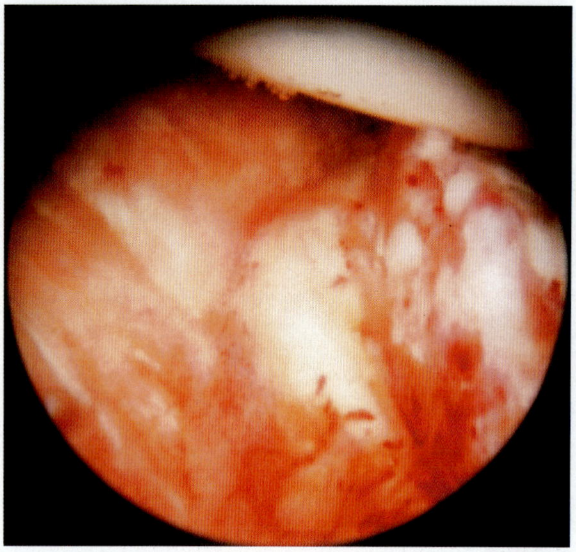

FIG. 3. An example of an anterior labroligamentous periosteal sleeve avulsion (ALPSA) lesion as viewed from the anterior portal in a right shoulder. Note how the anteroinferior glenohumeral ligament (AIGL) is in continuity with the labrum, which has healed medially along the glenoid margin.

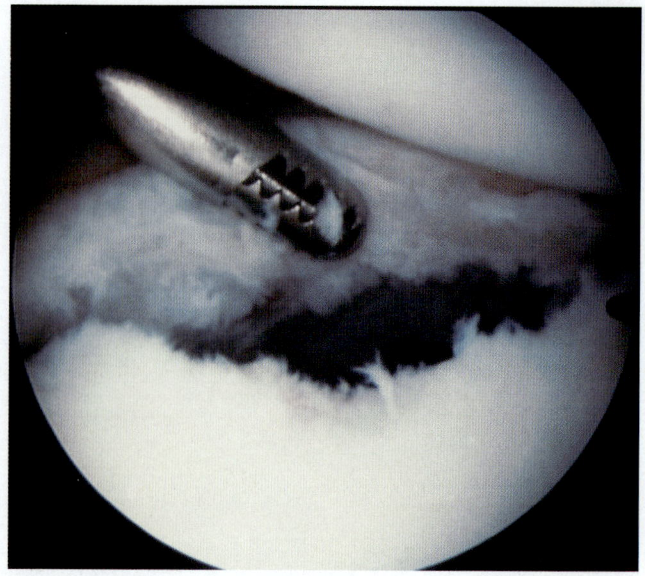

FIG. 5. An example of satisfactory preparation and mobilization of the anterior capsule, as viewed from the posterior portal in a right shoulder.

Transglenoid Multiple-Suture Repair

Bankart Repair

If a Bankart lesion is identified, the remaining labrum is debrided of fibrous tissue, and the anterior capsule is dissected free from the glenoid neck and subscapularis muscle. This step is essential to the success of the repair and generally is not thought to be completed until direct visualization of the subscapularis muscle belly is achieved (Fig. 5). The capsulolabral detachment is developed to its inferiormost extent (typically the 5:30 or 6 o'clock position in a right shoulder). A grasper is used to pull the capsule superiorly and confirm appropriate mobility. Extensive mobilization of the anterior capsule, including the middle and inferior glenohumeral ligaments, allows the capsule to be retensioned and shifted superolaterally to its anatomic insertion at the anterior glenoid margin. After dissection and mobilization of the anterior capsule, the glenoid neck is abraded with a motorized burr or rasp. Preparation of the

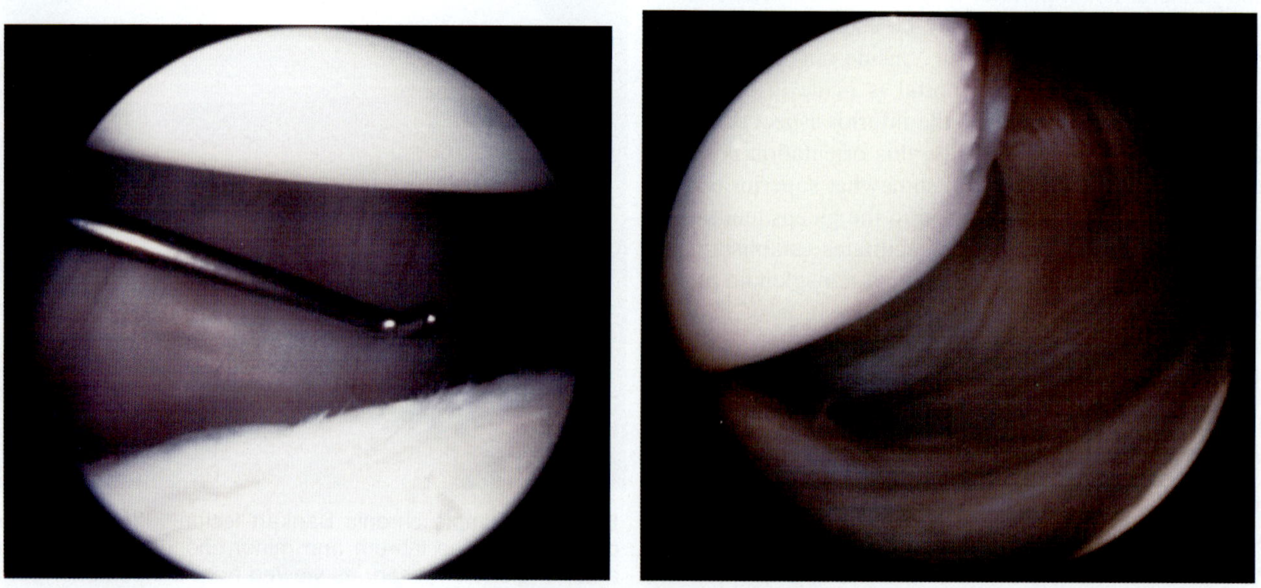

A B

FIG. 4. An example of capsular laxity without labral detachment in a right shoulder, as viewed from the posterior portal with the probe placed through the anterior portal **(A)**. The scope is in the axillary pouch, and the light source has been directed superiorly **(B)**.

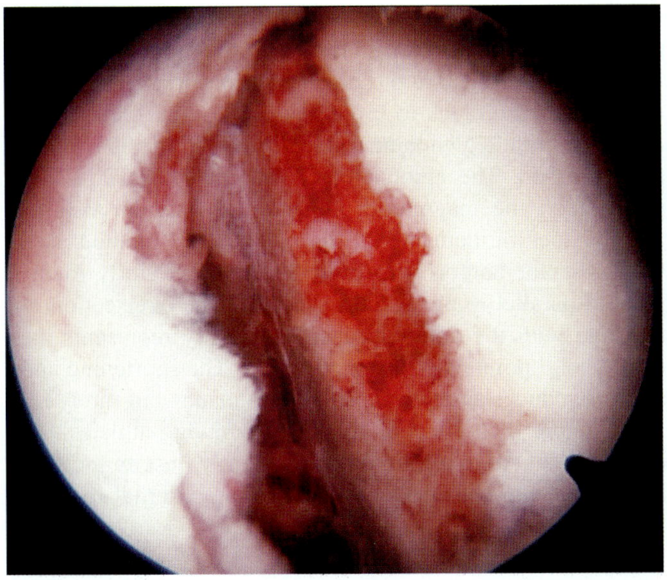

FIG. 6. An example of preparation of the glenoid neck into a bleeding bony surface to which the labrum and or capsule has the potential to heal.

glenoid neck inferiorly at or beyond the 6 o'clock position can be facilitated with curved shaver blades. The arthroscope is transferred to the anterior portal to confirm adequate preparation of a bleeding bony surface (Fig. 6). The anterior portal is enlarged to accept an oval cannula, through which the suture punch is placed. Once the suture punch is within the glenohumeral joint, the oval cannula can be withdrawn beyond the capsule to allow the fluid distention of the joint and optimal visualization. Multiple 2.0 PDS (polydioxanone suture; Ethicon, Somerville, NJ, U.S.A.) simple sutures are placed along the free edge of the anterior capsule and labrum (if present). In cases with Bankart lesions, mattress sutures can be placed by tying adjacent sutures together on the articular side of the capsule. When tensioned, this arrangement effectively reduces the labrum. The most superior stitch is placed approximately at the level of the middle glenohumeral ligament. Tension applied to this stitch by an assistant allows the entire anterior capsule to become taut and facilitates the placement of the remaining sutures (usually in a sequential fashion beginning superiorly and working inferiorly to the 6 o'clock position or beyond). Typically, between 6 and 10 size 2.0 PDS sutures are used. Placement of more sutures or the use of a larger diameter suture might seem desirable but makes transglenoid passage through the 3.65-mm hole difficult and sometimes impossible. Much like the open Bankart procedure, the depth of suture placement in the labrum or capsule determines to some extent the amount of capsular shortening or shifting (capsulorrhaphy). The magnitude of the capsulorrhaphy is dependent on the chronicity of the problem, the degree of laxity compared with the opposite shoulder, and the arthroscopic assessment of the amount of anterior capsular laxity. As each suture is placed, it is brought out of the anterior portal and tagged, together with the others, with a hemostat. Next, a drill guide is placed though the cannula and directed from the 2 o'clock position (in a right shoulder, or the 10 o'clock position in a left shoulder) toward the medial and inferior quadrant of the scapula. The starting position of the transglenoid hole is crucial (12,13,18). It should be placed not only superior enough to allow retensioning of the capsule, but also lateral enough (at the articular surface) to allow anatomic reduction of the labrum or capsule or both. A drill hole placed medially along the glenoid neck will result in residual medial displacement of the anterior capsule and less satisfactory reconstruction of the anterior inferior glenohumeral ligament (12,13,36,49). Next, a modified Beath pin with a 3.65-mm drill point and eyelet (Linvatec, Largo, FL, U.S.A.) is placed through the guide, drilled across the glenoid neck (well medial and inferior to the spinoglenoid notch), and exteriorized through a small posterior incision (Fig. 7). The sutures are passed (by using a loop of heavy

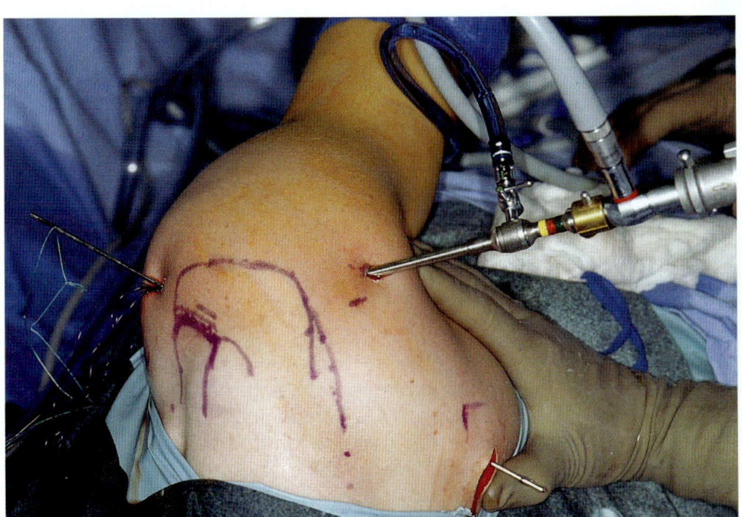

FIG. 7. The modified Beath pin has been drilled across the glenoid neck and exteriorized in the inferomedial quadrant of the scapula.

suture placed through the eyelet in the Beath pin as a suture passer), tensioned individually, and divided into two even bundles. The anterior capsule is visualized to confirm appropriate restoration of tension and apposition along the glenoid margin (Fig. 8A-C). The arm is released from traction and placed at the side in the internally rotated position while the sutures are tied over the infraspinatus fascia, taking care to avoid inclusion of subcutaneous tissue in the knot. If the sutures exit near the medial border of the scapula, periosteum can be used for fixation.

Anteroinferior Capsulorrhaphy

If no labral detachment is present and the primary pathoanatomy is capsular laxity (poorly defined glenohumeral ligaments and excessive capsular volume, as seen in Fig. 4), a capsulorrhaphy is performed. The anterior capsule is divided just lateral to the labrum (Fig. 9) from approximately the 2 o'clock to 6 o'clock position (in a right shoulder, or the 10 o'clock to 6 o'clock position in a left shoulder). The middle glenohumeral ligament and the labrum are not disturbed. The amount of capsule resected varies depending on the magnitude of perceived capsular volume and the specific demands of the patient. The method used by the senior author is to project a line anteriorly to the glenoid parallel to the articular surface. The intersection of this line with the anterior capsule typically represents the most lateral point of capsular resection. The shortening and shifting reduces anterior-capsular redundancy but rarely involves more than 1 cm of tissue. In throwing athletes, the resection is kept to a minimum; frequently, just an incision is made in the capsule to avoid limiting external rotation

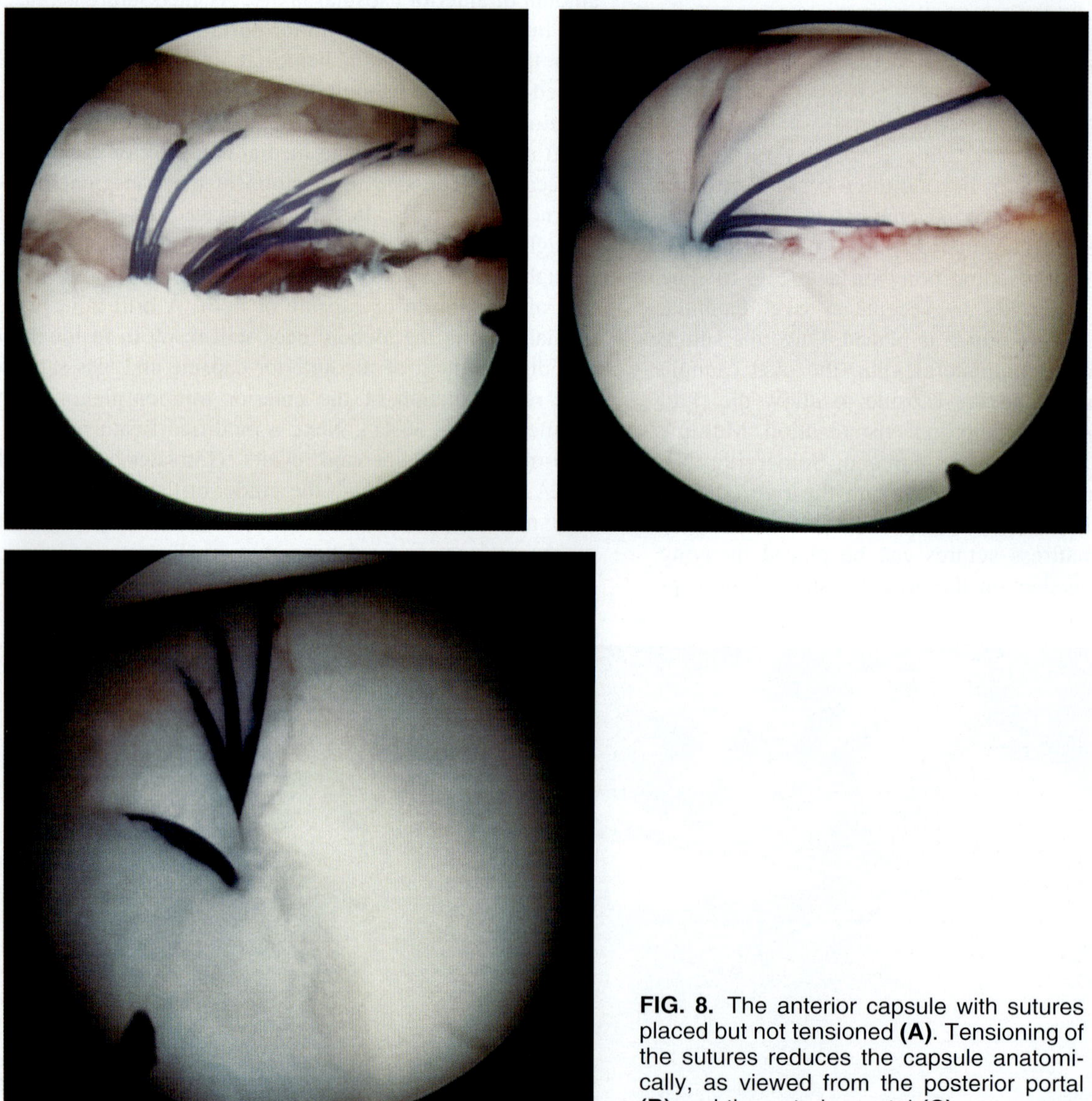

A B C

FIG. 8. The anterior capsule with sutures placed but not tensioned **(A)**. Tensioning of the sutures reduces the capsule anatomically, as viewed from the posterior portal **(B)** and the anterior portal **(C)**.

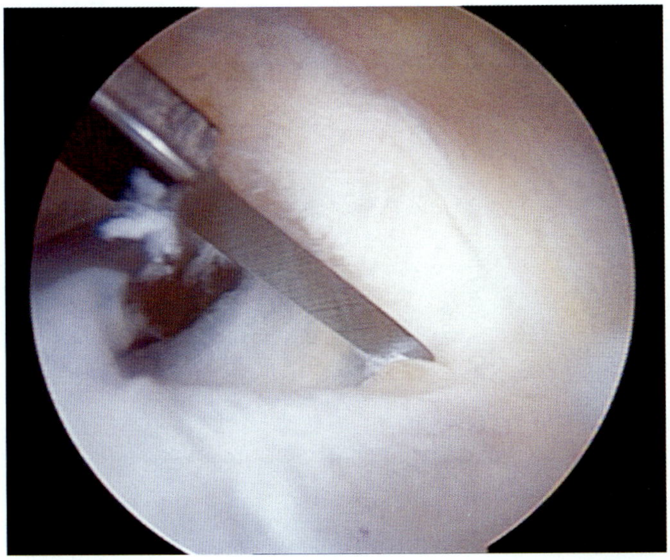

FIG. 9. During the capsulorrhaphy, the capsule is divided adjacent to the labrum with an arthroscopic knife.

with the arm in the abducted position. The free edge of the capsule is then mobilized and repaired to the glenoid neck in a manner identical to the transglenoid multiple-suture Bankart repair.

Postoperative Care

After the procedure, patients are discharged from the outpatient surgical center and seen in follow-up the next morning where dressings are changed and a written physical therapy protocol is provided and reviewed. The recommended length of immobilization with the arm in the internally rotated position is 3 weeks. Pendulum exercises and pain-free isometrics are performed immediately. Progressive mobilization is typically begun at 6 weeks. Combined abduction and external rotation are avoided for at least 8 weeks. Functional progression is initiated at 12 to 16 weeks.

RESULTS

Reported results of the transglenoid suture technique are outlined in Table 1. In this table, the rates of recurrent instability have been emphasized; however, in the overall scheme, of patient satisfaction, other factors such as range of motion, residual pain, and return to desired activity are often equally important (29). These measures of outcome are taken into account in the Rowe score, which some authors have included in their reports.

The results of the transglenoid mattress-suture technique or Morgan technique are included as a separate group because of our feeling that this method of repair is fundamentally different from the multiple-suture technique (19; see Advantages/Disadvantages section).

Senior Author's Experience

We reviewed the results of the transglenoid multiple-suture repair in 150 cases performed by the senior author (19). The mean follow-up interval was 4.1 years (range, 2 to 8.2 years). To our knowledge, this was the first study of arthroscopic stabilization for anterior glenohumeral instability in which patients were not preselected for the procedure on the basis of their desired activity (including collision sports), chronicity of symptoms, degree of instability or generalized laxity, prior surgery, or the pathologic findings encountered at the time of diagnostic arthroscopy. Although the patient group was heterogeneous, the technique was consistent (single surgeon). Thus, we were able to stratify the results according to multiple variables and identity key factors associated with both satisfactory and unsatisfactory outcomes.

Specific criteria were required for inclusion in the study. First, the diagnosis of chronic anterior instability had to be clear. The patient must have sustained multiple documented anterior dislocations. Alternatively, there had to be a strong clinical history of recurrent anterior subluxations combined with either classic arthroscopic findings or an EUA that confirmed the diagnosis. Second, the surgery had to be performed by the senior author. Third, the case had to be done before July 1, 1992, to allow a minimal postoperative follow-up interval of 2 years. Patients that had known multidirectional instability with a primary posterior component were excluded. Preoperatively, no effort was made to determine the presence or absence of a Bankart lesion with special imaging studies such as computed tomography (CT) arthrography or magnetic resonance imaging (MRI).

Recurrent Instability

During the follow-up interval, 11 (7.3%) shoulders redislocated. Another 14 (8.6%) shoulders had at least one episode of pain with the arm in the provocative position of abduction and external rotation. Although there often was no objective evidence to substantiate recurrent instability, we considered these episodes recurrent subluxations and included them in the group of failed repairs. A Kaplan–Meier survival analysis demonstrated a progressive increase in the probability of any recurrent instability over time that reached 18% after 5 years. Nearly half of the failures occurred more than 2 years after surgery.

In the multivariate analysis, two factors were found to have a statistically significant independent effect on the probability of failure: the type of pathology encountered at surgery and patient age. The 66 shoulders with an isolated Bankart lesion had a 27% probability of failure after 5 years versus only 6% for the 53 shoulders with capsular laxity and no Bankart lesion

TABLE 1. *Results reported with the transglenoid suture technique*

Author	Year published	Source	No. shoulders	Shoulders in series with a traumatic etiology (%)	Follow-up (mo)	Redislocation (%)	Resubluxation (%)	Any recurrent instability (%)	Reoperation for instability (%)	Other scoring	Comments
Multiple-suture technique											
Caspari and Savoie (3)	1991	*Operative Arthroscopy*	49	100	24–72	4	4	8	NR	96% satisfactory (Rowe scale)	Initial experience
Peterson and Newton (17)	1991	*Orthop Transactions*	25	NR	26	4	NR	4	NR	Successful in 24/25 shoulders, all returned to full activity	Used two transglenoid drill holes, "little experience with violent athletic activities"
Duncan and Savoie (4)	1993	*Arthroscopy*	10	100	12–36	NR	NR	NR	0	Mean Rowe score, 90 points	40% Bankart lesions, no patient had "congenital hyperelasticity"
Goldberg et al. (5)	1993	*AJSM*	38	100	36	0	11	16	8	90% "functionally stable"	Less satisfactory results with longer follow-up [see Organ, et al. (15)]
Neviaser (14)	1993	*Arthroscopy*	26	100	>24	4	NR	4	4	All patients returned to their normal athletic activities	All ALPSA lesions four acute, 22 chronic, nonabsorbable sutures used for repair
Uribe and Hechtman (20)	1993	*Orthopedics*	11	100	18–38	0	9	9	9		All cases of acute first-time dislocations
Youssef et al. (23)	1995	*Arthroscopy*	30	100	>24	20	7	27			Young patients (mean age, 26 years), 100% Bankart lesions

Marcacci et al. (Part I) (10)	1996	*Arthroscopy*	29	100	59	NR	NR	27		66% satisfactory (Rowe)	Initial experience, nonabsorbable sutures used
Marcacci et al. (Part II) (10)	1996	*Arthroscopy*	42	100	48	NR	NR	4.8		90% satisfactory (Rowe)	Technique "improved," 5–10 mm, capsular resection, Bankart lesion extended to 5 or 6 o'clock to improve mobility, nonabsorbable sutures tied to scapular spine
Molonge et al. (11)	1996	*AJSM*	49	100	12–49	20	16	41	20	47% fair or poor (Rowe)	Young active-duty military population, all had Bankart lesions, transglenoid hole made 5 mm medial to the glenoid articular surface, standard beath pin not used, two pins placed "parallel" in several cases, 38% noncompliant with postoperative immobilization
Organ et al. (15)	1996	*Orthop Transactions*	30	NR	>60	NR	NR	60	27	40% failures	Minimum 5-year f/u on series reported by Goldberg in 1993, risk factors: women, contact athletes, gen. lig. laxity, and absent labrum

Continued

TABLE 1. *Continued*

Author	Year published	Source	No. shoulders	Shoulders in series with a traumatic etiology (%)	Follow-up (mo)	Redislocation (%)	Resubluxation (%)	Any recurrent instability (%)	Reoperation for instability (%)	Other scoring	Comments
Yoneda et al. (22)	1996	*Arthroscopy*	28	86	27		14	18		83% successful (Rowe scale)	Sutures tied over PLLA button
Savoie (18)	1977	*Arthroscopy*	161	100	36–72	NR	NR	9	NR	91% satisfactory (Rowe)	26% failure in pts <18, all patients had at least two documented dislocations preoperatively
Torchia et al. (19)	In press	*Arthroscopy*	150	81	49	7	9	18 (at 5 yr by Kaplan–Meier survival analysis)	10		Unselected group, (includes revisions) 35% had capsular laxity alone, all had chronic recurrent instability documented by history, EUA, or arthroscopy
Mattress-suture technique											
Morgan and Bodenstab (12)	1987	*Arthroscopy*	25	100	17	0	0	0	0	All excellent	
Maki (9)	1991	*Op Tech Orthop Surg.*	15	100	NR	7	NR	7	NR	All returned to previous level of activity	No collision athletes included
Morgan (13)	1991	*Op Tech Orthop Surg.*	175	100	12–84	NR	NR	5	NR	95% excellent (Rowe)	Seven or 42 (16%) recurrence in collision athletes

Bendetto and Glötzer (2)	1992	*Arthroscopy*	22	100	29	0	0	0	0		"No degenerative changes in the labral tears," all returned to unrestricted activity
Landsiedl (8)	1992	*Arthroscopy*	65	91	35	14	2	15	NR		
Granna et al. (6)	1993	*AJSM*	27	NR	36	37	7	44			
Rose (35)	1993	*Arthroscopy*	50	NR	24–72	4	6	10	NR	Improvement from 2.6 to 9.3 postop on subjective instability scale	
Arcerio et al. (38)	1994	*AJSM*	21	100	15–45	5	10	14	5		Young active-duty military population, all acute, initial anterior dislocations that required reduction, 14% recurrence vs. 80% for a similar group treated nonoperatively
Green et al. (7)	1995	*AJSM*	47	100	41	38	6	42	NR	78% completely satisfied	Low failure rate 4.5% w/ simple labral detachment
Walch et al. (21)	1995	*Arthroscopy*	59		49	44	5	49		49% poor (Rowe)	Only AIGHL repaired
Pagnani et al. (16)	1996	*AJSM*	37	100	48–120	5	14	19	14	74% satisfactory	Selected population, two of three pts. w/o Bankart lesion failed, two of five revised open continued to complain of instability

AIGHL, anterior inferior glenohumeral ligament; ALPSA, anterior labroligamentous periosteal sleeve avulsion, NR, not recorded; EUA, examination under anesthesia; PLLA, poly-L-lactic acid.

Series of Weber (1990) not included (not all repairs were done with the suture technique); series of Wolin (1990) not included (specific technique used was not described in Abstract); and series of Altchek (1992) not included (not all repairs were done with the suture technique).

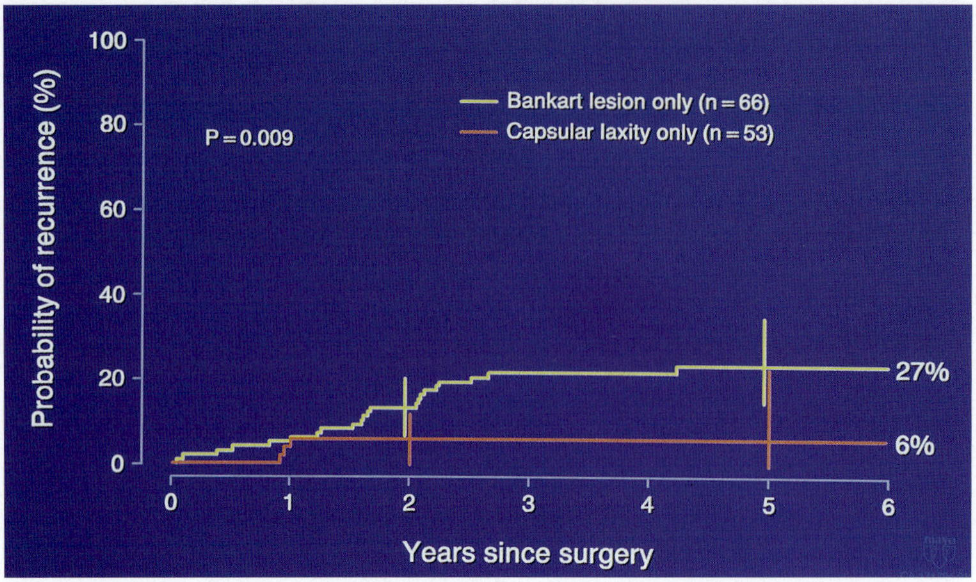

FIG. 10. Survival free of failure, stratified by pathologic anatomy, in patients who had an arthroscopic transglenoid multiple-suture repair for anterior glenohumeral instability.

(p = 0.009; Fig. 10). In fact, only three of the 53 shoulders without a Bankart lesion developed recurrent instability. In the group of 82 patients aged 25 years or younger, the recurrence rate was 29% versus only 4% for the group of 68 patients older than 25 years (p = 0.0003; Fig. 11). Of the 10 patients aged 16 years or younger with a Bankart lesion, six (60%) had developed recurrent instability at the time of final follow-up. None of the seven patients age 16 years or younger without a Bankart lesion failed. Although the numbers of patients were small, this difference was statistically significant (p = 0.02).

The presence of generalized ligamentous laxity and the type of postoperative sporting activity both had an effect on the probability of failure that was of borderline statistical significance ($p > 0.05$ and $p < 0.01$). Patients with generalized ligamentous laxity (25 shoulders) had a 28% probability of failure after 5 years versus 16% for the group with normal flexibility (125 shoulders; p = 0.059). For the 29 shoulders subjected to collision sports postoperatively (basketball, football, or rugby), the probability of failure was 29% versus 12% for the 75 shoulders of patients who participated in overhand athletic activity (swimming, base-

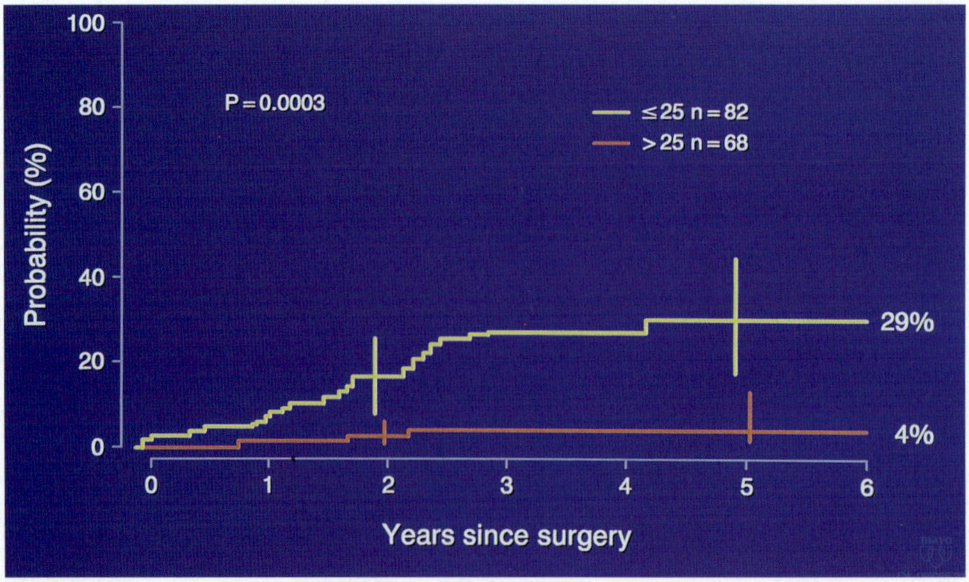

FIG. 11. Survival free of failure, stratified by age, in patients who had an arthroscopic transglenoid multiple-suture repair for anterior glenohumeral instability.

ball, softball, volleyball, tennis, racquetball, or handball), but no collision sports ($p = 0.07$).

Factors that had no significant effect on the probability of failure included the following: sex of the patient, extremity dominance, origin of the instability, the duration of symptoms, the degree of instability (preoperative subluxation vs. dislocation and degree of translation during the EUA), the size of the Bankart lesion, the presence of a Hill-Sachs lesion, minor deficiency of the anterior glenoid margin, the number of sutures used for the repair, the operative time, or the duration of postoperative immobilization. There were more early failures in the group of 12 shoulders immobilized for less than 21 days compared with the group of 138 shoulders immobilized for at least 21 days; however, the probability of failure after 5 years (25% vs. 17%, respectively) was not statistically significant ($p = 0.31$.)

Revision Stabilization

Revision surgery for recurrent instability was necessary in 12 cases (four because of recurrent dislocation and eight because of recurrent subluxation). The majority of cases that required revision stabilization had recurrent Bankart lesions related to a specific traumatic episode. Included in this group was one patient with initially unrecognized multidirectional instability who had a successful anterior capsulorrhaphy and later required a posterior repair for symptomatic posterior instability.

Rowe Scores

The mean estimated Rowe score increased significantly from 25 points preoperatively to 87 points postoperatively ($p = 0.0001$). At final follow-up, the results according to the Rowe scale were excellent in 120 (80%) shoulders, good in four (3%) shoulders, fair in eight (5%) shoulders, and poor in 18 (12%) shoulders. These figures included the 25 shoulders that developed any degree of recurrent instability postoperatively. For the group of 125 shoulders that did not have any recurrent instability, the mean Rowe score improved from 25.8 points preoperatively to 96.8 points at follow-up.

DISCUSSION

Analysis of the results of the transglenoid technique (multiple-suture and mattress-suture) revealed that the reported results are highly variable. The factors that seem to affect outcome are related to the patient populations, the anatomic pathology, the surgeon, the technical aspects of the procedure, the length of follow-up, and the definition of recurrent instability.

Patient Factors

Age, compliance with the necessary postoperative protection, and participation in high-risk collision sports affect the rate of recurrent instability after this operation (13,18,19).

Pathologic Factors

In most reported series, patients were carefully selected for the transglenoid technique based on the presence of traumatic, unidirectional (anterior) instability associated with a Bankart lesion. In this selected population, the results may be related to severity of the Bankart lesion (7, 29). Less commonly, anterior instability occurs in the absence of labral avulsion, and in this setting, the transglenoid multiple-suture capsulorrhaphy provided a very low rate of recurrent instability (19). This relative success may be related to the preservation of the labrum (28,46,47).

Surgeon Factors

The effect of surgeon experience should not be underestimated. Table 1 demonstrates the trend toward better results by the originators of the technique or by those who have extensive experience with this procedure. Although Morgan and Rose reported low recurrence rates (5.1% after 1 to 7 years and 4% after 2 years), others had less success with the transglenoid mattress-suture technique and reported recurrence rates more than 40%.

Technical Factors

The significance of other technical factors is evolving. The importance of shifting and retensioning the anterior capsule to the glenoid margin has been emphasized repeatedly in the literature (13,29,50). In our opinion, these maneuvers can be accomplished easily by using the multiple-suture technique but may be more challenging to accomplish with other methods (see Advantages section).

Recently Marcacci et al. (22) reported improved results when the multiple-suture technique was modified to include more attention to mobilization of the capsule, abrasion of the glenoid neck, and suture fixation to the scapular spine. The latter modification carries with it the significant disadvantage of potential injury to the main branch of the suprascapular nerve. Other methods of enhancing fixation have been proposed, including the use of a poly-L-lactic acid (PLLA) button (22). Nonabsorbable sutures seem to work well but have been associated with subcutaneous granulomas (see Complications section). Others have routinely drilled two transglenoid holes to increase the fixation points along the glenoid and have reconstructed the inferior and middle glenohumeral ligaments independently (Peterson, CA, personal communication, 1994).

Follow-up

Multiple studies documented that recurrence rates after surgery tend to increase over time (5,13,15,19,42). It is of interest that nearly half of the failures in our study occurred after more than 2 years. This suggests that when comparing the results of various techniques, a follow-up of longer than 2 years is desirable.

Definition of Recurrent Instability

To some extent, the results reported for various capsular procedures (arthroscopic or open) are dependent on the definition of recurrent instability. In the classic series of Rowe (51), the term "recurrence" was used to describe recurrent dislocation. Therefore, the redislocation rate in that series of 145 shoulders followed up for an average of 6 years (range, 1 to 30 years) was 3.5%. In the frequently quoted series of Morrey and Janes (42), long-term results (mean follow-up, 10.3 years; range 1 to 25 years) were reported for 176 cases (Putti–Platt and Bankart procedures). The redislocation rate was 11%, and in the 42 shoulders examined, external rotation was "limited" in all but five. In a similar series of modified Putti–Platt and Bankart procedures reported by Hovelius (52) (114 shoulders with 1- to 10.5-year follow-up), the redislocation rate was 12%. Thomas and Matsen (53) reported 97% satisfactory results in their series of 39 shoulders followed up for an average of 5.5 years (range, 2.2 to 11.3 years) after anatomic repair of traumatic avulsions of the glenohumeral ligaments. A single patient had recurrent dislocation; however, follow-up was available for only 39 (62%) of 63 repairs performed during the study period. Berg (54) reported an 8.6% rate of recurrent instability in 69 cases (one dislocation, five subluxations) after a mean of 6 years by using an identical "inside-out" technique. Paulos (55) reported redislocation in five (7%) of 69 shoulders, a mean of 3 years after treatment with a modified Bankart repair. In a recently published series of 42 Bankart repairs (56) followed up for 13 to 77 months, redislocation occurred in four (9.5%) cases, and recurrent subluxation occurred in another four cases, for an overall rate of recurrent instability of 19%. This is not dissimilar to the overall experience after open Bankart repairs in cadets at West Point (40; 3% redislocation and 20% resubluxation). Thus, when definitions are held constant, the results of the transglenoid multiple-suture technique (7.3% redislocation after 4.1 years; 19) can be comparable to those of traditional open procedures.

COMPLICATIONS

Complications reported with the transglenoid suture technique are outlined in Table 2. As recorded, there have been few serious joint-threatening complications. With the exception of one case of deep infection (39), other serious complications related to intra-articular hardware, brachial plexus injury, subscapularis insufficiency, and motion loss were conspicuously absent in these reports.

The most significant potential complication unique to the transglenoid method is related to errant pin placement that may result in scapulothoracic penetration or injury to the suprascapular nerve or both (11,12,57,58). To perform this technique safely, the surgeon must have a thorough knowledge of the anatomy of the scapula and suprascapular nerve. It has been the senior author's preference to direct the transglenoid pin from the anterior glenoid margin toward the inferomedial quadrant of the scapula well medial to the main trunk of the suprascapular nerve (Figs. 7 and 12). This practice has resulted in a very low incidence of nerve injury: of 150 consecutive cases done by the senior author, one partial nerve palsy occurred early in the series (sixth case) when a Beath pin broke as it was drilled across the glenoid. Removal required the use of a cannulated reamer. Postoperatively, atrophy of the infraspinatus was noted. The patient eventually recovered sufficient strength to continue working as a college professor and participate in recreational racquetball.

Others using similar transglenoid methods also have noted a low incidence of injury to the suprascapular nerve (10,14). Modifications of this technique may place the suprascapular nerve at higher risk (11). In the series reported by Yoneda et al. (22) in which a biodegradable PLLA button was used to enhance fixation, transient infraspinatus atrophy was noted in two of 28 patients.

Scapulothoracic penetration of the Beath pin was reported (58). This complication should not occur, provided motorized instruments are used to drive the pin into the bone of the glenoid neck under direct arthroscopic visualization. Other reported complications seem to be related to the use of nonabsorbable sutures (synovial fistulas and suture granulomas; 10). These problems were infrequent when absorbable PDS sutures were used (19).

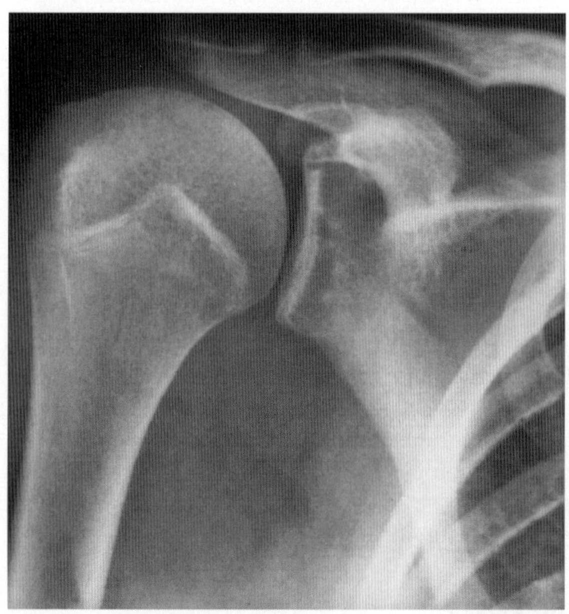

FIG. 12. A postoperative radiograph demonstrating the appropriate inferomedial trajectory of the transglenoid drill hole.

TABLE 2. *Complications reported with the transglenoid suture technique*

Author	Year published	Source	No. cases in series	Transglenoid pin problems (no. cases)	Suprascapular nerve injury (no. cases)	Subcutaneous suture problems (no. cases)	Loss of external rotation (degrees)	Infection (no. cases)	Comments
Multiple-suture technique									
Caspari and Savoie (3)	1991	*Operative Arthroscopy*	49	0	0	1	NR	0	Synovial fistula early in the series related to nonabsorbable sutures tied over a button outside the skin
Peterson and Newton (17)	1991	*Orthop Transactions*	25	0	0	0	"Nearly full ROM in all shoulders"	0	No complications
Duncan and Savoie (4)	1993	*Arthroscopy*	10	0	0	2	"Minimal"	0	
Goldberg et al. (5)	1993	*AJSM*	38	0	1	0	NR	1	Single infection was superficial
Neviaser (14)	1993	*Arthroscopy*	26	0	0	0	0	0	
Uribe and Hechtman (20)	1993	*Orthopedics*	11	0	0	0	0	0	No complications
Youssef et al. (23)	1994	*Arthroscopy*	30	0	0	0	0	0	No complications
Marcacci et al. (Part I) (10)	1995	*Arthroscopy*	29	0	0	3	43% lost at least 25% ER @ 90°abd relative to opposite side	0	Nonabsorbable surtures used
Marcacci, et al. (Part II) (10)	1996	*Arthroscopy*	42	0	0	5	31% lost at least 25% ER @ 90°abd relative to opposite side	0	Technique changed, nonabsorbable sutures tied to scapular spine
Molonge et al. (11)	1996	*AJSM*	39	0	3	0	NR	2	All three nerve injuries documented by EMG, transglenoid pin(s) not directed toward inferomedial quadrant of scapula, infections (one septic shoulder, one portal abscess) responded to debridement and antibiotics

Continued

TABLE 2. *Continued*

Author	Year published	Source	No. cases in series	Transglenoid pin problems (no. cases)	Suprascapular nerve injury (no. cases)	Subcutaneous suture problems (no. cases)	Loss of external rotation (degrees)	Infection (no. cases)	Comments
Organ et al. (15)	1996	*Orthop Transactions*	30	NR	NR	NR	NR	NR	Longer f/u on Goldberg series
Yoneda et al. (22)	1996	*Arthroscopy*	28	0	2 (transient)	0	6 @ 90°abd		Sutures tied over bioabsorbable button positioned directly in the scapula; no further nerve palsies with transglenoid pin directed to inferomedial quadrant of scapula
Savoie (18)	1997	*Arthroscopy*	161	0	0	5	31 throwers had >90° ER @ 90° abd	0	No neurovascular complications
Torchia et al. (19)	In press	*Arthroscopy*	150	1	1	0	three @ side, three @ 90° abd	0	
Mattress-suture technique									
Morgan and Bodenstab (12)	1987	*Arthroscopy*	25	0	0	0	0	0	No complications reported
Maki (9)	1991	*Op Tech Orthop Surg*	15	NR	NR	NR	NR	NR	
Morgan (13)	1991	*Op Tech Orthop Surg*	175	0	0	0	0	0	One treatment, cutaneous nerve palsy
Bendetto and Glötzer (2)	1992	*Arthroscopy*	22	0	0	0	2 pts > 20°	0	ER loss related to excessive capsulorrhaphy
Landsiedl (8)	1992	*Arthroscopy*	65	1	1	1	4 @ 0	0	
Granna et al. (6)	1993	*AJSM*	27	0	0	0	6	1	One superficial infection
Rose (35)	1993	*Arthroscopy*	50	0	0	0	4 @ side, 8 @ at 90°	0	No complications reported
Arcerio et al. (38)	1994	*AJSM*	21	0	0	1	NR	1	One superficial infection; two transient median neuropathies
Green et al. (7)	1995	*AJSM*	47	2	0	3	1	0	Pin/knot problems eliminated with improved technique
Walch et al. (21)	1995	*Arthroscopy*	59	0	0	0	0	0	
Pagnani et al. (16)	1996	*AJSM*	37	0	0	1	4	0	

ER, external rotation; abd, abduction; EMG, electromyogram; ROM, range of motion; NR, not reported.

ADVANTAGES UNIQUE TO THE MULTIPLE-SUTURE METHOD

The multiple-suture method has many inherent advantages. The suture punch allows multiple sutures to be placed in the inferior capsule without the need to create accessory anterior portals that may compromise the integrity of the subscapularis tendon, rotator interval capsule, axillary nerve, or musculocutaneous nerve (18,36,58–60). Compared with other techniques, this portion of the procedure is technically forgiving. In our experience and that of others (21,49), attempting to ''spear'' the inferior half of the labrum with a pin or guide wire placed through the anterior portal can be a difficult exercise because of the local anatomy. Moreover, if a Bankart lesion is absent, other techniques have limited application (16,29,37). In contrast, the multiple-suture technique can be used to address not only a Bankart lesion but also pathologic laxity of the capsule and lesions of the superior labrum (61,62). Thus, a wide spectrum of pathology can be treated with a single set of instruments working through a single anterior portal without the need to place hardware or tie intra-articular knots. The simplicity of the multiple-suture technique is highlighted by the senior author's mean operating room time of 63 minutes over a 150-case experience (19).

DISADVANTAGES UNIQUE TO THE SUTURE METHOD

The most substantial disadvantage of the transglenoid suture method is potential injury to the suprascapular nerve. In reality, this complication is rare and avoidable. All techniques, open or arthroscopic (if performed well), require effort to learn and substantial practice. Safety when performing open methods of capsular repair require a thorough knowledge of the anatomy of the inferior capsule and the axillary nerve; likewise, safety when performing transglenoid drilling depends on a thorough understanding of the anatomy of the scapula and the suprascapular nerve. It is generally agreed that directing the transglenoid pin to the inferior half of the scapula, well below the posterior portal and spine of the scapula, reduces the risk of injury to the main branch of the suprascapular nerve (3,12,13,16,57). The optimal mediolateral trajectory is not known (3,12,13, 16,22,37,57). Although anatomic studies that address this question have not been published, the authors' preference is to direct the pin as far medially and inferiorly as possible (Figs. 7 and 12). Typically, the pin penetrates the inferomedial aspect of the infraspinatus muscle. At this point, the branches of the suprascapular nerve have arborized, and clinically significant injury is avoided. An alternative approach (12,13) would be to direct the pin lateral to the main branch of the nerve. In practice, this pin trajectory can be difficult to achieve because of the regional anatomy and the usual position of the anterior portal. The anterior portal must stay lateral to the conjoined tendon to avoid injury to the musculocutaneous nerve. If this guideline is followed, it can be difficult to direct the pin lateral to the spinogleniod notch posteriorly.

Other disadvantages unique to the transglenoid multiple suture technique include the small posterior incision over the scapula and the temporary subcutaneous suture mass. In the authors' experience, these less-substantial disadvantages have not translated into clinically significant problems (19). Finally, there is some evidence that braided suture materials might perform better than monofilament sutures for soft-tissue repair to bone (63). New developments in suture-punch design and intra-articular suturing techniques (64) now allow the arthroscopic placement of any type of suture in the anterior labrum or capsule. Whether these theoretical advantages will improve outcomes remains to be determined.

REFERENCES

1. Arciero RA, Wheeler JH, Ryan JB, McBride JT. Arthroscopic Bankart repair versus nonoperative treatment for acute, initial anterior shoulder dislocations. *Am J Sports Med* 1994;22:589–594.
2. Bendetto KP, Glötzer W. Arthroscopic Bankart procedure by suture technique: indications, technique, and results. *Arthroscopy* 1992;8: 111–115.
3. Caspari RB, Savoie FH. Arthroscopic reconstruction of the shoulder: the Bankart repair. In: McGinty MB, et al. eds. *Operative arthroscopy.* New York: Raven Press, 1991;507–514.
4. Duncan R, Savoie FH. Arthroscopic inferior capsular shift for multidirectional instability of the shoulder: a preliminary report. *Arthroscopy* 1993;9:24–27.
5. Goldberg BJ, Nirschl RP, McConnell JP, Pettrone FA. Arthroscopic transglenoid suture capsulolabral repairs: preliminary results. *Am J Sports Med* 1993;21 (5):656–665.
6. Grana WA, Buckley PD, Yates CK. Arthroscopic Bankart suture repair. *Am J Sports Med* 1993;21 (3):348–353.
7. Green MR, Christensen KP. Arthroscopic Bankart procedure: two to five year follow-up with clinical correlation to severity of glenoid labral lesion. *Am J Sports Med* 1995;23 (3):276–281.
8. Landsiedl F. Arthroscopic therapy of recurrent anterior luxation of the shoulder by capsular repair. *Arthroscopy* 1992;8 (3):296–304.
9. Maki NJ. Arthroscopic stabilization: suture technique. *Oper Tech Orthop* 1991;1 (2):180–183.
10. Marcacci M, Zaffagnini S, Petitto A, Neri MP, Iacono F, Visani A. Arthroscopic management of recurrent anterior dislocation of the shoulder: analysis of technical modifications on the Caspari procedure. *Arthroscopy* 1996;12:144–149.
11. Mologne TS, Lapoint JM, Morin WD, Zilberfarb J, O'Brien TJ. Arthroscopic anterior labral reconstruction using a transglenoid suture technique: results in active-duty military patients. *Am J Sports Med* 1996;24:268–274.
12. Morgan CD, Bodenstab AB. Arthroscopic Bankart suture repair: technique and early results. *Arthroscopy* 1987;3 (2):111–122.
13. Morgan CD. Arthroscopic transglenoid Bankart suture repair. *Oper Tech Orthop* 1991;1 (2):171–179.
14. Neviaser TJ. The anterior labroligamentous periosteal sleeve avulsion lesion: a cause of anterior instability of the shoulder. *Arthroscopy* 1993;9 (1):17–21.
15. Organ SW, Siekanowicz AJ, Nirschl RP, Pettrone FA. Arthroscopic transglenoid suture capsulolabral repairs: five year follow-up. *Orthop Trans* 1996;20:79–80.
16. Pagnani MJ, Warren RF, Altchek DW, Wickiewicz TL, Anderson AF. Arthroscopic shoulder stabilization using transglenoid sutures: a four-year minimum follow-up. *Am J Sports Med* 1996;24:459–467.
17. Peterson CA, Newton SE. Arthroscopic Bankart repair. *Orthop Trans* 1991;15:49.
18. Savoie FH, Miller CD, Field LD. Arthroscopic reconstruction of traumatic anterior instability of the shoulder: the Caspari technique. *Arthroscopy* 1997;13 (2):201–209.

19. Torchia ME, Caspari RB. Arthroscopic transglenoid multiple suture repair: 2-8 year results in 150 shoulders. *Arthroscopy* 1997;13:609–619.
20. Uribe JW, Hechtman KS. Arthroscopically assisted repair of acute Bankart lesion. *Orthopedics* 1993;16:1019–1023.
21. Walch G, Boileau P, Levigne C, Mandrino A, Neyret P, Donell S. Arthroscopic stabilization for recurrent anterior shoulder dislocation: results of 59 cases. *Arthroscopy* 1995;11 (2):173–179.
22. Yoneda M, Hayashida K, Izawa K, Shimada K, Shino K. A simple and secure anchoring system for Caspari's transglenoid multiple suture technique using a biodegradable poly-L-lactic acid button. *Arthroscopy* 1996;12:293–299.
23. Youssef JA, Carr CF, Walther CE, Murphy JM. Arthroscopic Bankart suture repair for recurrent traumatic unidirectional anterior shoulder dislocations. *Arthroscopy* 1995;11:561–563.
24. Bach BR, Warren RF, Fronek J. Disruption of the lateral capsule of the shoulder: a cause of recurrent dislocation. *J Bone Joint Surg [Br]* 1988;70B:274–276.
25. Bigliani LU, Pollock RG, Soslowsky LJ, Flatow EL, Pawluk RJ, Mow VC. Tensile properties of the inferior glenohumeral ligament. *J Orthop Res* 1992;10:187–197.
26. Caspari RB, Geissler WB. Arthroscopic manifestations of shoulder subluxation and dislocation. *Clin Orthop* 1993;291:56–66.
27. Field LD, Bokar DJ, Savoie FH III. Humeral and glenoid detachment of the anterior inferior glenohumeral ligament: a cause of anterior shoulder instability. *J Shoulder Elbow Surg* 1997;6:6–10.
28. Harryman DT, Ballmer FP, Harris SL, Sidles JA. Arthroscopic labral repair to the glenoid rim. *Arthroscopy* 1994;10:20–30.
29. Johnson LL. *Diagnostic and surgical arthroscopy of the shoulder.* St. Louis: CV Mosby, 1993:231–364.
30. Oberlander MA, Morgan BE, Visotsky JL. Case report: the BHAGL lesion: a new variant of anterior shoulder instability. *Arthroscopy* 1996;12:627–633.
31. Ogawa K, Yoshida A. Extensive shoulder capsule tearing as a main cause of recurrent anterior shoulder dislocation. *J Shoulder Elbow Surg* 1997;6:1–5.
32. Speer CKP, Pagnani M, Warren RF. Arthroscopic anterior shoulder stabilization: 2-5 year follow-up using a bioabsorbable tack. *J Bone Joint Surg [Am]* 1996;78 (12):1801–1807.
33. Speer KP, Deng X, Borrero S, Torzilli PA, Altchek DA, Warren RF. Biomechanical evaluation of a simulated Bankart lesion. *J Bone Joint Surg [Am]* 1994;76 (12):1819–1826.
34. Warner JJP. Treatment options for anterior instability: open versus arthroscopic. *Oper Tech Orthop* 1995;5:233–237.
35. Rose DJ, Moyer RA, Sidor M. Arthroscopic transglenoid suture capsulorrhaphy for anterior shoulder instability. *Arthroscopy* 1993;9:356.
36. McIntyre LF, Caspari RB. The rationale and technique for arthroscopic reconstruction of anterior shoulder instability using multiple sutures. *Orthop Clin North Am* 1993;24 (1):55.
37. Altchek DW, Warren RF, Skyhar MJ. Shoulder arthroscopy. In: Rockwood CA, Matsen FA III, eds. *The shoulder*. Philadelphia: WB Saunders, 1990:258–277.
38. Arciero RA, Taylor DC, Snyder RJ, Uhorchak JM. Arthroscopic bioabsorbable tack stabilization of initial anterior shoulder dislocations: a preliminary report. *Arthroscopy* 1995;11:410–417.
39. McIntyre LF, Caspari RB, Savoie R. The arthroscopic treatment of anterior and multidirectional shoulder instability [Review]. *Instr Course Lect* 1996;45:47–56.
40. Uhorchak JM, Arciero RA, Taylor DC. Recurrent instability after open shoulder stabilization in athletes. Presented at The American Shoulder and Elbow Surgeons Tenth Open Meeting, New Orleans, LA, February 27, 1994.
41. Weber SC. A prospective evaluation comparing arthroscopic and open treatment of recurrent anterior glenohumeral dislocation. *Orthop Trans* 1991;15:763.
42. Morrey BF, Janes JM. Recurrent anterior dislocation of the shoulder: long-term follow-up of the Putti-Platt and Bankart procedures. *J Bone Joint Surg [Am]* 1976;58 (2):252–256.
43. Simonet WT, Cofield RH. Prognosis in anterior shoulder dislocation. *Am J Sports Med* 1984;12 (1):19–23.
44. Reeves B. Experiments on the tensile strength of the anterior capsular structures of the shoulder in man. *J Bone Joint Surg [Br]* 1968;50 (4):858–865.
45. Altchek DW, Wickiewicz TL, Warren RF, London K. Arthroscopic anterior stabilization in patients without labral detachment. Presented at the 11th annual meeting of the Arthroscopy Association of North America, Boston, April, 1992.
46. Howell SM, Galinat BJ. The glenoid-labral socket: a constrained articular surface. *Clin Orthop* 1989;243:122–125.
47. Lippitt SB, Vanderhooft, Harris SL, et al. Glenohumeral stability from concavity compression. *J Shoulder Elbow Surg* 1993;2:27–35.
48. Wolf EM, Cheng JC, Dickson K. Humeral avulsion of glenohumeral ligaments as a cause of anterior shoulder instability. *Arthroscopy* 1995;11:600–607.
49. Bacilla PB, Field LD, Savoie FH III. Arthroscopic Bankart repair in a high demand patient population. *Arthroscopy* 1997;13:51–60.
50. Post WR. Percutaneous tensioning of the glenohumeral ligaments during arthroscopic Bankart repair. *Arthroscopy* 1996;12:116–119.
51. Rowe CR, Patel D, Southmayd WW. The Bankart procedure: a long-term end-result study. *J Bone Joint Surg [Am]* 1978;60 (1):1–15.
52. Hovelius L, Thorling GJ, Fredin L, Fredin H. Recurrent anterior dislocation of the shoulder. *J Bone Joint Surg [Am]* 1979;61 (4):566–569.
53. Thomas SC, Matsen FA. An approach to the repair of avulsion of the glenohumeral ligaments in the management of traumatic anterior glenohumeral instability. *J Bone Joint Surg [Am]* 1989;71 (4):506–513.
54. Berg EE, Ellison AE. The inside-out Bankart procedure. *Am J Sports Med* 1990;18 (2):129–133.
55. Paulos LE, Evans IK, Pinkowski JL. Anterior and anterior-inferior shoulder instability: treatment by glenoid labrum reconstruction and a modified capsular shift procedure. *J Shoulder Elbow Surg* 1993;2 (6):305–313.
56. Ungersböck A, Markus M, Hertel R. Factors influencing the results of a modified Bankart procedure. *J Shoulder Elbow Surg* 1995;4 (5): 365–369.
57. Cash JD, Abrams JS. Arthroscopy for anterior instability. In: Hawkins RJ, Misamore GW, eds. *Shoulder injuries in the athlete: surgical repair and rehabilitation*. New York: Churchill Livingstone, 1996: 155–171.
58. Shea KP, Lovallo JL. Scapulothoracic penetration of a Beath pin: an unusual complication of arthroscopic Bankart suture repair. *Arthroscopy* 1991;7:115–117.
59. Davidson PA, Tibone JE. Anterior-inferior (5 o'clock) portal for shoulder arthroscopy. *Arthroscopy* 1995;11 (5):519–525.
60. Resch H, Wykypiel HF, Maurer H, Wambacher M. What would you do? The antero-inferior (transmuscular) approach for arthroscopic repair of the Bankart lesion: an anatomic and clinical study. *Arthroscopy* 1996;12:309–322.
61. Field LD, Savoie FH. Arthroscopic suture repair of superior labral detachment lesions of the shoulder. *Am J Sports Med* 1993;21 (6): 783–790.
62. Snyder SJ, Karzel RP, Del Pizzo W, Ferkel RD, Friedman MJ. SLAP lesions of the shoulder. *Arthroscopy* 1990;6:274.
63. Gerber C, Schneeberger AG, Beck M, Schlegel U. Mechanical strength of repair of the rotator cuff. *J Bone Joint Surg [Br]* 1994;76: 371–380.
64. Thal R. A technique for arthroscopic mattress suture placement. *Arthroscopy* 1993;9:605–607.

The Unstable Shoulder,
edited by R.F. Warren, E.V. Craig, and D.W. Altchek.
Lippincott–Raven Publishers, Philadelphia © 1999.

CHAPTER 21

Arthroscopic Labral Repair with Suture Anchors

Mark H. Field, Larry D. Field, and Felix H. Savoie III

Shoulder dislocation was described as early as *The Edwin Smith Surgical Papyrus,* circa 3,000 to 2,500 B.C. (1). Perthes (1906; 2) and Bankart (1938; 3) described the detachment of the glenoid ligament from the anterior margin of the glenoid cavity as the typical lesion found with recurrent anterior shoulder dislocations. Numerous studies documented the functional significance of the anterior–inferior capsulolabral structures in maintaining stability of the glenohumeral joint (3–7). Although previously classified as TUBS (Traumatic, Unidirectional, with Bankart lesion, responding to Surgery) versus AMBRI (Atraumatic, Multidirectional, Bilateral, Rehabilitation, Inferior capsular shift), instability actually is a spectrum between these extremes. Repair of the Bankart lesion has become the standard form of treatment for patients with traumatic anterior instability (8). Advances in technology have led to multiple arthroscopic techniques described to repair the Bankart lesion (9–22). The Johnson staple, an arthroscopic modification of the DuToit procedure, was the initial arthroscopic stabilization technique. Results were unsatisfactory, and a high incidence of complications related to use of metal implants adjacent to the joint were reported (10,11, 23,24). The next evolution using transglenoid suture-repair technique has had better results (90% to 93%; 9,16,17). This method was associated with risk of injury to the suprascapular nerve from the transosseous scapular drilling and the need for a second incision for tying sutures (9,16,17). More recently, the advent of suture anchors has allowed complete intra-articular repairs to be accomplished (18,22). This chapter is devoted to the indications for and technique, advantages, and published results of labral repair by using suture-holding screws and anchors.

M. H. Field: Mississippi Sports Medicine and Orthopaedic Center, Jackson, Mississippi 39202.

L. D. Field: Upper Extremity Service, Mississippi Sports Medicine and Orthopaedic Center, Jackson, Mississippi 39202; and Department of Orthopaedic Surgery, University of Mississippi Medical Center, Jackson, Mississippi 39216.

F. H. Savoie III: Upper Extremity Service, Mississippi Sports Medicine and Orthopaedic Center, Jackson, Mississippi 39202; and Department of Orthopaedic Surgery, University of Mississippi School of Medicine, Jackson, Mississippi 39216.

INDICATIONS

Patients with TUBS type of shoulder instability have a Bankart lesion most of the time (25). These patients are the ideal candidates for arthroscopic repair with suture anchors because they generally have normal labral tissue that can be reapproximated and secured. Recurrent dislocation in this type of patient is the primary indication for arthroscopic suture anchor repair.

The possibility of using arthroscopic reconstruction after an initial first-time dislocation is controversial. This may be an acceptable method of management in younger, high-risk athletes in whom recurrence would be expected and in whom such a recurrence would be functionally disabling. Results of this are not available and at best cannot be completely recommended.

CONTRAINDICATIONS

A lack of experience with open and arthroscopic shoulder surgery, as well as unfamiliarity with the use of suture-anchor techniques, should be considered a contraindication to arthroscopic reconstructive procedures. A poorly performed arthroscopic reconstruction will at best have a high failure rate and, at its worst, can result in significant neurologic or vascular complications.

PHYSICAL EXAMINATION

A complete history and physical examination is essential in the evaluation of shoulder instability. Some patients, es-

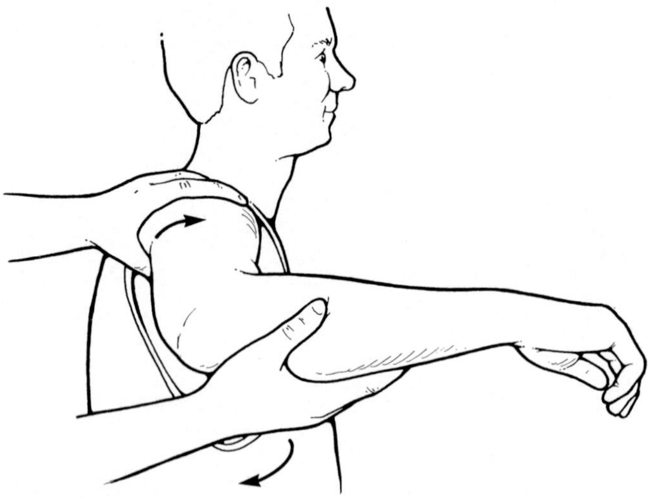

FIG. 1. When examining the right shoulder, the examiner uses the left hand to stabilize the scapula, the left thumb is placed behind the humeral head, and the right hand, while holding the patient's flexed elbow, is used to load the joint. By using this method, anterosuperior, anterior, and anteroinferior components of stability can be individually evaluated.

pecially in the athletic population, will have increased translation on examination, but only when this is symptomatic should instability be considered. Physical examination for anterior instability includes zone-specific load-and-shift maneuvers. Each maneuver is based on the examiner's thumb being used as a fulcrum for loading the anterior stabilizing structures. When examining the right shoulder, the examiner's left hand is used to stabilize the scapula, the left thumb is placed behind the humeral head, and the right hand, while holding the patient's flexed elbow, is used to load the joint (Fig. 1). By using this method, anterosuperior, anterior, and anteroinferior components of stability can be individually evaluated. If a patient found to have anterior instability, has failed nonoperative treatment, and is functionally impaired by the instability, surgical correction should be considered.

SURGICAL TECHNIQUE

After adequate induction of general or interscalene regional anesthesia, the patient is placed in the standard lateral decubitus position, rolled posteriorly 30 degrees. Alternately, the patient can be placed in the beach-chair position. Stability testing is then performed to confirm the degree and direction of instability. With one hand, the examiner applies an axial load at the elbow to center the humeral head on the glenoid. The other hand is then used to translate the humeral head anteriorly and posteriorly. Grading is recorded as 1+ when increased translation is present, as compared with the opposite extremity, but is insufficient to cause humeral head subluxation over the glenoid rim. An instability grading of 2+ is assigned when the examiner can subluxate the humeral head over the glenoid, and the head spontaneously reduces to its anatomic position when the force is removed. A 3+ grading signifies the ability of the examiner to lock the humeral head over the glenoid rim (26). After an examination under anesthesia, a standard sterile preparation and drape are then performed, and the arm suspended with 10 to 15 pounds of traction in 45 degrees of abduction and 20 to 30 degrees of forward flexion if the lateral decubitus position is used.

A posterior portal is initially established in the interval between the infraspinatus and teres minor tendons, and a diagnostic arthroscopic examination performed. The presence of a Bankart lesion is confirmed, and other pathology noted. A second portal is established anteriorly by using an outside–in technique to assure proper positioning of this anterior portal. The portal should be established so that the surgeon will have access at a proper angle in three planes to the glenoid rim for anchor placement at the 1, 3, and 5 o'clock positions, as well as access to the anterior and inferior capsulolabral ligamentous complex for suture placement at the 2, 4, and 6 o'clock positions (Fig. 2). Localization with a spinal needle before placement of the cannula ensures adequate placement. A cannula is then inserted into the joint at the upper edge of the subscapularis tendon and through the lower aspect of the rotator interval just lateral to or above the middle glenohumeral ligament, for instrumentation.

The labral edge is debrided of degenerative tissue, and the capsulolabral ligamentous complex completely released from the glenoid neck down to the 6 o'clock position (Fig. 3A and B). A high-speed burr is then used to abrade the anterior and inferior glenoid neck down to the 6 o'clock position. The debridement and abrasion are necessary to allow adequate vertical shift of the damaged capsulolabral structures as well as adequate healing of the repair once the reconstruction is completed. Often, the avulsed labrum has healed or partially healed medially on the glenoid neck, and extensive freeing of the labrum in this area must be performed to allow adequate mobilization. This may be accomplished with rasps, shavers, burrs, or knives.

Suture-First Technique

A Caspari suture punch (Linvatec) is then inserted through the anterior portal. A 48-inch doubled 2.0 polypropylene suture (Ethicon, Somerville, NJ) is loaded into a suture punch with the two free ends passed into the suture punch and the loop portion remaining proximal (Fig. 4A). The suture punch is inserted into the joint and used to pass this double suture through the inferior glenohumeral ligament, lateral to its labral attachment, at approximately the 6 o'clock position (Fig. 4A and B). The suture punch is withdrawn, pulling both the free ends and the loop end outside of the same cannula. A no. 2 braided polyester su-

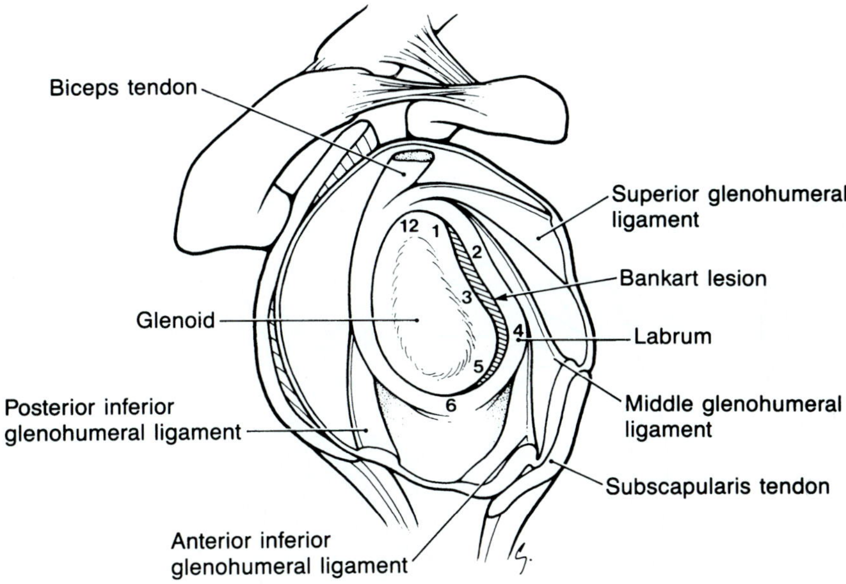

FIG. 2. The Bankart lesion, demonstrating the positioning of anchors *(1, 3, 5)* and sutures *(2, 4, 6)*.

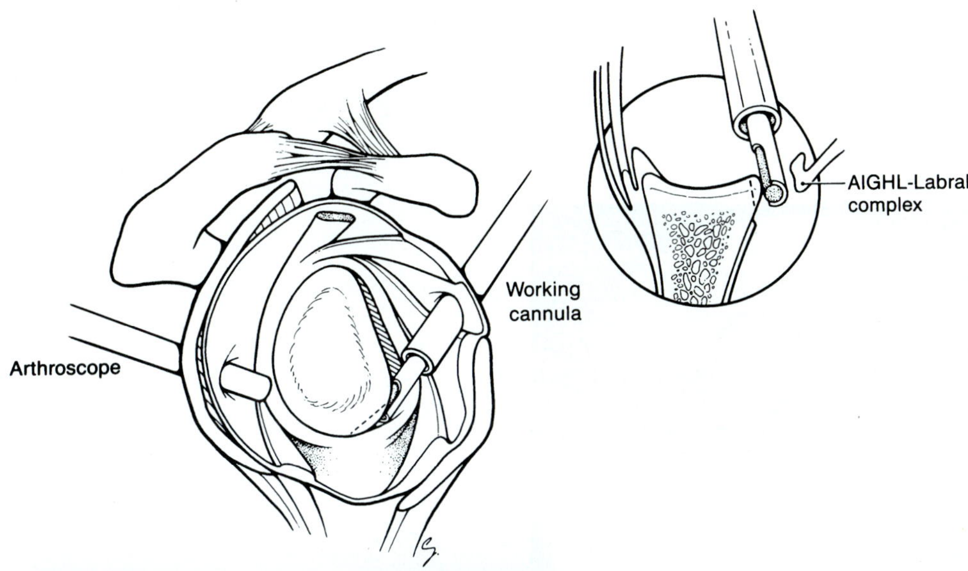

A

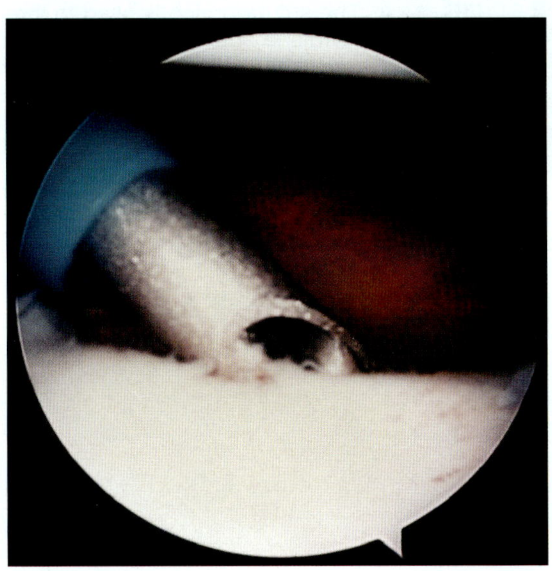

B

FIG. 3. A: Capsular release and glenoid neck abrasion taken to the 6 o'clock position inferiorly. **B:** The notchplasty abrader is taken across the anterior glenoid down to the 6 o'clock position.

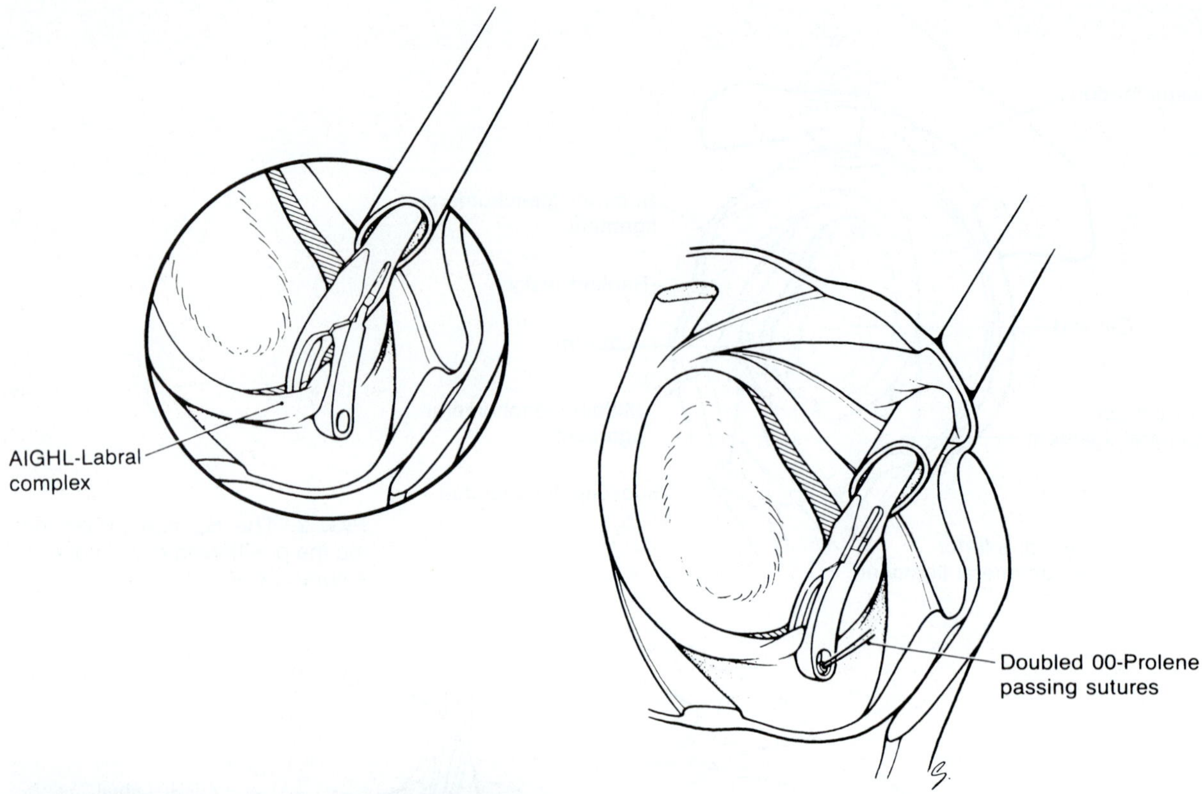

A

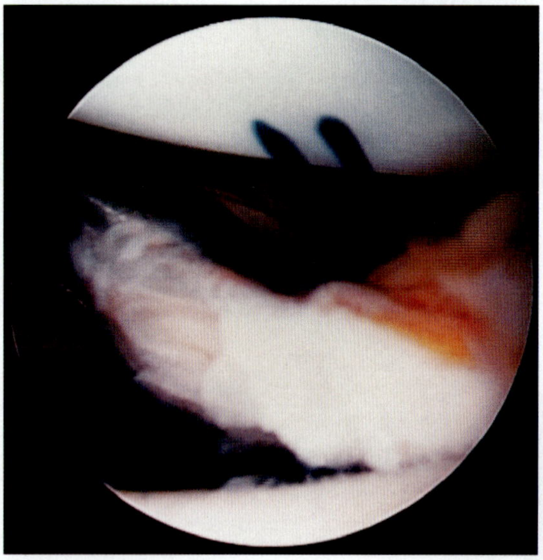

B

FIG. 4. A: The suture punch is used to thread a 48-inch doubled 2.0 Prolene suture through the inferior glenohumeral ligament complex at approximately the 6 o'clock position. **B:** The suture punch is positioned on the inferior capsule as it is pulled superiorly. The two strands of the 2.0 Prolene suture are then threaded into the glenohumeral joint.

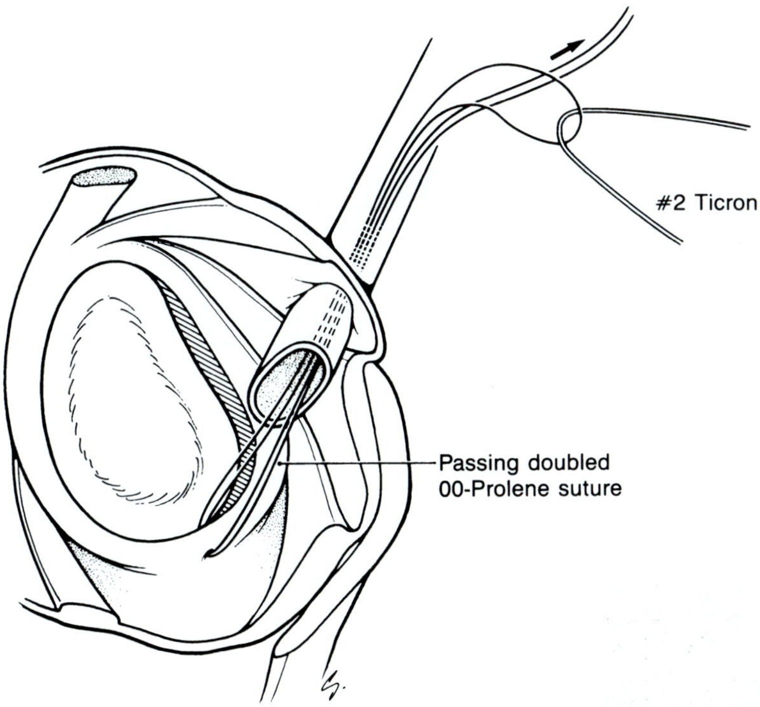

A

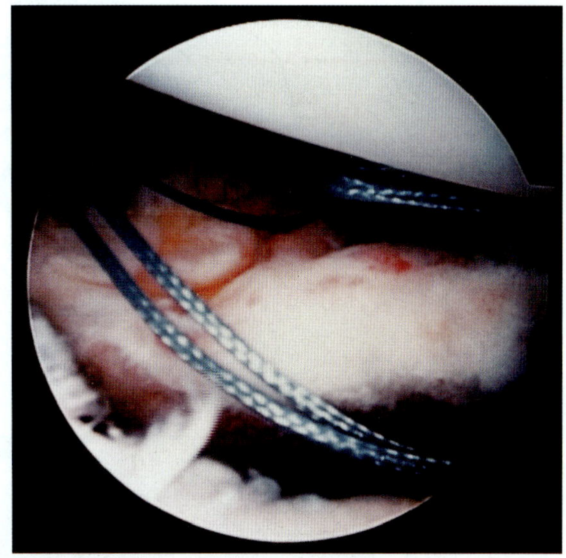

B

FIG. 5. A: The doubled 2.0 Prolene suture is used to retrieve a no. 2 Ticron braided nonabsorbable suture through the inferior glenohumeral ligament complex. **B:** The Prolene can be seen pulling the no. 2 Ticron suture through the inferior glenohumeral ligament and back out the anterior cannula.

ture is then placed in the loop, and by pulling on the two free ends, the suture is passed through the inferior glenohumeral ligament (Fig. 5A and B).

The drilling guide is placed into the joint through the suture punch cannula. The first or inferior hole is drilled at the edge of the glenoid articular surface at approximately the 5 o'clock position. The guide tip is wedged onto the glenoid neck–face junction and acts as a fulcrum downward against the soft tissues, so that the drill is perpendicular to the vertical axis of the glenoid (Fig. 6A and B). The pilot hole is drilled, maintaining adequate visualization from the posterior portal. While the surgeon is visualizing from the posterior portal, it is critical that the drill hole is placed with at least half the diameter of the hole into the edge of the articular surface of the glenoid, thereby assuring optimal anchor placement. The anchor is loaded on the inserter and held in position with an absorbable 2-0 polyglactin 10 (Vicryl) suture. The inner limb of the Ticron suture is threaded through the anchor, and the anchor inserted into the previously drilled pilot hole (Fig. 7A–C). The anchor is carefully tested by pulling on the 2-0 Vicryl suture, which is removed after adequate holding power is confirmed.

The suture punch is reinserted into the joint, and a second double Prolene placed through the inferior glenohumeral ligament ~5 mm more superior than the initial suture (5:30 to 5:45 position). This Prolene is used to pull the inner limb of the Ticron suture through the inferior glenohumeral ligament, creating a horizontal mattress suture and allowing capsular plication (Fig. 8A and B). An arthroscopic knot-tying device is used to tie the two ends of the Ticron suture, repairing the inferior glenohumeral ligament through the glenoid while advancing it superiorly and eliminating inferior capsular redundancy (Fig. 8C and D).

Each step is then repeated, and a second and third anchor are inserted in similar fashion (Fig. 9A–C). The sutures are generally placed at the 6, 4, and 2 o'clock positions into the capsule, with the anchors inserted at 5, 3, and 1 o'clock positions on the glenoid rim (Fig. 2). Placing the sutures inferior to the anchor allows a superior shift of the capsule, eliminating inferior redundancy and correcting any plastic deformity that may exist in the capsular or ligamentous tissues. Mattressing the suture allows plication of the capsule and also helps to eliminate redundancy.

Anchor-First Technique

An alternative method allows placement of the anchor into the glenoid first, followed by retrieval of both limbs of the suture through the capsule. This technique is used for preloaded anchors or for those with foramen of insufficient width to allow two sutures (holding suture and repair suture) to be placed into the anchor simultaneously.

In this variation, the 5 o'clock hole is placed, and the anchor with attached no. 2 nonabsorbable suture is inserted into the glenoid. The suture punch is used to place a doubled 40-in 2.0 Prolene passing suture through the capsule

(text continues on page 323)

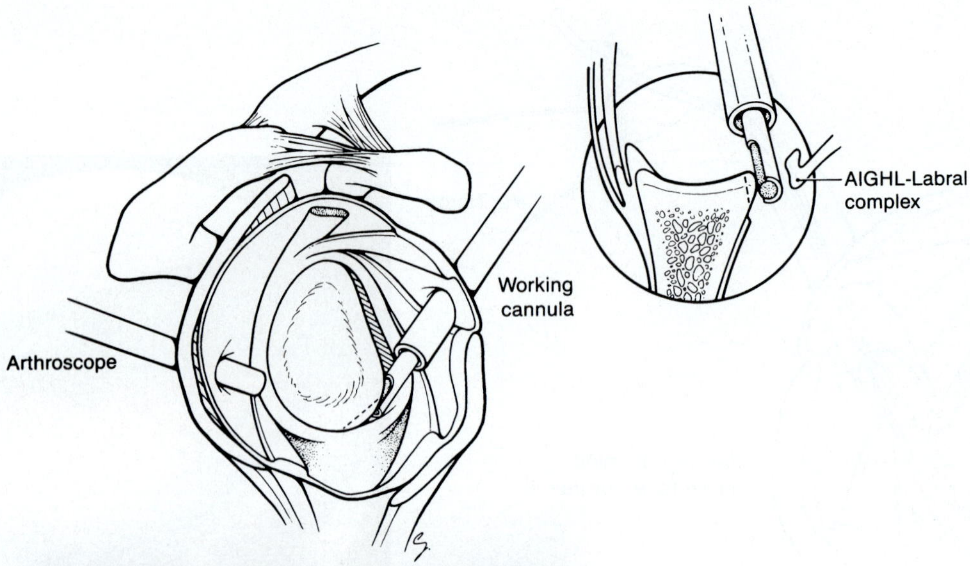

A

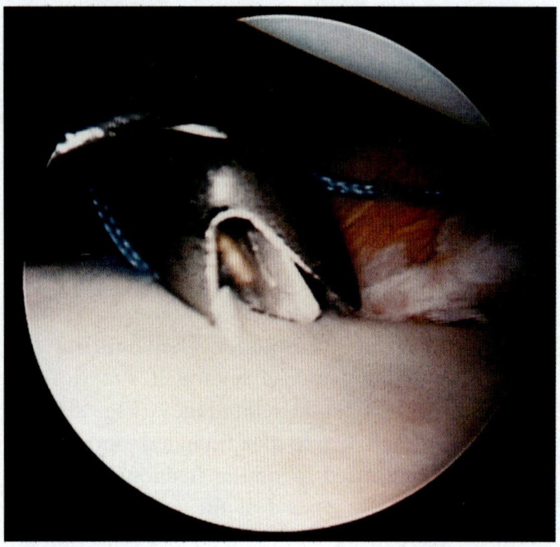

B

FIG. 6. A: The drill guide is placed on the glenoid neck face junction at approximately the 5 o'clock position. This should be placed so that approximately half the diameter of the whole is on the articular surface **(inset)**. **B:** In this view from the posterior portal, the drill guide and drill can be seen in position for the 5 o'clock anchor placement.

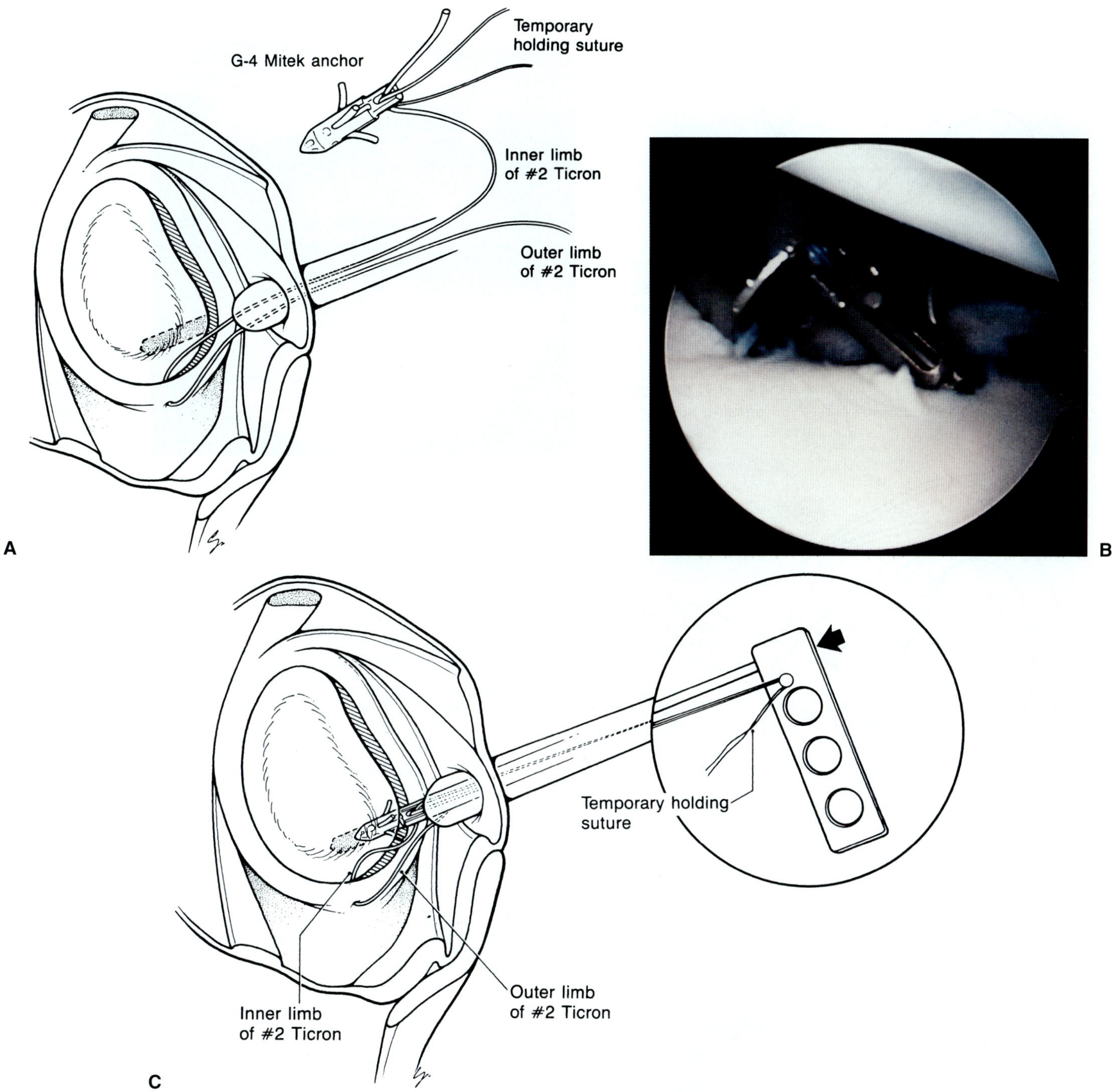

FIG. 7. A: The inner limb of the no. 2 Ticron is passed through the Mitek G4 anchor, along with a 2-0 Vicryl suture. The Vicryl is used to hold the anchor onto the guide. **B:** The Mitek G4 anchor is inserted into the drill hole previously made in the glenoid neck. **C:** The anchor is tapped into position.

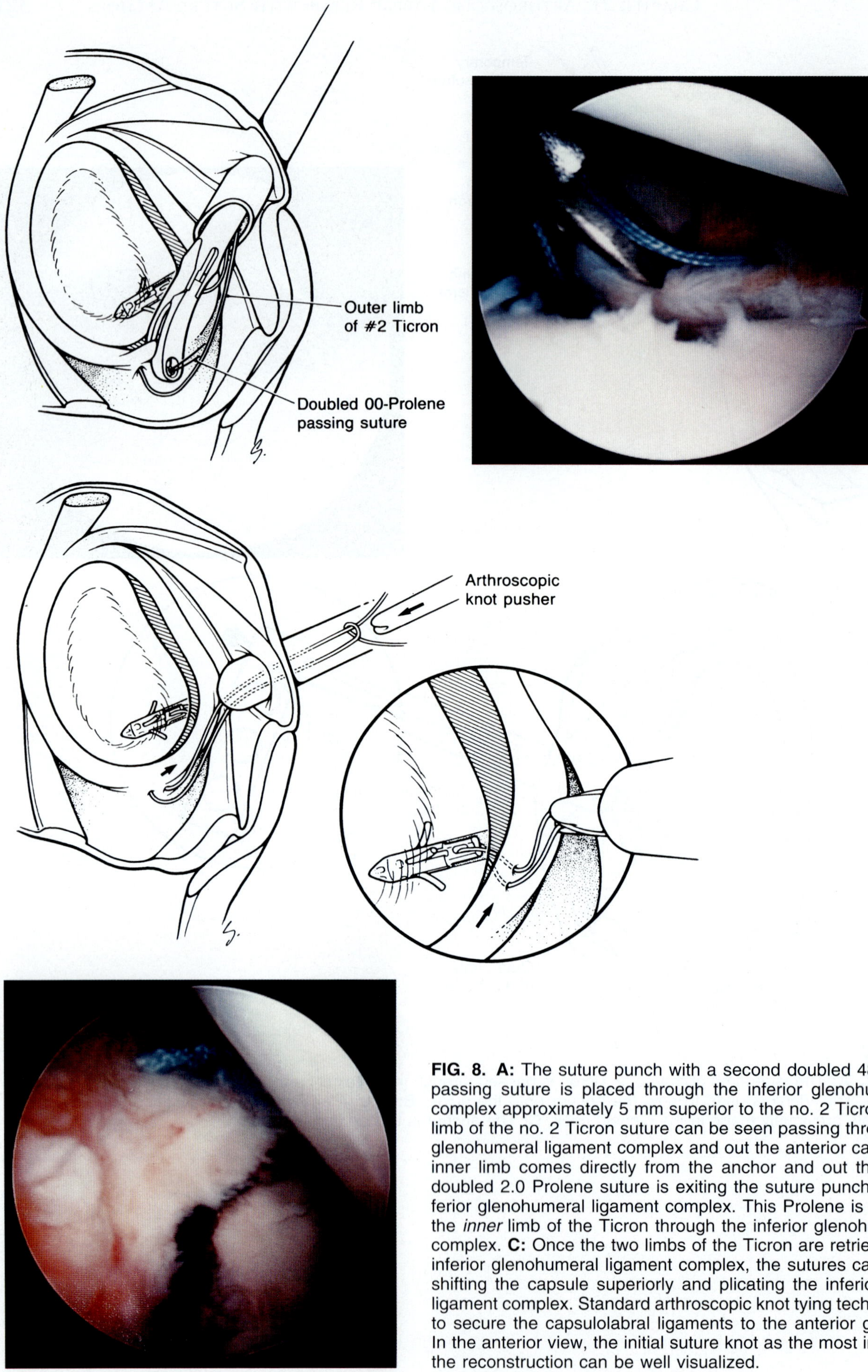

FIG. 8. A: The suture punch with a second doubled 48-in 2.0 Prolene passing suture is placed through the inferior glenohumeral ligament complex approximately 5 mm superior to the no. 2 Ticron. **B:** The outer limb of the no. 2 Ticron suture can be seen passing through the inferior glenohumeral ligament complex and out the anterior cannula, while the inner limb comes directly from the anchor and out the cannula. The doubled 2.0 Prolene suture is exiting the suture punch through the inferior glenohumeral ligament complex. This Prolene is used to retrieve the *inner* limb of the Ticron through the inferior glenohumeral ligament complex. **C:** Once the two limbs of the Ticron are retrieved through the inferior glenohumeral ligament complex, the sutures can be tensioned, shifting the capsule superiorly and plicating the inferior glenohumeral ligament complex. Standard arthroscopic knot tying techniques are used to secure the capsulolabral ligaments to the anterior glenoid neck. **D:** In the anterior view, the initial suture knot as the most inferior aspect of the reconstruction can be well visualized.

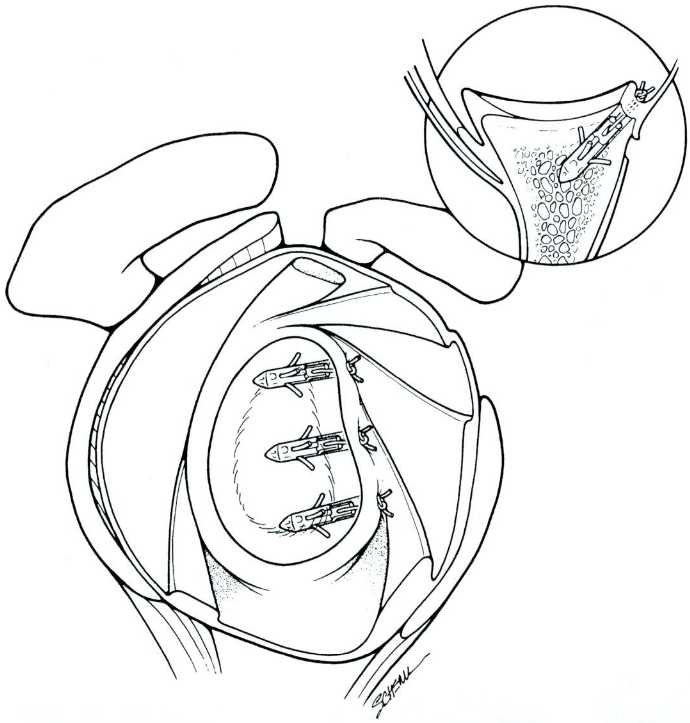

A

FIG. 9. **A:** In most cases, three anchors are inserted into the glenoid neck, shifting the capsule superiorly and repairing the avulsed capsulolabral structures to the glenoid. **B:** The view from the posterior portal demonstrates the repaired capsulolabral complex, restoring a normal buttress in the anterior aspect of the shoulder. **C:** In the view from the anterior portal, the repaired capsulolabral complex is noted.

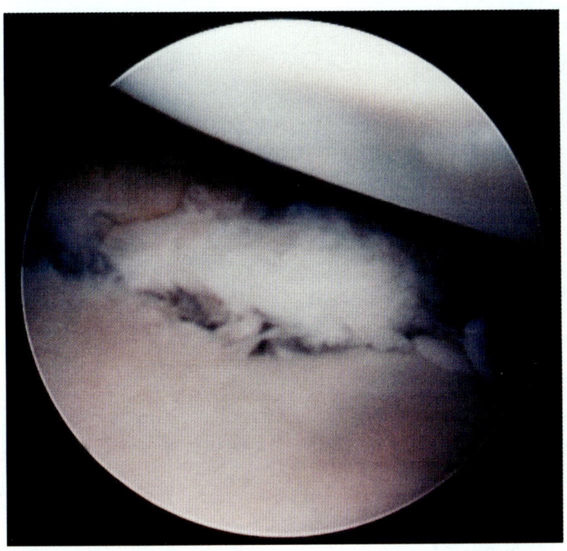

B

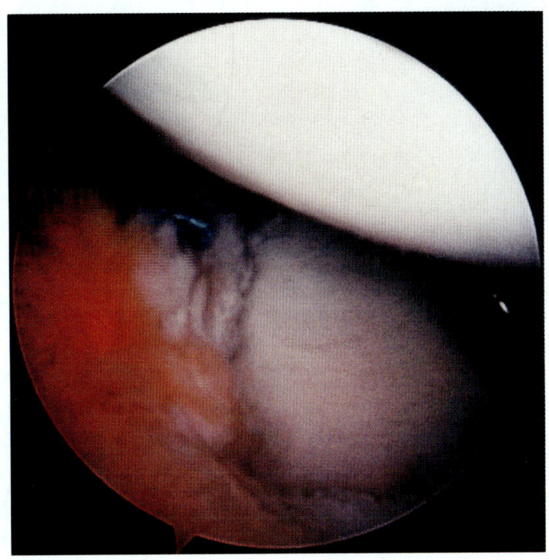

C

at the 6 o'clock position. The Prolene is used to retrieve one limb of the Ticron through the capsule and out the cannula. The suture-passing step is then repeated to create a mattress suture, thereby shifting the capsule superiorly and simultaneously plicating it. These strategies are then repeated for the 3 and 1 o'clock anchors.

Alternate Technique for 3 and 1 O'clock Anchors

As an alternative to the earlier techniques, the Ticron sutures of the 3 o'clock and 1 o'clock anchors can be pulled through the labrum with a retrograde suture retriever (Innovasive Devices, Marlborough, MA, U.S.A.) (Fig. 10). This is accomplished by placing the 15-, 30-, 45-, or 60-degree suture retriever through the anterior cannula and then passing it through the labrum at the same location described for the Caspari punch. This will reproduce the horizontal mattress suture and capsular plication required for the repair. This device simplifies the suture passing but is unable to reach efficiently the 6 o'clock position on the labrum required for the inferior suture.

Knot Tying

Harryman et al. (27) showed that the most secure knot configurations are achieved by reversing half-hitch throws while alternating the post (Fig. 11A). By using this technique, five throws are recommended. A modified slipknot

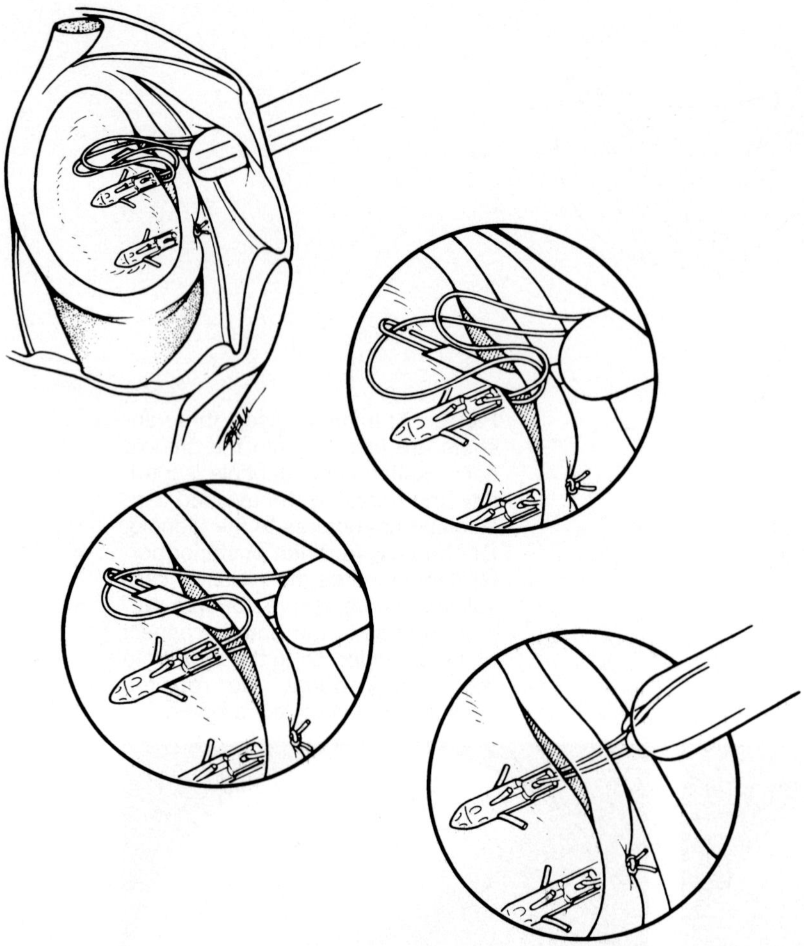

FIG. 10. An alternate method of passing sutures through the labrum for the 3 o'clock and 1 o'clock anchors using the 30° suture retriever (Linvotec).

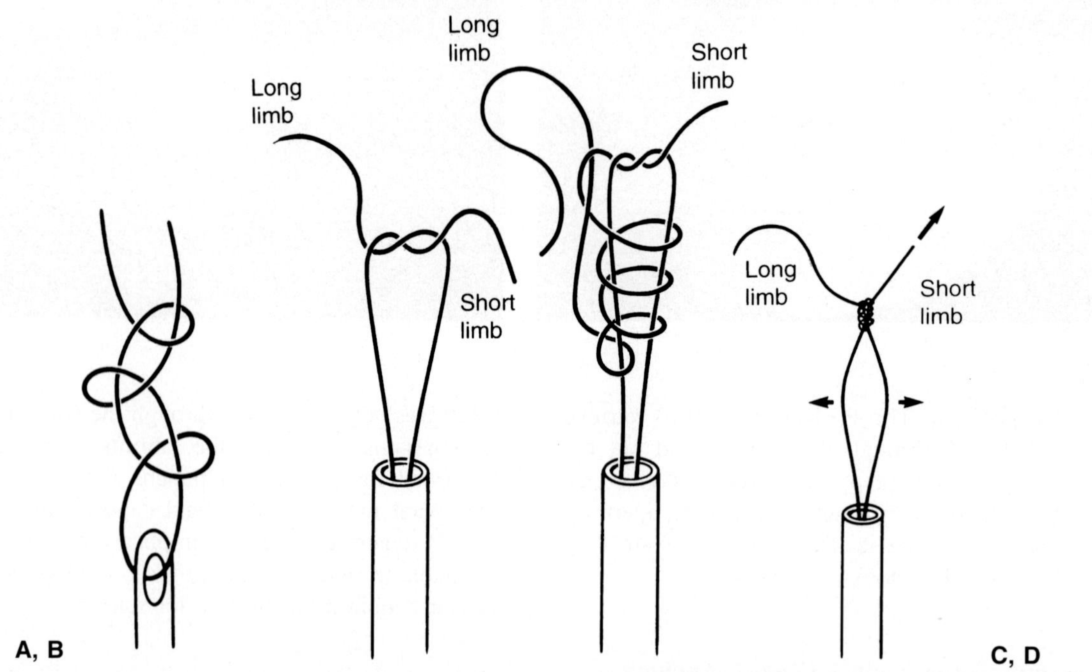

FIG. 11. A: The most secure knot configuration of reversing both throws and posts as described by Harryman et al. **B:** The Roeder knot is accomplished by first throwing the first half of a square knot, leaving one end long and one end short. **C:** The long end is then passed around both limbs of the suture three times, then once around the short limb. The long limb of the suture is then passed through the loop adjacent to the half square knot. **D:** The knot is then compressed by spreading the distal limbs while holding the short limb as a post.

called the Roeder knot can also be used. We prefer a modification of the Roeder knot; it is accomplished by first throwing the first half of a square knot, leaving one end long and one end short (Fig. 11B). The long end is then passed around both limbs of the suture 3 times and then once around the short limb. The long limb of the suture is then passed through the loop adjacent to the half-square knot (Fig. 11C). The knot is then compressed by spreading the distal limbs while holding the short limb as a post (Fig. 11D). The knot is then advanced by pulling on the short limb. It is imperative that the long limb not be pulled on until the knot is snug against the soft tissues and has approximated the Bankart lesion, because this will lock the knot. The knot is then secured by at least one single half-hitch with the short limb as a post.

Once the repair is completed, the shoulder is tested for adequate stability while visualizing the glenohumeral articulation from both the anterior and posterior portals. Specific attention is directed toward any laxity of the posterior inferior glenohumeral ligament and rotator interval. In most cases in which this technique has been performed correctly, there will be no laxity posterior (corrected by suture).

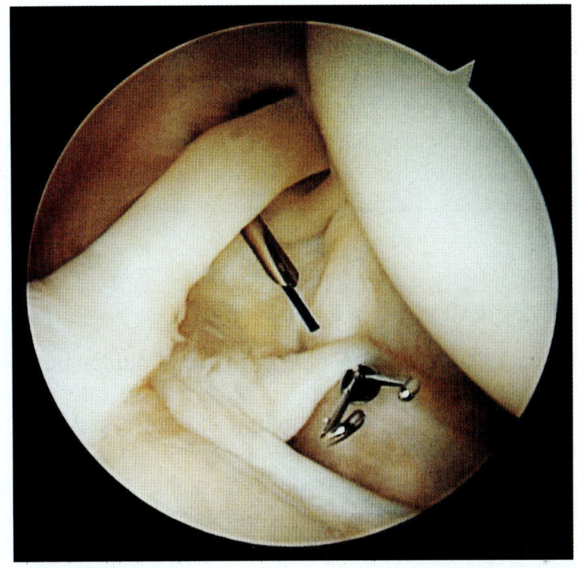

FIG. 12. Initiation of intra-articular rotator interval repair. Note the suture transport device through the subscapularis tendon and middle glenohumeral ligament and the spinal needle through the anterior margin of the supraspinatus tendon adjacent capsule. A zero Prolene suture is advanced through the spinal needle.

Rotator-Interval Closure

The importance of the rotator interval in shoulder instability has been established in cadaveric and clinical studies (26,28). Arthroscopic plication of the rotator interval is sometimes carried out after arthroscopic Bankart repair to supplement this labroligamentous reapproximation. The rotator interval may be plicated by one of the two methods (29). While the surgeon maintains the arthroscope in the posterior portal, a transporter or suture-retrieval device is inserted through the capsule adjacent to the subscapularis tendon and through the middle glenohumeral ligament. Occasionally, a small portion of the subscapularis may be included in this repair, but it is important to include the capsule anterior to the subscapularis as well as a portion of the middle glenohumeral ligament. A spinal needle is then placed through the anterior superior portal adjacent to the inferior lateral corner of the acromion and through the capsule adjacent to the anterior margin of the supraspinatus tendon. A no. 1 Prolene suture is then passed through the spinal needle and retrieved out the anterior portal, by using the transporter device (Fig. 12). This suture will close or plicate the more lateral portion of the rotator interval. The transporter can then be placed back down the anterior cannula and through the capsule medial and superior to the first stitch, a second or third time as necessary.

The arthroscope is then removed from the posterior portal and reinserted into the subacromial bursa. Repositioning of the anterior cannula into the bursa by following the line of suture facilitates identification of the anterior sutures. The superior sutures should be readily visualized at the anterior margin of the supraspinatus tendon. A crochet hook is then used to retrieve the more lateral of the sutures out of the anterior cannula, and arthroscopic knot tying is used to tighten the more lateral aspect of the rotator interval. In similar fashion, the second and third sutures are retrieved and tied down arthroscopically. The adequacy of each knot can be assessed arthroscopically in the bursa. Replacement of the scope into the posterior glenohumeral portal facilitates examination of the rotator interval from an intra-articular position.

A second method of closing the rotator interval can be performed exclusively on the bursal side of the rotator cuff and capsule. Once an adequate assessment of the rotator interval from within the glenohumeral joint has been performed, the arthroscope is placed into the subacromial bursa. The bursa is resected by using the standard shaver device, allowing adequate visualization of the rotator interval. A standard curved Caspari suture punch is loaded with a zero Prolene suture and introduced into the bursa through the lateral portal. The arm is slightly externally rotated, and a single bite of this most superior aspect of the subscapularis tendon or capsule adjacent to this tendon is taken. The suture punch is then opened, but the needle is maintained through the anterior capsule and tendinous structure. The arm is then internally rotated, bringing the anterior margin of the supraspinatus into the open jaw of the suture punch. Closure of the suture punch at this point creates a second bite through the more superior aspect of the rotator interval. The suture is then threaded within the bursa and removed through the lateral portal. The efficacy of the suture in plicating the rotator interval can be assessed under direct visualization. If the plication is thought to be adequate, an arthroscopic knot tying is then performed, tightening the more lateral aspect of the rotator interval. In this case, these steps are repeated, placing three sutures across the rotator interval. Each suture tightens the rotator interval, facilitating placement of the next stitch in a more medial position. The plication of the rotator interval can be checked on both the intra-articular and bursal sides to ensure adequate stability. Shifting of the shoulder under direct visualization ensures adequate stabilization of the rotator-interval plication (27–29).

POSTOPERATIVE CARE

The patient is asked to remain in the shoulder immobilizer for approximately 7 to 10 days postoperatively, removing it only for hygienic purposes and dressing. One week after surgery, the patient is placed in an arm sling in the daytime and the immobilizer at night. After the first week, the patient is asked to perform passive frontal flexion exercises with the arm held in internal rotation, as well as external rotation exercises to a neutral position. Four weeks after surgery, active rehabilitation is initiated and immobilization discontinued, although combined abduction and external rotation are avoided. Eight weeks after surgery, the patient is mobilized into full abduction and external rotation, aggressive strengthening is initiated, and plyometric conditioning for the throwing athlete is started. Full range of motion is expected by 12 weeks. Functional rehabilitation is started between 8 and 12 weeks and continued as needed. Overhead athletes begin throwing between 8 and 12 weeks and progress as tolerated, usually returning to throwing sports between 3 and 6 months postoperatively. Contact sports such as football, basketball, and volleyball are allowed 6 months postoperatively.

PUBLISHED RESULTS

The use of metallic suture anchors for Bankart repair was introduced by Wolf and Snyder (18,22). Wolf and Richmond (30) reported, with limited follow-up, no recurrences of instability in 50 patients by using Mitek GII suture anchors (Mitek products, Westwood, MA, U.S.A.) and absorbable polydioxanone sutures (PDSs). With a similar technique, Hoffman and Reif (31) reported a 12% redislocation rate in 26 patients treated for recurrent anterior dislocation. Although Snyder (18) initially used the Mitek anchor, he now uses a removable suture anchor and nonabsorbable suture. Development of the Shuttle Relay (Linvatec Corp., Largo, FL, U.S.A.) has allowed the passage of nonabsorbable sutures through the capsulolabral ligamentous complex but does necessitate the use of a third portal. This device, however, allows mattressing of the suture and plication of the capsule (18). By using this technique, Snyder et al. (32) reported an 11% recurrence of instability at 1 year.

In this chapter, we describe a technique similar to Snyder's but with several technical differences. Only two portals are required, minimizing damage to the rotator interval. The suture and instrumentation are readily available in most operating rooms. The use of nonabsorbable sutures in mattress fashion more closely mimics the open Bankart procedure. The suture punch allows each pass through the ligament to be tested for position and quality and also allows the suture to be placed inferior to the anchor site, providing for correction of the vertical component of the instability. Use of the original, unmodified suture punch allows each stitch to be retrieved through the same portal.

Our published experience with this technique includes 40 consecutive high-risk patients undergoing reconstruction between January 1993 and October 1994 for recurrent anterior shoulder instability (33). All patients in this study had sustained two or more dislocations, were younger than 23 years, and were involved in high-demand sporting activities, including football, basketball, overhead sports involving the throwing shoulder, and repetitive overhead work with heavy materials. At last follow-up (average, 30 months), the average postoperative Bankart score was 90 (range, 30 to 100). All patients regained more than 170 degrees of both frontal flexion and abduction. In 90 degrees of abduction, the average external rotation was 112 degrees (range, 95 to 135 degrees). Three patients had postoperative instability symptoms and were classified as failures. One of these patients returned to high school football practice 6 weeks postoperatively. The second patient was involved in a motor vehicle accident 5 weeks postoperatively and dislocated both the operative and contralateral, or normal, shoulder. The third patient resubluxated during baseball practice while attempting a sudden high-velocity throw.

The first two patients underwent a diagnostic arthroscopy, followed by an open reconstruction. At the time of surgery, a fresh Bankart lesion with both intact and ruptured sutures was found. The third patient was unable to throw after his subluxation and underwent diagnostic arthroscopy. He was noted to have completely healed his Bankart lesion but had avulsed the humeral attachment of his anterior capsule. All three patients resumed normal activities after revision stabilization.

Twenty-nine of 32 patients participating in sports had postoperative eligibility remaining at the high school or college level. Twenty-six (90%) of these 29 were able to return to sports at the same or higher level. This includes all five baseball players with dominant extremity involvement. Both of the older athletes in the study resumed their profession at the same level as before their injury.

ADVANTAGES

There are several advantages in using arthroscopically placed suture anchors in the treatment of anterior shoulder instability. First, the arthroscope allows the surgeon to visualize the labrum, glenohumeral ligaments, and capsule directly. This information, along with the physical examination, allows the surgeon to individualize the reconstruction. Second, in addition to this potential for improvement in surgical technique, Green and Christensen (34) showed a significant reduction in perioperative morbidity compared with open techniques. This includes a reduction in operative time, perioperative complications, and days of hospitalization.

Several arthroscopic techniques have been developed in an attempt to use these advantages. Transglenoid suturing techniques, arthroscopic stapling techniques, and more recently, use of suture anchors have all been described. Reports of using the transglenoid technique have demonstrated some clinical success, but it has not been shown to be effective in patients younger than 25 years. Concern over the potential for damage to the suprascapular nerve during transosseous drilling of the scapula and lack of reproducibility in several studies limited its acceptance (15,16,19). Arthroscopic stapling techniques have a poor success rate and are associated with a high incidence of complications related to the use of metal implants adjacent to the joint (10,11,23,24). The use of arthroscopically placed suture anchors avoids these technical pitfalls and appears to be the next step in the evolution of arthroscopic anterior shoulder reconstruction.

DISADVANTAGES

Any new operative procedure must be critically evaluated. The availability of instruments, the technical demands, operative time, perioperative morbidity, and ultimately the results must be considered. Although the instruments are readily available, this procedure is technically demanding. To perform this procedure, the surgeon must be an accomplished shoulder arthroscopist and familiar with suture-anchor techniques. Although perioperative morbidity has been shown to be decreased with arthroscopic shoulder reconstructions, the results of these procedures in general have not been as good or reproducible as open shoulder reconstructions (8,18,22,30,32,33). Although several authors have reported results from arthroscopically placed suture anchors for anterior shoulder reconstruction, follow-up has been short and patient numbers often small. Because of the technical demands of this procedure and the lack of published results, the ultimate role of arthroscopically placed suture anchors in the management of anterior shoulder instability has yet to be thoroughly defined.

CONCLUSION

The use of arthroscopically placed suture anchors is a viable alternative for anterior labral repair. The use of suture anchors provides the skilled arthroscopic surgeon with several options in anterior shoulder reconstruction. The labrum, glenohumeral ligaments, and capsule can be evaluated and treated on an individualized basis, based on the pathology found. There is definitely a learning curve associated with this procedure, and long-term follow-up is needed to better evaluate its true potential. However, arthroscopic shoulder reconstruction by using suture anchors will likely play an increasingly significant role in the future.

ACKNOWLEDGMENT

We thank Michael P. Schenk, M.S., CMI, Director of Medical Illustration, University of Mississippi Medical Center, Jackson, Mississippi.

REFERENCES

1. DuToit GT, Roux D. Recurrent dislocation of the shoulder: a twenty-four year study of the Johannesberg stapling operation. *J Bone Joint Surg [Am]* 1956;38:1–12.
2. Perthes G. Uber Operationen bei Habitueller Schulterluxation. *Dtsch Z Chir* 1906;85:199–227.
3. Baker CL, Uribe JN, Whitman C. Arthroscopic evaluation of acute initial anterior shoulder dislocations. *Am J Sports Med* 1990;18 (1): 25–28.
4. Galinat BN, Howell SM. The containment mechanism: the primary stabilizer of the glenohumeral joint. Presented at the 54th AAOS Meeting, San Francisco, CA, January 1987.
5. Moseley HF, Overgaard B. The anterior capsular mechanism in recurrent anterior dislocation of the shoulder: morphological and clinical studies with special references to the glenoid labrum and the glenohumeral ligaments. *J Bone Joint Surg [Br]* 1962;44:913–927.
6. O'Brien SJ, Neves MC, Arnoczky SP, et al. The anatomy and histology of the inferior glenohumeral ligament complex of the shoulder. *Am J Sports Med* 1990;18 (5):449–456.
7. Turkel SJ, Pavio MW, Marshall JL, et al. Stabilizing mechanisms preventing anterior dislocation of the glenohumeral joint. *J Bone Joint Surg [Am]* 1981;63 (8):1208–1217.
8. Rockwood CA, Matsen FA, eds. *The shoulder.* Philadelphia: WB Saunders, 1990;577–581.
9. Caspari RB. Arthroscopic reconstruction for anterior shoulder instability. In: Paulos LE, Tibone JE, eds. *Operative techniques in shoulder surgery.* Gaithersburg, MD: Aspen, 1991:57–63.
10. Coughlin L, Rubinovich M, Johansson J, et al. Arthroscopic staple capsulorrhaphy for anterior shoulder instability. *Am J Sports Med* 1992;20 (3):253–256.
11. Hawkins RB. Arthroscopic stapling repair for shoulder instability: a retrospective study of 50 cases. *Arthroscopy* 1989;5 (2):122–128.
12. McIntyre LF, Caspari RB. The rationale and techniques for arthroscopic reconstruction of anterior shoulder instability using multiple sutures. *Orthop Clin North Am* 1993;24 (1):55–58.
13. Maki NJ. Arthroscopic stabilization: suture technique. *Oper Tech Orthop* 1992;1:180–183.
14. Matthews LS, Vetter WL, Oweida SJ, Spearman J, Helfet DL. Arthroscopic staple capsulorrhaphy for recurrent anterior shoulder instability. *Arthroscopy* 1988;4 (2):106–111.
15. Morgan CD. Arthroscopic transglenoid Bankart suture repair. In: Paulos LE, Tibone JE, eds. *Operative techniques in shoulder surgery.* Gaithersburg, MD: Aspen, 1991:71–77.
16. Morgan CD, Bodenstab AB. Arthroscopic Bankart suture repair: technique and early results. *Arthroscopy* 1987;3 (2):11–22.
17. Savoie FH, Miller C. Technique of capsulorrhaphy (Caspari technique). In: Parisien M. ed. *Current techniques in arthroscopy.* Philadelphia: Current Medicine, 1996.
18. Snyder SJ, ed. *Shoulder arthroscopy.* New York: McGraw-Hill, 1994: 179–215.
19. Snyder SJ, Stafford BB. Arthroscopic management of instability of the shoulder. *Orthopedics* 1993;16 (9):993–1002.
20. Speer KP, Warren RF. Arthroscopic shoulder stabilization: a role for biodegradable materials. *Clin Orthop* 1993;291:67–74.
21. Warner JLP, Warren RF. Arthroscopic Bankart repair using a cannulated, absorbable fixation device. *Oper Tech Orthop* 1991;1:192–198.
22. Wolf EM. Arthroscopic capsulolabral repair using suture anchors. *Orthop Clin North Am* 1993;24 (1):59–69.
23. Zuckerman JD, Matsen FA III. Complications about the glenohumeral joint related to the use of screws and staples. *J Bone Joint Surg [Am]* 1984;66:175–180.
24. Lane JG, Sachs RA, Riehl B. Arthroscopic staple capsulorrhaphy: a long-term follow-up. *Arthroscopy* 1993;9:190–194.

25. Rowe CR, Patel D, Southmayd WW. The Bankart procedure: a long-term end-result study. *J Bone Joint Surg [Am]* 1978;60:1–16.
26. Field LD, Warren RF, O'Brien SJ, Altchek DW, Wickiewicz TL. Isolated closure of rotator interval defects for shoulder instability. *Am J Sports Med* 1995;23:556–563.
27. Loutzenheiser TD, Harryman DT, Yung SW, FRCS France MP, Sidles JA, eds. Optimizing arthroscopic knots. *Arthroscopy* 1995;11 (2): 199–206.
28. Harryman DT, Sidles JA, Harris LS, Matsen FA. The role of the rotator interval capsule in passive motion and stability of the shoulder. *J Bone Joint Surg [Am]* 1992;74:54–66.
29. Treacy SH, Field LD, Savoie FH. Rotator interval capsule closure: arthroscopic technique. *Arthroscopy* 1997;13 (1):103–106.
30. Wolf EM, Richmond JC. Arthroscopic Bankart repair using suture anchors. *Oper Tech Orthop* 1991;1 (2):184–191.
31. Hoffman F, Reif G. Arthroscopic shoulder stabilization using Mitek anchors. *Arthroscopy* 1995;3:50–54.
32. Snyder SJ, Banas MP, Belzer JP. Arthroscopic treatment of anterior shoulder instability using threaded suture anchors and nonabsorbable suture. *Instr Course Lect* 1996;71–81.
33. Bacilla P, Field LD, Savoie FH. Arthroscopic Bankart repair in a high demand patient population. *Arthroscopy* 1997;13:51–60.
34. Green MR, Christensen KP. Arthroscopic Bankart procedure by suture technique: indications, technique, and results. *Arthroscopy* 1992;8:111–115.

The Unstable Shoulder,
edited by R.F. Warren, E.V. Craig, and D.W. Altchek.
Lippincott–Raven Publishers, Philadelphia © 1999.

CHAPTER 22

Thermally-Assisted Arthroscopic Stabilization of the Shoulder Joint

Gary S. Fanton and Michael S. Wall

Arthroscopic stabilization techniques for the treatment of glenohumeral instability have recently gained considerable attention. Despite their appeal for smaller incisions, lower morbidity, and easier rehabilitation, the results to date for most arthroscopic techniques have failed to equal those of open procedures. In addition, the techniques for reducing excessive capsular volume associated with glenohumeral instability remain technically demanding. Recently, a procedure to tighten or ''shrink'' the glenohumeral ligaments and capsule thermally has gained popularity. A radiofrequency (RF) electrothermal arthroscopic probe with temperature-feedback capability was developed to deliver a specified amount of thermal energy to effect controlled and reproducible tissue shrinkage. This thermal energy source has shown considerable promise when used alone or in combination with arthroscopic Bankart repairs in the treatment of glenohumeral instability. We believe that this device will become an important addition to the surgeon's armamentarium in the treatment of glenohumeral instability.

SHOULDER INSTABILITY

Background

The magnitude of shoulder instability–related problems is reflected in its incidence in the general population. Glenohumeral instability (GHI) is estimated to affect between 2% and 8% of the population and represents one third of all shoulder-related emergency room visits (1–4). If we consider the spectrum of shoulder instability to include occult subluxations that produce activity-related pain, then the true incidence of GHI is grossly underestimated. Although any age group can be affected, GHI is primarily a disorder of the younger population. Numerous studies reported that the recurrence rate of instability is inversely proportional to the patient's age at the time of the original injury (5–7). Thus young, active individuals with shoulder instability can have a disability that significantly limits their ability to work and participate in sports. Often, these individuals will decrease their activity level to accommodate their functional instability. Shoulder-instability symptoms encompass a spectrum that includes frank dislocations, gross or occult subluxations, shoulder weakness/fatigue, ''dead-arm'' syndrome, and secondary impingement symptoms or rotator-cuff tears (1,8–14).

Glenohumeral stability is dependent on an intact capsulolabral complex and a neuromuscularly intact rotator cuff. Instability can occur from a single traumatic event that disrupts the capsulolabral complex, recurrent microtrauma, and atraumatic constitutional ligamentous laxity. Most cases of unidirectional and multidirectional GHI are associated with the common finding of excessive joint capsular volume (9,13,15). Recent evidence supported an increased role of the shoulder capsule/glenohumeral ligaments in providing joint stability (16–18). Bigliani et al. (19) demonstrated that plastic deformation of the capsule occurs with shoulder dislocation in a cadaveric model, whereas Speer (20) concluded that a Bankart lesion alone is insufficient to allow joint dislocation. We believe that the pathologic feature common to all forms of symptomatic GHI is a varying degree of interstitial damage or plastic deformation of the capsule/glenohumeral ligaments or both. Successful treatment of GHI relies on the identification of the direction of the instability and an assessment of the extent of the soft-tissue injury. The soft-tissue injury can include plastic deformation or redundancy of the capsule/glenohumeral ligaments with or without a Bankart lesion.

The current treatment of GHI is directed at repair of the

G. S. Fanton and M. S. Wall: Sports Orthopedic and Rehabilitation, Menlo Park, California 94025; and Division of Sports Medicine, Stanford University Medical Center, Stanford Health Services, Stanford, California 94305.

periarticular soft tissue with open and arthroscopic techniques. Strengthening exercises of the dynamic stabilizers, including the rotator cuff and periscapular muscles, is frequently prescribed. Strengthening exercises alone as a treatment for traumatic GHI often result in an unacceptably high recurrence rate in the young athletic individual (8,21). The open treatment of GHI is directed toward anatomic repair of the injured stabilizers (22–25). Although these techniques usually result in a stable joint, they carry a high morbidity (26–28). Postoperative rehabilitation can require extensive time, and some patients may not return to their preinjury level of activity. Fewer than 25% of overhead athletes appear to be able to achieve their preinjury level of function after ''anatomic'' capsular repairs (17,29–32). Arthroscopic-stabilization procedures have the potential benefits of improved range of motion, less risk of neurovascular injury, and easier rehabilitation (33). However, the recurrence rate of GHI after arthroscopic stabilization ranges from 0 to 42% and appears to be related to technique (34–41). Arthroscopic-suture techniques and suture-anchor techniques are technically demanding procedures with a steep learning curve and a risk of neurovascular injury. The technical difficulties associated with trying arthroscopically to address capsular/glenohumeral ligament laxity led many authors to state that arthroscopic stabilization in this patient population is contraindicated (12,29,36,42,43).

In summary, GHI is a common and recurring problem that current treatments do not satisfactorily address. Conservative treatment is associated with an unacceptable high recurrence rate in the young athletic individual. Open stabilizations carry a high morbidity, often require prolonged rehabilitation, and return a minority of overhead athletes to their preinjury levels of activity. Arthroscopic procedures have a higher rate of failure, are technique dependent, and may be contraindicated in cases of capsular/glenohumeral ligament redundancy–related shoulder instability. Whether an operative or nonoperative treatment program is chosen, prolonged physical therapy ranging from 3 to 6 months is often needed. There thus remains considerable room for improvement in the treatment of GHI. With increasing pressures to drive down the costs of medicine, many health-care plans severely restrict either access to physical therapy or the total number of visits available for patient treatment. For a new treatment alternative to gain acceptance, the technique must adequately address the pathology, be relatively easy to carry out, and ideally, must remain cost effective.

THERMAL MODIFICATION OF COLLAGEN

Joint laxity can result from capsular redundancy or ligamentous injury (i.e., partial tears with permanent deformation vs. complete disruption) or both. In the case of joint laxity producing clinical instability, resulting from either capsular redundancy or plastic deformation, shrinking the dense collagenous tissue may be an effective method for reducing excessive joint motion. Outcomes that make the shrinkage of densely collagenous tissue desirable for reducing joint laxity include the preservation of tissue mechanical properties and cell viability and an acceptable risk of complications.

Shrinkage of collagen can be achieved through thermal or chemical methods (i.e., extremes of pH, lyotrophic agents). The ability to ''shrink'' collagen through thermal or chemical methods has been known for many years. The earliest mention of the ability of collagen to shrink or contract appeared in the literature as early as 1871, although it was not until the early 1900s that several articles were published (44). It became well known to leather chemists in the early 1900s that different substances caused the contraction of collagenous tissue at room temperature (44). Despite these early descriptions in the literature, the classic example of applied collagen shrinkage is probably the shrinking of heads by South American headhunters (45).

Collagen is the most abundant protein in the human body (46). More than 90% of the organic matter in tendon, ligament, and bone is type I collagen (47). Mammalian collagen molecules in their native state possess a rod-like conformation and are aggregated into fibrils with their long axis oriented roughly parallel to the fibril axis (48). Hodge and Petruska (49) described the ultrastructural organization of collagen molecules based on electron-microscopic studies. Their description depicts the collagen molecules (4.4D in length, with D = 640 Angstrom) being aligned head to tail with a spacing of approximately 0.6D (49). The molecules are further organized into a linear array in which the molecules are staggered with respect to each other by a distance D or a multiple of D (49,50).

In their native state, collagen molecules are in a highly ordered or ''crystalline'' arrangement in which the molecules are oriented in an extended conformation (Fig. 1; 51–53). This extended conformation must be stabilized by both intra- and intermolecular forces because the preferred state is that of a contracted, random coil conformation (51–53). The molecular forces stabilizing the extended conformation consist primarily of hydrogen bonds and covalent cross-links (both reducible and irreducible; 52,53). The highly ordered or ''crystalline'' arrangement of collagen molecules in this extended conformation forms the structural basis for the relative *inextensibility* of densely collagenous tissues, such as tendon and ligament (52). This ultrastructural arrangement is illustrated by the short toe region and rather abrupt increase into the linear region in the stress–strain (mechanical) response that is characteristic of tendons and ligaments.

The ultrastructural basis underlying the shrinking of collagenous tissue is a conformational change from the crystalline, extended state to the random-coil, contracted state (52–55). In this case, the observed macroscopic tissue

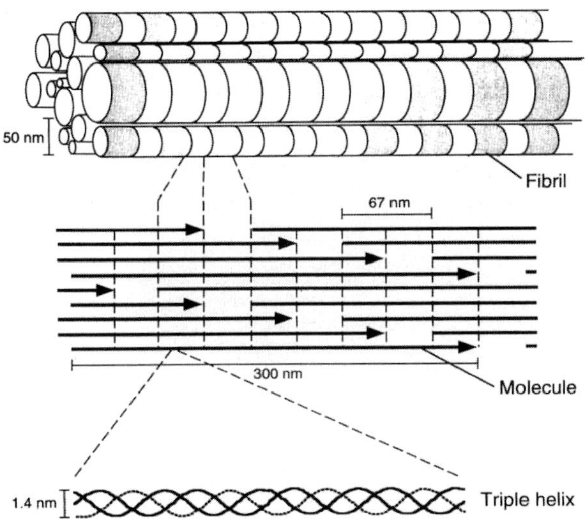

FIG. 1. Structural orientation of type 1 collagen. Collagen fibrils aggregate to form a collagen fiber. Molecules are packed in a staggered fashion that give rise to the striated appearance in transmission electron micrographs. Three polypeptide chains coil together to form a triple helix configuration. (From Hayashi K, Thabit G III, Bogdanske JJ, Mascio LN, Markel MD. The effect of nonablative laser energy on the ultrastructure of joint capsular collagen. *Arthroscopy* 1996;12:479, with permission.)

changes (tissue shrinkage) are related to the changes taking place at the molecular (ultrastructural) level. Flory (32) eloquently characterized this conformational change as a "phase transition" due to the "melting" of the crystalline extended conformation, which transforms the collagen molecule into an "amorphous contracted," random-coil conformation, which is more extendible and "rubber-like." The stabilizing forces that must be disrupted before this conformational change can occur are believed to be primarily the hydrogen bonds (53,56,57). When collagen exists in the random-coil conformation, it is said to be denatured.

The shrinkage temperature (T_s) of collagen has been variably defined as the temperature at which one half of the helical structure of collagen is lost (denatured), the temperature at which the shrinkage rate is greatest, and as the temperature causing one half shrinkage in 1 minute (58–60). Difficulty arises in that there is no single value for T_s, but rather a range of temperatures. Thermal shrinkage of collagen depends on the temperature and on the amount of time the tissue is heated. Thus, the same amount of shrinkage can be achieved through exposure to high temperature for short periods as with lower temperatures for longer periods. This concept of "instantaneous" shrinkage (high rate) versus "incipient" (low rate) of collagen was first recognized by Pankhurst (42). Thermodynamic considerations concerning the shrinkage of collagen were nicely outlined by Weir (60).

Several factors can affect the measurement of T_s. The shrinkage temperature is related to the total imino acid content (proline/hydroxyproline) of the collagen, which can vary significantly from species to species (11,53,61,62). For mammalian collagen, the T_s is in the neighborhood of 65°C, whereas that of codfish is closer to 40°C (1). Age of the animal also can affect the T_s (44,53,56,63,64). In general, the thermal stability of collagen increases with age and is thought to be related to the increase in (stabilizing) irreducible cross-links (65,66). Pre-tension on the collagenous tissue has also been shown to change T_s, with increasing pre-tension generally increasing T_s (53,60). In addition, the specific solute in which the tissue is bathed can profoundly affect T_s (44,53,54,60). An example of solutes that can reduce T_s include lyotrophic agents such as urea. Urea achieves this by breaking hydrogen bonds, thus destabilizing the extended conformation and allowing the molecule to seek the preferred contracted, random-coil conformation (53,57). Agents that dehydrate the collagen fibril will tend to increase the T_s (51,60). The effect on T_s of some agents will vary with concentration. For example, glucose in 2 *M* solution will decrease T_s by approximately 15°C by serving as a competitor to water in forming hydrogen bonds (53). At higher concentration, the dehydrating effect of the glucose solution predominates and actually increases T_s (53). Extremes of pH, such as those occurring with concentrated acidic or basic solutions, will also influence T_s, although no significant effect is seen in the pH range extending from approximately pH 3 to 10 (53,54,60). Finally, it also has been theorized that the proteoglycan content of the tissue may affect the T_s of the collagen in the specific tissue (i.e., tendon vs. articular cartilage), although this is not supported in the literature (67).

Microscopically, a variety of architectural arrangements have been found in collagenous tissues (47). These range from the densely aligned organization characteristic of ligament and tendon to the looser network seen in skin. The architectural arrangement of collagen plays an instrumental role in determining the mechanical properties of the tissue. Collagen density and packing orientation play a role in the amount of shrinkage possible; for example, dermis with a higher density of collagen has been shown to contract more than loosely packed dermis (25,40). This may explain why some regions of the shoulder capsule appear more "responsive" (shrink more) than do other areas.

To define broadly the relation between tissue mechanical properties and tissue shrinkage, uniaxial tensile testing of normal and heat-shrunken bovine tendons was carried out at the Hospital for Special Surgery. The experimental data was fitted to a mathematical model by using curve-fitting software as shown in Figure 2 (68). It was found that the mechanical properties decreased with increasing shrinkage. The change in the mechanical properties was found to be independent of the method used in achieving the shrinkage. In other words, the stress–strain response for a specimen

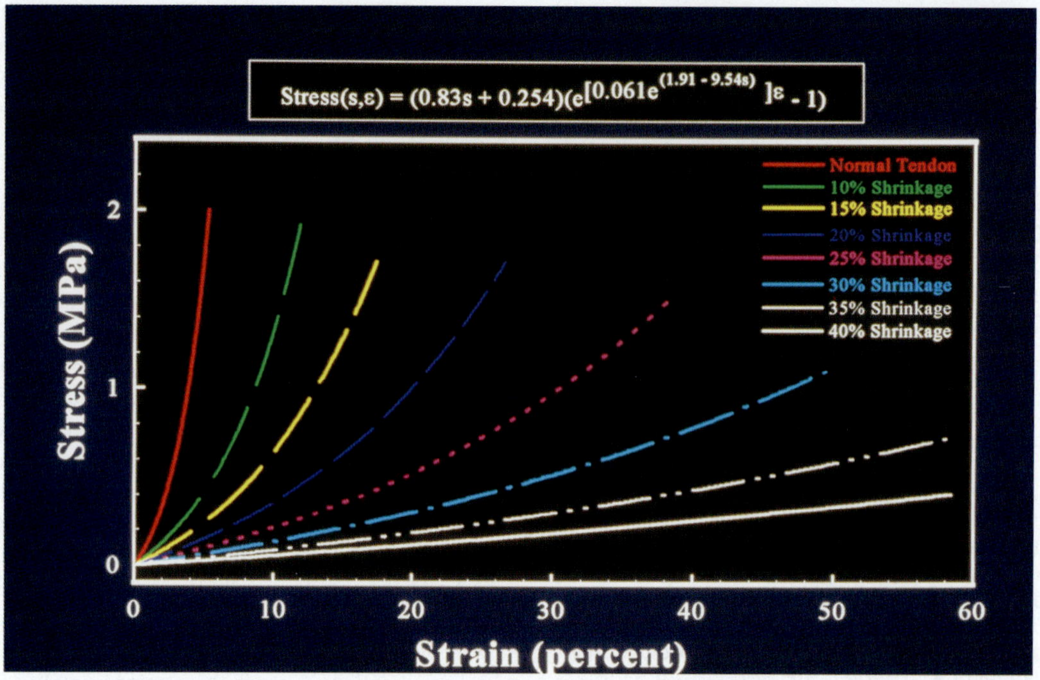

FIG. 2. Relation between tissue stress and strain as a function of increasing tissue shrinkage (immediately after shrinkage), as predicted by mathematical model fitted to experimental data for heat-shrunken bovine tendons ($n = 60$).

shrunken by 20% through heating at high temperature and for a short period was the same as that obtained by heating at lower temperatures for a longer period. The primary factor influencing changes in the mechanical response was the amount of tendon shrinkage and not the method used to achieve this shrinkage. Transmission electron microscopy (TEM) of normal tendon shows the classic cross-striations characteristic of collagen molecules in their native organized (''crystalline'') and extended conformation. With increasing shrinkage, a higher proportion of the collagen fibrils undergoes the conformation change from an extended, crystalline, inextensible state to that of a contracted, random-coil, extendible state (Fig. 3; 68). These TEM photographs provide evidence of the changes taking place at the ultrastructural level that are responsible for the observed mechanical property changes.

In addition, the relation between shrinkage, time, and applied temperature was also studied. Tendon shrinkage was found to be a function of time and temperature (Fig. 4; 68). At any given temperature, the shape of the shrinkage-versus-time response was sigmoidal, with an initial region of slow change, followed by an increase in shrinkage rate, and finally, a plateau to maximal shrinkage. The results from the experiments measuring the shrinkage rate as a function of temperature showed that the shrinkage process is extremely sensitive to temperature. This is in agreement with Weir (60), who reported that a 2° increase in temperature resulted in the shrinkage rate doubling. In contrast, an ordinary chemical reaction generally requires about a 10° increase to double the speed of reaction (60). Weir (60) also reported that shrinkage follows, at least in part, a first-order reaction rate, which is similar to what has been found for the denaturation of proteins in general.

Shrinkage occurs rapidly (''instantaneous shrinkage'') with higher temperatures. This is consistent with the observed effects of the holmium:yttrium aluminum garnet (YAG) laser. Lower rates of shrinkage (''incipient shrinkage'') occur at lower temperatures and longer exposures. Given that the mechanical properties of the tissue decrease (directly after shrinkage) with increasing shrinkage, our goal would be optimally to shrink the tissue without overshooting the maximal allowable shrinkage before unacceptable mechanical property changes occur. The shrinkage of tissue under conditions producing incipient shrinkage may provide better control with less risk of ''overshrinkage.'' The sensitivity of tissue shrinkage to temperature underscores the importance of a temperature-feedback mechanism in the design considerations of the safest arthroscopic device to administer the desired heat.

Several studies provide a foundation for the applicability of using thermal energy for the modification and tightening of densely collagenous tissue (69–72). By using the holmium:YAG laser as the thermal source, the effect of laser energy on the mechanical, biochemical, histologic, and ultrastructural properties of joint capsular tissue were studied (69–72). At three different power settings, the application of the laser thermal energy resulted in a 9%, 26%, and 36% reduction in capsular tissue length for the 5-, 10-, and 15-

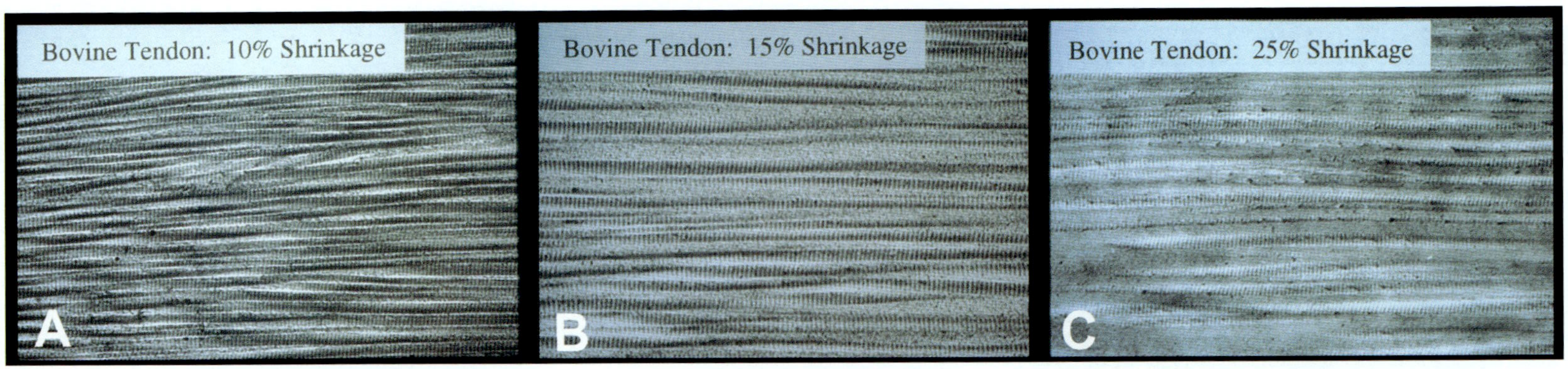

FIG. 3. Transmission electron microscopy of bovine tendon heat shrunk to variable percentages. **A:** 10% shrinkage. **B:** 15% shrinkage. **C:** 25% shrinkage. Note the progressive increase in relative proportion of fibrils denatured with increasing shrinkage (×19,800; 1 mm = 0.051 μm).

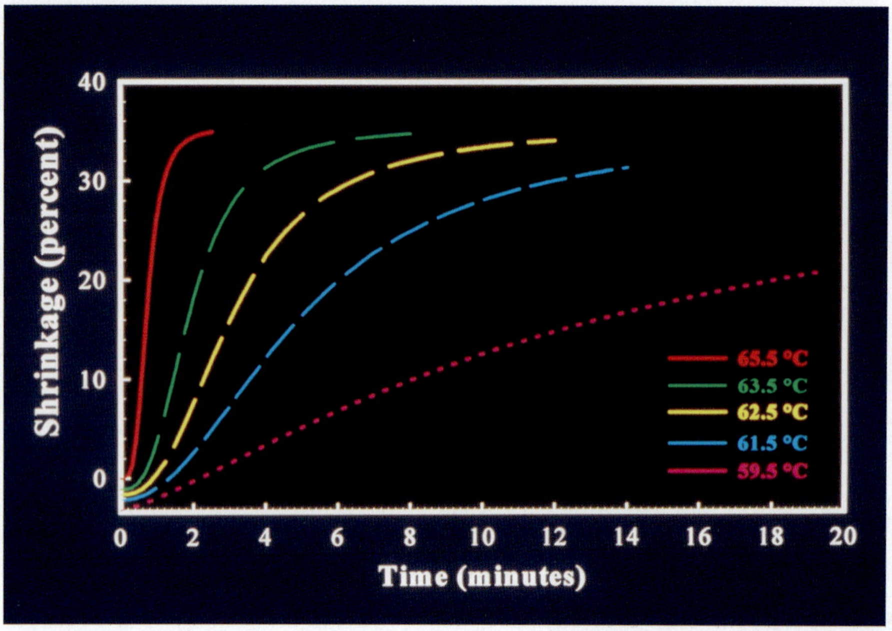

FIG. 4. Shrinkage versus time for various temperatures, as predicted by experimental mathematical model fitted to experimental data ($n = 60$). The slope of each line reflects the shrinkage "rate." Note the extreme sensitivity of shrinkage rate to temperature change.

W groups, respectively (Fig. 5; 69). Tissue shrinkage was significantly and strongly correlated with energy density. Laser thermal energy caused a significant decrease in tensile stiffness only at the higher energy level but did not change the relaxation properties of capsular tissue at any energy density when compared with pretreatment values. TEM revealed alteration of the collagen architecture with significantly increased fibril cross section for each of the treated groups compared with control (Fig. 6; 71). The fibrils began to lose their distinct edges and their cross-striations at higher energy densities. Each increase in energy level also caused a significant increase in collagen fibril diameter. These studies demonstrated that significant capsular shrinkage can be achieved with the application of laser thermal energy without a detrimental effect on the viscoelastic properties of the tissue, although at higher energy densities, laser energy did lessen the capsular stiffness (69). Application of laser thermal energy did not cause significant alteration of biochemical parameters evaluated, but significant changes in the histologic and ultrastructural properties of the collagen molecule were associated with thermal changes in the tissue.

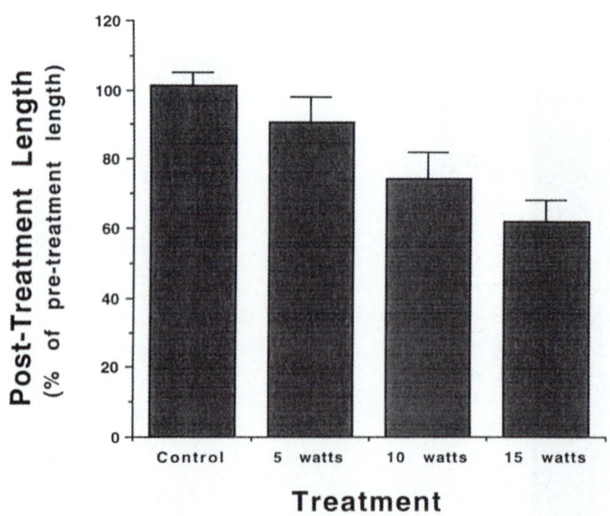

FIG. 5. Posttreatment joint capsular length normalized to pretreatment length, comparing control group with three laser-treatment groups. Each group is significantly different from the other ($p < 0.05$). (From Hayashi K, Thabit G III, Vailas AC, Bogdanske JJ, Cooley AJ, Markel MD. The effect of nonablative laser energy joint capsular properties: an in vivo histologic and biochemical study using a rabbit model. *Am J Sports Med* 1996;24:640, with permission.)

The healing response of thermal energy on joint capsular tissue was studied in an *in vivo* rabbit model (70). Both control and laser-treated samples showed normal response to tissue trauma resulting from standard surgical procedures, with initial fusion of collagen and nucleolar streaming of fibroblasts. By 30 days after treatment, the acellular hyalinized regions of collagen were infiltrated by fibroblasts, which appeared to use the fused collagen as a framework or "scaffold" for migration and secretion of a new collagen matrix for tissue repair to proceed. Studies detailing the healing response and change in mechanical properties with time are under way.

CLINICAL BACKGROUND OF ARTHROSCOPIC THERMAL STABILIZATION

The use of lasers in orthopedic surgery and arthroscopy has been investigated since the early 1980s (73–76). "Laser" is an acronym for **L**ight **A**mplification by the **S**timulated **E**mission of **R**adiation. Originally developed in the

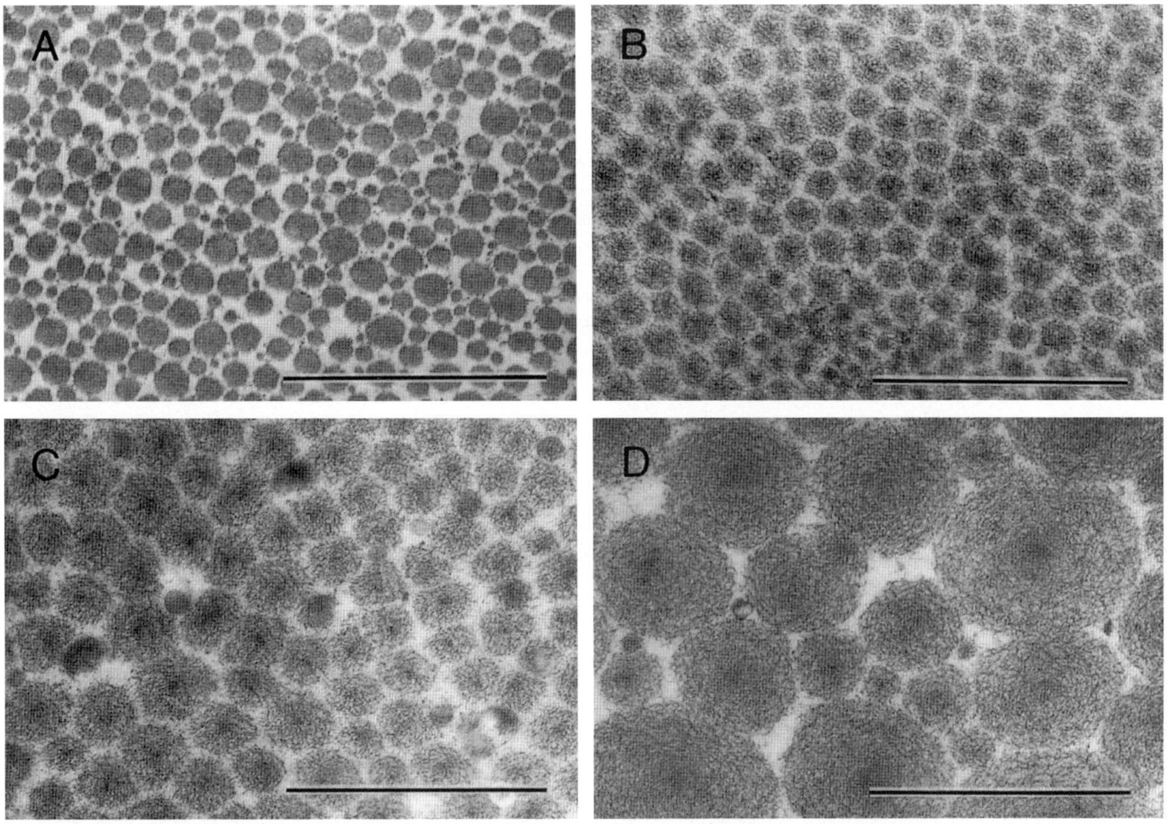

FIG. 6. Transmission electron microscopy of cross-sections of **(A)** control joint capsular tissue, demonstrating a variety of fibril sizes with tight fibril packing; **(B)** 5-W joint capsular tissue, demonstrating loss of fibrils' distinct edges; **(C)** 10-W joint capsular tissue, demonstrating changes similar to those of 5-W group but with significantly greater increases in fibril diameter; and **(D)** 15-W joint capsular tissue, demonstrating dramatic increases in fibril diameter (original magnification ×24,000; bar = 1 μm). (From Hayashi K, Thabit G III, Bogdanske JJ, Mascio LN, Markel MD. The effect of nonablative laser energy on the ultrastructure of joint capsular collagen. *Arthroscopy* 1996;12:477, with permission.)

early 1960s for research and industrial use, lasers soon found application in various medical specialties (76). In orthopedics, the most widely accepted lasers use the infrared potion of the electromagnetic spectrum—the neodymium:YAG and holmium lasers (41,74,77). These lasers generate an intense thermal-energy beam that can be directed through fiberoptic handpieces arthroscopically. How a particular tissue reacts to the laser beam depends on several variables including the laser wavelength, the power and energy output, the surgical technique, and the absorptive properties of the target tissue. As surgical instruments, arthroscopic laser systems have gained in popularity over the past several years, primarily as high-temperature cutting and ablation tools for thick or dense tissues such as the meniscus of the knee or the coracoacromial ligament. Only recently have some of the benefits of low-power thermal energy been studied, primarily to induce a morphologic change to the target tissue rather than to produce tissue destruction and vaporization (69–71).

In 1993, a multicenter clinical study reported a promising new treatment for patients with GHI without capsulolabral detachments or full-thickness rotator-cuff tears (78). This treatment used an arthroscopic approach for the application of low-power laser thermal energy to the synovial surface of the joint capsule (Fig. 7). The authors observed intraoperative shrinkage of the joint capsule that resulted in stabilization of the shoulder joint. Patients' subjective scores improved dramatically after surgery, with a majority returning to their previous levels of activity. Despite short-term follow-up and lack of a control group, this study demonstrated a novel approach for the treatment of joint instability through the application of thermal energy. Unpublished 2-year clinical data have supported the arthroscopic thermal approach to shoulder stabilization with more than 90% efficacy (G. Thabit, personal communication). Equally important, this study found few, if any, overt negative effects of this treatment. This approach was thought to show promise as a new treatment option for glenohumeral instability.

Basic science research on the thermal modification of collagen demonstrated that the thermal contraction of collagen is extremely sensitive to temperature and that the me-

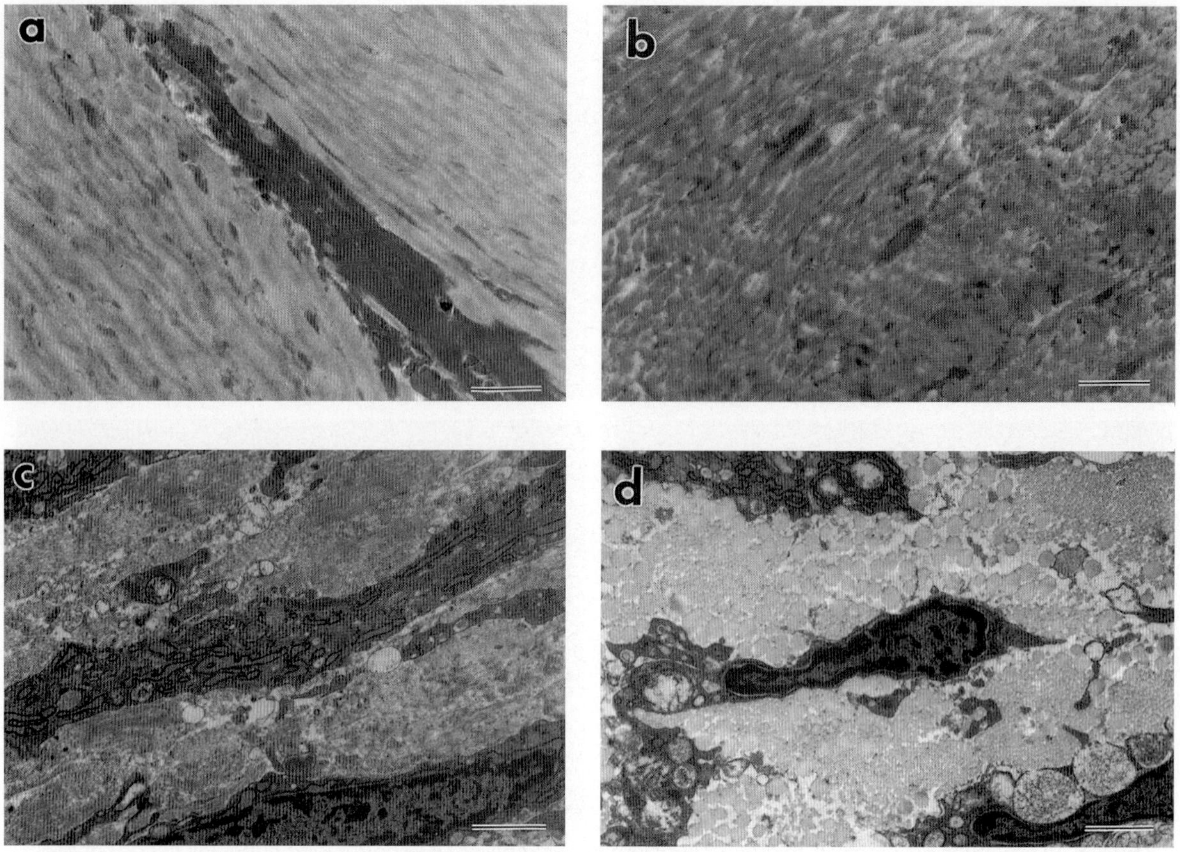

FIG. 7. Transmission electron microscopy of **(a)** laser-treated day 0 joint capsular tissue, demonstrating a pyknotic fibroblast and collagen fibrils with loss of striations; **(b)** laser-treated day 7 joint capsular tissue, demonstrating striated collagen fibrils and loss of cellularity; **(c)** laser-treated day 7 joint capsular tissue in the areas adjacent to the treated areas, demonstrating an increased number of active fibroblasts; and **(d)** laser-treated day 30 joint capsular tissue, demonstrating large and small collagen fibrils around active fibroblasts (×6,900; bar = 1 μm).

chanical properties of the tissue (at the time of shrinkage) decrease with increasing shrinkage. It is imperative that energy application to induce a thermally mediated response be accurately controlled. Unfortunately, limitations in current laser technology dictate that the surgeon visually titrate the tissue response to thermal treatment because there is no available method of reading the actual temperature delivered to the target tissue in an arthroscopic environment. Because the most widely used holmium laser is a noncontact device, energy delivery is largely dependent on surgical technique. If the probe tip is too far from the tissue, a suboptimal therapeutic effect is obtained. If the tip gets too close, there is risk of causing excessive thermal damage or cutting through the tissue. Because infrared lasers function primarily by heating intracellular water, the depth of thermal penetration is sometimes very limited and may be ineffective in situations in which deeper heating into the capsule is desired or in patients with scar formation from previous trauma or surgery. Finally, the capital outlay for an arthroscopic laser system can easily exceed $150,000, a cost profile that is becoming increasingly prohibitive in our rapidly changing medical-reimbursement environment. Design considerations of an ideal thermal probe thus dictate the requirement for temperature control/feedback. Ideally, the thermal-energy source should allow enough tissue penetration to affect the entire capsule, be safe and easy to direct to the target tissue arthroscopically, and be cost effective relative to other stabilization techniques. Radiofrequency devices developed for arthroscopic use meet or exceed the promise that arthroscopic lasers once offered, but with increased safety, ease of use, increased therapeutic reliability, and at a fraction of the cost.

BACKGROUND OF RADIOFREQUENCY ENERGY DEVICES

The concept of using RF energy in medicine is not new. The earliest investigators thought that passing currents through the body (diathermy) had certain healing properties. These therapies have enjoyed periodic interest over the past 100 years and include the use of diathermy and electromagnetic energy to accelerate soft-tissue healing and the resolution of tissue edema, as well as to promote bone healing. RF energy was first introduced as a cauterizing and cutting device for general surgery. This initiated the use of electrosurgical devices as we know them today. Electrosurgery was thought to provide less scar formation and improve hemostasis. Bovie (79) developed the cutting-wave forms in the early 1920s that led to the emergence of modern electrosurgery. RF energy was first used surgically in the late 1920s for transurethral resection of the prostate (TURP), but electrosurgery remained without significant change until the 1950s when RF energy found applications in the treatment of certain brain tumors and specific neurologic disorders (80,81). In the early 1980s, RF energy was used to ablate abnormal cardiac-conduction pathways.

Today, many endoscopic procedures use RF energy. RF generators are economic heat sources with a high degree of safety. The current literature describes numerous clinical applications for RF treatment, including tissue ablation and shrinkage in neurosurgery, gynecology, cardiology, oncology, urology, and ophthalmology (81–85). In orthopedics, RF energy has been used to remove unwanted tissue, achieve hemostasis, and accomplish denervation (1,86,87). The tip of the RF electrode comes in direct contact with the target tissue, and contact is maintained until the appropriate level of thermal energy is delivered to achieve the desired effect. The thermal effect on treated tissue is achieved through the excitation and oscillation of intracellular and extracellular electrolytes. The application of RF energy produces a well-defined area of tissue heating, with the effect on the tissue dictated by the power settings and the type of tissue treated.

An RF thermal-feedback arthroscopic probe (Oratec Interventions, Inc., Menlo Park, CA, U.S.A.) that the Food and Drug Administration has approved for soft-tissue coagulation has been developed and used successfully in performing electrothermally-assisted capsulorrhaphy of the shoulder. The RF probe can be set at a specific temperature, and a built-in thermocouple controls the current application at the probe tip. We believe that this provides the highest margin of safety and efficacy in the application of thermal energy for capsulorrhaphy. In addition, these temperature-controlled probes are malleable, which facilitates access to specific areas within a joint. Various sizes are under development for both small- and large-joint use with various tip designs to carry out specific applications, including capsule and ligament shrinkage, coagulation, or soft-tissue ablation and vaporization. More than 200 arthroscopic shoulder stabilizations have been performed with temperature-controlled RF instrumentation, and a new multicenter study is under way for further evaluation of its use alone and in conjunction with other arthroscopic procedures.

SURGICAL TECHNIQUE

Arthroscopic Thermal Shoulder Stabilization

Arthroscopic thermal stabilization of the shoulder requires no special set-up or alteration of arthroscopy fluids. Either the lateral decubitus or beach-chair position can be chosen based on the surgeon's preference. After the examination under anesthesia, a standard posterior arthroscopy portal is used to initiate a diagnostic arthroscopy. A standard anterior portal is created at the upper border of the subscapularis tendon through the rotator interval. A disposable cannula in this portal allows the easy introduction of the thermally-assisted capsulorrhaphy (TAC) probe but is not mandatory. The TAC probe is directed down into the axillary pouch. Typically, a 30-degree bend placed near the tip of the probe facilitates passage around the curved articular surfaces of the glenoid and humeral head (Fig. 8). With the RF generator set at 35 W and 65°C, the probe is deliv-

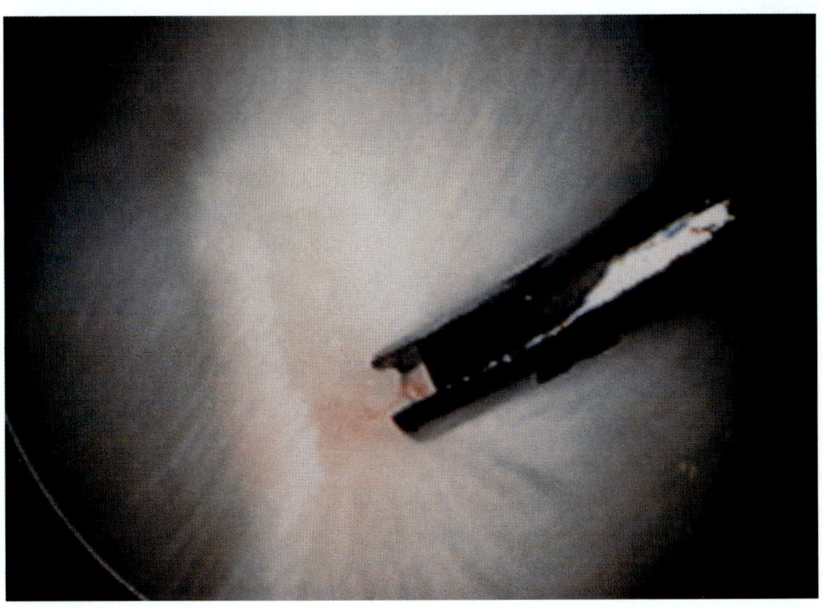

FIG. 8. Arthroscopic thermal plication of anterior inferior shoulder capsule by using holmium:yttrium aluminum garnet (YAG) laser at 10 W, 1.0 joules per pulse.

ered in a contact fashion along the capsule from the glenoid toward the humeral head and back toward the glenoid. The TAC probe is thus slowly swept back and forth along the capsule while the surgeon visually inspects for the capsular response. The probe, through tissue contact, delivers RF energy, which then heats the tissue. The thermocouple in the probe tip measures tissue temperature through conduction, and thus accurate tissue temperature is best obtained by leaving the probe in direct contact with the tissue. Moving the probe too quickly in the fluid medium makes it more difficult for the electrothermal generator to maintain the set temperature. Thus, in this setting, moving the probe tip slowly actually results in a quicker and more effective capsule response. Typically, after a 1- to 2-second lag, during which the treated tissue is heating up, the capsule dramatically shrinks, and the axillary recess is drawn up, eliminating some of the capsular redundancy (Fig. 9). This technique is then continued toward the anterior inferior and anterior portions of the capsule. Those areas of the capsule that have a higher collagen density respond more dramatically, especially the areas of the inferior and middle glenohumeral ligaments (Fig. 10). Some areas of the capsule near the axillary recess and between the ligament structures are fairly thin and do not contract so much. Capsular tightening is dependent on both heat and time. For greater capsular contraction, the probe is left stationary for a few seconds until the desired amount of shrinkage is obtained. The procedure continues anteriorly to the top of the middle glenohumeral ligament and to the rotator interval of the capsule if desired. In patients with multidirectional instability, the posterior and inferior portions of the capsule are tightened in a similar fashion. This can be done by creating an accessory posterior portal approximately 1.5 cm below the standard posterior portal and introducing the probe parallel to the arthroscope (Fig. 11). Alternatively, the arthroscope can be switched to an anterior portal, and the TAC probe brought in through the posterior portal. Areas of the capsule tighten variably depending on the collagen content/thickness of the capsule. The least responsive area is the posterior superior capsule. If a capsulolabral detachment is encountered, the TAC procedure can be used as an adjunct to arthroscopic capsulolabral-reattachment procedures. Arthroscopic repair of the Bankart lesion is typically performed after the TAC-shift procedure, although it may be done before as well. Prior studies of arthroscopic Bankart repairs implicated the inability to address capsular laxity effectively as being a cause of failure (33,36,37,43). The importance of addressing all of the pathology involved, including capsular laxity, was emphasized (88,89). If only a portion of the pathology is addressed, higher failure rates can be expected. The TAC procedure may be an easy and cost-effective means for enhancing joint stability when used alone or in combination with an arthroscopic Bankart repair. We believe its use will improve the success rate of arthroscopic-stabilization procedures.

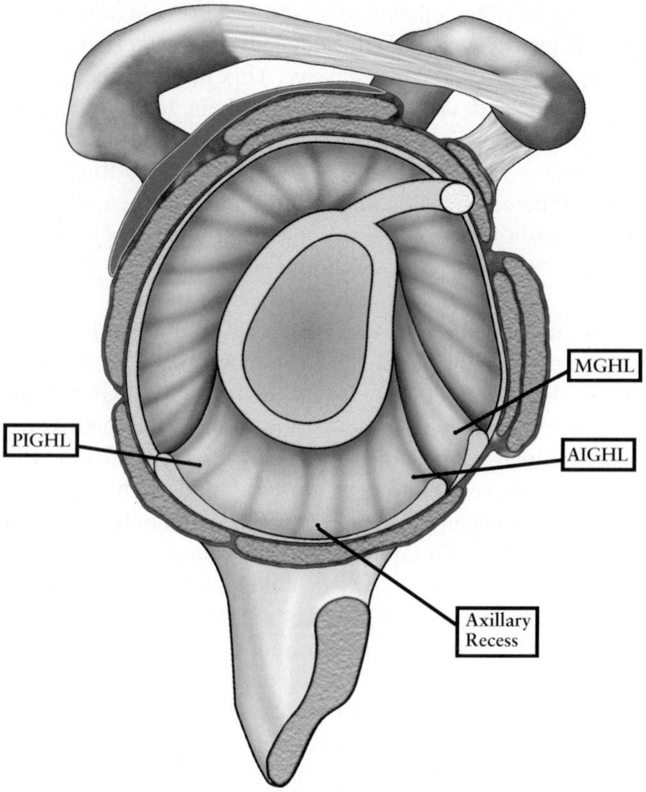

FIG. 10. Cross-section of glenohumeral joint capsule, demonstrating thick collagen condensations that correspond to the anterior and posterior ligament structures, with relatively thin collagen layering in the region of the central axillary pouch.

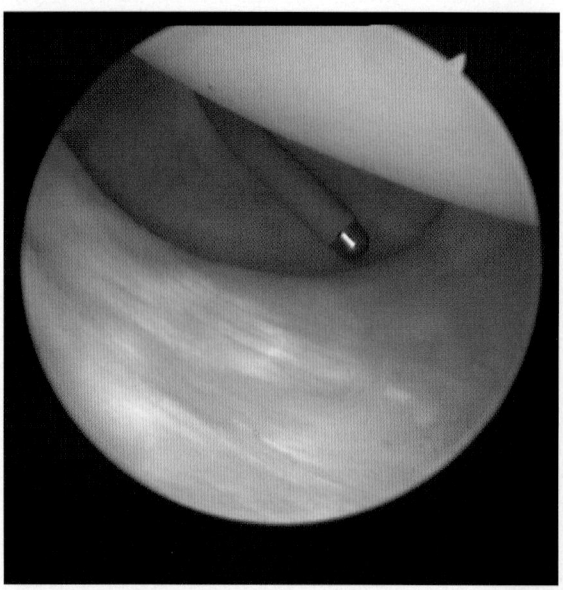

FIG. 9. Temperature-regulated radiofrequency thermal capsule shift of the anterior inferior glenohumeral ligament complex. Note shrinkage and advancement of redundant capsule tissue at 35 W, 65°C.

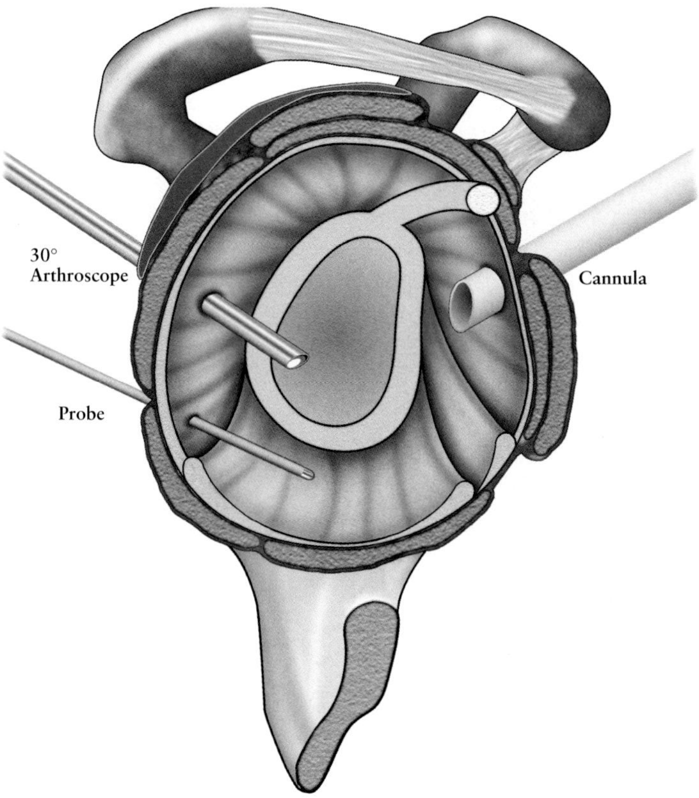

FIG. 11. Accessory posterior shoulder portal created 1.5 cm directly below the primary arthroscope portal to provide access to the inferiormost regions of the joint capsule.

EARLY CLINICAL RESULTS OF THE THERMALLY-ASSISTED CAPSULORRHAPHY PROCEDURE

Success with the TAC procedure has been reported at symposia in more than 500 patients with follow-ups ranging from 1 to 4 years (79,90). All procedures were performed with the holmium laser and more recently with the temperature-controlled RF probe. Clinical indications have included unidirectional and multidirectional instability in isolation or associated with other pathologies, most commonly capsulolabral avulsion or rotator-cuff inflammation. Because of mixed pathologies, many of these reports remain anecdotal. However, the consensus of physicians supports success rates of more than 90% in restoring stability and function with a minimum of 2 years' follow-up and a very high patient-satisfaction rate. Retrospective studies are under way. Thermal capsule shift appears especially useful in improving the results of arthroscopic capsule reattachment, in which tightening of the patulous anterior inferior capsule, the essential lesion in nearly all recurrent anterior instabilities, is technically very difficult and risky.

Thabit (78) performed an initial multicenter clinical trial that demonstrated improved stability and function in the vast majority of patients. Forty-one shoulders were treated in 40 patients for unidirectional or multidirectional instability without significant rotator-cuff pathology or capsule avulsion. These patients were reviewed by an independent examiner, who incorporated the data from five separate surgical practices. Laser energy was applied though a standard arthroscopic portal in a tangential, defocused manner by using 10 W (1 joule, 10 Hz) to shrink capsule ligamentous tissues of the glenohumeral joint without ablation. The laser probe was radically applied to the capsule in a paintbrush-like motion, beginning at the inferior capsule and working superiorly in a defocused manner. Standard arthroscopy portals were used. At a mean follow-up time after surgery of 6 months (range, 2 to 12 months), patients were subjectively and objectively scored by using the Carter–Rowe rating system with a total possible score of 100 points. Shoulder-evaluation scores improved from a preoperative average of 38 to a postoperative average of 88. The magnitude of luxation, including a history of recurrent dislocation, did not affect the frequency of good and excellent results, which were achieved in more than 95%. Patient satisfaction was extremely high, with 39 of 40 patients indicating they would have the procedure performed again. Thirty-one patients were competitive athletes, and all have returned to their previous levels of sports participation. Although this short-term pilot study had no comparable nonoperated-on control population or an operated-on open surgical repair group, the results indicated that instability symptoms improved dramatically after nonablative reduction of redundant glenohumeral joint capsule by using the holmium:YAG laser as the thermal energy source.

More than 150 patients have been treated with RF thermal capsulorrhaphy. Fifty-one patients have been followed up for more than 1 year, and of these, 34 patients had no associated

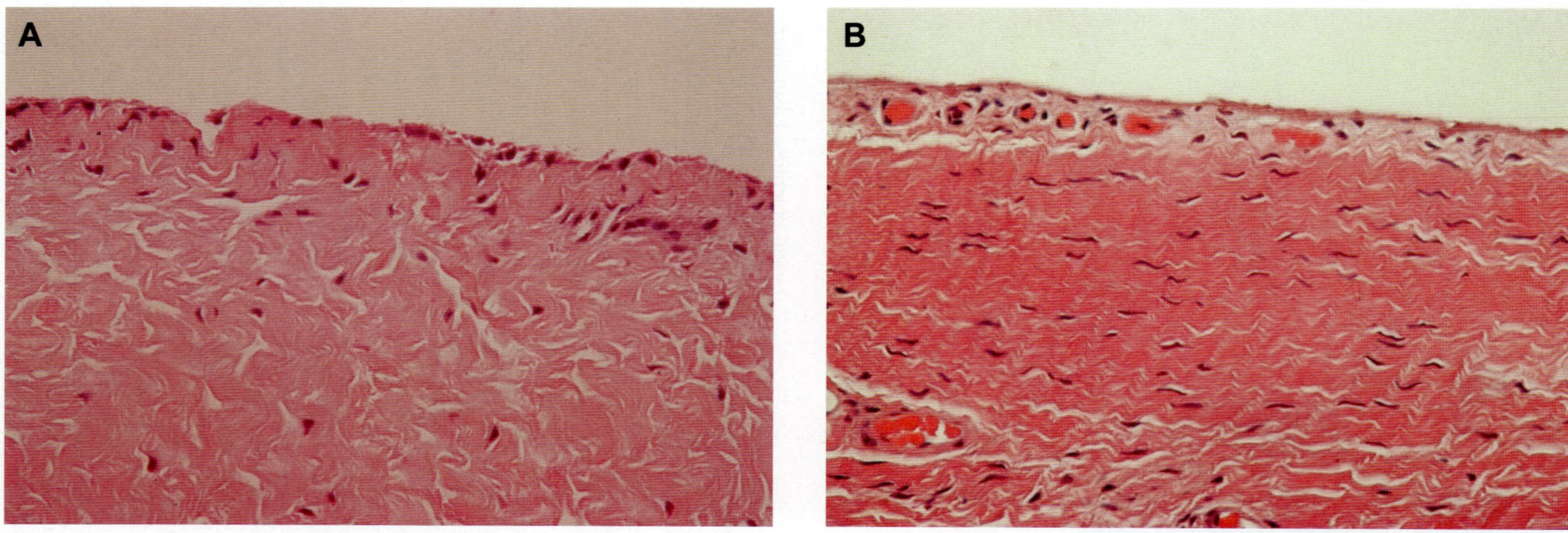

FIG. 12. A: Untreated area of capsule 9 months after thermal radiofrequency stabilization, demonstrating normal collagenous architecture. **B:** Biopsy of treated area of same shoulder capsule, revealing abundant and well-organized collagen fibrils with typical "crimping" that appears in type 1 collagen. Abundant fibroblasts are noted with no identifiable inflammatory cells.

pathology of the labrum or rotator cuff requiring additional surgical intervention. A prospective evaluation of these 34 patients was performed. The average patient age was 23 years (range, 15 to 35 years), and all patients had a minimum follow-up of 1 year, with an average follow-up of 16 months (12 to 34 months). The dominant shoulder was involved in 20 patients and the nondominant shoulder in 14. A nonoperative program of exercise and strengthening had failed for all patients before surgical intervention. The average preoperative Bankart score was 24 (range, 0 to 55), and the average postoperative Bankart score was 93 (range, 65 to 100). Patient-satisfaction rate was 97%, and 33 of 34 patients indicated that they would have the same procedure performed again under the same circumstances. Nearly all patients gained full range of motion and had improved function (91). Thirty-two of 34 patients have returned to their previous levels of work or sports, including four professional and four collegiate football players.

Postoperative capsulitis was noted in fewer than 3% of our patients and is consistent with the frequency noted with other shoulder-stabilization procedures. In this instance, rehabilitation can take up to 6 months but does not appear to affect the final outcome. One case of axillary neuritis took approximately 3 weeks to resolve. This patient had a very thin joint capsule with multidirectional instability. Only the sensory portion of the nerve was involved, and there has been no sequel. However, any surgical procedure performed at or near the 6 o'clock position at the inferior capsule warrants special precautions to avoid injury to the axillary nerve where it passes closest to the joint capsule and the inferior glenoid rim. In patients undergoing thermal stabilization of any type, it is recommended that the arm not be abducted interoperatively beyond 30 degrees to avoid pulling up the axillary nerve closer to the inferior capsule. Additionally, in patients with a very hypermobile multidirectional instability and thin joint capsule, the temperature and power settings on the RF generator should be turned down to 60° and 25 W and gradually increased until the desired capsule response is observed. Alternatively, the inferior capsule between the 5 o'clock and 7 o'clock position can be left untreated in these patients.

One patient in our series had a recurrence of instability that required a subsequent open stabilization. Biopsy specimens from the treated and untreated portions of the capsule at 9 months after the initial TAC procedure showed a significant increase in dense collagenization, increased fibroblasts, and increased vascularization along the synovial surface of the treated capsule, evidence of a "scaffold-like" function of the tightened capsule (Fig. 12). Further animal studies to elucidate better the contribution of the healing response to improved shoulder stability are under way. There have been no reported infections, instrument breakage, or damage to non-target tissue associated with the RF instrumentation. Overall, the risks and complications of performing the RF TAC procedure appear to be equal to or better than those with other arthroscopic-stabilization techniques.

SUMMARY

The TAC procedure appears to be a safe and effective technique for enhancing shoulder stability, either in isolation or when used in combination with an arthroscopic Bankart repair. The thermal contraction of collagen is a result of a conformational change in the collagen protein that occurs when sufficient energy is delivered to disrupt the stabilizing bonds. The relations between tissue shrinkage, time, and temperature, as well as the change in initial mechanical properties, have been studied. Other studies and biopsy specimens have suggested that the thermally contracted tissue may serve as a scaffold for new tissue ingrowth. Work is under way to assess the healing response and time needed to restore mechanical properties. Clinical experience has suggested that 4 to 6 weeks of relative protection is sufficient, with normal strength and range of motion being reasonable goals at 3 months.

Increased shrinkage at temperatures above the "therapeutic" range may significantly alter mechanical properties. A thermocouple-controlled RF device developed for soft-tissue coagulation may provide an arthroscopic method for addressing pathologic capsular laxity that is technically straightforward, cost-effective, and reproducible. Further study is needed to determine the long-term biomechanical properties of thermally treated ligaments, and investigations are under way to evaluate clinical efficacy in other joints that are subject to instability.

REFERENCES

1. Cofield RH, Kavanagh BF, Frassica FJ. Anterior shoulder instability. *Instr Course Lect* 1985;34:210–217.
2. Hovelius L. Anterior dislocation of the shoulder in teenagers and young adults. *J Bone Joint Surg [Am]* 1987;69:393–399.
3. Hovelius L, Eriksson K, Fredin H, et al. Recurrences after initial dislocation of the shoulder: results of a prospective study of treatment. *J Bone Joint Surg [Am]* 1983;65:343–349.
4. Rowe CR, Sakellarides HT. Factors related to recurrences of anterior dislocation of the shoulder. *Clin Orthop* 1961;20:40–48.
5. Henry JH, Genung JA. Natural history of glenohumeral dislocation, revisited. *Am J Sports Med* 1982;10:135–137.
6. McLaughlin HL, Cavallaro WW. Primary anterior dislocation of the shoulder. *Am J Surg* 1950;80:615.
7. Rowe CR. Dislocations of the shoulder. In: Rowe CR, ed. *The shoulder*. New York: Churchill Livingstone, 1988:165.
8. Burkhead WZ, Rockwood CA. Treatment of instability of the shoulder with an exercise program. *J Bone Joint Surg [Am]* 1992;74:890–896.
9. Collins HR, Wilde AH. Shoulder instability in athletics. *Orthop Clin North Am* 1973;4:759–774.
10. Flatow EL, Miller SR, Neer CS II. Chronic anterior dislocation of the shoulder. *J Shoulder Elbow Surg* 1993;2:2–10.
11. Gustavson KH. The function of hydroxyproline in collagens. *Nature* 1955;175:70–74.
12. Pollock RG, Bigliani LU. Glenohumeral instability: evaluation and treatment. *J Am Acad Orthop Surg* 1993;1:24–32.
13. Rockwood CA Jr. Subluxation of the shoulder: the classification, diagnosis and treatment. *Orthop Trans* 1979;3:306.
14. Simonet WT, Cofield RH. Prognosis in anterior shoulder dislocation. *Am J Sports Med* 1984;12:19–24.
15. Rowe CR, Zarins B. Recurrent transient subluxation of the shoulder. *J Bone Joint Surg [Am]* 1981;63:863–872.

16. Cooper RA, Brems JJ. The inferior capsular-shift procedure for multidirectional instability of the shoulder. *J Bone Joint Surg [Am]* 1992; 74:1516–1521.
17. Jobe FW, Giangarra CE, Kvitne RS, et al. Anterior capsulolabral reconstruction of the shoulder of athletes in overhand sports. *Am J Sports Med* 1991;19:428–434.
18. O'Driscoll SW. Atraumatic instability: pathology and pathogenesis. In: *The shoulder: a balance of mobility and stability*. Rosemont, IL: American Academy of Orthopedic Surgeons, 1993:305–316.
19. Bigliani LU, Kurzweil PR, Schwartzbach CC, Wolfe IN, Flatow EL. Inferior capsular shift procedure for anterior-inferior shoulder instability in athletes. *Am J Sports Med* 1994;22:578–584.
20. Speer KP. Anatomy and pathomechanics of a shoulder joint. *Clin Sports Med* 199514:751–760.
21. Arciero RA, Wheeler JH III, Ryan JB, McBride JT Jr. Arthroscopic Bankart repair for acute, initial anterior shoulder dislocations. Presented at the American Academy of Orthopedic Surgeons annual meeting, 1993.
22. Clarke HO. Habitual dislocation of the shoulder: the Putti-Platt operation. *J Bone Joint Surg [Br]* 1948;30:19–25.
23. Helfet AJ. Coracoid transplantation for recurring dislocation of the shoulder. *J Bone Joint Surg [Br]* 1958;40:198–202.
24. Magnuson PS, Stack JK. Recurrent dislocations of the shoulder. *JAMA* 1943;123:889–892.
25. Neer CS II, Foster CR. Inferior capsular shift for involuntary inferior and multidirectional instability of the shoulder: a preliminary report. *J Bone Joint Surg [Am]* 1980;62:897–908.
26. Hawkins RH, Hawkins RJ. Failed anterior reconstruction for shoulder instability. *J Bone Joint Surg [Br]* 1985;67:709–714.
27. Rowe CR, Zarins B, Ciullo JV. Recurrent transient subluxation of the shoulder after surgical repair. *J Bone Joint Surg [Am]* 1984;66:159–168.
28. Warner JP, Marks PH. Management of complications of surgery for anterior shoulder instability. *Sports Med Arthrosc Rev* 1933;1:272–292.
29. Altchek DW, Warren RF. Arthroscopic anterior stabilization in patients without labral detachment. Presented at Annual Meeting of Arthroscopy Association of North America, Boston, Massachusetts, 1992.
30. Altchek DW, Warren RF, Skyhar MJ, Ortiz G. T-Plasty modification of the Bankart procedure for multidirectional instability of the anterior and inferior types. *J Bone Joint Surg [Am]* 1991;73:105–112.
31. Bigliani LU. Anterior and posterior capsular shift for multidirectional instability. *Tech Orthop* 1989;3:36–45.
32. Rowe CR, Patel D, Southmayd WW. The Bankart procedure: a long-term end-result study. *J Bone Joint Surg* 1978;60:1–16.
33. Green MR, Christensen KP. Arthroscopic versus open Bankart procedures: a comparison of early morbidity and complications. *J Arthrosc Rel Surg* 1993;9 (4):371–374.
34. Altchek DW. Arthroscopic shoulder stabilization using a biodegradable fixation device. *Sports Med Arthrosc Rev* 1993;1:266–271.
35. Altchek DW, Skyhar MJ, Warren RF. Shoulder arthroscopy for shoulder instability. *Instr Course Lect* 1989;38:187–198.
36. Caspari RB, Savoie FH. Arthroscopic reconstruction of the shoulder: the Bankart repair. In: McGinty JB, Caspari RB, Jackson RW, Poehling GG, eds. *Operative arthroscopy*. New York: Raven Press, 1991: 507–515.
37. Green MR, Christensen KP. Arthroscopic Bankart procedure: two to five year follow-up with clinical correlation to severity of glenoid labral lesion. *Am J Sports Med* 1995;23 (3):276–282.
38. Johnson LL. Arthroscopic management of shoulder instability: stapling. Presented at the Arthroscopy Association of North America annual meeting, 1988.
39. Matthews LS, Vetter WL, Oweida SJ, Spearman J, Helfet DL. Arthroscopic staple capsulorrhaphy for recurrent anterior shoulder instability. *Arthroscopy* 1989;4:106–111.
40. Morgan CD, Bodenstab AB. Arthroscopic Bankart suture repair: technique and early results. *Arthroscopy* 1987;3:111–122.
41. Smith JB, Nance TA. Laser energy in arthroscopic surgery. In: *Orthopedic Surgery*. New York: McGraw-Hill, 1989:44–67.
42. Pankhurst K. Incipient shrinkage of collagen and gelatin. *Nature* 1947;159:538.
43. Thomas SC, Matsen FA III. An approach to the repair of avulsion of the glenohumeral ligaments in the management of traumatic anterior glenohumeral instability. *J Bone Joint Surg* 1989;71:506–513.
44. Verzar F. Aging of the collagen fiber. In: Hall DA, ed. *International review of connective tissue research*, vol. 2. New York: Academic Press, 1964:243–300.
45. Rasmussen DM, Khalil GW, Winkelmann RK. Isotonic and isometric thermal contraction of human dermis. I. Technique and controlled study. *J Invest Dermatol* 1964;43 (5):333–339.
46. Tanzer ML. Cross-linking of collagen: endogenous aldehydes in collagen react in several ways to form a variety of unique covalent cross-links. *Science* 1973;180 (86):561–566.
47. Birk, DE, Silver FH, Trelstad RL. Matrix assembly. In: Hay ED, ed. *Cell biology of extracellular matrix*. 2nd ed. New York: Plenum Press, 1991;221.
48. Katz EP, Li ST. The intermolecular space of reconstituted collagen fibrils. *J Mol Biol* 1973;73:351–369.
49. Hodge AJ, Petruska JA. In: Ramachandran GN, ed. *Aspects of protein structure*. London: Academic Press, 1963:239.
50. Smith JW. Packing arrangement of tropocollagen molecules. *Nature* 1965;205:356–8.
51. Bear RS. The structure of collagen fibrils. In: Anson ML, Bailey K, Edsall JT, eds. *Advances in protein chemistry*, vol. VII. New York: Academic Press, 1952:69–160.
52. Flory PJ. Role of crystallization in polymers and proteins. *Science* 1956;124 (3211):53–60.
53. Gustavson KH. *The chemistry and reactivity of collagen*. New York: Academic Press, 1956.
54. Lennox FG. Shrinkage of collagen. *Biochim Biophys Acta* 1949;3: 170–187.
55. Weiderhorn NM, Reardon GV, Browne AR. Studies concerned with the structure of collagen: stress strain behavior of thermally contracted formaldehyde tanned collagen. *J Am Leather Chemists Assoc* 1959; 48:7–18.
56. Brown PC, Consden BR, Glynn LE. Observations on the shrink temperature of collagen and its variations with age and disease. *Ann Rheum Dis* 1958;17:196–208.
57. Rigby BJ. Two-stage contraction in rat tail tendon. *Biochim Biophys Acta* 1961;47:534–538.
58. Compton, ED. Effect of tannage on strength of collagen fibers. *J Am Leather Chemists Assoc* 1949;44:140–151.
59. Stryer L. *Biochemistry*. 3rd ed. San Francisco: WH Freeman, 1988: 191.
60. Weir CE. Rate of shrinkage of tendon collagen: heat, entropy and free energy of activation of the shrinkage of untreated tendon; effect of acid salt, pickle, and tannage on the activation of tendon collagen. *J Am Leather Chem Assoc* 1949;44:108–138.
61. Berg RA, Prockop DJ. The thermal transition of a nonhydroxylated form of collagen: evidence for a role for hydroxyproline in stabilizing the triple helix of collagen. *Biochem Biophys Res Commun* 1973;52 (1):115–120.
62. Rigby BJ. Hydroxyproline and the shrinkage temperature of collagen. *Nature* 1960;187–9:150–1.
63. Brown PC, Consden R. Variations with age of shrinkage temperature of human collagen. *Nature* 1958;181:349–356.
64. Rasmussen DM, Khalil GW, Winkelmann RK. Isotonic and isometric thermal contraction of human dermis. II. Age-related changes. *J Invest Dermatol* 1964;43 (5):341–348.
65. Allain JC, Le Lous M, Bazin S, Bailey AJ, Delaunay A. Isometric tension developed during heating of collagenous tissues: relationships with collagen cross-linking. *Biochim Biophys Acta* 1978;533:147–155.
66. Kohn RR, Rollerson E. Relationship of age to swelling properties of human diaphragm tendon in acid and alkaline solutions. *J Gerontol* 1958;13:241–247.
67. Rigby BJ. Thermal transition in different mammalian collagen-bearing structures. *Biochim Biophys Acta* 1963;75:279–281.
68. Wall MS, Deng XH, Torzilli PA, Doty SB, O'Brien SJ, Warren RF. Thermal modification of collagen. *J Shoulder Elbow Surg*.
69. Hayashi K, Markel MD, Thabit G III, et al. The effect of nonablative laser energy on joint capsular properties: an in vitro mechanical study using a rabbit model. *Am J Sports Med* 1995;23:482–487.
70. Hayashi K, Nieckarz JA, Thabit G III, Bogdanske JJ, Cooley AJ, Markel MD. Effect of nonablative laser energy on the joint capsule:

an in vivo rabbit study using a Holmium:YAG laser. *Lasers Surg Med* 1997;20:164–171.
71. Hayashi K, Thabit G III, Bogdanske JJ, Mascio LN, Markel MD. The effect of nonablative laser energy on the ultrastructure of joint capsular collagen. *Arthroscopy* 1996;12:474–481.
72. Hayashi K, Thabit G III, Vailas AC, Bogdanske JJ, Cooley AJ, Markel MD. The effect of nonablative laser energy joint capsular properties: an in vivo histologic and biochemical study using a rabbit model. *Am J Sports Med* 1996;24:640.
73. Fanton GS, Dillingham MF. Arthroscopic menisectomy using holmium: YAG laser: a double-blind study. Presented at the Arthroscopy Association of North America Annual Meeting, 1990.
74. Fanton GS, Dillingham MF. The use of the holmium:YAG laser in arthroscopic surgery. *Semin Orthop* 1992;7:102–116.
75. O'Brien SJ, Fealy S, Miller DV. Nd:YAG laser arthroscopy. *Semin Orthop* 1992;7:117–124.
76. Sherk HH. Current concepts review: the use of lasers in orthopedic procedures. *J Bone Joint Surg* 1993;75:768–776.
77. Miller DV, O'Brien SJ, Arnoczky SS, Kelly A, Fealy SV, Warren RF. The use of the contact Nd:YAG laser in arthroscopic surgery: effects on articular cartilage and meniscal tissue. *Arthroscopy* 1989;5: 245–253.
78. Thabit G. Treatment of unidirectional and multidirectional glenohumeral instability by an arthroscopic holmium:YAG laser-assisted capsular shift procedure: laser application in arthroscopy. Presented at the 1st Congress of International Musculoskeletal Laser Society, 1994.
79. Bovie WT. A preliminary note on a new surgical-current generator. *Surg Gynecol Obstet* 1928;47:751–784.
80. Aronow S. The use of radio-frequency power in making lesions in the brain. *J Neurosurg* 1960;17:431.
81. Sweet WH, Wepsic JG. Controlled thermocoagulation of trigeminal ganglion and rootlets for differential destruction of pain fibers. Part 1: Trigeminal neuralgia. *J Neurosurg* 1974;40:143–156.
82. Aquavella JV, Smith RS, Shaw EL. Alterations in corneal morphology following thermokeratoplasty. *Arch Ophthalmol* 1976;94:2082–2085.
83. Goldwasser B, Ramon J, Engelberg S, et al. Transurethral needle ablation (TUNA) of the prostate using low-level radiofrequency energy: an animal experimental study. *Eur Urol* 1993;24:400–405.
84. Haines DE. The biophysics of radiofrequency catheter ablation in the heart. *PACE Pacing Clin Electrophysiol* 1993;16:586–591.
85. LeVeen HH, Ahmed N, Piccone VA, Shugaar S, Falk G. Radio-frequency therapy: clinical experience. *Ann N Y Acad Sci* 1980;335:363–371.
86. Sherk HH, Black JD, Prodoehl JA, Diven J. The effects of lasers and electrosurgical devices on human meniscal tissue. *Clin Orthop* 1995;310:14–20.
87. Voyles CR, Petro AB, Meena AL, Haick AJ, Koury AM. A practical approach to laparoscopic cholecystectomy. *Am J Surg* 1991;161L: 365–371.
88. Lebar RD, Alexander AH. Multidirection shoulder instability. Clinical results of inferior capsular shift in the active-duty population. *Am J Sports Med* 1992;20:193–198.
89. Matsen FA III, Zuckerman JD. Anterior glenohumeral instability. *Clin Sports Med* 1983;2:379–348.
90. Savoie FH. Thermal stabilization of the shoulder joint. Presented at the Workshop Symposium on Thermal Shoulder Surgery, San Diego, California, April 1997.
91. Fanton GS. Electrothermally-assisted capsule shift (ETAC) procedure for shoulder instability. Presented at the Australia Orthopedic Association, closed shoulder session, October 1997.
92. Cobb CA, Fung D. Quantitative analysis of lesion parameters in radiofrequency trigeminal rhizotomy. *J Neurosurg* 1983;58:388–391.
93. Pagnani MJ, Warren RF. Multidirectional instability: medial T-plasty and selective capsular repairs. *Sports Med Arthrosc Rev* 1939;1:249–258.

Section 5

Special Considerations

The Unstable Shoulder,
edited by R.F. Warren, E.V. Craig, and D.W. Altchek.
Lippincott–Raven Publishers, Philadelphia © 1999.

CHAPTER 23

SLAP Lesions and Lesions of the Long Head of the Biceps Tendon

Treatment Considerations

Mark H. Getelman and Stephen J. Snyder

Shoulder arthroscopy is now routinely used by orthopedic surgeons. Consequently, we can often recognize intra-articular pathology that was previously not appreciated with open surgical techniques. Arthroscopy allows the visualization of the entire glenoid labrum, and our knowledge of this structure has advanced dramatically. Tears of the superior labrum from anterior to posterior, SLAP lesions, are now well recognized. With the improved techniques of magnetic resonance imaging (MRI) and with the advent of magnetic resonance arthrography (MRA), these lesions can be diagnosed more accurately. This understanding has led to improved techniques for treatment. Presently, SLAP lesions can be treated arthroscopically with a high success rate. In this chapter, we review the normal and pathologic labral anatomy, discuss the biomechanics of the labrum and biceps tendon, and outline the diagnosis, classification, and treatment of SLAP lesions. In addition, we describe the latest information regarding lesions involving the long head of the biceps tendon and outline our approach to treatment.

ANATOMY AND BIOMECHANICS

In 1953, Gardner and Gray (1) detailed the embryologic development of the glenohumeral joint and glenoid labrum. In early fetal development, they identified an area of condensed precartilage cells called the interzone (Fig. 1). This three-layered area eventually forms the joint line and subsequently develops into the biceps tendon, glenoid labrum, capsule, and subscapularis muscle. The labrum then further changes from the primitive mesenchymal tissue to a fibrocartilaginous structure during the first decade of life (2).

The fully developed glenoid labrum is composed of fibrocartilage distinct from the adjacent articular hyaline cartilage of the glenoid and the fibrous tissue of the joint capsule (2). The labrum is often more developed posteriorly than anteriorly, and the superior labrum attachment may be meniscal in nature, attaching loosely to the underlying glenoid (3). On the inner side, the labrum becomes continuous with the hyaline cartilage of glenoid, and the outer side becomes continuous with the fibrous tissue of the capsule. The capsule then covers the periphery of the labrum and attaches broadly to the scapular neck. Histologic examination reveals the labrum to have delicate, short elastin fibers interspersed within the fibrocartilaginous matrix. The fibrocartilaginous interzone is routinely seen in the superior, anterior, and posterior labrum, but is not seen inferiorly (4).

Several different authors performed cadaveric dissections to look at the anatomy of the labrum (3,5,6). They all noted that there can be some variability in the gross labral appearance. Typically, the posterior and inferior labrum have the most consistent appearance (4). However, in the anterosuperior (AS) quadrant, consistent anatomic variables have been described and can be visualized arthroscopically. First, a meniscoid labrum may be noted superiorly. In these cases, a free edge on the labrum can extend onto the glenoid surface (Fig. 2). Although this can appear pathologic, careful examination reveals that the articular cartilage of the superior glenoid will extend onto the glenoid neck where the labrum is attached.

There can also be variability with the insertions of the middle glenohumeral ligament (MGHL). The usual appear-

M. H. Getelman and S. J. Snyder: Southern California Orthopedic Institute, Van Nuys, California 91405.

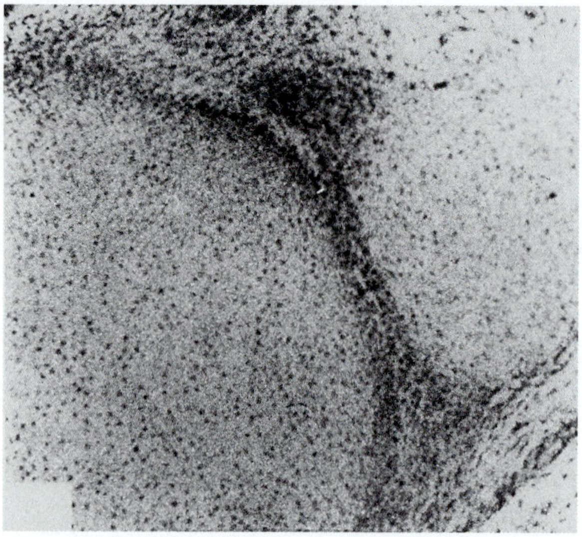

FIG. 1. Three-layered interzone. The early formation of the glenoid labrum can be seen. (From Gardner E, Gray DJ. Prenatal development of the human shoulder and acromioclavicular joint. *Am J Anat* 1953;92:219, with permission.)

ance of the MGHL is a sheet-like structure that drapes over the subscapularis tendon at a 45-degree angle (Fig. 3). However, in approximately 19% of shoulders, there is thickening of the ligament rather than the usual sheet-like structure (7). We describe this as a cord-like MGHL. The cord may attach to its usual position at the neck of the superior glenoid, or it may be associated with a sublabral hole where there is a bare area on the glenoid in the 2 o'clock position (Fig. 4). A Buford complex is another variant seen in approximately 1.5% of shoulders (7,8). This involves a cord-like MGHL that attaches to the base of the biceps anchor with the absence of labral tissue on the anterior superior glenoid (Fig. 5). This is important to recognize as a normal variant. It can be quite striking and may mistakenly appear to be an avulsion of the anterior superior labrum or MGHL or both.

The vascularity of the labrum has been well studied. Branches of the suprascapular, circumflex scapular, and posterior circumflex humeral arteries all contribute to the labrum. The blood supply arises from the capsular or periosteal vessels rather than from the underlying bone (3). The vessels are concentrated more peripherally and penetrate the labrum both radially and circumferentially (9). The blood supply to the superior labrum is less abundant; with increasing age, the blood supply has been shown to decrease (2). These findings help explain the degeneration of the labrum that occurs with aging and the limited healing potential for SLAP lesions.

The long head of the biceps tendon arises from the supraglenoid tubercle and the superior glenoid labrum (3,10). It is common for a significant portion of the biceps tendon to be attached to the glenoid labrum, with only a small portion attached to the supraglenoid tubercle. The attachment is often toward the posterior aspect of the labrum from the 12 o'clock position. The tendon is covered by a synovial membrane reflection in the intertubercular groove, making it intra-articular but extrasynovial (3). It is stabilized in the groove by the coracohumeral ligament proximally. The transverse humeral ligament and fibers of the subscapularis tendon stabilize the biceps more distally in the groove.

BIOMECHANICS

The shoulder is the least constrained joint in the body and thus is highly dependent on the surrounding soft-tissue envelope to provide stability. The humeral head is maintained in the glenoid fossa by compressive muscular forces and the concave glenoid structure, which act in concert to provide stability. This is commonly referred to as the concavity–compression mechanism. It is most important with

A

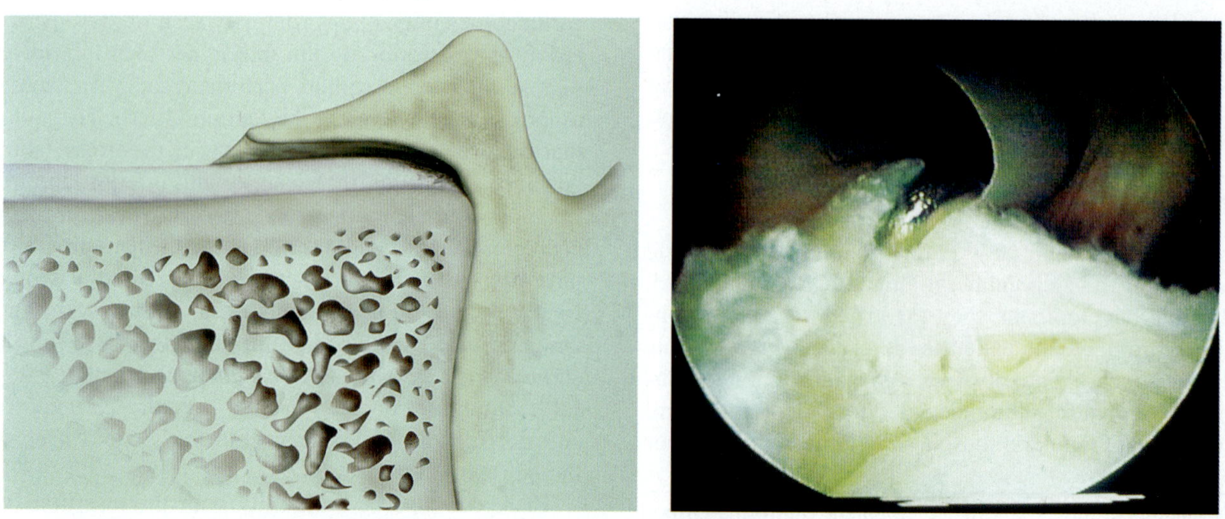

B

FIG. 2. Artist's rendition **(A)** and arthroscopic photograph **(B)** demonstrating a normal meniscoid labrum.

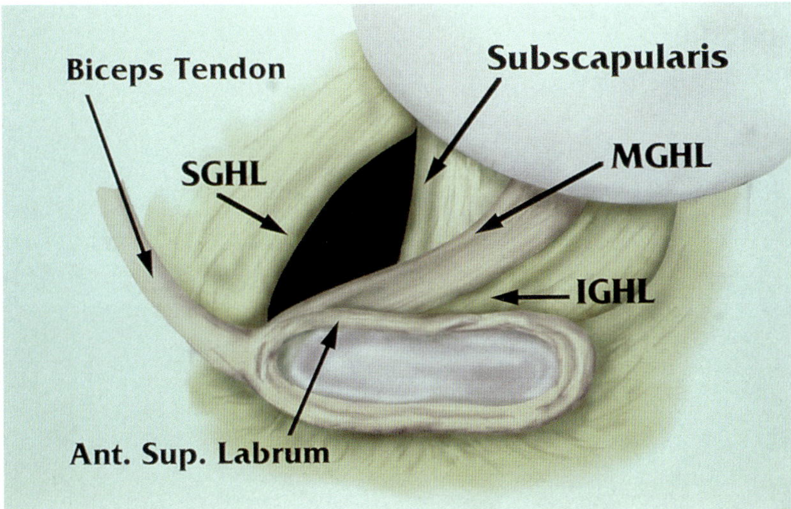

FIG. 3. Classic glenohumeral ligament pattern. *SGHL*, superior glenohumeral ligament; *MGHL*, middle glenohumeral ligament; *IGHL*, inferior glenohumeral ligament.

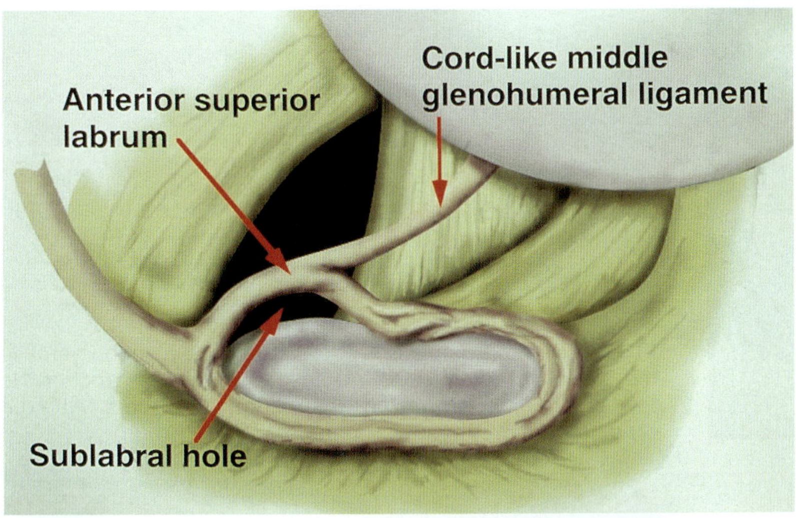

A

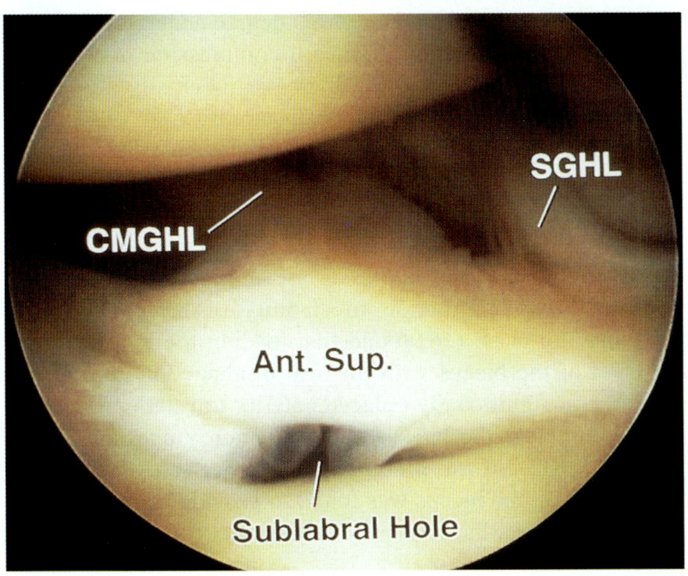

B

FIG. 4. Cord-like middle glenohumeral ligament and associated sublabral hole. **A:** Artist's rendition. **B:** Intraoperative photograph.

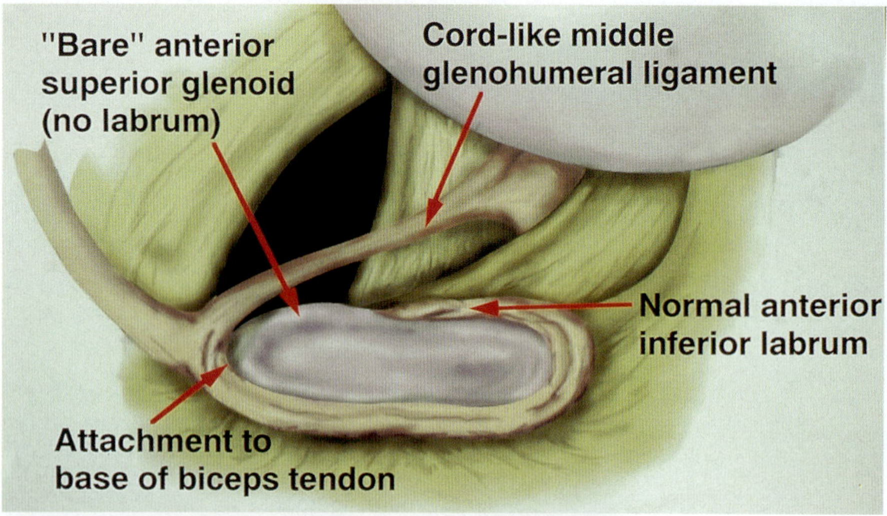

A

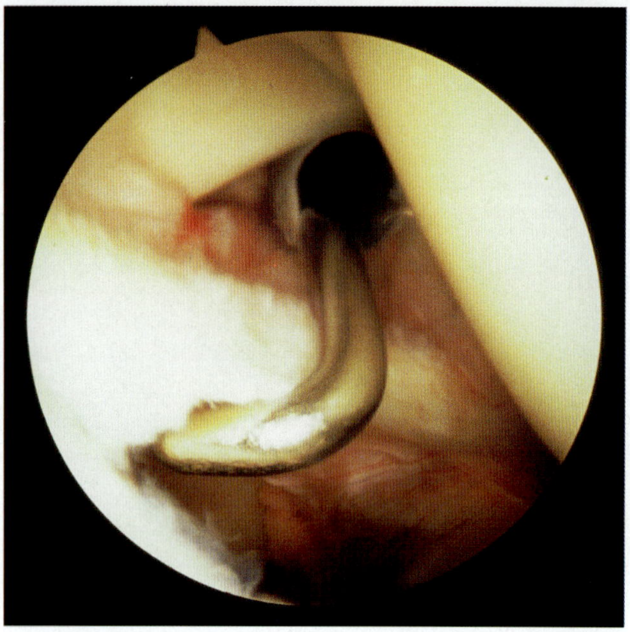

B

FIG. 5. Buford complex. A cord-like middle glenohumeral ligament (MGHL) attaches to the base of the biceps anchor. Note the absence of labrum on anterosuperior glenoid. **A:** Artist's rendition. **B:** Intraoperative photograph.

the joint in functional midrange, as the capsule and ligaments are slack in that position (11). The labrum contributes stability as well (12,13). It acts to increase the depth of the glenoid. In fact, the diameter of the glenoid surface with the attached labrum increases to 75% of the humeral head vertically and to 57% in the transverse plane, and the labrum contributes approximately 50% of the total depth of the socket (13). The combination of the glenoid–labral socket aided by the concavity–compression mechanism provides a constraining effect on the joint, thereby providing stability. A cadaveric study that created a chondral–labral defect showed an approximately 80% loss of glenoid height and an approximately 65% loss in the stability ratio for translation in the direction of the defect (11).

With regard to the superior labrum specifically, Jobe (14, 15) demonstrated that impingement of the rotator cuff may occur onto the superior labrum and lead to tearing. By using cadaveric specimens fixed in 70-degree abduction and maximal external rotation, he noted compression of the posterior superior labrum by the greater tuberosity and the interposed cuff. When anterior instability also was present, the posterior labral impingement increased. This observation may help explain the posterior labral tears commonly observed in throwers (4,14).

Whereas the long head of the biceps has been regarded as a humeral-head depressor, several recent studies confirmed its contribution to stability of the glenohumeral joint. Itoi et al. (16) found that loading the long and short head of the biceps with the arm in abduction and external rotation significantly reduced anterior translation. The loading effect of the biceps was even more important when a Bankart lesion was present. In a cadaver study by Rodosky et al. (17), the biceps was found to provide anterior stability by increasing the resistance to torsional forces in abduction and external rotation and by diminishing the stress on the inferior glenohumeral ligament (IGHL). When a superior labral lesion was created, the glenohumeral joint developed anterior instability and was less able to withstand external rotation forces in the abducted and externally rotated position. They concluded that the lack of an intact superior labrum resulted in greater stress demands on the IGHL, which could theoretically result in damage to the IGHL and allow subsequent anterior instability. Warner and McMahon (18) evaluated patients after removal of the proximal attachment of the biceps tendon with tenodesis. They noted 2 to 6 mm of superior translation of the humeral head in positions of humeral abduction. Thus, they concluded that the long head of the biceps acts as an important humeral stabilizer during shoulder abduction. Additionally, Pagnani et al. (19) found that the long head of the biceps reduced both anteroposterior (AP) and superoinferior humeral translations, suggesting that, in addition to aiding in stability, the biceps acts to center the humeral head on the glenoid, thereby providing a fulcrum to allow arm elevation.

CLASSIFICATION

The initial description of a lesion involving the superior labrum was offered by Andrews et al. (20) in 1985. They reported on a group of high-level throwing athletes, and they described changes in the AS labral tissue, which included fraying, detachment, and sometimes partial tearing of the biceps tendon. In 1990, Snyder et al. (21) at the Southern California Orthopedic Institute (SCOI) described a similar, more extensive type of injury to the superior glenoid labrum. The lesions began posterior to the biceps tendon anchor and extended anteriorly, stopping at or above the midglenoid notch. They labeled this specific injury a SLAP lesion. The arthroscopic appearance of these lesions was reviewed and then classified into four distinct types.

Type I: The superior labrum demonstrates fraying and degeneration. The attachment of the labrum to the glenoid is intact. The biceps anchor is intact (Fig. 6).

Type II: The superior labrum and biceps anchor are detached from the insertion on the superior glenoid, allowing the complex to arch away from the glenoid neck (Fig. 7).

Type III: There is a bucket-handle tear of the meniscoid superior labrum. The remaining biceps tendon and labral rim attachment are intact. This is similar to a bucket-handle tear of the knee meniscus (Fig. 8).

Type IV: There is a bucket-handle tear of the superior labrum with extension into the biceps anchor. The torn biceps tendon and the labral flap are displaced into the joint (Fig. 9).

Complex: A combination of two or more SLAP types, most commonly a combination of types II and III or types II and IV.

Recently, other investigators described three variations based on this classification of SLAP lesions (22). These include an anteroinferior Bankart lesion, which also has separation of the biceps tendon, biceps tendon separation with an unstable labral flap tear, and finally, a superior labrum–biceps lesion that extends anteriorly inferior to the middle glenohumeral ligament (MGHL). We have seen these variations; however, we prefer to use the classification based on the four basic types and describe any additional labral pathology separately.

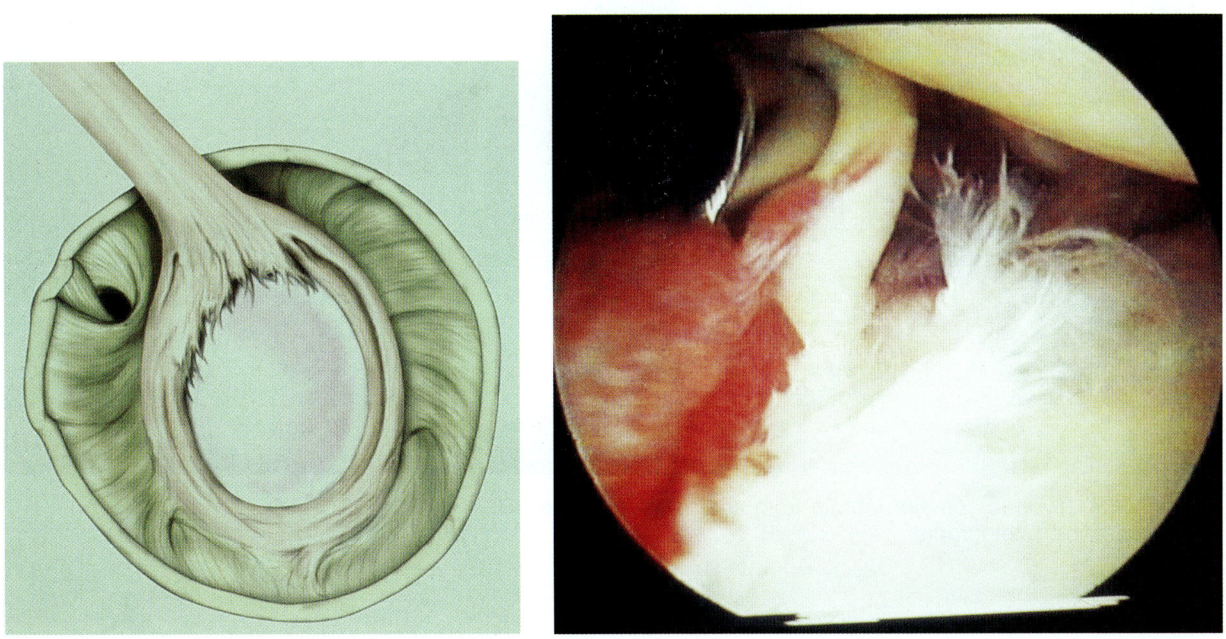

A B

FIG. 6. Type I superior labrum from anterior to posterior (SLAP) lesion. **A:** Artist's rendition. **B:** Arthroscopic photograph.

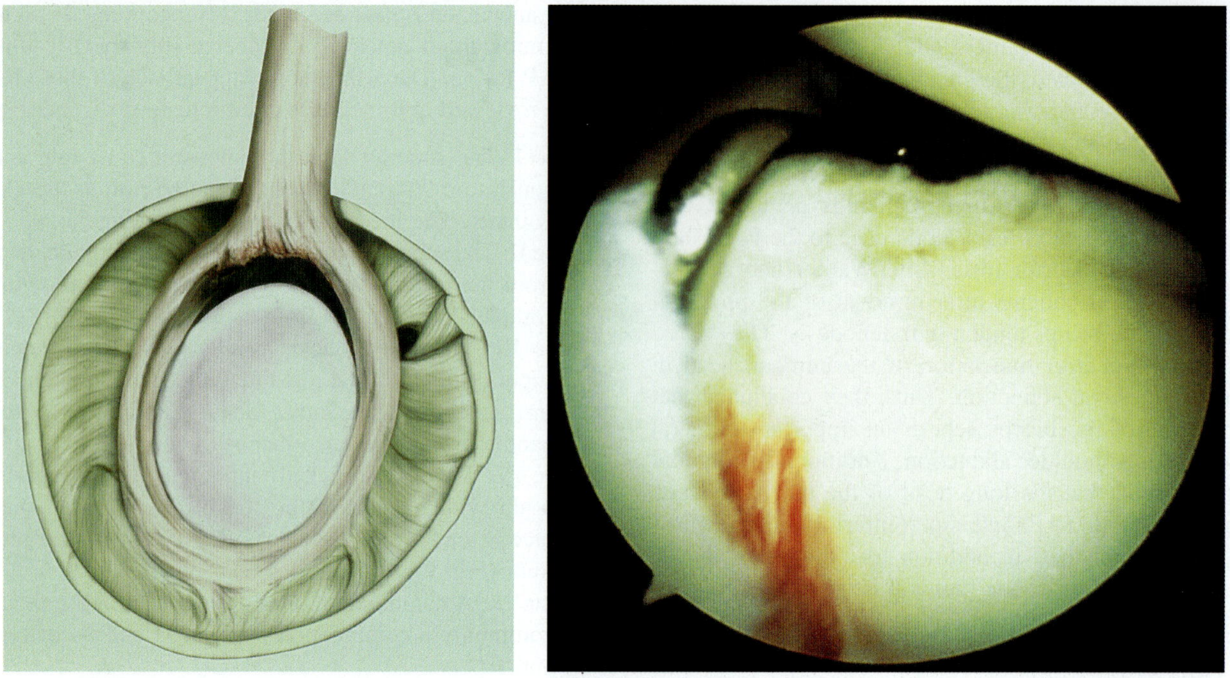

A B

FIG. 7. Type II superior labrum from anterior to posterior (SLAP) lesion. **A:** Artist's rendition. **B:** Arthroscopic photograph.

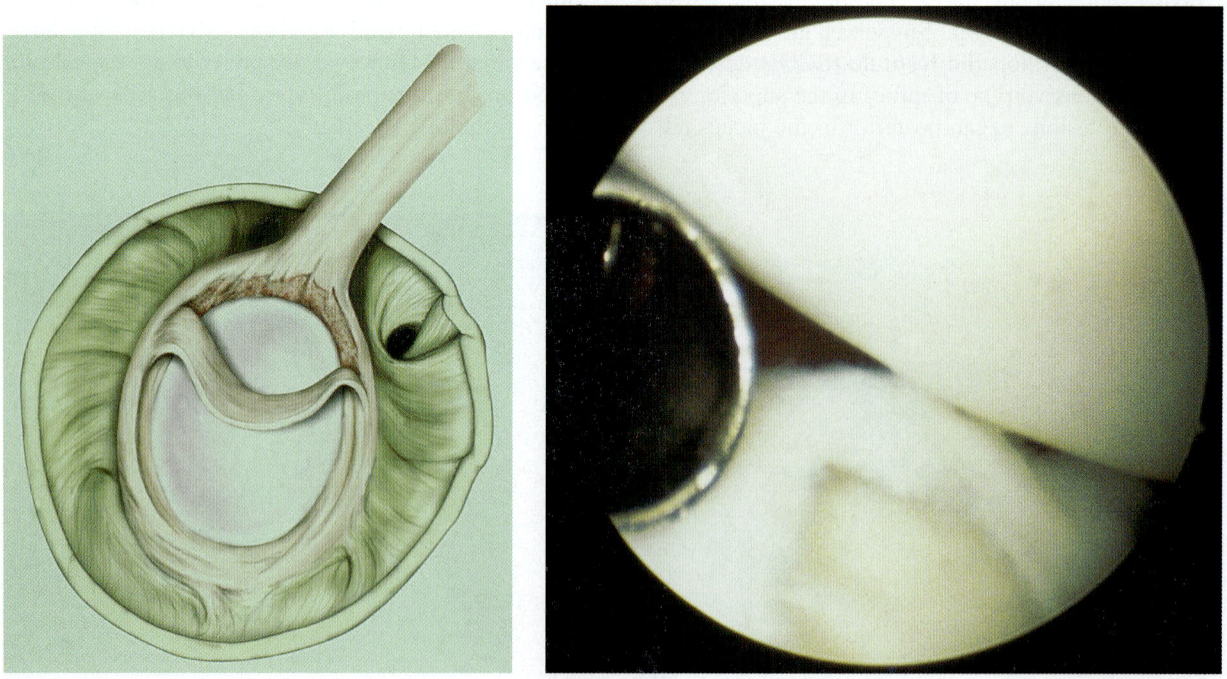

A B

FIG. 8. Type III superior labrum from anterior to posterior (SLAP) lesion. **A:** Artist's rendition. **B:** Arthroscopic photograph.

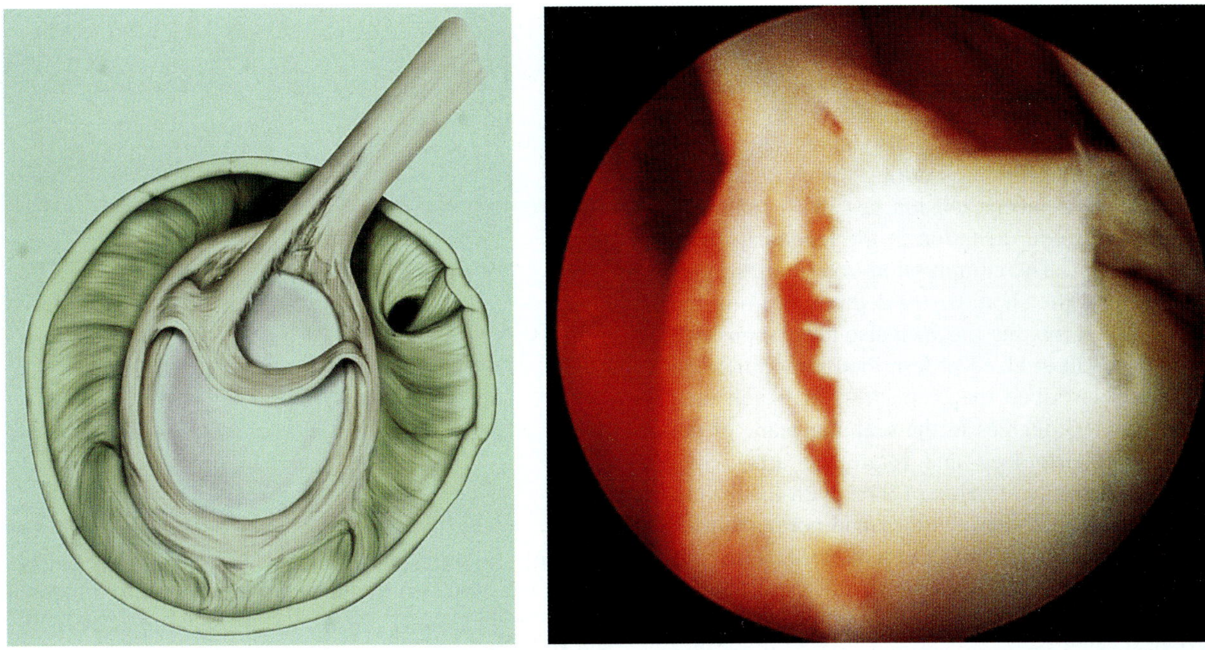
A B

FIG. 9. Type IV superior labrum from anterior to posterior (SLAP) lesion. **A:** Artist's rendition. **B:** Arthroscopic photograph.

MECHANISM OF INJURY

No controlled cadaveric studies have proved biomechanically the origin of SLAP lesions. However, several mechanisms of injury are commonly found clinically. In the original article on SLAP lesions, many patients were noted to have fallen onto an abducted and extended arm (21). This produced a compression force with impaction of the superior joint surface and proximal subluxation of the humeral head. In many cases, there was an associated impaction defect on the superior articular surface of the humeral head, analogous to a Hill–Sachs defect. The second mechanism is due to traction with a sudden pull on the arm, which causes the biceps tendon to tear and avulse the superior labrum. Similarly, repetitive impaction or repetitive biceps tension from either throwing or overhead sports motion can produce a SLAP lesion (14,20).

A study of 140 SLAP lesions by Snyder et al. (23) demonstrated the most common cause of injury to be a fall or direct blow to the shoulder. This was reported in 31% of cases. Nineteen percent had an episode of glenohumeral subluxation or dislocation, and 16% related the onset of pain to lifting a heavy object. Six percent developed symptoms while participating in overhead racquet sports, and an additional 6% had pain with throwing. Fourteen percent had an insidious onset of pain in which no clear mechanism was identified.

DIAGNOSIS

Shoulder pain may result from numerous causes. Often, the presenting symptoms do not clearly lead to the diagnosis. There may be a combination of pathologies. In addition to a SLAP lesion, there may be associated glenohumeral instability, rotator-cuff, or biceps pathology. Although imaging modalities continue to improve, they are not always accurate. Presently, the diagnosis of a SLAP lesion is made by arthroscopy; however, several factors may increase the diagnostic accuracy.

History

A careful history may be suggestive of a labral tear. As described earlier, the mechanism of injury may yield important information. Traction and compression are the most common injuries that lead to SLAP lesions (21,23). A sudden pull can occur in many instances, such as losing grip on a heavy object or grasping an object in an attempt to avoid a fall. Throwing and overhead racquet activities, particularly during deceleration, also can lead to traction injuries. A history of a fall onto an abducted outstretched arm or of a direct blow to the shoulder is also suggestive.

The most common complaints are pain and mechanical symptoms that include catching, locking, popping, or grinding. These occur most commonly with overhead activities. Patients may also complain of limited range of motion (ROM), pain while lying on the shoulder, loss of strength, and symptoms likened to dead-arm syndrome.

Physical Examination

It is essential to perform a thorough shoulder examination accurately to diagnose shoulder pathology. It is important to diagnose instability and impingement, but unfortunately, there is no specific physical finding for patients with SLAP lesions. A trapped labral tear can cause pain, and a sensation of catching or locking can be appreciated. Popping, snapping, and crepitus may also be present. Often, patients will demonstrate findings during the evaluation of the biceps tendon. The biceps tension test or Speed's test will be painful, suggesting irritation in the tendon itself or in the superior anchor. The compression–rotation test, performed by abducting the shoulder 90 degrees, loading the joint axially, and then rotating the arm, also may be positive (21). Additionally, Liu et al. (24) described a modification of this test. They described the crank test, in which they elevate the arm to 160 degrees in the scapular plane of the body and then similarly load and rotate the arm. They claimed a positive predictive value of 94% with the arm in 160 degrees of abduction, although they had not performed the compression–rotation test with the arm at 90 degrees to compare the two tests.

At the SCOI, we recently reviewed 23 patients with isolated SLAP lesions. The most common physical finding was a painful impingement sign (52%, impingement I with flexion; 35%, impingement II with abduction and internal rotation), leading to an initial diagnosis of impingement in more than half the patients. Forty-three percent had audible popping and snapping on shoulder motion, and 39% had pain in the provocative apprehension position. Pain also was noted with biceps tension testing and with resisted supraspinatus testing in 35% of patients (25).

DIAGNOSTIC IMAGING

Standard conventional radiographs are helpful in initially evaluating patients with shoulder abnormalities and may yield important information suggesting arthrosis, impingement, or instability. They are not usually helpful in diagnosing SLAP lesions. However, Ianotti (26) recently described two cases of supraglenoid tubercle fractures with documented SLAP lesions (Fig. 10). Although rare, this radiographic finding may increase the clinical suspicion of a SLAP lesion.

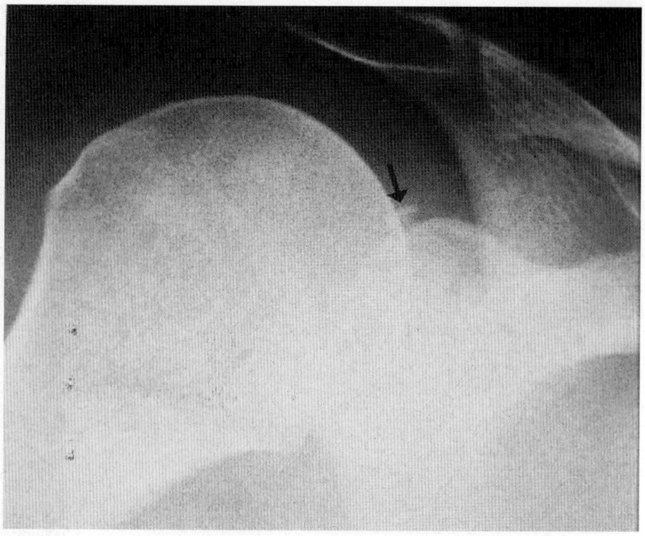

FIG. 10. Supraglenoid tubercle fracture. (From Ianotti JP, Wang ED. Avulsion fracture of the supraglenoid tubercle: a variation of the SLAP lesion. *J Shoulder Elbow Surg* 1992;1: 26, with permission.)

Computed tomography (CT) arthrography is helpful for the detection of some labral pathology, particularly when Bankart lesions are present, but the CT is generally more useful for bony pathology. The MRI has revolutionized soft-tissue imaging. With the use of surface coils and high-strength magnets and new software packages, we can now generate excellent images of the soft tissues. With multiplanar images, our evaluation of the rotator cuff, biceps tendon, and superior labrum have improved immensely. However, it often remains difficult to see the labrum well. The addition of gadolinium allows improved imaging. This highly magnetic contrast agent allows the use of a short T_1 imaging time and yields excellent images with low signal-to-noise ratio (SNR) and excellent spatial resolution. The intra-articular use of gadolinium is presently not approved by the Food and Drug Administration (FDA). However, the required dose is quite small compared with the intravenous dose, which is FDA approved. Studies demonstrated no accumulation in rabbit synovium and cartilage, and no reports have demonstrated adverse results in human use (6,27).

At our institution, the present MRI protocol involves the use of proton density and T2-weighted images in an oblique coronal plane along the long axis of the supraspinatus tendon, sagittal oblique images perpendicular to the supraspinatus long axis, and axial images perpendicular to the long axis of the humerus. If labral pathology is suspected but not detected with these images, then MRI with gadolinium (MRA) is performed. Twelve to 20 ml of diluted gadopentetate dimeglumine (Magnevist, Berlex Laboratories, Wynne, NJ, U.S.A.) is injected into the glenohumeral joint under fluoroscopic control, and additional images are obtained (9).

Findings indicative of superior labral pathology include bright signal in the biceps labral anchor or in the superior glenoid labrum and the superior portion of the glenoid fossa (Fig. 11). Displacement of the labrum from its usual anatomic position is highly suggestive. The presence of a glenoid labral cyst also can be suggestive (Fig. 12) (28). In a study of 20 glenoid labral cysts, nine were located in the superior glenoid area. All patients had a SLAP lesion at the time of arthroscopy. Additionally, all cysts involving the suprascapular and the spinoglenoid notch were found to have associated superior labral lesions.

The reported sensitivities for detecting labral pathology are 96% for MRA and 93% for MRI (29). However, the specificities are likely not so high. The anatomy can be rather variable, and pathology can be overdiagnosed. Thus glenohumeral arthroscopy ultimately remains the only tool for diagnosing SLAP lesions accurately.

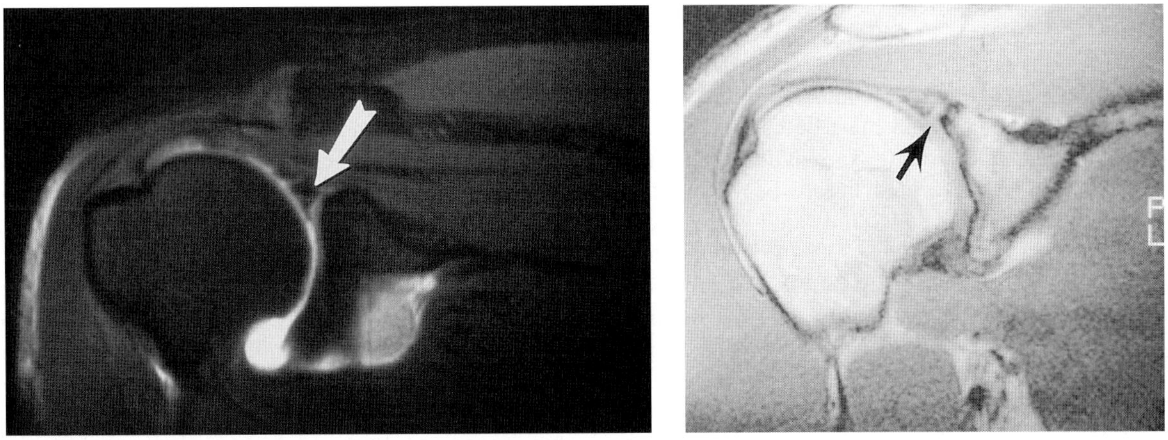

A B

FIG. 11. Coronal magnetic resonance imaging (MRI) scans with **(A)** and without **(B)** gadolinium, demonstrating bright signal in the biceps labral anchor *(arrows)* indicative of a superior labrum from anterior to posterior (SLAP) lesion.

DIAGNOSTIC ARTHROSCOPY

With the limitations in the clinical and radiographic examinations, it is important to maintain a high index of suspicion for a possible superior labral tear. Many patients with persistent shoulder symptoms that do not accompany usual shoulder pathology will often be found to have a superior labral injury at the time of arthroscopy (30). Thus, the ultimate diagnosis of a SLAP lesion requires an accurate arthroscopic evaluation. However, it can sometimes be difficult to differentiate a SLAP lesion from normal anatomic variation. Consequently, it is imperative that the operating surgeon have a thorough understanding of the arthroscopic anatomy and variations in the superior labral region. It is important to recognize a normal sublabral hole or Buford complex and not to label incorrectly these variations pathologic.

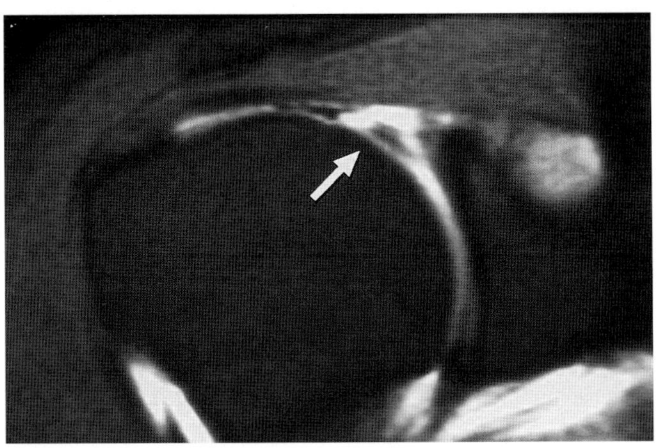

FIG. 12. Coronal magnetic resonance imaging (MRI) scan, demonstrating supraglenoid cyst *(arrow)*. This may suggest the presence of an associated superior labrum from anterior to posterior (SLAP) lesion.

Differentiating between a type II SLAP lesion and a normal meniscoid variant can be difficult. In an acute lesion, the diagnosis is relatively clear, as there is hemorrhage in the area of the avulsed labral tissue. Chronic lesions are more difficult to differentiate. The normal superior labrum often has a meniscoid appearance with a free edge, which can give the appearance of pathologic detachment. With a chronic lesion, the attempted healing process may result in fibrous tissue that conceals the pathologic detachment along the superior glenoid neck. In a normal shoulder, the superior glenoid articular cartilage extends to the labral attachment. However, with type II SLAP lesions, there will usually be a space between the glenoid articular cartilage edge and the attachment of the superior biceps. The torn superior labrum will often arch away 3 to 4 mm from the underlying bone when tension is applied to the biceps tendon. The normal superior labrum can be loosely attached, and as long as it remains in the normal position, it is considered a normal variant rather than a SLAP lesion.

ASSOCIATED INJURIES

In a review of 2,375 shoulder arthroscopies performed at our institution between 1985 and 1993, we found 140 who had injuries to the superior glenoid labrum (23). Thus, our incidence of SLAP lesions was 6%. Of those, 28% had isolated superior labral pathology, whereas the remaining 72% had associated injuries. Most commonly, we detected partial rotator-cuff tears (29%), and 11% had complete cuff tears. Twenty-two percent had associated Bankart lesions, 16% had acromioclavicular joint arthrosis, and 10% had glenohumeral articular injuries. The associated rotator-cuff pathology (40%) also was reported by other authors (31). Others reported subacromial bursitis, glenohumeral ligament tears, and additional anterior, inferior, and posterior labral tears associated with SLAP lesions (31–33).

TREATMENT

Many SLAP lesions occur in association with other glenohumeral pathology. However, glenohumeral instability has implications for treatment and must be carefully evaluated and documented. A thorough examination under anesthesia (EUA) must be performed before beginning the arthroscopy. In several cases, we recommended video fluoroscopic documentation. In one study, 70% of patients with superior labral lesions had instability on EUA despite no history or clinical evidence of instability (34). At our institution, shoulder arthroscopy is performed in the lateral decubitus position. The procedure always begins with a comprehensive video-recorded 15-point examination (7).

When a SLAP lesion has been correctly identified and classified, the surgeon is faced with determining proper treatment. The treatment performed is based on the type of SLAP lesion present. For a type I lesion, the superior labrum is debrided back to a stable rim by using a combination of basket forceps and motorized shaver. The torn tissue is debrided to prevent mechanical catching within the joint, similar to the debridement of a degenerative meniscus in the knee. Type III lesions, with a bucket-handle tear, are carefully probed to ensure that the biceps anchor and remaining labral rim are stable. The torn fragment is then resected, taking care to leave a smooth transition zone in the remaining tissue. With both types of lesions, it is important to inspect carefully the remaining superior labrum to be sure that the rim is well anchored to the glenoid and the biceps anchor is functional.

Truly isolated tears with normal glenohumeral stability can be treated effectively with debridement alone. Glasgow et al. (37) reported a 91% good or excellent result at 2-year follow-up in patients with normal shoulder stability. However, in the presence of glenohumeral instability, 75% had fair or poor results when debridement alone was performed. Payne and Jokl (33) evaluated the results of debridement based on tear location. Whereas results were initially quite good, with 93% good to excellent at 6 months, their results deteriorated to 71% at 2 years. Three patients with superior and anteroinferior lesions did well, but patients with anterosuperior lesions were found to be at risk for the delayed development of glenohumeral instability despite having a stable joint preoperatively. Altchek et al. (38) also found that the results of debridement deteriorated with time when instability was present. Whereas 72% initially reported good results, only 7% had satisfactory long-term relief. Cordasco et al. (36) looked specifically at arthroscopic debridement of superior lesions and found that 78% had excellent pain relief at 1 year. However, at 2 years, only 45% were able to return to their previous levels of athletic performance, and the good results had deteriorated to 63%. They attributed the declining results to the fact that 70% had occult instability. Thus, particularly in high-level athletes, instability must be considered present until proven otherwise with a thorough ligamentous examination and possibly arthroscopy.

TYPE II LESIONS

In the type II lesion, the superior labrum is detached from the glenoid, resulting in instability of the biceps anchor. The superior labrum–biceps complex must be restored to preserve normal glenohumeral stability and biceps function. The early treatment of these lesions consisted of debridement of interposed tissue and decortication of the superior glenoid neck in an attempt to stimulate healing. However, the healing was often incomplete, and the required immobilization prevented early motion, which is so desirable, particularly when additional pathology is present. Most authors now agree that lesions that disrupt the superior labrum biceps anchor be repaired. Several arthroscopic techniques have been reported and include the use of staples, tacks, transosseous sutures, and various suture anchors.

Yoneda (39) used a 5.5-mm staple to treat 10 athletes with type II lesions. The lesions were arthroscopically abraded and then stapled. Repeated arthroscopy was performed at 3 to 6 months for staple removal. All lesions appeared healed, and 80% had good or excellent results. The relative failures were due to one case of subacromial bursitis and one of multidirectional instability. Field and Savoie (34) used transosseous suture fixation for 15 type II and five type IV lesions. Follow-up ranged from 12 to 42 months, and all 20 patients had good to excellent results. All patients returned to work, and the athletes were able to return to their sports without limitation. One patient developed adhesive capsulitis. He was treated with manipulation under anesthesia, but he still had a good long-term result. Resch et al. (40) stabilized 14 cases. In six, he used a cannulated titanium screw with a 5.0-mm washer, and in eight, he used the Suretac (Smith Nephew Dyonics, Andover, MA, U.S.A.) absorbable tack. At a mean follow-up of 18 months, eight patients had returned to their sports, four were somewhat improved but unable to return completely, and two had failures. Four patients were debrided alone without repair, and only one had improvement.

In our series, type II lesions were identified in 55% of 140 cases (23). The early cases were treated with debridement and abrasion as described earlier. However, to allow early mobilization and promote healing, fixation has since been used. Both bioabsorbable tacks and suture anchors were used for fixation. However, five patients treated with the polylactic acid (PLA) bioabsorbable tacks required a repeated arthroscopic procedure to remove a symptomatic loose head fragment of the tack. Because of this finding, we no longer use an absorbable tack device. We have since used a retrievable screw in suture anchor. At an average follow-up of 9 months we arthroscopically reinspected six type II and two complex type II and III lesions. At second look, seven of the eight were firmly healed to the underlying bone (30).

Pagnani et al. (31) presented their results after using a polyglyconate (PGA) absorbable tack (Suretac). Twenty-two patients underwent repair, and at 2-year average follow-up, 86% had satisfactory results. They had no complications related to the use of the PGA implant. These results differ from our experience with a PLA tack. The difference appears to be related to the absorption profile. The PGA absorbs within weeks, reaching zero strength at 4 weeks. The PLA implants degrade over a period of months. If the head becomes sheared off, the PLA implant remains as a loose body, causing symptoms. With the PGA implant's more rapid degradation, loose-body symptoms do not seem to be a problem (32). We currently prefer suture-anchor fixation with permanent braided no. 2 suture. However, PGA biodegradable implants can be used as an alternative.

TECHNIQUE OF TYPE II SLAP REPAIR

Once diagnostic arthroscopy has confirmed the presence of a type II lesion, the surgeon must create a total of three glenohumeral portals. The standard posterior portal is used to guide the creation of an AS portal. The arthroscope is directed into position just anterior to the biceps tendon. A transarticular Wissinger rod is then passed inside-out, and a cannula is then advanced back into the joint. A third portal is placed anteroinferiorly. This portal is created outside-in with the use of a spinal needle. Under direct vision, the needle is placed approximately 2 cm inferior to the AS portal. The portal should enter the joint just above the superior border of the subscapularis tendon just lateral to the articular surface of the glenoid. The portal should always be made lateral to the coracoid process.

While the surgeon is viewing from the posterior portal, the fibrous membrane over the superior glenoid neck is debrided with a motorized shaver through the AS portal. The torn labrum and biceps are carefully debrided. A 4.0-mm ball-tip burr is used lightly to decorticate the bone beneath the superior labrum and biceps anchor (Fig. 13). A shallow pilot hole can then be made with the burr to guide positioning of the punch or drill. This should be located directly below the normal biceps tendon insertion. A drill bit or punch is then inserted through the AS portal, and the tip is placed into the pilot hole. The drill is then angled 45 degrees away from the articular surface and 45 degrees posteriorly and advanced to its hub (Fig. 14).

A suture anchor (4 mm Revo Screw or recently a 3.5-mm bioresorbable Bio-Anchor; Fig. 15) is then loaded with no. 2 braided permanent suture (Ethibond) and is inserted via the AS portal into the predrilled hole. After the anchor has been seated, tension is applied to the suture to assess security. One limb of the suture is then pulled out the anterior midglenoid (anteroinferior; AI) portal by using a crochet hook (Fig. 16).

A 6-inch spinal needle or a crescent suture hook (Linvatec Corp., Largo, FL, U.S.A.) is then inserted through the AS portal, piercing the labrum and biceps anchor near the anterior edge of the biceps origin (Fig. 17). A suture Shuttle Relay (Linvatec) is then passed through the needle/suture hook and is retrieved out the AI portal by using an arthroscopic grasper. The Shuttle is then advanced out the AI portal until the central eyelet has exited the cannula. The limb of the suture that is outside the AI portal is then placed through the eyelet of the Shuttle. The Shuttle is then pulled back through the tissue from the AS portal, delivering the limb of the suture through the labrum back through the AS cannula (Fig. 18).

The same process is then repeated with the other suture limb to create a mattress stitch. This time the needle/suture hook should pass through the labrum approximately 8 mm posterior to the other suture. The Shuttle is again retrieved

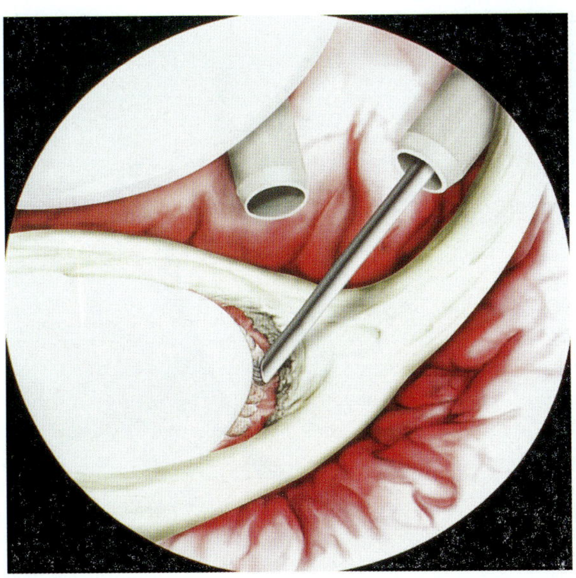

FIG. 13. A 4.0-mm ball burr is used to decorticate the underlying bone.

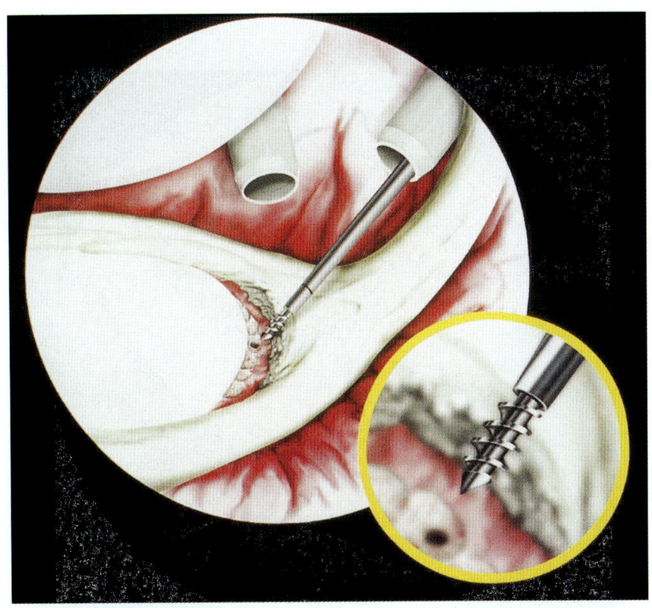

FIG. 14. Revo drill or punch is used to create a pilot hole. The drill is angled 45 degrees from the articular surface and 45 degrees posteriorly.

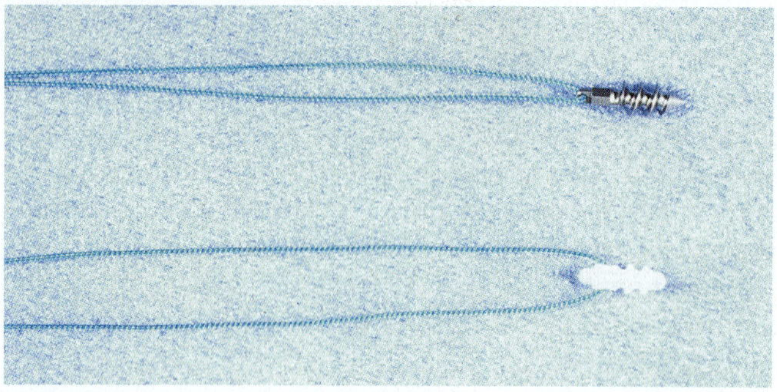

FIG. 15. Suture anchors: 4.0-mm Revo screw (superior) and 3.5-mm BioAnchor (inferior).

through the AI portal, the suture is loaded through the eyelet, and the Shuttle is again removed via the AS portal. Consequently, both limbs of the suture are now on the superior side of the labrum and exit the joint from the AS portal. The two suture limbs are then tied together with an arthroscopic knot-pusher through the AS cannula (Fig. 19). A minimum of five knots are placed, alternating the post after the third and fourth knots (Revo knot); a sliding knot may be used if the suture glides easily through the tissue. An arthroscopic probe is then used to check the security of the repair (Fig. 20). The suture tails are cut and removed. Additional suture anchors can be used if the tear is excessively large.

TYPE IV LESIONS

Type IV lesions have tearing of the biceps tendon in addition to the tearing of the labrum. Usually, the remaining biceps anchor remains firmly attached to the superior labrum. The treatment is based on the extent of tearing in the biceps tendon. If the torn segment composes less than 30% of the tendon, then the detached labral and biceps tissue can be simply resected. However, when more than 30% of the tendon is involved, the treatment considerations differ. If the patient is older, and particularly with signs of biceps irritation, then the labrum is debrided, and a primary biceps tenodesis is performed. In younger patients with extensive tears found in conjunction with a bucket-handle tear in the superior labrum, we recommend preserving the tendon, and we perform an arthroscopic suture repair. Suture anchors

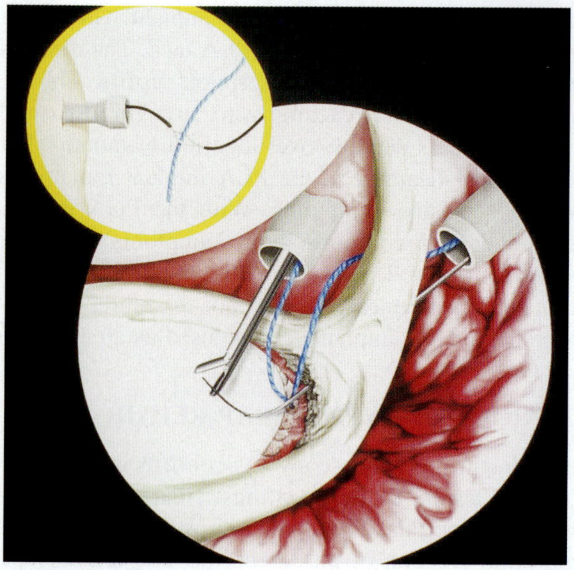

FIG. 17. Crescent suture hook pierces the biceps anchor, and suture shuttle is passed and retrieved out through the midglenoid portal.

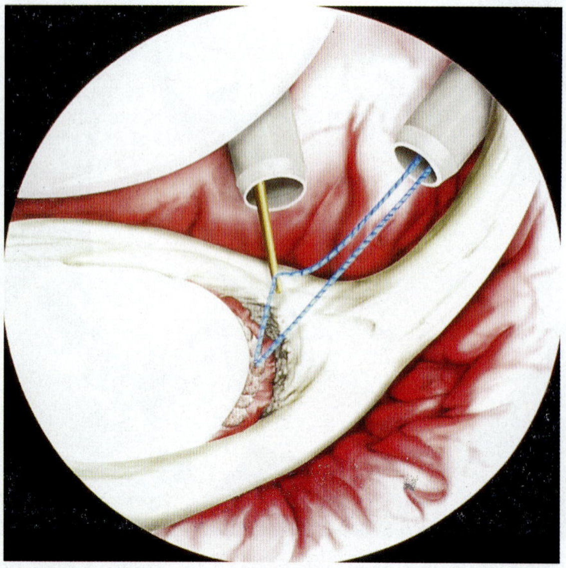

FIG. 16. Crochet hook is used to pull one limb of suture out through the midglenoid portal.

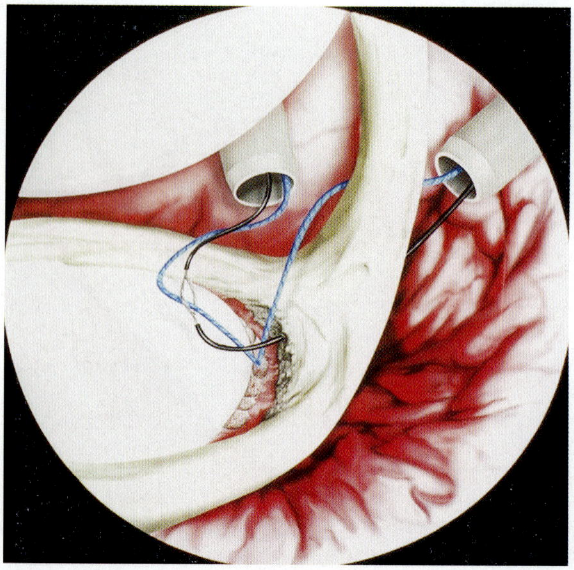

FIG. 18. Suture Shuttle Relay advancing the suture back through the labrum and out through the superior cannula.

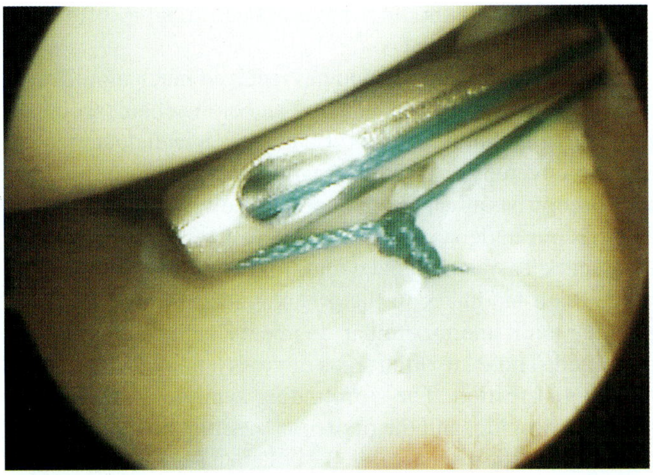

FIG. 19. Completed knot affixing the superior labrum.

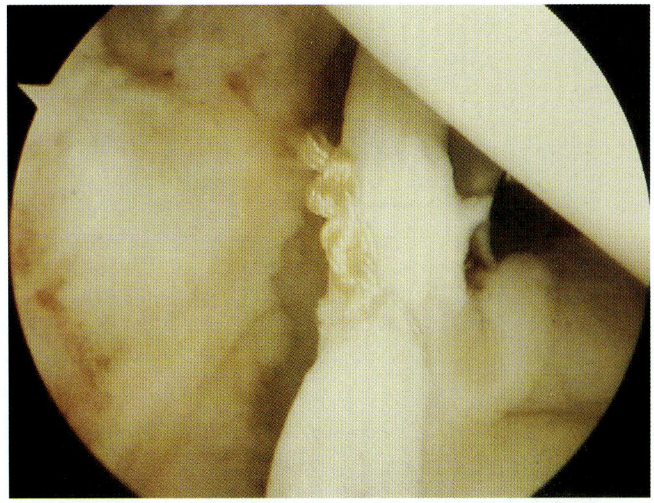

FIG. 21. Arthroscopic photograph demonstrating completed repair of a type IV superior labrum from anterior to posterior (SLAP) lesion.

are not required because the remaining tissue is well anchored to the glenoid.

With this lesion, multiple mattress sutures are used to complete the repair. This can often be accomplished with a posterior and AS portal alone. A 6-inch, 17-gauge epidural needle is passed percutaneously adjacent to the anterolateral acromial edge into the joint across the intact biceps tendon and then through the split portion. A Shuttle relay is then passed through the needle and retrieved through the AS portal. The spinal needle is withdrawn, the Shuttle is loaded with a nonabsorbable suture on the percutaneous side, and the suture is carried across the torn biceps by pulling the Shuttle out the AS cannula. The needle is then reinserted, entering the biceps 3 to 4 mm away from the other suture, and the Shuttle is again passed through the needle and retrieved through the AS portal. The limb of the suture exiting the AS portal is loaded into the Shuttle and advanced through the tissue by pulling the Shuttle out the percutaneous end. This leaves both limbs of the suture outside the skin. A crochet hook is then used to retrieve both limbs through the AS cannula. The arthroscopic knot-pusher is then used to tie the suture limbs together in a mattress fashion. The process is repeated anteriorly and posteriorly until the entire labral tear has been repaired (Fig. 21). In some cases, the tear may extend so far posteriorly that the arthroscope needs to be shifted to the AS portal so that the instruments can be passed posteriorly to complete the repair.

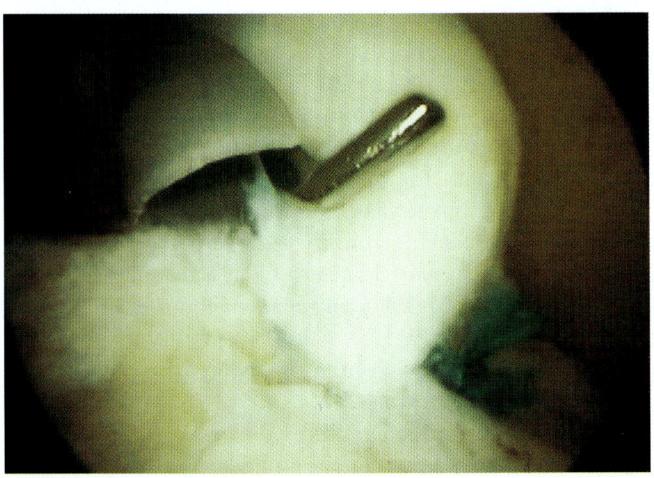

FIG. 20. Security of repair is confirmed with an arthroscopic probe.

Two type IV lesions treated with suture repair were arthroscopically reevaluated. Follow-up was an average of 14 months after repair. Both cases demonstrated a healed tendon and labrum (30).

COMPLEX TEARS

In some cases, complex tears are seen. These usually consist of combined type II and III or combined II and IV lesions. The previously described treatment principles should be followed to effect repair. In combined II and IV lesions, the first step is to reattach the superior labrum to the glenoid. The remaining detachment can then be either resected or repaired as described earlier.

REHABILITATION

For type I and III lesions, patients are placed in a neutral rotation sling (UltraSling, Smith & Nephew DonJoy Inc., Carlsbad, CA, U.S.A.; Fig. 22) for comfort and then treated with early mobilization. For type II and IV repairs, the rehabilitation is more conservative. The patient is protected in the UltraSling for 3 weeks. During this time, patients are allowed to perform elbow, wrist, and hand exercises. After the first week, they may remove the sling for gentle pen-

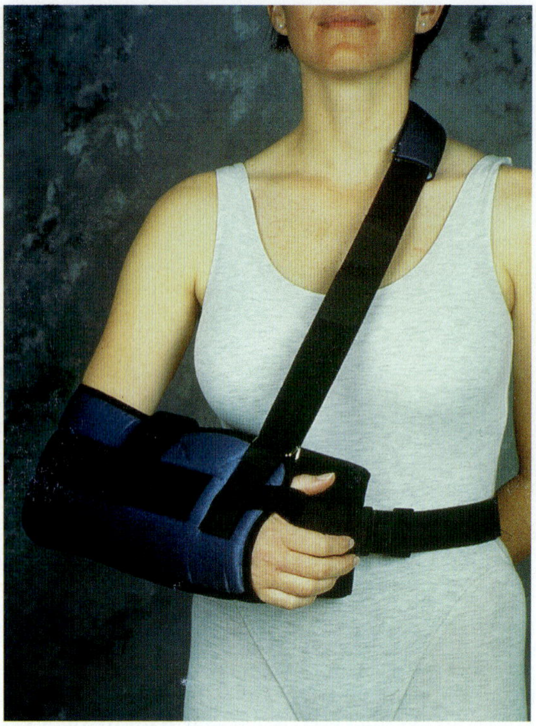

FIG. 22. Neutral rotation sling (UltraSling; Smith and Nephew DonJoy, Inc., Carlsbad, CA, U.S.A.).

dulum exercises. They are instructed, however, to avoid external rotation beyond neutral and extension of the arm behind the body with the elbow extended. This precaution is continued for 4 weeks to prevent tension on the biceps tendon. Therapy is then progressed with protected biceps strengthening. No stressful biceps activity is allowed for 3 months.

BICEPS TENDON INJURIES

Biceps tendon pathology has been an enigma for the orthopedic surgeon for many years. The historic literature has largely ignored the role of the biceps tendon as a source of shoulder pain. Codman, writing in his classic textbook (41), thought that the biceps tendon played a limited role as a primary source of shoulder pain. In 1972, Neer (42) revolutionized the approach to shoulder pain with his description of impingement syndrome. He stated that the primary cause of shoulder pain was impingement and that biceps tendinitis was a secondary phenomenon. Burkhead (43) similarly believed that 95% to 98% of patients with the diagnosis of biceps tendinitis had in reality an impingement with the biceps involvement occurring secondarily.

Other authors supported the role of the biceps as a primary source of shoulder pain. In 1938, Schrager (44) first described the anatomic findings of biceps tenosynovitis and established it as a distinct clinical entity. Hitchcock and Bechtol (45) similarly believed that biceps tendinitis was a primary source of shoulder pain and described a soft-tissue tenodesis for treatment.

Recently, the biceps tendon has received much more attention in the literature. The anatomy and biomechanical contribution to glenohumeral stability have been well documented and are covered in the earlier part of this chapter. Shoulder arthroscopy has advanced our knowledge of the biceps tendon as it has our understanding of SLAP lesions. The biceps tendon can be easily visualized and, for many arthroscopists, it is the main landmark in the glenohumeral joint. The intra-articular and intertubercular segments can be thoroughly evaluated. There are often signs of gross tendon damage with fraying or attrition. The surrounding synovium is inflamed and hypertrophic, and the peritenon vasculature may be congested (44). Microscopically, the collagen fibrils become disorganized bundles, having lost their lamellar alignment. Leukocytes and macrophages are seen to occupy the normally acellular environment. However, when the arthroscope is placed into the subacromial space, there are seldom signs of impingement, and the bursae often appear pristine. In such cases, it is impossible to believe that the visualized and microscopic changes are due to impingement. Primary or intrinsic biceps tendinitis is thus becoming more widely accepted as a source of shoulder pathology.

Other forms of biceps pathology also are recognized. The most common biceps pathology remains secondary tendinitis. As described earlier, this may account for 95% to 98% of the tendinitis seen. The primary impingement can be identified and the acromial structure can be classified. Associated rotator-cuff tears are common, and treatment must address the impingement, rotator-cuff pathology, and the biceps tendinitis to effect successful treatment.

Biceps tendon instability also has been addressed. The biceps tendon is stabilized by the coracohumeral ligament proximally and the transverse humeral ligament and fibers of the subscapularis distally within the groove (Curtis AS, Snyder SJ, unpublished data). Meyer (47) and Paavolainen et al. (48) showed that the rotator-cuff interval is the principal restraint to instability. Instability may occur in older individuals or in young throwing athletes. In such cases, the treatment must be directed at the interval. Stability should result if the rotator-cuff interval is imbricated in the area of the tendon's exit from the joint (44).

Patients with full-thickness subscapularis tears should be carefully evaluated for the presence of biceps instability. The medial restraint to dislocation is disrupted, and the biceps can then dislocate from the groove (44). The subscapularis should be repaired back to the lesser tuberosity. The biceps may be stabilized with repair of the rotator-cuff interval if detected early. However, if instability remains, especially if the groove is rough or hypoplastic, then a tenodesis should be performed.

Finally, biceps tendon ruptures do occur. They may be acute or chronic and can often go undetected. The ruptured tendon results in a deformed muscular contour. The associated loss of strength has been reported to be 16% for loss of elbow flexion and 11% for loss of forearm supination strength (47). Surgical treatment can be recommended for younger individuals, manual laborers or athletes, or rarely for cosmetic reasons. Patients with symptoms due to a remaining proximal tendon stump may also be candidates for arthroscopy.

CLINICAL DIAGNOSIS

A careful history should be obtained. Patients frequently describe pain over the anterior aspect of the shoulder with radiation down the biceps muscle. The pain is exacerbated by repetitive overhead or lifting activities and is relieved by rest. Night pain may occur and can be quite severe. Antecedent trauma should be identified. A tearing sensation after a fall or forceful internal-rotation contracture against resistance may indicate a subscapularis tear and concomitant biceps subluxation. Patients with subluxation may complain of pain in the intertubercular groove, especially with internal and external rotation, that can be exacerbated by throwing activities. Acute ruptures may be preceded by a long history of shoulder pain, which can actually be relieved after rupture. The patient then complains of deformity and pain more distally in the arm.

Upon physical examination, tenderness will be noted in the region of the intertubercular groove. Specific tests for the biceps tendon should be performed and include Speed's or biceps tension test, Yergason's sign, Luddington's test, and the biceps instability test (Curtis AS, Snyder SJ, unpublished data). Evaluation for impingement and rotator-cuff pathology should be performed on all patients.

Routine radiographs should include a supraspinatus outlet view to rule out impingement. A biceps groove view, as described by Cone et al. (50), can be obtained. It may reveal spurring or trauma to the groove, which may help in cases of presumed primary tendinitis. MRI can be very helpful. The tendon can be well visualized on the oblique coronal and axial views. Additionally, the MRI can similarly evaluate the rotator cuff and the biceps anchor.

TREATMENT

For impingement-related or primary tendinitis, treatment begins with rest and discontinuing those activities that exacerbate the symptoms. Antiinflammatory agents may be helpful. For refractory cases, an injection or two may be attempted into the subacromial space for impingement and into the biceps tendon sheath for primary tendinitis. Therapy is instituted as the acute symptoms abate.

If the patient's symptoms fail to resolve after a prolonged trial of conservative management, then arthroscopic evaluation of the glenohumeral joint and subacromial space is indicated. The usual 15-point arthroscopic glenohumeral examination is performed to identify pathology. The biceps tendon is placed under tension with a probe to allow visualization of the intertubercular component of the tendon. The integrity of the tendon should be examined and graded. Grade I is minor fraying, involving less than 25% of the fibers. Grade II fraying involves less than 50% of the tendon. Grade III is greater than 50%, and grade IV is a complete rupture (Curtis AS, Snyder SJ, unpublished data). For grade I or II lesions, shaving of the tendon followed by subacromial decompression is performed to treat the primary impingement syndrome if present. For grade III and IV lesions, a subacromial decompression is followed by a biceps tenodesis. Cases of primary biceps tendinitis can be treated with a tenodesis alone, assuming that the subacromial bursoscopy demonstrates no evidence of impingement.

Results after isolated biceps tenodesis have been somewhat variable in the past. In 1982, Dines et al. (51) reported failure in six of 20 patients who underwent isolated tenodesis for a diagnosis of primary tendinitis. Of the failures, four underwent an additional procedure. They recommended that the tenodesis be accompanied by acromioplasty and coracoligament release. Becker and Cofield (52) reported a long-term failure rate of 46% with an average of 7-year follow-up. They concluded that isolated biceps tenodesis was rarely indicated. Depalma and Callery (53) and Post and Benca (54) had higher success rates (82% and 94%, respectively) after tenodesis for primary tendinitis.

When evaluating these results, it must be remembered that these studies were all done before the routine use of shoulder arthroscopy. With present techniques, proper diagnosis of intrinsic versus secondary tendinitis should more readily be made. If any evidence of impingement exists, then an arthroscopic subacromial decompression should always be done concomitantly to avoid failure.

For treatment of biceps tendon instability without associated subscapularis tears, patients should initially be treated conservatively. Rest and discontinuation of the inciting activities should be attempted. If this is unsuccessful, then arthroscopy should be performed. The area of the rotator interval and coracohumeral ligament should be carefully addressed. Closure of a rotator interval defect may stabilize the tendon (44). If not, tenodesis should be performed.

Treatment for complete ruptures must be individualized, as we discussed earlier. Patients who are willing to accept the cosmetic deformity and functional deficit can be treated nonoperatively. Younger and athletic individuals and especially those who perform tasks that require supination strength should be offered a biceps tenodesis and subacromial decompression if indicated.

SOUTHERN CALIFORNIA ORTHOPEDIC INSTITIUTE TECHNIQUE FOR BICEPS TENODESIS

Several different techniques were described for tenodesis of the biceps tendon. Our technique is a modification of those previously described. We perform an arthroscopically assisted biceps tenodesis by using a subpectoral approach. It allows removal of the biceps stump from the joint, secure fixation of the distal tendon to the bone, does not disrupt the deltoid, and maintains the normal tension in the muscle–tendon unit.

The procedure begins with a complete arthroscopic examination of the shoulder. Any necessary debridement is then performed. The arthroscopic irrigating solution is changed to glycine, and the subacromial electrosurgical tool is inserted through an anterior insulated cannula. The biceps tendon is then transected just above the labrum (Fig. 23). A few remaining fibers are left intact to maintain the tendon in its position. A routine bursal examination is performed, and any necessary subacromial surgery is performed. The arthroscope is then removed, and the arm is removed from the traction device. The table is tilted 30 degrees posteriorly, and the arm and shoulder are reprepped with povidone–iodine (Betadine).

A 3- to 4-cm incision is made in the anterior axilla, centered on and perpendicular to the lower border of the pectoralis major tendon. The subcutaneous and areolar tissue are carefully dissected to allow visualization of the pectoral insertion into the humerus. A sharp Hohmann retractor is placed medially around the humerus to retract the conjoined tendon. The pectoralis tendon is retracted proximally with a second pointed-tip, curved Hohmann retractor. The biceps groove is then palpated, and the sheath is opened to expose the tendon.

A marker suture is placed through the tendon at the level of the inferior portion of the biceps groove. The electrosurgical tool is then used to mark a corresponding spot on the underlying bone. This mark will serve as a guide for setting the tension in the tendon at the time of fixation. Tension is then applied to the marker suture to sever the remaining few biceps fibers and deliver the proximal tendon from the joint. The degenerated tendon is then resected, leaving approximately 2 cm of tendon proximal to the marker suture. A double whip stitch is then placed into the biceps tendon by using a no. 2 braided nonabsorbable suture. This should begin in the free end, extend down the tendon to the level of the marker stitch, and then return up the tendon to the free edge (Fig. 24). This will serve as the lead suture for the tenodesis.

A central hole is then created in the lower portion of the biceps groove where the previous electrosurgical mark was made (Fig. 25). The hole diameter should be similar to the size of the biceps tendon. Two additional holes are then created with a 7/64-inch drill bit. These should be 1.5 cm distal to the original hole with one positioned medial and one lateral to the central hole (Fig. 26).

A crescent suture hook is then used to pass a Shuttle Relay through the inferior medial drill hole. The Shuttle end is retrieved out the central hole by using an arthroscopic grasper. One of the suture ends from the biceps tendon is loaded into the Shuttle eyelet and carried down through the central hole and out the medial inferior hole. The second limb is passed in a similar fashion through the central hole and out the inferior lateral drill hole (Fig. 27).

The biceps stump is then directed into the central hole by pulling distally on the suture limbs. The tendon is advanced distally into the medullary canal until the original marker suture is near the level of the central hole (Fig. 28). This will ensure that the resting length of the biceps tendon remains physiologic. The patient's elbow is then extended, and the forearm is supinated. The two limbs of the suture are tied together, fixing the tendon in the proper position (Fig. 29). The fixation is then tested by pulling distally on the biceps tendon. The subcutaneous tissue is closed in the standard fashion.

Postoperatively, the arm is placed in a neutral rotation sling immobilizer (UltraSling), and gentle biceps exercises are begun immediately. A Shoulder Therapy Kit (Breg, Inc., Vista, CA, U.S.A.) is used to begin forward elevation and gentle internal and external rotation strengthening. Full activity is delayed for 3 to 4 months to allow the tenodesis to heal completely.

(text continues on page 366)

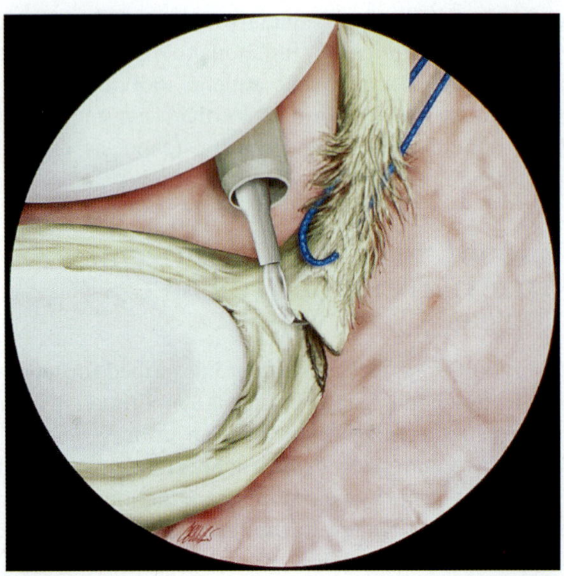

FIG. 23. Biceps anchor is transected by using electrosurgery.

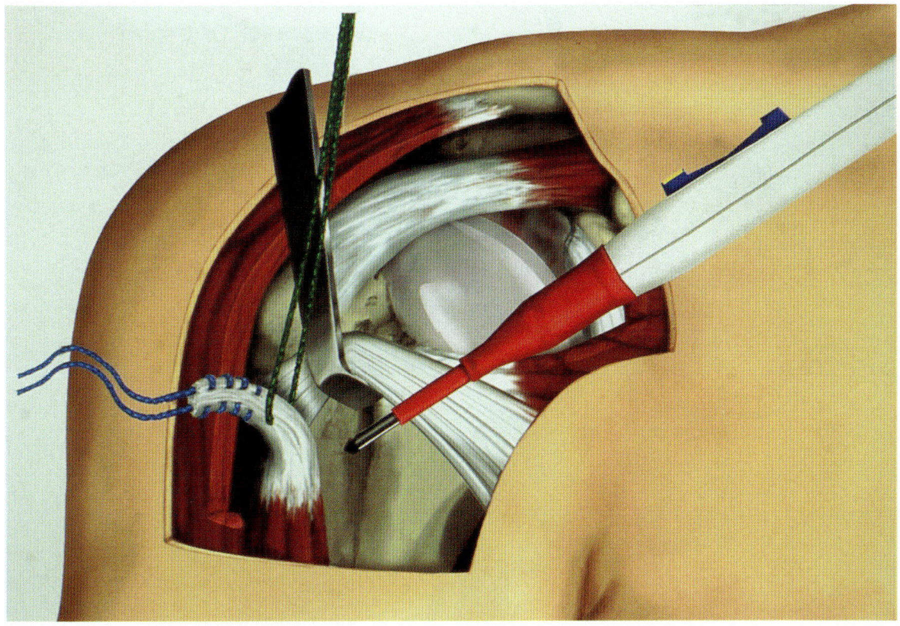

FIG. 24. Marker suture, whip stitch, and electrocautery being used to mark the bone at the level of the marker suture.

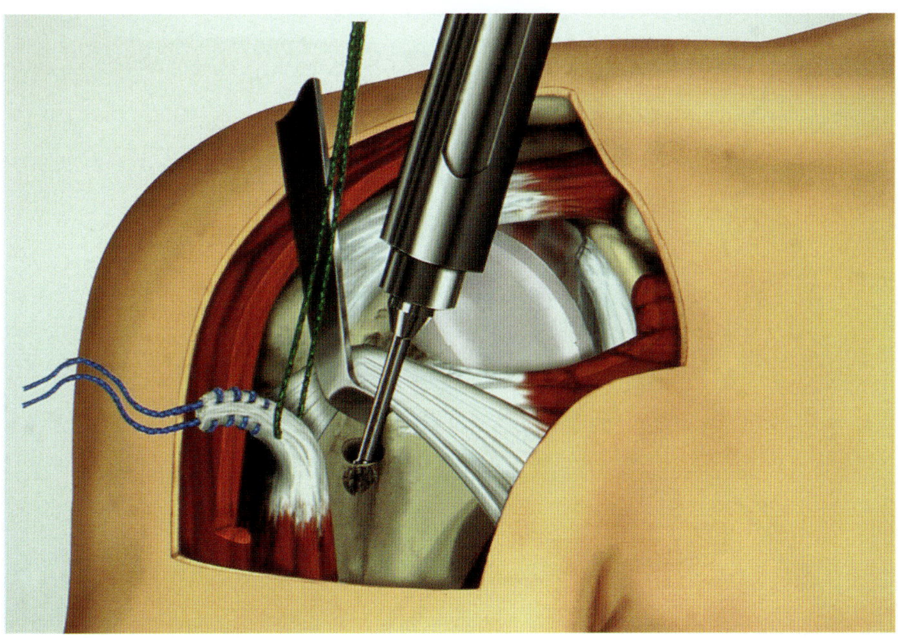

FIG. 25. Central hole created at inferior end of biceps groove at the level where the electrosurgery mark was made.

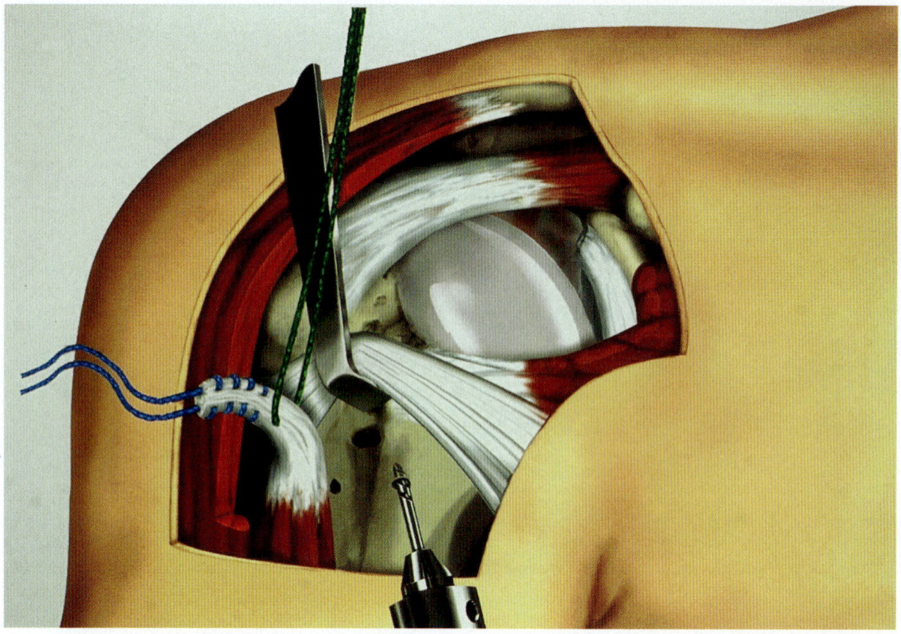

FIG. 26. Distal 7/64-inch drill holes made 1.5 cm distal to the original hole.

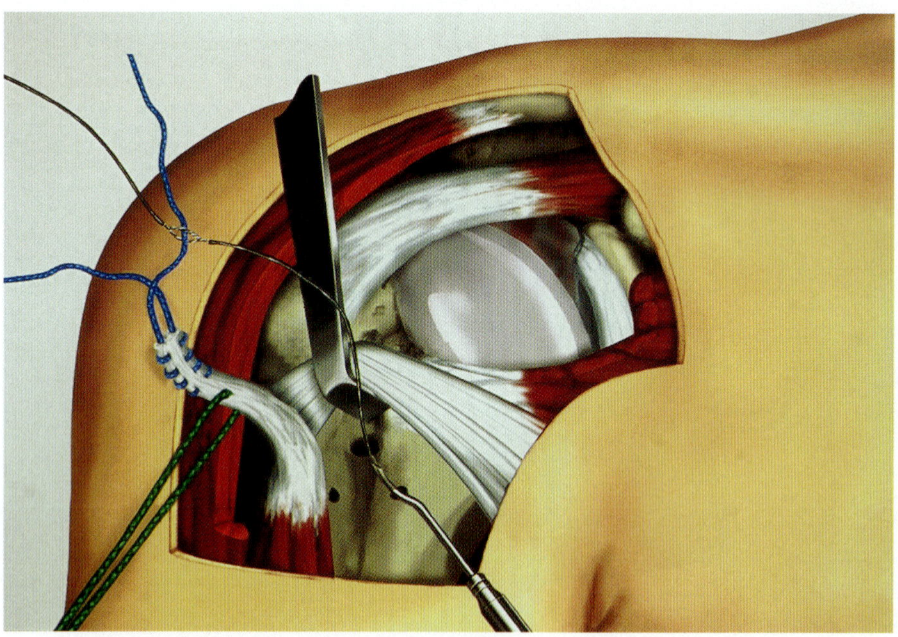

FIG. 27. Crescent suture hook is used to pass a suture Shuttle Relay from the inferior hole at the proximal central hole.

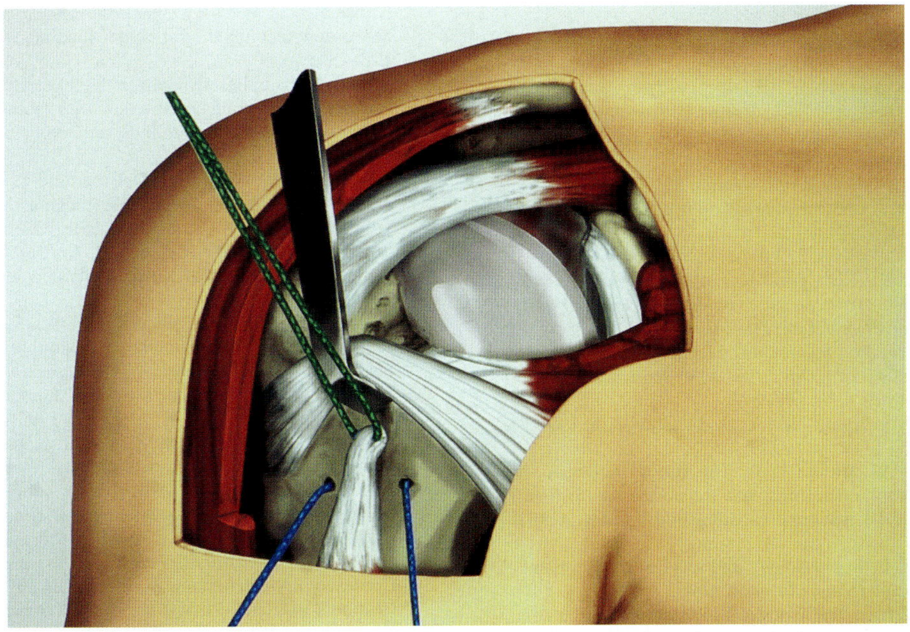

FIG. 28. Biceps tendon is advanced into central hole by pulling distally on the suture limbs.

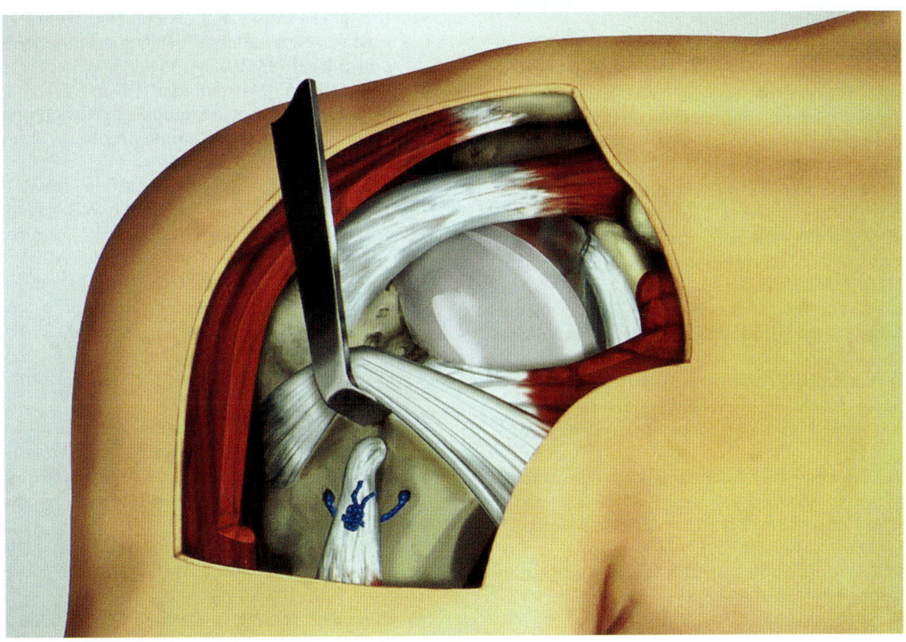

FIG. 29. The result: the tenodesis is secured by tying the two distal limbs together over the tendon with the forearm in full extension and supination.

REFERENCES

1. Gardner E, Gray DJ. Prenatal development of the human shoulder and acromioclavicular joint. *Am J Anat* 1953;92:219–276.
2. Prodromos CC, Ferry JA, Schiller AL, Zarins B. Histological studies of the glenoid labrum from fetal life to old age. *J Bone Joint Surg [Am]* 1990;72:1344–1348.
3. Cooper DE, Arnoczky SP, O'Brien SJ, Warren RF, DiCarlo E, Allen AA. Anatomy, histology, and vascularity of the glenoid labrum. *J Bone Joint Surg [Am]* 1992;74:46–52.
4. Snyder SJ, Rames RD, Wolbert E. Labral lesions. In: McGinty JB, ed. *Operative arthroscopy*. New York: Raven Press, 1991:491–499.
5. Detrisac DA, Johnson LL. *Arthroscopic shoulder anatomy: pathologic and surgical implications*. Thorofare, NJ: Slack, 1986.
6. Karzel RP, Snyder SJ. Labral lesions. In: McGinty JB, Caspari RB, Jackson RW, Poehling GG, eds. *Operative arthroscopy*. 2nd ed. Philadelphia: Lippincott-Raven, 1996:663–675.
7. Snyder SJ. *Shoulder arthroscopy*. New York: McGraw-Hill, 1993:31–33.
8. Williams MM, Snyder SJ, Buford D Jr. The Buford complex—the "cord-like" middle glenohumeral ligament and absent anterosuperior labrum complex: a normal anatomic capsulolabral variant. *Arthroscopy* 1994;10:241–247.
9. Mileski RA, Snyder SJ. Pathophysiology and surgical management of SLAP lesions. *J Am Acad Orthop Surg* (in press).
10. Vangsness CT Jr, Jorgenson SS, Watson T, Johnson DL. The origin of the long head of the biceps from the scapula and glenoid labrum. *J Bone Joint Surg [Br]* 1994;76:951–954.
11. Lazarus MD, Sidles JA, Harryman DT, Matsen FA III. Effect of a chondral-labral defect on glenoid concavity and glenohumeral stability. *J Bone Joint Surg [Am]* 1996;78:94–102.
12. Pagnani MJ, Deng XH, Warren RF, Torzilli PA, Altchek DW. Effect of lesions of the superior portion of the glenoid labrum on glenohumeral translation. *J Bone Joint Surg [Am]* 1995;77:1003–1010.
13. Howell SM, Galinat BJ. The glenoid-labral socket: a constrained articular surface. *Clin Orthop* 1989;243:122–125.
14. Jobe CM. Evidence linking posterior superior labral impingement and shoulder instability. Presented at the American Shoulder and Elbow Surgeons Meeting, Seattle, Washington, September 1991.
15. Jobe CM. Posterior superior glenoid impingement: expanded spectrum. *Arthroscopy* 1995;11:530–536.
16. Itoi E, Kuechle DK, Newman SR, Morrey BF, An KN. Stabilising function of the biceps in stable and unstable shoulders. *J Bone Joint Surg [Br]* 1993;75:546–550.
17. Rodosky MW, Harner CD, Fu FH. The role of the long head of the biceps muscle and superior glenoid labrum in anterior stability of the shoulder. *Am J Sports Med* 1994;22:121–130.
18. Warner JJP, McMahon PJ. The role of the long head of the biceps brachii in superior stability of the glenohumeral joint. *J Bone Joint Surg [Am]* 1995;77:366–372.
19. Pagnani MJ, Deng XH, Warren RF, Torzilli PA, O'Brien SJ. Role of the long head of the biceps brachii in glenohumeral stability: a biomechanical study in cadavera. *J Shoulder Elbow Surg* 1996;5:255–262.
20. Andrews JR, Carson WG, McLeod WD. Glenoid labrum tears related to the long head of the biceps. *Am J Sports Med* 1985;13:337–341.
21. Snyder SJ, Karzel RP, Del Pizzo W, Ferkel RD, Friedman MJ. SLAP lesions of the shoulder. *Arthroscopy* 1990;6:274–279.
22. Maffet MW, Gartsman GM, Moseley B. Superior labrum-biceps tendon complex lesions of the shoulder. *Am J Sports Med* 1995;23:93–98.
23. Snyder SJ, Banas MP, Karzel RP. An analysis of 140 injuries to the superior glenoid labrum. *J Shoulder Elbow Surg* 1995;4:243–248.
24. Liu SH, Henry MH, Nuccion SL. A prospective evaluation of a new physical examination in predicting glenoid labral tears. *Am J Sports Med* 1996;24:721–725.
25. Stetson WB, Snyder SJ, Karzel RP, Banas MP, Rahhal SE. Long term clinical follow-up of isolated SLAP lesions of the shoulder. Presented at the Annual Meeting of the American Academy of Orthopaedic Surgeons, San Francisco, 1997.
26. Ianotti JP, Wang ED. Avulsion fracture of the supraglenoid tubercle: a variation of the SLAP lesion. *J Shoulder Elbow Surg* 1992;1:26–30.
27. Karzel RP, Snyder SJ. Magnetic resonance arthrography of the shoulder: a new technique of shoulder imaging. *Clin Sports Med* 1993;12:123–135.
28. Tirman PFS, Feller JF, Janzen DL, Peterfy CG, Bergman AG. Association of glenoid labral cysts with labral tears and glenohumeral instability: radiologic findings and clinical significance. *Radiology* 1994;190:653–658.
29. Chandnani VP, Yeager TD, DeBerardino T, et al. Glenoid labral tears: prospective evaluation with MR imaging, MR arthrography and CT arthrography. *Am J Radiol* 1993;161:1229–1235.
30. Snyder SJ, Banas MP, Belzer MP. Arthroscopic evaluation and treatment of injuries to the superior glenoid labrum. *Instr Course Lect* 1996;45:65–70.
31. Pagnani MJ, Speer KP, Altchek DW, Warren RF, Dines DM. Arthroscopic fixation of superior labral lesions using a biodegradable implant: a preliminary report. *Arthroscopy* 1995;11:194–198.
32. Speer KP, Warren RF. Arthroscopic shoulder stabilization: a role for biodegradable materials. *Clin Orthop* 1993;291:677–74.
33. Payne LZ, Jokl P. The results of arthroscopic debridement of glenoid labral tears based on tear location. *Arthroscopy* 1993;9:560–565.
34. Field LD, Savoie FH III. Arthroscopic suture repair of superior labral detachment lesions of the shoulder. *Am J Sports Med* 1993;21:783–790.
35. Martin DR, Garth WP Jr. Results of arthroscopic debridement of glenoid labral tears. *Am J Sports Med* 1995;23:447–451.
36. Cordasco FA, Steinmann S, Flatow EL, Bigliani LU. Arthroscopic treatment of glenoid labral tears. *Am J Sports Med* 1993;21:425–431.
37. Glasgow SG, Bruce RA, Yacobucci GN, Torg JS. Arthroscopic resection of glenoid labral tears in the athlete: a report of 29 cases. *Arthroscopy* 1992;8:48–54.
38. Altchek DW, Warren RF, Wickiewicz TL, Ortiz G. Arthroscopic labral debridement: a three year follow-up study. *Am J Sports Med* 1992;20:702–706.
39. Yoneda M, Hirooka A, Saito S, Yamamoto T, Ochi T, Shino K. Arthroscopic stapling for detached superior glenoid labrum. *J Bone Joint Surg [Br]* 1991;73:746–750.
40. Resch H, Golser K, Thoeni H, Sperner G. Arthroscopic repair of superior glenoid labral detachment (the SLAP lesion). *J Shoulder Elbow Surg* 1993;2:147–155.
41. Codman EA. *The shoulder*. Boston: Thomas Todd, 1934.
42. Neer CS. Anterior acromioplasty for chronic impingement syndrome in the shoulder: a preliminary report. *J Bone Joint Surg [Am]* 1972;4:41–50.
43. Burkhead WZ. The biceps tendon. In: Rockwood CA, Matsen FA, eds. *The shoulder*. Philadelphia: WB Saunders, 1990; 791–836.
44. Schrager VL. Tenosynovitis of the long head of the biceps humeri. *Surg Gynecol Obstet* 1965;66:785–790.
45. Hitchcock HH, Bechtol CO. Painful shoulder: observations on the role of the tendon of the long head of the biceps brachii in its causation. *J Bone Joint Surg [Am]* 1948;30:263–273.
46. Bell RH, Noble JS. Biceps disorders. In: Hawkins RJ, Misamore GW, eds. *Shoulder injuries in the athlete*. New York: Churchill Livingstone, 1996:267–282.
47. Meyer AW. Spontaneous dislocation and destruction of the tendon of the long head of the biceps brachii. *Arch Surg* 1928;17:493–506.
48. Paavolainen P, Bjorkenheim JM, Slatis P, Paulku P. Operative treatment of severe proximal humeral fractures. *Acta Orthop Scand* 1983;54:374–379.
49. Sturzenegger M, Beguin D, Brunig B, Jakob RP. Muscular strength after rupture of the long head of the biceps. *Arch Orthop Trauma Surg* 1986;105:18–23.
50. Cone RO, Danzig L, Resnick D, Goldman AB. The bicipital groove: radiographic, anatomic, and pathologic study. *Am J Roentgenol* 1983;41:781–788.
51. Dines D, Warren RF, Inglis AE. Surgical treatment of lesions of the long head of the biceps. *Clin Orthop* 1982;164:165–171.
52. Becker DA, Cofield RH. Tenodesis of the long head of the biceps brachii for chronic bicipital tendinitis. *J Bone Joint Surg [Am]* 1989;71:376–380.
53. DePalma AF, Callery GE. Bicipital tenosynovitis. *Clin Orthop* 1954;3:69–85.
54. Post M, Benca P. Primary tendinitis of the long head of the biceps. *Clin Orthop* 1989;246:117–125.

The Unstable Shoulder,
edited by R.F. Warren, E.V. Craig, and D.W. Altchek.
Lippincott–Raven Publishers, Philadelphia © 1999.

CHAPTER 24

Rehabilitation After Shoulder Stabilization Surgery

Kevin E. Wilk

Rehabilitation plays a vital role in the ultimate functional outcome after shoulder stabilization surgery. The ultimate goal of the postoperative rehabilitation program is to return the patient to unrestricted functional activities, and in some instances, the goal is to return to sport activities. After shoulder stabilization surgery, the emphasis is early restricted motion, protected strengthening, and a functional rehabilitation program. There are numerous surgical procedures to stabilize the shoulder—more than 150 different surgical techniques have been described. There are numerous factors that should be considered when designing the postoperative rehabilitation program. Additionally, specific rehabilitation programs are discussed for several of the most common surgical procedures.

Numerous complications can develop as a result of shoulder stabilization surgery (1). Some of these postoperative complications such as recurrent instability, limitation of motion, inability to return to previous level of sport, and development of osteoarthritis and pain may be prevented with a well-designed and implemented postoperative rehabilitation program. Probably the most common complication after shoulder stabilization surgery is loss of motion, particularly external rotation (ER) after anterior stabilization (2–8). The goals of the ideal postoperative rehabilitation program are (a) to maintain the surgically corrected stability, (b) to restore the full functional range of motion (ROM) gradually, (c) to enhance dynamic stability, and (d) to return to full unrestricted activities.

Rehabilitation after shoulder stabilization surgery should proceed in a progressive and sequential fashion, organized in multiple phases with each phase comprising specific goals. The ultimate goal of this process is to return the patient to the desired activity as quickly and safely as possible without complications. The rehabilitation programs I will discuss are based on several factors. These factors include the classification of the type of instability exhibited by the patient (see Table 1) and the unique characteristics of the patient (see Table 2). Thus, classifying the patients into specific types may prevent some postoperative complications. Additionally, the rehabilitation programs should be modified to the individual, based on tissue type, healing rate, and specific surgical procedure.

K. E. Wilk: Department of Physical Therapy, Marquette University, Milwaukee, Wisconsin 53201; and Healthsouth Rehabilitation Corporation, Birmingham, Alabama 35205.

PRINCIPLES OF REHABILITATION

Before designing a postsurgery rehabilitation program, the clinician should always consider six basic principles of rehabilitation (see Table 3). First, healing tissue should never be overstressed. Thus, the program must be progressive and sequential, with each phase building from the prior phase. Frequently, attempting to have a patient progress too quickly may result in tissue failure, inflammation, and soreness. Second, the effects of immobilization must be minimized. Often after shoulder stabilization surgery, a short period of immobilization may be indicated to allow initial healing. During the immobilization period, the clinician should give serious thought to performing mild dynamic stabilization drills, gentle restricted passive motions, and submaximal isometrics to enhance dynamic stability, assist in collagen organization, and prevent loss of motion. Third, the patient must fulfill specific criteria to progress from one phase to the next phase; this allows the rehabilitation program to be individualized, based on the patient's unique healing rate and constraints. Fourth, the rehabilitation program should be based on current clinical and scientific research. Thus, the rehabilitation program should be updated periodically. Next, the rehabilitation program must not be a cookbook; rather, it should be adaptable to the patient's

TABLE 1. *Shoulder instability classification*

Onset
Traumatic, atraumatic, repetitive microtrauma
Frequency
Acute, recurrent, chronic (fixed)
Direction
Anterior, posterior, multidirectional
Degree
Dislocation, subluxation, silent subluxation
Volition
Voluntary, involuntary

TABLE 3. *Basic principles of rehabilitation*

Healing tissue should never be overstressed
The effects of immobilization must be minimized
The patient must fulfill specific criteria to progress
The rehabilitation program should be based on current scientific and clinical research
The rehabilitation program must not be a cookbook
Team approach—physician, therapist, and patient

goals and unique tissue characteristics. A successful outcome is directly related to a team effort, with the physician, therapist, athletic trainer, and patient all working together toward a common goal. The key to the team approach is communication; it is the role of the physician to communicate with the rehabilitation specialist, providing information regarding the type of surgical procedure used, the method of fixation, the integrity and quality of the patient's tissue, and the expectations of the physician for that specific patient. This information is invaluable to the rehabilitation specialist in designing and implementing a rehabilitation program.

FACTORS AFFECTING THE REHABILITATION PROGRAM

Before designing and implementing a postsurgical rehabilitation program, the clinician must contemplate several factors that directly affect it (See Table 4).

The first factor is the type of surgical procedure performed. The type of surgical exposure (open or arthroscopy), type of surgical procedure (Bankart-type repair, capsular shift, etc.), and the method of fixation (bioabsorbable tack, suture anchors, sutures, etc.) should be carefully considered. In addition, the rehabilitation program should consider whether a muscle, such as the subscapularis, is resected off the insertion or split (to gain exposure to the capsule). The method of fixation is a very important factor for the therapist in designing a program.

The second factor is the type of instability exhibited by the patient. This factor should be considered carefully by the surgeon before performing any surgical procedure—thus it is closely related to the first factor. The rate of the rehabilitation program's progression will be significantly different for an individual with atraumatic instability compared with an individual with instability from a traumatic injury.

The patient's tissue status is the third factor that should be considered. This is another critical factor, upon which the rate of progression of the rehabilitation program is based. If the patient has significant tissue laxity or hyperlaxity, the rate of progression should be slower than that of an individual with "normal" collagen tissue. It was noted by Hawkins and Bell (9) that patients with congenital atraumatic laxity have an element of collagen deficiency that may contribute to their instability and collagen formation after surgery. For that reason, we suggest moving patients with atraumatic (congenital) instability much more slowly than a young athletic patient who has trauma or acquired laxity (overhead athlete) and has "normal" collagen tissue, as well as an excellent postsurgical healing response. To that end, the program of someone who forms collagen rapidly after surgery (i.e., "fast healer") should be monitored and accelerated to prevent loss of motion and contractures. Figures 1 and 2 illustrate two significantly different patients who have both undergone capsular-shift surgical procedures. The rate of progression for each would be dramatically different. The patient's response to the surgical procedure should be carefully monitored by the rehabilitation specialist and the person must be properly adjusted.

The next factor to be considered is the status of the patient's dynamic stabilizers. An individual who has good to

TABLE 2. *Patient variables and factors*

Patient's tissue status
Hyperelasticity ↔ hypermobility
Dynamic stabilizers status
Muscle–bone
Muscular strength and balance
Proprioceptive ability
Classification of instability
Previous activity level
Desired activity level (expectations)
Healing abilities
Rapid healers, slow healers

TABLE 4. *Factors affecting the rehabilitation program*

- Type of surgical procedure
  (Exposure, specific procedure, tissue used)
- Method of fixation
- Type of instability
  (Instability classification)
- Patient's tissue status
  (Hyperelasticity, normal, hypoelasticity)
- Patient's response to surgery
- Patient's dynamic stabilization
  (Muscular strength, dynamic stability, proprioception)
- Patient's activity level
  (Past, present, desired goals)
- Physician's philosophical approach

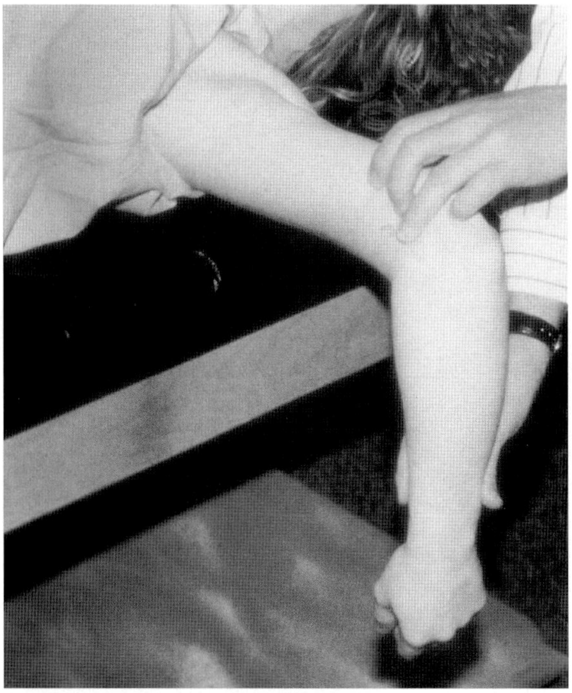

FIG. 1. This patient exhibits significant external rotation motion, in excess of 175 degrees, and an example of atraumatic congenital hypermobility.

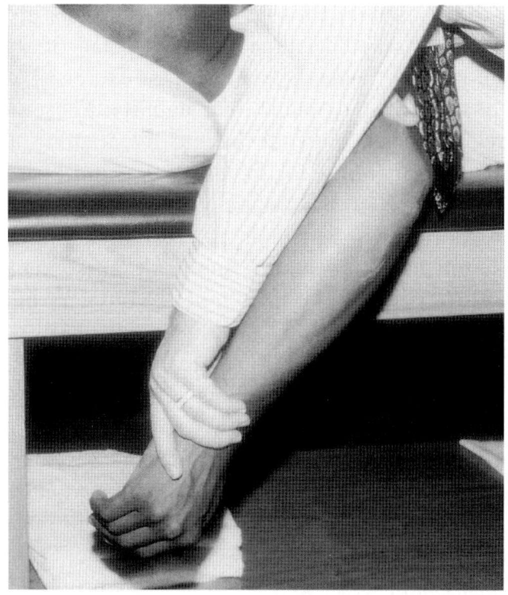

FIG. 2. The motion exhibited by this overhead athlete is due to inherent hypermobility and superimposed adaptive stretching.

excellent muscular development, muscular strength, dynamic stability, and proprioceptive abilities should progress more rapidly than someone who has an underdeveloped, slender body type and nonathletic shoulder girdle musculature. The patient's proprioceptive status should also be carefully assessed.

Finally, the patient's activity level should be considered, including past, present, and desired goals: whether the patient is athletic or nonathletic, whether the patient is an overhead athlete (thrower, tennis player, swimmer, etc.), or whether the patient leads a sedentary lifestyle.

The philosophical approach of the surgeon should be considered. Often, the surgeon's philosophy has been shaped by the training site, mentor, and previous personal experiences. All of these factors should be carefully considered before implementing a postsurgical rehabilitation program because they can significantly affect the outcome.

GENERAL REHABILITATION GUIDELINES AFTER SURGERY

In all of our rehabilitation programs after shoulder stabilization surgery, we have a multiple-phase approach, with each phase consisting of specific goals and exercises (see Table 5). We also use a criteria-based rehabilitation approach.

In the first phase, the immediate postoperative period, the rehabilitation goals are to (a) protect the healing soft tissues, (b) prevent the negative effects of immobilization, (c) reestablish dynamic joint stability, and (d) diminish postoperative pain and inflammation. Thus, during this maximal protection phase, we use early motion in a restricted and protected arc of motion. This early motion is intended to nourish the articular cartilage, assist in collagen tissue synthesis and collagen organization, and promote healing. Early motion will assist in decreasing the patient's pain through neuromuscular modulation (10–13). Depending on the type of surgical procedure, method of fixation, and the patient's tissue status, a prescribed ROM is outlined. The primary goal of this phase is to prevent excessive scarring but not allow too aggressive motion to compromise the surgical repair. Often after anterior stabilization, motions such as extension and ER are limited or restricted

TABLE 5. *General rehabilitation guidelines*

Phase I: Intermediate postoperative phase	
Goals:	Protect the healing tissue (maintain static stability
	Prevent the negative effects of immobilization
	Reestablish dynamic joint stability
	Diminish postoperative pain and inflammation
Phase II: Intermediate phase	
Goals:	Reestablish full range of motion
	Normalize arthrokinematics
	Enhance neuromuscular control
	Improve muscular strength
Phase III: Advanced strengthening phase	
Goals:	Enhance strength, power, and endurance
	Improve muscular balance
	Monitor functional motion
Phase IV: Return-to-activity phase	
Goals:	Return gradually to functional sport or work activities or both
	Maintain muscular strength and flexibility

because of the anterior capsule, whereas shoulder elevation in the plane of scapula is encouraged instead of shoulder abduction (ABD). Dynamic stabilization exercises are performed to reestablish dynamic joint stability. These stability drills are performed with the patient maintaining a static position as the therapist facilitates a muscular co-contraction (Figs. 3 and 4). The static joint position should be carefully chosen by the therapist to prevent excessive stress on the stabilization procedure. Submaximal isometrics are performed for the rotator cuff to initiate voluntary muscular contractions of these muscles, which aids in preventing muscular atrophy and a loss of motor control. Wickiewicz et al. (14) reported that most human shoulder musculature is roughly a 50:50 mixture of slow- and fast-twitch muscle fibers. Immobilization has been shown to have a greater effect on slow-twitch fibers; thus it is important for the patient to perform submaximal isometrics to prevent muscular atrophy. During this first week, we attempt to control the patient's pain and inflammation through guarded motion and isometric exercises and the judicious use of various therapeutic modalities (ice, etc.)

Phase II, the intermediate phase, emphasizes the advance of shoulder mobility. Before the patient enters phase II, the following criteria must be met: (a) satisfactory static stability, (b) diminishing pain and inflammation, and (c) adequate muscular control and dynamic stability. During this phase, the patient's ROM is gradually increased by using active–assisted and passive ROM (AAROM and PROM) exercise, stretching, and joint-mobilization techniques. Guidelines for motion progression are based on the surgical procedure, method of fixation, the patient tissue status, and are discussed throughout this chapter. Additionally, the rate of progression is based on the clinician's assessment of the quantity of motion at that time and the patient's end feel. For example, a patient with less motion than desirable at that timeframe and with a firm or hard-end feel is stretched more aggressively than a patient who has a capsular or soft-end feel. Joint-mobilization techniques are used to normalize the arthrokinematics of the glenohumeral joint. The primary goal of the joint-mobilization techniques is to restore normal motion and to correct asymmetric capsular tightness; thus the anterior capsule and posterior capsule should exhibit comparable flexibility. If one side of the capsule is excessively tight compared with the opposite side, this will result in the humeral head displacing excessively in the opposite direction (15,16). Thus, if the anterior capsule is excessively tight compared with the posterior capsule (after anterior stabilization surgery), the humeral head will tend to displace posteriorly during arm movements (17). Correcting asymmetric capsular tightness should be a critical goal for the therapist. Other goals during this phase include improving muscular strength and enhancing neuromuscular control. To achieve these goals, we use proprioceptive neuromuscular facilitation (PNF) techniques with rhythmic stabilization (18,19), neuromuscular control drills (20,21), and isolated muscular strengthening exercises for the rotator

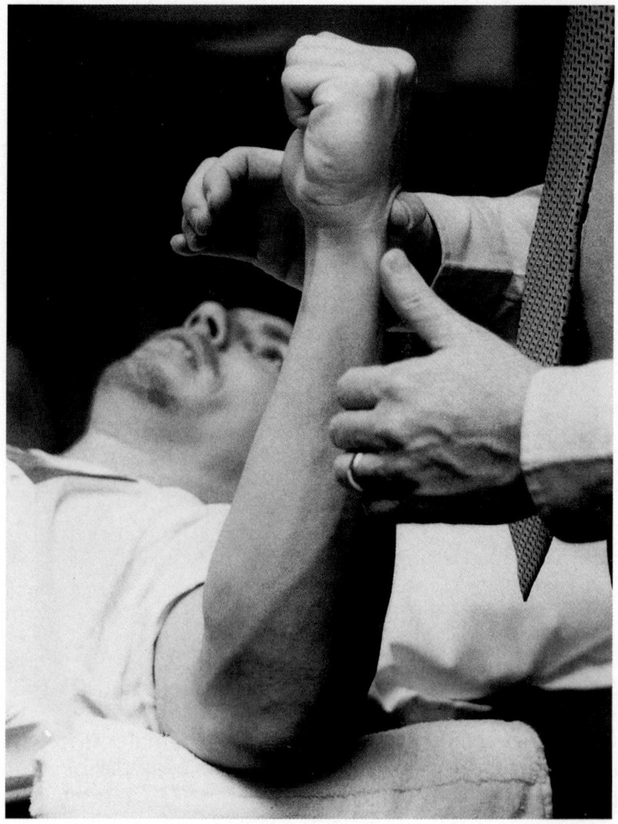

FIG. 4. Dynamic stabilization drill performed during external/internal rotation motions.

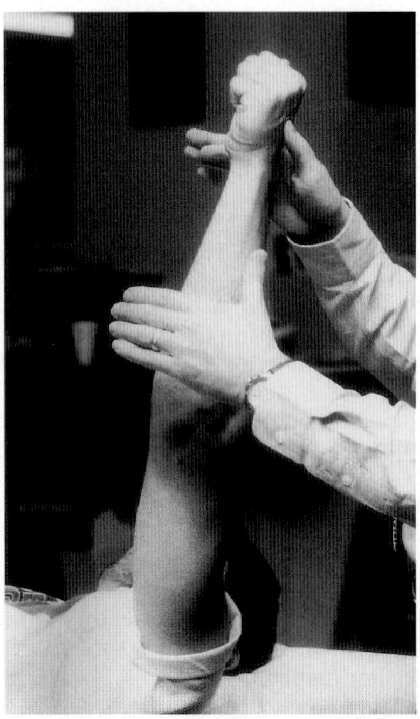

FIG. 3. Dynamic stabilization drills are performed at various arm positions. This drill is performed during shoulder flexion in the scapular plane.

cuff and scapular muscles. In the overhead athlete, toward the end of this phase, the therapist can begin aggressive stretching techniques gradually to increase motion past 90 degrees of ER. External rotation of 115 to 125 degrees is necessary for the thrower to be able to begin throwing. Strengthening exercises are focused on reestablishing muscular balance.

The third phase, the dynamic strengthening phase, is directed toward improving the patient's strength, power, and endurance while maintaining a functional ROM of the shoulder joint. The criteria that should be met before entering phase III are (a) full nonpainful functional motion, (b) muscular strength of at least 4 over 5 or of the good grade (manual muscle test), (c) satisfactory static stability on clinical examination, and (d) dynamic joint stability. Resistance exercises are progressed during this phase. The goal of this phase is to reestablish significant strength for the desired functional activities but also to reestablish muscular balance. Thus, a suitable ratio should exist between the posterior and anterior rotator-cuff muscles, rotator-cuff and deltoid muscles, and scapular muscles. The muscular ratios we strive for are ER/ internal rotation (IR) ratios of 62% to 70%, rotator cuff (ER) to deltoid (ABD) ratio of 66% to 72%, and scapular retractor to protractor ratio of approximately 100% (22–25). Muscular balance and dynamic joint stability should be achieved before initiating aggressive strengthening exercises such as plyometrics or functional activities such as throwing and swimming to ensure that dynamic joint stability has been accomplished. During this phase, eccentric muscle training and proprioceptive training are emphasized (26). Muscular endurance training also is emphasized in this phase. This is a critical element in the rehabilitation program. Wickiewicz et al. (27) showed that once the rotator-cuff muscles have reached a significant level of fatigue, the humeral head displaces superiorly with simple arm movements such as shoulder ABD. The rehabilitation program should emphasize muscular endurance training to enhance dynamic functional joint stability and to prevent fatigue-induced subluxation.

Phase IV is referred to as the return-to-activity phase. The goal of this phase is to increase gradually and progressively the functional demands on the shoulder to return the patient to full unrestricted sport or daily activities. The criteria established before a patient's return to sport activities are (a) full functional ROM, (b) adequate static stability, (c) satisfactory muscular strength and endurance, (d) adequate dynamic stability, and (e) a satisfactory clinical examination. Once these criteria are successfully met, the patient may initiate a gradual return to sport activity in a controlled manner. Healing constraints based on surgical technique and fixation, as well as the patient's tissue status, should be considered before a functional program can be initiated. Other goals of this phase are to maintain the patient's muscular strength, dynamic stability, and shoulder functional motion established in the previous phase. A stretching and strengthening program should be performed on an ongoing basis to maintain and continue to improve on these goals.

REHABILITATION AFTER SHOULDER STABILIZATION SURGERY FOR TRAUMATIC INSTABILITY

The rehabilitation program after surgical repair of an injured capsule or capsulolabral complex due to a traumatic injury is based on several factors. The most important factor is the type of surgical procedure performed, and subsequently whether the surgery was performed via an open incision or an arthroscopic technique. Another important factor is the exact surgical procedure performed; this is important for the therapist to understand. Third, the method of fixation of the injured tissue is extremely important to consider when designing the rehabilitation program (i.e., was the repair accomplished by using suture anchors, bioabsorbable tacks, sutures, or staples). The fixation method is important because each fixation type has different strengths; thus the rate of the rehabilitation progression must be adjusted to match each fixation device. Fourth, consider the extent of the injury. Was a Bankart procedure performed with a capsular tensioning or capsular-shift procedure? Or was an isolated Bankart procedure performed? Fifth, the tissue status of the patient must be carefully considered. Does the patient have a capsule that is thick and robust or a capsule that is thin and pouchous? The status of the patient's dynamic stabilizers, muscle tone, and muscle mass surrounding the shoulder complex is important to consider. The patient's desired activity level and expectations should be taken into consideration. To what activities is the patient returning? It is important to determine the degree of motion required to perform the desired activities (i.e., whether the patient is an overhead athlete who requires excessive motion or a sedentary office worker who participates in light recreational sports such as golf). In addition, the patient's response to the surgery must be cautiously monitored during the rehabilitation process and the process and the program adjusted accordingly.

REHABILITATION AFTER OPEN STABILIZATION PROCEDURES

Numerous operative procedures correct anterior instability; more than 250 different operative procedures have been described. Payne and Altchek (28) classified the most popular current techniques into four basic groups:

1. Anatomic repairs: reconstruction of the disrupted anatomy anteroinferior capsulolabral structure (Bankart, Bankart-type procedures, capsulolabral reconstructions and modifications).
2. Bony block procedures: coracoid-process transfer procedures such as a Bristow procedure.
3. Procedures that tighten the anterior structures: Magnusson–Stack, Putti–Platt procedures.
4. Osteotomies: designed to change the bony rotational alignment of the glenoid or the humerus or both.

This is a useful classification scheme by which a therapist can design rehabilitation programs. In this chapter, I discuss the rehabilitation approach for several of these surgical procedures.

Several authors described the postoperative rehabilitation program after a Bankart procedure (14,28,29) or a capsulolabral reconstruction (30–32).

A Bankart procedure or capsulolabral reconstruction often includes not only restoring the correct anatomic attachment site of the capsule but also restoring the proper tension of the inferior glenohumeral ligament through a selective capsular repair (28–30,32). The primary goal of the surgical procedure is regaining glenohumeral joint stability while preserving adequate ROM to resume functional activities. The primary goal of the rehabilitation program is restoring adequate ROM, enabling the patient to resume desired sport and functional activities while preserving the integrity and stability of the surgical procedure. This can represent a significant challenge in rehabilitating the overhead athlete or patients who require more than 90 degrees of ER for functional activities.

At our center, the surgical technique is performed by using suture anchors to fixate the capsule to bone. The subscapularis muscle is either split (in overhead athletes; 32,33) or is particularly divided from the lateral tendon insertion (in nonoverhead athletes). In my opinion, it appears most patients have significantly less postoperative muscular spasm and soreness after the muscle-splitting procedure. The capsular repair is performed with the arm in ER. The amount of ER varies depending on the degree of capsular laxity and the functional demands of the patient. Overhead athletes are positioned in 60 degrees of ABD, neutral forward flexion, and 60 to 75 degrees of ER. Conversely, nonoverhead athletes are positioned in 45 to 60 degrees of ABD and 30 degrees of ER.

The rehabilitation program after an open Bankart procedure is divided into four phases (see Table 6). In the first

TABLE 6. *Open anterior capsulolabral reconstruction*

I. Phase I: Immediate postoperative phase
   Goals: Protect the surgical procedure
   Minimize the effects of immobilization
   Diminish pain and inflammation

   Weeks 0–2
   - Sling for comfort (1 week)
   - May wear immobilizer for sleep (2 weeks) **Physician decision
   - Elbow/hand ROM
   - Gripping exercises
   - Passive ROM and active assistive ROM (L-bar)
     - Flexion to tolerance
     - Abduction to tolerance
     - ER/IR in scapular plane
   - Submaximal isometrics
   - Rhythmic stabilization
   - Cryotherapy, modalities as needed

   Weeks 3–4
   - Gradually progress ROM
     - Flexion to 120–140 degrees
     - ER in scapular plane to 35–45 degrees
     - IR in scapular plane to 45–60 degrees
     - Shoulder extension
   - Initiate light isotonics for shoulder musculature
     - Tubing for ER/IR
     - Dumbells; deltoid, supraspinatus, biceps, scapular
     - Continue dynamic stabilization exercises, PNF
   - Initiate self-capsular stretching

   Weeks 5–6
   - Progress ROM as tolerated
     - Flexion to 160 degrees (maximum)
     - ER/IR at 90 degrees abduction:
       - IR to 75 degrees
       - ER to 70–75 degrees
     - Shoulder extension to 30–35 degrees
   - Joint mobilization, stretching, etc.
   - Continue self-capsular stretching
   - UBE arm at 90 degrees abduction
   - Progress all strengthening exercises
     - Continue PNF diagonal patterns (rhythmic stabilization techniques)
     - Continue isotonic strengthening
     - Dynamic stabilization exercises

(continued)

TABLE 6. *Continued*

Weeks 6–7
- Progress ROM to
  - ER at 90 degrees abduction: 80–85 degrees
  - ER at 90 degrees abduction: 70–75 degrees
  - Flexion: 165–175 degrees

II. Phase II: Intermediate phase
Goals: Reestablish full ROM
Normalize arthrokinematics
Improve muscular strength
Enhance neuromuscular control

Weeks 8–10
- Progress to full ROM (weeks 7–8)
- Continue all stretching exercises
  - Joint mobilization, capsular stretching, passive and active stretching
- In overhead athletes, progress ER past 90 degrees
- In nonoverhead athletes, maintain 90-degree ER
- Continue strengthening exercises
  - Throwers Ten Program (for overhead athlete)
  - Isotonic strengthening for entire shoulder complex
  - PNF manual technique
  - Neuromuscular control drills
  - Isokinetic strengthening

Weeks 10–14
- Continue all flexibility exercises
- Continue all strengthening exercises
- May initiate "light" plyometric exercises
- May initiate "controlled" swimming, golf swings, etc
- May initiate light isotonic machine weight training (weeks 12–14)

III. Phase III: Advanced strengthening phase (months 4–6)
Goals: Enhance muscular strength, power and endurance
Improve muscular endurance
Maintain mobility

Criteria to enter Phase III:
1) Full range of motion
2) No pain or tenderness
3) Satisfactory stability
4) Strength 70–80% of contralateral side

Weeks 14–20
- Continue all flexibility exercises
  - Self-capsular stretches (anterior, posterior, and inferior)
  - Maintain ER flexibility
- Continue isotonic strengthening program
- Emphasize muscular balance (ER/IR)
- Continue PNF manual resistance
- May initiate and continue plyometrics
- Initiate interval throwing program (physician approval necessary)

Weeks 20–24
- Continue all exercises listed earlier
- Continue and progress all interval sport program (throwing, etc.)

IV. Phase IV: Return-to-activity phase (months 6–9)
Goals: Gradual return to sport activities
Maintain strength and mobility of shoulder

Criteria to enter Phase IV:
1) Full nonpainful ROM
2) Satisfactory stability
3) Satisfactory strength (isokinetics)
4) No pain or tenderness

Exercises:
- Continue capsular stretching to maintain mobility
- Continue strengthening program
  - Either Thrower's Ten or fundamental shoulder-exercise program
- Return to sport participation (unrestricted)

ER, external rotation; IR, internal rotation; PNF, proprioceptive neuromuscular facilitation; ROM, range of motion; UBE, upper body ergometer.

phase, the immediate postoperative period, the goals are to protect the surgical procedure while minimizing the effects of immobilization. During this phase, approximately 6 weeks in duration, the goal is to increase gradually the patient's shoulder motion in a safe and expeditious manner, while preserving the integrity of the stabilization procedure. Early protected and guarded motion is essential for collagen tissue synthesis, organization, and the prevention of excessive scarring, which may restrict motion (34). Additionally, isometric strengthening exercises are performed to minimize muscular atrophy and to reestablish dynamic joint stability.

The postoperative rehabilitation program begins on the day after surgery with the patient performing gripping exercises and active motion at the elbow and wrist. The shoulder is passively moved through an arc of motion for shoulder ABD, flexion, and ER and IR in the scapular plane. Additionally, the patient performs AAROM exercises by using an L-bar (Breg Corp., Vista, CA, U.S.A.) (Figs. 5 and 6). Submaximal isometrics and rhythmic stabilization exercises are performed to prevent muscular atrophy and improve proprioception, this to promote dynamic stability through muscular co-contraction. The patient is placed in a sling for comfort but is encouraged to remove the sling daily to perform shoulder exercises. ROM exercises are performed 3 times per day and isometric strengthening twice per day.

ROM gradually progresses, and at 3 to 4 weeks, shoulder flexion should be 120 to 140 degrees, IR, 45 to 60 degrees, and ER, 35 to 45 degrees with the arm in the scapular plane. Shoulder extension and horizontal ABD/adduction stretching are initiated at this time. Shoulder-strengthening exercises progress by using exercise tubing for the internal and external rotators (Fig. 7) and isotonic dumbbell (low-weight) strengthening for deltoid and scapular muscles.

At four weeks after surgery, we allow the overhead athlete to perform IR/ER stretching at 90 degrees of ABD (see Fig. 8), and at week 5, we expect the patient to have approximately 70–75 degrees of ER and IR and 160 degrees of flexion. At 6 weeks, the patient is expected to have 80–85 degrees of ER and full IR and shoulder flexion. The shoulder-strengthening exercises progress with special emphasis on the rotator-cuff, deltoid, and scapular muscles. In addition, techniques to enhance dynamic stability such as PNF exercises (Fig. 9), neuromuscular control drills, and co-contractions also are performed.

Full functional ROM is expected by week 8, when the second phase, the intermediate phase, is initiated. The focus of this phase is the advancement of shoulder mobility to match the functional demands of the patient. It is important for the therapist now to balance the capsular mobility anteriorly and posteriorly. Joint mobilization and stretching are useful techniques to accomplish this goal. This prevents asymmetric capsular tightening. During this phase (between weeks 8 and 10), aggressive stretching techniques are implemented to reestablish the amount of ER necessary to perform overhead sports. During this phase, all strengthening exercises progress; in the overhead athlete, the ''Thrower's Ten program'' is implemented (see Table 7). At approximately weeks 12 to 14, plyometrics can be initiated in a gradual fashion. During this phase, stretching exercises are performed by the patient twice daily until full motion is comfortable, and then stretching exercises are performed once daily.

The third phase, the advanced strengthening phase, is initiated once the patient has met the specific criteria necessary to advance (see Table 6). Once these criteria are achieved, the patient may begin an aggressive sports-specific or a functional strengthening program. Exercises such as plyometrics, eccentrics, fast-speed isotonics, PNF, isotonics, and functional drills are emphasized.

During this phase, the goals are to enhance the patient's strength, power, and endurance, and to maximize the efficiency of the dynamic stabilizers. Specific exercises based on the specific demands of the patient are emphasized. In

(Text continues on page 381)

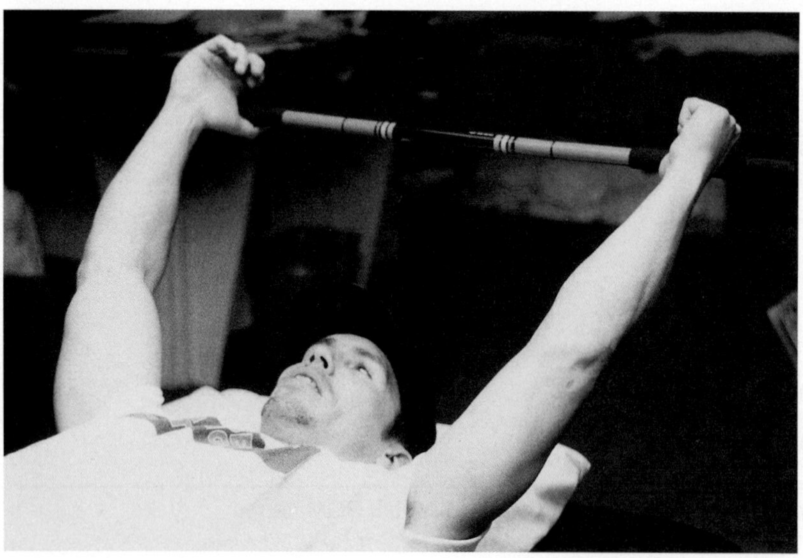

FIG. 5. Active–assisted flexion motion performed with an L-bar (Breg Corp., Vista, CA, U.S.A.).

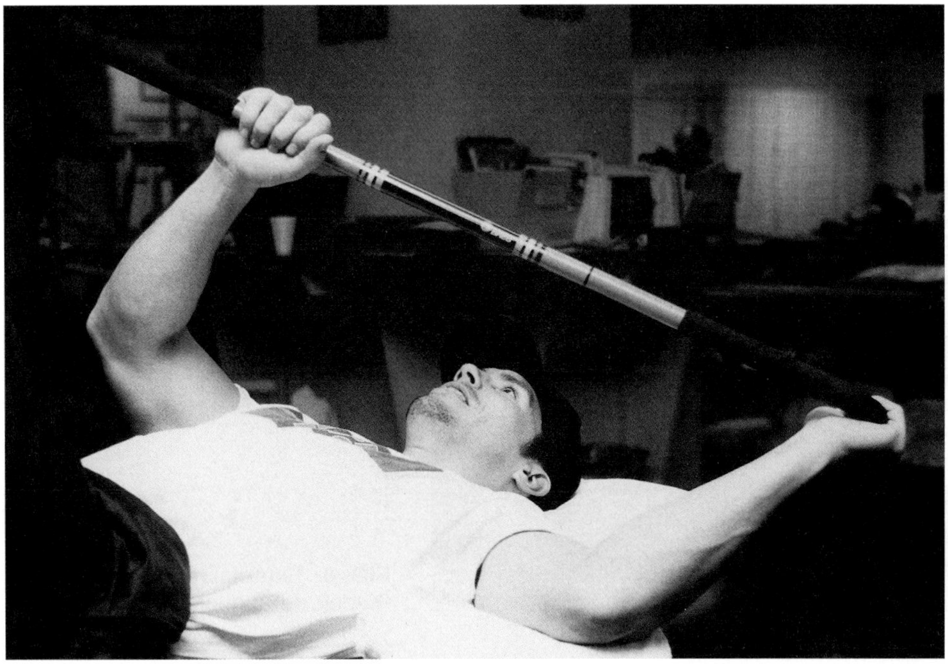

FIG. 6. Active–assisted external/internal rotation performed with an L-bar in the scapular plane.

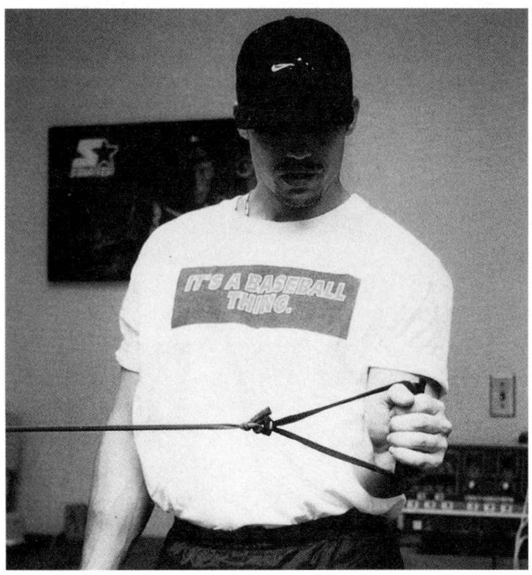

FIG. 7. Shoulder external rotation is performed by using exercise tubing.

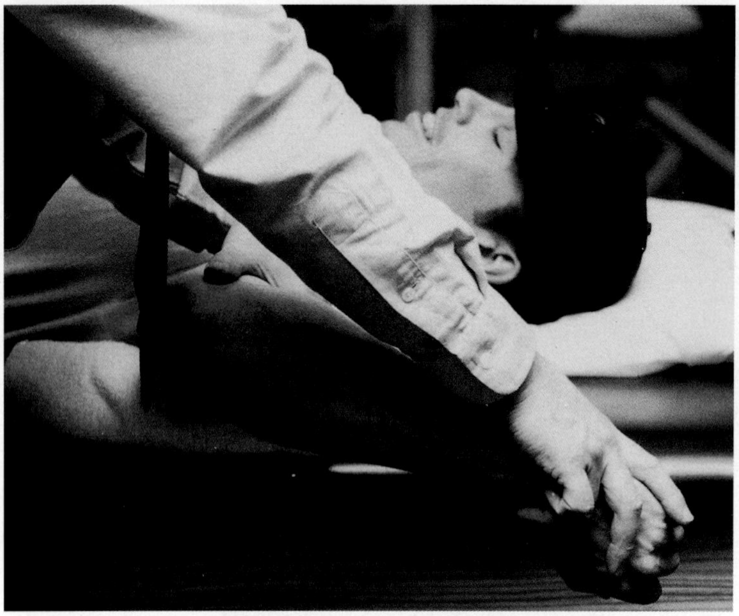

FIG. 8. External rotation stretching is performed in the 90-degree abducted position.

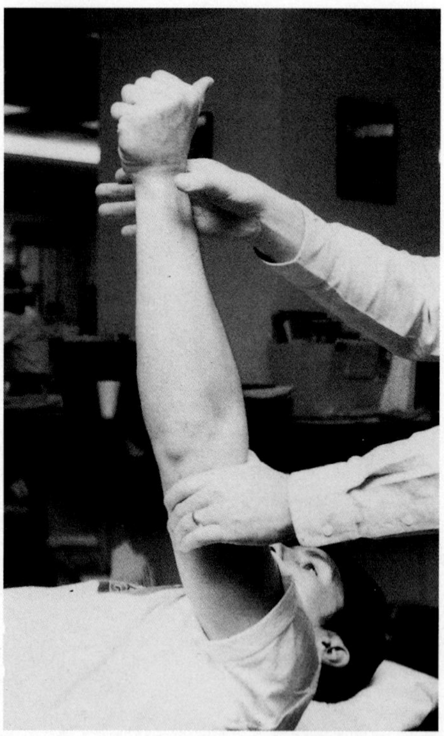

FIG. 9. Dynamic stabilization is enhanced by using a proprioceptive neuromuscular facilitation (PNF) D_2 flexion pattern with rhythmic stabilization performed at 75 degrees of arm elevation.

TABLE 7. *Thrower's Ten program*

The Throwers Ten Program is designed to exercise the major muscles necessary for throwing. The program's goal is to be an organized and concise exercise program. In addition, all exercises included are specific to the thrower and are designed to improve strength, power and endurance of the shoulder complex musculature.

1. A. Diagonal Pattern D2 Extension: Involved hand will grip tubing handle overhead and out to the side. Pull tubing down and across your body to the opposite side of leg. During the motion lead with your thumb. Perform _ sets of _______ repetitions _______ daily.

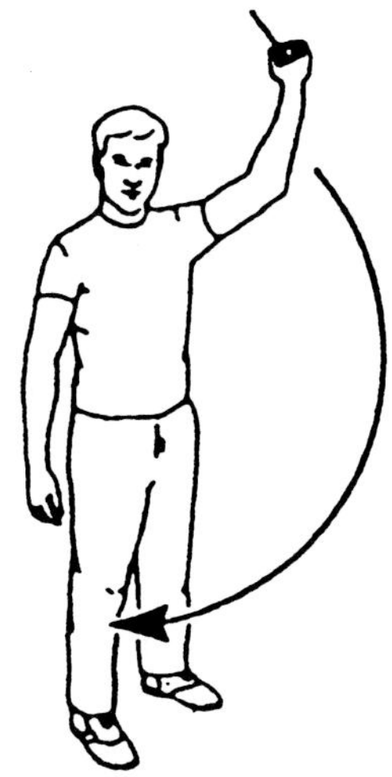

1. B. Diagonal Pattern D2 Flexion: Gripping tubing handle in hand of involved arm, begin with arm out from side 45° and palm facing backward. After turning palm forward, proceed to flex elbow and bring arm up and over uninvolved shoulder. Turn palm down and reverse to take arm to starting position. Exercise should be performed in controlled manner. Perform _______ sets of _______ repetitions _______ daily.

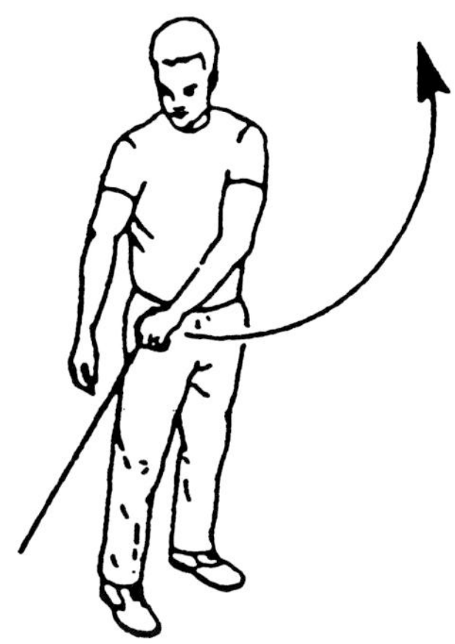

2. A. External Rotation at 0 degrees Abduction: Stand with involved elbow fixed at side, elbow at 90° and involved arm across front of body. Grip tubing handle while the other end of tubing is fixed. Pull out with arm, keeping elbow at side. Return tubing slowly and controlled. Perform _______ sets of _______ repetitions _______ times daily.

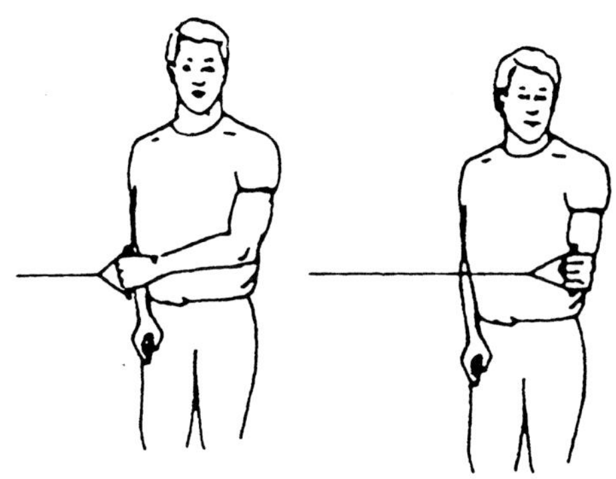

2. B. Internal Rotation at 0 degrees Abduction: Standing with elbow at side fixed at 90° and shoulder rotated out. Grip tubing handle while other end of tubing is fixed. Pull arm across body keeping elbow at side. Return tubing slowly and controlled. Perform _______ sets of _______ repetitions _______ times daily.

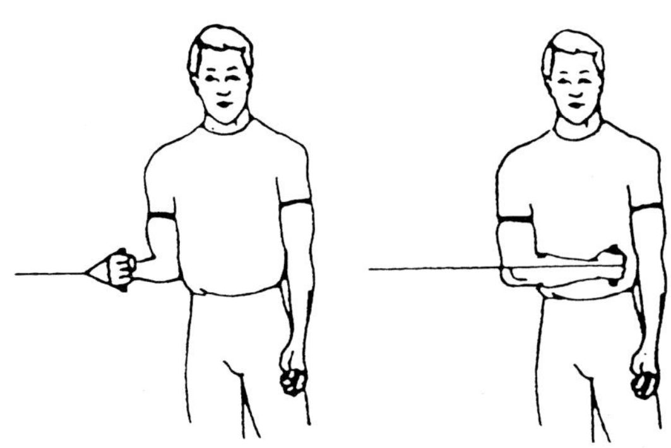

(*continued*)

TABLE 7. *Continued*

2\. C. External Rotation at 90 degrees Abduction:
Stand with shoulder abducted 90 degrees and elbow flexed 90 degrees. Grip tubing handle while the other end is fixed straight ahead, slightly lower than the shoulder. Keeping shoulder abducted, rotate shoulder back keeping elbow at 90 degrees. Return tubing and hand to start position.
I. *Slow Speed, Sets:* (Slow and Controlled): Perform _______ sets of _______ repetitions _______ times daily.
II. *Fast Speed Sets:* Perform _______ sets of _______ repetitions _______ times daily.

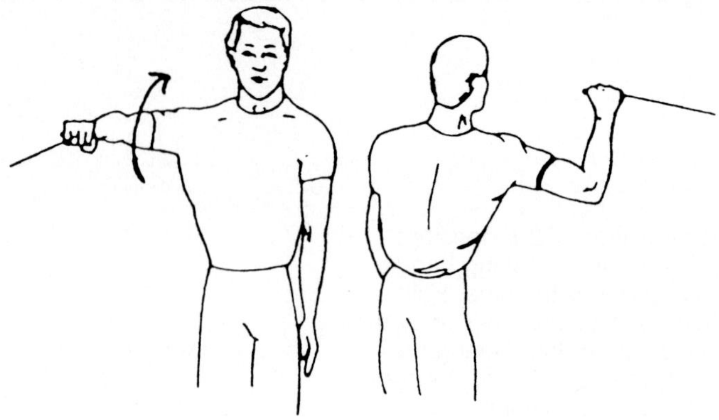

2\. D. Internal Rotation at 90 degrees Abduction:
Stand with shoulder abducted to 90 degrees, externally rotated 90 degrees and elbow bent to 90 degrees. Keeping shoulder abducted, rotate shoulder forward, keeping elbow bent at 90°. Return tubing and hand to start position.
I. *Slow Speed Sets:* (Slow and Controlled): Perform _______ sets of _______ repetitions _______ times daily.
II. *Fast Speed Sets:* Perform _______ sets of _______ repetitions _______ times daily.

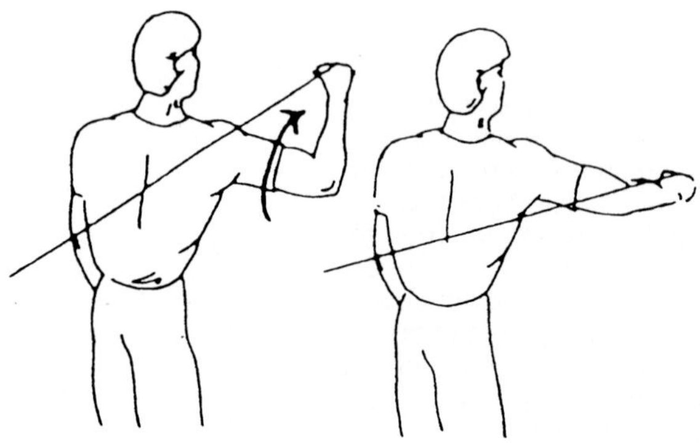

3\. Shoulder Abduction to 90 degrees:
Stand with arm at side, elbow straight, and palm against side. Raise arm to the side, palm down, until arm reaches 90 degrees (shoulder level). Hold 2 seconds and lower slowly. Perform _______ sets of _______ repetitions _______ times daily.

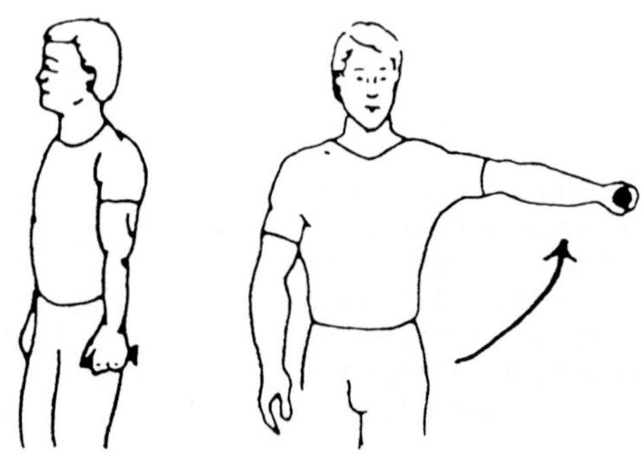

4\. Scaption, "Full can":
Stand with elbow straight and thumb up. Raise arm to shoulder level at 30 degrees in front of body. Do not go above shoulder height. Hold 2 seconds and lower slowly. Perform _______ sets of _______ repetitions _______ times daily.

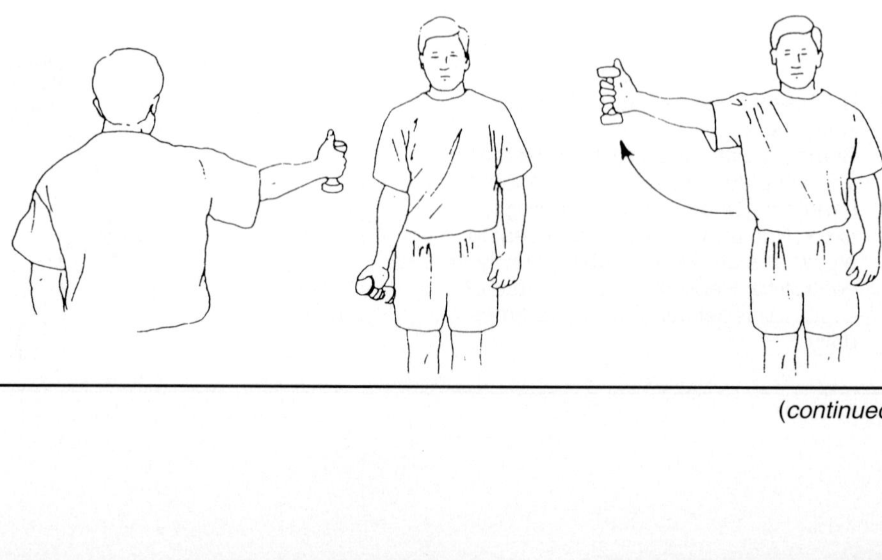

(*continued*)

TABLE 7. *Continued*

5. A. Prone Horizontal Abduction (Neutral):
Lie on table, face down, with involved arm hanging straight to the floor, and palm facing down. Raise arm out to the side, parallel to the floor. Hold 2 seconds and lower slowly. Perform ________ sets of ________ repetitions ________ times daily.

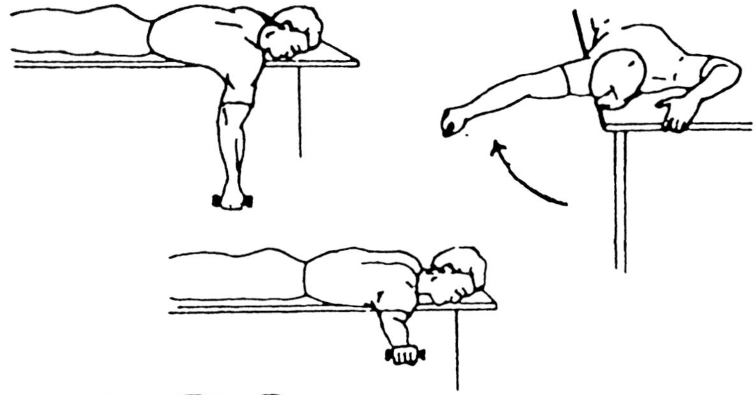

5. B. Prone Horizontal Abduction Full ER, 100 degrees ABD):
Lie on table, face down, with involved arm hanging straight to the floor, and thumb rotated up (hitchhiker). Raise arm out to the side with arm slightly in front of shoulder, parallel to the floor. Hold 2 seconds and lower slowly. Perform ________ sets of ________ repetitions ________ times daily.

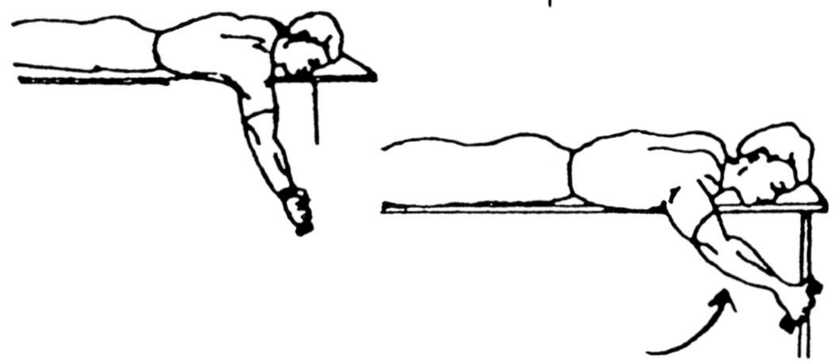

6. Press-Ups:
Seated on a chair or on a table, place both hands firmly on the sides of the chair or table, palm down and fingers pointed outward. Hands should be placed equal with shoulders. Slowly push downward through the hands to elevate your body. Hold the elevated position for 2 seconds and lower body slowly. Perform ________ sets of ________ repetitions ________ times daily.

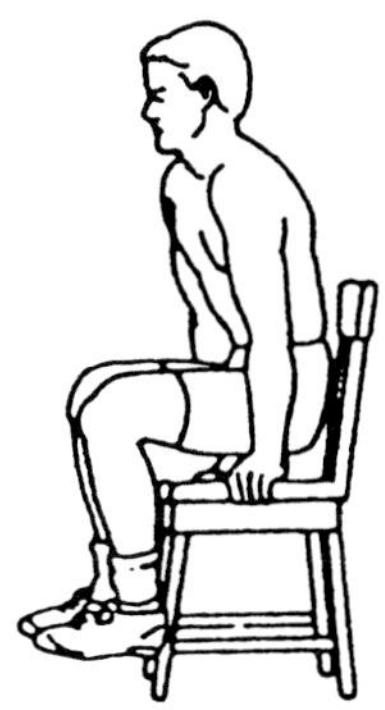

7. Prone Rowing:
Lying on your stomach with your involved arm hanging over the side of the table, dumbbell in hand and elbow straight. Slowly raise arm, bending elbow, and bring dumbbell as high as possible. Hold at the top for 2 seconds, then slowly lower. Perform ________ sets of ________ repetitions ________ times daily.

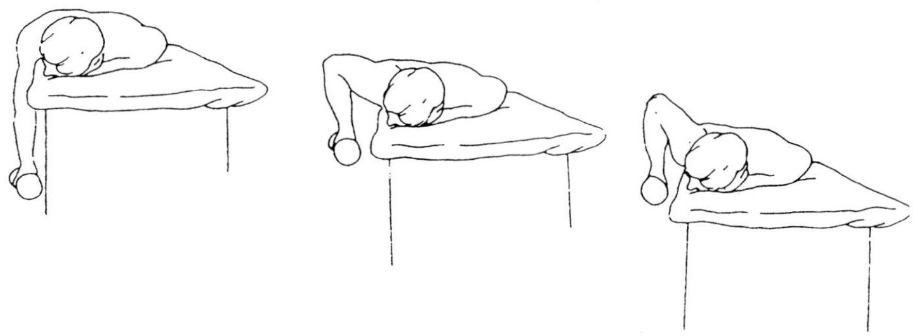

8. Push-Ups:
Start in the down position with arms in a comfortable position. Place hands no more than shoulder width apart. Push up as high as possible, rolling shoulders forward after elbows are straight. Start with a push-up into wall. Gradually progress to table top and eventually to floor as tolerable. Perform ________ sets of ________ repetitions ________ times daily.

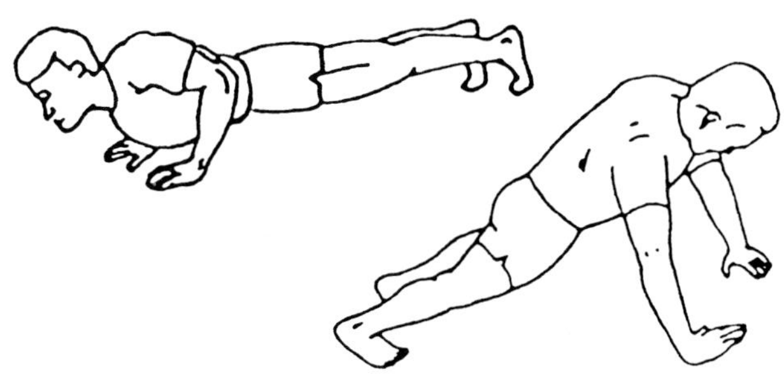

(*continued*)

TABLE 7. *Continued*

9. A. Elbow Flexion:
Standing with arm against side and palm facing inward, bend elbow upward turning palm as you progress. Hold 2 seconds and lower slowly. Perform ____ sets of ________ repetitions ________ times daily.

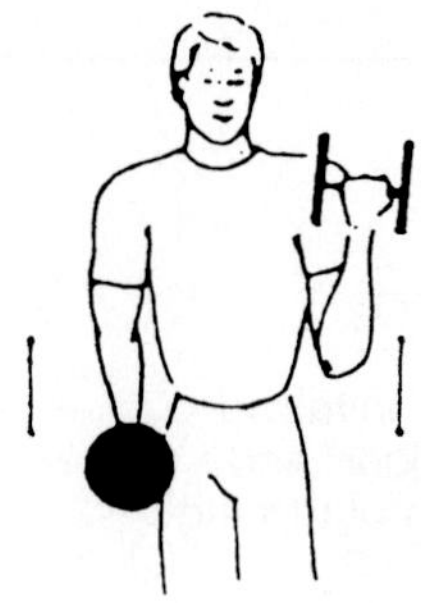

9. B. Elbow Extension:
Abduction:
Raise involved arm overhead. Provide support at elbow from uninvolved hand. Straighten arm overhead. Hold 2 seconds and lower slowly. Perform ________ sets of ________ repetitions ________ times daily.

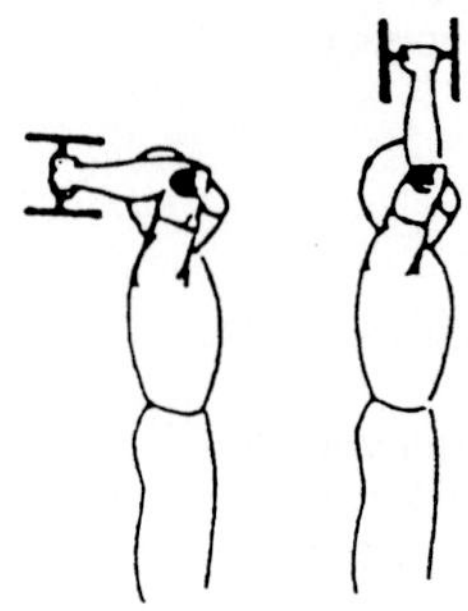

10. A. Wrist Extension:
Supporting the forearm and with palm facing downward, raise weight in hand as far as possible. Hold 2 seconds and lower slowly. Perform ________ sets of ________ repetitions ________ times daily.

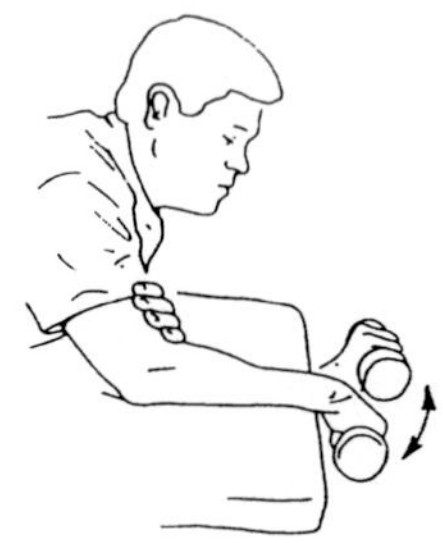

10. B. Wrist Flexion:
Supporting the forearm and with palm facing upward, lower a weight in hand as far as possible and then curl it up as high as possible. Hold for 2 seconds and lower slowly. Perform ________ sets of ________ repetitions ________ times daily.

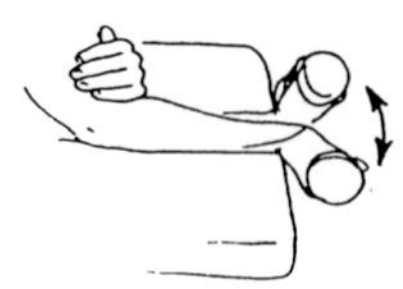

10. C. Supination:
Forearm supported on table with wrist in neutral position. Using a weight or hammer, roll wrist taking palm up. Hold for a 2 count and return to starting position. Perform ________ sets of ____ repetitions ________ times daily.

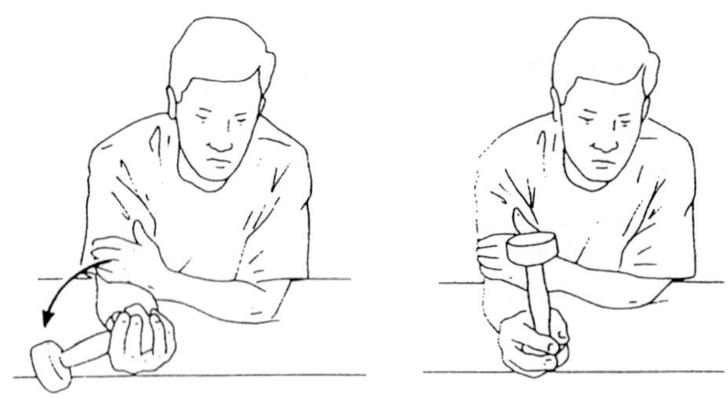

10. D. Pronation:
Forearm should be supported on a table with wrist in neutral position. Using a weight or hammer, roll wrist taking palm down. Hold for a 2 count and return to starting position. Perform ________ sets of ________ repetitions ________ times daily.

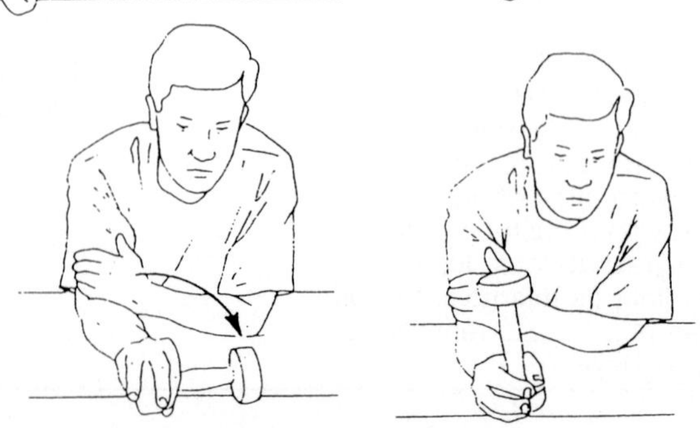

the overhead athlete, an interval sport program (throwing, tennis, swimming, etc.) may be initiated. It is critical that the patient continue a stretching program to maintain shoulder motion and to address any residual stiffness.

The last phase is the return-to-activity phase. During this period, athletes may gradually return to their specific sports once the established criteria have been met. A return to overhead sports usually occurs between 6 and 7 months. Other sports can usually be initiated in 5 to 6 months. A strengthening and flexibility program should be continued for all patients for at least 12 to 18 months.

This surgical procedure and rehabilitation program has been extremely successful in providing stability and regaining functional mobility at the glenohumeral joint. Previous authors reported a recurrence rate of shoulder instability of less than 5% by using an open Bankart repair procedure (35,36). However, regaining full ROM and functional activities has been variable in athletes. Rowe and Patel (36) reported that only 33% of the athletes in their series were able to return to the preoperative competitive level. Kvitne et al. (37) reported 97% good to excellent results with a capsulolabral reconstruction and similar rehabilitation program. They noted a 90% return to athletics at the previous level of competition and approximately 64% return to competitive baseball. Rosenberg et al. (38) reported a 15-year follow-up on 33 shoulders that underwent a Bankart procedure. The average restriction in ER was 15 degrees. The investigators noted a positive correlation between loss of ER motion and degenerative changes noted on plain radiographs. This emphasizes the importance of restoring full motion, especially symmetric capsular mobility.

In summary, the rehabilitation program after an open Bankart-type procedure after trauma is rapid in the restoration of motion and strength. The therapist should restore balance in the degree of mobility of the anterior and posterior capsule. If balance is not achieved, or the anterior capsule exhibits significant tightness, the humeral head will tend to displace posteriorly or to the most lax portion of the capsule during functional activities. Asymmetric capsular tightness contributes to osteoarthritic changes to the glenohumeral joint. Strengthening should be restored to normal muscular strength for that patient. A bilateral comparison is usually sufficient, with the dominant arm exhibiting 5% to 10% greater strength (39). Once these goals have been accomplished, a gradual program that returns the patient to strenuous functional activities or sports or both may be initiated.

REHABILITATION AFTER ARTHROSCOPIC STABILIZATION PROCEDURES

Although the open Bankart procedure has been considered by some as the "gold standard," some authors have suggested arthroscopic stabilization techniques for certain patients under specific conditions. The arthroscopic technique has been suggested by some physicians because there appears to be less residual stiffness, less loss of motion, and improved cosmesis. There are numerous arthroscopic stabilization procedures, in which the method of soft-tissue fixation used is the major difference. These procedures include the use of arthroscopic staples (40–42), implantable suture anchors (43,44), and transosseous suturing (45,46).

At our center, the arthroscopic stabilization technique for repair of a Bankart lesion uses either a suture-anchor device or a cannulated absorbable fixation device (Suretac, Acufex Microsurgical Inc., Mansfield, MA, U.S.A.) as described by Warner and Warren (47). Although some authors have reported unacceptable high recurrence rates for arthroscopic stabilization (48–50), we have noted that, with proper selection criteria, this surgical technique is extremely beneficial. The selective criteria include a history of a traumatic anterior subluxation or dislocation with a discrete Bankart lesion, robust capsuloligamentous structures, no evidence of multidirectional hyperlaxity, and no rotator-cuff pathology.

The rehabilitation program after arthroscopic stabilization is significantly different from that of the open stabilization. The rate of progression immediately after surgery is much slower in the arthroscopically stabilized shoulder because of the method of fixation used. Shall and Crowley (51) reported the pull-out strength of various soft-tissue fixation devices. The Acufex Suretac was found ultimately to fail at approximately 122 N (27 lb), with the majority of failures (94%) occurring because of the tack pulling out from the bone. The investigators reported that the suture anchor (Mitek super-anchor) was almost twice as strong (failing at 217 N). The Suretac is made of polyglyconate polymer that loses its strength over a 4- to 6-week period and gradually becomes reabsorbed during the next several months (52). It is important for the clinician to realize that the strength of the arthroscopic tissue-fixation method is somewhat tenuous for the first 4 to 6 weeks, and care should be taken not to disturb the soft-tissue repair. For that reason, the initial postoperative rehabilitation is much slower for the arthroscopically stabilized shoulder compared with the open procedure.

Several authors briefly outlined their postoperative rehabilitation programs after arthroscopic stabilization (14,46, 53–56). Some authors advocated postoperative immobilization for 4 to 6 weeks and a guarded-motion program with a gradual restoration of motion. Wieckiewicz et al. (14) suggested 4 weeks of immobilization followed by AAROM and PROM from week 4, and full motion by approximately 2.5 months. Immobilization was reported to be critical in the immediate postoperative phase (46) because the repair is of soft tissue to bone. Various authors suggested several time frames for immobilization. Some authors suggested 3 weeks (53–55), others 4 weeks (14,46,52,56), and others 6 weeks (57,58) of immobilization after arthroscopic stabilization. Johnson (59) reported a dramatic decrease in recurrent instability after arthroscopic stapling by increasing the period of immobilization from 1 to 3 weeks. Grana et al. (53) noted that some patients may not comply with long periods of strict immobilization because of minimal pain and less operative morbidity. These patients may return to some activities prematurely. Grana et al. (53) reported on

27 patients who underwent arthroscopic suture stabilization. The authors noted that 10 patients admitted removal of the immobilizer after the first week; eight of the 10 were rated as poor results because of recurrent instability. Most authors agree on restricting or limiting shoulder ABD and ER for several weeks (4 to 6 weeks), initiating a strengthening program at 4 to 8 weeks, and restricting contact sports or strenuous sports for 6 months (14,51,52,57).

Our rehabilitation program is divided into four specific phases (see Table 8). The first phase is considered the maximal protection phase or restricted motion phase. Immediately postoperatively, the patient is placed in an immobilizer brace; this brace is used consistently for the first 7 days and is worn during sleep for 2 to 4 weeks after surgery. The patient will use a sling during daily activities from weeks 2 to 3. During the first 2 weeks, the patient is allowed to perform AAROM and PROM. The active–assisted motion is restricted to 60 degrees of forward flexion, 45 degrees of IR, and 5 to 10 degrees of ER with the arm placed in 20 degrees of ABD. Additionally, PROM is performed for shoulder flexion and ABD to a maximum of 90 degrees, and IR and ER, with the arm at 20 degrees of ABD to tolerance. These ranges are strictly enforced to prevent potentially deleterious forces on the anteroinferior aspect of the glenohumeral capsule where the surgical procedure has been performed. During this phase, the patient also performs submaximal and subpainful isometrics for the shoulder musculature. Additionally, cryotherapy and other modalities may be used to reduce postoperative pain and inflammation.

At weeks 3 to 4, the sling is usually discontinued; this is based on the clinical assessment of the patient's stability, response to surgery, and pain level. Occasionally, the patient is encouraged to continue the use of the shoulder immobilizer while sleeping to restrict excessive uncontrolled shoulder motions and positioning. At this time, AAROM and PROM exercises are continued gradually to improve ABD and ER, as well as flexion and IR. At 4 weeks, we increase but restrict active–assisted and passive ABD and flexion motion to 90 degrees to prevent excessive tension on the repaired capsule. The ER and IR motions are performed at 20 to 30 degrees of shoulder ABD and are limited to 15 to 20 and 60 degrees, respectively. In addition, the patient will perform light strengthening exercises such as rhythmic stabilization exercises for the ER/IR muscles and submaximal isometrics for all the shoulder musculature, both to restore dynamic joint stability.

At weeks 5 to 6, the goal is gradually to restore motion. The ER/IR stretching and motion exercises are performed at 45 degrees of ABD, which produces a mild stretch on the inferior capsule (during ER motion). The patient is encouraged gradually to improve shoulder flexion, progressing to 135 to 140 degrees at 6 weeks. Also at this time, we will allow the patient to begin light resistance isotonic strengthening exercises. The ER/IR muscles are exercised by using exercise tubing. Additionally, a light weight (1 to 2 lb) can be used to perform ABD to 90 degrees, flexion to 90 degrees, and scapular musculature strengthening.

During the first 6 weeks, we restrict motion to prevent overloading or overstressing the repaired capsule. Furthermore, I attempt to allow gradual restoration of motion, which helps prevent the negative effects of immobilization and assists in collagen formation and organization. During these first 6 weeks, care must be taken by the therapist not to overstress the healing tissue and the soft-tissue fixation.

Phase II, the moderate protection phase, begins at week 6 and progresses to week 14. The goals of this phase are to (a) gradually restore full, nonpainful ROM, (b) preserve the integrity of the surgical repair, (c) restore muscular strength and endurance, and (d) allow some functional activities.

During this phase, all motions gradually progress. Shoulder flexion and ABD progress to 180 degrees. Shoulder IR and ER motion exercises are performed at 90 degrees of ABD, and at 7 to 8 weeks, the patient should have 75 to 80 degrees of ER and full IR (70 to 75 degrees). At weeks 9 to 10, we expect full ROM; ER should be approximately 85 to 90 degrees. At week 12, we begin aggressively to stretch the thrower's shoulder past 90 degrees of ER with the goal of 115 to 125 degrees of ER. During this phase, all strengthening exercises gradually progress with the goal of improving rotator-cuff and scapular strength, restoring muscular balance, and enhancing dynamic stabilization of the glenohumeral joint complex. The patient is not allowed to perform isotonic exercises on weight-lifting equipment such as the bench press, pull-overs, and so on.

Phase III is the minimal-protection phase, extending from weeks 14 through 20. The goals of this phase are to (a) establish or maintain full ROM, (b) improve strength and endurance, and (c) initiate functional activities gradually. At approximately 14 to 16 weeks, activities such as light swimming exercises at 90 degrees of ABD, plyometrics, and golf swings are permitted. An interval throwing program or other interval sport programs may be initiated at week 18 if the criteria (see Table 8) have been met by the patient.

The advanced strengthening phase extends from weeks 22 through 26. This phase is characterized by aggressive strengthening exercises such as plyometrics, PNF drills, isotonic strengthening, and functional sports activities. In the overhead athlete, throwing from the pitching mound may be initiated. Contact sports may also be permitted during this period. Competitive throwing is usually not permitted until 7 to 9 months after surgery.

In summary, the rehabilitation program after arthroscopic stabilization for a capsulolabral lesion from a traumatic injury is much slower than the rehabilitation after open stabilization, especially during the early phase, which allows soft-tissue healing to bone. A period of immobilization is often advocated and has been shown to be a critical factor in preventing recurrent instability (53,59,60). I have noted significantly less postoperative scarring after arthroscopic stabilization than with open stabilization procedures. Ad-

TABLE 8. *Arthroscopic stabilization rehabilitation*

I. Phase I: Immediate postoperative phase "restrictive motion"
  Goals: Protect the anatomic repair
  Prevent negative effects of immobilization
  Promote dynamic stability
  Diminish pain and inflammation

Weeks 0–2
- Sling for 2 weeks
- Sleep in immobilizer for 2–4 weeks
- Elbow/hand ROM
- Hand gripping exercises
- Passive and gentle active assistive ROM exercise
  - Flexion to 60 degrees
  - Elevation in scapular plane to 60 degrees
  - ER/IR with arm in 20 degrees of abduction
  - ER to 5–10 degrees
  - IR to 45 degrees

  **NO active ER or extension or abduction
- Submaximal isometrics for shoulder musculature
- Cryotherapy, modalities as indicated

Weeks 3–4
- Discontinue use of sling
- May use immobilizer for sleep (physician decision)
- Continue gentle ROM exercises (PROM and AAROM)
  - Flexion to 90 degrees
  - Abduction to 75–85 degrees
  - ER in scapular plane to 15–20 degrees
  - IR in scapular plane to 55–60 degrees

  **NOTE: Rate of progression based on evaluation of the patient
- No active ER, extension or elevation
- Continue isometrics and rhythmic stabilization (submax)
- Continue use of cryotherapy

Weeks 5–6
- Gradually improve ROM
  - Flexion to 135–140 degrees
  - ER at 45 degrees abduction: 25–30 degrees
  - ER at 45 degrees abduction: 55–60 degrees
- May initiate stretching exercises
- Initiate exercise tubing ER/IR (arm at side)
- PNF manual resistance

II. Phase II: Intermediate phase: moderate protection phase
  Goals: Gradually restore full ROM (week 10)
  Preserve the integrity of the surgical repair
  Restore muscular strength and balance

Weeks 7–9
- Gradually progress ROM
  - Flexion to 160 degrees
  - ER at 90 degrees abduction: 70–75 degrees
  - IR at 90 degrees abduction: 70–75 degrees
- Continue to progress isotonic strengthening program
- Continue PNF strengthening

Weeks 10–14
- May initiate slightly more aggressive strengthening
- Progress isotonic strengthening exercises
- Continue all stretching exercises

  **Progress ROM to functional demands (i.e., overhead athlete)

III. Phase III: Minimal protection phase
  Goals: Establish and maintain full ROM
  Improve muscular strength, power, and endurance
  Gradually initiate functional activities

  Criteria to enter Phase III:
  1) Full nonpainful ROM
  2) Satisfactory stability
  3) Muscular strength (good grade or better)
  4) No pain or tenderness

Weeks 15–18
- Continue all stretching exercises (capsular stretches)
- Continue strengthening exercises:
  - Throwers Ten Program or fundamental exercises
  - PNF manual resistance
  - Endurance training
  - Initiate light plyometric program
  - Restricted sport activities (light swimming, half golf swings)

Weeks 18–21
- Continue all exercise listed earlier
- Initiate interval sport program (throwing, etc.)

IV. Phase IV: Advanced strengthening phase
  Goals: Enhance muscular strength, power, and endurance
  Progress functional activities
  Maintain shoulder mobility

  Criteria to enter Phase IV:
  1) Full nonpainful ROM
  2) Satisfactory static stability
  3) Muscular strength 75–80% of contralateral side
  4) No pain or tenderness

Weeks 20–24
- Continue flexibility exercises
- Continue isotonic strengthening program
- PNF manual-resistance patterns
- Plyometric strengthening
- Progress interval sport programs

V. Phase V: Return-to-activity phase (months 6 1/2 to 9)
  Goals: Gradual return to sport activities
  Maintain strength, mobility, and stability

  Criteria to enter Phase V:
  1) Full functional ROM
  2) Satisfactory isokinetic test that fulfills criteria
  3) Satisfactory shoulder stability
  4) No pain or tenderness

Exercises
- Gradually progress sport activities to unrestrictive participation
- Continue stretching and strengthening program

ER, external rotation; IR, internal rotation; PNF, proprioceptive neuromuscular facilitation; ROM, range of motion.

ditionally, slower rehabilitation and progression are encouraged because of the somewhat weaker fixation methods currently used in arthroscopic stabilization procedures, and appear significantly weaker than the normal capsulolabral complex tissue. This reinforces the necessity for adequate postoperative immobilization (61,62). A period of strict immobilization of at least 3 to 4 weeks appears to be sufficient to allow adequate tissue healing after arthroscopic stabilization (63–65). I advocate relative immobilization with early restricted and protected motion to expedite the functional return of the arm. We expect full motion at approximately 10 weeks after arthroscopic stabilization. The ultimate goals are similar to those of the open stabilization technique. A return to strenuous and contact sports is usually permitted at 6 to 7 months after surgery, with a return to competitive throwing slightly later (7 to 9 months).

The Bristow procedure, although not performed as commonly as in previous years, is an open procedure that may be occasionally seen by the rehabilitation specialist. It is for this reason that the postoperative rehabilitation program is included in this chapter. Several complications of the Bristow procedure or a modification of the Bristow have been reported by several authors (66–68). This procedure may have limited indications for the nonoverhead athlete or for the nondominant arm, where limitation in ROM (i.e., ER) is not so detrimental. Several authors have described their surgical techniques with a brief overview of the postoperative rehabilitation (69–73). Functionally, ER motion is most commonly limited by the Bristow procedure, with reported limitations of 20 degrees (68), 11 to 12 degrees (66), 18 to 23 degrees (74), and 10 degrees (75). Thus, the goal of the rehabilitation program is to restore full functional mobility and movement while maintaining the surgically restored stability.

In the early phases of the rehabilitation program, the therapist must not overstress the anterior structures (with excessive ABD and ER) because this may place excessive stress on the metal screw used to fix the bony block. Loosening, migration, or failure of the screw may result.

The rehabilitation process after a Bristow procedure is outlined in Table 9. The first phase lasts from day 1 to day 5. A sling is used for 2 to 3 days for patient comfort. During this phase, ROM exercises are performed 3 times daily, with ice being used before and after exercise. The ROM exercises are performed to tolerance with the arm positioned in the scapular plane. The goals of the motion exercises are gradually to improve motion, diminish pain, and reestablish neuromuscular control of the glenohumeral joint. Strengthening exercises consist of submaximal isometrics for all shoulder motions.

Phase II begins during the second week and lasts until the sixth week. The goals of this phase are to reestablish full motion, diminish the patient's pain/inflammation, and improve muscular control. ROM exercises (active–assisted, passive, and active) are performed by using an L-bar, and ER/IR motions are performed with the arm at 45 degrees of ABD. Progression of motion during the second and third weeks is based on the patient's tolerance. During the second week, joint mobilization and gentle isotonic strengthening can be initiated.

At week 4, motion is pursued more aggressively. ER and IR are performed with the arm at 90 degrees of ABD. All motions are continued to tolerance; however, at the end of week 4, we expect 50 to 60 degrees of ER. At week 6, the patient should have nearly full ROM. Usually IR is full, and there may be a limitation of ER of 10 to 15 degrees.

Phase III begins at week 7 and progresses until week 12. All stretching exercises, joint mobilization, and ROM exercises progress with the goal of full, unrestricted shoulder motion in all movement planes. All strengthening exercises progress, and the patient may become more involved in an aggressive isotonic weight-training program with some restrictions. The patient is allowed to bench press with light weight but not through a full arc of motion (shoulder horizontal ABD is restricted); exercises such as shoulder pullovers and pectoralis fly exercises are prohibited until 5 months after surgery. Usually during this phase, once the athletes obtain full functional motion, normal strength, and functional stability, they may return to sport participation.

As mentioned previously, the most common complication from the Bristow-type procedure is loss of motion. We have found that, by using a criteria-based protocol as discussed earlier, the goal of full ROM is emphasized and thus accomplished by weeks 6 to 8. If full motion is not obtained, the patient must stay in the intermediate phase (phase II) until the patient has acceptable motion. It should be noted that the Bristow procedure is not indicated for overhead athletes; thus only a functional ROM should be emphasized. Often 80 to 85 degrees of ER is satisfactory and appears functional in most cases after this procedure.

REHABILITATION AFTER POSTERIOR STABILIZATION

The rehabilitation program after stabilization surgery for posterior instability is a significant challenge to the clinician because of the inherent weakness and the thin capsular structures of the posterior compared with anterior shoulder. There are significantly fewer capsuloligamentous structures posteriorly, so most physicians prefer a period of relative immobilization to allow sufficient healing of the capsular structure.

Posterior instability is less common than anterior instability but can occur in athletic and nonathletic populations. Specific sports movements such as a tennis backhand, the pull-through phase of swimming, the follow-through phase in throwing, and blocking by offensive linemen in football can all produce episodes of posterior instability.

Once the diagnosis of posterior instability has been established, the patient is most often placed on a nonoperative rehabilitation program in an attempt to avoid surgical intervention. The nonoperative program emphasizes glenohumeral joint muscular strengthening, neuromuscular control to promote dynamic joint stability, co-contraction of

does any other postoperative rehabilitation program. This is due to the presence of greater degrees and directions of instability and many times also includes congenital laxity. The therapist is often faced with the fine line between increasing or restricting motion. The clinician must consider numerous factors related to patients with multidirectional unstable shoulder before a postoperative rehabilitation regimen can be established. These factors determine the type and aggressiveness of the rehabilitation program (Table 10).

The first factor is the type of capsular shift performed (anterior vs. posterior). We generally advise progress for the patient with posterior capsular shift much more slowly than for the patient with anterior capsular shift because of poorer capsular quality and strength disparity. The specific surgical technique should also be thoroughly understood by the clinician (80–85).

The next factor to be considered is the type of instability exhibited by the patient. The concept of MDI was introduced by Neer and Foster (82) in 1980; it describes glenohumeral subluxation or dislocation in three different directions: anterior, inferior, and posterior. The primary abnormality in MDI is a loose and redundant inferior pouch (80). The patient with MDI is often characterized as a young sedentary patient with generalized ligamentous laxity who often has significant capsular looseness and laxity because repetitive excessive motions selectively "stretch-out" through the shoulder capsule. This has been referred to as "acquired laxity" by Andrews and Satterwhite (84). This general "stretch-out" can be seen in overhead throwers, butterfly swimmers, and gymnasts (86). In addition, patients with MDI may also have a Bankart lesion (83). The rate of progression (aggressiveness of the rehabilitation program) varies based on the underlying instability pattern with patients with acquired laxity progressing much more aggressively than do the congenitally unstable patients.

The third and fourth factors are closely related and address the patient's tissue status and efficiency of the dynamic stabilizers. Patients with atraumatic, congenital instability due to significant capsular redundancy and generalized laxity progress at a slower rate. This is due to the concern about capsular stretch-out. Conversely, the overhead athlete with acquired laxity due to repetitive microtrauma usually has better capsular structure, less-generalized laxity (unidirectional or bidirectional instability), and much better dynamic stabilizers than the previously described patient with MDI; thus the rehabilitation rate is much more aggressive. The patient's activity level is also considered (i.e., athletic compared with orthopedic patient), and the rehabilitation program is tailored accordingly.

TABLE 10. *Factors affecting the rehabilitation program after capsular shift surgery*

Type of shift performed
Anterior or posterior
Type of instability
Acquired or congenital
Patient's tissue status
Patient's dynamic stabilizers status
Patient's response to surgery
Desired activity level

The postoperative rehabilitation program is based on the type of patient and his or her unique tissue characteristics. The overhead athlete is treated aggressively because our concern is that the patient may become too tight anteroinferiorly, which will restrict ABD and ER motion, which is necessary to throw, swim, and so on. In contrast, the general orthopedic patient with generalized laxity often desires pain-free daily activities without recurrent instability. This patient rarely has difficulty gaining motion; our concern is that this patient will develop increased capsular laxity. During the rehabilitation course of treatment, the assessment of the patient's end feel will provide vital information as to the rate of progression.

We advocate the clinical use of two different rehabilitation approaches after a capsular-shift procedure. The first approach is for the overhead athlete. The emphasis is on motion, dynamic stability, and early functional activities (see Table 11). In comparison, the general orthopedic patient (generalized laxity) progresses more slowly because of inadequate capsular structures and poor dynamic stabilization (see Table 12).

THE ACCELERATED APPROACH

The accelerated approach is based on immediate restricted motion and a gradual return to the motion necessary for sporting activities. Immediately after surgery, the patient's shoulder is passively moved, and the patient performs active–assisted motion. In the first phase, the protected motion phase, from weeks 1 through 6, the primary goals are to (a) restore motion gradually, (b) protect the repaired capsule, and (c) reestablish dynamic stability. During weeks 1 through 3, AAROM for ER/IR is performed with the arm in 30 degrees of ABD and is performed to patient tolerance. Shoulder flexion also is performed to tolerance, usually to 100 to 125 degrees by week 2. During the first 2 weeks, isometrics and rhythmic-stabilization exercises also are performed.

During weeks 2 to 4, ROM and stretching gradually progress. Active–assisted ER and IR ROM exercises are performed at 45 degrees of ABD, with the goal of 45 degrees of motion (ER and IR) by week 4. During this time, tubing exercises may be initiated for the shoulder internal and external rotators; rhythmic-stabilization drills and co-contraction also are performed.

At weeks 4 to 5, ER/IR stretching is performed at 90 degrees of ABD. This progression is based on clinical assessment (degrees of motion and end feel). At approximately 4.5 to 5 weeks, ER motion progresses more aggressively. By the end of week 6, our goal is 75 degrees of ER in the overhead athlete. The rate of progression (aggres-

TABLE 11. *Anterior capsular-shift rehabilitation protocol, accelerated for acquired instability*

I. Phase I: Protection phase (weeks 0–6)
  Goals: Allow healing of sutured capsule
    Begin early protected range of motion
    Retard muscular atrophy
    Decrease pain/inflammation
  A. Weeks 0–2
    Precautions
    1. Sleep in immobilizer for 2 weeks
    2. No overhead activities for 4–6 weeks
    3. Wean from immobilizer and into sling as soon as possible (orthopedist or therapist will tell you when)
    Exercises:
      Gripping exercises
      Elbow flex/extension and pronation/supination
      Pendulum exercises (nonweighted)
      Rope and pulley active-assisted exercises
        Shoulder flexion to 90 degrees
        Shoulder abduction to 60 degrees
      L-Bar exercises
        External rotation to 15–20 degrees with arm in scapular plane
        Shoulder flexion/extension to tolerance
      AROM cervical spine
      Isometrics
        Flexors, extensors, ER, IR, ABD
    Criteria for hospital discharge
    1. Shoulder range of motion (AAROM) flexion, 90 degrees; abduction, 45 degrees; ER, 40 degrees
    2. Minimal pain and swelling
    3. "Good" proximal and distal muscle power
  B. Weeks 2–4
    Goals: Gradual increase in ROM
      Normalize arthrokinematics
      Improve strength
      Decrease pain/inflammation
    1. Range-of-motion exercises
      L-Bar active-assisted exercises
      ER at 45 degrees ABD to 45 degrees
      IR at 45 degrees ABD to 45 degrees
      Shoulder flex/ext to tolerance
      Shoulder abduction to tolerance
      Shoulder horizontal ABD/ADD
      Rope and pulley flex/ext
      *All exercises performed to tolerance
        Take to point of pain or resistance or both and hold
        Gentle self-capsular stretches
    2. Gentle joint mobilization to reestablish normal arthrokinematics to
        Scapulothoracic joint
        Glenohumeral joint
        Sternoclavicular joint
    3. Strengthening exercises
        Isometrics
        May initiate tubing for ER/IR at 0 degrees of shoulder abduction
    4. Conditioning program for
        Trunk
        Lower extremities
        Cardiovascular
    5. Decrease pain/inflammation
        Ice, NSAID, modalities
  C. Weeks 4–5
      AAROM flexion to tolerance (approx. 145 degrees)
      IR/ER at 90 degrees ABD to tolerance
      Initiate isotonic (light wt.) strengthening
      Gentle joint mobilization (grade III)
  D. Week 6
      AAROM; continue all stretching exercises
      Progress ER/IR at 90 degrees abduction
        ER at 90 degrees ABD, 75 degrees
        IR at 90 degrees ABD, 75 degrees
        Flexion to 165–170 degrees
        Extension to 30 degrees

(*continued*)

TABLE 11. *Continued*

II. Phase II: Intermediate phase (weeks 7–12)
  Goals: Full nonpainful ROM at week 8
    Normalize arthrokinematics
    Increase strength
    Improve neuromuscular control
 A. Weeks 7–9
  1. Range-of-motion exercises
   L-Bar active-assisted exercises
   Continue all exercises listed earlier
   Gradually increase ROM to full ROM week 8
    ER at 90 degrees ABD, 85–90 degrees
    IR at 90 degrees ABD, 70–75 degrees
   Continue self-capsular stretches
   Continue joint mobilization
  2. Strengthening exercises
   Initiate isotonic dumbbell program
    Side-lying ER
    Side-lying IR
    Shoulder abduction
    Supraspinatus
    Latissimus dorsi
    Rhomboids
    Biceps curls
    Triceps curls
    Shoulder shrugs
    Push-ups into chair (serratus anterior)
   Continue tubing at 0 degrees and at 90 degrees abduction for ER/IR
  3. Initiate neuromuscular control exercises for scapulothoracic joint
 B. Weeks 10–12
  1. Continue all exercises listed earlier
  2. Initiate tubing exercises for rhomboids, latissimus dorsi, biceps, and triceps
  3. Initiate aggressive stretching and joint mobilization, if needed
    Progressive ROM for overhead thrower to functional ROM
III. Phase III: Dynamic strengthening phase (weeks 12–20)
 A. Advanced strengthening phase (Weeks 12–16)
   Goals: Improve strength/power/endurance
     Improve neuromuscular control
     Maintain shoulder mobility
     Prepare athlete to begin to throw
   Criteria to enter phase III
    a. Full nonpainful ROM
    b. No pain or tenderness
    c. Strength 70% or better compared with contralateral side
    d. Satisfactory shoulder-joint stability
   Emphasis of phase III
    High-speed, high-energy strengthening exercises
    Eccentric exercises
    Diagonal patterns
    Functional positions of stretching and strengthening
   Exercises
  1. Continue self-capsular stretches (very important)
  2. Throwers Ten exercises
   Tubing exercises in 90/90 position for IR and ER (slow sets, fast sets)
   Isotonics for
    Rhomboids
    Latissimus dorsi
    Biceps
    Diagonal patterns D2 extension
    Diagonal patterns D2 flexion
   Continue dumbbell exercises for supraspinatus and deltoid
   Continue serratus anterior strengthening exercises, push-ups floor
   Continue all isotonic strengthening
  2. Continue trunk/LE strengthening exercises
  3. Continue neuromuscular exercises
  4. Initiate plyometric training program

(*continued*)

TABLE 11. *Continued*

B. Weeks 16–20
  Initiate interval sport programs
  Continue all exercises
  Progress plyometrics for shoulder
    ER at 90 degrees ABD
    IR at 90 degrees ABD
    D2 extension plyometrics
    Biceps plyometrics
    Serratus anterior plyometrics

IV. Phase IV: Throwing phase (weeks 20–26)
  Goals: Progressively increase activities to prepare patient for full functional return
  Criteria to progress to phase IV
  1. Full ROM
  2. No pain or tenderness
  3. Isokinetic test that fulfills criteria to throw
  4. Satisfactory clinical examination
 Exercise
    Progress interval throwing program
    Continue Throwers Ten exercises
    Continue plyometric five exercises
    Continue all flexibility exercises
 A. Interval throwing program
  1. Interval throwing program phase II, 22nd week
 B. Return to sports, 26–30 weeks

AAROM, active–assisted range of motion; ABD, abduction; ADD, adduction; ER, external rotation; IR, internal rotation; NSAID, nonsteroidal antiinflammatory drugs.

This rehabilitation program's goal is to return the patient/athlete to the activity/sport as quickly and safely as possible, while maintaining a stable shoulder. The program is based on muscle physiology, biomechanics, anatomy, and the healing process after surgery for a capsular shift.

The capsular-shift procedure is one in which the orthopedic surgeon makes an incision into the ligamentous capsule of the shoulder, pulls the capsule tighter, and then sutures the capsule together.

The ultimate goal is a functional stable shoulder and a return to a presurgery functional level.

TABLE 12. *Anterior capsular-shift rehabilitation protocol: regular program for general orthopedic patient*

I. Phase I: Protection phase (weeks 0–6)
  Goals: Allow healing of sutured capsule
    Begin early protected and restricted range of motion
    Retard muscular atrophy and enhance dynamic stability
    Decrease pain/inflammation
     Brace: Patients with bidirectional instability are placed in sling for 4–6 weeks
     Patients with multidirectional instability are placed in abduction brace for 4–6 weeks
     **Physician will make determination
 A. Weeks 0–2
  Precautions:
  1. Sleep in immobilizer for 4 weeks
  2. No overhead activities for 6–8 weeks
  3. Compliance with rehab program is critical
  Exercises:
   Gripping exercises with putty
   Elbow flex/extension and pronation/supination
   Pendulum exercises (nonweighted)
   Rope and pulley active-assisted exercises
    Shoulder flexion to 90 degrees
    Shoulder elevation in scapular plane to 60 degrees
   L-Bar exercises
    External rotation to 15 degrees with arm abducted at 30 degrees
    No shoulder abduction or extension
   AROM cervical spine
   Isometrics
    Flexors, extensors, ER, IR, ABD
  Criteria for hospital discharge
  1. Shoulder range of motion (AAROM): flexion, 90 degrees; abduction, 45 degrees; external rotation, 20 degrees
  2. Minimal pain and swelling
  3. "Good" proximal and distal muscle power

(*continued*)

TABLE 12. *Continued*

B. Weeks 2–4
  Goals: Gradual increase in ROM
  Normalize arthrokinematics
  Improve strength
  Decrease pain/inflammation
  1. Range-of-motion exercises
    L-Bar active-assisted exercises, gentle PROM exercises
      ER to 25–30 degrees in scapular plane
      IR to 30–35 degrees in scapular plane
      Shoulder flexion to 105–115 degrees
      Shoulder elevation in scapular plane to 115 degrees
      Rope and pulley flexion
    *All exercises performed to tolerance and therapist/physician motion guidelines
    *Take to point of pain or resistance or both and hold
    **Gentle* self-capsular stretches
  2. Gentle joint mobilization to reestablish normal arthrokinematics to
      Scapulothoracic joint
      Glenohumeral joint
      Sternoclavicular joint
  3. Strengthening exercises
      Isometrics
      Rythmic stabilization exercises
      May initiate tubing for ER/IR at 0 degrees
  4. Conditioning program for
      Trunk
      Lower extremities
      Cardiovascular
  5. Decrease pain/inflammation
      Ice, NSAID, modalities
C. Weeks 4–6
  1. Continue all exercises listed earlier
  2. Range-of-motion exercises
    L-Bar active-assisted exercises
      ER to 25–35 degrees at 45 degrees of shoulder ABD
      Continue all others to tolerance (based on end feel)
  3. Continue stabilization exercises.
      PNF with rythmic stabilization, neuromuscular exercises

II. Phase II: Intermediate phase (weeks 6–12)
  Goals: Full nonpainful ROM at weeks 10–12
  Normalize arthrokinematics
  Increase strength
  Improve neuromuscular control
A. Weeks 6–8
  1. Range-of-motion exercises
    L-Bar active-assisted exercises at 90 degrees ABD
    Continue all exercises listed earlier
    Gradually increase ROM to full ROM, week 12
    Continue self-capsular stretches
    Continue joint mobilization
    May initiate IR/ER ROM at 90 degrees of abduction
  2. Strengthening exercises
    Initiate isotonic dumbbell program
      Side-lying ER
      Side-lying IR
      Shoulder abduction
      Supraspinatus
      Latissimus dorsi
      Rhomboids
      Biceps curls
      Triceps curls
      Shoulder shrugs
      Push-ups into chair (serratus anterior)
    Continue tubing at 0 degrees for ER/IR
    Continue stabilization exercises for the glenohumeral joint
  3. Initiate neuromuscular control exercises for scapulothoracic joint

(*continued*)

TABLE 12. *Continued*

B. Weeks 8–10
 1. Continue all exercises listed earlier, emphasis on neuromuscular control drills, PNF stabilization drills, and scapular strengthening.
 2. Initiate tubing exercises for rhomboids, latissimus dorsi, biceps, and triceps
 3. Progress ROM to full ROM
  ER at 90 degrees ABD: 80–85 degrees
  IR at 90 degrees ABD: 70–75 degrees
  Flexion to 165–170 degrees.

III. Phase III: Dynamic strengthening phase (weeks 12–20) Advanced strengthening phase
**Aggressive strengthening or stretching program based on type of patient. Therapist and/or physician will determine.

A. Weeks 12–17
 Goals: Improve strength/power/endurance
  Improve neuromuscular control
  Prepare athletic patient for gradual return to sports
 **Criteria to enter phase III
 1. Full nonpainful ROM
  **Patient must fulfill this criterion before progressing to this phase
 2. No pain or tenderness
 3. Strength 70% or better compared with contralateral side
 Emphasis of Phase III
  Dynamic stabilization exercises
  Eccentric exercises
  Diagonal patterns, functional movements
 Exercises
  Fundamental shoulder exercises
   Emphasis: neuromuscular control drills, PNF rhythmic stabilization, rotator-cuff strengthening, scapular strengthening
  Continue tubing exercises for IR/ER at 0 degrees ABD (arm at side)
  Continue isotonics for
   Rhomboids
   Latissimus dorsi
   Biceps
   Diagonal patterns D2 extension
   Diagonal patterns D2 flexion
  Continue dumbbell exercises for supraspinatus and deltoid
  Continue serratus anterior strengthening exercises, push-ups floor
  Continue trunk/LE strengthening exercises
  Continue neuromuscular exercises
  Continue self-çapsular stretches

B. Weeks 17–20
  Continue all exercises
  Emphasis on gradual return to recreational activities

IV. Phase IV: Return to activity (weeks 20–28)
  Goals: Progressively increase activities to prepare patient for full functional return
  Criteria to progress to phase IV
   1. Full ROM
   2. No pain or tenderness
   3. Isokinetic test that fulfills criteria
   4. Satisfactory clinical examination
 Exercise
  Initiate interval sports programs (if patient is a recreational athlete)
  Continue tubing exercises as listed in phase III
  Continue all strengthening exercises
  Continue ROM exercises

AAROM, active–assisted range of motion; ABD, abduction; ER, external rotation; IR, internal rotation; LE, lower extremity; NSAID, nonsteroidal antiinflammatory drug; PNF, proproprioceptive neuromuscular facilitation.

This rehabilitation program's goal to return the patient/athelete to the activity/sport as quickly and safely as possible, while maintaining a stable shoulder. The program is based on muscle physiology, biomechanics, anatomy, and the healing process after surgery for a capsular shift.

The capsular-shift procedure is one in which the orthopedic surgeon makes an incision into the ligamentous capsule of the shoulder, pulls the capsule tighter, and then sutures the capsule together.

The ultimate goal is a functional stable shoulder and pain-free return to presurgery functional level.

Compliance with the rehabilitation program is critical to the patient's ultimate outcome.

siveness) of the stretching is determined by the clinical assessment and is based on the assessment of motion, stability, and end feel. If the patient appears to be progressing slowly toward these goals, the program must be adjusted at week 6. Several stretches that have proven successful in restoring anterior flexibility are illustrated in Figures 10 to 13. Figure 10 illustrates a horizontal ABD stretch at 90 degrees of elevation; Figure 11, an ER stretch with horizontal ABD; Figure 12, an anterior joint mobilization technique at end range; and Figure 13, a low-load, long-duration stretch. In my opinion, all of these stretches are safe if performed with a gradual force, and force should not be applied rapidly. Stretches are usually initiated during week 7, and the therapist should consult the physician before their use. During this phase, isotonic strengthening exercises are performed for the entire shoulder complex. During weeks 3 to 4, rhythmic-stabilization drills are emphasized with the goal of restoring dynamic stability. At week 5, ER/IR strengthening may be performed at 90 degrees of ABD.

The intermediate phase, weeks 7 through 12, is characterized by establishing full motion at week 8 and improving muscular strength and endurance. At week 8, the patient should exhibit full motion (90 degrees of ER and 45 to 55 degrees of horizontal ABD). From weeks 8 to 12, the overhead athlete's stretching exercises progress to the amount of ER necessary to throw, usually a minimum of 115 to 120 degrees of ER. This is usually accomplished through physiologic stretching, capsular stretching, low-load, long-duration stretches, and controlled plyometric activities. During this phase, all strengthening exercises progress, with emphasis on functional strengthening exercises, muscular balance, scapular strengthening, and endurance.

The advanced strengthening phase begins at week 12 and progresses through week 20. The primary goals are to enhance muscular strength, power and endurance, while maintaining capsular mobility and glenohumeral joint stability. The patient is instructed to continue stretching (Figs. 14–16) to prevent capsular or muscular tightening or both caused by the aggressive strengthening exercises. The strengthening exercises consist of PNF, the Thrower's Ten program, plyometrics, and neuromuscular-control drills (86, 87). At this time, the patient is carefully evaluated and a determination made as to when a throwing program can be initiated. A gradual throwing or sport program can usually be initiated between 14 and 16 weeks, depending on patient variables and progression in rehabilitation.

The return-to-activity phase is initiated at 21 weeks after surgery and represents a gradual return to sport activities.

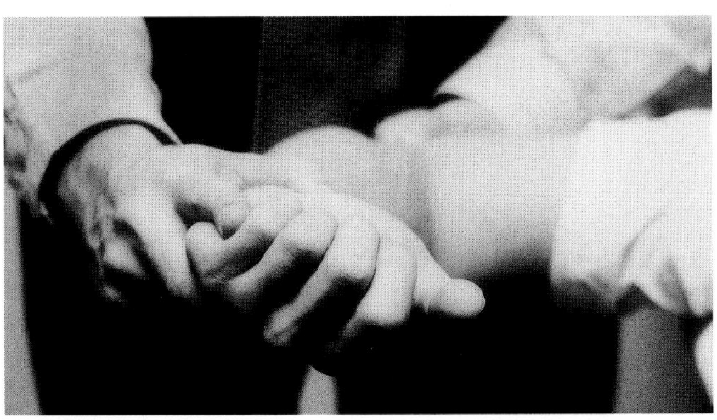

FIG. 10. Stretching the anterior shoulder capsule. The patient's arm is positioned at 90 degrees of abduction, and then the arm is stretched into horizontal abduction.

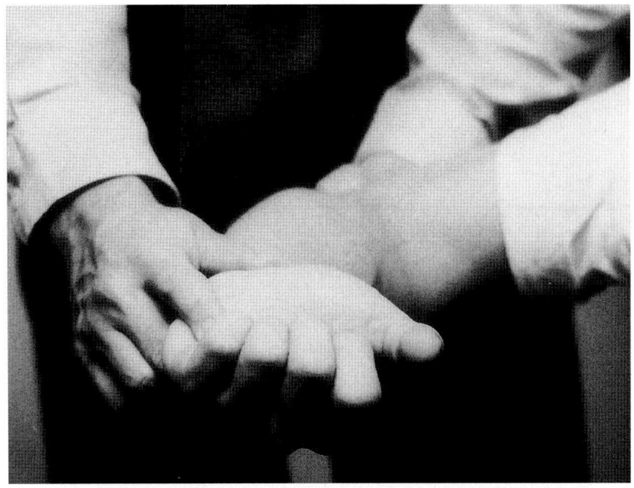

FIG. 11. Stretching the anterior shoulder capsule. The patient's arm is positioned in 90 degrees of abduction and full external rotation; the stretch is performed as the arm is gently stretched into horizontal abduction.

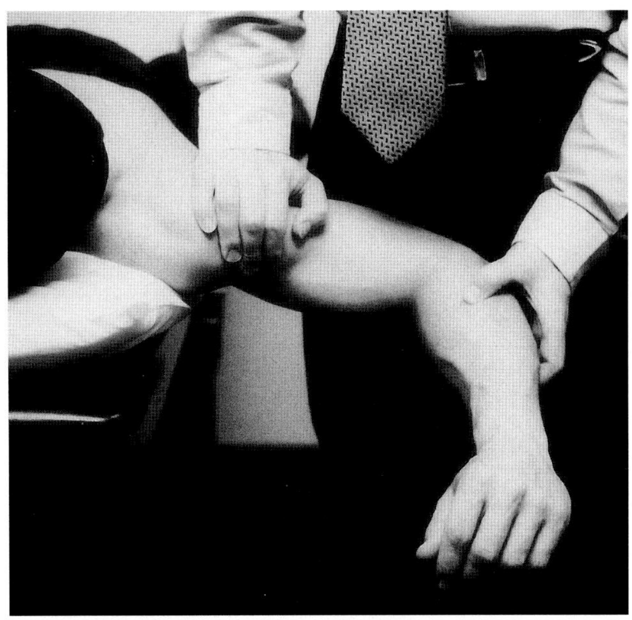

FIG. 12. Stretching the anterior shoulder capsule. Joint mobilization is performed to stretch the anteroinferior capsule. A gradual glide is performed to take the capsule to end range and then is held at that position to produce a stretch on the capsule.

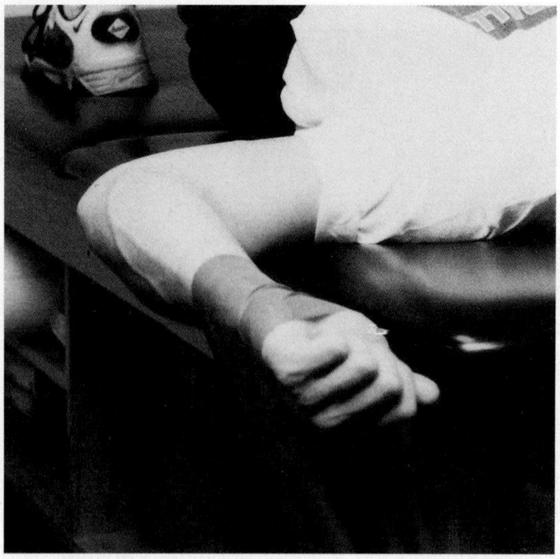

FIG. 13. Stretching the anterior shoulder capsule. A low-load, long-duration stretch is performed. The patient's arm is placed in 90 degrees of abduction and a tolerable degree of external rotation. A piece of low-resistance Theraband is secured around the patient's wrist and to the base of the treatment table, thus producing a stretch into external rotation. The stretch should be mild, sustained for 10 to 12 minutes.

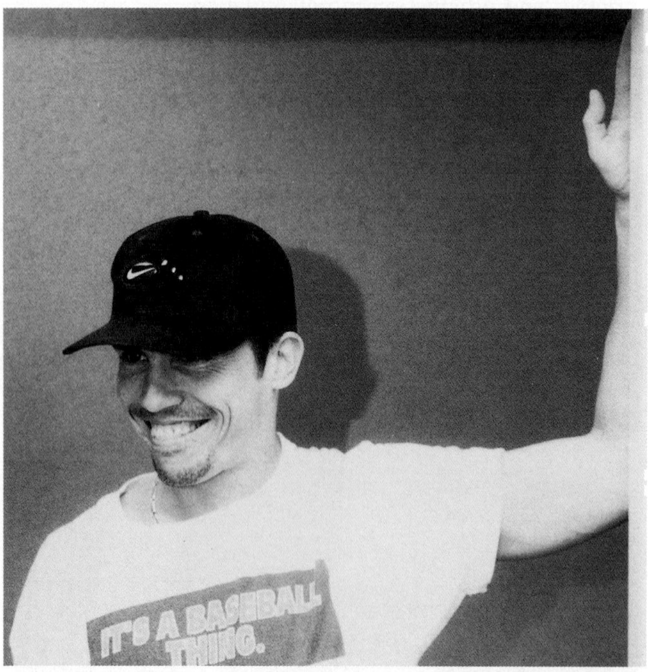

FIG. 14. Self-capsular stretch for the anterior shoulder capsule.

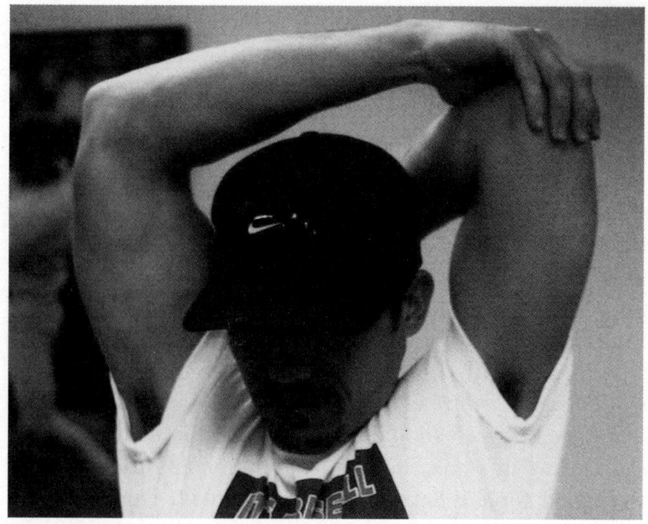

FIG. 15. Self-capsular stretch for the anteroinferior shoulder capsule.

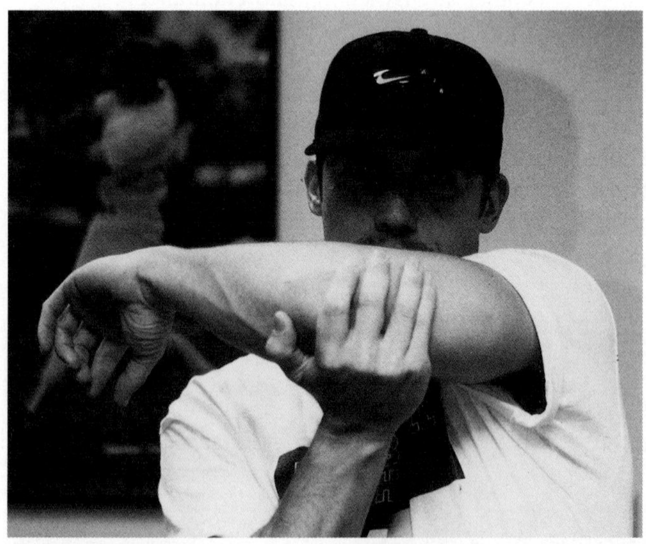

FIG. 16. Self-capsular stretch for the posterior shoulder capsule.

During this time, it is imperative that the athlete continue all strengthening and stretching exercises outlined in the previous phase. A return to unrestricted sports usually occurs between 6 and 9 months, depending on the patient's sport, position, skill level, and rate of progression.

Altchek et al. (83) reported on 40 patients (42 shoulders) who were surgically stabilized by using a T-plasty modification for MDI. Thirty-eight of 40 patients returned to sports, at an average of 6.5 months (range, 5 to 10 months). Only three patients in the series were throwers; all three reported that they were unable to throw as fast as before the operation. Bigliani et al. (81) reported the results of an anteroinferior capsular shift performed on 63 athletic patients (68 shoulders). Of the 63 patients, 31 were overhead athletes, consisting of 16 baseball players. The results indicated that 50% returned to the same competition level. Kvitne and Jobe (88) reported on 105 patients who had undergone anterior capsulolabral reconstruction. In this series, 52 were baseball players, 35 of whom were pitchers. The investigator noted that 64% of the baseball players returned to the same level of competition; 69% of all pitchers and 60% of the professional baseball pitchers were able to return to the same level. LeBar and Alexander (89) reviewed the results of the capsular-shift procedure in an active-duty military population. Three patients were unable to return to full active duty.

The rehabilitation process after capsular tensioning in the overhead athlete is challenging to the clinician. Success rates vary greatly, depending on the sport and position. The reasons for failure are multifactorial. One reason frequently seen is a loss of ER. The rehabilitation program must be aggressive in restoring ER and IR motion in the throwing athlete. Fleisig (90) determined the total arc of motion [late cocking (ER) to follow through] as one of the critical factors in the pitcher's effectiveness. The optimal treatment for the overhead thrower remains a well-structured nonoperative rehabilitation program. The only patients who should be considered as possible surgical candidates are those for whom a well-structured nonoperative rehabilitation program that has been attempted for a minimum of 3 months has failed.

THE GENERAL ORTHOPEDIC APPROACH

The rehabilitation approach after an inferior capsular shift performed on a patient with generalized ligamentous laxity is considerably slower than the approach for the overhead athlete. The program is slower because of collagen deficiency (9), less-developed and efficient dynamic stabilizers, and an activity level that generally does not involve competitive athletics. The ultimate goal of the program is to restore stability and functional mobility. The key to successful rehabilitation is to individualize the program to the patient's tissue status and healing response.

Neer and Foster (82) in 1980 first described the postoperative regimen after inferior capsular-shift surgery. They suggested the arm being immobilized at the side, elbow flexed to 90 degrees, and approximately 10 degrees of ER for 5 to 6 weeks. At week 6, gentle active–assisted motion is instituted; at week 8, isometrics are initiated; and at 12 weeks, isotonics are initiated. The authors noted that most patients tend to recover motion rapidly. The authors also recommended 9 months of recovery before heavy lifting or sports are initiated.

Since Neer and Foster's article, several authors have described their rehabilitation guidelines after capsular-shift surgery (80,81,83,91,92). Bigliani (80) suggested using a shoulder immobilizer that supports the arm in slight ABD and neutral rotation for 6 weeks for patients with ''classic'' MDI. He continued to recommend no motion exercises for 6 weeks and then a gradual progression of motion. For patients with bidirectional (anterior and inferior) instability without significant posterior instability, he recommended protection in a sling for 6 weeks. After 10 days, the arm was removed from the sling for gentle ROM exercises and isometrics. ER motion slowly progressed and may be less than 50 degrees after 3 months. Wickiewicz et al. (14) pointed out that they had formerly placed patients in an orthoplast splint in slight ABD and IR but have since found it unnecessary if the inferior instability was eliminated when the repair was treated surgically. Altchek et al. (83) recommended 6 weeks of immobilization in a brace. Gentle rotational motion began at 3 weeks with passive flexion to 90 degrees. At 6 weeks, active–assisted motion can be performed, and isotonic strengthening can be started once full motion has been established.

Our rehabilitation program is similar to those described earlier. In patients with classic MDI, a spica brace with a circumferential waist belt is worn for 6 weeks. In patients with gross generalized laxity, occasionally an immobilizer brace is used with the arm abducted to 25 to 30 degrees and neutral rotation. In patients with bidirectional instability, a sling is worn for 4 to 6 weeks, depending on the rate of recovery, shoulder stability, and pain level.

At approximately 7 to 10 days, passive motion and gentle active–assisted motion are initiated for patients with bidirectional instability. The motion guidelines are discussed but are based on the patient's response to surgery, which is evaluated through the assessment of the end feel. Motion is restricted to 115 degrees of flexion and 15 degrees of ER. Motion is restricted for 8 to 10 weeks (depending on quantity of motion and end feel); then motion is gradually increased. By 12 weeks, the patient should have 160 degrees of flexion, 85 degrees of ER, and 70 degrees of IR. The rate of recovery of motion is based on the clinician's assessment of the end feel. If the patient exhibits a soft feel and motion greater than the guidelines, motion is slowed; conversely, if the patient exhibits a hard or firm end feel and less motion than the guidelines, motion is accelerated to meet the criterion.

Patients with classic MDI progress slightly more slowly than described earlier (see Table 12). Motion is not initiated for 3 to 4 weeks and progresses extremely slowly. IR and ER movements are performed with the arm positioned in the scapular plane and are restricted to 5 to 10 degrees at week 4, 15 to 25 degrees at week 6, and 25 to 35 degrees at week 8; after week 8, motion progresses. The goal is to restore motion approximately 10 to 15 degrees less than the normal ROM of the shoulder at 10 to 12 weeks.

Neuromuscular training drills are initiated early in the program for both patient groups. The goals of the exercises are to enhance dynamic stabilization through muscle-reeducation training and to enhance proprioception. Exercises such as rhythmic stabilization, co-contractions, and neuromuscular drills are performed with the arm placed in the scapular plane to minimize capsular stress. Isometrics also are performed. The use of biofeedback is extremely beneficial in these patients in muscle-reeducation and activation patterns. An isotonic strengthening program is not initiated until the patient has sufficient dynamic stability. The emphasis of the isotonic program is on rotator-cuff and scapular muscle training. Muscular-endurance training is emphasized in this patient population and is a critical element to improve. A gradual return to strenuous work or light sport activity is usually not allowed until 6 to 9 months from surgery. I attempt to match a recreational activity, such as light swimming (restricted swimming stroke), to this type of patient. This is to maintain muscular strength, tone, and activation through a lifetime leisure sport that does not reproduce symptoms.

REHABILITATION AFTER LASER CAPSULORRHAPHY

At our center, the laser capsulorrhaphy procedure is considered for a specific patient population. In general, these are patients who have generalized ligamentous laxity, redundant capsule, no distinct Bankart lesion, and moderate instability. The postoperative rehabilitation of these patients is initially conservative, with a gradual progression of ROM.

The postoperative rehabilitation program is outlined in Table 13. Immediately after surgery, the patient is placed in a sling for 10 to 14 days. During this time, the patient performs wrist, hand, and elbow exercises, but no exercises for the shoulder, to allow an initial healing period of the capsule. At 14 days after surgery, ROM exercises are initiated with the arm at the side or in the scapular plane. Shoulder-flexion motion is limited to 90 degrees (at 4 weeks), and the patient performs isometrics and rhythmic-stabilization exercises. At weeks 4 to 6, the patient is permitted to perform ER/IR AAROM exercises at 45 degrees of ABD, and flexion is limited to 145 degrees. During this time, light isotonics are initiated.

The intermediate phase, from weeks 6 to 12, focuses on gradual restoration of motion and dynamic stability. During this period, the patient is allowed to perform ER/IR AAROM at 90 degrees of ABD. Our goal is to restore functional motion, enabling the patient to perform daily activities, but not enough mobility to challenge stability. We usually strive for motion restoration that is 15 degrees less than "normal motion" and encourage the patient to obtain that motion through daily activities. Emphasis is on protected ROM for 6 to 8 weeks. The emphasis during this phase is on dynamic stability exercise, proprioception scapular strengthening, and rotator-cuff exercises.

The advanced strengthening phase begins from week 12 and progresses to week 18. During this period, the patient is encouraged to continue strengthening exercises that emphasize dynamic stability. The patient is instructed that no heavy lifting or strenuous sports are allowed until at least 4 months after surgery.

REHABILITATION AFTER THERMAL-ASSISTED CAPSULAR SHRINKAGE

A relatively new procedure is the thermal-assisted capsular shrinkage (TACS) procedure. At our center, we have used this procedure since May of 1997 for specific patients, such as the overhead athlete. The procedure is designed arthroscopically to remove the capsular hypermobility commonly seen in the overhead athlete without the potential risks of loss of motion after an open capsular shift. Often this procedure is performed concomitant with an arthroscopic rotator-cuff debridement and labral debridement, repair or removal. From May 1997 to February 1998, 56 procedures were performed with 75% occurring in the overhead athlete. The early results are extremely encouraging.

The postoperative rehabilitation program is slightly more aggressive than the rehabilitation program after a laser capsulorrhaphy (see Table 14). Immediately after surgery, a sling is used for approximately 7 to 10 days. Additionally, the patient is initiated on AAROM and PROM exercises in a prescribed ROM. IR and ER ROM exercises are initially performed in the scapular plane for the first 4 weeks and then progress at 5 weeks after surgery to 90 degrees of ABD. We expect 90 to 100 degrees of ER at 90 degrees of ABD at week 8. Beginning at week 9 and progressing to week 12, ER motion progresses to the overhead athlete's demands of 115 to 125 degrees.

Muscle training is performed immediately after surgery in the form of isometric muscular contractions for the first 2 weeks. Then the strengthening program progresses to isotonic strengthening exercises (beginning with light weights and progressing gradually). Aggressive strengthening exercises such as plyometrics and specific weight machines can usually be initiated at 10 to 12 weeks after surgery.

A gradual return to specific sport activities such as an interval throwing program, tennis, or swimming is generally initiated at week 14 to 16. A return to competitive sports is permitted at 6 months after surgery or once the patient has met our specific criteria.

Overall, we have been extremely encouraged by the early results in overhead athletes with this procedure at our cen-

TABLE 13. *Rehabilitation after laser capsulorrhaphy*

I. Phase I: Protection phase (day one to week 6)
   Goals: Allow soft-tissue healing
   Diminish pain and inflammation
   Initiate protected motion
   Retard muscular atrophy
   Weeks 0–2
   - Sling/immobilizer for 10–14 days
   - Sleep in sling/immobilizer for 2 weeks
   - Avoid abduction and external rotation for 2 weeks

   Exercises
   - Hand-gripping exercises
   - Elbow and wrist range-of-motion exercises
   - AROM cervical spine
   - Passive range of motion (begin at 10 days)
     - Elevation in scapular plane (0–60 degrees)
     - ER/IR in scapular plane (5–10 degrees)
   - Cryotherapy to control pain

   Weeks 3–4
   - Range-of-motion exercises (AAROM and PROM only)
     - Elevation in scapular plane (0–90 degrees)
     - IR in scapular plane (0–30 degrees)
     - ER in scapular plane (0–15 degrees)
   - Strengthening exercises
     - Isometrics in all planes
     - Rhythmic stabilization exercises in mid range
   - Continue use of cryotherapy and modalities to control pain

   Weeks 5–6
   - Continue all exercises listed above
   - Progress ROM to the following
     - Elevation in scapular plane (0–135 degrees)
     - ER/IR in scapular plane (to tolerance)
       - ER to maximum of 0–25 degrees
       - IR to maximum of 45 degrees
   - May initiate active range-of-motion exercises (ER/IR)
   - Tubing ER/IR
   - Tubing biceps
   - Initiate scapula-strengthening program

II. Phase II: Intermediate phase (weeks 7–12)
   Goals: Restore functional ROM (weeks 7–12)
   Normalize arthrokinematics
   Improve dynamic stability, muscular strength
   Weeks 7–8
   - Initiate ER/IR at 90 degrees abduction
     - ER motion to maximum of 65 degrees
     - IR motion to maximum of 50 degrees
     - Flexion to maximum of 160 degrees
   - Continue AAROM and gentle stretching
   - Initiate joint mobilization to balance capsule
   - Strengthening exercises
     - ER/IR with exercise tubing
     - Prone rowing
     - Prone horizontal abduction
     - Prone extension
     - Biceps curls
     - Light shoulder abduction
     - Continue rhythmic stabilization drills

   Weeks 10–12
   - Continue to progress all ROM exercises and strengthening drills
   - Restore functional ROM by weeks 10–12
   - Motion restoration in 15 degrees less than "normal motion"
     **(Remaining motion will be obtained through functional activities)
   - Continue all exercises listed earlier

III. Phase III: Advanced activity and strengthening phase (weeks 12–20)
   Goals: Improve strength, power, and endurance
   Enhance neuromuscular control
   Prepare for increased activities
   Criteria to enter phase III
   - Functional range of motion (85% of normal motion)
   - No pain or tenderness
   - Muscular strength 75% or greater than contralateral side

   Weeks 12–16
   - Continue stretching and ROM exercises if ROM is not acceptable
   - Continue all strengthening exercises listed in weeks 7–9
   - Initiate push-ups into wall or table
   - Progress deltoid, rotator cuff, and scapular strengthening

   Weeks 16–20
   - Continue all exercises listed earlier
   - May initiate light swimming, etc. (if physician approves)

IV. Phase IV: Return-to-activity phase (weeks 20–26)
   Goals: Maintain static and dynamic stability of shoulder joint
   Gradual return to unrestricted activities
   Criteria to enter phase IV
   - Full functional ROM
   - No pain or tenderness
   - Muscular strength which is satisfactory
   - Statisfactory clinical examination

   Exercises
   - Continue maintance for ROM (stretches)
   - Continue strengthening program
   - Initiate interval sport program

AAROM, active–assisted range of motion; ER, external rotation; IR, internal rotation; PROM, passive range of motion.

TABLE 14. *Thermal-assisted anterior capsulorrhaphy for the overhead athlete*

I. Phase I: Protection phase (day 1 to week 6)
   Goals: Allow soft-tissue healing
   Diminish pain and inflammation
   Initiate protected motion
   Retard muscular atrophy
  Weeks 0–2
  - Sling use for 7–10 days
  - Sleep in sling/brace for 7 days
    Exercises
    - Hand-gripping exercises
    - Elbow and wrist range-of-motion exercises
    - AROM cervical spine
    - Passive and AAROM exercises
      - Elevation to 75–90 degrees
      - IR in scapular plane (45 degrees by 2 weeks)
      - ER in scapular plane (25 degrees by 2 weeks)
    - Rope and pulley (flexion) AAROM
    - Cryotherapy to control pain
    - Submaximal Isometrics
    - Rhythmic stabilization exercises at 7 days
    - Proprioception and neuromuscular control drills
  Weeks 3–4
  - Range-of-motion exercises (AAROM, PROM, AROM)
    - Elevation to 125–135 degrees
    - IR, in scapular plane, full motion
    - ER, in scapular plane, 45–50 degrees by week 4
    - At week 4, begin ER/IR at 90 degrees abduction
  - Strengthening exercises
    - Initiate *LIGHT* isotonic program
    - ER/IR exercise tubing (zero degrees abduction)
    - Continue dynamic stabilization drills
    - Scapular strengthening exercises
    - Biceps/triceps strengthening
    - PNF D2 flex/ext manual resistance
  - Continue use of cryotherapy and modalities to control pain
  Weeks 5–6
  - Continue all exercises listed earlier
  - Progress ROM to the following
    - Elevation to 145–160 degrees by week 6
    - ER at 90 degrees abduction (75–80 degrees)
    - IR at 90 degrees abduction (65–70 degrees)
  - Initiate Throwers Ten strengthening program

II. Phase II: Intermediate phase (weeks 7–12)
   Goals: Restore full ROM (week 7)
   Restore functional ROM (weeks 10–11)
   Normalize arthrokinematics
   Improve dynamic stability, muscular strength
  Weeks 7–8
  - Progress ROM to the following
    - Elevation to 180 degrees
    - ER at 90 degrees abduction to 90–100 degrees by week 8
    - IR at 90 degrees abduction to 70–75 degrees
  - Continue stretching program
  - Strengthening exercises
    - Continue Throwers Ten program
    - Continue manual resistance, dynamic stabilization drills
    - Initiate plyometrics (two-handed drills)
  Weeks 9–12
  - Progress ROM to the overhead athlete's demands
    - Gradual progression from weeks 9 to 12
  - Strengthening exercises
    - Progress isotonic program
    - May initiate more aggressive strengthening
      - Push-ups
      - Shoulder press
      - Bench-press
      - Pull-downs
      - Single-arm plyometrics

III. Phase III: Advanced activity and strengthening phase (weeks 12–20)
   Goals: Improve strength, power, and endurance
   Enhance neuromuscular control
   Functional activities
   Criteria to enter phase III
   - Full range of motion
   - No pain or tenderness
   - Muscular strength 80% of contralateral side
  Weeks 12–16
  - Continue all stretching exercises
    Self-capsular stretches, AROM passive stretching
  - Continue all strengthening exercises
    - Isotonics
    - Plyometrics
    - Neuromuscular control/dynamic stabilization drills
  - Initiate interval sport program (throwing, tennis, swimming, etc.)
  Weeks 16–20
  - Progress all exercises listed earlier
  - May resume normal training program
  - Continue specific strengthening exercises
  - Progress interval program (throwing program to phase II)

IV. Phase IV: Return-to-activity phase (weeks 22–26)
   Goals: Gradual return to unrestricted activities
   Maintain static and dynamic stability of shoulder joint
   Criteria to enter phase IV
   - Full functional ROM
   - No pain or tenderness
   - Satisfactory muscular strength (isokinetic test)
   - Satisfactory clinical examination
  Exercises
  - Continue maintenance for ROM
  - Continue strengthening exercises
  - Gradual return to competition

AAROM, active–assisted range of motion; ER, external rotation; IR, internal rotation; PROM, passive range of motion.

ter. The overall rate of progression is based on the patient's response to the procedure and the patient's unique tissue characteristics. After this procedure, it is not uncommon for patients to report shoulder capsular soreness for 8 to 12 weeks after surgery. We believe that this has contributed to capsular inflammation after the thermal effects. Most patients report improved stability immediately after surgery and throughout their rehabilitation course.

FUNCTIONAL SHOULDER BRACES

Frequently, shoulder braces have been prescribed to help prevent recurrent anterior instability of the glenohumeral joint either after traumatic injury or during the early return to sports after surgery. Because of the complexity of the glenohumeral joint, no device or taping procedure is guaranteed to protect the unstable shoulder. Because the most frequent mechanism of anterior instability is ER and ABD of the shoulder, many braces have been designed to limit these motions while allowing an athlete to return to competition. Thus, athletes who require significant ABD and ER to perform their sports are not viable candidates for bracing. Athletes who can benefit from bracing are those who play a sport and position that does not require 90 degrees or greater of ABD and more than 70 degrees of ER. Often, these athletes are linemen in football, hockey players, or soccer players (93).

Numerous types of shoulder braces are available to the clinician. The Shoulder Subluxation Inhibitor (SSI; Physical Support Systems Inc., Windham, NM, U.S.A.) is a custom-fitted brace made of low- and high-density polyethylene. The Dennison-Duke Wyre Shoulder Vest (C.D. Dennison Orthopedic Appliance Co., Baltimore, MD, U.S.A.) is constructed of sturdy canvas and straps that limit ABD and ER. The SAWA shoulder orthosis (Brace International, Scottsdale, AZ, U.S.A.) is an off-the-shelf brace constructed of a blend of cotton and rubber materials; straps are applied to the humerus that limit ABD, ER, and extension (94; Fig. 17). The Sully Brace (The Saunders Corp., Chaska, MN, U.S.A.) is a neoprene brace that also uses straps to limit motion (Fig. 18).

DeCarlo et al. (95) compared three braces (SAWA, Duke Wyre, and SSI) in controlling active ABD, flexion, and ER at 90 degrees of ABD. Measurements were taken before and after active resisted exercise. The investigators reported that all three braces limited motion in the sagittal and frontal planes (flexion and ABD), but none of the braces controlled ER. The authors went on to recommend specific braces for specific sports and positions.

The efficacy of shoulder braces remains controversial. In my opinion, some braces used in specific patients and conditions can be useful. The brace may restrict specific motion and provide proprioceptive and joint awareness to the patient. However, because of the complexity of the glenohumeral joint, no brace or device could restore dynamic stability during full motion in an unstable shoulder. Thus, bracing may be useful under specific conditions and guidelines and may be used as a valuable adjunct for returning an athlete to competition.

SUMMARY

A well-developed and properly administered postoperative rehabilitation program after shoulder stabilization surgery is a vital component of a successful outcome. The ultimate goal of the program is to restore full functional ROM and activities while maintaining the static stability of the glenohumeral joint. Numerous variables and conditions

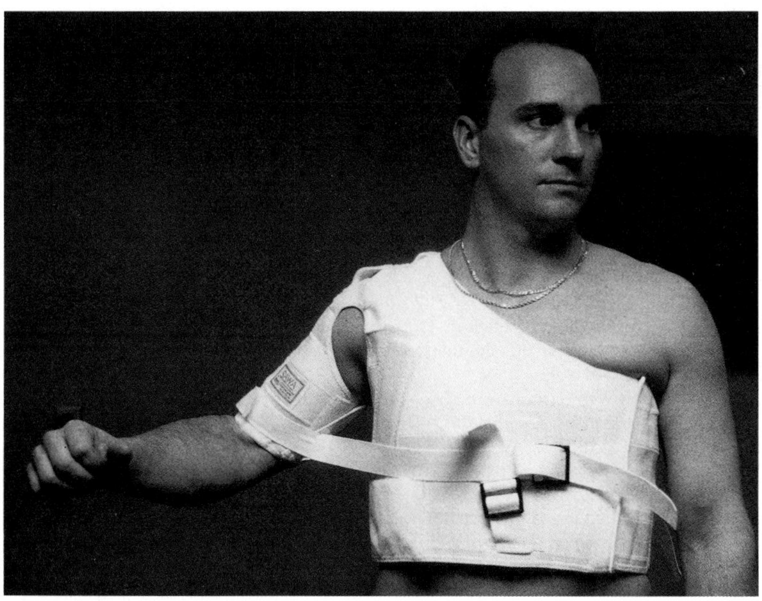

FIG. 17. The SAWA Shoulder Orthosis (Brace International, Scottsdale, AZ, U.S.A.)

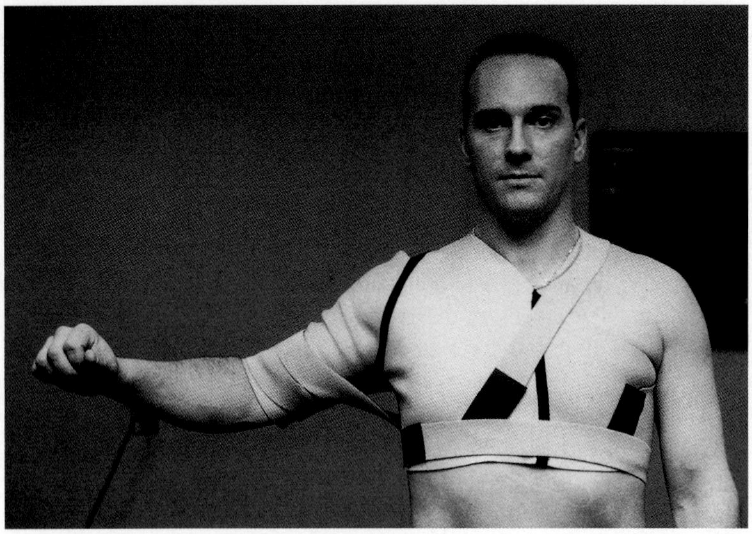

FIG. 18. The Sully Shoulder Brace. (The Saunders Group, Chaska, MN, U.S.A.)

affect the rehabilitation program; these have been discussed in this chapter. These variables must be carefully considered by the rehabilitation team before and during the post-surgery rehabilitation process. The rehabilitation specialist must adjust the rate of progression to the patient's healing response to the surgical procedure. The assessment of the patient's end feel can render vital information regarding the rate of progression of motion. Furthermore, the rehabilitation specialist should always attempt to correct asymmetric capsular tightness and muscular imbalance to prevent long-term complications. The rehabilitation specialist should emphasize dynamic stability before initiating an isotonic strengthening program to prevent humeral head displacement. The two most common complications seen after shoulder stabilization are loss of motion and recurrent instability. Loss of motion should be prevented with a proper, well-developed, and supervised rehabilitation program. Factors such as accidental stress, noncompliance, and inappropriate rehabilitation contribute to the recurrence of instability. Each rehabilitation program should be tailored to the type of instability, type of surgical procedure, patient tissue status, healing response, and desired goals—this will ensure a successful result.

REFERENCES

1. Wall MS, Warren RF. Complications of shoulder instability surgery. *Clin Sports Med* 1995;14:973–1000.
2. Brav EA. Recurrent dislocation of the shoulder: ten years experience with the Putti-Platt reconstruction procedure. *Am J Surg* 1960;100: 423–430.
3. Bryan RS, DiMichele JD, Ford QJ. Anterior recurrent dislocations of the shoulder: report of a series of the Augustine variation of Magnusson-Stack repair. *Clin Orthop* 1969;63:177–180.
4. Halley DK, Olix ML. A review of the Bristow operation for recurrent anterior shoulder dislocations in athletes. *Clin Orthop* 1975;106:175–179.
5. Hovelius L, Thorling J, Fredin H. Recurrent anterior dislocation of the shoulder: results after the Bankart and Putti-Platt operations. *J Bone Joint Surg [Am]* 1979;61:566–569.
6. May JR. A modified Bristow operation for anterior recurrent dislocation of the shoulder. *J Bone Joint Surg [Am]* 1970;52:1010–1016.
7. Rowe CR. Acute and recurrent dislocations of the shoulder. *J Bone Joint Surg [Am]* 1962;44:998–1008.
8. Cofield RH, Kavanaugh BF, Frassion FJ. Anterior shoulder instability. *Instr Course Lect* 1985;36:210–227.
9. Hawkins RJ, Bell R. Collagen analysis in patients with multidirectional instability. Presented at American Shoulder and Elbow Surgeons Specialty Day, Anaheim, CA, March 1991.
10. Dehre E, Tory R. Treatment of joint injuries by immediate mobilization based upon the spinal adaption concept. *Clin Orthop* 1971;77: 218–232.
11. Salter RB, Hamilton HW, Wedge JH. Clinical application of basic science research on continuous passive motion for disorders of injuries and synovial joints. *J Orthop Res* 1984;1:325–333.
12. Tipton CM, Mattes RD, Maynard JA. The influence of physical activity on ligaments and tendons. *Med Sci Sports Exerc* 1975;7:165–175.
13. Haggmark T, Eriksson E, Jansson E. Muscle fiber type changes in human muscles after injuries and immobilization. *Orthopaedics* 1986;9:181–189.
14. Wickiewicz TL, Pagnani MJ, Kennedy K. Rehabilitation of the unstable shoulder. *Sports Med Arthrosc Rev* 1993;1:227–235.
15. Harryman DT, Sidles JA, Clark JM, et al. Translation of the humeral head on the glenoid with passive glenohumeral motion. *J Bone Joint Surg [Am]* 1990;72:1334–1338.
16. Wilk KE, Andrews JR. Rehabilitation following arthroscopic subacromial decompression. *Orthopaedics* 1993;16:349–358.
17. Hawkins RJ, Angelo RL. Glenohumeral osteoarthrosis: a late complication of the Putti-Platt procedure. *J Bone Joint Surg [Am]* 1990;72: 1193–1197.
18. Knott M, Voss DE. *Proprioceptive neuromuscular facilitation.* 2nd ed. New York: Harper & Row, 1968.
19. Wilk KE, Arrigo CA. Current concepts in the rehabilitation of the athlete's shoulder. *J Orthop Sports Phys Ther* 1993;18:365–375.
20. Davies GJ, Dickoff-Hoffman S. Neuromuscular testing and rehabilitation of the shoulder complex. *J Orthop Sports Phys Ther* 1993;18: 449–456.
21. Wilk KE, Arrigo CA. An integrated approach to upper extremity exercises. *Orthop Phys Ther Clin North Am* 1992;9:337–349.
22. Wilk KE, Arrigo CA, Andrews JR. The strength characteristics of the internal and external rotator muscles in professional baseball pitchers. *Am J Sports Med* 1993;21:61–69.
23. Davies GJ. Macrotraumatic shoulder injuries. In: Davies GJ, ed. *A compendium of isokinetics in clinical usage.* 4th ed. Onalaska, WI: S & S Publishers, 1992:433–480.
24. Paine RM, Voight M. The role of the scapula. *J Orthop Sports Phys Ther* 1993;18:385–391.
25. Wilk KE, Andrews JR, Arrigo CA. The abductor and adductor

strength characteristics of professional baseball pitchers. *Am J Sports Med* 1995;23 (3):307–311.
26. Lephart SM, Warner JP, Borsa PA, Fu FH. Proprioception of the shoulder joint in healthy, unstable surgically repaired shoulders. *J Shoulder Elbow Surg* 1994;3:371–380.
27. Wickiewicz TH, Chen SK, Otis JC, Warren RF. Glenohumeral kinematics in a muscle fatigue model: a radiographic study. *Orthop Trans* 1995;18:126.
28. Payne LZ, Altchek DW. The surgical treatment of anterior shoulder instability. *Clin Sports Med* 1995;14 (4):863–883.
29. Altchek DW, Dines DW. The surgical treatment of anterior instability: selective capsular repair. *Oper Tech Sports Med* 1993;1:285–292.
30. Jobe FW, Glousman RE. Anterior capsulolabral reconstruction. *Tech Orthop* 1989;3:29–35.
31. Brewster CE, Seto JL, Moynes DR, Jobe FW. Capsulolabral reconstruction and rehabilitation. In: Andrews JR, Wilk KE, eds. *The athlete's shoulder.* New York: Churchill Livingstone, 1994:221–227.
32. Jobe FW, Giangarra CE, Kvitne RS, Glousman RE. Anterior capsulolabral reconstruction of the shoulder in overhead sports. *Am J Sports Med* 1991;19:428–434.
33. Andrews JR, Satterwhite YS. Anatomic capsular shift. *J Orthop Tech* 1993;1:151–160.
34. Akeson WH, Amiel D, Woo Sh-Y. Immobilization effects on synovial joints. The pathomechanics of joint contractures. *Biorheology* 1980; 17:95–107.
35. Dickson JW, Devas MB. Bankart's operation for recurrent dislocation of the shoulder. *J Bone Joint Surg [Br]* 1957;19:114–119.
36. Rowe CR, Patel D. The Bankart procedure: a long term end result study. *J Bone Joint Surg [Am]* 1978;60:1–16.
37. Kvitne RS, Jobe FW, Jobe CM. Shoulder instability in the overhead or throwing athlete. *Clin Sports Med* 1995;14 (4):917–935.
38. Rosenberg BN, Richmond JC, Levine WN. Long term follow-up of Bankart reconstruction: incidence of late degenerative glenohumeral arthrosis. *Am J Sports Med* 1995;23:538–544.
39. Schexeider MA, Catlin PA, Davies GJ, Mattson PA. An isokinetic estimation of total arm strength. *Isokin Exerc Sci* 1991;1 (3):117–121.
40. Gross R. Arthroscopic staple capsulorrhaphy: does it work? *Am J Sports Med* 1989;17:459–500.
41. Hawkins R. Arthroscopic stapling repair for shoulder instability: a retrospective study of 50 cases. *Arthroscopy* 1989;5:122–128.
42. Lane J, Sachs R, Riehl B. Arthroscopic staple capsulorrhaphy: a long term follow-up. *Arthroscopy* 1993;9:190–194.
43. Grana W, Buckley P, Yates C. Arthroscopic Bankart suture repair. *Am J Sports Med* 1993;21:348–353.
44. Snyder S. Arthroscopic technique for the anterior shoulder stabilization using the suture shuttle relay and implantable bone anchors. Presented at the 13th Annual Meeting of the Arthroscopy Association of North America, Orlando, FL, April 1994.
45. Wolf E, Wilk R, Richmond J. Arthroscopic Bankart repair using suture anchors. *Oper Tech Orthop Surg* 1991;1:184–191.
46. Morgan CD. Arthroscopic transglenoid suture repair. *Oper Tech Orthop Surg* 1991;1:171–179.
47. Warner JP, Warren RF. Arthroscopic Bankart repair using a cannulated absorbable fixation device. *Oper Tech Orthop Surg* 1991;1:192–198.
48. Geiger D, Hurley J, Tovey J. Results of arthroscopic vs. open Bankart suture repair. *Orthop Trans* 1993;17:973.
49. Pagnani M, Warren RF. Arthroscopic shoulder stabilization. *Oper Tech Sports Med* 1993;1:276–284.
50. Rose D, Moyer R, Marchetto P. Arthroscopic suture capsulorrhaphy for anterior shoulder instability. *Orthop Trans* 1990;14:597.
51. Shall LW, Crowley PW. Soft tissue reconstruction in the shoulder: comparison of suture anchors, absorbable staples and absorbable tacks. *Am J Sports Med* 1994;22 (5):715–718.
52. Warner JJP, Miller M, Marks P. Arthroscopic Bankart repair with Suretac device: clinical and experimental observations. *Arthroscopy* 1995;11:2–20.
53. Grana W, Buckley P, Yates C. Arthroscopic Bankart suture repair. *Am J Sports Med* 1993;21:348–353.
54. Acerio RA, Wheeler JH, Ryan JB. Arthroscopic Bankart repair vs. non-operative treatment for acute, initial anterior shoulder dislocations. *Am J Sports Med* 1994;22:589–594.
55. Wolf E, Wilk R, Richmond J. Arthroscopic Bankart repair using suture anchors. *Oper Tech Orthop Surg* 1991;1:184–191.
56. Altchek DW. Arthroscopic shoulder stabilization using a bioabsorbable fixation device. *Sports Med Arthrosc Rev* 1992;1:266–271.
57. Caspari R. Arthroscopic reconstruction for anterior shoulder instability. *Oper Tech Orthop Surg* 1988;3:59–66.
58. Hawkins R. Arthroscopic stapling repair for shoulder instability: a retrospective study of 50 cases. *Arthroscopy* 1989;5:122–128.
59. Johnson LL. The shoulder joint: an arthroscopist's perspective of anatomy and pathology. *Clin Orthop* 1987;223:113–125.
60. Johnson LL. Shoulder arthroscopy. In: Johnson LL, ed. *Arthroscopic surgery: principles and practice.* St. Louis: CV Mosby, 1986:1301–1304.
61. O'Keefe RM, Shea KP, Fulkerson JP. Initial failure strength of orthoscopic Bankart suture and staple repairs. *Arthroscopy* 1990;6:158–161.
62. Lane JG, Sachs RA, Riehl B. Arthroscopic staple capsulorrhaphy: a long term follow up. *Arthroscopy* 1993;9:190–194.
63. Altchek DW, Skybar MJ, Warren RF. Shoulder arthroscopy for shoulder instability. *Instr Course Lect* 1989;37:187–198.
64. Caspari RB, Savoie F. Arthroscopic reconstruction of the shoulder: the Bankart repair. In: McGinty J, ed. *Operative arthroscopy.* New York: Raven Press, 1991:507–515.
65. Morgan CD, Bodenstab AB. Arthroscopic Bankart suture repair: technique and early results. *Arthroscopy* 1987;3:111–122.
66. Hovelius L, Korner GL, Lundberg GB. The coracoid transfer for recurrent dislocation of the shoulder: technical aspects of the Bristow-Laterjet procedure. *J Bone Joint Surg [Am]* 1983;65:926–934.
67. Young D, Rockwood CA. Complications of a failed Bristow procedure and their management. *J Bone Joint Surg [Am]* 1991;73:969–975.
68. Norris TR. Complications following anterior instability repairs. In: Bigliani LU, ed. *Complications of shoulder surgery.* Baltimore: Williams & Wilkins, 1993:96–116.
69. Ferlic DC, DiGiovine NM. A long term retrospective study of the modified Bristow procedure. *Am J Sports Med* 1988;16:469–474.
70. Hill JA, Lombardo SJ, Kerlan RF. The modified Bristow-Helfet procedure for recurrent anterior shoulder subluxations and dislocations. *Am J Sports Med* 1981;9:283–287.
71. Lombardo'SJ, Kerlan RK, Jobe FW. The modified Bristow procedure for recurrent dislocation of the shoulder. *J Bone Joint Surg [Am]* 1976;58:256–261.
72. Shively J, Johnson J. Results of modified Bristow procedure. *Clin Orthop* 1984;187:150–153.
73. Hovelius L, Akermark C, Albrektsson B. Bristow-Laterjet procedure for recurrent anterior dislocation of the shoulder: a 2–5 year follow-up study on the results of 112 cases. *Acta Orthop Scand* 1983;54: 284–290.
74. Torg JS, Baldvini FC, Bonci C. A modified Bristow-Helfet-May procedure for recurrent dislocation and subluxation of the shoulder. *J Bone Joint Surg [Am]* 1987;69:904–913.
75. Craythorne CB, Glasgow MT, Glasgow SG. Long term evaluation of the modified Bristow procedure for anterior glenohumeral instability. Presented at the American Academy of Orthopaedic Surgery 60th Annual Meeting, San Francisco, CA, February 19, 1993.
76. Fronek J, Warren RF, Bowen M. Posterior subluxation of the glenohumeral joint. *J Bone Joint Surg [Am]* 1989;71:205–216.
77. Hurley JA, Anderson TE, Dear W. Posterior shoulder instability: surgical versus conservative results in the evaluation of glenoid version. *Am J Sports Med* 1992;20:396–400.
78. Dehne E, Tory R. Treatment of joint injuries by immediate mobilization, based upon the spinal adaption concept. *Clin Orthop* 1971;77: 218–232.
79. Woo SLY, Matthews SU, Akeson WH. Connective tissue response to immobility. *Arthritis Rheum* 1975;18:257–264.
80. Bigliani U. Anterior and posterior capsule shift for multi-directional instability. *Tech Orthop* 1989;3 (4):36–45.
81. Bigliani LU, Kurzweil PR, Schwartzback CC, Wolfe I, Flatow EL. Inferior capsular shift procedure for anterior-inferior shoulder instability in athletes. *Am J Sports Med* 1994;22:578–584.
82. Neer CS, Foster CR. Inferior capsular shift for involuntary inferior and multi-directional instability of the shoulder: a preliminary report. *J Bone Joint Surg [Am]* 1980;62:897–908.
83. Altchek DW, Warren RF, Skybar MJ, Oritz G. T-Plasty modification of the Bankart procedure for multi-directional instability of the anterior and inferior types. *J Bone Joint Surg [Am]* 1991;73:105–112.

84. Andrews JR, Satterwhite YS. Anatomic capsular shift. *J Orthop Tech* 1993;1:151–160.
85. Jobe FW, Tibone JE, Jobe CM, Kvitne RS. The shoulder in sports. In: Rockwood CA, Matsen FA, eds. *The shoulder.* Philadelphia: WB Saunders, 1990:961–990.
86. Wilk KE, Arrigo CA. Current concepts in the rehabilitation of the athletic shoulder. *J Orthop Sports Phys Ther* 1993;18 (1):365–378.
87. Wilk KE. Shoulder injuries in baseball. In: Andrews JR, Wilk KE, eds. *The athlete's shoulder.* New York: Churchill Livingstone, 1994: 369–390.
88. Kvitne RS, Jobe FW, Jobe CM. Shoulder instability in the overhead or throwing athlete. *Clin Sports Med* 1995;14:917–935.
89. LeBar RD, Alexander AH. Multi-directional shoulder instability. *Am J Sports Med* 1992;20:193–198.
90. Fleisig GS. Ten years in twenty minutes: conclusions from ASMI's research. Presented at 15th Annual Injuries in Baseball Course, American Sports Medicine Institute, Birmingham, AL, January 24, 1997.
91. Cooper RA, Brems JJ. The inferior capsular procedure for multi-directional instability of the shoulder. *J Bone Joint Surg [Am]* 1992;7: 1516–1522.
92. Yamuguchi K, Flatow EL. Management of multi-directional instability. *Clin Sports Med* 1995;14:885–902.
93. Konin JG, McCue FC. Taping, strapping and bracing of the shoulder complex. In: Andrews JR, Wilk KE, eds. *The athlete's shoulder.* New York: Churchill Livingstone, 1994:679–689.
94. Sawa TM. An alternative conservative management of shoulder dislocations and dislocations. *J Athlet Train* 1992;27:366–369.
95. DeCarlo M, Malone K, Gehrig B, Hunker M. Evaluation of shoulder instability braces. *J Sports Rehabil* 1996;5:143–150.

The Unstable Shoulder,
edited by R.F. Warren, E.V. Craig, and D.W. Altchek.
Lippincott–Raven Publishers, Philadelphia © 1999.

CHAPTER 25

Contracture and Other Complications

Paul A. Dowdy, Lucio S. Ernlund, and Jon J.P. Warner

LOSS OF SHOULDER MOTION

Causes

Surgical Technique

Successful surgery for shoulder instability has traditionally been defined as the elimination of instability episodes (1–4). However, the functional demands of the overhead athlete have led shoulder surgeons to broaden the definition of successful surgery to include the restoration of stability with a complete, functional, painless range of motion (ROM) and adequate strength (5).

Surgery to stabilize the unstable shoulder may result in a certain degree of ROM loss. The procedures to stabilize the shoulder form two basic categories: those anatomic procedures that identify and treat pathology, such as the Bankart and capsular-shift procedures (1,3,4,6–16), and those nonanatomic repairs that attempt to provide an external-rotation (ER) block or check-rein, such as the Putti–Platt, Magnuson–Stack, and Bristow procedures (2,3,17–26). The anatomic repairs, when they result in motion loss, do so by producing a capsular or intra-articular contracture (Fig. 1A; 27). The nonanatomic repairs may produce both an intra- and an extra-articular contracture (Fig. 1B and C). In fact, the goal of some of these nonanatomic repairs is to limit ER so that the arm cannot reach the provocative position to produce instability. Thus, loss of motion is an expected consequence of these procedures, and this may be problematic in some patients if ER loss is excessive (8,21,27–29). In addition, the nonanatomic repairs distort normal anatomy and cause scarring throughout the tissue planes dissected during surgery (both intra- and extra-articular). This can make revision surgery extremely difficult, as well as perilous, because of the altered anatomy and proximity of neurovascular structures (30).

Bristow–Latarjet Procedure

In the modified Bristow procedure, the distal 1 to 1 ½ cm of the coracoid process, along with the conjoined tendons of the coracobrachialis and short head of the biceps, is transferred to the scapular neck to serve as a bony buttress anteriorly and to act as a dynamic soft-tissue sling (18). The coracoid process is fixed to the scapular neck with a screw through either a longitudinal split in the subscapularis muscle or a vertical division of its fibers (2,5,18, 20,21,30). Loss of motion can result from scarring and entrapment of the subscapularis muscle/tendon (30). Extra-articular scarring from transposing the conjoined tendon adds to the restriction of motion (5). The screw used to fix the coracoid process must be the appropriate length. If it is too long, it may irritate the infraspinatus muscle, which further contributes to decreased motion (5,30; Fig. 2A). In a significant number of cases, the screw used to fix the coracoid process leads to progressive articular cartilage damage from inadvertent intra-articular screw placement (30,31; Fig. 2B). This articular cartilage damage produces arthrosis, which causes joint contracture, not unlike primary osteoarthritis (32). If the graft is secured too prominently, the humeral head can abut the graft (Fig. 2C and D). This will occur especially if the procedure was performed in the presence of a redundant capsule (30) or if the graft is placed superior to the equator of the glenoid (2), both instances allowing unchecked humeral head subluxation (Fig. 2D). Young and Rockwood (30) demonstrated that if a Bristow procedure is performed in multidirectional instability (MDI), then posterior subluxation of the humeral head can result if loss of ER is severe. This situation can result in

P. A. Dowdy: Central Florida Sports Medicine Institute and Central Florida Bone and Joint Institute, Davenport, Florida 33837.

L. S. Ernlund: Department of Orthopaedic Surgery, University of Pittsburgh, Center for Sports Medicine, Pittsburgh, Pennsylvania 15213.

J. J. P. Warner: Department of Orthopaedic Surgery, Harvard Medical School; and Harvard Shoulder Service, Department of Orthopaedic Surgery, Massachusetts General Hospital, Boston, Massachusetts 02114.

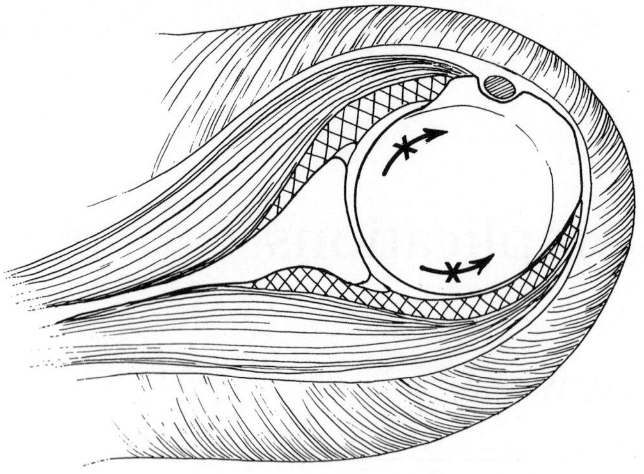

A

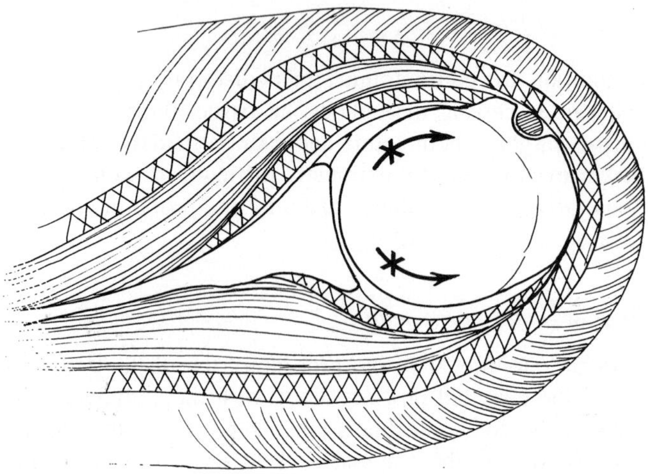

B

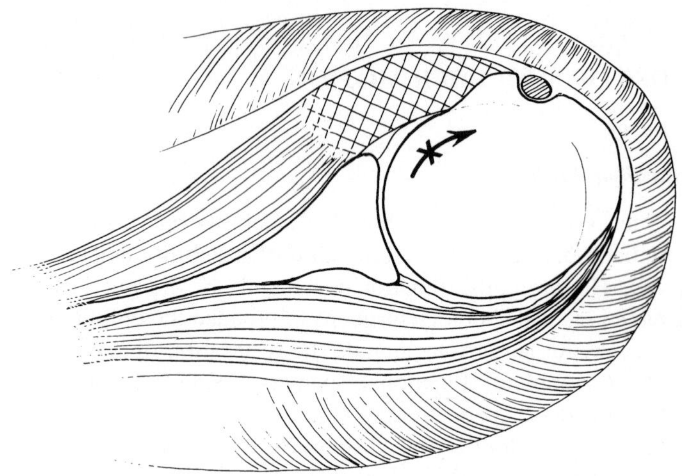

C

FIG. 1. Anatomic causes of shoulder stiffness. **A:** Global capsular contracture *(cross-hatching).* **B:** Scarring between tissue planes as well as global capsular contracture *(cross-hatching).* **C:** Shortened and scarred subscapularis tendon *(cross-hatching).* (From Warner JJP. Acquired shoulder stiffness. In: Warner JJP, Iannotti JP, Gerber C, eds. *Complex and revisions problems in shoulder surgery.* Philadelphia: Lippincott–Raven, 1997:131–147, with permission.)

abnormal joint mechanics that lead to arthritis from increased posterior joint compression (Fig. 3A and B). Finally, nonunion of the coracoid bone graft may or may not be associated with shoulder pain (Fig. 4).

Series that report successful results after Bristow repair describe an average of 9 to 15 degrees of loss of ER (18–21,24,26). However, loss of ER of a greater magnitude has been reported with this procedure (30). To avoid motion loss, the surgical technique must avoid entrapping the subscapularis. The initial postoperative course must include early ROM to avoid adhesions between the subscapularis and the transferred conjoined tendon.

Putti–Platt Repair

The Putti–Platt procedure treats anterior instability by shortening the subscapularis to limit ER. In this procedure, the subscapularis tendon is detached 2.5 cm medial to its insertion, and it is repaired in a vest-over-pants fashion with the lateral limb sutured to the glenoid rim (5,23,27). This leads to both an extra-articular and intra-articular (from capsular plication and scarring) contracture of the glenohumeral joint (24,27). A general rule is that 20 degrees of ER is lost for every 1 cm of subscapularis imbrication (33). As with other procedures that constrain ER, arthritis from abnormal joint forces is a real risk in this procedure (Fig. 3A and B; 29).

Magnuson–Stack

The Magnuson–Stack procedure also acts as an extra-articular check-rein to anterior instability by blocking ER. In this procedure, the subscapularis insertion is transferred from the lesser tuberosity about 1 cm across the bicipital groove and repaired into the humerus (17,22). The purpose of this procedure is to limit ER by shortening the subscapularis and creating an extra-articular restraint (33). As with other procedures that constrain joint rotation, this surgery can lead to arthritis (29). Because a lax capsule may remain despite this ER loss, revision surgery often requires a capsular shift in addition to release and mobilization of the subscapularis tendon.

Bankart Repair

The classic Bankart repair (1) and its many modified forms (4,7,8,10–13,34) involve repair of the avulsed anteroinferior glenoid labrum with its attached inferior and mid-

(text continues on page 408)

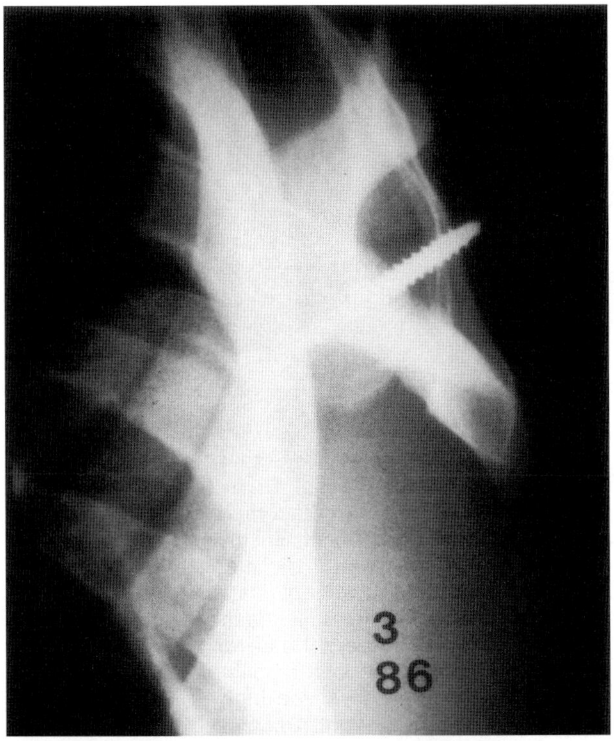

A

FIG. 2. A:. Excessively long screw used to fix coracoid bone graft in Bristow procedure. The screw protrudes into the infraspinatus fossa. Errors in placement of coracoid bone graft with Bristow procedure. **B:** Intra-articular screw from Bristow procedure seen on plane radiograph **(left)** and computed tomography (CT) scan **(right)**. *(figure continues)*

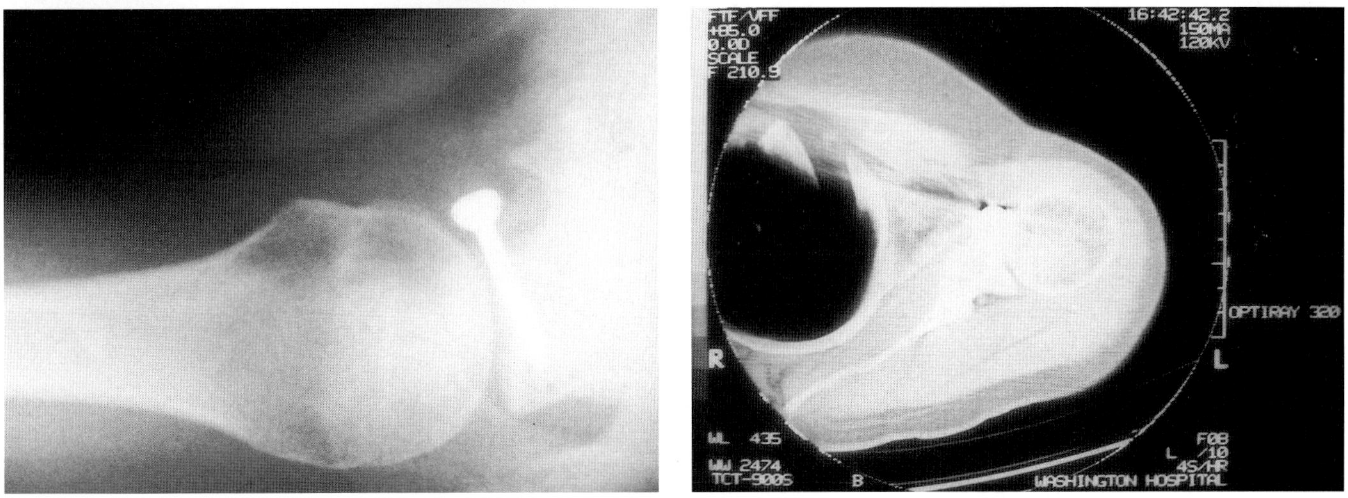

B

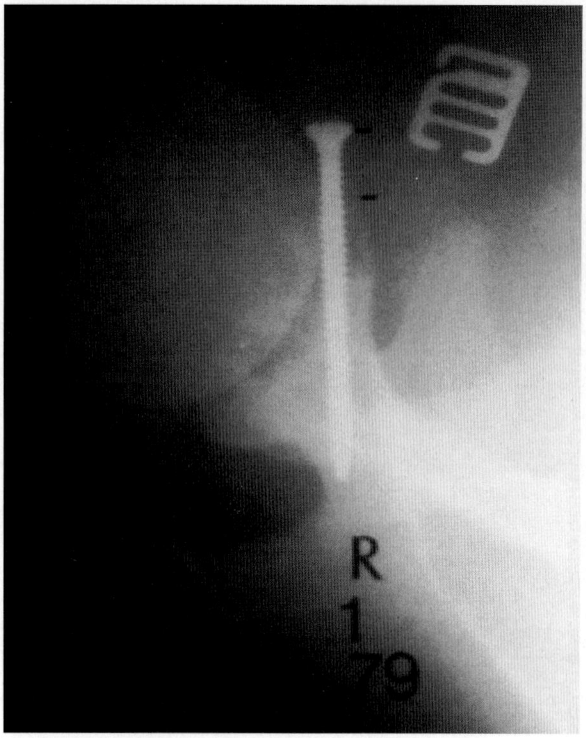

C

FIG. 2. *Continued.* **C:** Screw contacting the humeral head. **D:** Schematic drawing of errors in placement of coracoid bone graft with Bristow procedure. *A*, Graft placed too medially results in residual anterior instability. *B,* Graft placed too laterally results in contact with the humeral head *(arrow)*. *C*, Correct placement of the bone graft. **Inset:** Graft placement too high *(1)*, too low *(2)*, and just right *(3)*.

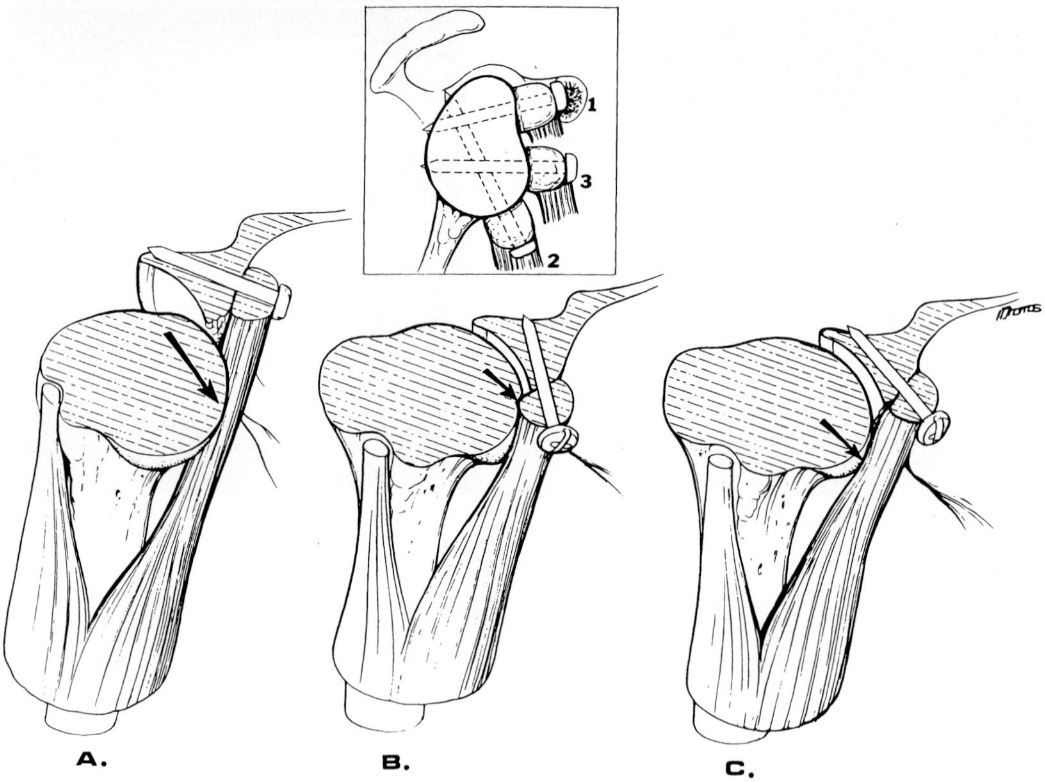

D

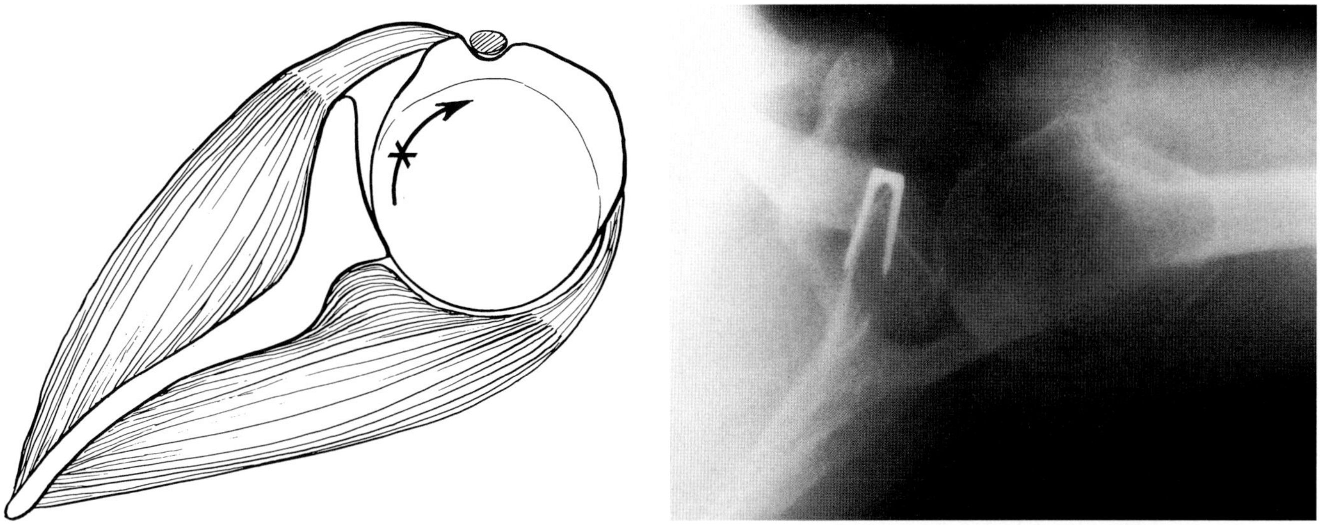
A B

FIG. 3. A: Posterior subluxation of the humeral head in a patient with multidirectional instability and an overly tight anterior instability repair. **B:** Radiograph of a patient who had an anterior staple capsulorrhaphy, which has resulted in posterior subluxation of the humeral head. Also note intra-articular placement of staple.

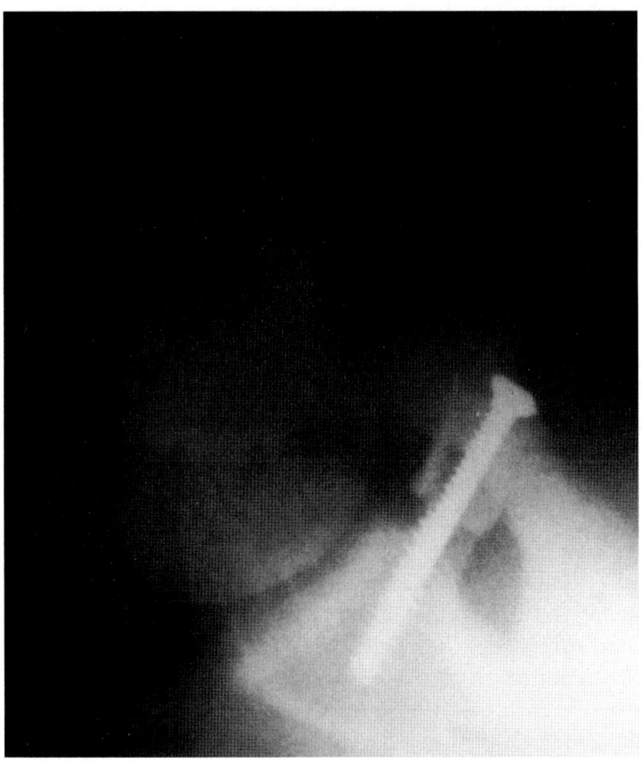

FIG. 4. Patient with asymptomatic coracoid bone graft nonunion.

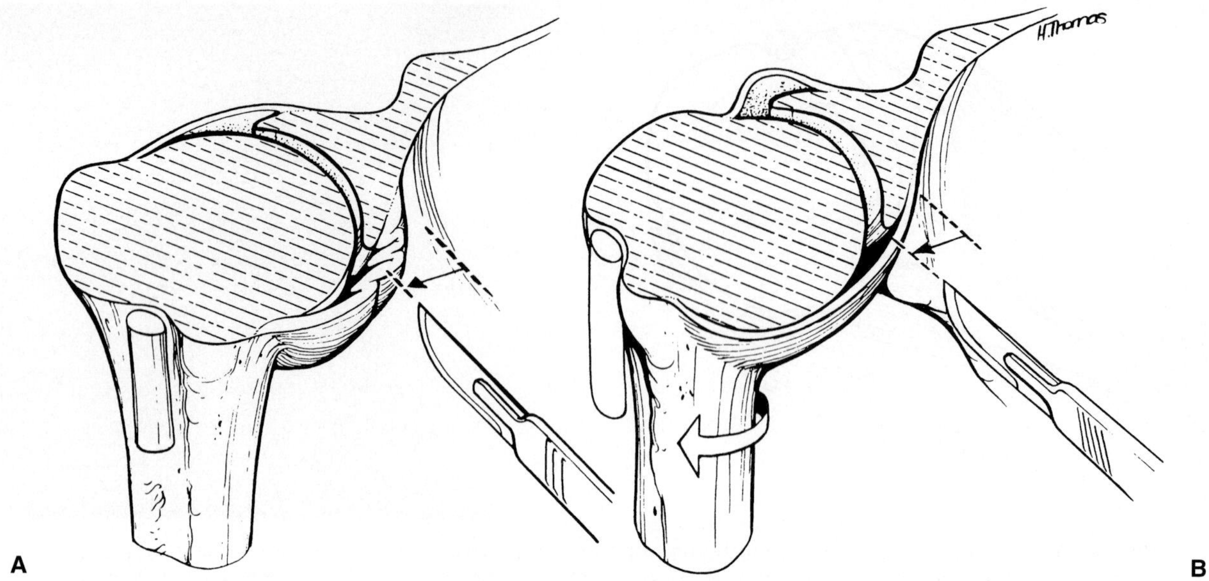

FIG. 5. Capsulotomy incision for Bankart repair. If the vertical paraglenoid capsular incision is made with the arm in internal rotation, the capsule may be divided laterally **(A)**. Its repair medially can then result in loss of external rotation **(B)**. If the arm is externally rotated before capsular division, the capsule is divided at the glenoid rim, and direct repair will minimize loss of external rotation.

dle glenohumeral ligaments. Reported loss of motion after Bankart repair has varied from 0 (1) to 18 degrees (7).

Technical errors can lead to motion loss with this procedure. First, if the vertical capsular incision is made too laterally and the lateral end of the capsule is imbricated into the glenoid margin, ER will be limited (Fig. 5). This usually occurs if the vertical paraglenoid capsulotomy incision is made with the arm in internal rotation (IR). Second, shortening of the subscapularis tendon may limit motion (5). Finally, even with an anatomic Bankart repair, gradual motion loss may occur in patients who develop arthritis as a result of articular injury from prior recurrent dislocations. Rosenberg et al. (7) found a significant rate of arthrosis in long-term follow-up of the Bankart repair.

Capsular Shift

Significant loss of motion after capsular shift (either posterior, anterior, or anteroinferior) can result if the repair is made too tight. A technical error may be to assume that physiological laxity is pathologic in a given individual and then perform a capsular shift that overshifts the capsule. This can occur if one detaches the capsular insertion from the neck of the humerus and then performs a capsular shift with the patient's arm at the side. Capsular length will be shortened and thus motion may be constrained globally (Fig. 6). The key to avoiding this error is to identify the type of instability properly. Patients with classic MDI rarely become stiff after a capsular shift; however, patients with posttraumatic instability who may require a capsular shift need careful attention to tensioning of the capsular repair. In general, in these patients, the senior author (J.P.W.) prefers to place the shoulder in abduction and ER when shifting the inferior capsule and then in adduction and ER when shifting the superior capsule (13). Bigliani et al. (28) were able to achieve return to sports and minimal loss of ER (average, 7 degrees) in the majority of their patients after capsular shift.

Arthroscopic Repair

One of the proposed advantages of arthroscopic stabilization is that there should be less loss of motion because there is minimal dissection between normal tissue planes (5,12,14–16,33,35–45). Uribe et al. (41), in treating 11 young athletes with acute traumatic initial anterior dislocation with an arthroscopic Bankart reconstruction, found one case of stiffness, which eventually resolved, giving maintenance of full ROM. Green et al. (36) reported an average 2-degree loss of ER after arthroscopic Bankart repair. Walch et al. (42) had two of 59 patients with postoperative stiffness that lasted 8 and 10 months, respectively, after arthroscopic transglenoid Bankart repair. Lane et al. (38) reported an average 5-degree ER loss and loss of one spinal segment IR after arthroscopic staple capsulorrhaphy. Yoneda et al. (43) reported an average 6-degree loss of ER with the arm in 90 degrees of abduction after arthroscopic transglenoid stabilization. Speer et al. (9) found an average 3-degree loss in elevation, 3-degree ER with the arm at the side, and 6-degree ER loss with the arm abducted 90 degrees after arthroscopic Bankart repair with a bioabsorbable tack. Goldberg et al. (44), by using arthroscopic transglenoid capsulolabral suture repairs, found that 37% of their 38 shoulders lost less than 10 degrees of ER, whereas 5%

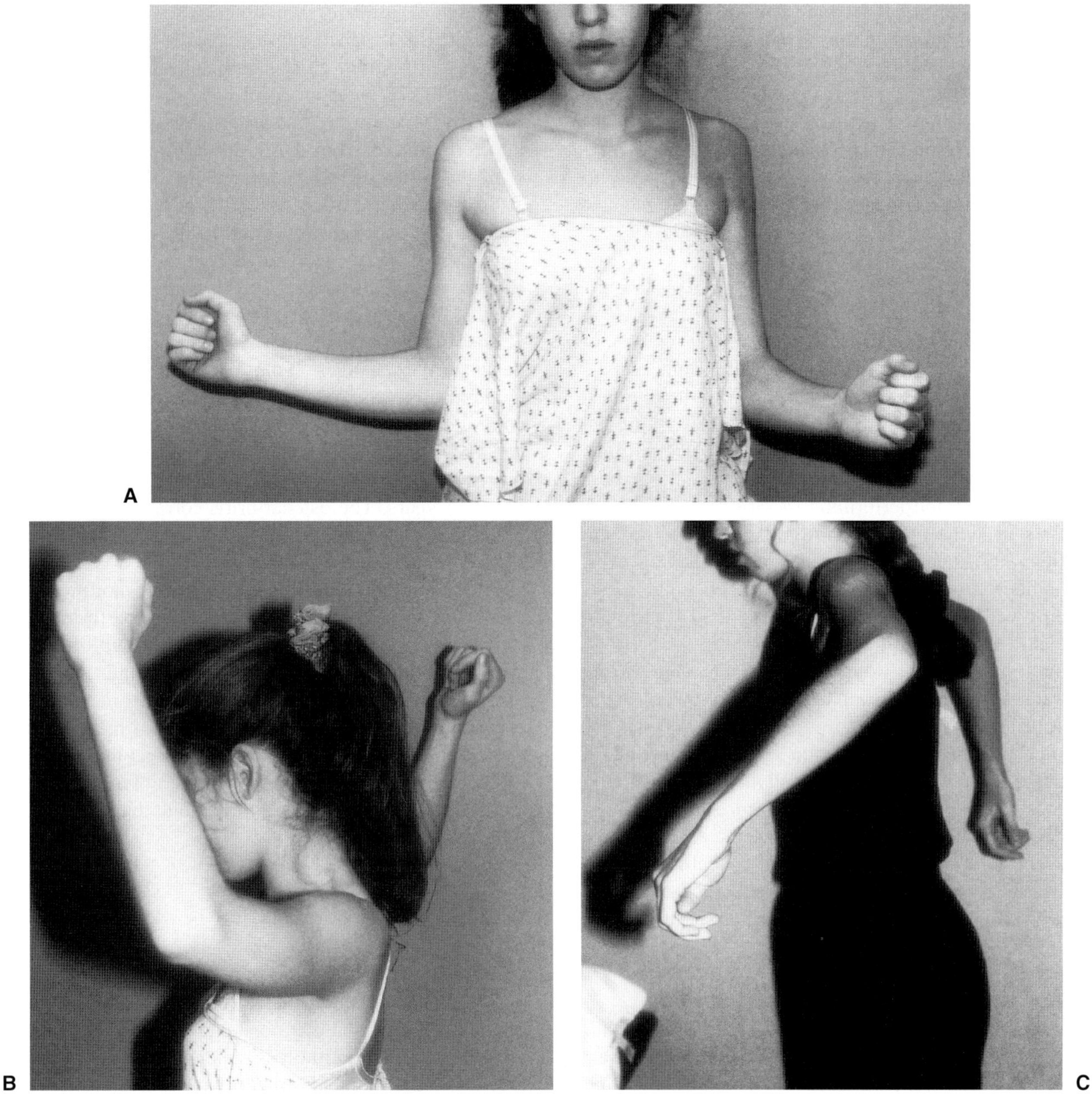

FIG. 6. A 21-year-old woman who underwent an anteroinferior capsular shift for atraumatic instability. The capsule was overshifted, resulting in mild but noticeable loss of external rotation with the arm in adduction **(A)** and abduction **(B)**. Internal rotation also is limited **(C)**.

had a greater than 10-degree loss in ER. One patient had greater motion than preoperative values. The senior author (J.P.W.) encountered four cases of motion restriction requiring intervention in 130 patients undergoing an arthroscopic repair with an absorbable fixation device. These four cases had global refractory motion loss and had the appearance of an acquired adhesive capsulitis. All were refractory to therapy of 6 to 12 months, and all recovered motion after an arthroscopic release. None of these patients had recurrent instability.

Infection

Shoulder infections can lead to both intra- and extra-articular loss of motion after instability surgery. If an open stabilization was performed, then any tissue plane that was violated from the surgery can be involved with the diffuse inflammatory reaction associated with the infection (46). The magnitude of pressure that the purulent material is subjected to can make it break across tissue planes, thus contaminating surrounding structures. These reactions can cause a severe extra-articular contracture. Contracture also can be caused by pain inhibition of motion, causing or exacerbating further contracture. Once bacterial infection is established in the joint, the release of bacterial toxins and the subsequent cascade of cytokine-mediated events leads to intense inflammation and cartilage degradation (46). Destructive enzymes are released by the synoviocytes and inflammatory cells (46,47). Once started, this self-propagated response leads to severe intra-articular contracture.

Rehabilitation

In an open Bankart or capsular-shift repair, the senior author's (J.P.W.) preference is to assess the limits of passive motion after the repair and then to allow the therapist to perform passive motion, moving the shoulder within the safe zone defined by this surgical observation. These limits are maintained for 3 weeks, during which time the patient wears a sling when not performing therapy. After 3 weeks, active–assisted motion is begun with an attempt to recover full motion. Resistance exercises are delayed for 8 weeks. If the shoulder is overly stiff, we recommend supplementing therapy with a pool program, as described by Liotard and Walch (48). The patient is encouraged actively to stretch the shoulder in the water. The buoyancy and warmth of the water may help recover motion by allowing better muscle relaxation.

In an arthroscopic repair, motion is not begun until 4 weeks after surgery, because historically such early motion has been associated with a higher recurrence rate (49). Because scarring is usually limited only to the region of the Bankart repair, motion loss from adhesions between tissue planes is less a concern. In these patients, active motion and strengthening is begun at 4 weeks after surgery.

Arthritis

Arthritis after instability surgery occurs in two settings (7, 25,29,50,51). The trauma from instability (dislocation arthropathy; 49,50) or surgery (capsulorrhaphy arthropathy; 7,25,29,50) can cause the arthritis, which subsequently causes contracture. In the latter case, if the stabilization procedure is made too tight, then arthritis and further contracture result (27,29). In a Putti–Platt (29) or capsulorrhaphy that shortens the anterior capsule (27), there is markedly decreased ER. This tends to displace the humeral head posteriorly, leading to a smaller articular contact area and greater compressive forces (5). Lusardi et al. (27) found 16 of 20 shoulders with severe ER loss after capsulorrhaphy to have degenerative arthritis. Young and Rockwood (30) found, in patients after a Bristow procedure and unrecognized MDI, that the patients would have unmasked and symptomatic/painful posterior instability from the captured joint anteriorly. This was associated with posterior chondrosis. Of the 31 patients with a failed Bristow procedure that were operated on, 52% demonstrated osteoarthritic changes (30).

Articular cartilage chondrosis releases proinflammatory cytokines (52), which causes capsular contracture and further loss of motion. This same mechanism of capsular contracture caused by arthrosis also occurs if the arthritis is the result of infection, trauma from surgery, metal penetration into the joint, or from the initial trauma of dislocation.

In the series of Samilson and Prieto (51) of dislocation arthropathy of the shoulder, 39% of the 74 shoulders had never had a surgical procedure. In the report by Rowe and Southmayd (4) at an average follow-up of 6 years after Bankart repair, there were no cases of osteoarthritis. However, Rosenberg et al. (7), at an average 15-year follow-up of the Bankart repair, found 18 of 33 shoulders to have degenerative changes. Fourteen cases were mild, three moderate, and one severe. They found that the osteoarthritis correlated with ER loss and length of follow-up. Dowdy and O'Driscoll (50) found a high rate of shoulder osteoarthritis after open staple capsulorrhaphy at average follow-up of 15 years. The osteoarthritis correlated with traumatic initial dislocation, length of follow-up, and loss of motion, especially IR. At average follow-up of 8.6 years, Banas et al. (18) found three of 45 shoulders after modified Bristow procedure to have mild-to-moderate osteoarthritis. In contrast, Singer et al. (25), at average follow-up of 20.5 years after the modified Bristow procedure, found that 10 (71%) of 14 demonstrated osteoarthritic changes in the operated-on shoulder. They found that the patients had significantly decreased ER, but believed that this was the result of the osteoarthritis and not its cause, as in the report of Hawkins and Angelo (29), in which the patients had severe restriction in ER.

Treatment

Early

Stiffness may occur after all types of instability repairs, especially those that are nonanatomic. However, the consequence of this motion loss depends on its magnitude and the functional demands of the patient. Now, there are no guidelines to the acceptable degree of motion loss. There does not appear to be any threshold of motion loss beyond which joint deterioration and arthritis are assured. Therefore, the senior author's approach is to consider motion that is less than 80% that of the contralateral extremity to be significant. The aggressiveness of treatment depends on the patient and the degree of pain and disability.

Lesser degrees of motion loss may be a significant disability to a throwing athlete. The prognosis for a throwing athlete to return to a preinjury level of throwing is optimized by performing an anatomic repair (4,8,21,24,26,28, 40).

The exact incidence of motion loss after surgery for recurrent shoulder instability is difficult to determine from the literature because of several methodologic problems. First, many patients may report no symptoms and good satisfaction with the repair, and they may not notice any motion loss. Second, the analysis of postoperative motion may be quite variable from study to study, with qualitative methods and eyeball measurements in some cases, whereas in others, more quantitative and independent review may be used. Careful measurement with a goniometer and control of scapulothoracic motion is not clearly detailed in the methods of most clinical reports. In fact, many studies are retrospective chart reviews; therefore the degree of motion loss is probably underestimated in the literature. In fact, most articles report a small prevalence of motion loss that does not require treatment. Tibone and Ting (53) reported that two of their 20 athletes, after posterior staple capsulorrhaphy for recurrent posterior instability, had significant stiffness requiring further intervention. Ungersbock et al. (11) had one case of frozen shoulder in 42 open modified Bankart procedures. Uribe and Hechtman (42) noted one case of stiffness with eventual resolution not requiring surgical intervention in their 11 cases of arthroscopic stabilization for initial acute anterior dislocations. Walch et al. (43) reported two cases of postoperative stiffness in their 59 cases of arthroscopic transglenoid capsulolabral repair. Goldberg et al. (45) reoperated on one of the 38 arthroscopic transglenoid capsulolabral repairs for shoulder stiffness. The senior author's experience has been that about 2% to 4% of patients with open instability repair develop motion loss that results in less than 80% of the motion of the contralateral extremity.

In a patient with a shoulder that is overly stiff in the initial 3 months after surgery, we use an aggressive stretching program, but one that does not lead to severe pain. If the therapist stretches the shoulder repeatedly beyond the pain tolerance of the patient, reflex muscle guarding may become a progressive problem, and soft-tissue trauma may lead to additional scarring. Nonsteroidal antiinflammatory medications are used with oral narcotic medications. An aquatherapy program may help these patients. This approach was described by Liotard and Walch (48). The warmth and buoyancy of the water help to reduce muscle guarding, and the patient can often more effectively regain motion by active self-assistance exercises in the water.

Although many patients will improve and follow a course similar to that of adhesive capsulitis (54,55), some may have refractory stiffness (56). Although our goal is to achieve full functional motion by 12 weeks after surgery, we will continue with this therapy program if the patient is making slow progress.

If, 6 months after surgery, there is still marked motion loss and pain despite patient compliance with the previously described program, then we will consider operative intervention to regain motion. In all cases, preoperative evaluation must demonstrate that no articular incongruity or bony block is contributing to motion loss. In patients who have had an anatomic procedure such as a Bankart repair or a capsular shift, but who have severe motion loss after therapy, our preference is to perform an arthroscopic capsular release of the contracted capsular tissues. This technique is described in the following text. A closed manipulation is usually not performed, as it is our impression that this can place the subscapularis repair at significant risk in the first 6 months after surgery. Arthroscopic release allows precise section of adhesions and controlled, gentle manipulation.

Arthroscopic Release

This technique is appropriate only for those patients in whom contracture and scarring of the capsule are the primary causes of motion loss. It is contraindicated in those that have known extra-articular contracture, or for those with known shortening of the subscapularis tendon (e.g., Putti–Platt or Bristow procedure). An indwelling interscalene catheter is used for anesthesia as well as complete and long-lasting analgesia and muscle relaxation. We use 30 ml of 0.05% bupivacaine with 1:200,000 epinephrine, which provides approximately 12 hours of analgesia (57,58).

The procedure is performed with the patient in a beach-chair position, as this allows the arm to be freely manipulated and also permits conversion to an open approach if extra-articular adhesions must be treated by nonarthroscopic means (59).

The technique of arthroscopic release was described in detail previously (56,59,60). The technical pitfalls of this procedure are an atraumatic insertion of the arthroscope into a stiff joint and adequate release of adhesions (56,61–65). A spinal needle is first introduced from a posterior position so that it enters the joint over the humeral head. The joint is then insufflated with sterile saline. This distends the joint, and the hydrostatic pressure tends to push the articular surfaces apart. The arthroscope is then carefully inserted into the joint following the course of the spinal needle. A palpable "pop" is usually accompanied by reflux of saline out of the open port of the arthroscopic sheath, thus confirming placement of the arthroscope in the joint. Forceful insertion of the arthroscope is to be avoided, or significant chondral injury can occur. The anterosuperior region of the shoulder is usually seen, and this area is usually obscured by a dense layer of scar tissue and synovitis. A 6-mm cannula is then inserted through an anterosuperior portal so that it enters the joint just underneath the biceps tendon. A motorized shaver and an electrocautery device then release this scar tissue beginning just underneath the biceps tendon (Fig. 7A). The upper border of the subscapularis will be seen as the capsular adhesions are released. As the anterosuperior capsular scar in the rotator-interval region is released, the humeral head will move laterally and inferiorly away from the glenoid, and it will become easier to move the arthroscope into the joint (Fig. 7B and C). The entire upper border of the subscapularis tendon is "skeletonized" by releasing all capsular adhesions from it. The capsule is usually released in its midportion. This may be

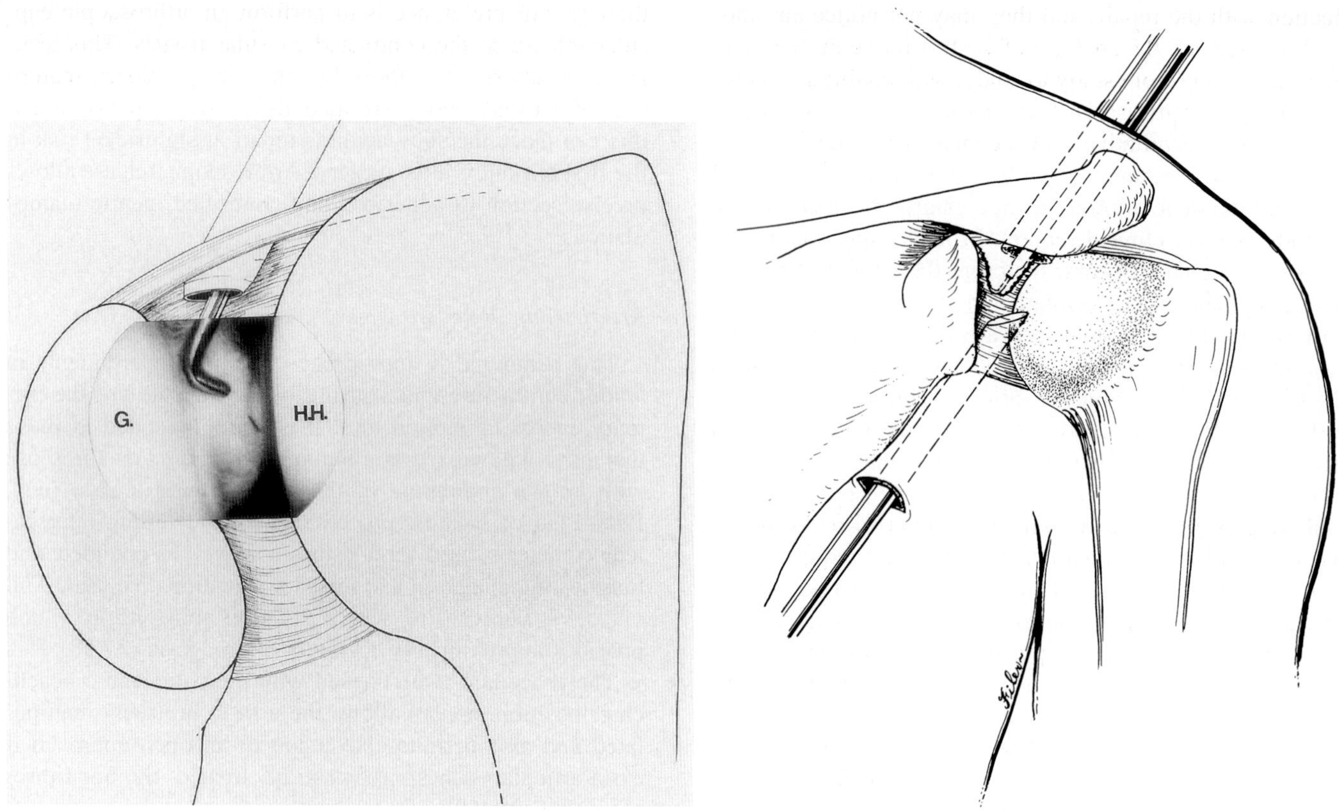

A

B

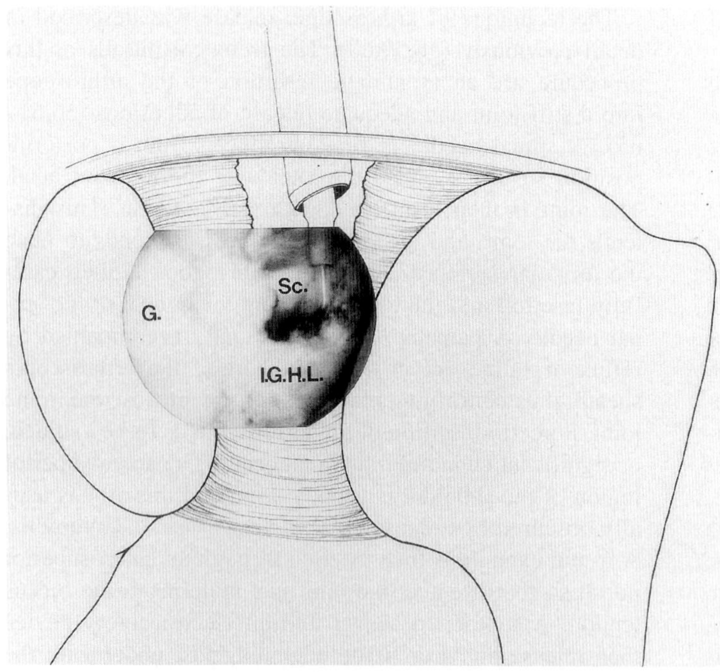

C

FIG. 7. Arthroscopic anterior capsular release. **A:** An arthroscopic probe has been placed through a small cannula and onto the thickened and contracted rotator interval capsule. The glenoid *(G)* and humeral head *(HH)* have been labeled. **B:** Release of the contracted rotator-interval region of the capsule allows the humeral head to move laterally away from the glenoid. **C:** After release of the contracted rotator interval capsule the normal subscapularis tendon *(Sc)* is demonstrated. The scarred and thickened inferior glenohumeral ligament *(IGHL)* is labeled, as is the glenoid *(G)*.

done with either an electrocautery device or a basket forceps (66). It is critical in this portion of the procedure to confirm the location and integrity of the subscapularis tendon. Failure to do this may result in its division. The consequences of subscapularis division are insufficiency of that muscle's function, as well as injury to the more superficial brachial plexus (67,68). Some authors recommended release of the intra-articular portion of the subscapularis tendon (69); however, our feeling is that this technique is neither necessary nor safe.

Once the subscapularis tendon has been defined, the anterior capsule is carefully ''peeled'' off the subscapularis and released down to the inferior glenoid (Fig. 7D and E). The axillary nerve is not at risk above the axillary pouch, as the subscapularis is interposed between it and the electrocautery or basket forceps.

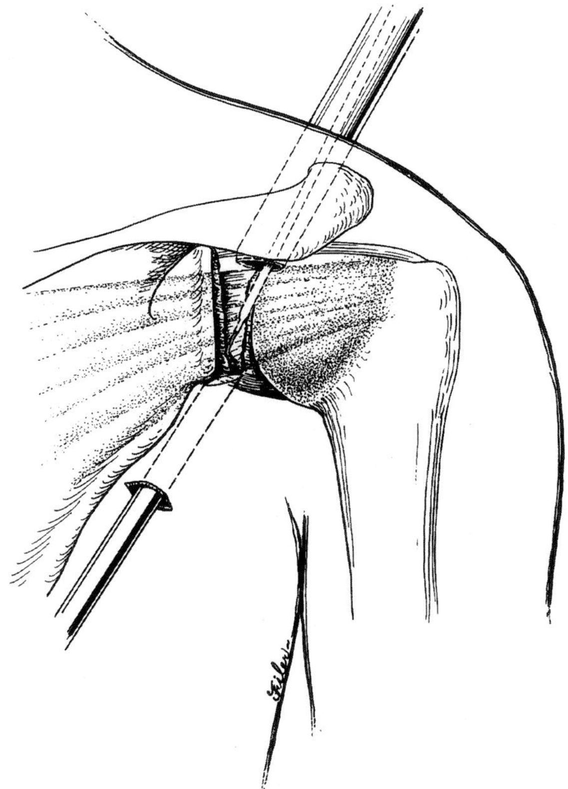

D

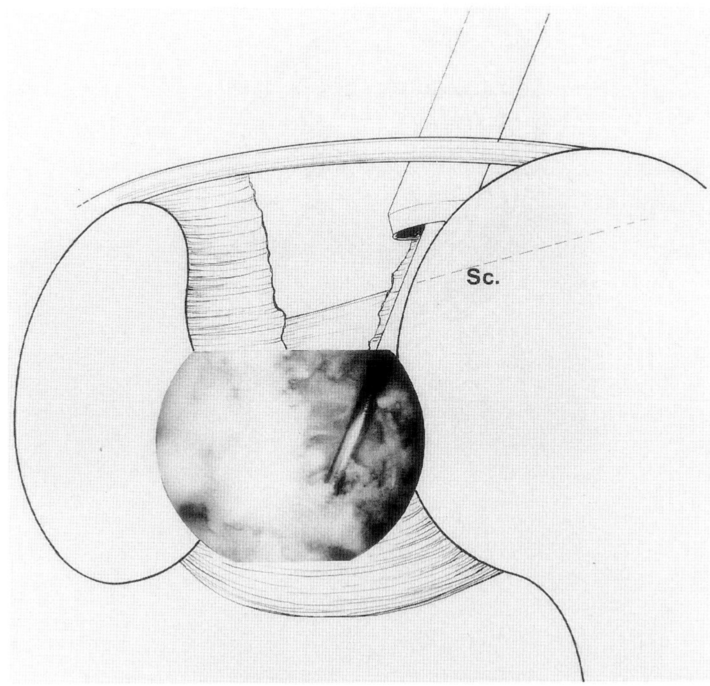

E

FIG. 7. *Continued.* **D:** The anterior capsule can be released down to the inferior glenoid as the subscapularis protects the axillary nerve. **E:** The scarred anterior capsule has been resected off the subscapularis tendon and muscle to the inferior glenoid. (From Warner JJP. Acquired shoulder stiffness. In: Warner JJP, Iannotti JP, Gerber C, eds. *Complex and revisions problems in shoulder surgery.* Philadelphia: Lippincott–Raven, 1997:131–147, with permission.).

Once the entire capsule has been released, the arthroscope is removed, and a gentle manipulation is performed. Usually ER is restored to a degree similar to that of the other side, with little or no force required. Flexion, abduction, and IR are then restored with additional gentle manipulation that causes both audible and palpable yielding of adhesions.

Some patients will continue to have limitation in IR and flexion, despite improvement of ER. In these patients, the arthroscope is reinserted, and a posterior capsular release is performed (64). The arthroscope is placed through the anterosuperior cannula while the arthroscopic sheath in the posterior portal is removed over a switching stick and replaced by an operative cannula (Fig. 8A). An electrocautery device and motorized shaver are used to release the posterior capsule from just posterior to the biceps tendon origin down to the posteroinferior rim of the glenoid. In these cases with severe loss of IR, the posterior capsule is markedly thickened (Fig. 8B and C). After the posterior release is performed, the arthroscopic instruments are removed, and a gentle manipulation is performed once again (Fig. 8D). Flexion and IR are usually restored with gentle manipulation, although this motion gain is not usually accompanied by palpable or audible tissue release.

When the subscapularis tendon cannot be clearly visualized or if the arthroscopic release does not produce acceptable motion, the procedure is converted to an open release through a deltopectoral approach. This technique is described in the following text.

Postoperative Treatment

The patient remains in the hospital for 48 hours, during which time analgesia and partial anesthesia are given through an indwelling interscalene catheter. Alternatively, a repeated interscalene block may be given by using bupivacaine on the morning of the first and second postoperative days. A therapist then performs passive motion exercises in the morning and the afternoon of each day. Continuous passive motion may be used, although the senior author (J.P.W.) has not found that this improves the gains achieved by therapy alone. The patient does not wear a sling and is encouraged to use the arm as much as possible. On the afternoon of the second postoperative day, the

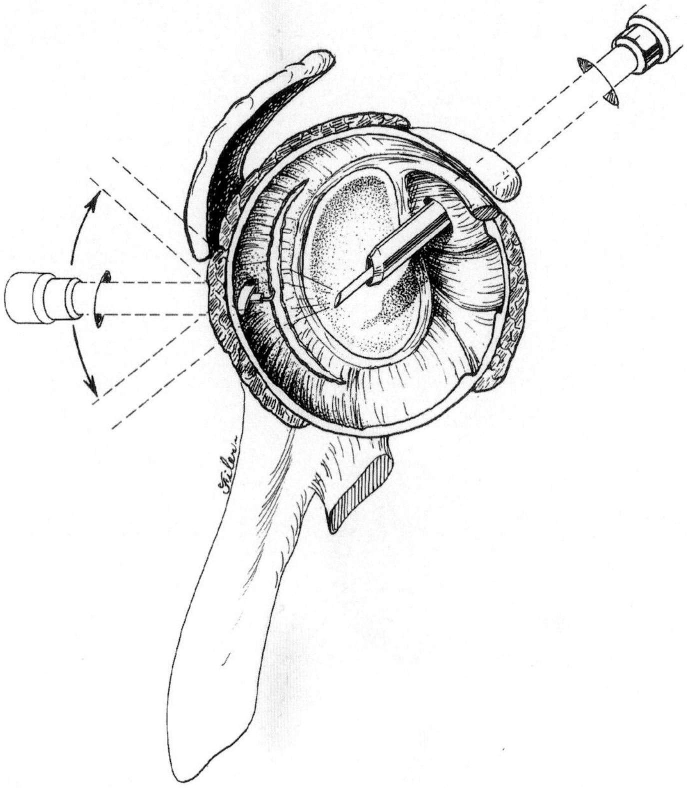

A

FIG. 8. **A:** Posterior capsular release (see text for additional explanation). **B:** View of thickened posterior capsule *(PC)* in a left shoulder. The rotator cuff *(RC)*, glenoid *(G)*, and humeral head *(HH)* have been labeled. (From Warner JJP. Acquired shoulder stiffness. In: Warner JJP, Iannotti JP, Gerber C, eds. *Complex and revisions problems in shoulder surgery.* Philadelphia: Lippincott–Raven, 1997:131–147, with permission.) **C:** Appearance after release of the thickened posterior capsule *(PC)* along the glenoid rim *(G)*. After posterior capsular release, gentle manipulation restores internal rotation. (From Warner JJP, Allen AA, Marks PH, Wong P. Arthroscopic release of postoperative capsular contracture of the shoulder. *J Bone and Joint Surg* 1997; 79:1151–1158, with permission.)

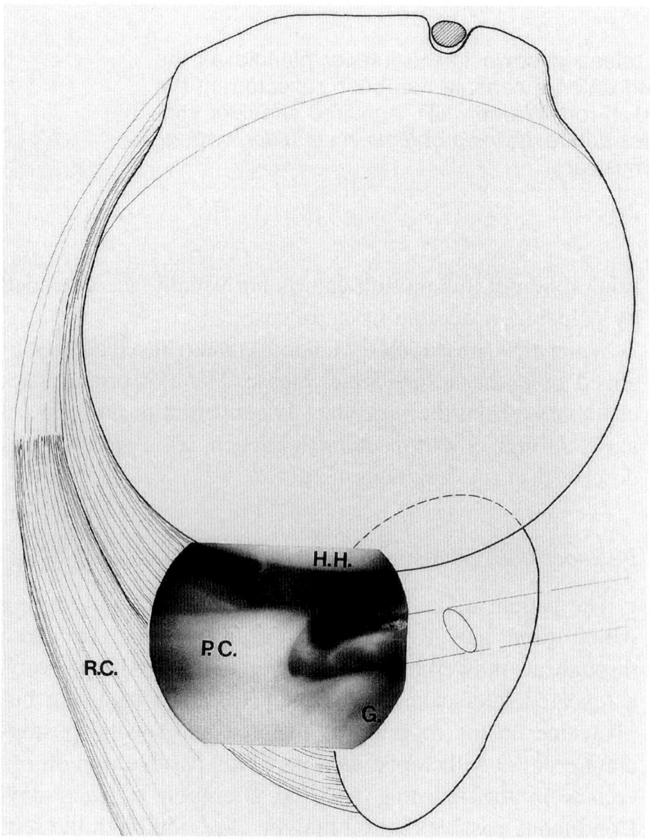

B

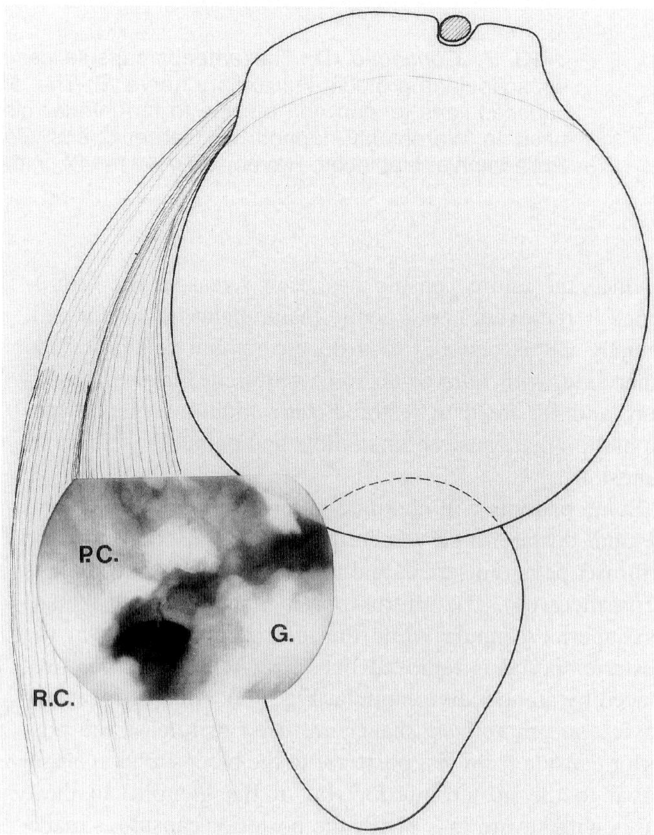

C

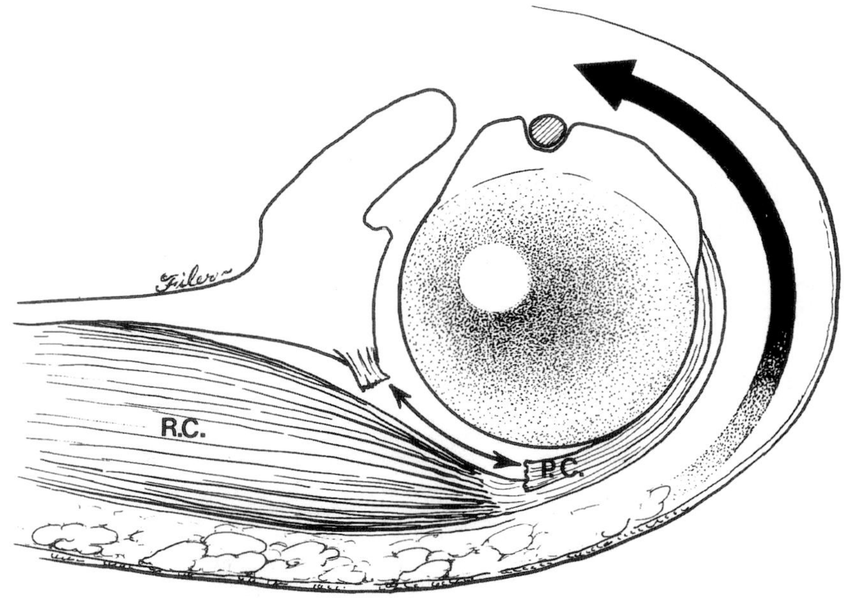

D

FIG. 8. *Continued.* **D:** Following posterior capsular release, gentle manipulation restores internal rotation.

patient is discharged after the second therapy session. Therapy is then performed on an outpatient basis 5 days/week for 2 weeks and then 3 days/week for 2 weeks. The patient is given a home pulley and performs exercises at home as well. Pool therapy is used, if available, as described earlier. After 4 weeks, the patient's progress is assessed, and further therapy is recommended, if necessary.

Author's Experience. The senior author (J.P.W.) performed an arthroscopic release on 12 patients with motion loss after open or arthroscopic instability repair (Fig. 9). This successfully restored motion in nine cases. In the remaining three cases, the procedure was converted to an open approach to release extra-articular adhesions and entrapment of the subscapularis tendon. Injury to the neurovascular structures had not occurred, and only one patient developed recurrent instability after arthroscopic release. This patient had voluntary instability, which recurred after resolution of her shoulder stiffness.

Zanotti and Kuhn (70) performed a cadaveric study of arthroscopic capsular release, and they noted that during the release, they were at least 5 mm away from any neurovascular structures. Harryman et al. (66) successfully performed arthroscopic release starting posteriorly first and then releasing anteriorly, if needed. In patients after instability surgery, the scarring is mainly in the rotator interval and anterior capsule, so we find releasing anteriorly first more effective. Segmuller et al. (71) used two posterior portals at first because of the difficulty in establishing an anterior portal in the face of capsular contracture.

Late (Longer Than 6 Months)

Severe chronic shoulder stiffness, especially if there is asymmetric loss of motion as the result of an instability repair, can result in the premature development of arthritis (25,27,29,50). This can be a devastating situation for an otherwise young and healthy individual. It is, therefore, the surgeon's responsibility to treat this problem aggressively, before this kind of situation develops.

If a patient has shoulder stiffness after an anatomic procedure and has not had a course of physical therapy after this surgery, then we recommend formal therapy and carefully assess the progress. In most cases of chronic motion loss, the patient has never made any gains with therapy after surgery. In these cases, surgical release of the contracted tissues is recommended. The type of prior surgery, the physical examination, and proper radiographic study will determine the most appropriate method for surgical release. For example, a patient with known shortening or entrapment of the subscapularis tendon, as the result of a Bristow or Putti–Platt procedure, will usually require an open release and reconstruction of this muscle–tendon unit. However, a patient who is stiff after a Bankart or capsular-shift procedure, may be a good candidate for arthroscopic release, because the subscapularis is usually uninvolved. The technique of arthroscopic release was described earlier; open release is described in the following text.

Open Release

The prior deltopectoral incision is used. There is usually marked scarring in the deltopectoral interval as well as in the subdeltoid plane. In the former case, the coracoid process is used as the landmark to locate the plane of dissection between the pectoralis major and the deltoid. Release of adhesions between the deltoid and the humerus is facilitated by abducting and flexing the arm to take tension off the deltoid muscle. A retractor is then placed underneath the

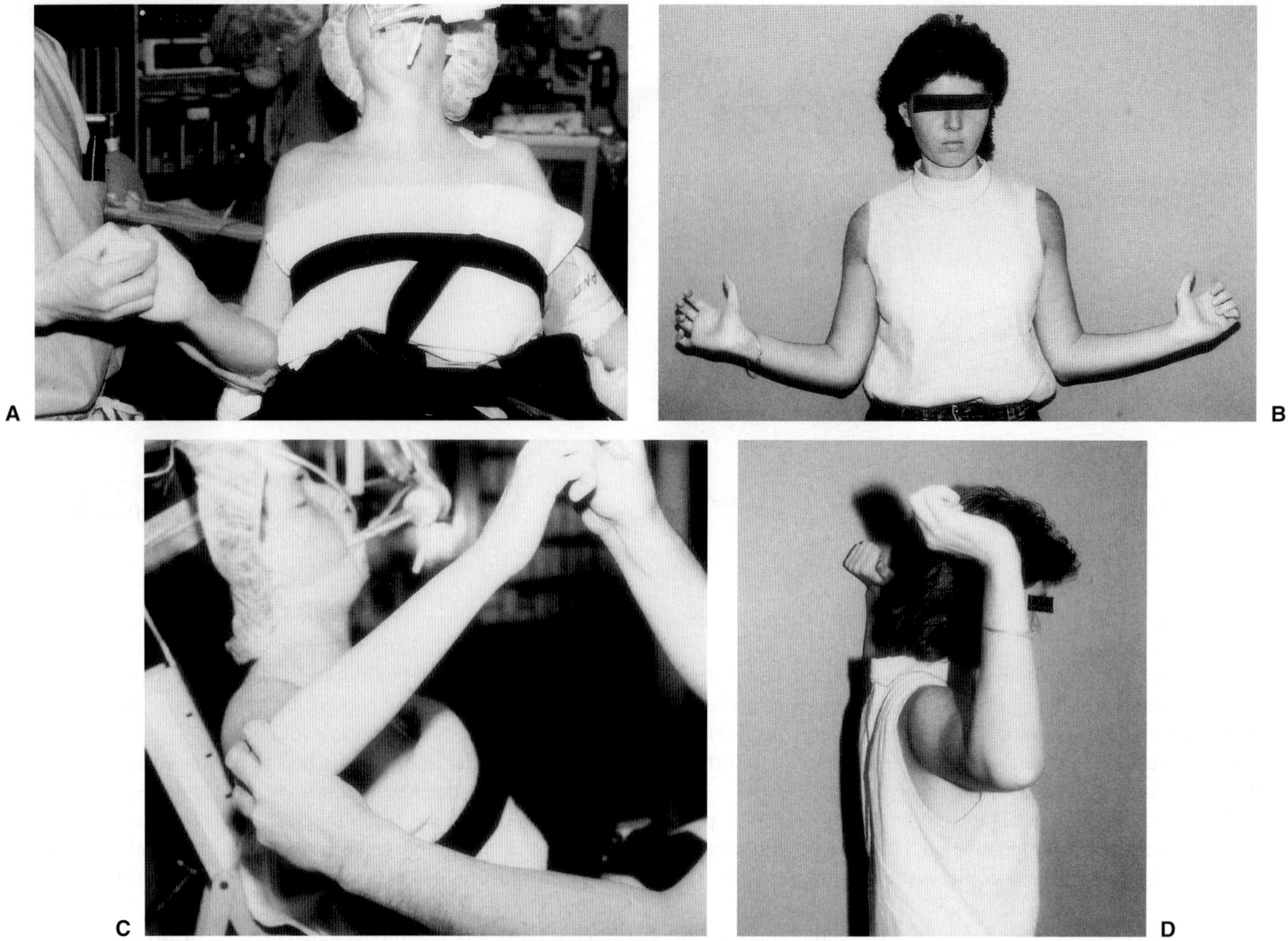

FIG. 9. A 22-year-old woman with loss of motion 1 year after an arthroscopic Bankart repair. Before arthroscopic release, external rotation with the arm in adduction is only 10 degrees **(A)**, and 2 years after release, it is 45 degrees **(B)**. Before arthroscopic release, external rotation of the abducted shoulder is 10 degrees **(C)**, and 2 years after arthroscopic release, it is 90 degrees **(D)**.

deltoid, and it is lifted off the humerus. Adhesions are sharply divided as the humerus is internally rotated (Fig. 10A and B). The entire deltoid should be freed from the humerus, although this must be done with care, as the axillary nerve is at risk where it courses onto the deep surface of the deltoid once it exits the quadrilateral space. The axillary nerve can be palpated and visualized on the deep surface of the deltoid muscle approximately 3 to 5 cm below the lateral border of the acromion.

After the subdeltoid interval is completely freed and the humerus is seen to glide freely underneath the deltoid, the dissection proceeds medially, and the coracoacromial ligament is excised. The subacromial space may be restricted by a dense scar between the rotator cuff and the acromion. This scar is released by gently retracting the deltoid with the arm in abduction and then sharply dividing the scar off the undersurface of the acromion. Care must be taken with handling the deltoid, as overzealous retraction can injure the muscle at its origin or insertion.

The conjoined tendon and its muscles are separated from the underlying subscapularis and are retracted medially. This may need to be done by a combination of sharp and blunt dissection. The location of the musculocutaneous nerve should be borne in mind. Even in an individual with extensive scarring between the subscapularis and the conjoined tendon, there is usually some fat surrounding the nerve. The surgeon should look for this fat when dissecting on the undersurface of the conjoined tendon. If the patient has had a previous Bristow procedure, then we expose the musculocutaneous nerve throughout its length.

The remainder of the deeper dissection depends on the degree of distortion of anatomy by the prior operative procedure. In cases in which the subscapularis has not been shortened by a prior surgery (i.e., Bankart or capsular shift),

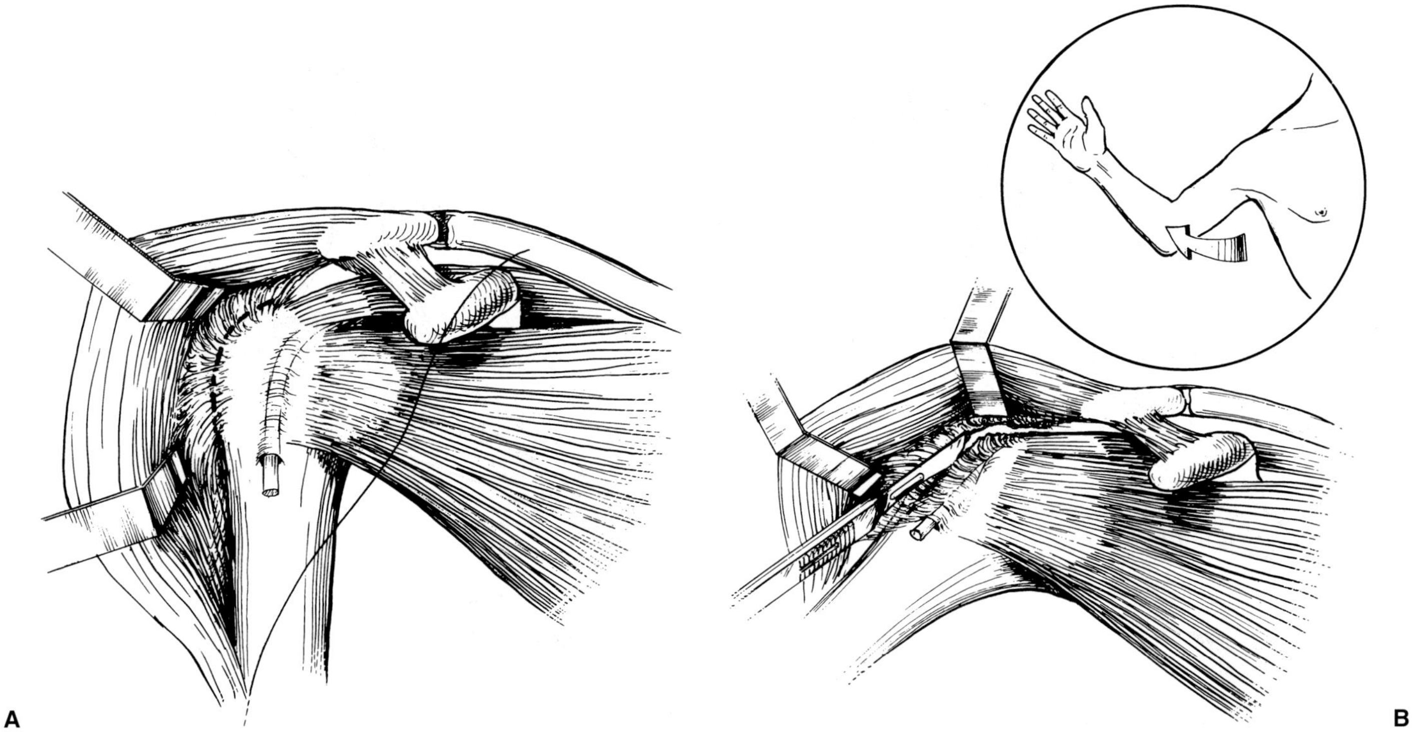

FIG. 10. A: Subdeltoid and subacromial adhesions limit humeral rotation. **B:** Abduction and external rotation allow relaxation of the deltoid and make sharp division of subdeltoid and subacromial adhesions easier. (From Warner JJP. Acquired shoulder stiffness. In: Warner JJP, Iannotti JP, Gerber C, eds. *Complex and revisions problems in shoulder surgery.* Philadelphia: Lippincott–Raven, 1997:131–147, with permission.)

the interval between it and the underlying capsule is developed. In some of these patients who have marked limitation of ER with the arm at the side, release of the rotator interval will markedly improve this motion. This may often be due to closure of this capsular region with the arm in IR and adduction. The rotator interval can be identified as the region from the coracoid process to the top of the lesser tuberosity. There may be dense scarring and sutures here from the prior surgery. If possible, the superior border of the subscapularis tendon is identified, and the rotator interval is released from the coracoid process to the humerus (72,73). With each step, as the dissection releases adhesions between tissue layers, the shoulder is gently manipulated to regain motion. Remaining limitation of ER is caused by shortening of the subscapularis tendon or its adhesion to the underlying capsule or both (74). In some cases, it may be possible to improve ER without releasing the subscapularis from its insertion on the humerus. This is done by splitting it in its midportion in line with its fibers and then by using an elevator to develop the interval between it and the underlying capsule. This may allow it to have mobility, so that the arm can be externally rotated. In most such cases, however, a coronal Z-plasty lengthening of the subscapularis and capsule is performed. This is done by dividing the scarred capsule and subscapularis tendon in the coronal plane so that the superficial half of the tendon remains attached to the muscle, while the remaining deep half is divided at the glenoid and remains attached to the lesser tuberosity (Fig. 11A and B). A helpful technique is to judge the thickness of the tissue by visualizing and palpating through the rotator interval. This will allow the surgeon to release the tissue with robust tissue flaps rather than creating a tissue flap that is too thin. The next step is to mobilize the subscapularis muscle from adhesions. The axillary nerve is first identified and a vessel loupe placed around it. The subscapularis muscle is then globally mobilized by releasing any remaining adhesions superiorly, inferiorly, and on its deep surface (Fig. 11C and D). These steps will usually allow an increase of 30 to 60 degrees of ER.

If abduction and IR are still limited, the inferior and posterior capsule can be released through the joint; thus a global capsulotomy is performed. To do this, a humeral head retractor is placed to displace the humeral head posteriorly, and a blunt retractor is inserted underneath the inferior capsule to protect the axillary nerve. The capsule is then released from an inferior to a posterosuperior direction under direct vision (Fig. 11E). The retractors are removed, and the shoulder is placed through a ROM to determine motion gains. The humeral head is relocated, and the arm is positioned in the maximum ER that can allow secure closure of the Z-plasty of the anterior capsule and subsca-

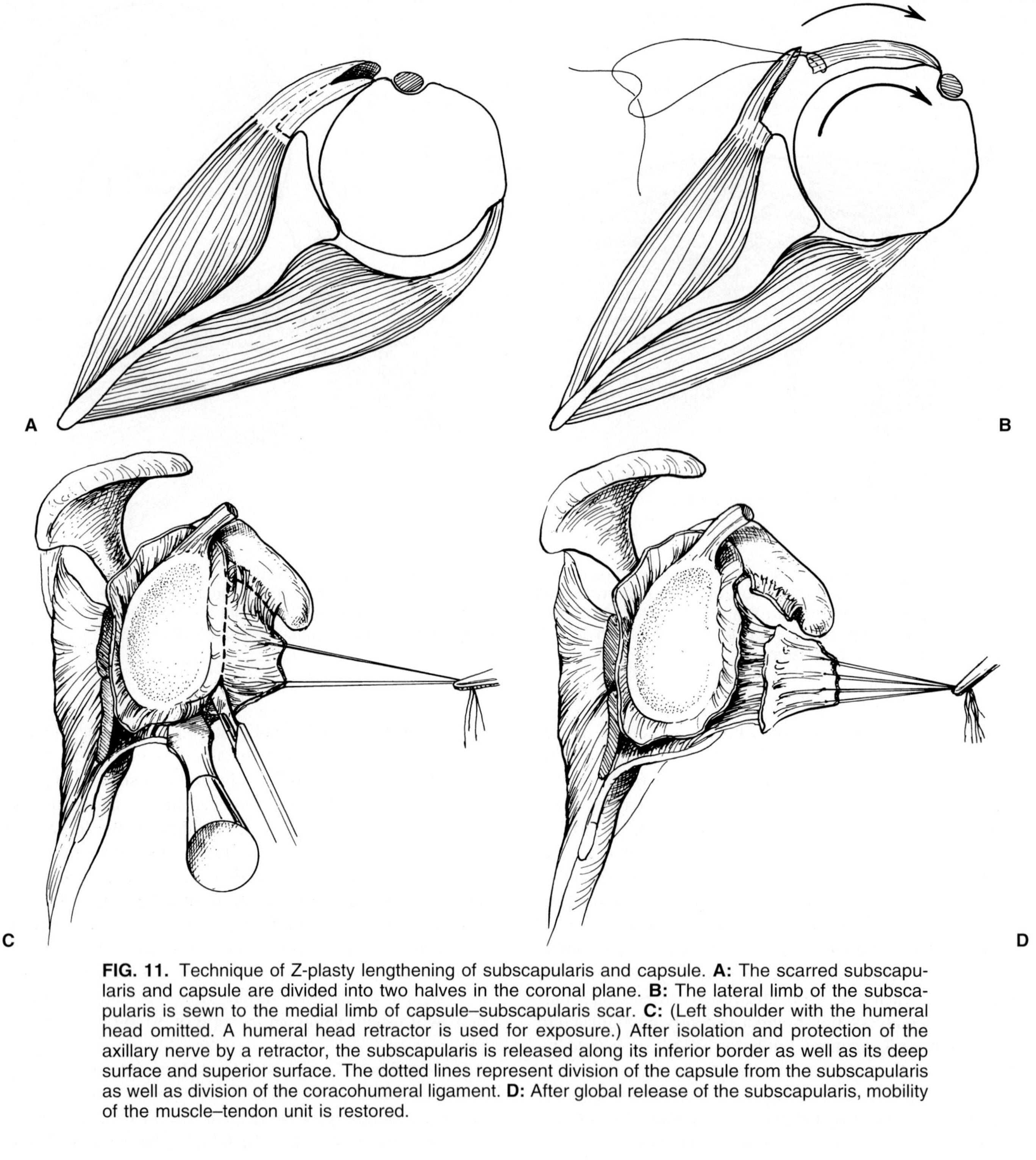

FIG. 11. Technique of Z-plasty lengthening of subscapularis and capsule. **A:** The scarred subscapularis and capsule are divided into two halves in the coronal plane. **B:** The lateral limb of the subscapularis is sewn to the medial limb of capsule–subscapularis scar. **C:** (Left shoulder with the humeral head omitted. A humeral head retractor is used for exposure.) After isolation and protection of the axillary nerve by a retractor, the subscapularis is released along its inferior border as well as its deep surface and superior surface. The dotted lines represent division of the capsule from the subscapularis as well as division of the coracohumeral ligament. **D:** After global release of the subscapularis, mobility of the muscle–tendon unit is restored.

pularis tendon by using no. 2 nonabsorbable, braided suture.

Passive ROM is assessed to determine where there is tension on the soft-tissue repair, and this defines a ''safe zone'' for early passive ROM. This information is communicated to the therapist who assists the patient in the immediate postoperative period.

In cases in which the subscapularis has been distorted or shortened (i.e., Bristow, Putti–Platt, Magnuson–Stack procedures), additional dissection is necessary to mobilize and reconstruct the tissue. Young and Rockwood (30) described the steps in dissection of the subscapularis after a Bristow procedure. Our preference is to define the conjoined tendon, locate the musculocutaneous and axillary nerve, and then

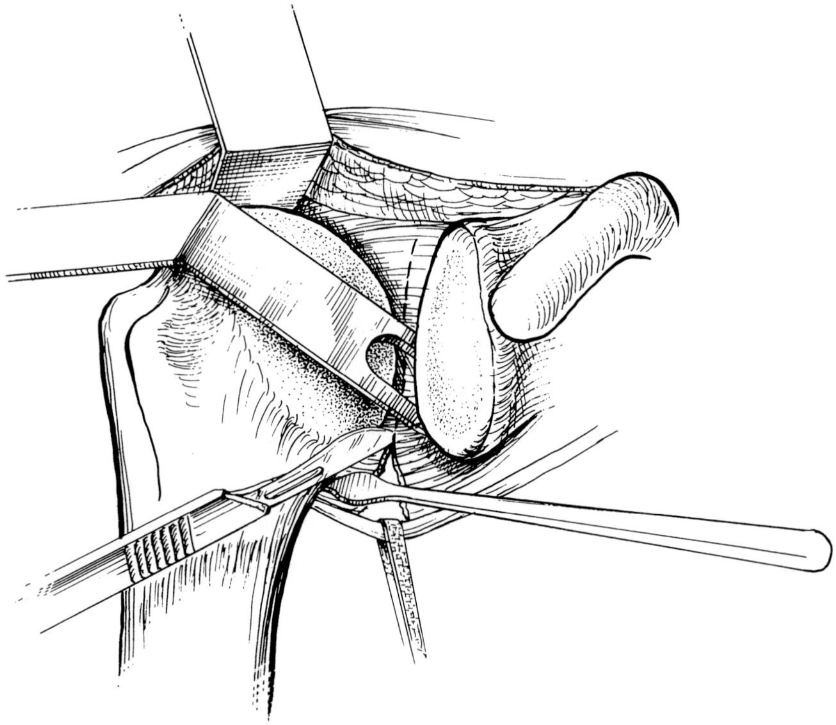

E

FIG. 11. *Continued.* **E:** The posterior capsule can be released if necessary to restore internal rotation. The axillary nerve *(AN)* is isolated with a vessel loop and a retractor. A humeral head retractor displaces the humeral head to allow access to the posterior capsule. (From Warner JJP. Acquired shoulder stiffness. In: Warner JJP, Iannotti JP, Gerber C, eds. *Complex and revisions problems in shoulder surgery.* Philadelphia: Lippincott–Raven, 1997:131–147, with permission.)

dissect the conjoined tendon from the subscapularis. The conjoined tendon is removed with or without its transferred bone, and then the subscapularis tendon is mobilized as described earlier.

In a Putti–Platt procedure, a coronal plane Z-plasty lengthening is usually required, as previously described.

When revising a stiff shoulder after a Magnuson–Stack procedure, the subscapularis is identified and dissected to its transferred location lateral to the bicipital groove. Care should be taken to assess the biceps tendon, as we frequently noted that these patients may have injury to this tendon from the staple commonly used to fix the subscapularis tendon. The tendon of the subscapularis may be quite thin as well. Once the subscapularis tendon has been defined and separated from the capsule, the shoulder should be assessed to determine the laxity of the capsule. Some of these individuals may have had MDI and may require a capsular shift in addition to a subscapularis reconstruction. The subscapularis tendon is then repaired to its anatomic location.

Postoperative Treatment

As with the arthroscopic-release technique, regional interscalene blocks or an indwelling interscalene catheter are used for the first 48 hours after surgery, and the patient undergoes two daily sessions of therapy while remaining in the hospital during this time. The aggressiveness of postoperative treatment depends on the degree of soft-tissue repair and reconstruction necessary. For the first 6 weeks after surgery, the patient undergoes passive motion by a therapist who moves the shoulder within the "safe zone" of the soft-tissue repair. After this, active–assisted motion is begun, and a pulley is used by the patient as well.

As soon as the sutures are removed, a pool-therapy program is commenced, as described previously.

After arthroscopic or open release, the strengthening phase of the postoperative therapy program is usually delayed until a nearly full, pain-free arc of motion has been achieved. This usually takes at least 3 months.

Author's Experience. Over a 3-year period, the senior author (J.P.W.) performed an open release in 15 cases after anterior instability repair. In all cases, motion was improved, although severe tissue distortion and shortening tended to limit these gains (Fig. 12).

NERVE INJURY

Nerve injuries associated with shoulder instability can occur either with the initial dislocation or in iatrogenic injuries resulting from surgical treatment. Nerve injuries associated with shoulder instability can affect any portion of the brachial plexus (75,76) but most commonly involve the axillary, musculocutaneous, or suprascapular nerves (75–77).

After acute initial anterior shoulder dislocation, nerve injuries are reported to occur in between 1 in 3 and 1 in 20 cases (75,77–80). The most common injury is to the axillary nerve (75,77–80). The axillary nerve is predisposed to injury during anterior dislocation because it is tethered in the quadrilateral space (81), so that during an anterior dislocation, it is stretched around the humerus. The incidence

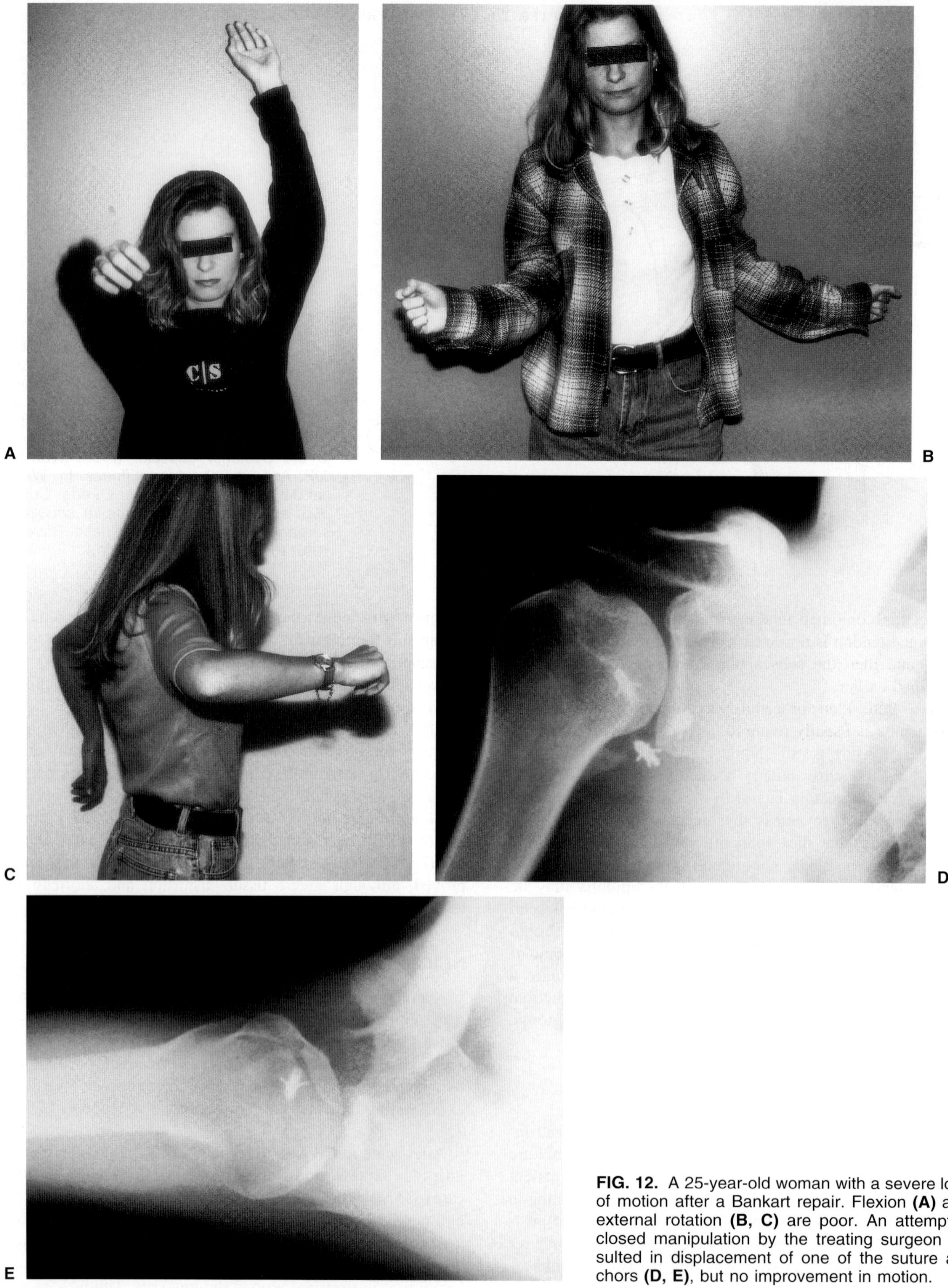

FIG. 12. A 25-year-old woman with a severe loss of motion after a Bankart repair. Flexion **(A)** and external rotation **(B, C)** are poor. An attempted closed manipulation by the treating surgeon resulted in displacement of one of the suture anchors **(D, E)**, but no improvement in motion.

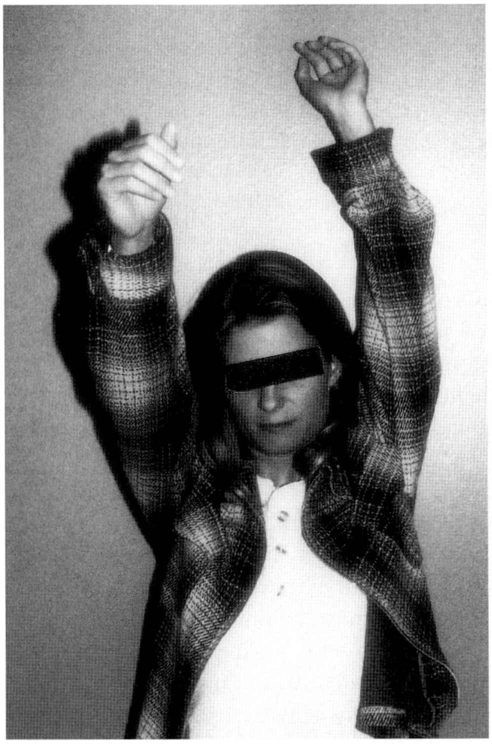

F

FIG. 12. *Continued.* After an open release and Z-plasty lengthening, motion is improved but still limited **(F–H)** because of severe shortening and scarring of tissue.

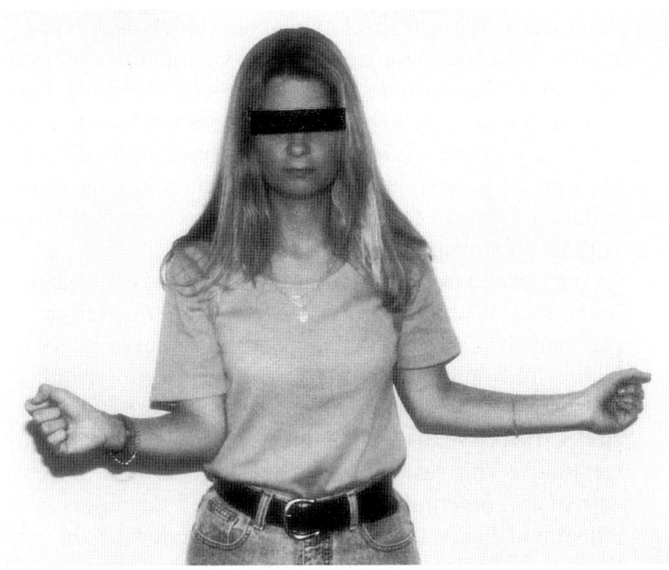

G

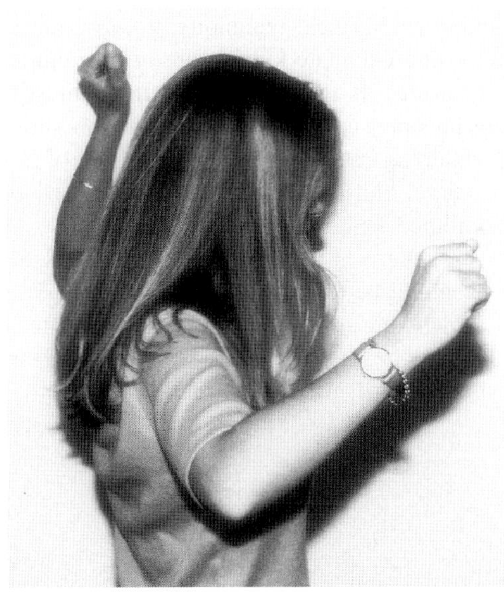

H

of axillary nerve injury increases with age of the patient, the duration of the dislocation, and the amount of trauma that caused the dislocation (75,79).

Iatrogenic nerve injury is dependent on surgical technique, as certain procedures place different nerves at risk. With a Bristow procedure, the musculocutaneous nerve is at greatest risk for injury (18,30,82,83). Young and Rockwood (30) reported one musculocutaneous nerve and one axillary nerve injury (both permanent) in their review of 40 failed cases of the Bristow procedure. Banas et al. (18) reported two transient musculocutaneous nerve palsies in reviewing 86 Bristow procedures. Flatow et al. (84), in an anatomic study of the musculocutaneous nerve, showed that its course is quite variable and can come within 2.5 cm of the coracoid process. Richards et al. (85) recommended that the musculocutaneous nerve be explored in each case of the Bristow procedure. They further cautioned that if the nerve enters the conjoined tendon close to the coracoid process (i.e., within 2.5 cm) that the nerve be freed to the level of the lateral cord, or the procedure abandoned. After the modified Bankart procedure, Ungersbock et al. (11) reported one case of musculocutaneous nerve neuropraxia.

The axillary nerve is predisposed to injury during dissection around the inferior capsule. Morrey and Janes (3) reported on long-term follow-up of the Putti–Platt and Bankart procedures and found that there was axillary neuropathy in four and deltoid atrophy in seven. Altchek and Warren (86) reported one neuropraxia of each of the musculocutaneous and median nerves after a modified inferior capsular shift. Neer and Foster (6) had three cases of neuropraxia of the axillary nerve after inferior capsular shift.

During arthroscopic transglenoid capsulolabral repair, the suprascapular nerve is predisposed to injury when bringing the Beath pin out through the back of the shoulder. Injury to this nerve can occur from either direct compression from the pin or from tying the sutures down on the deltoid fascia in the back of the shoulder. Suprascapular palsy occurred in three of 49 cases of arthroscopic transglenoid labral reconstruction performed by Mologne et al. (87). Two temporary suprascapular nerve palsies were reported by Yoneda et al. (44), and one permanent injury to the suprascapular branch of the infraspinatus in 38 cases reported by Goldberg et al. (45). To eliminate the complication of suprascapular nerve palsy after arthroscopic transglenoid capsulolabral repair, it has been recommended that the Beath pin be directed inferiorly to the equator of the glenoid (87). Finally, Lane et al. (39) reported three cases of neuropraxia after arthroscopic staple capsulorrhaphy, but did not state which nerve(s) was/were involved.

The key to avoiding nerve injuries during surgery on the shoulder is meticulous surgical technique, good retraction and visualization, and adequate knowledge of the regional neurovascular anatomy. If the conjoined tendon must be retracted during an open approach, such retraction should be gentle. Self-retaining retractors increase the risk of neuropraxia to the nerve, and these should never be used underneath the conjoined tendon.

If a Bristow procedure is performed, then the musculocutaneous nerve should be identified and protected (85). In procedures in which the subscapularis tendon or inferior capsule is involved, the axillary nerve should be clearly palpated and visualized, if necessary.

Evaluation

A comprehensive examination of the brachial plexus is performed. The attitude in which the extremity is held indicates whether the scapular suspensory muscles (serratus anterior, trapezius, rhomboids, levator scapulae) are properly functioning. The entire upper extremities are examined for sensation, motor strength, and reflexes. In a musculocutaneous nerve palsy, there is decreased sensation along the distribution of the lateral cutaneous nerve of the forearm, and there may be weakness of elbow flexion strength. With suprascapular nerve palsy, there is paralysis of the supraspinatus and infraspinatus muscles, with subsequent weakness of ER. In chronic cases, there will be wasting of these muscles in the supraspinatus and infraspinatus fossae, respectively. Usually the infraspinatus wasting is easier to appreciate because the bulky trapezius muscle overlies the supraspinatus. Axillary nerve palsy is detected clinically by anesthesia over the lateral shoulder or inability to initiate a deltoid contraction (Fig. 13; 88). Wasting of the deltoid in chronic cases will produce the classic squaring of the shoulder with loss of the normal deltoid contour.

Classification of Nerve Injury

Seddon's classification of nerve injuries into three clinical degrees of severity (89) is the most useful of the classification systems (90). This classification is based on the pathologic change to the nerve and thus gives insight into the prognosis and helps us to direct an individualized treatment plan.

The first degree of injury is a conduction block called a neuropraxia. This is the most benign type of nerve injury. This typically results from a mild blunt contusion, compression, or traction injury, in which there is no loss of nerve continuity. The most common cause is traction or compression from a retractor during open instability surgery. It is clinically manifested as a motor loss that may be quite profound, yet usually is also accompanied by a partial sensory deficit and little or no disturbance in sympathetic function. There is a focal conduction block with no axonal injury. Electromyographic (EMG) examination may or may not fail to demonstrate any spontaneous electrical activity at rest, so there will be no fibrillations or positive sharp waves seen if the patient is still paralyzed at 3 weeks from the time of injury. These injuries traditionally have an excellent prognosis for complete recovery within 12 weeks without treatment.

The second degree of injury to the nerve is called axonotmesis. With this injury, a more severe traction or crush mechanism is the cause. Damage to the nerve is confined to loss of continuity of the axon and myelin sheath. The supporting stroma of the nerve, including the endoneurium and perineurium, as well as the Schwann cell basal lamina, are intact. This lesion results in complete loss of sensory and motor function below the level of the injury and is indistinguishable from complete transection of the nerve. Wallerian degeneration takes place with this injury. The appropriate electrical changes of denervation are found 3 weeks after this injury. These lesions usually spontaneously recover because the supporting stroma of the nerve is intact (75). Return of neurologic function occurs at a rate of 1 mm/day after an initial 30-day delay. Functional recovery usually follows neurologic recovery (75).

In the third degree of injury, there has been complete loss of all structural elements of the nerve, called neurotmesis. This is analogous to complete transection of the nerve. It requires surgical intervention to reestablish the continuity of the peripheral nerve with the fascicular alignment sufficiently correct to allow regeneration and functional recovery. The EMG findings at 3 weeks will be identical to those changes seen in axonotmesis. These include

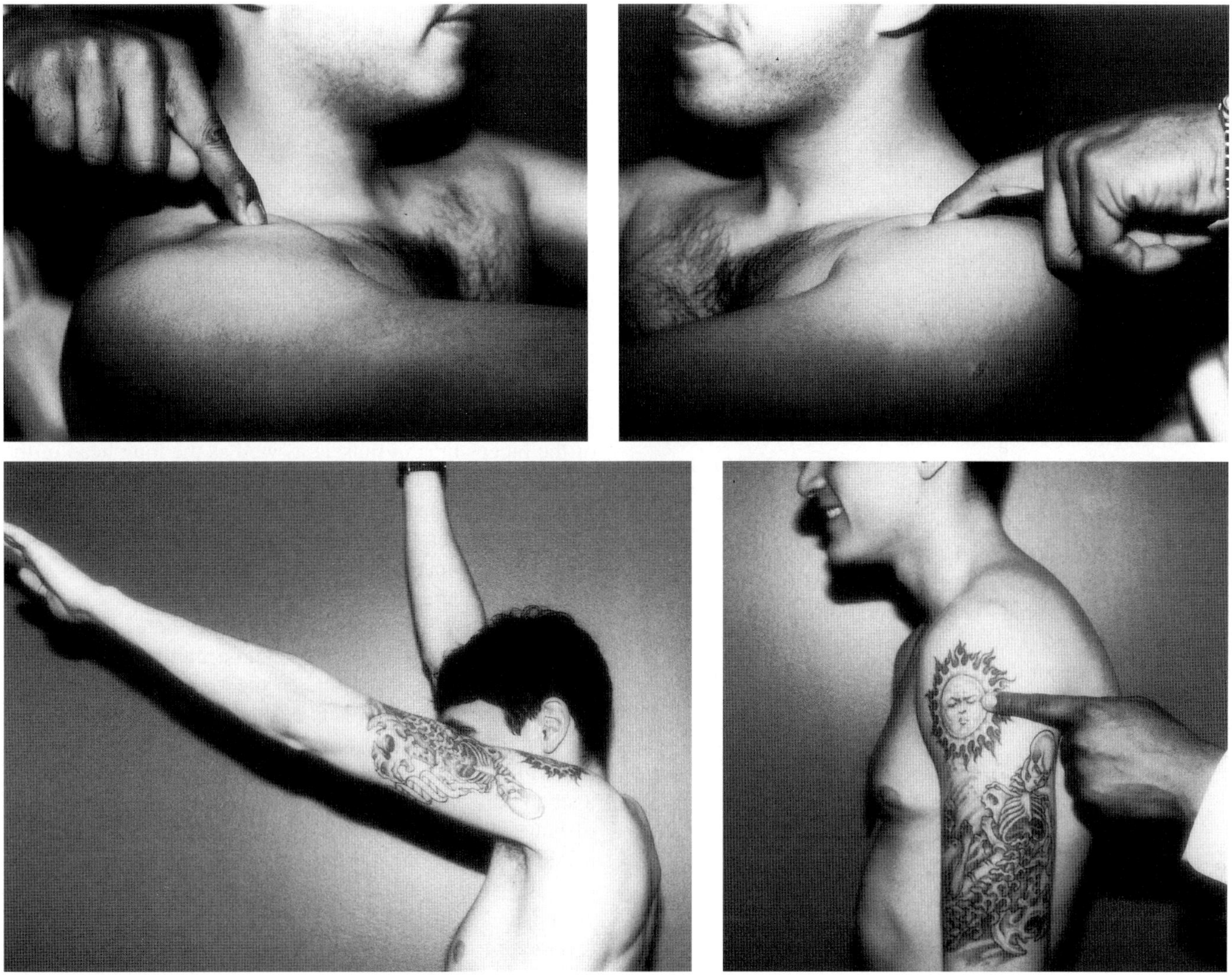

FIG. 13. Two patients with an axillary nerve palsy in anterior shoulder dislocation. Note loss of anterior deltoid muscle contour in this chronic case (**A:** normal; **B:** side with axillary nerve palsy). Acute case with limited flexion **(C)** and anesthesia over deltoid **(D)**.

fibrillation potentials at rest and no action potentials seen on attempted voluntary contractions. The prognosis for neurotmesis is guarded, at best. The mechanism of injury will often help to differentiate between the two lesions.

Role of Electromyography

Appropriately timed electrodiagnostic testing is important for defining the extent of nerve injury. Electrodiagnostic testing may further reveal the extension of the pathologic process beyond the confines of a single peripheral nerve, or it may indicate that the observed neuropathy is part of a generalized peripheral neuropathy. An EMG can be important in evaluating which muscles are involved and the extent of involvement. The use of nerve-conduction velocities can help to localize a specific lesion along the length of the motor unit and peripheral nerve. An EMG can give objective evidence of nerve injury. This is particularly important in the clinical situation in which it has been shown that sensory loss, such as in the axillary patch for axillary nerve injuries, is unreliable in the diagnosis of axillary nerve injury (75).

Although rarely practical, an EMG performed 1 day after nerve injury will demonstrate whether the nerve is in continuity; however, it will not differentiate between neuropraxia and axonotmesis. Thus, unless there is suspicion that a nerve may be transected, EMGs are not performed until Wallerian degeneration has taken place (at least 3 weeks after the injury). At this time, the absence of spontaneous electrical activity at rest, such that there is no fibrillation potentials or positive sharp waves, indicates a neuropraxia. A finding of fibrillation potentials at rest and no action potentials on attempted voluntary contraction indicates axonotmesis or neurotmesis.

Management

Axillary Nerve Injury

Early

Axillary nerve palsy associated with a traumatic anterior dislocation of the shoulder is usually a traction injury, and this is either a neuropraxia or axonotmesis (75,77). It is important to diagnose correctly this condition and not to confuse it with a rotator-cuff tear. The latter condition is not uncommon in patients older than 40 years who have an anterior shoulder dislocation (91–93). In an axillary nerve injury, there is typically abduction weakness but no weakness of ER, whereas in a rotator-cuff tear, there is usually ER weakness as well. In those cases in which the patient is weak, magnetic resonance imaging (MRI) may be useful to rule out a full-thickness rotator-cuff tear (94,95). In a patient with an axillary nerve palsy after an anterior dislocation, we immobilize the shoulder briefly and then begin active–assisted motion exercises. The first electrodiagnostic evaluation is performed at the 3-week mark from injury to document whether Wallerian degeneration is taking place, differentiating neuropraxia from axonotmesis and neurotmesis. Of 15 cases of dislocation of the shoulder associated with axillary nerve palsy, Watson-Jones (96,97) noted that 10 recovered spontaneously within 6 months, three recovered between 6 and 12 months from the time of injury, and two had permanent deltoid paralysis (96,97).

An axillary nerve palsy noted after instability surgery is treated more aggressively. Because there may be a concern about transection of the nerve, an EMG performed in the first 24 hours after surgery will document whether the nerve remains in continuity. In practice, such a study is usually not practical, and thus if there is a high degree of suspicion for direct injury to the nerve, an immediate re-exploration should be performed by a surgeon proficient in management of these kinds of injuries.

The axillary nerve is explored through the same incision that was used to perform the instability surgery. If the nerve has a suture around it or is transected, any strangulating material is removed, and nerve repair or grafting is performed according to the guidelines for treatment of peripheral nerve injuries (98–100). If the emergency EMG shows no conduction block or if the surgeon is confident that the nerve has not been cut or entrapped in a suture, then management is expectant. Another EMG is repeated at the 3-week mark from nerve injury to evaluate whether the nerve injury is neuropraxia or axonotmesis.

Late

Patients with chronic axillary nerve dysfunction are functionally disabled because of deltoid weakness. They have difficulty flexing and abducting their affected shoulder. Spontaneous recovery of axillary nerve function has been documented up to 7 months after injury (101); therefore optimistic expectant management may be continued over that period. After this period, recovery is unlikely. Occasionally, a patient may be able to compensate for the deltoid weakness by rotator-cuff substitution and trunk rotation (102).

Several surgical options are available to treat this injury. Some surgeons recommended transferring part of the deltoid to compensate for partial loss of the deltoid, but in nerve injury, this is not possible. Petrucci et al. (103,104) reported good results with nerve grafting and neurolysis, with the best results obtained if performed within 6 months of injury. This procedure, however, has not become popular in the United States. Several tendon transfers have also been described. These include transfer of the long head of the triceps to the acromion (105), transfer of the short head of the biceps brachii muscle as well as the long head of the triceps to the central part of the acromion (106–108), pectoralis major transfer (109), and free pectoralis major transfer (110). Several surgeons recommended transfer of the trapezius for paralysis of the deltoid (111–114). Even though these surgeons were only able to attach the trapezius to the capsule covering the humerus, they noted fair to good results. Mayer (115–117) described a transfer of the insertion of the trapezius muscle to the acromion and clavicle to near the deltoid tuberosity of the humerus by lengthening the tendon with a strip of fascia lata. Bateman's modification (118) of this trapezius muscle transfer was to remove a small part of the spine of the scapula and to fix the piece of bone with screws to the proximal humerus; Saha (119) added mobilization of the superior and middle part of the trapezius muscle lateral of its origin. These modifications established a greater length of muscle and increased the leverage of the transfer on the humerus with solid fixation. However, trapezius transfer provides a lever arm shorter than that of the normal deltoid (120). The trapezius transfer cannot be performed if the rotator cuff is not functional because the acromion can no longer buttress against superior migration of the humeral head with contraction. Itoh et al. (120) developed a free latissimus muscle transfer for paralysis of the deltoid, noting that the lever arm is as long as that of the deltoid, the muscle volume and width of the latissimus transfer is sufficient to cover and stabilize the humeral head, the strength of the transferred muscle is sufficient for normal activities of daily living, and it adequately restores the normal deltoid contour (as compared with the trapezius transfer).

Musculocutaneous Nerve Injury

Early

If a patient in the immediate postoperative period has a musculocutaneous nerve palsy after an open Bankart or capsular-shift procedure, demonstrated by decreased elbow flexion and anesthesia in the distribution of the lateral cutaneous nerve of the forearm, this is usually a neuropraxia from compression or traction by a retractor underneath the conjoined tendon. In these cases, this will usually recover over several weeks. If, however, musculocutaneous nerve function is absent after a Bristow procedure, then there may be a greater index of suspicion for axonotmesis or neurotmesis affecting the nerve. In these cases, immediate exploration or an EMG in the first 24 hours may determine whether the nerve is in continuity. If the surgeon is confident that the nerve is not entrapped in a suture and is not cut, or if the initial EMG is normal, then another EMG is performed at 3 weeks to differentiate neuropraxia from axonotmesis.

Late

The prognosis for recovery from a musculocutaneous nerve injury is good in most cases. Leffert (121) noted excellent recovery in four of five patients with musculocutaneous nerve or lateral cord injury. The one patient who did not recover significantly still had powerful elbow flexion because of an intact brachioradialis. Richards et al. (85) also noted this. If neurologic recovery was not evident by 3 months, Richards et al. (85) performed neurolysis or nerve grafting with good motor recovery but inconsistent sensory recovery.

INFECTION

Septic arthritis after instability surgery is produced by bacterial seeding at the time of surgery, by secondary spread of a superficial infection, or by hematogenous inoculation. Bacterial adherence is characterized by the production of an extracellular polysaccharide glycocalyx, known as "slime." This glycocalyx allows the bacteria to modify their local environment. It is inhibitory of certain aspects of the immune system and inflammatory response, including T-cell and B-cell function, chemotaxis, opsonization, and phagocytosis (46,122).

Infection after instability surgery is relatively rare. The shoulder has a well-developed soft-tissue envelope, and it is well vascularized. This contributes to the low infection rates. The increasing use of metallic foreign objects, such as suture anchors, does not seem to increase the infection rates, although it is a concern. There were four infections (two deep) in the long-term follow-up of the Putti–Platt and Bankart procedure by Morrey and Janes (3). Torg et al. (24) noted one deep infection caused by *Staphylococcus aureus* after 212 Bristow procedures. Bigliani et al. (28) noted two superficial wound infections after 68 inferior capsular shifts. There were no deep infections. Most other reports noted no infections (8,10,11,18,35,123). In immunocompetent hosts, the most common infecting organisms are staphylococcal species (124–127).

The major problem with infection, in addition to injury to the articular cartilage of the shoulder joint, is the development of adhesions between tissue planes as well as destruction of normal capsular and tendon tissue. Those patients who recover from such an infection often have residual stiffness, and tissue quality may be poor.

Prevention of Infection

Meticulous skin preparation, draping, and atraumatic tissue handling is critically important in the prevention of infection. Prophylactic antibiotics are effective in preventing infection because bacteria are more susceptible to antibiotics before adherence and production of slime (128). An antibiotic that is effective against skin organisms is used: typically cefazolin because of its effectiveness, low cost, and relatively long half-life.

Treatment

Superficial

If the infection is superficial and diagnosed promptly, then the patient is treated with local wound care, antibiotics (tailored to the culture and sensitivities), and daily observation by the attending surgeon. If the infection clears, then the antibiotics are continued for 2 weeks and the patient's routine postoperative protocol is resumed.

Deep

In an established deep infection, or if a superficial infection does not get better within a day or two, the patient is taken back to the operating room, where a formal irrigation and debridement is performed. All contaminated and devitalized tissue is excised. All implants (such as suture anchors) are assessed, and if they are loose, they are removed. Multiple intraoperative cultures are taken for aerobic and anaerobic bacteria, fungi, and acid-fast staining. The wound is closed over a drain, and the patient is given intravenous broad-spectrum antibiotics, pending the results of the cultures. The patient is given intravenous antibiotics specific to the culture and sensitivity results for 6 weeks. We prefer to involve our infectious diseases colleagues to assist us in this determination. In this period, the patient is carefully observed for recurrence of the infection clinically, and serial sedimentation rates and C-reactive protein levels are measured.

HEMATOMA

Significant hematoma formation after surgery for shoulder instability is relatively uncommon, although the exact incidence is hard to determine from the literature. Rowe and Southmayd (4) reported five hematomas after 162 Bankart procedures. Four of these resolved spontaneously, whereas one required surgical drainage. Bigliani et al. (28) noted one small hematoma, which drained spontaneously with no sequelae, after 68 open inferior capsular shifts.

Banas et al. (18) noted one hematoma after 86 modified Bristow procedures. This resolved spontaneously, with no sequelae. A postoperative hematoma can be painful for the patient and can act as a nidus for infection if present for a long time (especially if draining). We estimate the incidence of postoperative hematoma after an open anterior instability repair is between 2% and 5%, but this is dependent on surgical technique and the exact procedure performed. If a postoperative hematoma develops, then we recommend applying a sterile compressive dressing, ice packs, and watching the patient's clinical course carefully. Consideration should be given to prophylactic antibiotics. If the hematoma is expanding, the patient is becoming febrile, or if the hematoma is not improving significantly over 1 to 2 days, then the patient is brought back to the operating room where the hematoma is evacuated, and the wound explored, irrigated, and closed over suction drain(s). Cultures (anaerobic and aerobic) are taken intraoperatively. The patient is given intravenous antibiotics to cover skin organisms pending culture results.

REFLEX SYMPATHETIC DYSTROPHY

Reflex sympathetic dystrophy (RSD) is characterized by pain out of proportion to physical findings, swelling, limited ROM with associated signs of vasomotor instability, trophic skin changes, and diffuse osteopenia (129). The incidence of RSD after instability surgery is hard to determine. Morrey and Janes noted two cases of RSD in reviewing the results of Putti–Platt or Bankart reconstruction performed on 183 shoulders (3). Many cases of frozen shoulder after instability surgery may have a component of RSD (130–132).

Treatment

The key to treatment of RSD is early diagnosis. Once the diagnosis is made, we prefer the administration of sympathetic blocks performed in conjunction with the pain team service at our institution. The sympathetic block is both diagnostic and therapeutic. It interrupts the pain cycle, allowing the patient to overcome the pain and start to increase shoulder motion (133).

REFERENCES

1. Bankart ASB. The pathology and treatment of recurrent dislocation of the shoulder-joint. *Br J Surg* 1938;26:23–29.
2. Hovelius L, Korner GL, Lundberg GB, et al. The coracoid transfer for recurrent dislocation of the shoulder: technical aspects of the Bristow-Latarjet procedure. *J Bone Joint Surg [Am]* 1983;65:926–934.
3. Morrey BF, Janes JM. Recurrent anterior dislocation of the shoulder: long-term follow-up of the Putti-Platt and Bankart procedures. *J Bone Joint Surg [Am]* 1976;58:252–256.
4. Rowe CR, Southmayd WW. The Bankart procedure: a long-term end-result study. *J Bone Joint Surg [Am]* 1978;60:1–16.
5. Warner JJP, Marks PH. Management of complications of surgery for anterior shoulder instability. *Sports Med Arthrosc Rev* 1993;1:272–292.
6. Neer CS II, Foster CR. Inferior capsular shift for involuntary inferior and multidirectional instability of the shoulder: a preliminary report. *J Bone Joint Surg [Am]* 1980;62:897–908.
7. Rosenberg BN, Richmond JC, Levine WN. Long-term follow-up of Bankart reconstruction: incidence of late degenerative glenohumeral arthrosis. *Am J Sports Med* 1995;23:538–544.
8. Rubenstein DL, Jobe FW, Glousman RE, Kvitne RS, Pink M, Giangarra CE. Anterior capsulolabral reconstruction of the shoulder in athletes. *J Shoulder Elbow Surg* 1992;1:229–237.
9. Speer KP, Warren RF, Pagnani M, Warner JJP. An arthroscopic technique for anterior stabilization of the shoulder with a bioabsorbable tack. *J Bone Joint Surg [Am]* 1996;78:1801–1807.
10. Thomas SC, Matsen FA III. An approach to the repair of avulsion of the glenohumeral ligaments in the management of traumatic anterior glenohumeral instability. *J Bone Joint Surg [Am]* 1989;71:506–513.
11. Ungersbock A, Michel M, Hertel R. Factors influencing the results of a modified Bankart procedure. *J Shoulder Elbow Surg* 1995;4:365–369.
12. Warner JJP. Treatment options for anterior instability: open versus arthroscopic. *Oper Tech Orthop* 1995;5:233–237.
13. Warner JJP, Johnson D, Miller MD, Caborn DN. Technique for selecting capsular tightness in repair of anterior-inferior shoulder instability. *J Shoulder Elbow Surg* 1995;4:352–364.
14. Warner JJP, Kann S, Marks PH. Arthroscopic repair of combined Bankart and superior labral detachment anterior and posterior lesions: technique and preliminary results. *Arthroscopy* 1994;10:383–391.
15. Warner JJP, Miller MD, Marks P, Fu FH. Arthroscopic Bankart repair with the Suretac device. Part I: clinical observations. *Arthroscopy* 1995;11:2–13.
16. Warner JJP, Schulte KR, Imhoff AB. Current concepts in shoulder instability. *Adv Oper Orthop* 1995;3:217–248.
17. Ahmadain AM. The Magnuson-Stack operation for recurrent anterior dislocation of the shoulder. *J Bone Joint Surg [Br]* 1987;69:111–114.
18. Banas MP, Dalldorf PG, Sebastianelli WJ, DeHaven KE. Long-term followup of the modified Bristow procedure [See comments]. *Am J Sports Med* 1993;21:666–671.
19. Barry TP, Lombardo SJ, Kerlan RK, et al. The coracoid transfer for recurrent anterior instability of the shoulder in adolescents. *J Bone Joint Surg [Am]* 1985;67:383–387.
20. Ferlic DC, DiGiovine NM. A long-term follow-up retrospective study of the modified Bristow operation. *Am J Sports Med* 1988;16:469–474.
21. Lombardo SJ, Kerlan RK, Jobe FW, et al. The modified Bristow procedure for recurrent dislocation of the shoulder. *J Bone Joint Surg [Am]* 1976;58:256–261.
22. Magnuson PB, Stack JK. Recurrent dislocation of the shoulder. *JAMA* 1943;123:889–892.
23. Osmond-Clarke H. Habitual dislocation of the shoulder: the Putti-Platt operation. *J Bone Joint Surg [Br]* 1948;30:19–25.
24. Regan WD, Webster-Bogaert S, Hawkins RJ, Fowler PJ. Comparative functional analysis of the Bristow, Magnuson-Stack, and Putti-Platt procedures for recurrent dislocation of the shoulder. *Am J Sports Med* 1989;17:42–48.
25. Singer GC, Kirkland PM, Emery RJH. Coracoid transposition for recurrent anterior instability of the shoulder: a 20-year follow-up study. *J Bone Joint Surg [Br]* 1995;77:73–76.
26. Torg JS, Balduini FC, Bonci C, et al. A modified Bristow-Helfet-May procedure for recurrent dislocation and subluxation of the shoulder: report of two hundred and twelve cases. *J Bone Joint Surg [Am]* 1987;69:904–913.
27. Lusardi DA, Wirth MA, Wurtz D, Rockwood CAJ. Loss of external rotation following anterior capsulorrhaphy of the shoulder. *J Bone Joint Surg [Am]* 1993;75:1185–1192.
28. Bigliani LU, Kurzweil PR, Schwartzbach CC, Wolfe IN, Flatow EL. Inferior capsular shift procedure for anterior-inferior shoulder instability in athletes. *Am J Sports Med* 1994;22:578–584.
29. Hawkins RJ, Angelo RL. Glenohumeral osteoarthrosis: a late complication of the Putti-Platt repair. *J Bone Joint Surg [Am]* 1990;72:1193–1197.

30. Young DC, Rockwood CA Jr. Complications of a failed Bristow procedure and their management. *J Bone Joint Surg [Am]* 1991;73: 969–981.
31. Zuckerman JD, Matsen FA III. Complications about the glenohumeral joint related to the use of screws and staples. *J Bone Joint Surg [Am]* 1984;66:175–180.
32. Neer CS II, Watson KC, Stanton FJ. Recent experience in total shoulder replacement. *J Bone Joint Surg [Am]* 1982;64:319–337.
33. Matsen FA III, Harryman DT II, Sidles JA. Mechanics of glenohumeral instability. *Clin Sports Med* 1991;10:783–788.
34. Allen AA, Warner JJP. Shoulder instability in the athlete. *Orthop Clin North Am* 1995;26:487–504.
35. Levine WN, Richmond JC, Donaldson WR. Use of the suture anchor in open Bankart reconstruction: a follow-up report. *Am J Sports Med* 1994;22:723–726.
36. Arciero RA, Wheeler JH, Ryan JB, McBride JT. Arthroscopic Bankart repair versus nonoperative treatment for acute, initial anterior shoulder dislocations. *Am J Sports Med* 1994;22:589–594.
37. Green MR, Christensen KP. Arthroscopic versus open Bankart procedures: a comparison of early morbidity and complications. *Arthroscopy* 1993;9:371–374.
38. Jobe FW, Moynes DR, Brewster CE. Rehabilitation of shoulder joint instabilities. *Orthop Clin North Am* 1987;18:473–482.
39. Lane JG, Sachs RA, Riehl B. Arthroscopic staple capsulorrhaphy: a long-term follow-up. *Arthroscopy* 1993;9:190–194.
40. Pavlik A, Csepai D, Hidas P, Banoczy A. Sports ability after Bankart procedure in professional athletes. *Knee Surg Sports Traumatol Arthrosc* 1996;4:116–120.
41. Swenson TM, Warner JJP. Arthroscopic shoulder stabilization: overview of indications, technique, and efficacy. *Clin Sports Med* 1995;14:841–862.
42. Uribe JW, Hechtman KS. Arthroscopically assisted repair of acute Bankart lesions. *Orthopedics* 1998;16:1019–1023.
43. Walch G, Boileau P, Levigne C, Mandrino A, Neyret P, Donell S. Arthroscopic stabilization for recurrent anterior shoulder dislocation: results of 59 cases. *Arthroscopy* 1995;11:173–179.
44. Yoneda M, Hayashida K, Izawa K, Shimada K, Shino K. A simple and secure anchoring system for Caspari's transglenoid multiple suture technique using a biodegradable poly-L-lactic acid button. *Arthroscopy* 1996;12:293–299.
45. Goldberg BJ, Nirschl RP, McConnell JP, Pettrone FA. Arthroscopic transglenoid suture capsulolabral repairs: preliminary results. *Am J Sports Med* 1993;21:656–665.
46. Sawyer JR, Esterhai JJL. Shoulder infections. In: Warner JJP, Iannotti JP, Gerber C, eds. *Complex and revision problems in shoulder surgery.* Philadelphia: Lippincott–Raven, 1997:385–398.
47. Ward WG, Goldner RD. Shoulder pyarthrosis: a concomitant process. *Orthopaedics* 1994;17:591–595.
48. Liotard JP, Walch G. Nonsurgical management of shoulder stiffness. In: Warner JJP, Iannotti JP, Gerber C, eds. *Complex and revision problems in shoulder surgery.* Philadelphia: Lippincott–Raven, 1997:149–157.
49. Johnson LL. *Arthroscopic surgery: principles and practice.* St. Louis: CV Mosby, 1986:1405–1445.
50. Dowdy PA, O'Driscoll SW. Osteoarthritis following stabilization for recurrent anterior shoulder instability. *J Bone Joint Surg [Br]* 1995;77(suppl III):311–312.
51. Samilson RL, Prieto V. Dislocation arthropathy of the shoulder. *J Bone Joint Surg [Am]* 1989;65:456–460.
52. Mankin HJ, Mow VC, Buckwalter JA, Iannotti JP, Ratcliffe A. Form and function of articular cartilage. In: Simon SR, ed. *Orthopaedic basic science.* Rosemont, IL: American Academy of Orthopaedic Surgeons, 1994:1–44.
53. Tibone J, Ting A. Capsulorrhaphy with a staple for recurrent posterior subluxation of the shoulder. *J Bone Joint Surg [Am]* 1990;72: 999–1002.
54. Miller MD, Wirth MA, Rockwood CA Jr. Thawing the frozen shoulder: the ''patient'' patient. *Orthopedics* 1996;19:849–853.
55. Shaffer B, Tibone JE, Kerlan RK. Frozen shoulder: a long-term follow-up. *J Bone Joint Surg [Am]* 1992;74:738–746.
56. Warner JJP. Acquired shoulder stiffness. In: Warner JJP, Iannotti JP, Gerber C, eds. *Complex and revision problems in shoulder surgery.* Philadelphia: Lippincott–Raven, 1997:131–147.
57. Brown AR, Weiss R, Greenberg C, et al. Interscalene block for shoulder arthroscopy: comparison with general anaesthesia. *Arthroscopy* 1993;9:295–300.
58. Kinnard P, Truchon R, St-Pierre A, Montreuil J. Interscalene block for pain relief after shoulder surgery. *Clin Orthop* 1994;304:22–24.
59. Warner JJP. Shoulder arthroscopy in the beach-chair position: basic setup. *Oper Tech Orthop* 1991;1:147–154.
60. Warner JJP. Frozen shoulder: diagnosis and management. *J Am Acad Orthop Surg* 1997;5:130–140.
61. Allen AA, Warner JJP. Management of the stiff shoulder. *Oper Tech Orthop* 1995;5:238–247.
62. Bradley JP. Arthroscopic treatment for frozen capsulitis. *Oper Tech Orthop* 1991;1:248–252.
63. Warner JJP, Allen A, Marks PH, Wong P. Arthroscopic release for chronic, refractory adhesive capsulitis of the shoulder. *J Bone Joint Surg [Am]* 1996;78:1808–1816.
64. Warner JJP, Iannotti JP. Treatment of a stiff shoulder after posterior capsulorrhaphy: a report of three cases. *J Bone Joint Surg [Am]* 1996;8:1419–1421.
65. Wiley AM. Arthroscopic appearance of frozen shoulder. *Arthroscopy* 1991;7:138–143.
66. Harryman DT II, Matsen FA III, Sidles JA. Arthroscopic management of refractory shoulder stiffness. *Arthroscopy* 1997;13:133–147.
67. Gerber C, Krushell R. Isolated rupture of the tendon of the subscapularis muscle: clinical features in 16 cases. *J Bone Joint Surg [Br]* 1991;73:389–394.
68. Warner JJP, Allen AA, Gerber C. Diagnosis and management of subscapularis tendon tears. *Tech Orthop* 1994;9:116–125.
69. Ogilvie-Harris DJ, Myerthall S. The diabetic frozen shoulder: arthroscopic release. *Arthroscopy* 1997;13:1–8.
70. Zanotti RM, Kuhn JE. Arthroscopic capsular release for the stiff shoulder: description of technique and anatomic considerations. *Am J Sports Med* 1997;25:294–305.
71. Segmuller HE, Taylor DE, Hogan CS, Saies AD, Hayes MG. Arthroscopic treatment of adhesive capsulitis. *J Shoulder Elbow Surg* 1995;4:403–408.
72. Neer CS II. Frozen shoulder. In: Neer CS II, ed. *Shoulder reconstruction.* Philadelphia: WB Saunders, 1990:422–427.
73. Reeves B. Arthrographic changes in frozen and post-traumatic stiff shoulders. *Proc R Soc Med* 1966;59:827.
74. MacDonald PB, Hawkins RJ, Fowler PJ, Miniaci A. Release of the subscapularis for internal rotation contracture and pain after anterior repair for recurrent anterior dislocation of the shoulder. *J Bone Joint Surg [Am]* 1992;74:734–737.
75. Blom S, Dahlback LO. Nerve injuries in dislocations of the shoulder joint and fractures of the neck of the humerus. *Acta Chir Scand* 1970;136:461–466.
76. Liveson JA. Nerve lesions associated with shoulder dislocation: an electrodiagnostic study of 11 cases. *J Neurol Neurosurg Psychiatry* 1984;47:742–744.
77. Brown JT. Nerve injuries complicating dislocation of the shoulder. *J Bone Joint Surg [Br]* 1952;34:526.
78. Leffert RD, Seddon HJ. Infraclavicular brachial plexus injuries. *J Bone Joint Surg [Br]* 1965;47:9–22.
79. Pasila M, Jaroma H, Kiviluoto O, Sundholm A. Early complications from primary anterior shoulder dislocations. *Acta Orthop Scand* 1978;49:260–263.
80. Rowe CR. Instabilities of the glenohumeral joint. *Bull Hosp Joint Dis* 1978;39:180–186.
81. Burkhead WZ II, Scheinberg RR, Box G. Surgical anatomy of the axillary nerve. *J Shoulder Elbow Surg* 1992;1:31–36.
82. Frankin TH. Injury to the musculocutaneous nerve as a complication of operations for recurrent dislocation of the shoulder. *J Bone Joint Surg [Br]* 1984;66:449.
83. Wall MS, Warren RF. Complications of shoulder instability surgery. *Clin Sports Med* 1995;14:973–1000.
84. Flatow EL, Bigliani LU, April EW. An anatomic study of the musculocutaneous nerve and its relationship to the coracoid process. *Clin Orthop* 1989;244:166–171.
85. Richards RR, Hudson AR, Bertoia JT, Urbaniak JR, Waddell JP. Injury to the brachial plexus during Putti-Platt and Bristow procedures: a report of eight cases. *Am J Sports Med* 1987;15:374–380.
86. Altchek DW, Warren RF, Skyhar MJ, Ortiz G. T-Plasty anterior

repair for anterior and inferior instability of the shoulder. *J Bone Joint Surg [Am]* 1991;73:105–111.
87. Mologne TS, Lapoint JM, Morin WD, Zilberfarb J, O'Brien TJ. Arthroscopic anterior labral reconstruction using a transglenoid suture technique: results in active-duty military patients. *Am J Sports Med* 1996;24:268–274.
88. Wiener DN, Speer KP. The deltoid sign [Letter]. *Anesth Analg* 1994;79:192.
89. Seddon HJ. Three types of nerve injury. *Brain* 1943;66:237.
90. Sunderland S. *Nerve and nerve injuries.* New York: Churchill Livingstone, 1978.
91. Hawkins RJ, Bell RH, Hawkins RH, Koppert GJ. Anterior dislocation of the shoulder in the older patient. *Clin Orthop* 1986;206:192–195.
92. Neviaser RJ, Neviaser TJ, Neviaser JS. Anterior dislocation of the shoulder and rotator cuff ruptures. *Clin Orthop* 1993;291:103–106.
93. Neviaser RJ, Neviaser TJ, Neviaser JS. Concurrent rupture of the rotator cuff and anterior dislocation of the shoulder in the older patient. *J Bone Joint Surg [Am]* 1988;70:1308–1311.
94. Iannotti JP, Zlatkin MB, Esterhai JL, et al. Magnetic resonance imaging of the shoulder: sensitivity, specificity, and predictive value. *J Bone Joint Surg [Am]* 1991;73:17–29.
95. Miniaci A, Dowdy PA, Willits K, Vellet AD. Magnetic resonance imaging evaluation of the rotator cuff tendons in the asymptomatic shoulder. *Am J Sports Med* 1995;23:142–145.
96. Watson-Jones R. *Fractures and joint injuries.* Edinburgh: Churchill Livingstone, 1976.
97. Watson-Jones R. Fractures in the region of the shoulder joint. *Proc R Soc Med* 1930;29:1058.
98. Merle M, Amend P, Cour C, Foucher G, Michon J. Microsurgical repair of peripheral nerve lesions. *Peripheral Nerve Repair Regen* 1986;2:17–26.
99. Seddon HJ. Nerve grafting. *J Bone Joint Surg [Br]* 1963;45:447–461.
100. Seddon HJ. *Surgical disorders of the peripheral nerves.* Baltimore: Williams & Wilkins, 1972.
101. Hirsch S. Paralysis of the axillary (circumflex) nerve with spontaneous recovery after 7 months. *JAMA* 1936;106:705.
102. Leffert RD. Neurological problems. In: Rockwood CA Jr, Matsen FA III, eds. *The shoulder.* Philadelphia: WB Saunders, 1990:750–790.
103. Alnot JY, Valenti PH. Surgical reconstruction of the axillary nerve. In: Post M, Morrey BF, Hawkins RJ, eds. *Surgery of the shoulder.* St. Louis: Mosby Year Book, 1990:330–333.
104. Petrucci FS, Morelli A, Raimondi PL. Axillary nerve injuries: 21 cases treated by nerve graft and neurolysis. *J Hand Surg* 1982;7:271–278.
105. Slomann W. Ueber die behandlung der deltoidenslahmheit. *Z Orthop Chir* 1916;35.
106. Davidson WD. Traumatic deltoid paralysis treated by muscle transplantation. *JAMA* 1936;106:2237.
107. Moore BH. A new operation to relieve paralysis of the deltoid muscle. *JAMA* 1932;99:2182.
108. Ober FR. An operation to relieve paralysis of the deltoid muscle. *JAMA* 1932;99:2182.
109. Mustard WT. Muscle transposition for paralysis of the deltoid muscle. *J Bone Joint Surg [Br]* 1956;38:778.
110. La Chapelle EH. Pectoralis major transfer for deltoid paralysis. *J Bone Joint Surg [Br]* 1961;43:192.
111. Gersuny B. Eine operation bei motorischen lahmungen. *Wien Klin Wochenschr* 1906;263.
112. Hoffa A. Ueber die end-resultate der sehnenplastiken. *Arch F Klin Chir* 1906;79:493.
113. Kiliani OGT. An operation for the paralytic shoulder joint due to infantile paralysis. *Ann Surg* 1910;49:79.
114. Lewis DD. Trapezius transplantation in the treatment of deltoid paralysis. *JAMA* 1910;55:2211–2213.
115. Haas S. The treatment of permanent paralysis of the deltoid muscle. *JAMA* 1935;104:99.
116. Mayer L. The physiologic method of tendon transplantation. *Surg Gynecol Obstet* 1916;22:182.
117. Mayer L. Transplantation of the trapezius for paralysis of the abductors of the arm. *J Bone Joint Surg* 1927;9:412–420.
118. Bateman JE. Transplant of the trapezius for abductor paralysis of the shoulder. *J Bone Joint Surg [Br]* 1948;30:221.
119. Saha AK. Surgery of the paralyzed and flail shoulder. *Acta Orthop Scand Suppl* 1967;97:85–90.
120. Itoh Y, Sasaki T, Ishiguro T, Uchinishi K, Yabe Y, Fukuda H. Transfer of the latissimus dorsi to replace a paralysed anterior deltoid: a new technique using an inverted pedicle graft. *J Bone Joint Surg [Br]* 1987;69:647–651.
121. Leffert B, ed. *Brachial plexus injuries.* New York: Churchill Livingstone, 1985.
122. Ho G, Toder JS, Zimmermann B. An overview of septic arthritis and septic bursitis. *Orthopedics* 1984;7:1571.
123. Field LD, Warren RF, O'Brien SJ, Altchek DW, Wickiewicz TL. Isolated closure of rotator interval defects for shoulder instability. *Am J Sports Med* 1995;23:557–563.
124. Esterhai JJL, Gelb I. Adult septic arthritis. *Orthop Clin North Am* 1991;22:503–514.
125. Gelberman RH, Menon J, Austerlitz MS, Weisman MH. Pyogenic arthritis of the shoulder in adults. *J Bone Joint Surg [Am]* 1980;62:550.
126. Leslie BM, Harris JM, Driscoll D. Septic arthritis of the shoulder in adults. *J Bone Joint Surg [Am]* 1989;71:1516.
127. Toby EB, Webb LX, Voytec A, Gristina AG. Septic arthritis of the shoulder. *Orthop Trans* 1987;11:230.
128. Petty W. Prevention of infections of skeletal prostheses. *Compr Orthop* 1994;78.
129. van Laere M, Claessens M. The treatment of reflex sympathetic dystrophy syndrome: current concepts. *Acta Orthop Belg* 1992;58:259–261.
130. Adebajo AO, Hazleman BL. Shoulder pain and reflex sympathetic dystrophy. *Curr Opin Rheumatol* 1990;2:270–275.
131. Uhthoff HK, Sarkar K. Shoulder pain and reflex sympathetic dystrophy. *Curr Opin Rheumatol* 1991;3:240–246.
132. Waldburger M, Meier JL, Gobelet C. The frozen shoulder: diagnosis and treatment: prospective study of 50 cases of adhesive capsulitis. *Clin Rheumatol* 1992;11:364–368.
133. Lankford LL. Reflex sympathetic dystrophy. In: Green DP, ed. *Operative hand surgery.* New York: Churchill Livingstone, 1993:627–660.

The Unstable Shoulder,
edited by R.F. Warren, E.V. Craig, and D.W. Altchek.
Lippincott–Raven Publishers, Philadelphia © 1999.

CHAPTER 26

Recurrent Instability

Surgical Failures

Stephen J. Zabinski, Peter T. Simonian, Jon J. P. Warner, and Russell F. Warren

Recurrent instability after a previous shoulder repair remains among the most difficult problems confronting shoulder surgeons. There are few reported series in the literature to assist in the management of these patients, and additional factors such as contracture, nerve injury, and glenohumeral arthritis also may be present and further complicate treatment.

The management of contracture, nerve injury, glenohumeral arthritis, and other complications of shoulder-stabilization surgery are detailed elsewhere in the text. The central focus of this chapter is to review the management of patients in whom the primary cause of pain and disability is recurrent instability of the glenohumeral joint after prior repair.

Two groups of patients have this complication: the first typically have a traumatic and unidirectional dislocation with an anatomic lesion, whereas the second typically have atraumatic or multidirectional dislocations or both without any anatomic lesion. The outcome of treatment is most closely related to the particular group the patient is in; however, other factors are important as well. Through a careful history, physical examination, and appropriate diagnostic imaging, it is possible fully to define the cause of recurrence.

Proper treatment necessitates this understanding, as repeated surgical stabilization may be a reliable intervention in patients with traumatic unidirectional recurrence but should be avoided until rehabilitative efforts have been exhausted in patients with recurrent atraumatic multidirectional instability (MDI). The nature of the prior repair also influences outcome. Revision of a prior arthroscopic repair is often easier because of less scarring and soft-tissue disruption than a prior open repair, whereas revision of nonanatomic procedures such as the Putti–Platt or Bristow is often technically more demanding because of the disruption of normal anatomy and constraint of glenohumeral motion. Coexistent problems such as arthrosis and contracture may further complicate management and must be considered as well before initiating treatment.

LITERATURE REVIEW

There are few reports of recurrent dislocation after surgical stabilization. Additionally, the majority of reported cases are solely of the traumatic unidirectional type. In other reports, there is not a clear distinction or classification of the cause or type of instability present, making comparisons among these series difficult.

Morrey and Janes in 1976 (1) reviewed 176 patients among 223 who underwent 232 Putti–Platt or Bankart repairs for recurrent anterior shoulder dislocation. There was an 11% recurrence rate with an average follow-up of 10.2 years. Redislocation occurred two or more years after op-

S. J. Zabinski: Department of Orthopaedic Surgery, Thomas Jefferson University, Philadelphia, Pennsylvania 19107; and Department of Orthopaedic Surgery, Shore Memorial Hospital, Somers Point, New Jersey 08224.

P. T. Simonian: Department of Orthopaedic Surgery, University of Washington, Seattle, Washington 98195.

J. J. P. Warner: Department of Orthopaedic Surgery, Harvard Medical School; and Harvard Shoulder Service, Department of Orthopaedic Surgery, Massachusetts General Hospital, Boston, Massachusetts 02114.

R. F. Warren: Department of Orthopaedics, Cornell University Medical College, New York, New York 10021; and Department of Orthopaedics, The Hospital for Special Surgery, New York, New York 10021.

eration in seven of the 20 patients with recurrence. At the time of revision surgery, 60% had a Bankart lesion or inadequate glenoid rim. Surgical repair permitted good function without significant pain in most cases.

Rowe et al. in 1984 (2) analyzed 39 patients who were treated for recurrent anterior dislocation of the shoulder after unsuccessful surgery for the same condition. The most common pathologic lesion associated with the recurrence of the dislocation after prior repair was a Bankart lesion. Excessive capsular laxity, and a Hill-Sachs lesion of the humeral head also were present in some patients. Other factors associated with recurrence were scarring of the subscapularis, generalized ligamentous laxity, technical errors at surgery, and severe reinjury.

Hawkins and Hawkins (3) retrospectively reviewed 46 patients with continuing difficulties after anterior reconstruction for shoulder instability. The primary complaint was continued instability in 31 patients. Of these, 12 had unrecognized posterior or MDI, whereas 11 had an uncorrected anatomic defect. They concluded that "recurrence of symptoms may imply that the direction of the instability was not recognized, that an anterior repair should not be too tight, and that pain after successful stabilization is often due to impingement." This study was the first to identify such a large proportion of patients with MDI in their surgical-failure group.

In 1986 Walch et al. (4) reported 79 recurrences after surgical procedures for recurrent dislocation of the shoulder. They concluded that recurrences are more common in younger patients. Distal displacement or lengthening of the coracoid process was the most common treatment of the initial instability. The main cause of recurrence was failure of the "anteroinferior part of the joint."

Young and Rockwood in 1991 (5) retrospectively evaluated 40 shoulders in 39 patients who had undergone a Bristow procedure. Complications included recurrent painful anterior dislocation (primarily due to capsular laxity), injury to the articular cartilage, failure of the coracoid bone-block to unite with the glenoid, loosening of the screw, neurovascular injury, and posterior instability. MDI was identified in more than half of the patients, and an untreated Bankart lesion was present in 20% of the shoulders. They concluded that revision surgery for a failed Bristow procedure was difficult and often unsuccessful.

Finally, Wirth et al. in 1996 (6) reported good to excellent results in 86% of patients with failed prior stabilizations treated with a capsular imbrication procedure. Unfortunately, this study did not evaluate the revision group in any detail and considered patients with traumatic instability and MDI together in the analysis of results.

FEATURES OF AN IDEAL SURGICAL REPAIR

To better understand surgical failure, it is helpful first to define the ideal surgical repair. Foremost among the qualities of an ideal repair is the *restoration of shoulder stability through anatomic repair of only the pathology within the shoulder*. Anatomically stated, this goal is to secure any detached capsular ligamentous structures (i.e., a Bankart lesion) firmly to the bony attachment and to reset the tension within any lax capsular ligamentous structures back to a normal level. Nonanatomic repairs (such as the Bristow or Putti–Platt) do not achieve this standard because they do not address the capsular ligamentous system and instead constrain the joint to achieve stability. Additionally, even though Bankart repairs reliably obtain a good result in most patients with traumatic anterior instability, untreated capsular-stretching injury may be a cause of failure in some patients after Bankart repair (2,4,5).

The ideal repair would have a *low recurrence rate* and would not stretch or loosen with time. Unfortunately, even with a technically perfect repair, other factors such as recurrent trauma and patient-specific factors such as the quality of the capsular tissue do not allow an absolute zero recurrence rate.

Additionally, the ideal surgical repair would *preserve full glenohumeral motion*. Again most "nonanatomic procedures" such as the Magnuson–Stack and Putti–Platt do not achieve this goal (1,7,8). However, some loss of motion may accompany all stabilization procedures. Indeed, capsular tensioning is inexact and performed most commonly in a position of some loss of external rotation to allow extension of the repair in the postoperative period. Clinical experience justifies this approach; however, even with optimal technique, some patients may lose significant range of motion (9).

The ideal repair would also allow *return to full functional activities*. Certainly many patients do return to vigorous and even overhead activities after shoulder stabilization. However, results in certain groups, such as overhead-throwing athletes and patients with globally lax, MDI, are not so reliable (10,11). In both cases, patients frequently must modify their functional goals postoperatively to accommodate the limitations of the surgical repair.

Finally, the ideal surgical repair would *avoid complications related to hardware and to injury caused by the surgical approach itself*. Hardware complications played a major role in the history of shoulder repairs and despite recent attempts to minimize such complications, concerns remain about the use of metal about the shoulder (5,12,13). Recent suture-anchor designs as well as bioabsorbable implants represent steps toward addressing these concerns. Similarly, the increase in arthroscopic stabilization techniques clearly represents an attempt to diminish the potential soft-tissue risk (nerve injury, musculotendinous violation) associated with open shoulder procedures. Each "advance" has brought with it, however, its own set of complications (i.e., synovitis or osteolysis with bioabsorbable products and higher recurrence rates with arthroscopic techniques), which remain to be resolved (14).

In summary, the ideal surgical repair would stabilize the

shoulder through restoration of the anatomy and tension of the glenohumeral capsular ligamentous system. The repair would allow full return of shoulder motion and strength and would stand up to all functional demands placed on it. It could be effected safely, with minimal invasiveness and no compromise of musculotendinous or neurovascular structures and without complications related to implants used. Although current techniques continue to approach these goals, the ideal stabilization procedure has yet to be defined.

CAUSES OF RECURRENT INSTABILITY AFTER SURGERY

The causes of recurrent instability after a previous stabilization may be broadly divided into problems related to preoperative incorrect diagnosis, problems related to surgical technique or anatomy, and problems related to postoperative rehabilitation, activity, and other patient-specific variables.

Preoperative Factors

Preoperative diagnostic error may lead to postoperative recurrence of instability in a number of ways. Obviously, *incorrect or incomplete identification of the direction of instability* will lead to operative failure. This problem concerns especially patients with multidirectional and posterior instability, in whom inferior subluxation may be noted as well. It may be avoided simply through appropriate history and provocative physical examination, as well as through complete examination under anesthesia for all patients.

Additionally, *failure to recognize psychological causes of glenohumeral subluxation, including the problem of voluntary instability*, will lead to surgical failure. This problem is especially of concern in patients with multidirectional and posterior instability. There is no doubt that some patients with MDI demonstrate abnormal behavioral patterns and responses in regard to their shoulder. This affects both the perception of the shoulder problem and the ability to comply with rehabilitation and activity restrictions. Avoiding surgical intervention in patients with significant voluntary instability is paramount and, if significant concerns about their psychological status are present, a psychological profile may be obtained preoperatively. Some patients with posterior instability, which begins *involuntarily*, learn with time to subluxate their shoulders *voluntarily* (15). This has led to a differentiation between those patients who learn posturally to translate their shoulders posteriorly (in a position of forward flexion and internal rotation) and those who, through selective activation of glenohumeral internal rotators, muscularly subluxate their shoulders. The first group is thought to have a better prognosis in regard to surgical outcome. However, in a patient with a purely muscular type of voluntary posterior dislocation, surgical intervention should be avoided.

Finally, shoulder pain is a predominant complaint in many patients whose shoulder stabilization failed. Although this pain is often related to the recurrence of instability, *other causes of pain must be considered, such as subacromial impingement, glenohumeral arthritis, biceps tendonitis, cervical radiculopathy, and reflex sympathetic dystrophy.* Failure to identify these problems will lead to certain postoperative failure of any revision stabilization.

Operative Technique

Inadequate tensioning of the capsular ligamentous structures is foremost among causes of recurrence. Cadaveric studies demonstrated that detachment of the anteroinferior capsulolabral complex is not sufficient by itself to allow glenohumeral anterior dislocation (16–18). Some element of capsular injury/stretching is required for recurrent anterior instability to develop. This capsular laxity, if neglected by the surgeon performing the initial repair, may lead to surgical failure. The capsule should be tensioned with the arm abducted approximately 30 to 45 degrees in the scapular plane and externally rotated a similar degree, depending on the patient's activity level and goals (10). Slightly greater values of external rotation are allowed for overhead athletes. The difficulty in adequately shifting and accurately tensioning the capsule is likely the main reason for the higher incidence of recurrence after arthroscopic repairs despite a seemingly good reattachment of the Bankart lesion.

Failure to repair a Bankart lesion certainly contributes to recurrence after nonanatomic and bone-block procedures, rarely encountered currently (2,5,19). However, the technique of Bankart repair is often overlooked and is vital to preventing failure. The glenoid neck must be prepared to bleeding bone, a step often overlooked during arthroscopic repairs. Similarly, it is vital to reattach the capsulolabral complex precisely at the articular margin (not medial to it). Fixation with staples or tacks is less secure than with suture techniques, and it is significant that nearly all staple or tack procedures carry higher rates of recurrence than do suture techniques. This may relate to lower mechanical strength or to necrosis of the tissue under the staple or tack.

Rupture of the subscapularis has been increasingly recognized as a cause of recurrence, and it remains important to be meticulous during repair of this tendon (20). We occasionally use subscapularis-splitting techniques (particularly in overhead athletes and for capsular reefing procedures) and routinely attempt to leave the lower one third of the subscapularis attached to the humerus. Overzealous early rehabilitation may also play a role in subscapularis rupture.

Anatomic factors encountered intraoperatively may predispose to failure. Patients with a *large Hill-Sachs lesion* (greater than 30% of the humeral articular surface) are at a distinct mechanical disadvantage and are at some higher risk of recurrence (2). In patients with severe humeral head deformity, consideration of the use of an allograft bone–tendon graft may be given.

Significant anterior glenoid bone loss (greater than 30%) also predisposes to recurrence through loss of the normal glenoid concavity. Repair of the bony Bankart, as well as willingness to augment a capsular procedure with some anterior bone "grafting" procedure if glenoid loss in excess of 30% is present, is important to prevent recurrence.

Error in operative technique is an especially important cause of failure in patients with MDI. The primary mistake made in these patients is *failure to address all elements of capsular laxity* (2,3,5). Because of the inferior component in these patients, rotator interval defects must be looked for and closed (21). If the interval capsule is merely lax, it should be imbricated, or recurrent inferior subluxation will occur. Similarly, failure to carry the capsular incision adequately inferiorly into the axillary recess and past the 6 o'clock position will result in inadequate shifting of the inferior flap and inadequate tensioning of the opposite limb of the inferior glenohumeral ligament. This will predispose to recurrent instability in a posterior direction. Rarely, combined approaches (both anterior and posterior) may be required if residual laxity exists in the opposite capsular ligaments.

Postoperative and Patient-Specific Factors

Appropriate postoperative immobilization and rehabilitation is a vital and often overlooked factor in ensuring good outcome after shoulder stabilization. Immobilization must be in an appropriate position to protect the repair and must be maintained for a sufficient time to allow healing of the repair. If any significant element of posterior laxity was corrected at the time of operation, immobilization should be in an orthoplast brace in neutral rotation rather than in internal rotation. In patients in whom compliance is a concern, we have occasionally used a shoulder spica cast rather than a removable orthosis. In patients with significant inferior laxity, the arm should not be allowed to "hang free," as this downward force may stress the rotator interval repair. Although pendulum exercises are initiated early in the postoperative period, it is vital to increase mobilization slowly, and some protection of the repair should be maintained for 6 to 8 weeks. Return to overhead activities must be delayed until both healing of the repair and rehabilitation of the shoulder musculature are complete, often 4 to 6 months postoperatively.

Recurrent trauma does play a role in failure in some patients. This "trauma" may be a discrete dislocation event, such as might occur after return to contact sports or in a motor vehicle accident. Recurrent trauma also may be unrelated to sporting activities or unfortunate accidents, such as in patients with poorly controlled seizures, Tourette's syndrome, or other neuromuscular disorders. Pharmacologic management of these disorders must be optimized during the postoperative period to prevent failure of the repair. Repetitive microtrauma also contributes to failure. In the case of the overhead athlete (thrower, swimmer, or volleyball player), the return to repeated high-demand shoulder activities may precipitate recurrent instability.

In certain patients, especially those with MDI, the treatment may fail because of *idiopathic recurrent capsular laxity* in the absence of any trauma. In these patients, simple activities of daily life result in stretching of the repair and recurrent instability. The precise cause of this phenomenon remains to be defined. It is known that skin fibroblasts in patients with MDI demonstrate increased collagen production (22). At revision, rather than finding a thin attenuated capsule, we often noted the capsular tissue to be markedly thick, redundant, and loose. These two findings imply an overproduction of deficient collagen in some patients. The nature of this deficiency, however, is uncertain, and investigations now center on possible abnormalities in collagen cross-linking in these patients. Unfortunately, it remains impossible to identify reliably before surgery those patients at risk for this mode of failure (23).

PATIENT EVALUATION

In a patient with recurrent symptoms after a previous shoulder stabilization, the initial and most important step in evaluation is to determine whether the patient's symptoms are related to the recurrence of shoulder instability or to some other cause. Occasionally, this distinction will be obvious, as in the patient who has a repeated dislocation or who complains of the sensation of recurrent instability. Often, however, the patient complains of pain within the shoulder, and it is up to the surgeon to determine whether this pain is related to the recurrence of instability.

Although the differentiation of pain related to instability and pain related to other causes is difficult, a thorough history and physical examination will accurately guide the surgeon in most cases. During the evaluation, it is important to keep in mind other causes of shoulder pain after instability surgery. These include glenohumeral or acromioclavicular (AC) arthritis, rotator cuff/biceps tendonitis or tear, capsular contracture and inflammation, scapulothoracic disorders, hardware complications, and neurologic syndromes (reflex sympathetic dystrophy, cervical radiculopathy, or brachial plexopathy). A variety of key elements of pain related to instability assist in differentiating it from these other causes. These include its positional nature (typically in a position of apprehension rather than impingement) and its associated mechanical symptoms (such as "slipping," "falling off," or "dead arm"). Additionally, the patient will often describe a manipulative popping of the shoulder to relieve the pain.

Examination must include careful evaluation of the cervical spine and neurologic examination to rule out a neurologic cause of the patient's pain. Palpation should evaluate areas of tenderness (AC joint, subdeltoid region, or bicipital groove) or crepitus (subacromial, glenohumeral, or scapulothoracic) that suggest other shoulder pathology. It is vital then to confirm with the patient that these areas of tenderness or crepitus correspond to the site and type of pain and are not incidental findings. Both active and passive range of motion must be carefully assessed and compared with the opposite shoulder, as well as with previous follow-ups. Significant loss of motion typically suggests pain related to capsular contracture or glenohumeral arthritis, although infrequently instability opposite the contracture may exist as well. Anterior, inferior, and posterior apprehension should be assessed individually and correlated with the patient's presenting symptoms. Apprehension alone does not confirm that instability has recurred. Shoulder-stability testing (anterior and posterior drawer, sulcus sign) may confirm the suspicion of recurrent glenohumeral laxity; however, it may be difficult in the apprehensive patient. Again, laxity must be correlated with patient symptoms to provide meaningful direction to treating the patient. Rotator-cuff and deltoid function should be evaluated for evidence of dysfunction related to mechanical causes (rotator-cuff tear, deltoid detachment) or neurologic causes (axillary or suprascapular neuropathy). The lift-off test should be used to assess subscapularis integrity (24).

Radiographic evaluation should include a true anteroposterior (AP) view of the glenohumeral joint in internal rotation, a Y-lateral scapular view, and an axillary view. It is vital to assess for degenerative changes, hardware loosening or joint penetration, glenoid bone loss, or other factors that may affect the patient's symptoms or outcome. Magnetic resonance imaging (MRI) of the shoulder is indicated to rule out other causes of pain (i.e., rotator-cuff tear) and to define the cause of recurrent instability (Bankart lesion, subscapularis rupture). Unfortunately, the presence of metal implants from prior surgery may limit the diagnostic usefulness of MRI in some patients, but proper software techniques will generally provide helpful images. Electromyography and nerve-conduction studies should be obtained if there is suspicion of a neurologic cause of the patient's pain or if examination suggests axillary neuropathy. Stellate ganglion blockade may be used to confirm the diagnosis if reflex sympathetic dystrophy is suspected.

Finally, we found it important to review the operative note(s) from prior surgeries. These records frequently contain important information regarding the patient's examination under anesthesia, the status of the glenohumeral articular cartilage and labrum, the quality of the capsular tissue and rotator cuff, and the specifics of the repair performed. This information is often of assistance in confirming the cause of the patient's recurrent symptoms; however, it also is valuable in guiding subsequent treatment decisions and in preoperative planning of any revision procedure that may be required.

TREATMENT AND RESULTS

After the examination and work-up of a patient with recurrent shoulder instability after a prior repair, careful consideration to treatment should be given. It is vital to remember that the prognosis of revision treatment varies greatly, based primarily on the *direction* of instability present. It is helpful, therefore, to consider treatment options and expected results separately, based on this distinction.

Unidirectional Anterior Instability

Nonoperative Treatment

The nonoperative treatment of recurrent unidirectional anterior instability after a prior repair is similar to the treatment of first-time dislocators. If a traumatic dislocation has occurred, immobilization is presently recommended only until the patient is comfortable enough to begin therapy, as longer periods of immobilization have not been shown to affect outcome. Rehabilitation begins with restoration of full glenohumeral motion. Although internal rotation is often neglected, it remains an important component of therapy, as the fixed loss of internal rotation, particularly at 90 degrees, may lead to a coupled increase in anterior humeral translation. Motion restoration is followed by a gradual strengthening regimen aimed at both the shoulder musculature and the periscapular stabilizers. Return to activity may begin once shoulder strength has returned, and in some sports, protective bracing may be helpful in preventing future injury.

Revision Operative Treatment

Indications

The indications for operative management in a patient with recurrent unidirectional anterior instability after operative repair depend on a variety of factors. Many patients will initially be managed nonoperatively, and the recurrence of instability or dislocation despite appropriate rehabilitation is a clear indication for operative management. Not all patients must first undergo a trial of conservative management, however. Certainly in young active patients engaged in overhead activities, nonoperative treatment will often fail, and consideration to early operative treatment of these patients is reasonable. Additionally, if the prior stabilization has a documented history of poor results (i.e., staple capsulorrhaphy) or was an arthroscopic procedure that appears to have failed, consideration to moving directly to operative treatment is indeed reasonable. Also, if an obvious anatomic lesion, such as rupture of the subscapularis or a large Bankart/bony Bankart is present, the patient may be strongly advised to consider revision surgery.

Techniques

At present, the indications for and expected results of arthroscopic revision stabilization are not known, and therefore our preference is to perform nearly all revision stabilization procedures open. Diagnostic arthroscopy may be valuable at the beginning of the case to provide information important to the revision repair, such as the presence of a Bankart lesion, metal penetration into the joint, or subscapularis rupture.

The technique of revision surgery is similar to that used in primary repairs in this group. A deltopectoral approach is used. The interval between the deltoid and pectoralis muscle may be defined more distally with the arm in abduction if scar or loss of the cephalic vein related to the prior surgery obscures this interval. If a Magnuson–Stack or Putti–Platt procedure was performed previously, we give consideration to a Z-plasty lengthening of the subscapular tendon only if less than 30 degrees of external rotation at zero degrees exists. Typically, if instability has recurred, this is not the case, and no subscapularis lengthening will be required. Reestablishing the tissue plane between the capsule and the subscapularis remains the most difficult step, particularly after prior Putti–Platt. To gain access to the subscapularis/capsular plane, it is helpful to divide longitudinally the subscapularis tendon in line with its fibers at the junction between the upper two thirds and the lower third. A small elevator may then be passed inferiorly in the plane between the subscapularis and capsule to protect the axillary nerve (Fig. 1). Alternatively, the nerve may be dissected out and directly visualized for protection. Superiorly, the subscapularis/capsular plane is best defined *medially* at the musculotendinous junction of the subscapularis. A blunt clamp may then be passed along the plane and, by using the clamp as a dissector, the plane developed further laterally. The tendon is then tagged near the musculotendinous junction and divided just lateral to the tagging sutures as the clamp is cut down onto. Alternatively, the subscapularis division may be started laterally, and a small portion of the inferior layer of the tendon left with the capsule to reinforce it as the dissection is carried medially. This technique was originally advocated by Neer (26) for his inferior capsular-shift procedure. If the capsular tissue is deficient or markedly scarred to the subscapularis tendon, the capsule and subscapularis may be taken down together, and the capsule then either dissected off, or the entire unit shifted together (Fig. 2).

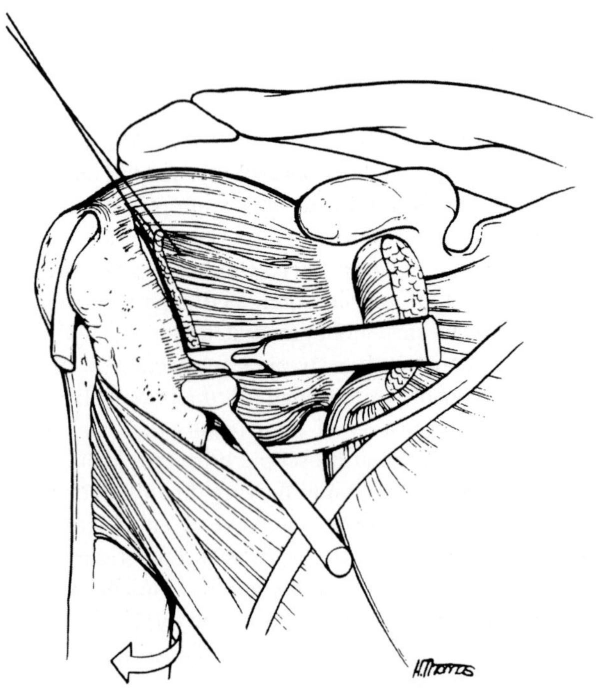

FIG. 1. Dissection of the inferior capsular flap is facilitated by traction sutures in the capsule, progressive external rotation, and protection of the axillary nerve with a periosteal elevator so that the capsule may be divided under direct vision. (From Warner JP, Marks PH. Management of complications of surgery for anterior shoulder instability. *Sports Med Arthrosc Rev* 1993;1:272–292, with permission.)

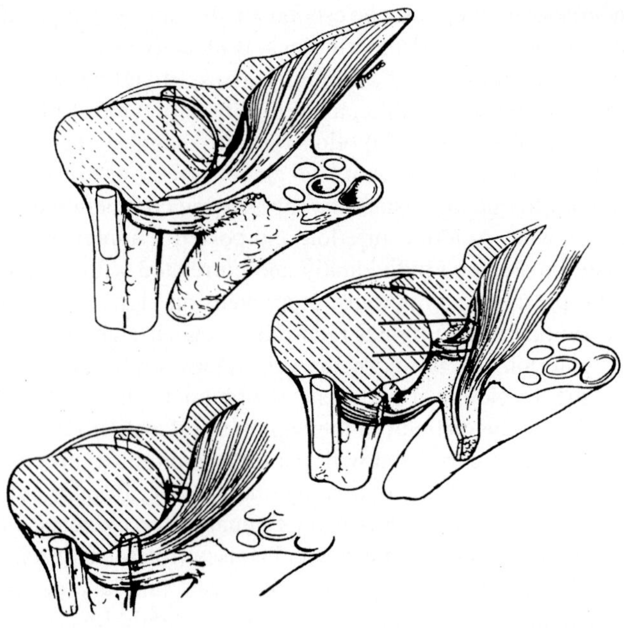

FIG. 2. In revision cases in which marked medial scarring may place the neurovascular structures at risk, both the subscapularis and capsule may be detached laterally. A Bankart repair may then be effected by placing the repair sutures in an inside–out fashion, or alternatively, the capsule may then be dissected off the subscapularis after detachment. (From Warner JP, Marks PH. Management of complications of surgery for anterior shoulder instability. *Sports Med Arthrosc Rev* 1993;1:272–292, with permission.)

Once the capsule has been defined, the anterior capsule and its glenoid attachment must be inspected. If an open rotator interval is encountered, this may be used as an entry point through which to insert a humeral head retractor and inspect the joint. Alternatively, the capsule may be divided horizontally along its midportion just between the middle and inferior glenohumeral ligaments. The majority of these patients *will* demonstrate a Bankart lesion. Additionally, most will demonstrate significant capsular laxity. A medially or laterally based capsular shift (T-plasty) should then be performed in conjunction with Bankart repair. If only capsular laxity is demonstrated, a lateral shift is typically

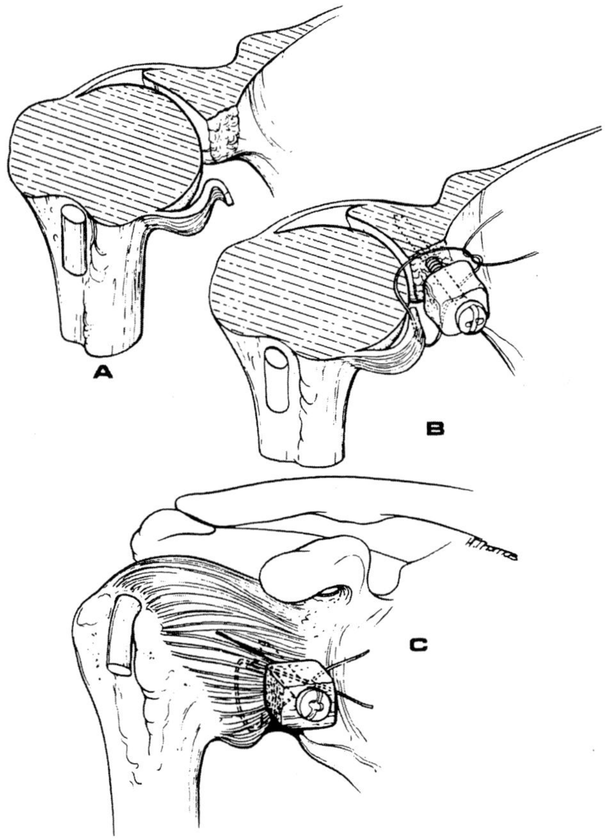

FIG. 3. A–C: If a bone block is necessary for anterior glenoid insufficiency, it must be placed extra-articularly. If suture anchors cannot be placed because of glenoid bone loss, then the suture may be anchored under the screw holding the bone block. (From Warner JP, Marks PH. Management of complications of surgery for anterior shoulder instability. *Sports Med Arthrosc Rev* 1993;1:272–292, with permission.)

performed. Closure of the rotator interval and superior capsular reefing should be performed if these structures are open or appear lax. Anatomic subscapularis closure is recommended. At present, because of operative complications and higher risk of recurrent instability, the Bristow procedure is not recommended in a large majority of these patients. However, with significant anterior/inferior glenoid bone loss, a Bristow or bone-grafting procedure may be used to augment the earlier described capsular procedures. If necessary, the graft must be placed external to the capsular repair, at about the 4 o'clock position, just far enough medial to the glenoid rim so that impingement with the humeral head does not occur (Fig. 3). Fortunately, instances requiring a bone graft are quite rare.

Results

A review of 23 patients with recurrent anterior instability after prior repair treated with this protocol by one of the senior authors was recently completed (25). A Bankart lesion was identified in 83% of patients at the time of index revision and in all three patients who underwent reoperation for repeated dislocation after revision surgery. Additionally, 83% had significant capsular laxity. Reflecting these findings, a Bankart procedure coupled with capsular shift was performed most commonly at reoperation. Four patients had only capsular laxity as a source of recurrent instability, and in these patients, a laterally based capsular shift was performed. The final clinical rating was excellent or good in 78% of patients, and even among those patients whose initial revision failed, good results were obtained with reoperation.

Overview

In summary, careful attention to precise Bankart repair, adequate capsular tensioning, reliable surgical implants, and appropriate rehabilitation will help to avoid primary surgical failure in patients with unidirectional anterior instability. With recurrent anterior instability or dislocation after a prior repair, nonoperative management may be indicated initially, depending on the patient's functional status and the type of previous surgery. Revision surgery in this setting is reliable and should be directed at the specific pathology of instability in the shoulder. Most often, a Bankart repair coupled with a capsular shift will be required. Successful results may be expected in 80% of patients or more.

Multidirectional Instability

Nonoperative Treatment

In a patient with MDI who demonstrates symptomatic recurrent instability after a prior repair, the most important issue to determine is whether this recurrence is on a traumatic or atraumatic basis. This seemingly straightforward issue is not always easily determined. Many patients *report* that some traumatic event led to the recurrence of their symptoms. However, often the "trauma" of this event is quite minimal. A good rule to apply is that only if the event seems sufficient in itself to have caused a subluxation or dislocation in a normal shoulder should the recurrence be designated traumatic. The importance of this determination is that only with truly traumatic recurrent dislocations in a patient with MDI should early revision surgery be considered. All other patients should be entered in an aggressive rehabilitation program, with revision reserved for those with continuing problems.

Conservative management of these patients begins with an appropriate rehabilitation program. If a redislocation has occurred, the arm should be immobilized only until pain and swelling have subsided enough to allow exercises to begin. Initial stages of therapy should be aimed at restoring motion, particularly rotational movements opposite to a direction of apprehension in the patient. Conversely, no aggressive attempts at restoring motion that produces apprehension or subluxation should be attempted in these patients. Strengthening programs must be directed at both the rotator cuff and periscapular muscles. Strengthening must be performed in the individual patient's ''safe zone'' (those glenohumeral positions that do not provoke apprehension). Strengthening is typically started with rubber tubing exercises and then progresses to Nautilus and isokinetic exercises. Free weights must be used cautiously early in rehabilitation, as they may cause symptomatic inferior subluxation in some patients. Isometric strengthening may be used, as well as teaching patients to ''hold'' their shoulders in place. Exercises performed in the plane of the scapula will stabilize the joint and avoid apprehension. Dependent weights that create inferior subluxation should be avoided.

Scapulothoracic mechanics are often disturbed in these patients, and in some, these abnormalities may worsen their glenohumeral instability. For this reason, in addition to strengthening of the scapular stabilizers, scapular-positioning exercises should be reviewed with the patient. These exercises assist patients in ''setting'' the entire shoulder girdle in a safe position during physical activities.

In the overhead athlete who has had recurrent subluxation events despite prior surgery, in addition to rehabilitation, some consideration must be given to changing the athlete's mechanics to continue in the particular sport. The overhead thrower may need to drop down to a lower delivery trajectory and attempt to incorporate greater leg and thoracic components in the pitching motion. Stroke change in persistently symptomatic swimmers may allow them to continue in their desired sport without painful subluxation. Ultimately, in some athletes for whom both rehabilitation and surgery have failed, removal from sport may be necessary, typically with resolution of their symptoms.

Finally, especially in the atraumatic globally lax patient, counseling in regard to the nature of the shoulder problem is vital. Activity modification is a vital tool in helping to limit subluxation events and shoulder pain. Apprehensive positions should be avoided in nearly all activities of daily living. This may require avoidance of all overhead activities for patients with anterior and anteroinferior subluxation. Objects weighing more than 5 to 10 pounds normally carried at the side (such as a heavy briefcase) must be abandoned by patients with significant inferior subluxation. Similarly, crossed-arm and forward-flexion activities must be avoided in patients with posterior subluxation. Patients with painful nocturnal subluxation events may be given an immobilizer to wear at night. In summary, the more patients are able to understand their shoulder-instability problems, the more they are able to avoid provocative activities in daily life.

Revision Operative Treatment

Indications

Revision stabilization in recurrent instability in patients with MDI should be undertaken only after careful consideration of anatomic and functional factors. In patients in whom a traumatic redislocation has disrupted a previously well-functioning repair or in whom an obvious anatomic lesion (such as subscapularis rupture) exists, consideration to early revision surgery may be given. In the majority of patients with MDI, however, the indication for revision surgery is the persistence of painful shoulder subluxation, affecting activities of daily life, that has failed to respond both to a supervised rehabilitation program and to activity modification. This conservative approach is vital, given the technical demands and unpredictable results of revision surgery in this patient group.

Techniques

The goal of revision surgery in this difficult setting is to stabilize the glenohumeral joint in all directions. This mandates that translation be diminished symmetrically at the completion of the repair. Although repair must not be so tight as to restrain glenohumeral motion excessively, given the capsular deficiency inherent to many of these patients, ''a little too tight is better than a little too loose,'' as long as the tightness is both functional and concentric.

Arthroscopic techniques now play little role in revision surgery in patients with MDI. Certainly laser capsular shrinkage and suture capsular imbrication procedures are now being used on an investigational basis in some patients. However, because of limitations in addressing the rotator interval capsule and in control of the magnitude and direction of capsular shift, they are not recommended for revision cases in which no less than an ideal repair must be achieved.

The surgical approach is determined by the pattern of instability present. This determination is based on the patient's symptoms, provocative awake examination, as well as the examination under anesthesia. In the absence of posterior-predominant pattern (type II), an anterior approach is generally chosen. Positioning is typically in the modified beach-chair position with the posterior portion of the shoulder fully accessible, should a combined approach be required. The technique of the anterior approach is carried out as outlined earlier in the section on revision in unidirectional anterior instability. Recurrent anteroinferior instability (type I) is managed by anterior capsular shift coupled with repair of any identifiable anatomic instability lesion (i.e., Bankart repair). A laterally based T-plasty is most commonly used, except when an accompanying Bankart repair is to be performed, in which case, the capsular shift may be based either medially or laterally (Fig. 4). Arm positioning during the shift is typically 30 to 40 degrees of external rotation with the arm abducted about 40 degrees in the scapular plane. The T-plasty is performed in the manner described by Neer (26,27) for primary MDI repairs. The inferior instability component must be addressed by superior capsular reefing and rotator interval closure, in addition to the inferior capsular tightening achieved through the cap-

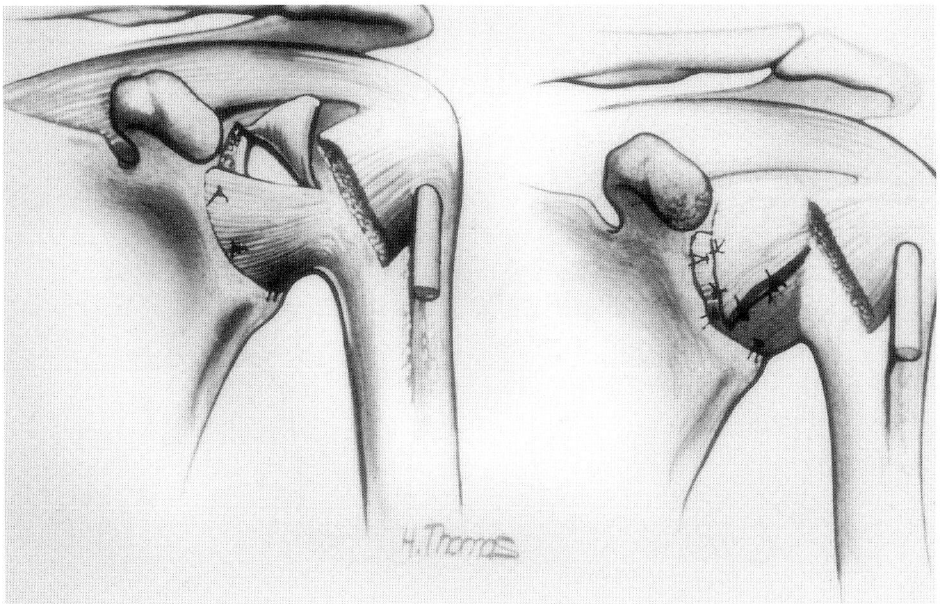

FIG. 4. T-Plasty repair shifts the inferior capsular flap superiorly and medially and the superior capsular flap inferiorly and medially. When a Bankart lesion is present, the vertical limb of the capsular incision may be placed medially (as demonstrated here) and fixed to the glenoid rim. Alternatively, in cases of capsular laxity without Bankart lesion, the vertical limb of the T-plasty may be placed laterally and fixed to the humerus. (From Altchek DW, Warren RF, Skyhar MJ, Ortiz G. T-Plasty anterior repair for anterior and inferior instability of the shoulder. *J Bone Joint Surg [Am]* 1991;73:105–111, with permission.)

sular T-plasty. If inferior translation remains increased despite these maneuvers, we found that reefing the superior capsular structures into the coracoacromial ligament will typically serve to dampen this motion.

In global instability (type III), stabilization is begun through superior capsular reefing and rotator interval closure in addition to the anterior and inferior capsular tightening through the capsular T-plasty. To tighten the posterior capsule through this technique, the capsular incision must be taken down past the 6 o'clock position to a point through the insertion of the posterior band of the inferior glenohumeral ligament. Obviously, care must be taken during this maneuver to protect actively the axillary nerve, either by direct identification or through placement of an elevator inferiorly. Arm positioning during the shift is similar to that used in type I patients, however, with slightly less external rotation. At the completion of the anterior procedure, glenohumeral translation must be critically assessed, specifically in regard to posterior translation. Rarely, if posterior translation remains excessive because of marked capsular laxity, posterior approach and capsular shift should be performed as outlined later. In rare cases in which capsular tissue is markedly deficient, anterior and posterior reconstruction may be performed with a hamstrings tendon graft passed through bone tunnels in the glenoid and humerus (Fig. 5). The tendon graft functions both as a posterior check rein and as an anterior reconstruction of the middle and inferior glenohumeral ligaments. Bone-block procedures are reserved for significant glenoid erosion or bone loss. Glenoid or humeral osteotomy would not appear to offer much success in this patient group, except in some patients with bony dysplasia.

As stated earlier, the posterior approach is indicated in MDI-revision cases in patients with a posterior-predominant instability pattern (type II) and in patents with global MDI (type III) in whom anterior and inferior capsular procedures fail to reduce posterior instability adequately. Currently, a vertical skin incision is used. The incision is created midway between the lateral border of the acromion and the posterior axillary skin crease. The superficial deltoid fascia is identified, and the deltoid is then split from the scapular spine inferolaterally, along the line of its fibers.

Deeper dissection now reveals the infraspinatus and teres minor tendons. If tissue quality is good and no significant scar from prior surgery exists, the interval between these two tendons may now be developed to expose the posterior capsule (Fig. 6). If tissue quality is poor or scarring prevents definition of this interval, the infraspinatus tendon may be incised in a manner similar to that of the subscapularis during anterior exposure to gain access to the posterior capsule.

A T-shaped capsular incision is then made. The vertical limb of this incision is placed medially near the glenoid to facilitate repair of any posterior capsular stripping (a ''reverse'' Bankart lesion). The capsule must be incised from the glenoid down past the insertion of the posterior band of the inferior glenohumeral ligament. The arm is then po-

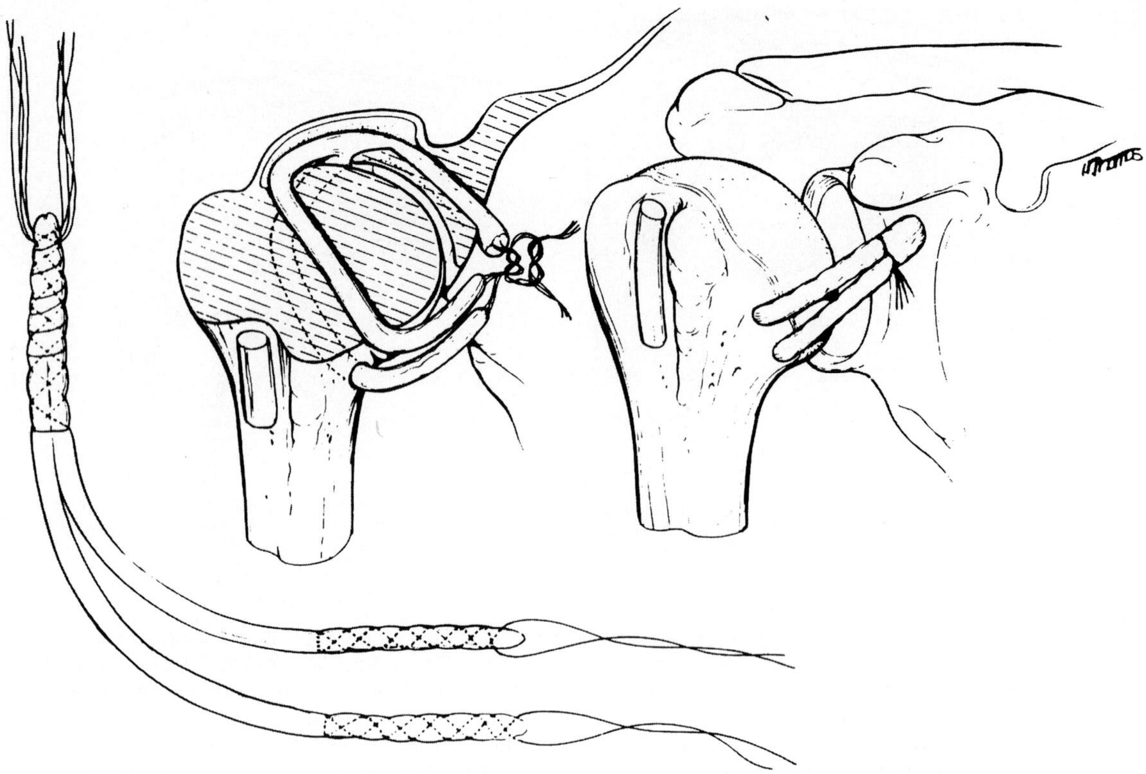

FIG. 5. In cases with recurrent refractory shoulder instability with marked capsular insufficiency after multiple operative procedures, a semitendinosus–gracilis autograft may be formed and placed as a reconstruction of the glenohumeral ligaments. (From Warner JP, Cooper RA, Warren RF. Pitfalls and complications of surgery for anterior shoulder instability. *Tech Orthop* 1997;12:7–32, with permission.)

sitioned in neutral rotation and 30 to 40 degrees of abduction, and the T-plasty capsular shift effected. The inferior capsular limb is shifted superiorly and medially and reattached to the glenoid (typically by using suture anchors). The superior limb is then overlapped to reinforce the repair (Fig. 7). If residual laxity exists after shift of the inferior capsular limb, a lateral vertical capsular incision may be created to effect an H-plasty, which will then allow further tightening of the posterior inferior capsule.

The capsular repair may be reinforced with the infraspinatus tendon if the tissue is markedly deficient or if separation of the capsule from this structure during exposure was impossible. If a large bony defect is found on the posterior glenoid, a bone-block procedure may be used to augment capsular repair with tricortical graft obtained from the scapular spine. The bone graft must be placed *external* to the capsular repair, in the posterior inferior glenoid quadrant, to increase the articulating surface of the glenoid at a point contiguous with its curvature. Glenoid osteotomy is rarely used because of both a high complication rate and a failure to control instability. We have not found humeral osteotomy to be helpful in the management of patients with MDI.

Finally, as discussed previously, it is vital to assess stability after the capsular procedure is completed. Occasionally, the inferior component of instability will not be reduced sufficiently by the posteroinferior capsular shift. In these instances, a combined approach must again be used with an anterior approach to close the rotator interval and reef the anterosuperior capsule to reduce inferior subluxation.

Results

A review of patients with MDI treated with this protocol by one of the senior authors was recently completed (25). The patient group consisted of 21 shoulders in 20 patients. Recurrent instability had developed at a mean of only 16 months after the initial stabilization and was traumatic in only two patients. Revision surgery included selective capsular shift in 11 patients, Bankart repair in five, anterior/posterior graft reconstruction in three, and posterior bone block/capsular shift in two. Of patients, 100% demonstrated significant capsular laxity. A Bankart lesion was found in only 24% of patients. At a mean follow-up of 61.5 months, there were only nine (39%) good or excellent results despite multiple reoperations. Four patients ultimately went on to glenohumeral fusion.

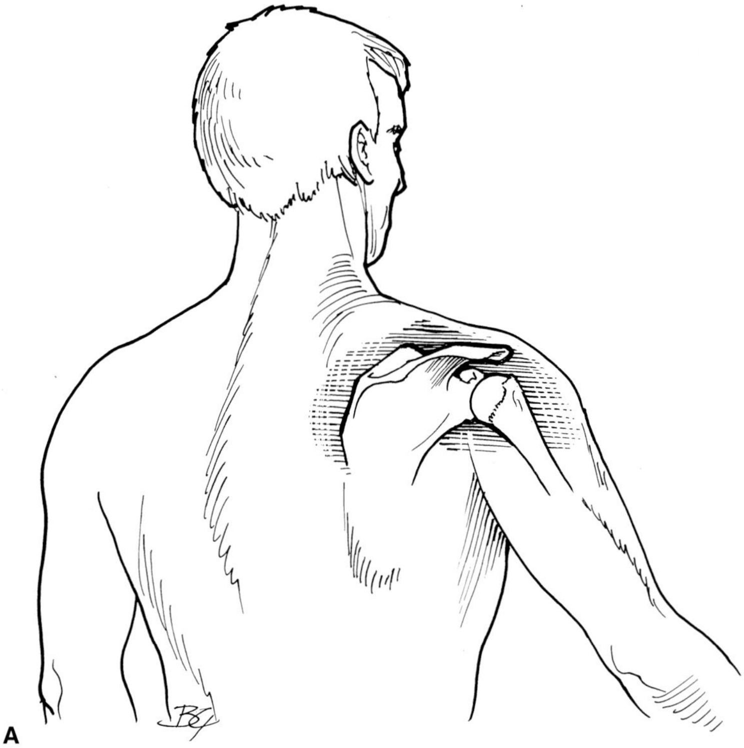

FIG. 6. A, B: When a posterior approach is required, a vertical skin incision is created midway between the lateral border of the acromion and the posterior axillary skin crease. After the deltoid is split along the line of its fibers, the interval between the infraspinatus and teres minor tendons is developed to expose the posterior capsule.

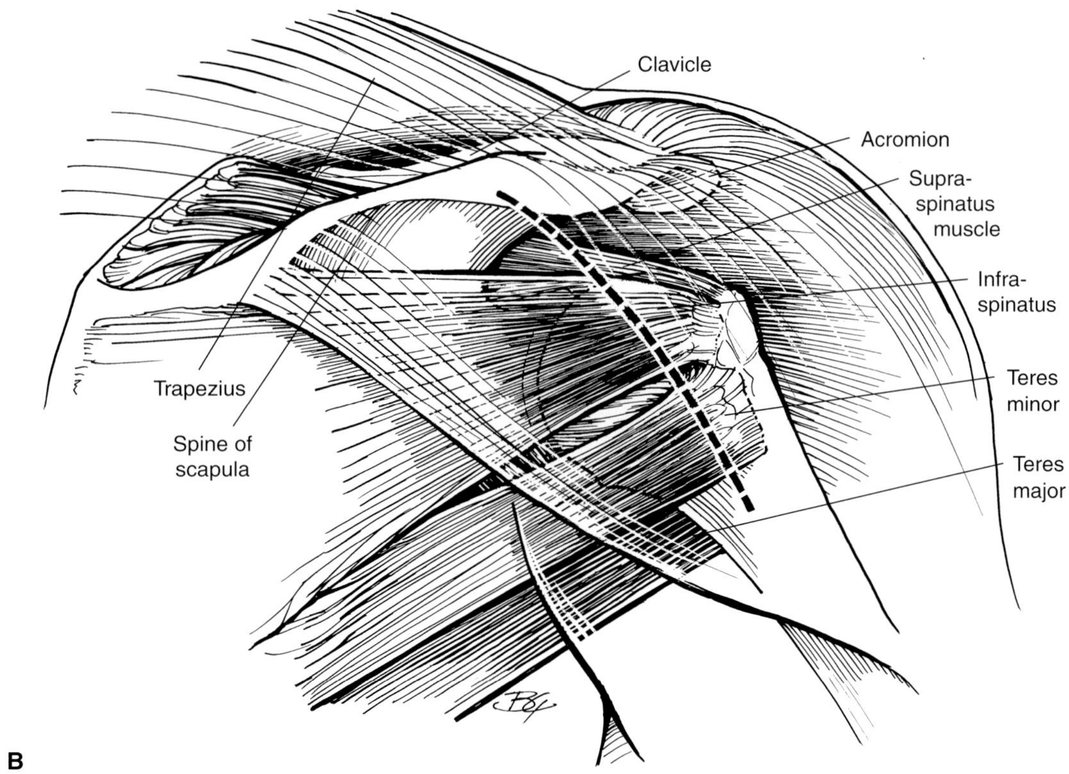

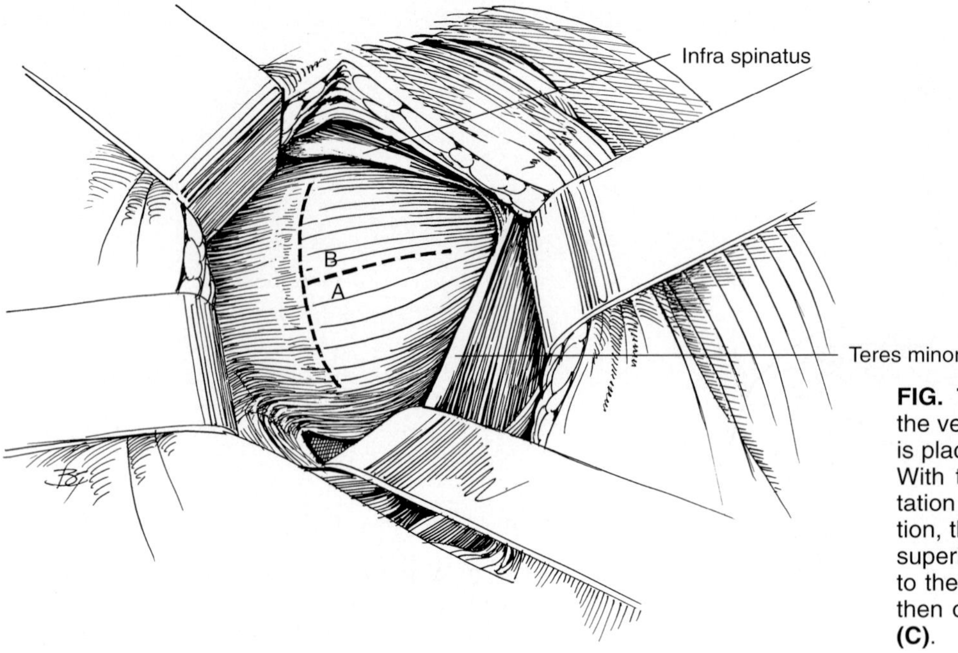

FIG. 7. A–E: In a posterior T-plasty, the vertical limb of the capsular incision is placed medially near the glenoid **(A)**. With the arm positioned in neutral rotation and 30 to 40 degrees of abduction, the inferior capsular limb is shifted superiorly and medially and reattached to the glenoid **(B)**. The superior limb is then overlapped to reinforce the repair **(C)**.

A

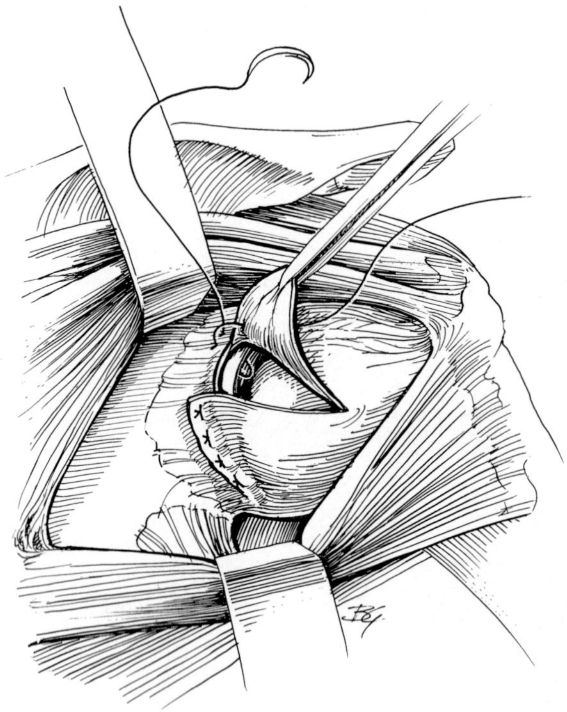

B

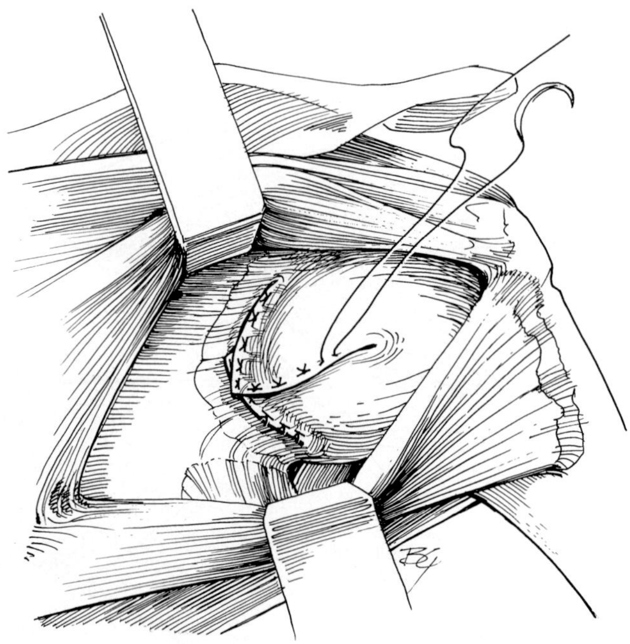

C

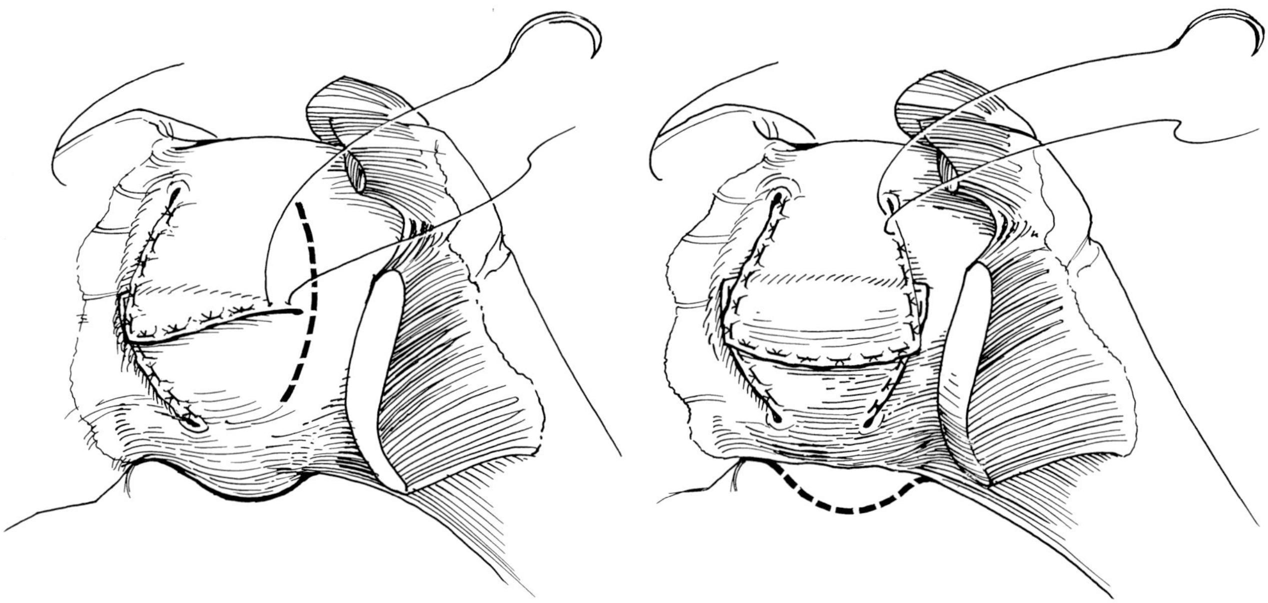

D E

FIG. 7. *Continued.* If residual laxity exists after shift of the inferior capsular limb, a lateral vertical capsular incision may be created to effect an H-plasty, which will then allow further tightening of the posterior inferior capsule **(D, E)**.

When compared with our revision results in patients with unidirectional anterior instability, many illustrative differences between the groups were noted. Our failures in the MDI group occurred much earlier postoperatively, at an average of 16 months, in contrast to 35.5 months for the unidirectional group. Trauma played a role in recurrence in only two (9.5%) of 21 MDI shoulders in comparison with 12 (54%) of 23 in the unidirectional group.

Revision surgery failure was much more common and difficult to treat in the MDI group than in the unidirectional anterior group. In the anterior-dislocator group, only four patients (17%) recurred at an average of 51 months after revision. Each was in a traumatic athletic event, and certainly, because of their good postoperative function, they may have been exposed to repeated trauma in sports. Three of these four patients are functioning well after reoperation.

In contrast, in the MDI group, we had 13 revision surgery failures (62%) at an average of only 11 months. None of these involved a traumatic event. Some 24 reoperations were subsequently performed in these patients, including 14 for instability. Whereas ultimate improvements in five patients were noted, early repeated failure was common, and four patients required fusion for refractory instability coupled with glenohumeral arthrosis. Overall, 47% of patients with MDI had radiographic evidence of degenerative joint changes at most recent follow-up.

Overview

In summary, primary repair failure is higher in the patients with MDI, particularly in those with "atraumatic" instability. Inherent capsular deficiency does play a major role in failure, although lack of attention to degree and technique of capsular tightening also leads to recurrent instability after primary repair. An aggressive rehabilitation program as well as patient counseling in regard to activity modification is the best treatment for the majority of these patients. In patients for whom nonoperative management fails, it is imperative that both the patient and the surgeon understand the goals and potential complications of revision surgery because of the high rate of failure and need for repeated revision surgery.

When revision stabilization is undertaken, symmetric capsular tightening is the goal. It is vital to address *all* existent directions of instability at one operative procedure, as any instability left alone is likely to become symptomatic in the postoperative period. The patient should be willing to accept moderate motion loss in exchange for glenohumeral stability.

Unidirectional Posterior Instability

Nonoperative Treatment

Most patients with recurrent posterior subluxation after an operative repair should be entered initially into an aggressive rehabilitation program aimed at strengthening the rotator-cuff musculature and deltoid while selectively "ignoring" the more powerful internal rotators of the glenohumeral joint. The periscapular muscles must also be strengthened, and scapular-stabilization techniques reviewed with the patient. Avoidance of the activity precipitating the painful posterior subluxation events (i.e., the bench press in weight-lifters, pass-blocking drills in football linemen, and the butterfly stroke in swimmers) may help to alleviate symptoms. Occasionally, protective strapping, limiting forward flexion of the shoulder, may be useful as well.

Revision Operative Treatment

Indications

The indication for revision operative management in this group is recurrent *symptomatic* episodes of posterior involuntary subluxation that has failed to improve despite high-level compliance with an appropriate rehabilitation program. In patients with no significant pain or disability related to their shoulder instability, a concern of significant voluntary muscular instability, poor rehabilitation compliance, or persistence of a marked risk factor for recurrence (i.e., poorly controlled seizure disorder), revision surgery should be avoided.

In a minority of patients with recurrent instability after a prior repair, consideration of early revision may be appropriate. These patients include those with an obvious traumatic failure of a previously well-functioning repair. Additionally, if the prior stabilization had a documented history of poor results (i.e., staple capsulorrhaphy or reverse Putti–Platt) or was an arthroscopic procedure that appears to have failed, consideration to moving directly to operative treatment is indeed reasonable if symptomatic instability exists.

Techniques

Arthroscopic techniques play little to no role in the treatment of recurrent posterior instability revision surgery. However, diagnostic arthroscopy may be helpful to note the labral status and degree of detachment before opening. The surgical approach of open revision surgery is as outlined earlier in the section on MDI. The reverse Bankart lesion, although uncommon, does occur and may be persistently painful if not addressed. The majority of patients in this group will be treated with capsular shift. The capsular-shift technique also was outlined previously. The key to the technique is adequate dissection of the capsule inferiorly into the axilla to allow subsequent advancement (Fig. 8). Bone-block or grafting procedures are used only with posterior glenoid bone loss and are rarely indicated. The repair should be assessed critically at completion and consideration given to an anterior approach and tightening of the anterosuperior capsule if stability after an appropriate posterior procedure remains unacceptable. Although it is uncommonly needed, this may be a useful adjunct in some patients.

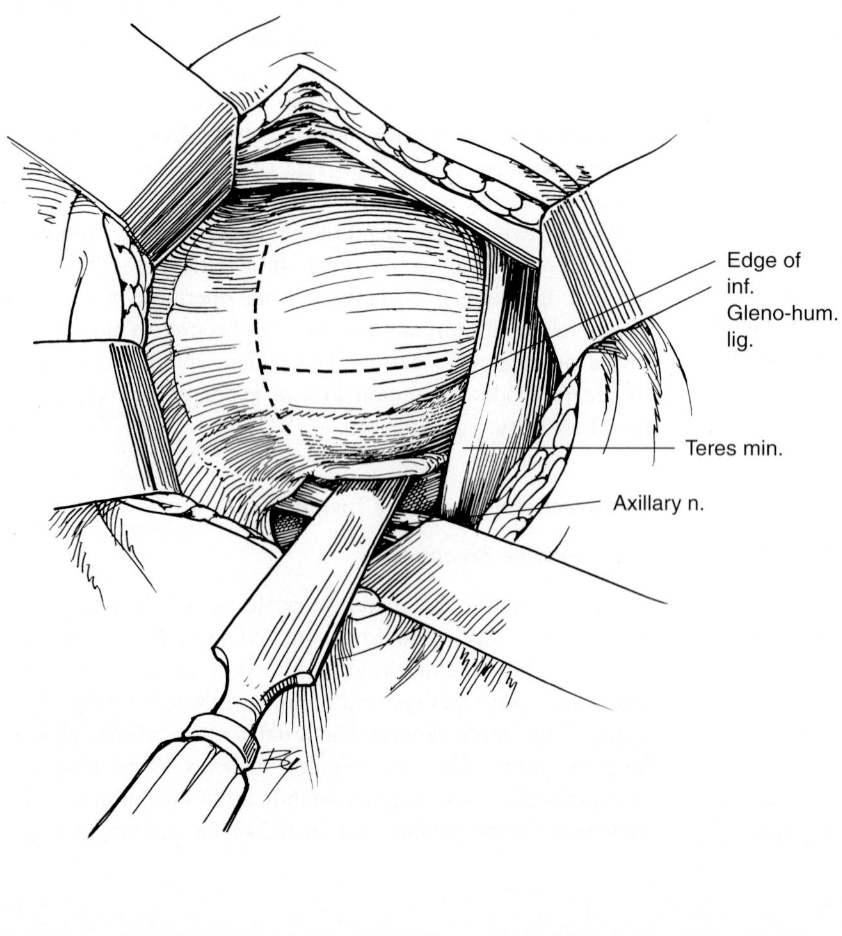

FIG. 8. In a posterior capsular shift, the capsule must be incised inferiorly *past* the insertion of the posterior band of the inferior glenohumeral ligament. Adequate dissection of the capsule inferiorly into the axilla is vital to allow subsequent capsular advancement. The axillary nerve may be protected with a periosteal elevator to allow capsular incision under direct vision.

Results

Few data are found in the literature regarding the results of revision posterior stabilization. Both Hawkins (28) and Bigliani (29) did not report the results of revision surgery separately from those patients who underwent primary repair in their studies on posterior instability. In the study of Fronek et al. (15), one patient had undergone a prior posterior repair and was treated successfully with posterior capsulorrhaphy and posterior bone block. In a recent review of one of our senior author's revision population (25), we identified three patients with recurrent posterior instability after a prior posterior repair. One patient had a successful outcome, and one a fair outcome after posterior capsulorrhaphy (combined with bone block in one). Multiple procedures failed in a third patient with Tourette's syndrome who developed painful arthritic change and ultimately underwent salvage glenohumeral fusion.

Overview

In summary, although primary repair failure is more common with unidirectional posterior instability, careful patient selection and the use of newer posterior capsular-shift procedures can limit this problem. With recurrent posterior instability or dislocation after a prior repair, nonoperative management is indicated in the majority of patients. Revision surgery typically consists of posterior capsular shift secured to a well-adhered labrum or directly to bone. Glenoid and humeral osteotomies have not been successful in our hands. With appropriate techniques and patient selection, improvement may be expected, although there remain few published series of posterior revision stabilizations.

SPECIAL CONSIDERATIONS

Instability Opposite to the Direction of a Prior Repair

Incidence

The problem of instability *opposite* to the direction of a prior repair is fortunately a rare cause of recurrent *instability* after shoulder stabilization. Instead, most patients with a fixed loss of external rotation after a repair have painful glenohumeral *arthritis* associated with posterior glenohumeral subluxation.

Reports in the literature regarding this problem are rare, and almost all document posterior instability after prior anterior repair. Rowe et al. (19), in his long-term review of 162 shoulders treated anteriorly with Bankart repair, reported no cases of posterior instability at follow-up. In contrast, symptomatic posterior instability has been reported to complicate Putti–Platt procedures, although more typically, this subluxation is asymptomatic on its own and reflective instead of glenohumeral arthritis (8). Young and Rockwood (5) documented posterior instability complicating the Bristow procedure in four patients. Similarly, seven patients in Hawkin's series (28) of 50 shoulders had undergone prior anterior repair. Finally, three of Altchek's (10) four failures in patients with anteroinferior MDI treated with anterior capsular T-plasty developed recurrent *posterior* subluxation.

Etiology

Although these reports are limited, they highlight the etiology of instability opposite in direction to a prior repair. *Overtightening* of the primary repair certainly plays an important role, as some element of contracture is seen in many of these patients, particularly those with previous unidirectional anterior instability. This contracture may affect capsular or extracapsular structures or both. Capsular overtightening typically relates to arm malposition at the time of capsular shift or Bankart repair and subsequent overly aggressive shortening of the capsule. Closure of the rotator interval can result in a fixed loss of external rotation if it is performed with the arm internally rotated. Extracapsular contracture typically relates to nonanatomic closure and shortening of either the subscapularis or infraspinatus tendon during repair. *Misdiagnosis* of the direction of instability at the time of primary repair also plays a role in some failures and is a mistake that should be avoidable in all patients, given an appropriate history and physical examination. Finally, in patients with MDI, *the failure to recognize and address all directions of glenohumeral instability* at primary repair may result in recurrence opposite to it. Contracture related to the repair plays a smaller role in these patients, and instead, subluxation develops in response to appropriately tightened opposite structures. This again highlights the importance of critically assessing glenohumeral laxity in all directions intraoperatively after capsular shift in patients with MDI. Laxity in the opposite direction is addressed by the capsular shift if performed properly in most patients. Symmetrically restrained glenohumeral translation must be present at the completion of the primary procedure to avoid this complication.

Nonoperative Treatment

The results of operative treatment in this group are frequently poor. For this reason, every attempt at maximal rehabilitation should be made in this group before considering revision surgery. Additionally, patients should be educated in regard to the avoidance of provocative apprehension positions through activity modification whenever feasible.

Revision Operative Treatment

Indications

Revision surgical management is indicated only in patients with recurrent painful episodes of subluxation that have failed to respond to appropriate rehabilitation and activity modification. Surgical intervention requires both correcting any contracture that exists from the prior repair and then effectively stabilizing the new direction of subluxation.

Techniques

Contracture release is typically undertaken first. If the contracture is capsular, arthroscopic release may be feasible and more controlled than formal open release. In extracapsular or combined contracture, formal open release may be required. Tendons may be lengthened through a variety of techniques including Z-plasty or V-Y lengthening. If a prior Magnuson–Stack has been performed, osteotomizing the lesser tuberosity is *not* recommended, and instead, subscapularis lengthening should be performed. It is vital that contracture release be controlled, as overzealous release may result in recurrent instability in this direction as well. General guidelines are to achieve external rotation to 30 degrees at zero degrees of elevation for an anterior release and internal rotation to 30 degrees at 90 degrees of elevation for a posterior release.

After contracture release, stabilization should be undertaken as described earlier. Procedures will be primarily directed at reducing capsular laxity and addressing any anatomic concerns (Bankart lesion, glenoid bone loss), as described previously. Once again it is vital to assess stability in all directions at the completion of the repair. Symmetrically restrained glenohumeral translation must be obtained before completing the repair.

Results

Reports of revision surgery for instability opposite a prior repair are extremely limited in the literature. The Young and Rockwood (5) report included four patients with posterior instability after a Bristow. Only one patient had a successful initial revision surgery. The other three patients required multiple operations, with one patient requiring arthroplasty for arthritic change. In contrast, Fronek et al. (15) reported satisfactory results in three patients undergoing posterior stabilization for posterior instability after prior anterior repair.

In a recent review of our revision population, we identified six patients with recurrent instability opposite a prior repair (25). In two, the new instability was anterior, and in four, posterior. Two patients from Fronek's earlier article were included in this study; one could not be located. Revision operative management consisted of combined release and capsulorrhaphy, as detailed earlier. At present follow-up, satisfactory results were found in only one patient. Five of the six required one or more further operations subsequent to their first revision. Persistent contracture and instability coupled with arthritic change were the primary reasons for the poor results. Two patients in this group required salvage glenohumeral fusion.

Overview

In summary, instability opposite a prior repair is fortunately a rare cause of failure of shoulder stabilization. Contracture frequently accompanies the instability when it occurs. Careful attention to surgical technique and critically assessing the adequacy of primary surgery may help to limit this complication. Depending on the degree of contracture, early release may prevent the complication of arthritis and new instability. In most patients, treatment should initially be through rehabilitation and activity modification. In patients for whom nonoperative modalities fail, revision stabilization may be attempted. Revision surgery must address both contracture and the instability. Results are often poor, with recurrent instability, contracture, and arthrosis all occurring in some patients.

Arthrodesis and Arthroplasty as Salvage Procedures

Unfortunately, despite following the indications and techniques outlined, revision shoulder stabilization surgery will fail in some patients. Infrequently, this failure may be attributed to a discrete, traumatic event (most commonly in anterior dislocators involved in contact sports), causing a recurrent dislocation. In the majority of cases, however, surgical failure is much more difficult both to define and to treat.

Most patients for whom revision surgery fails, rather than having one recurrent traumatic dislocation, have complaints of pain and episodic subluxation. Frequently, some element of contracture and glenohumeral arthritis may be present. Additionally, thoracic outlet–type neuropathy may be present in this patient group. These lower trunk brachial plexus symptoms may be caused by traction related to persistent inferior shoulder instability or soft-tissue contracture about the plexus from previous surgeries or both.

Aside from the patients with truly traumatic repeated dislocations, operative management in this group is not likely to be rewarding, and all attempts at a comprehensive conservative management program, as outlined earlier, should be given. In patients with a reflex sympathetic dystrophy–type presentation, sympathetic blockade may offer some assistance in pain control.

With disabling, painful instability that has not responded to well-performed revision surgery, coupled with glenohumeral degenerative change and contracture, both arthroplasty and arthrodesis play some role as salvage procedures.

Indications and Techniques

The indications for shoulder arthroplasty after a failed revision stabilization are pain related to contracture and arthrosis of the glenohumeral joint. Arthroplasty is not used if a significant element of persistent instability is present in the shoulder or if prior surgeries have led to a severely deficient rotator cuff or significant neurologic injury. Even in the absence of instability, shoulder arthroplasty in this group is a technically demanding procedure because of the contracture often associated with postdislocation arthritis. The results in this patient group are inferior to those obtained in patients with inflammatory arthritis or osteoarthritis because of problems with contracture, glenoid erosion, and possible instability of the prosthesis. Technical considerations regarding arthroplasty techniques are detailed in Chapter 29.

Shoulder arthrodesis is primarily indicated in the multiply operated-on patient with a painful and persistently unstable shoulder despite appropriate revision surgery. Additionally, it may be indicated in patients for whom prosthetic replacement has failed. A variety of techniques for arthrodesis have been described; however, the AO technique is primarily used today (30). The patient is positioned in the beach-chair position. A long incision is made posteriorly along the scapular spine and extended laterally over the acromion and humeral head down to the level of the deltoid insertion. After appropriate preparation of the humeral head, glenoid, and acromion, combined with autogenous bone grafting, the humeral head is preliminarily fixed to the glenoid by using cancellous screws and washers. A pelvic reconstruction or dynamic compression plate is then fashioned and fixed superiorly to the scapular spine, acromion, and laterally to the humerus. A second plate may be added posteriorly if needed for rotational control.

The ideal position for arthrodesis should allow the hand to reach both the mouth, the neck line, and the pants pocket. This approximates 15 to 20 degrees of abduction, 25 degrees of flexion, and 45 degrees of internal rotation. It is important to note that many different positions have been recommended, in part because of the difficulty of defining the exact relation of the humerus to the scapula at the time of surgery. For this reason, after preliminary fixation of the arthrodesis, it is vital to check that the hand may reach both the mouth and greater trochanter. This is best done in a beach-chair position as it makes it easier to determine the ultimate range of motion.

Results

Results from fusion, although far from optimal, can be rewarding (31). Reported fusion rates with present techniques are greater than 90%, and patient acceptance is fair (25,30,31). Thoracic outlet–type neuropathy due to persistent inferior subluxation is typically eliminated by arthrodesis. Pain syndromes, not related to degenerative changes or subluxation, may, however, persist despite successful fusion. Functional level in regard to activities of daily life may be improved yet still remain substantially limited.

REFERENCES

1. Morrey BF, Janes JM. Recurrent anterior dislocation of the shoulder: long term follow-up of the Putti-Platt and Bankart procedures. *J Bone Joint Surg [Am]* 1976;58:252–256.
2. Rowe CR, Zarins B, Ciullo JV. Recurrent anterior dislocation of the shoulder after surgical repair. *J Bone Joint Surg [Am]* 1984;66 (2): 159–168.
3. Hawkins RH, Hawkins RJ. Failed anterior reconstruction for shoulder instability. *J Bone Joint Surg [Br]* 1985;67:709–714.
4. Walch G, Charret P, Pietro-Paoli H, Dejour H. La luxation recidivante anterieure de l'epaule. Le recidives post-operatoires. *Rev Chir Orthop* 1986;72:541–555.
5. Young DC, Rockwood CA. Complications of a failed Bristow procedure and their management. *J Bone Joint Surg [Am]* 1991;73 (7): 969–981.
6. Wirth MA, Blatter G, Rockwood CA. The capsular imbrication procedure for recurrent anterior instability of the shoulder. *J Bone Joint Surg [Am]* 1996;78:246–259.
7. Miller LS, Donohue JR, Good RP, et al. The Magnuson-Stack procedure for recurrent glenohumeral dislocation. *Am J Sports Med* 1984;12:133–137.
8. Brav EA. An evaluation of the Putti-Platt procedure for recurrent dislocation of the shoulder. *J Bone Joint Surg [Am]* 1985;37:731–741.
9. Lusardi DA, Wirth MA, Wurtz D, Rockwood CA. Loss of external rotation following anterior capsulorrhaphy of the shoulder. *J Bone Joint Surg [Am]* 1993;75:1185–1192.
10. Altchek DW, Warren RF, Skyhar MJ, Ortiz G. T-Plasty modification of the Bankart procedure for multidirectional instability of the anterior and inferior types. *J Bone Joint Surg [Am]* 1991;73 (1):105–112.
11. Lebar RD, Alexander AH. Multidirectional instability: results of inferior capsular shift in an active-duty population. *Am J Sports Med* 1992;20:193–198.
12. O'Driscoll SW, Evans DC. Long-term results of staple capsulorrhaphy for anterior instability of the shoulder. *J Bone Joint Surg [Am]* 1993;75 (2):249–258.
13. Banas MP, Dalladorf PG, Sebastianelli WJ, Dehaven KE. Long-term follow-up of the modified Bristow procedure. *Am J Sports Med* 1993;21 (5):666–671.
14. Speer KP, Warren RF, Pagnani M, Warner JP. An arthroscopic technique for stabilization of the shoulder with a bioabsorbable tack. *J Bone Joint Surg [Am]* 1996;78:1801–1807.
15. Fronek J, Warren RF, Bowen M. Posterior subluxation of the glenohumeral joint. *J Bone Joint Surg [Am]* 1989;71:205–216.
16. Warner JJ, Deng XH, Warren RF, Torzilli PA. Static capsuloligamentous restraints to superior-inferior translation of the glenohumeral joint. *Am J Sports Med* 1992;20 (6):675–685.
17. Weber SC, Caspari RB. A biomechanical evaluation of the restraints to posterior shoulder dislocation. *Arthroscopy* 1989;5 (2):115–121.
18. O'Brien SJ, Neves MC, Arnoczky SP, et al. The anatomy and histology of the inferior glenohumeral ligament complex of the shoulder. *Am J Sports Med* 1990;18 (5):449–456.
19. Rowe CR, Patel D, Southmayd WW. The Bankart procedure: a long-term end-result study. *J Bone Joint Surg [Am]* 1978;60 (1):1–16.
20. Greis PE, Dean M, Hawkins RJ. Subscapularis tendon disruption after Bankart reconstruction for anterior instability. *J Shoulder Elbow Surg* 1996;5 (3):219–222.
21. Harryman DT, Sidles JA, Harris SL, Matsen FA. The role of the rotator interval capsule in passive motion and stability of the shoulder. *J Bone Joint Surg [Am]* 1992;74:53–65.
22. Bell RH, Hawkins RJ. Collagen typing and production in MDI. *Orthop Trans* 1991;15:188.
23. Marshall JL, Johanson N, Wickiewicz TL, Tischler HM. Joint looseness: a function of the person and the joint. *Med Sci Sports Exerc* 1980;12:189–194.
24. Gerber C, Hersche O, Farron A. Isolated rupture of the subscapularis tendon. *J Bone Joint Surg [Am]* 1996;78:1015–1023.
25. Zabinski SJ, Callaway GH, Cohen S, Warren RF. Long-term results of revision shoulder stabilization. Presented at the Annual Meeting of the American Academy of Orthopaedic Surgeons, Orlando, Florida, February 1995.
26. Neer CS II, Foster CR. Inferior capsular shift for involuntary inferior and multidirectional instability of the shoulder: a preliminary report. *J Bone Joint Surg [Am]* 1990;62:897–908.
27. Cooper RA, Brems JJ. The inferior capsular-shift procedure for mul-

tidirectional instability of the shoulder. *J Bone Joint Surg [Am]* 1992;74 (10):1516–1521.

28. Hawkins RJ, Koppert G, Johnston G. Recurrent posterior instability (subluxation) of the shoulder. *J Bone Joint Surg [Am]* 1984;66 (2): 169–174.
29. Bigliani LU, Pollack RG, McIlveen SJ, Endrizzi D, Flatow EL. Shift of the posteroinferior aspect of the capsule for recurrent posterior glenohumeral instability. *J Bone Joint Surg [Am]* 1995;77:1011–1020.
30. Richards RR, Sherman RM, Hudson AR, Waddell JP. Shoulder arthrodesis using a pelvic reconstruction plate. *J Bone Joint Surg [Am]* 1988;70:416–421.
31. Cofield RH. Arthrodesis: operative and long-term functional results. *J Bone Joint Surg [Am]* 1979;61:668–677.

The Unstable Shoulder,
edited by R.F. Warren, E.V. Craig, and D.W. Altchek.
Lippincott–Raven Publishers, Philadelphia © 1999.

CHAPTER 27

Fracture—Dislocations of the Shoulder

David S. Pereira and Joseph D. Zuckerman

DEFINITION OF PATHOLOGY

Fracture–dislocations of the glenohumeral joint are characterized by a fracture of the proximal humerus in the presence of a complete loss of contact between the articular surfaces of the humeral head and glenoid. These injuries are usually associated with significant disruption of the soft tissues. Such traumatized tissues are prone to develop periarticular scarring and heterotopic bone formation. Repeated forceful attempts at closed reduction will increase the risk and severity of these problems. Therefore, although the first goal of treatment is prompt definitive reduction of the dislocation, multiple manipulations are to be avoided. Excessive force should never be used in the manipulation of fracture–dislocations, because it adds to the amount of soft-tissue injury, endangers the adjacent neurovascular structures, and risks displacing previously nondisplaced fractures.

Classification

Fracture–dislocations are classified by the direction of the dislocation (anterior versus posterior) and the type of proximal humerus fracture. The most systematic method to categorize these injuries is the Neer classification of proximal humeral fractures. Although the validity of this classification system has come under scrutiny recently because of reports of suboptimal interobserver reliability and intraobserver reproducibility (1,2), it remains the most widely used system. This classification, described by Neer in 1970 (3), built on the prior teachings of Codman (4), who divided the proximal humerus into four distinct fragments coinciding with the epiphyseal lines: the humeral head, the greater tuberosity, the lesser tuberosity, and the humeral shaft. It was Codman's belief that all fractures of the proximal humerus were some combination of these different fracture fragments.

Neer's classification, based on this premise, was the first to relate the anatomic and biomechanical considerations to prognosis and treatment guidelines. Emphasis was placed on determining the vascular viability of the humeral head, because osteonecrosis is a complication of which the incidence increases in direct proportion to fracture comminution and soft-tissue displacement (i.e., increasing number of displaced segments). Neer's classification, summarized in Figure 1, is based on the accurate identification on plain radiographs of the four segments of the proximal humerus and their relation to each other. A comprehensive series of radiographs in several planes, the trauma series, is therefore essential to proper evaluation. This classification system describes two-, three-, or four-part fractures and fracture–dislocations based on the number of displaced segments. A fracture is not considered displaced unless the fragment is displaced more than 1 cm or angulated more than 45 degrees. The dislocation is described by the direction of displacement of the humeral head (i.e., anterior or posterior). Comminution and the number of fracture fragments are significant only if they fulfill the displacement criteria. All fractures without displaced fragments are considered minimally displaced or ''one-part fractures.'' Neer also added a category of intra-articular fractures of the humeral head, which includes not only ''head-splitting'' fractures but also the much more common impression fractures frequently associated with dislocations. Posterolateral impression fractures occur in association with anterior dislocations, whereas anterolateral impression fractures occur in cases of posterior dislocation.

Last, because of the relevance to the vascular supply of the humeral head, Neer distinguished between intracapsular ''anatomic neck'' fractures (very high risk of osteonecrosis) and extracapsular ''surgical neck'' fractures (much lower risk of osteonecrosis).

D. S. Pereira: Department of Orthpaedics, Hospital for Joint Diseases, New York, New York 10003.

J. D. Zuckerman: Department of Orthopaedic Surgery, New York University School of Medicine, New York, New York 10016; and Department of Orthpaedic Surgery, Hospital for Joint Diseases, New York, New York 10003.

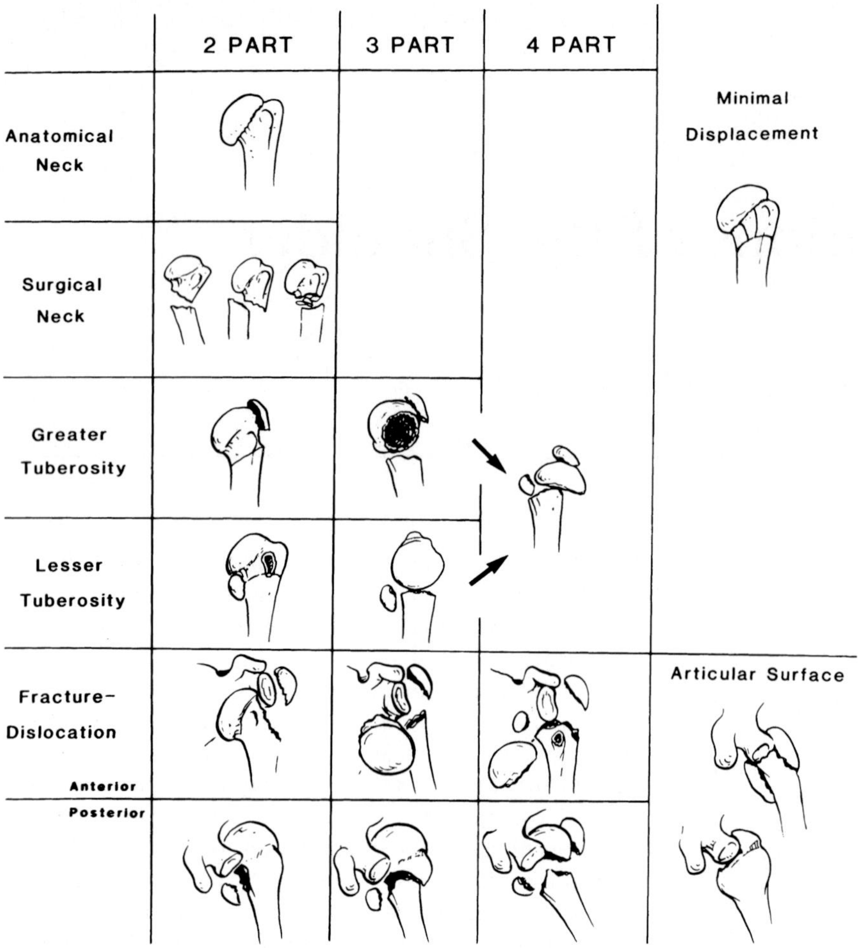

FIG. 1. The Neer classification of proximal humeral fractures.

CLINICAL AND RADIOGRAPHIC EVALUATION

Clinical Evaluation

Fracture–dislocations of the shoulder may occur at any age and by either indirect or direct mechanisms. In general, fracture–dislocations represent higher energy injuries than do simple dislocations or fractures alone. The history may indicate as much. The most common indirect mechanism involves a simple fall onto the outstretched upper extremity. Seizures and electroconvulsive therapy are other potential indirect causes of fracture–dislocations. The direct mechanism of injury involves a direct blow to the proximal humerus, and usually is the result of a fall directly onto the shoulder. With these common mechanisms in mind, patients should be asked about the circumstances surrounding the injury. If a fall was involved, patients should be asked about any head trauma, possible loss of consciousness, other injuries to the ipsilateral upper extremity, any subjective numbness or tingling involving that extremity, or any other focal sites of pain and tenderness. Other important history facts include patient age, occupation, hand dominance, and length of time since the injury.

Common presenting complaints include pain and swelling about the shoulder, especially with attempted motion. On examination, patients will typically exhibit crepitus and severe pain with minimal active or passive range of motion (ROM). Ecchymosis generally does not occur until 24 hours or more after the injury but can occur sooner in elderly patients. Eventually ecchymosis may involve the entire extremity (Fig. 2) as well as the axilla and down along the chest wall.

As with simple dislocations, there will be a change of the normal contour of the shoulder. In anterior fracture–dislocations, there is an anterior prominence in the shoulder, the lateral acromion becomes more prominent, and the coracoid more difficult to palpate. There is a flattening of the posterior aspect of the joint. Conversely, in cases of posterior fracture–dislocations, the posterior aspect of the shoulder will be full, the anterior aspect of the shoulder hollow, and the coracoid more prominent. These findings can be quite subtle in large, muscular individuals, especially if considerable swelling is present.

Most fracture–dislocations result in the affected arm's being held in a very characteristic manner. If anteriorly dislocated, the arm will usually be held in a position of relative abduction and external rotation; there can be a firm, painful block to passive internal rotation as the posterior aspect of the humeral head abuts the anterior glenoid. Conversely, in posterior dislocations, the arm may be in internal rotation,

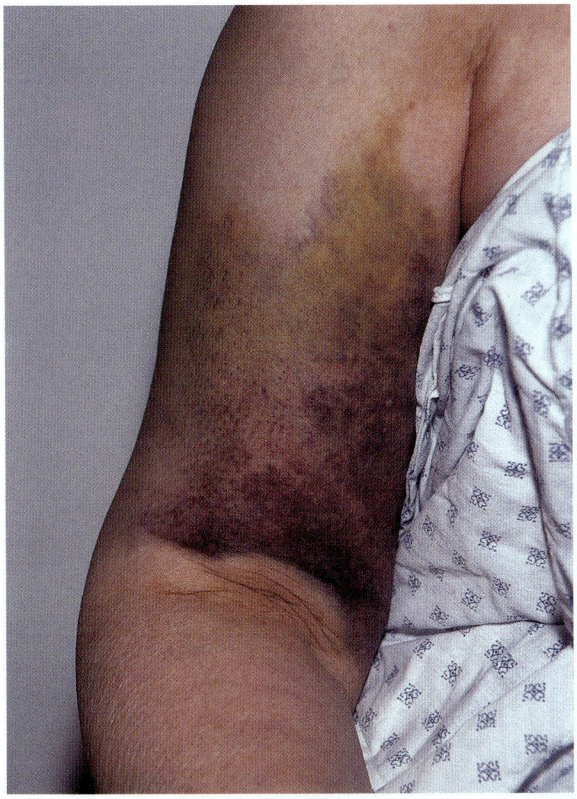

FIG. 2. A 72-year-old woman, 2 days after closed reduction of a two-part greater tuberosity fracture–dislocation; the area of ecchymosis has extended to the elbow.

with a firm, painful block to passive external rotation as the anterior aspect of the humeral head impacts the posterior rim of the glenoid. The primary exception to these findings occurs when a surgical neck fracture is present, in which case, motion in any plane may be possible through the fracture site rather than at the articulation.

A thorough neurovascular examination of the involved extremity is of paramount importance in cases of glenohumeral fracture–dislocation because of the increased risk of associated vascular or neurologic complications. Vascular injuries, although rare, are devastating when they occur and usually involve injury to atherosclerotic axillary vessels in the elderly. Signs to look for include diminished distal pulses, rapidly expanding axillary hematoma, pallor, and associated neurologic deficits. In suggestive cases, there should be a low threshold to conduct further studies such as side-to-side brachial blood pressure comparisons, Doppler flow studies, or an angiogram, or a combination of these.

Neurologic injuries are much more common sequelae of fracture–dislocations, with the incidence reported ranging from 2% to 30% (5–10). The axillary nerve is the most commonly involved, although the entire brachial plexus or any component thereof may be affected. These injuries almost always represent traction neuropraxias, and most resolve clinically within 5 months (11,12). However, it is critical that a thorough neurologic examination of the entire extremity be documented both before and after any attempted manipulations. In regard to evaluation of axillary nerve function, electromyographic studies have shown that the commonly used method of testing sensation over the lateral aspect of the shoulder is quite unreliable (11). A much more reliable method is to test for isometric deltoid motor function, which can be performed even in the context of the acute injury.

Despite the numerous signs and symptoms described, glenohumeral fracture–dislocations may be difficult to diagnose and can be missed by the initial examiner, particularly those involving posterior dislocations (13–15). It is estimated that up to 50% of these injuries are initially misdiagnosed (16). To avoid this pitfall, it is important to maintain a high level of suspicion for these relatively uncommon injuries, and to obtain a thorough and accurate radiographic evaluation.

Radiographic Evaluation

The plane of the glenohumeral articulation lies approximately 40 degrees anterior to the sagittal plane of the body. This must be taken into account if precise radiographs of this joint are to be obtained. Misdiagnosis of shoulder injuries is often attributed to radiographs being obtained in the plane of the body rather than in the plane of the scapula, centered on the glenohumeral joint. This results in overlapping structures, which can be confusing and preclude accurate assessment of the injuries.

The minimal radiographic requirement for the evaluation of any trauma to the shoulder consists of three views centered on the glenohumeral joint, with each projection at right angles to each other. This is collectively referred to as the ''trauma series.'' These radiographs are taken in the sagittal, coronal, and axial scapular planes, as shown in Figure 3. The anteroposterior (AP; Fig. 3A) view and lateral (scapular Y; Fig. 3B) view in the scapular plane can be taken with the patient's arm still in a sling and should cause no discomfort. These can be done in either a sitting or standing position. The AP view in the scapular plane is taken with the posterior aspect of the injured shoulder on the x-ray plate and the contralateral shoulder rotated anteriorly about 40 degrees. The lateral view in the scapular plane is performed by placing the anterior aspect of the involved shoulder against the x-ray plate and rotating the contralateral shoulder out 40 degrees. The x-ray tube is then placed posteriorly and parallel with the spine of the scapula.

The axillary view (Fig. 3C) is essential for evaluating glenoid and humeral articular surfaces and for identifying displaced tuberosities and is the most sensitive view for detecting glenohumeral dislocations and subluxations. This view is most easily obtained with the patient in the supine position and the affected arm gently abducted to at least 30 degrees. If possible, the arm can be supported in this position by the patient holding onto an intravenous (i.v.) pole. If the patient is unable to assist, the arm should be posi-

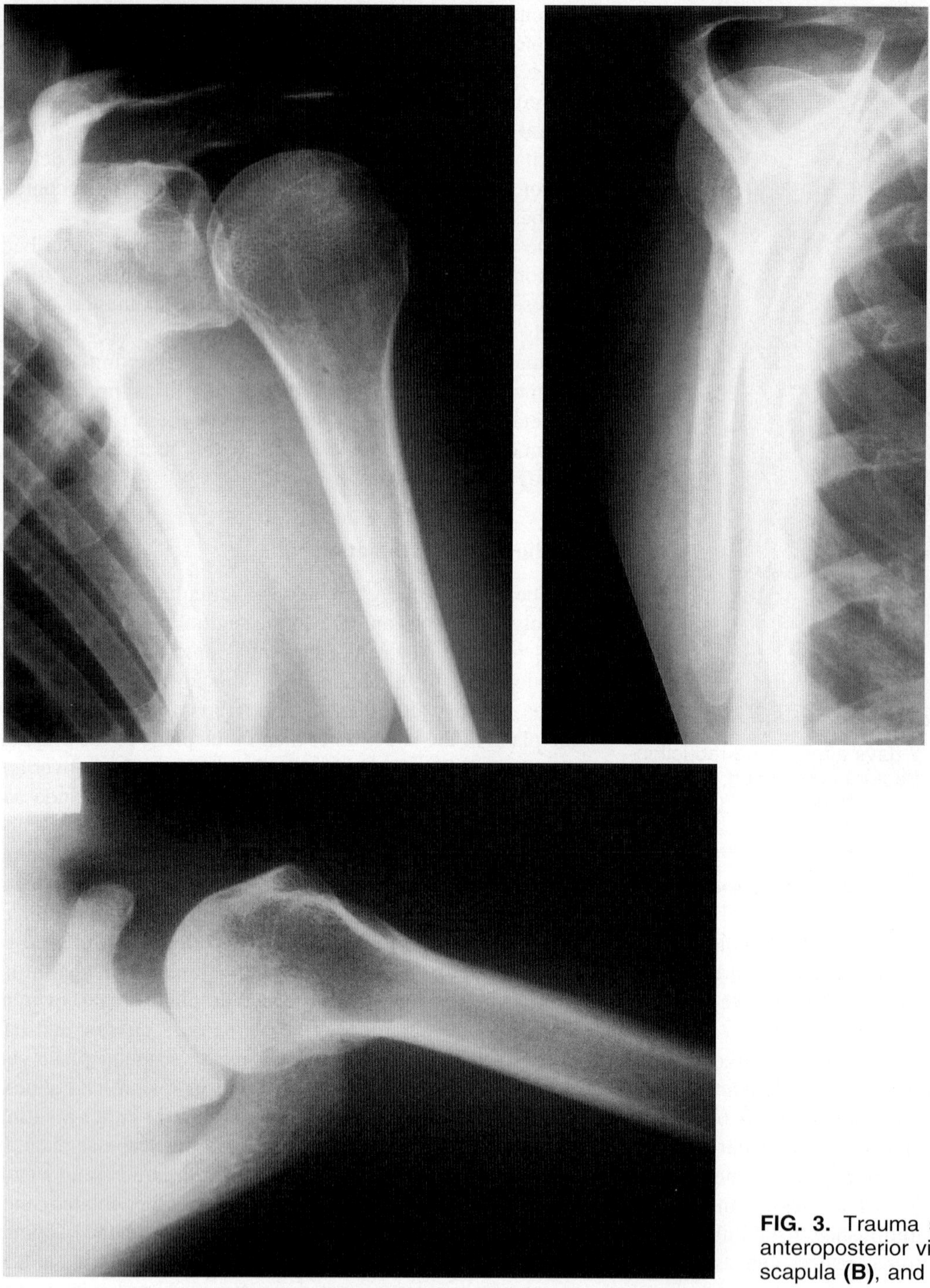

A B C

FIG. 3. Trauma series of radiographs includes anteroposterior view **(A)**, lateral view in plane of scapula **(B)**, and axillary view **(C)**.

tioned by someone wearing a lead gown. The x-ray plate is placed superior to the shoulder and against the base of the neck. The x-ray tube is positioned alongside the patient's hip with the beam directed cephalad and medially into the apex of the axilla.

Although the axillary view is the most difficult of the three views to obtain and requires moving the patient's painful arm, if done carefully, the great majority of patients will be able to tolerate the procedure. For those few patients who are unable to do so, however, the Velpeau axillary view has been described as a suitable substitute that does not require removing the arm from the sling (17). This radiograph is obtained with the patient leaning backward obliquely at 45 degrees over the plate positioned horizontally on top of the x-ray table. The x-ray beam is then shot straight downward through the shoulder and onto the plate.

Computed tomography (CT) is another imaging modality that can be used in the more complex or comminuted cases. This test provides unparalleled resolution for bony detail and therefore provides the most accurate assessment of fragment displacement, amount of articular involvement with a head-splitting or impression fracture (Fig. 4), glenoid

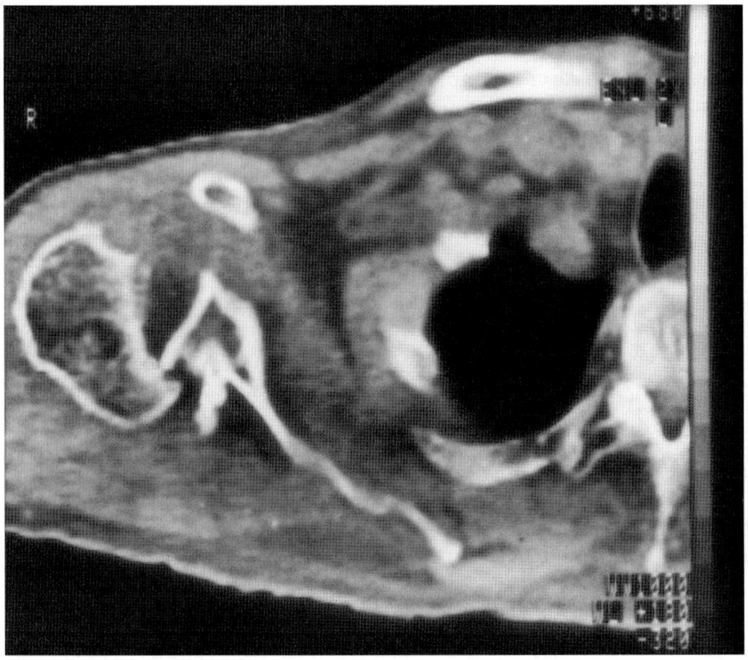

FIG. 4. Computed tomography scan of right shoulder in 56-year-old man with chronic posterior dislocation of the right shoulder. Image clearly shows impression fracture of anterolateral portion of the humeral head, as well as the amount of articular surface involvement. Calcification about posterior glenoid neck provides further evidence of chronic nature of dislocation.

rim fractures, and chronic fracture–dislocations. Castagno et al. (18) reported in their study that CT findings added so much more information than that provided by standard radiographs, that they altered the treatment of 15 of 17 patients in their series. One disadvantage of CT scans is that they provide imaging in only one plane. However, recent development of 2-D and 3-D reconstructions have the potential to provide useful information.

Although it is not as precise in assessing bony detail as a CT scan, magnetic resonance imaging (MRI) plays a very important role in evaluating traumatic shoulder injuries. MRI is the test of choice for evaluating soft-tissue injuries about the shoulder and so can be used in cases in which associated glenoid labral or rotator-cuff tears are suspected. It also can assess injuries involving the axillary vessels and brachial plexus, and it remains the most sensitive method to detect osteonecrosis, a potential sequela of fracture dislocations.

ASSOCIATED INJURIES

Rotator-Cuff Tears

All fracture–dislocations in which either or both tuberosities are significantly displaced will, of necessity, have a longitudinal split in the rotator cuff, often along the "rotator interval" between the supraspinatus and the subscapularis. In these cases, rotator-cuff repair should be performed when open reduction and internal fixation (ORIF) is performed (19). In cases in which the tuberosities do not fulfill the criteria for "displacement," associated cuff tears are not uncommon as a result of the gradual deterioration that occurs with advancing age. Therefore, the elderly are particularly susceptible to this injury because their already degenerated cuff tendons are less able to withstand the high tensile forces generated during dislocation.

Neurologic Injuries

Injury to peripheral nerves and the brachial plexus accompany fracture–dislocations of the shoulder with a reported incidence of between 2% and 30%. This variability reflects, in part, age differences of the groups studied, as well as the method of assessing neurologic deficits: physical examination versus electromyography (EMG). The axillary nerve, which courses anteriorly along the inferior border of the subscapularis, is especially vulnerable to traction injury during an anterior dislocation. It is the most commonly injured nerve in shoulder fracture–dislocations (5–10), and the likelihood of injury increases with the age of the patient, the duration of the dislocation, and the severity of the trauma producing the injury (5,20). The vast majority of these injuries represent traction neuropraxias and usually resolve spontaneously within 5 months (11,12). Other isolated nerve injuries to the musculocutaneous, radial, and ulnar nerves are much less common.

When a neurologic injury is suspected, the initial physical examination findings should be carefully documented. An EMG should be obtained 3 weeks after the injury for further documentation. This is a much more sensitive method of assessing a neurologic injury than the physical examination.

The difficulties in assessing axillary neuropathy based on physical examination are twofold. First, dermatomal sensory testing has been shown to be very unreliable (5). Second, the high incidence of rotator-cuff tears associated with these shoulder injuries confuses the picture somewhat. Clinical findings of weak abduction can be due to rotator-cuff tear, axillary neuropathy, or the acute pain associated with the injury.

Vascular Injuries

Fracture–dislocations of the shoulder can, on rare occasions, be associated with vascular injuries, usually involving the axillary artery, its branches, or the axillary vein. These injuries can occur either during the injury itself or during the reduction maneuver. Attempted reductions of chronic dislocations are particularly risky and should be discouraged. Invariably, too many attempts are made, and too much force used. Vascular damage most frequently occurs in elderly patients with fragile, atherosclerotic vessels, and in patients whose soft tissues (and vessels) may be adherent as a result of previous dislocations or other injuries (21–23). When a vascular injury occurs, it is an emergency and must be addressed immediately. These injuries are associated with a mortality rate of up to 50% (24,25).

Different types of arterial damage can occur, including intimal damage followed by thrombosis, avulsion of a large arterial branch, and laceration of the artery itself. Anatomic studies have shown the axillary artery to be relatively fixed at the lateral border of the pectoralis minor muscle (26). The artery becomes taut with abduction and external rotation of the arm and is vulnerable to injury when the humeral head dislocates anteriorly, and the pectoralis minor acts as a fulcrum over which the artery is compressed. The further risk with fracture–dislocations is that the artery can be impaled or lacerated by the fracture fragments.

The clinical findings of axillary artery injury may include severe pain, rapid swelling of the shoulder, diminished pulses distally, and neurologic deficits in the arm. The finding also may be quite subtle, consisting of a limited neurologic deficit and diminished blood pressure of the involved extremity compared with that of the uninvolved side. When an arterial rupture is recognized clinically, an attempt should be made to slow the bleeding by direct pressure. Surgical exploration should be carried out immediately through a subclavian–axillary approach. An intraoperative angiogram is preferred because of the emergency nature of the problem. The damaged segment of artery is generally resected, followed by a vascular anastomosis or interposition graft. Ligation of the axillary artery is contraindicated, especially in the elderly, because the limited collateral circulation is insufficient to maintain a functional arm.

In more subtle cases of suspected axillary artery injury, the shoulder should be reduced promptly and gently. If this fails to relieve the vascular compromise, the status of the vessel and the need for surgical intervention should be determined urgently with an angiogram.

Impression Fractures of the Humeral Head

All shoulder dislocations impact the humeral head against the glenoid to some extent. An anteriorly dislocated humeral head is compressed against the anterior glenoid by the concomitant muscular contraction, thereby causing an impression fracture of the posterolateral humeral head. This defect, referred to as a Hill-Sachs lesion, can be quite large, especially in cases of chronic dislocation.

Posterior dislocations frequently result in impression fractures of the anterolateral portion of the humeral head, referred to as a ''reverse Hill-Sachs lesion'' (Fig. 4). These impression fractures can be quite large, especially in chronic posterior dislocations. In general, the larger the size of the defect, the more difficult it is to obtain a successful closed reduction. These impression fractures play a much more prominent role in the treatment of chronic dislocations, and as such, they are discussed in greater detail in Chapter 17.

TREATMENT

Two-part Fracture–Dislocations

Surgical Neck

Two-part surgical neck fracture–dislocations are very uncommon, but when they occur, the dislocation is almost always anterior.

In general, the approach to these injuries is first to achieve a gentle, closed reduction of the dislocation, and then to determine the appropriate treatment for the fracture based on the evaluation of the postreduction radiographs. Although conscious sedation is usually sufficient, if closed reduction is unsuccessful, general anesthesia should be used to cover multiple attempts. Closed reduction of the anteriorly dislocated humeral head can often be accomplished with gentle fingertip mobilization of the humeral head while longitudinal traction is applied to the arm. There are a few circumstances in which open reduction is indicated:

1. Vascular injury.
2. Open fracture.
3. Failed or difficult closed reduction.
4. Anterior or posterior dislocation associated with a nondisplaced surgical neck fracture. (Closed manipulation risks fracture displacement).

After successful closed or open reduction, the operative approach is essentially the same as that used for two-part surgical neck fractures without dislocation. The deltopectoral interval is opened, and the clavipectoral fascia is divided lateral to the conjoint tendon. When open reduction is necessary, the dislocated humeral head should be carefully dissected free of the glenoid rim and away from the brachial plexus. Opening the rotator interval will improve visualization of the humeral head and glenoid and facilitate mobilization of the humeral head. This should permit a gentle reduction of the humeral head into the glenoid fossa. Once this has been accomplished, ORIF of the surgical neck can be performed by using a number of described techniques. Selection of technique should be based on bone quality as well as on the surgeon's experience and prefer-

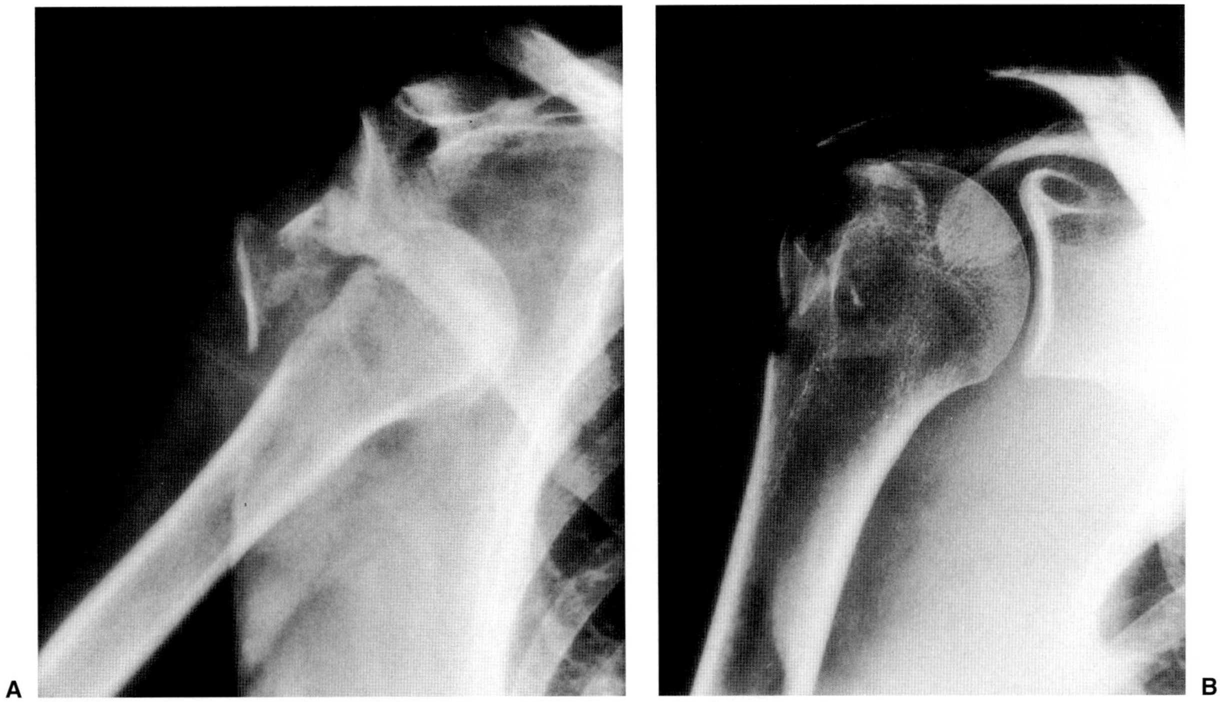

FIG. 5. A 61-year-old woman who fell onto the outstretched right upper extremity, causing a two-part anterior greater tuberosity fracture–dislocation **(A)**. After closed reduction, there is near-anatomic reduction of the greater tuberosity fragment **(B)**.

ence. If significant osteoporosis is present, the treatment of choice uses a combination intramedullary nail and tension-band technique. This consists of modified Ender rods inserted antegrade through the greater tuberosity and into the shaft with a tension-band wire or heavy nonabsorbable suture passed through the proximally prepared eye of the rods, through the rotator cuff, and through drill holes in the shaft fragment. This generally will provide stable fixation sufficient to allow early ROM. In selected younger patients with good bone quality, internal fixation of the fragments by using a plate and screws provides a viable option that should permit early ROM.

Postoperatively, the arm is protected in a sling and swath for 1 to 2 days. A simple sling can then be used for support for 4 to 6 weeks while a rehabilitation program is initiated, consisting of passive ROM of the shoulder. Active ROM begins at 4 to 6 weeks, depending on the progress of fracture healing. Stretching and strengthening are usually begun 10 to 12 weeks after surgery.

Greater Tuberosity

Greater tuberosity fractures have been reported to occur in up to 33% of anterior shoulder dislocations (27). This is the most common type of fracture–dislocation. The initial step in treatment of these injuries should always be gentle, closed reduction of the dislocation, followed by a complete set of postreduction radiographs. In many cases, the reduction restores the greater tuberosity fragment to near-anatomic position (Fig. 5). When this occurs, nonoperative management is preferred, consisting of sling immobilization for approximately 4 weeks. However, passive ROM exercises should be started as soon as discomfort subsides. Frequent follow-up radiographs are essential in the postreduction period to ensure that the tuberosity has not redisplaced with the early motion program.

In cases in which the greater tuberosity remains displaced by more than 5 mm, operative management is indicated unless the patient's medical condition or limited functional demands indicate otherwise (28). In most patients, ORIF of the greater tuberosity with tension-band suture fixation is performed to prevent the painful, limited ROM that results from malunion. The associated split in the rotator cuff also should be repaired. This procedure can usually be performed through a deltoid-splitting approach, thereby avoiding potential compromise of the deltoid insertion.

Postoperatively, the patient is placed in a sling and is started on an early passive motion program. Active ROM is started at 4 weeks when tuberosity healing has progressed sufficiently. Prognostically, dislocations associated with a greater tuberosity fracture rarely go on to become recurrent, because the anterior soft tissues are usually spared, and the joint stability is restored once fracture healing occurs.

Lesser Tuberosity

Posterior glenohumeral dislocations are sometimes accompanied by lesser tuberosity fractures (Fig. 6). This is an

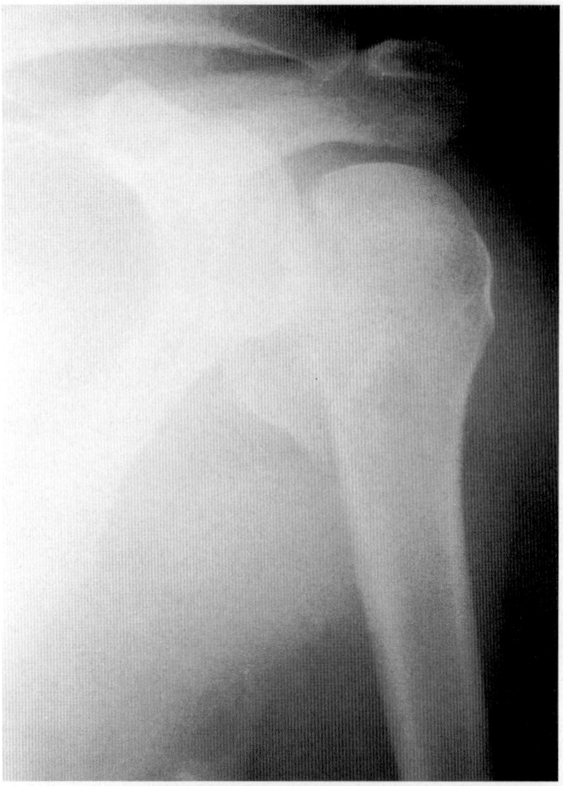

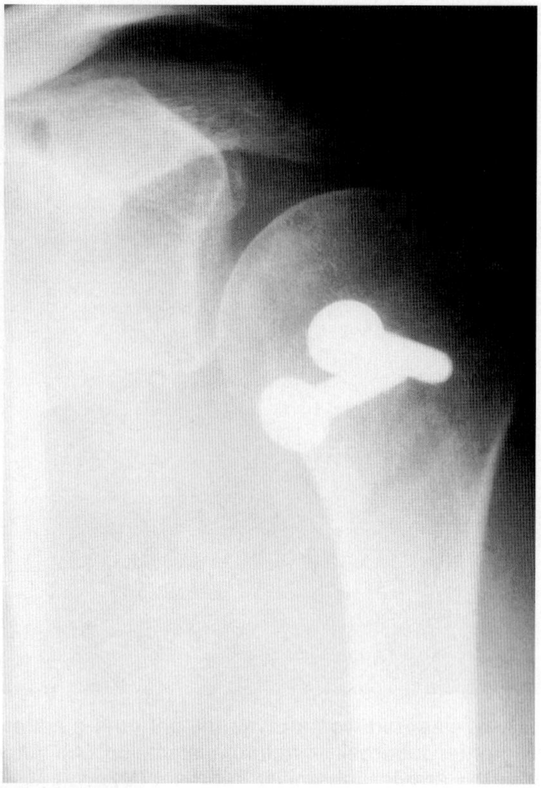

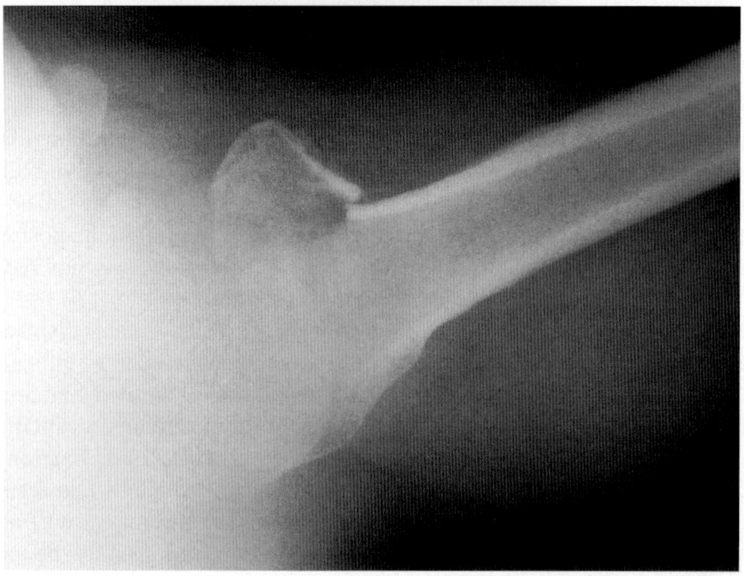

FIG. 6. A 44-year-old woman had a left two-part lesser tuberosity posterior fracture–dislocation after a seizure **(A, B)**. After closed manipulation, the humeral head was found to be quite unstable. Open reduction and internal fixation with two cancellous screws was performed **(C)**. The patient was maintained in a shoulder orthosis for 4 weeks after surgery.

avulsion-type fracture as a result of the strong pull of the attached subscapularis tendon and anterior capsule. When these injuries are acute or recent (within 2 weeks), the first step in treatment should be attempted closed reduction of the dislocation. This can be accomplished with the patient supine, by application of longitudinal traction to the arm while it is held in 90 degrees of forward flexion. The arm should then be gradually adducted across the chest while maintaining traction, in an effort to unlock the head from behind the glenoid. The maneuver can sometimes be facilitated by application of digital pressure on the humeral head from behind or a laterally directed force on the proximal humerus.

Postreduction radiographs should then be obtained to document reduction of the glenohumeral joint, to assess the position of the lesser tuberosity fragment, and to ensure that no other fractures have been displaced by the reduction maneuver. If the reduction is stable and residual tuberosity displacement is less than 1 cm, then the patient should undergo 4 weeks of immobilization in a modified shoulder spica cast or orthosis that maintains the arm at the side in 10 to 15 degrees of external rotation, 10 to 15 degrees of extension, and 10 to 15 degrees of abduction. When residual instability is present or the displacement of a large lesser tuberosity fragment exceeds 1 cm, operative management is indicated (29–31) (Fig. 6). The goals of operative management are to restore stability and anatomically reduce and securely fix the lesser tuberosity fragment. However, the decision to proceed with operative management should be based on a careful assessment of all factors, not the least of which is the patient's own functional expectations.

Fixation of the lesser tuberosity can be achieved by use of transosseous sutures or cancellous screws (Fig. 6C), depending on the bone quality. The rotator interval also should be repaired. Postoperatively, an orthosis should be used for up to 4 weeks if there is concern about the fixation. If stability is achieved, a simple sling can be used for 4 weeks. As early as postoperative day 1, passive ROM is begun with pendulum exercises, advancing to supine assisted overhead elevation and pulley exercises. The patient is advanced to active exercises at approximately 6 weeks when fracture union is ensured.

Three-part Fracture–Dislocations

Anterior

Three-part anterior fracture–dislocations consist of anterior dislocation of the humeral head with displaced fractures of the surgical neck and greater tuberosity (Figs. 7 and 8). The lesser tuberosity remains attached to the humeral head and provides some blood supply to the articular surface through the subscapularis and anterior capsule attachments. However, the arcuate artery of Laing, which carries the majority of the direct blood supply to the head, is at risk with this injury, as it penetrates the medial portion of the greater tuberosity, with the resulting risk of osteonecrosis (32).

Open reduction of the dislocation should be performed, as it can be done much more gently, thus reducing the risk of further soft-tissue injury. Our preferred treatment for this injury consists of open reduction of the dislocation followed by fixation of the displaced fragments. A deltopectoral approach is preferred. The biceps tendon may be used as a helpful guide to the tuberosities and the rotator interval. After reduction of the dislocation, if the remaining soft-tissue attachments to the head appear secure and the bone is not severely osteoporotic or comminuted, ORIF should be performed by using the tension-band technique alone or in combination with an intramedullary device, as previously described (Fig. 7). A repair of the rotator-cuff interval also should be performed.

When osteoporotic bone or comminution preclude stable fixation, proximal humeral replacement (PHR) is preferred, in combination with reconstruction of the tuberosities (Fig. 8). The prosthesis should be inserted with cement with the goal of achieving proper version and humeral length because both are critical to the function and stability of the shoulder. After-care and rehabilitation protocols are as described for two-part fracture–dislocations.

Posterior

Three-part posterior fracture–dislocations are characterized by posterior dislocation of the humeral head with the

A

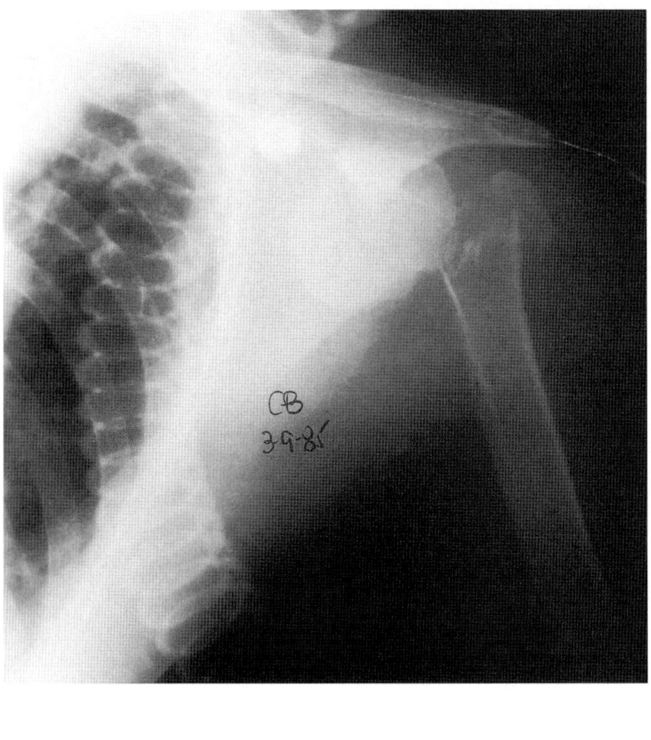

FIG. 7. A 32-year-old woman had a three-part anterior fracture–dislocation of the left shoulder **(A)**. *(figure continues)*

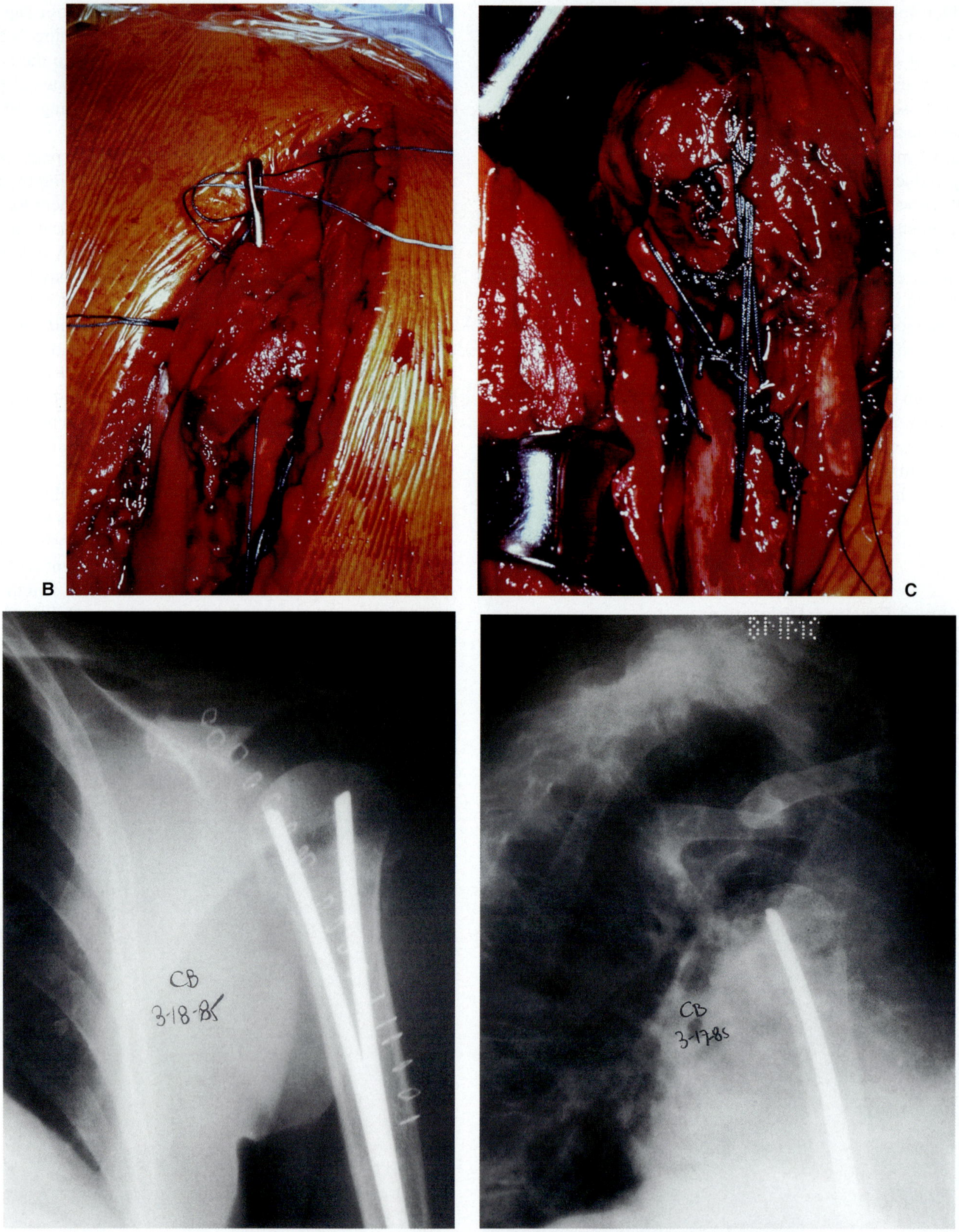

FIG. 7. *Continued.* The patient was treated with open reduction and internal fixation by using Ender rods in combination with tension-band sutures **(B, C)**. Postoperative radiographs **(D, E)** show excellent alignment and reduction of the fracture–dislocation.

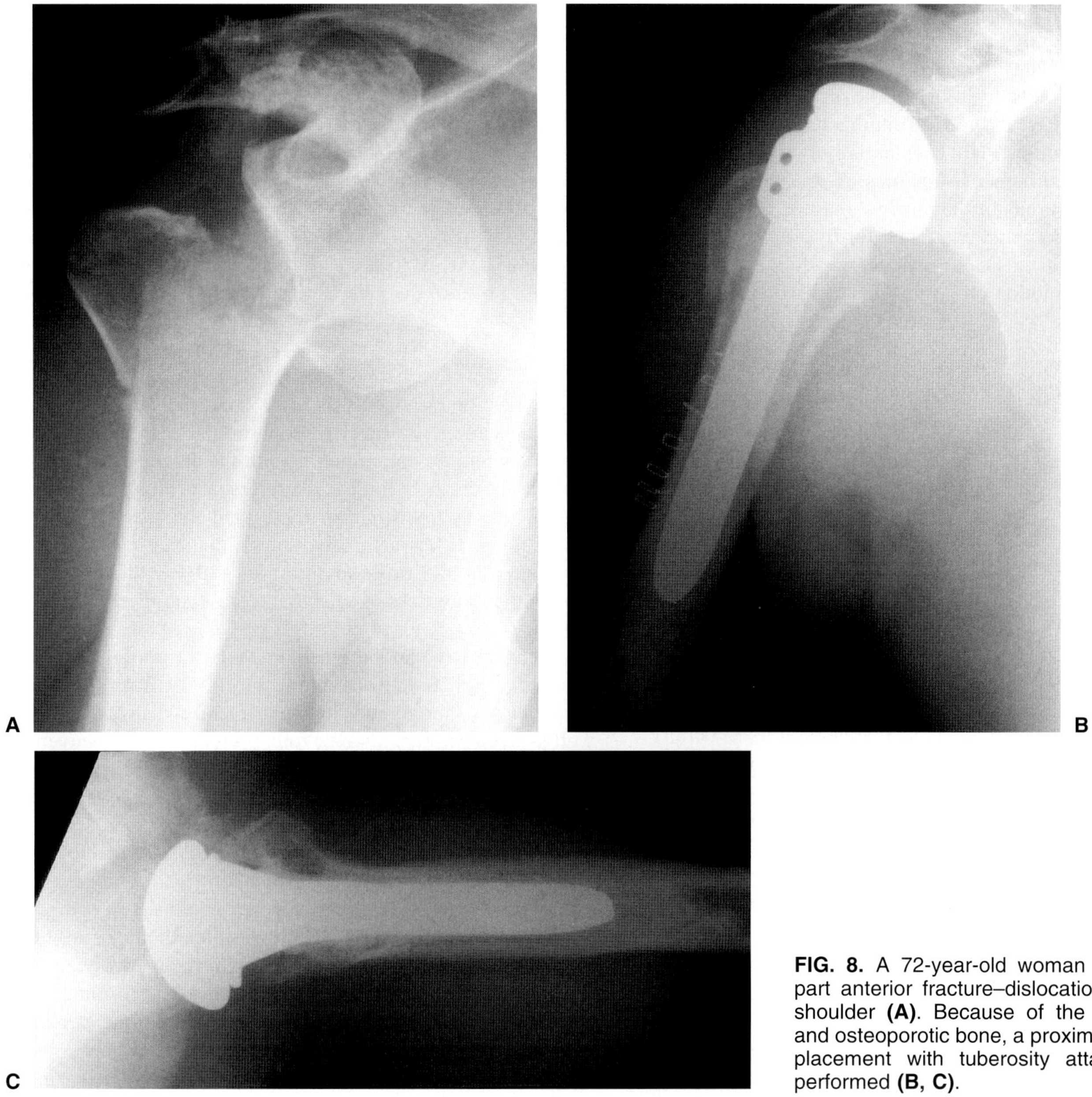

FIG. 8. A 72-year-old woman with a three-part anterior fracture–dislocation of the right shoulder **(A)**. Because of the patient's age and osteoporotic bone, a proximal humeral replacement with tuberosity attachment was performed **(B, C)**.

greater tuberosity attached in combination with displaced fractures of the surgical neck and lesser tuberosity. Complete radiographs (trauma series) are essential to accurately assess this injury and to avoid overlooking the posterior dislocation.

As with three-part anterior dislocations, these injuries require open reduction of the dislocation performed as soon as possible after the injury. Once again, the deltopectoral approach is preferred. The shaft should also be mobilized to allow visualization of the posteriorly dislocated articular segment. Gentle manipulation and a levering-type retractor should be used to reduce the dislocated segment. The decision to proceed with ORIF (by using the tension-band technique described) *or* PHR should be based on bone quality, comminution, and soft-tissue integrity.

Four-part Fracture–Dislocations

All four-part fracture–dislocations, whether anterior or posterior, are associated with significant disruption of the blood supply to the humeral head. Osteonecrosis of the articular segment is almost inevitable, and for this reason, (PHR) is the treatment of choice. ORIF is considered only in young patients with good bone quality. A deltopectoral approach is preferred, and the articular segment is removed. The prosthesis should be cemented in place with special focus on restoring proper version and humeral length. However, proper version may not necessarily mean anatomic version. In cases of subacute fracture–dislocations, stability can be enhanced by either decreasing retroversion (for posterior dislocations) or increasing retroversion (for anterior dislocations). The tuberosities should be reconstructed such that they are securely fixed to each other, to the prosthesis, and to the shaft. It is very important that the tuberosities be brought down to a level below the articular head of the prosthesis to avoid subacromial impingement.

Rehabilitation after PHR is essentially the same as after ORIF of proximal humerus fractures. A passive ROM program within the limits of the repair should be initiated 1 or 2 days after surgery and continued for 6 to 8 weeks. After this point, tuberosity healing should be stable enough to allow an active motion program.

COMPLICATIONS

Nonunion

Nonunions of the proximal humerus can occur between any or all of the four fragments but are most commonly encountered after two-part surgical neck fractures. Predisposing factors include severity of the original trauma and degree of displacement, residual distraction at the fracture site, inadequate immobilization or fixation, and overly aggressive physical therapy before secure fracture healing. Soft-tissue interposition, most often involving the deltoid or long head of the biceps, also can interfere with healing and lead to nonunion.

The treatment of surgical neck nonunion is generally more difficult than that of the original injury. If ORIF is undertaken, fixation options include a combined intramedullary rod/tension-band technique of the nonunion site or plate-and-screw fixation if bone quality is sufficient. In situations in which the bone is severely osteoporotic or the humeral head has collapsed, PHR with tuberosity reconstruction is preferred.

Malunion

Malunions result either from inadequate reduction of fracture fragments or from loss of reduction or fixation after operative management. This also can result from overly aggressive early therapy, which should obviously be avoided. Another method to decrease the possibility of significant malunion is obtaining frequent follow-up radiographs so that loss of reduction can be detected and addressed early.

Malunions involving the greater tuberosity often cause restricted motion and mechanical impingement if there is encroachment of the subacromial space. If it is symptomatic, the tuberosity can be osteotomized, advanced laterally and inferiorly from its displaced position, and secured to a cancellous bed by using a tension-band suture technique.

Malunions of the surgical neck, if significant, may restrict shoulder elevation. However, because this is rarely painful and motion is usually functional, reconstructive osteotomy is very uncommon. If corrective osteotomy is being considered, it is essential to carefully consider the contribution of soft-tissue contraction to the restriction of motion and to proceed with appropriate releases at the time of osteotomy.

Malunions of three-part and four-part fractures present very challenging problems. In most cases, the treatment of choice is PHR and tuberosity reconstruction. The most difficult aspect of these cases is the mobilization of the displaced tuberosities. This is especially true with long-standing malunions. Extensive soft-tissue releases are often needed to restore the tuberosities to near-anatomic position.

Osteonecrosis

The risk of osteonecrosis after proximal humeral fracture–dislocations is directly proportional to the degree of displacement, the comminution, and the associated soft-tissue disruption. It is logical, therefore, that this would primarily be a complication of three- and four-part fracture–dislocations. It has also been shown that the incidence of osteonecrosis is 5 times greater after ORIF with plate and screws than after less extensive internal fixation techniques (33).

Osteonecrosis can best be avoided by minimizing the amount of soft-tissue disruption during ORIF procedures, particularly of three- and four-part fracture–dislocations, as well as avoiding repetitive or forceful reduction maneuvers.

The treatment of osteonecrosis of the humeral head depends on the extent of symptoms. Some patients, even after head collapse, have only mild to moderate symptoms and can be treated with mild analgesics and modification of activity. Many, however, have disabling pain and loss of motion. In these cases, the treatment of choice is prosthetic replacement with either a PHR or a total shoulder arthroplasty (TSA), based on the degree of glenoid involvement (Fig. 9). There are two major advantages to performing the prosthetic replacement early rather than late: (a) the glenoid can be preserved, and (b) the humeral head collapse and soft-tissue contractures are less severe, thereby decreasing the necessity for extensive soft-tissue releases.

Neurovascular Injuries

Neurovascular injury may occur at the time of injury, during closed reduction, or during operative treatment. The incidence of brachial plexus and vascular injury in four-part fractures has been reported as 6% and 5%, respectively (34). Although these injuries are often unavoidable, the key to proper management is early detection. To avoid iatrogenic neurovascular injury, it is essential not to add to the soft-tissue trauma with reduction maneuvers that are excessive in either force or number.

If a vascular injury occurs, effective management depends on prompt vascular consultation and emergency surgical intervention. The damaged segment of the vessel is

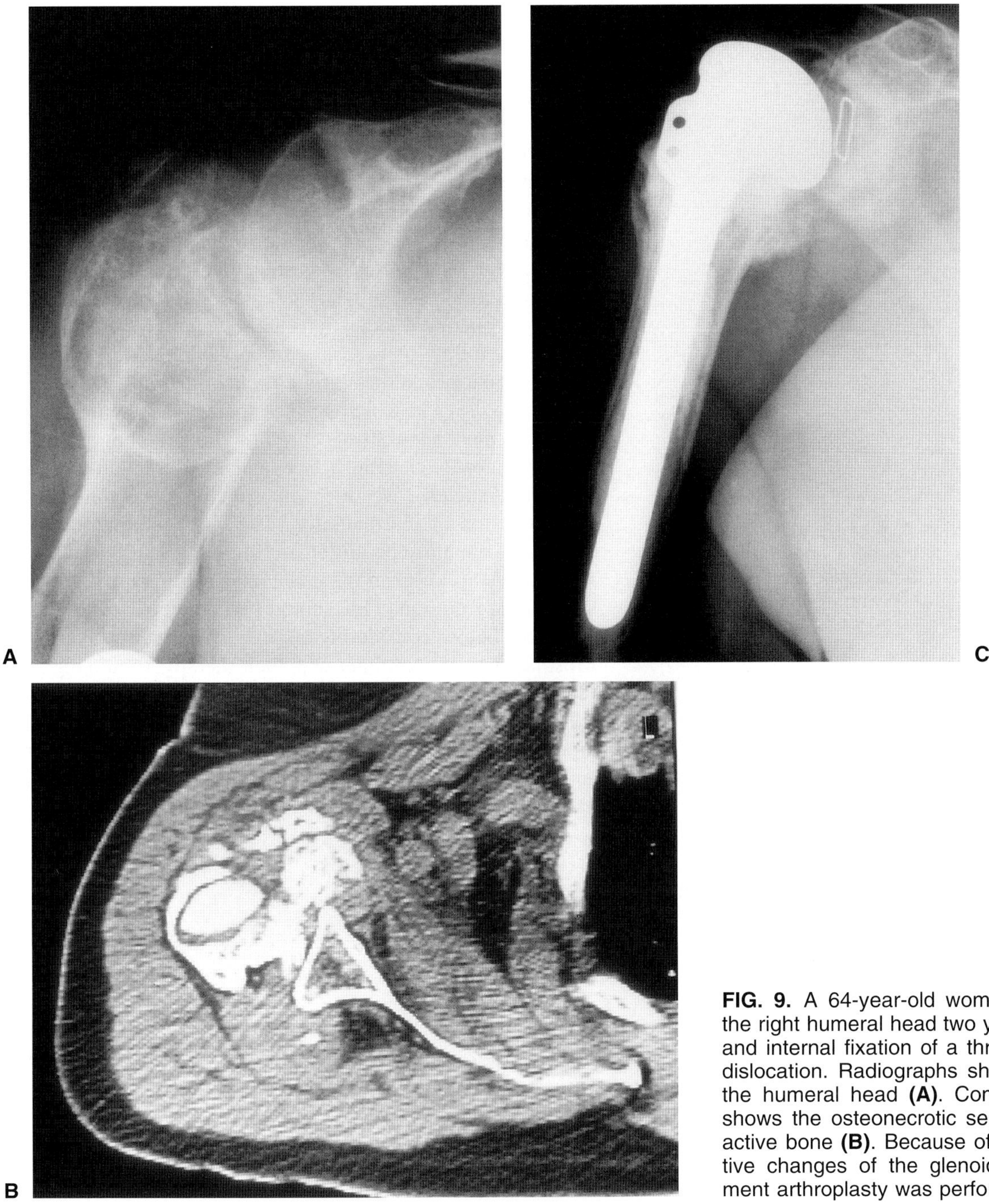

FIG. 9. A 64-year-old woman with osteonecrosis of the right humeral head two years after open reduction and internal fixation of a three-part anterior fracture–dislocation. Radiographs show extensive collapse of the humeral head **(A)**. Computed tomography scan shows the osteonecrotic segment surrounded by reactive bone **(B)**. Because of the extensive degenerative changes of the glenoid, total shoulder-replacement arthroplasty was performed **(C)**.

usually resected, and a primary repair or interposition graft is performed. Ligation of the axillary artery, even with collateral circulation present, is not indicated because of the potential for acute ischemic changes or, at best, chronic claudication with increased use.

Neurologic injury is much more forgiving and rarely warrants open exploration. These injuries are almost always traction neuropraxias and usually resolve spontaneously within 5 months (11,12). However, if a neurologic deficit occurs after operative management, early exploration should be considered if there is concern about intraoperative laceration or compromise by an encircling suture or wire.

Heterotopic Ossification

Fracture–dislocations are much more likely to develop heterotopic ossification than are the corresponding proximal humerus fractures without dislocation (Fig. 10). This is attributed to the higher degree of soft-tissue injury. When the

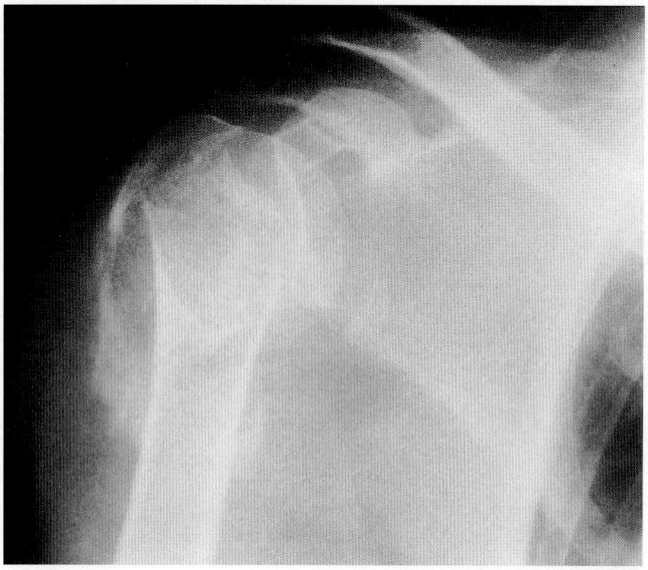

FIG. 10. After closed reduction of a two-part surgical neck anterior fracture–dislocation of the right shoulder in a 45-year-old man, significant heterotopic ossification developed. This resulted in significant stiffness with approximately 50% global loss of motion.

humeral head is dislocated, callus formation is stimulated around the head fragment. After the reduction, the ossification potential remains in the periarticular area. In the majority of cases, heterotopic bone is not extensive and is rarely functionally significant. In the uncommon event that it does cause severe restriction of motion and disability, then surgical excision is a consideration but is rarely pursued for a variety of reasons. First, the bone is often in close proximity to neurovascular structures. Second, excision of bone would often require excision of soft tissues that may significantly compromise glenohumeral stability. Third, it is uncommon for heterotopic ossification to be the isolated cause of restricted motion such that resection would be of significant benefit.

If resection of heterotopic ossification is anticipated, it should not be performed until the following criteria are met: (a) gains in motion with physical therapy have completely halted, and (b) the ossification has completely matured, as documented by a ''cold'' bone scan.

Joint Stiffness

Stiffness and restricted ROM are perhaps the most common complications after proximal humeral fracture–dislocations. The potential causes of this loss of motion are numerous and include the trauma to the soft tissues at the time of injury, prolonged immobilization, noncompliance with physical therapy protocols, and malunion of the fracture fragments. Prevention is the best treatment for many of these causes. Treatment of the initial injury should focus on expeditious reduction of the dislocation without use of excessive force or multiple attempts. There should be no hesitation to performing an open reduction to avoid repeated forceful manipulations. After reduction of the fracture–dislocation, the patient's shoulder should be sufficiently stable to permit early passive motion. If it is not, operative stabilization should be considered to avoid the need for prolonged immobilization. Patients should be informed about the importance of compliance with the rehabilitation program early in the treatment and that it is essential for a good functional outcome. The incidence of malunions as a cause of restricted motion can be minimized by proper operative indications and by careful, frequent radiographic follow-up to assess for possible loss of reduction as the patient progresses through rehabilitation.

In those cases in which stiffness occurs despite these efforts, treatment should be focused on the underlying cause. If a malunion is causing a mechanical obstruction to motion, recommended treatment may include osteotomy and reconstruction of the malunion. The most common cause, however, remains periarticular fibrosis. These patients should be started on an intensive physical therapy regimen to maximize motion. This should be continued for at least 6 months before considering any other treatment approach. Most patients, if compliant with their therapy, should regain functional shoulder motion. It is very uncommon to consider open or arthroscopic lysis of adhesions. Closed manipulation of these shoulders should be avoided as there is an unacceptable risk of refracture or further soft-tissue damage (33,35).

REFERENCES

1. Sidor ML, Zuckerman JD, Lyon T, et al. The Neer classification system for proximal humeral fractures: an assessment of interobserver reliability and intraobserver reproducibility. *J Bone Joint Surg [Am]* 1993;75:1745.
2. Siebenrock KA, Gerber C. The reproducibility of classification of fractures of the proximal end of the humerus. *J Bone Joint Surg [Am]* 1993;75:1751.
3. Neer CS. Displaced proximal humerus fractures. Part I: classification and evaluation. *J Bone Joint Surg [Am]* 1970;52:1077.
4. Codman EA. Rupture of the supraspinatus tendon and other lesions in or about the subacromial bursa. In: Codman EA, ed. *The shoulder.* Boston: Thomas Todd, 1934:313–333.
5. Wirth MA, Rockwood CA. Complications of treatment of injuries to the shoulder. In: Epps CH, ed. *Complications in orthopaedic surgery.* 3rd ed, vol 1. Philadelphia: JB Lippincott, 1994:229.
6. Gristina AG, Bigliani LU, Neviaser RJ, et al. Symposium: management of displaced fractures of the proximal humerus. *Contemp Orthop* 1987;15:61.
7. Depalma AF. *Surgery of the shoulder.* 2nd ed. Philadelphia: JB Lippincott, 1973.
8. Leffert RD, Seddon H. Infraclavicular brachial plexus injuries. *J Bone Joint Surg [Br]* 1965;47:9.
9. Ferkel RD, Hedley AK, Eckhardt JJ. Anterior fracture-dislocations of the shoulder: pitfalls in treatment. *J Trauma* 1984;24:363.
10. Watson-Jones R. Dislocation of the shoulder joint. *Proc R Soc Med* 1936;29:1060.
11. Blom S, Dahlback LO. Nerve injuries in dislocations of the shoulder joint and fractures of the neck of the humerus. *Acta Chir Scand* 1970;136:461.
12. Brown JT. Nerve injuries complicating dislocation of the shoulder. *J Bone Joint Surg [Br]* 1952;34:526.

13. Rowe CR, Zarins B. Chronic unreduced dislocations of the shoulder. *J Bone Joint Surg [Am]* 1982;64:494.
14. Wilson JC, McKeever FM. Traumatic posterior (retroglenoid) dislocation of the humerus. *J Bone Joint Surg [Am]* 1949;31:160.
15. Blasier RB, Burkus JK. Management of posterior fracture-dislocations of the shoulder. *Clin Orthop* 1988;232:197.
16. Clancy WG, Brand RL, Bergfeld JA. Upper trunk brachial plexus injuries in contact sports injuries. *Am J Sports Med* 1977;5:209.
17. Bloom MH, Obata W. Diagnosis of posterior dislocation of the shoulder with use of velpeau axillary and angle-up roentgenographic views. *J Bone Joint Surg [Am]* 1967;49:943.
18. Castagno AA, Shuman WP, Kilcoyne RF, et al. Complex fractures of the proximal humerus: role of CT in treatment. *Radiology* 1987;165 (3):759.
19. Bassett RW, Cofield RH. Acute tears of the rotator cuff. *Clin Orthop* 1983;175:18.
20. Asila M, Jaroma H, Kiviluoto O, et al. Early complications of primary shoulder dislocations. *Acta Orthop Scand* 1978;49:260.
21. Baratta JB, Lim V, Mastromonaco E, Edillon EL. Axillary artery disruption secondary to anterior dislocation of the shoulder. *J Trauma* 1983;23:1009.
22. Curr JF. Rupture of the axillary artery complicating dislocation of the shoulder: report of a case. *J Bone Joint Surg [Br]* 1970;52:313.
23. Henson GF. Vascular complications of shoulder injuries. *J Bone Joint Surg [Br]* 1956;38:528.
24. Jardon OM, Hood LT, Lynch RD. Complete avulsion of the axillary artery as a complication of shoulder dislocation. *J Bone Joint Surg* 1973;55:189.
25. Corley FG, Williams GR, Pearce JC, Rockwood CA. The management of nonunions of the humerus. *Instr Course Lect* 1990;38: 277.
26. Brown FW, Navigato WJ. Rupture of the axillary artery and brachial plexus associated with anterior dislocation of the shoulder: report of a case with successful vascular repair. *Clin Orthop* 1968;60:195.
27. Rowe CR. Prognosis in dislocations of the shoulder. *J Bone Joint Surg [Am]* 1956;38 (5):957.
28. Warren R. Symposium: management of displaced fractures of the proximal humerus. *Contemp Orthop* 1987;15 (1):61.
29. Jakob RP, Kristiansen T, Mayo K, et al. Classification and aspects of treatment of fractures of the proximal humerus. In: Bateman JE, Welsh RP, eds. *Surgery of the shoulder.* Philadelphia: BC Dekker, 1984.
30. Neer CS. Fractures about the shoulder. In: Rockwood CA, Green DP, eds. *Fractures in adults.* 2nd ed, vol 1. Philadelphia: JB Lippincott, 1984:675–721.
31. Neer CS, ed. *Shoulder reconstruction.* Philadelphia: WB Saunders, 1990.
32. Gerber C, Schneeberger A, Vinh TS. The arterial vascularization of the humeral head: an anatomic study. Presented at the American Shoulder and Elbow Surgeons Sixth Open Meeting, New Orleans, Louisiana, February 11, 1990.
33. Sturzenegger M, Fornaro E, Jakob RP. Results of surgical treatment of multi-fragmented fractures of the humeral head. *Arch Orthop Trauma Surg* 1982;100:249.
34. Bigliani LU. Fractures of the proximal humerus. In: Rockwood CA, Green DP, Bucholz RW, eds. *Fractures in adults.* 3rd ed, vol 1. Philadelphia: JB Lippincott, 1991:281–334.
35. Post M. *The shoulder: surgical and nonsurgical management.* 2nd ed. Philadelphia: Lea & Febiger, 1988:535.

The Unstable Shoulder,
edited by R.F. Warren, E.V. Craig, and D.W. Altchek.
Lippincott–Raven Publishers, Philadelphia © 1999.

CHAPTER 28

Dislocations Associated with Rotator-Cuff Tears

Robert J. Neviaser and Leesa M. Galatz

The relation between instability and rotator-cuff disease is poorly appreciated in spite of periodic reminders (1–13) that have appeared in the literature over the past 70 or more years. Recent emphasis has been focused on the cause-and-effect connection between instability in the athletically active population and tendinitis of the rotator cuff. The correlation between dislocations of the glenohumeral joint and injury to the rotator cuff has not received comparable attention, resulting in the diagnosis often being missed, to the detriment of the patient.

The detachment of the labrum from the anterior/inferior portion of the glenoid, representing a disruption of the anteroinferior glenohumeral ligament, has been assumed to be the result of a primary anterior glenohumeral dislocation and the cause in most cases of recurrent anterior dislocations. The remainder are thought to be due to capsular laxity. There is much evidence to support these concepts as true for the younger patient (i.e., younger than 40 years). This, however, does not appear to be the case for the patient older than 40 years.

In this chapter, the cause-and-effect relation between glenohumeral dislocations and injuries to the rotator cuff will be explored. Attention will be given to age factors, the pathologic anatomy and pathomechanics, the differential diagnosis, the decision making involved in the treatment options, and the appropriate therapeutic approach.

DISLOCATIONS AND PARTIAL-THICKNESS TEARS

This is a topic on which very little, if anything, of substance has been written. In light of the discussion that will follow on full-thickness tears, it seems logical that some deep surface tearing at the insertion of the cuff is inevitable. The deepest third of the rotator cuff is the least resistant to shear forces, accounting for the enthesopathy seen in the rotator-cuff tendons. Thus, with the tremendous forces that accompany a traumatic dislocation, deep surface tearing must occur. This can account for the insertional fraying often seen at arthroscopy of an unstable shoulder. Its clinical significance, if any, has yet to be established, and at this time, it can only be considered an interesting observation that does not require treatment.

There was recently some investigation of impingement of the greater tuberosity and the attached rotator cuff on the posterior aspect of the rim of the glenoid, known as internal impingement (14–16), seen in overhead athletic activities such as throwing or serving at tennis or volleyball. It also can occur in those who use their arms repetitively in the overhead position.

The pathomechanics involve the arm in a position of extreme abduction and external rotation, placing the greater tuberosity, the cuff, and the posterior superior glenoid in intimate proximity. As the arm abducts, the tuberosity and the deep surface of the cuff come in contact with the edge of the glenoid (Fig. 1). When the arm is in the "cocked" position (90 degrees of abduction and maximal external rotation), the articular side of the posterior aspect of the supraspinatus and the anterior aspect of the infraspinatus are pinched between the humerus and the glenoid. Static (anteroinferior glenohumeral ligament) and dynamic (subscapularis) stabilizers of the joint provide protection against this mechanism in the well-conditioned shoulder. In the fatigued shoulder or one with stretched glenohumeral ligaments, subtle anterior translation or instability can occur, increasing the effect of this internal impingement, causing articular side damage to the tendons.

The diagnosis can be suspected by applying an anterior translating force to the shoulder while holding the arm in 90 degrees of abduction and maximal external rotation. Production of posterior superior pain with this maneuver suggests internal impingement. If one then applies a posterior

R. J. Neviaser: Department of Orthopaedic Surgery, George Washington University, Washington, D.C. 20037; and Department of Orthopaedic Surgery, The George Washington University Medical Center, Washington, D.C. 20037.

L. M. Galatz: Department of Orthopaedic Surgery, The George Washington University Medical Center, Washington, D.C. 20037.

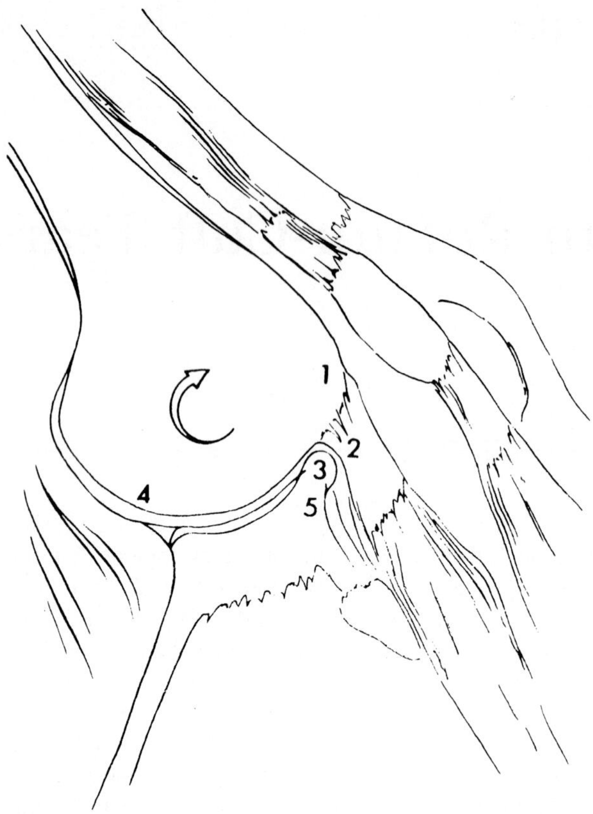

FIG. 1. The at-risk position for internal impingement. *1*, greater tuberosity; *2*, rotator cuff; *3*, labrum and biceps origin; *4*, the bony glenoid. (From Jobe CM. Superior glenoid impingement. *Orthop Clin North Am* 1997;28:137–143, with permission.)

force to the shoulder in this position (the so-called relocation test) the pain should disappear (15). Early treatment involves rehabilitation and conditioning to provide stability against anterior translation. In the few cases in which this program is not successful and the individual is not willing to change life style, a surgical approach to restore anterior stability can be helpful.

DISLOCATIONS AND FULL-THICKNESS TEARS

Although the first reports of rotator-cuff tears occurring in relation to anterior dislocations were of patients in their twenties (3,12,13), the majority of the subsequent discussion of this entity focused on its occurrence in the older population (9–11). Primary dislocations after age 40 years are much less common than in the teenage years and the twenties, and the pathologic anatomy is generally different. Tissues usually fail at their weakest site. As noted earlier, in the younger patient who sustains his first anterior dislocation, that site is the attachment of the anteroinferior glenohumeral ligament through the glenoid labrum. This, of course, is the Bankart lesion. Its failure to heal contributes to recurrence.

In the patient older than 40 years, however, the weakest link is the aging, less elastic rotator cuff. Thus, the site of failure is often the cuff, an entity referred to by McLaughlin (5) as the posterior mechanism. When the cuff fails, it does so either through its tendinous portion or through its insertion as represented by a fracture of the greater tuberosity, whichever is weaker, or both. In the patient with osteoporosis, a fracture of the tuberosity is more common, although rupture of the tendons of the cuff also can occur without fracture. It is noteworthy that an undisplaced tuberosity fracture can be associated with deep surface tearing only or with complete tearing of the tendons. A greater tuberosity fracture can only displace significantly with associated tearing of the cuff, but it is unwise to assume that if the fracture is undisplaced, the rotator cuff cannot be completely torn. This can result in undue delay in appropriate treatment and a potential poor result for the patient.

Recurrent dislocation in the patient older than 40 years is quite uncommon. The rate of recurrence for those whose primary dislocation occurred after age 40 years is between 10% and 16%. Although a Bankart lesion can occur in a primary dislocation after age 40 years, a recent report showed that a rupture of the subscapularis and underlying anterior capsule from the lesser tuberosity (Fig. 2) also can be the cause of recurrence (9–11). In the latter group, with subscapularis and capsular tearing, the onset of recurrence is usually within the first week, if not immediately. When the Bankart lesion is the underlying cause, the onset of recurrence is usually not so rapid. The true incidence of subscapularis and anterior capsular rupture is not known. Of 31 patients older than 40 years reported with previously unrecognized rupture of the rotator cuff as a result of a primary anterior dislocation of the shoulder, eight (25.8%) involved the subscapularis and anterior capsule (9). This, of course, does not reflect the true incidence of occurrence of such a lesion in the primary dislocator older than 40 years, but does suggest that one of every four patients who rupture the cuff at the time of dislocation might sustain this injury as opposed to a supraspinatus tear. As previously noted, tissues fail at their weakest point. In these patients, the weak link is not the attachment of the anterior/inferior glenohumeral ligament to the glenoid through the labrum but through its attachment to the humerus at the lesser tuberosity. Because the tendon of the subscapularis is so intimately blended with the capsule laterally and is less elastic in the older patient, it, too, ruptures with the capsule. This is effectively a failure through an anterior mechanism, but at a different part of the anterior stabilizing structures than with the common Bankart lesion.

Posterior dislocations of the shoulder are rare in any age group. The incidence of associated rotator-cuff tears is almost unheard of, as there is no series of such cases reported in the English literature. Personal experience has included only two cases. One was in a 38-year-old man who had a single posterior dislocation but had persistent pain despite recovery of function. He was later discovered to have a tear

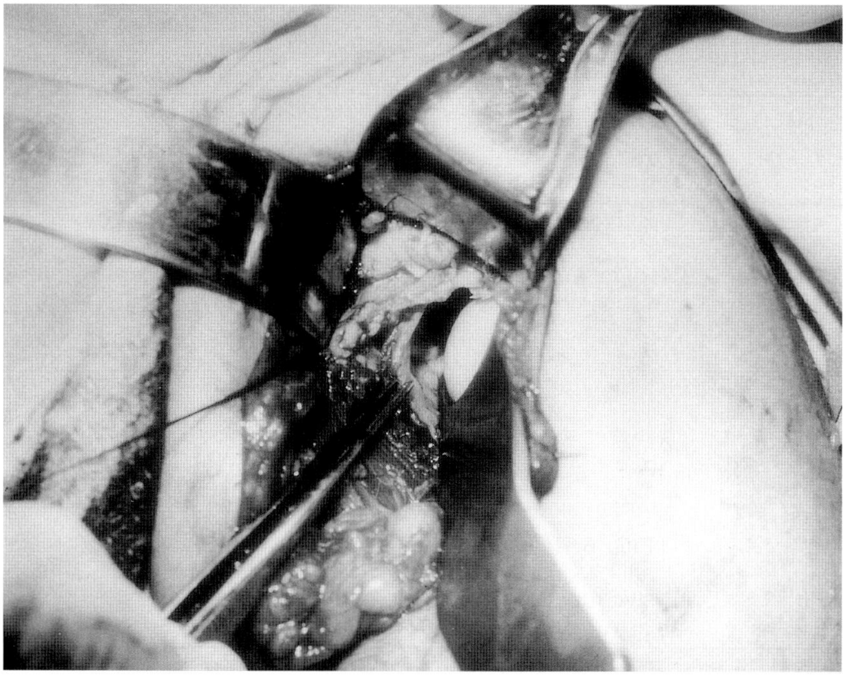

FIG. 2. Rupture of the subscapularis and anterior capsule from the lesser tuberosity in a case of recurrent anterior dislocation of the left shoulder in a 67-year-old woman. Those structures are tagged with a suture (to the *left*) and the humeral head is to the *right*. (From Neviaser RJ, Neviaser TJ. Recurrent instability of the shoulder with onset after age forty. *J Shoulder Elbow Surg* 1995;4:216–418, with permission.)

of the supraspinatus. The other, reported as part of a series of recurrent dislocations in the older patient (11), was in an 84-year-old woman who sustained her dislocation while swinging a golf club. She had immediate, multiple recurrences and at surgery was found to have ruptured infraspinatus, teres minor, and underlying posterior capsule from the greater tuberosity (Fig. 3). No labral lesion was found. Although it is not in the purview of this discussion, the only other known cause for recurrent posterior dislocation of the shoulder is a large, reverse Hill-Sachs lesion. If that is not present, then a rupture of the posterior cuff and capsule should be suspected.

The diagnosis of the initial, as well as recurrent, dislocation is made through physical examination and confirmed by radiograph. The patient's function should be assessed immediately before and after reduction. Over the next 2 to 3 weeks, function should be reevaluated every few days. If, over this time, the patient is not able to elevate the involved arm actively, then confirmatory diagnostic studies are indicated. If active elevation does return, the urgency of intervention is less, and the progress can continue to be monitored.

The implication behind the failure to regain elevation is that there has been a massive rupture of the rotator cuff and that there is not sufficient intact tendinous tissue to provide the glenohumeral stability or fixed fulcrum necessary to raise the arm at the shoulder. Continued observation under these circumstances risks creating a difficult or impossible cuff reconstruction later with a significantly reduced chance for a good outcome. If function does return, it suggests that enough of the tendons is still attached to stabilize the joint. Under these conditions, one may be able to wait to see whether rehabilitation will provide a comfortable, useful extremity.

Postreduction radiographs may give a clue as well to the extent of the rupture of the rotator cuff. With an associated fracture of the greater tuberosity, if the tuberosity fragment is retracted superiorly under the acromion (Fig. 4), or if it is externally rotated and retracted posteriorly (Fig. 5A), the tearing of the cuff is significant. The best view for the pos-

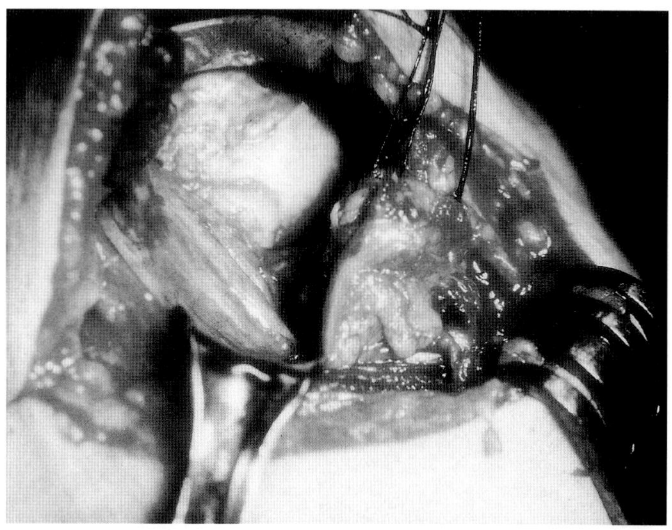

FIG. 3. Rupture of the infraspinatus and upper teres minor in recurrent posterior dislocation of the left shoulder in an 84-year-old woman. The tendon and capsule are tagged with sutures (*right*). (From Neviaser RJ, Neviaser TJ. Recurrent instability of the shoulder with onset after age forty. *J Shoulder Elbow Surg* 1995;4:216–418, with permission.)

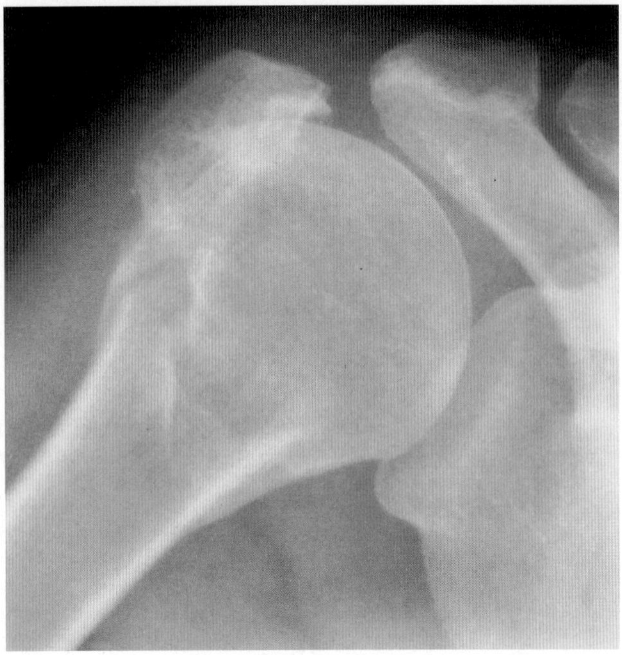

FIG. 4. Fracture of the greater tuberosity, which remains retracted superiorly after reduction of an anterior dislocation.

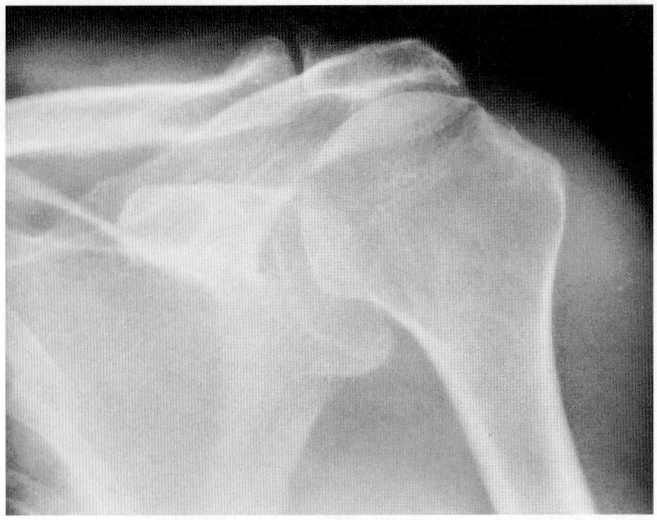

FIG. 6. Marked superior subluxation of the humeral head after reduction of an anterior dislocation, suggesting a massive rupture of the rotator cuff.

terior displacement is the axillary view (Fig. 5B). For the dislocation without fracture, if the postreduction film shows that the humeral head is markedly superiorly displaced directly under the acromion, it suggests that a massive rupture of the cuff is present (Fig. 6). The superior displacement is not just a result of the loss of the tendinous tissue between the head and the acromion, but more important, from the upward pull of the unopposed deltoid on the humerus.

The differential diagnosis of rotator-cuff rupture resulting from glenohumeral dislocations is limited. Neurologic injury is the only significant possibility (17,18). Complete brachial plexus palsy can occur with a particularly violent dislocation. A careful physical examination directed specifically toward neurologic assessment should be helpful in making this diagnosis. Isolated suprascapular nerve injury with dislocations mimicking a cuff rupture is extremely rare. Isolated axillary nerve injury is the most likely differential diagnosis. In the patient younger than 40 years, axillary neuropathy must be considered more likely. In the

A

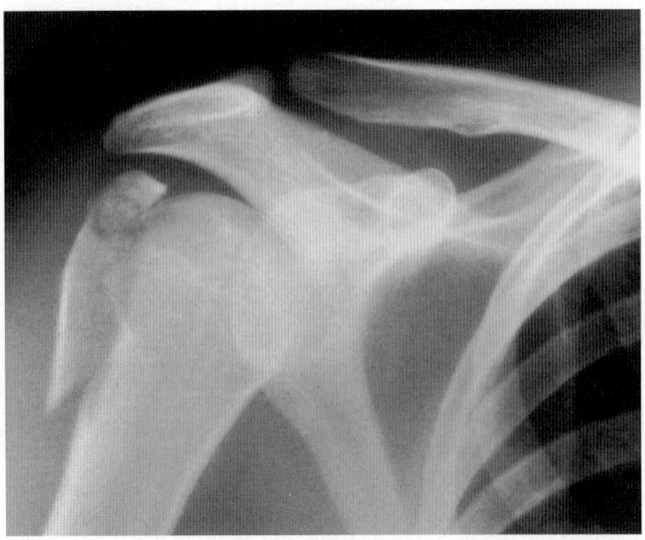

B

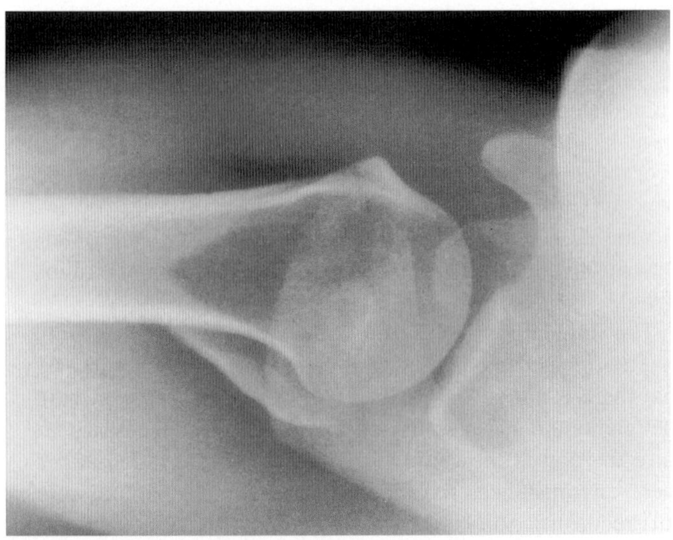

FIG. 5. A: Residual externally rotated fracture of the greater tuberosity after reduction of an anterior dislocation. B: The axillary view demonstrates the posterior position of this fragment in addition to the external rotation.

patient older than 40 years, rupture of the cuff must always be considered. In a series of 238 patients with primary dislocations, specifically looking for complications, Pasila et al. (18) reported that axillary nerve injury occurred in 21 cases, an incidence of 8.8% compared with 28 cases with concomitant rotator-cuff ruptures, all of whom were older than 50 years, an occurrence rate of 11.7%. In a smaller group studied by Blom and Dahlbeck (17), complete nerve injury was found by electromyogram (EMG) in 14.3%, but they did not look for cuff tears. In our series of 31 cases of concurrent dislocations and cuff tears in older patients, all had cuff ruptures, whereas only four (7.8%) had documented axillary neuropathy. This also highlights the fact that these two lesions can coexist. Therefore, even though a patient may have an axillary nerve injury resulting from a dislocation, there can be a concomitant rotator-cuff tear. The older the patient, the more likely the existence of the cuff injury regardless of the status of the nerve.

DECISION MAKING

Closed Treatment

As was suggested earlier, there are some indications for nonoperative treatment. In the case in which there is an associated fracture of the greater tuberosity, which on reduction of the dislocation also reduces anatomically, one should gently test the external rotation strength of the extremity with the arm at the side. If it is at least four out of five, as it often is, one can continue to observe the patient with the expectation that the fracture will heal and functional recovery will be good. It should be remembered that, even though the tuberosity is undisplaced or reduces well, we should not assume that there is no cuff lesion.

If there is no fracture of the tuberosity, but the patient can raise the arm in the forward plane after reduction of the dislocation, and the strength in external rotation at the side is four out of five or better, then we can treat the injury nonoperatively and with continued close observation with the reasonable expectation that the recovery will be good. Sometimes, because one is dealing with older patients, the immediate examination is not as clear cut as just described. Closely monitoring of the patient over the first 2 weeks with appropriate physical examination will usually clarify the extent of injury, at least to the degree that one can decide whether to consider surgical intervention or to continue with the rehabilitation program.

The nonoperative management of this injury, after reduction of the dislocation, consists initially of immobilization for comfort. Because it is usually a patient older than 40 years, the concern is not that recurrence will develop but that function may be impaired either through tendon rupture or stiffness. As noted earlier, in this age group, if recurrence develops because of subscapularis and anterior capsular tearing (or teres minor and posterior capsular tearing for recurrent posterior dislocation), it will generally appear quite promptly, and prolonged immobilization does not control it.

After immobilization for not more than 2 to 3 weeks for comfort, the nonoperative approach proceeds with a passive program of elevation in the forward or scapular planes and external rotation at the side, either by using the opposite hand to move the injured extremity or through careful, gentle assistance by someone else, not necessarily a physical therapist. During the next week or two, passive function should show progressive improvement, so active rehabilitation begins.

Initially, this means simply actively raising the arm, progressing from the active–assistive stage by using a stick and pulley to elevate the arm under control of the cuff and deltoid. Stretching exercises are integrated throughout the program. As with all conditions in the shoulder involving the strength of healing of the tendons, exercises designed to strengthen the cuff and deltoid are not instituted for 3 months, when collagen maturation is 90% complete. Return to activities such as swimming, golf, and tennis ground strokes is permitted at 3 months. By 6 months, full activity should be possible.

Open Treatment

When a fracture of the greater tuberosity remains displaced either superiorly or posteriorly after the dislocation is reduced, the decision to replace it surgically is easy to reach. Leaving the fracture fragment in such positions will block the ability to elevate the arm by abutting on the acromial arch or leave significant weakness in rotation and elevation or both.

The procedure can be done either through an anterior superior approach with a deltoid split or a deltopectoral approach. After the fragment is identified, it is often useful to extend the tear in the cuff longitudinally in line with the anterior margin of the supraspinatus. This will allow seeing the articular surface and aligning the fragments better when reducing them. It also gives a better appreciation of the relation of the height of the tuberosity to the top of the head. The tuberosity should not project above the head. Trying to reduce the tuberosity by keying it into the defect in the cortex and not seeing the articular surface may not always result in an anatomic replacement of the fragment. The tuberosity can be secured with a cannulated screw, by using intraoperative radiographs to confirm the reduction, guide-wire placement, and final screw position (Fig. 7). If the quality of the bone is not good, but the fragment is large, fixation also can be achieved by using a figure-of-eight tension-band principle. One can use either wire or heavy nonabsorbable suture, passed under the cuff where it attaches to the tuberosity fragment, reduce the tuberosity, cross the suture over the fragment, and anchor the suture distal to the fracture through drill holes and a bony bridge in the lateral aspect of the humerus. After fracture fixation, the tear in the rotator cuff must be sutured with a nonab-

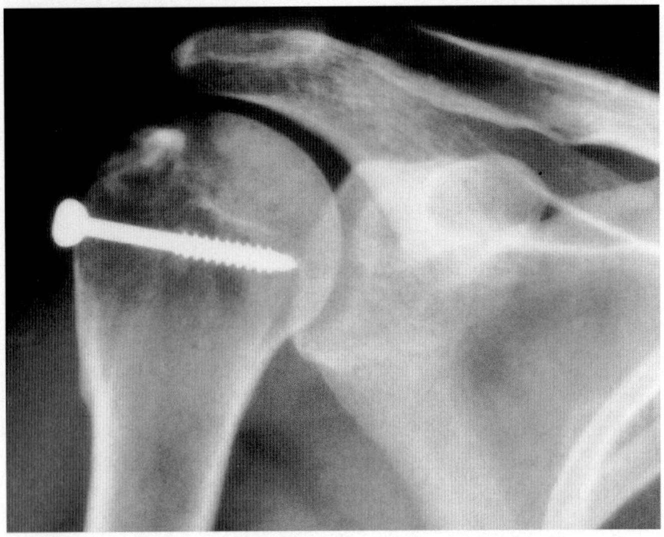

FIG. 7. Tuberosity fracture is reduced properly and secured with a cancellous screw.

sorbable no. 1 or 2 suture. If, however, the tuberosity fragment is thin, comminuted, or otherwise not usable, it can be dissected from the tendon and discarded. The tendon itself is then secured to the fracture defect with a screw and washer or with multiple sutures, securing the tendon to the adjacent bone.

For the patient with no fracture but with inability to elevate the arm without improvement over the first 2 weeks, consideration should then be given to operative intervention. Although we can proceed without further diagnostic studies, it is useful to obtain a confirmatory test to rule out the possibility of a neuropathy, even though a rotator-cuff tear is far and away the most likely underlying cause of the functional loss. It can also help in assessing the extent of the cuff disruption.

Arthrography has been the gold standard for many years and can not only establish the presence of a tear but, when done properly, also give a sense of the extent of the rupture. Over the past several years, magnetic resonance imaging (MRI) has replaced arthrography as the diagnostic study of choice. It, too, can confirm the presence of a tear. It also can show the extent of the rupture both in the medial/lateral and the anterior/posterior planes (Fig. 8A and B).

The issue arises of what to do if there is both a cuff tear and a neuropathy. Because the majority of nerve injuries are neuropraxias, it seems reasonable to repair the cuff before recovery of the nerve occurs. This philosophy provides the advantage of having an intact cuff when the nerve recovers and also minimizes the chance of having a difficult challenge in the reconstruction of the cuff, which can result from a prolonged delay in surgically addressing the cuff problem. As suggested earlier, if the ability to elevate the arm does not improve within the first 2 to 3 weeks, early surgical repair should be easier and should yield a better result than a late one.

Assuming that one is not dealing with a recurrent dislocating shoulder, then the repair of the rotator cuff should be done. As noted, there is not likely to be a Bankart lesion because this is a failure of the posterior, not the anterior, mechanism. With the patient in the sitting position, an anterior superior incision is made. The deltoid is split and reflected subperiosteally from the acromioclavicular joint and anterior acromion (8,19,20). After resection of the coracoacromial ligament and an anterior/inferior acromioplasty, blunt mobilization of the subacromial space is performed. The tear in the cuff should be visible. The edges are trimmed just enough to provide

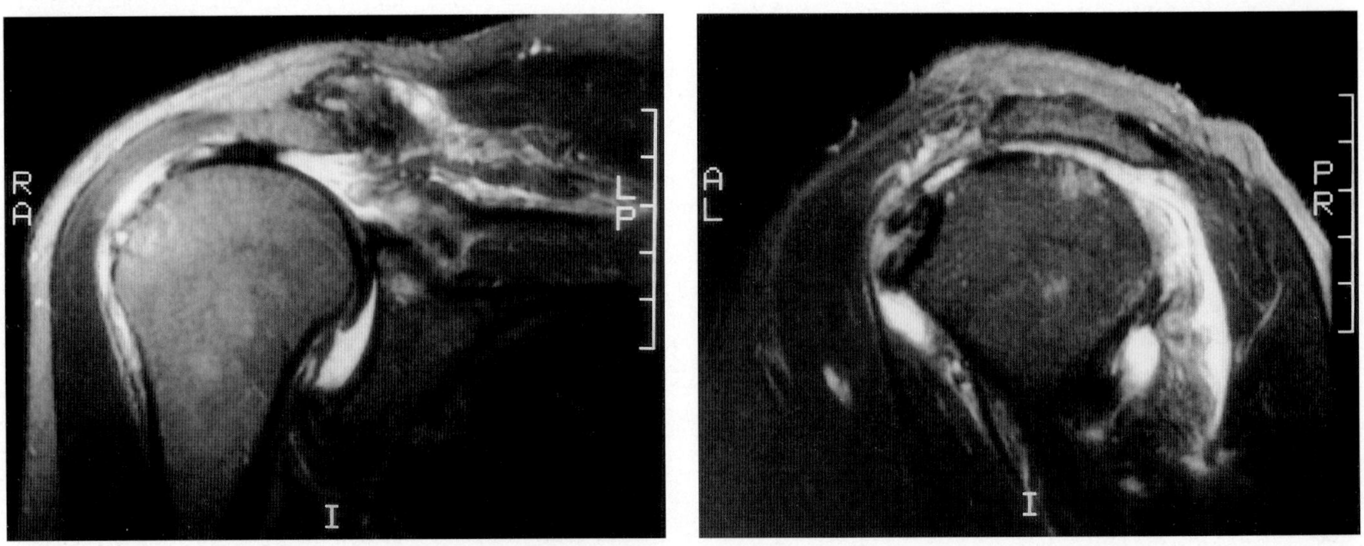

A B

FIG. 8. A: Magnetic resonance imaging (MRI) of a ruptured rotator cuff, demonstrating the lateral-to-medial defect in the cuff. B: MRI showing the extent of the rupture in the anterior/posterior plane.

The Unstable Shoulder,
edited by R.F. Warren, E.V. Craig, and D.W. Altchek.
Lippincott–Raven Publishers, Philadelphia © 1999.

CHAPTER 29

Shoulder Instability and Arthritis

Peter T. Simonian and David M. Dines

HISTORY AND ETIOLOGIC FACTORS

Arthritis after instability can be devastating because the population typically affected is young and active. Although there is little information on the epidemiology of glenohumeral arthropathy after dislocation, Samilson and Prieto (1) found that a significant number of patients with dislocations treated either operatively or nonoperatively went on to develop arthritis.

Three general groups of patients are predisposed to this condition: those with recurrent or missed dislocations, those who have had complications after surgical stabilization, and finally, those with the rare case of refractory multidirectional instability. The exact mechanism for the development of degenerative changes after dislocation is not known but is thought to be multifactorial (2), including traumatic articular damage, soft-tissue contracture, operative complications, and anatomic variants.

Articular Damage

Anterior Dislocations

Articular damage at the time of dislocation could contribute to the development of arthritis. In 1861, Flower (3) described the pathologic changes that occur in the shoulder joint after traumatic dislocation. He described the anatomic and pathologic changes found in 41 traumatically dislocated shoulder specimens in London museums. He wrote, ''where the head of the humerus rests upon the edge of the glenoid fossa absorption occurs, and a groove is evacuated, usually between the articular head and the greater tuberosity.'' In 1880, Eve (4) reported an autopsy on a patient who died 12 hours after an acute anterior dislocation in which he found a deep groove in the posterolateral aspect of the head. This was later confirmed by Joessel (5).

In 1940, Hill and Sachs (6) published a review of available information on humeral head compression-fracture defects resulting from dislocation. They reported a number of studies that described the finding of a posterolateral defect in the humeral head caused by the anterior glenoid rim after chronic or recurrent trauma (7–13).

Recurrent instability and reduction of the dislocation can increase the risk of articular damage. With increased recurrence, impression defects can become larger, ultimately affecting the articular surfaces. Reduction, especially if difficult, can also cause articular damage, especially to the glenoid.

Posterior Dislocations

There is little information regarding the development of arthritis after posterior dislocation (14). In 1839, Cooper (15) described a posterior dislocation of the shoulder. The dislocation occurred during an epileptic seizure; pain was greater than with the usual anterior dislocation; external rotation of the arm was entirely impeded, and the patient could not elevate his arm from his side. The shoulder had an anterior void or flatness and a posterior fullness, and the patient was unable to use or move the arm. A reduction could not be accomplished, and the patient never recovered the use of his shoulder. A postmortem examination of the shoulder, performed 7 years later, revealed that the subscapularis tendon was detached and the infraspinatus muscles were stretched posteriorly about the head of the humerus. Cooper further described a resorption of the anterior aspect of the humeral head where it was in contact with the posterior glenoid, probably the first description of the so-called reversed Hill-Sachs lesion.

P. T. Simonian: Department of Orthopaedic Surgery, University of Washington; Seattle, Washington 98195.

D. M. Dines: Department of Orthopaedic Surgery, Albert Einstein College of Medicine; and The Hospital for Special Surgery, New York, New York 10021; and Department of Orthopaedic Surgery, Long Island Jewish Medical Center, Great Neck, New York 11201.

Malgaigne in 1855 (16) reported 37 cases of posterior dislocations of the shoulder. This series of cases was collected 40 years before the discovery of x-rays, and it points out that with adequate physical examination of the patient, the correct diagnosis can be made. Subsequently, several studies reported on the different aspects of the posterior dislocation (14,17–24).

Samilson et al. (1) reviewed 70 patients with a history of single or multiple dislocations with radiographic evidence of glenohumeral arthropathy. In every patient, radiographs of the contralateral shoulder failed to reveal any abnormality (except, of course, in patients with bilateral dislocation). There were 62 anterior, 11 posterior, and one multidirectional dislocations. Shoulders with a posterior dislocation had a much higher incidence of moderate and severe arthrosis than those that had an anterior dislocation. This seemed to be related to delay in diagnosis.

Often in cases of unsuspected posterior instability, no axillary radiograph is taken, leading to misdiagnosis and failure to recognize posterior instability, glenoid fractures, or impression defects on the humeral head. The diagnosis is often made too late, requiring hemi or total shoulder arthroplasty for significant bone defects (Fig. 1).

Surgical Complications

Most reports of glenohumeral arthropathy after dislocation have occurred after some form of surgical intervention. Most procedures address the more common recurrent anterior dislocations. Hippocrates (25) described the use of a white-hot poker to scar the anteroinferior capsule. Since then, hundreds of operative procedures have been described for the management of recurrent anterior dislocations.

Various operative techniques were designed to address the posterolateral defect and the soft-tissue disruptions on the front of the shoulder. Capsular plication and shrinking were described in the late 1800s and early 1900s (26–28). Other procedures described during the same period included arthrodesis (29), deepening of the glenoid (30), muscle sling myoplasty (31,32), and a number of different check-rein operations (31–41). In 1906, Perthes (42) gave the first description of repair of the anterior labrum and capsule to the anterior glenoid rim. In 1923, Bankart (43) first published his operative technique. He stated that the essential lesion was the detachment or rupture of the capsule from the glenoid ligament and recommended repair between the free edge of the capsule and the glenoid ligament. In his 1939 article, Bankart (44) described the essential lesion as a detachment of the glenoid ligament from the anterior margin of the glenoid cavity. He recommended the repair of the lateral capsule down to the raw bone of the anterior glenoid and held it in place with suture through drill holes made in the anterior glenoid.

The development of arthritis after shoulder-stabilization surgery has been seen in the early and late postoperative period and has been related to different causes. In the early postoperative period, it is usually related to improperly placed hardware or hardware that has migrated (Fig. 2; 45,46). Sisk and Boyd (47), in 239 stapling procedures, found five cases of humeral grating on the staple. Impingement with mechanical wear may also result from bone-block procedures because of inadvertent impingement on the articular surface (48).

Glenoid osteotomies have been recommended for posterior instability; however, technical problems after this procedure can also be a source of arthritis. Glenoid osteotomies that either penetrate or excessively tilt the glenoid surface can lead to degeneration (49). Glenoid osteotomies that are also performed too close to the articular margin will create a slice that is too thin, which may result in avascular necrosis or nonunion and subsequent joint degeneration.

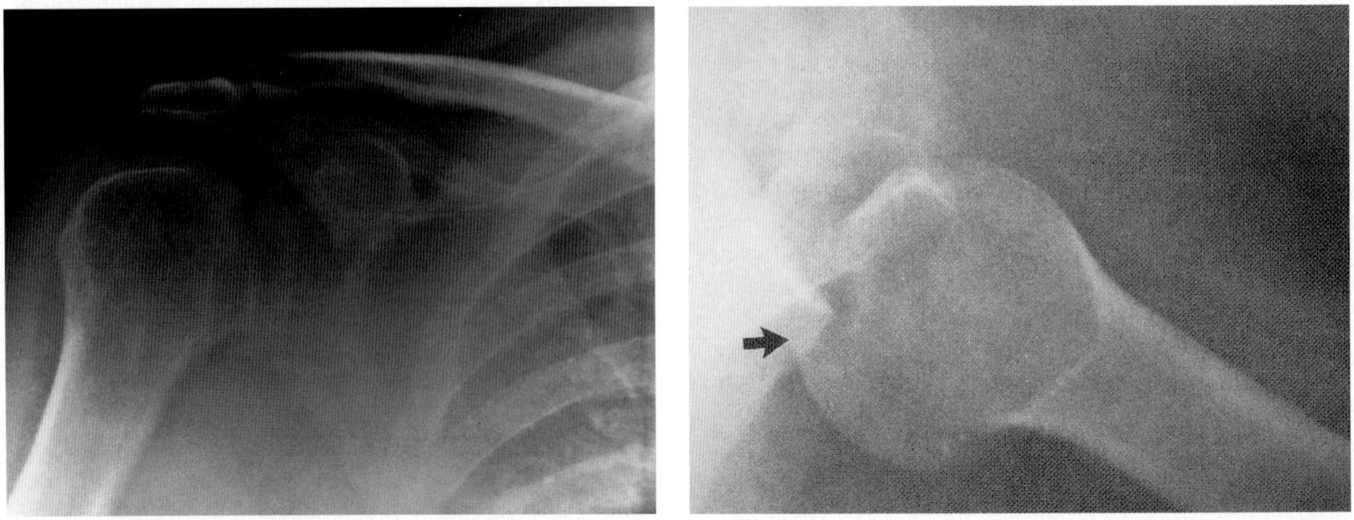

A B

FIG. 1. Anteroposterior **(A)** and lateral **(B)** radiographs demonstrating humeral head defect and glenoid damage after a "missed" posterior dislocation.

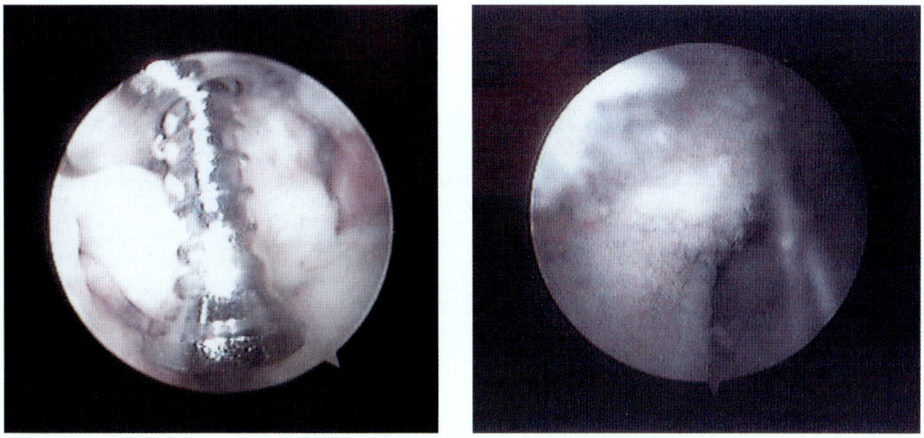

FIG. 2. Arthroscopic views demonstrating intra-articular hardware after shoulder stabilization **(A),** and subsequent articular damage **(B)**.

Secondary arthritic changes after instability repairs have been reported after many procedures, including the Magnuson–Stack procedures (1), duToit capsulorrhaphy (1,45, 46), Bristow procedures (45), Putti–Platt procedures (50), and Bankart repairs (1,51; Fig. 3). Hawkins and Hawkins in 1985 (52) retrospectively reported 46 patients with continuing difficulties after anterior reconstruction of a shoulder for instability. Osteoarthritis was the cause in seven, and implant irritation the cause in four of the patients. Hindmarsh and Lindberg (53) studied 119 patients after the Eden–Hybbinette procedure for recurrent anterior instability and found an incidence rate of 72% of moderate to severe arthrosis. In patients who were treated nonoperatively, the incidence was 7%. Solonen and Rokkanen (54) found an 11% incidence of arthritis after the Eden–Hybbinette in 95 patients with recurrent anterior dislocations. Lindholm (55) reported that 10 of 118 patients who underwent Bankart stabilization developed prominent arthritic changes. Lombardo et al. (56) reported two of 51 patients undergoing the Bristow procedure developed arthritis. Hastings and Coughlin (57) stated that 34 of 50 shoulders with recurrent anterior subluxation showed radiologic changes consisting mainly of infraglenoid new bone formation.

Stabilizations that result in significant limitation of motion, particularly external rotation, are associated with the delayed onset of arthritis (48,58). Hawkins and Angelo (48) speculated that an excessively tight Putti–Platt capsulorrhaphy repair could lead to limitation of external rotation. They reported 10 patients who had arthritis of the shoulder after Putti–Platt repair for recurrent anterior instability. Any attempt at rotating beyond the limit would result in increased joint force, leading to deterioration of the joint (Fig. 3; 48). Overtightening of the anterior repair leading to a substantial limitation of motion was thought to contribute to the arthritis. If at the time of surgery, excessive tightness is created on one side of the joint, a fixed subluxation or dislocation can occur in the opposite direction (49). This could result in uneven glenoid wear and degeneration (59).

Rotator-Cuff Injury

Another possible contributing factor to arthropathy is rotator-cuff injury that might occur at the time of dislocation. Instability may be associated with rotator-cuff tears and injury to articular surfaces, especially in older patients. Some of these patients might go on to chronic rotator-cuff insufficiency and subsequent cuff-tear arthropathy. Rotator-cuff tears are known to occur with traumatic instability, especially in the elderly (60). In 1880, Joessel (5) reported on his careful postmortem studies of four cases of known recurrent dislocations of the shoulder. In all cases, he found a rupture of the posterolateral portion of the rotator cuff from the greater tuberosity, which resulted in a greatly increased shoulder joint capsule volume. He found fractures of the humeral head and the anterior glenoid rim. He concluded that cuff disruptions that did not heal predisposed to recurrence of the problem, that recurrences were facilitated by the enlarged capsule, and that fractures of the glenoid or head of the humerus resulted in a smaller articular surface, which may tend to produce recurrent dislocation. However, his four patients were elderly and may have had the degenerative cuff changes before the dislocation. Neer et al. in 1983 (61) reported on the occurrence of cuff-tear arthropathy and specifically the relation of superior migration of the humeral head after rotator-cuff tear and the development of subsequent arthritis.

DIAGNOSTIC CONSIDERATIONS

History

Osteoarthritic changes in the glenohumeral joint will be seen as they may in any other major joint. Progressive pain is nearly always a component, with a variable degree of progressive functional deficit over a long period. Patients may complain of pain in the shoulder and upper arm, but they may also complain of parascapular and trapezius pain because of the need for increased scapular rotation to compensate for the limitation in glenohumeral motion. The pain

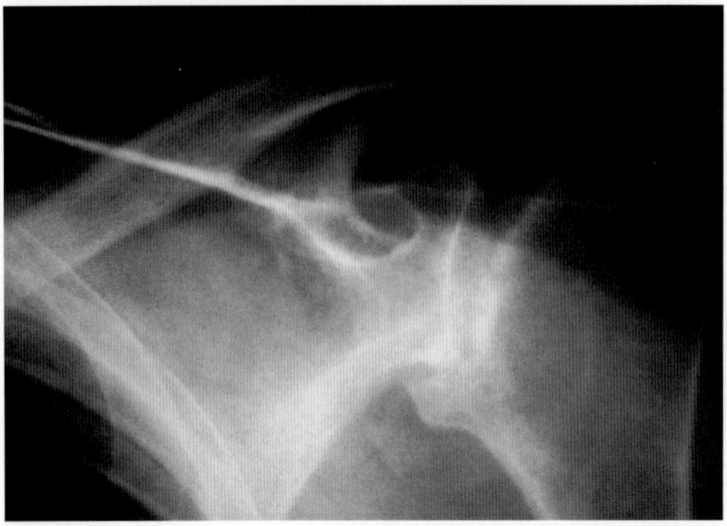

A

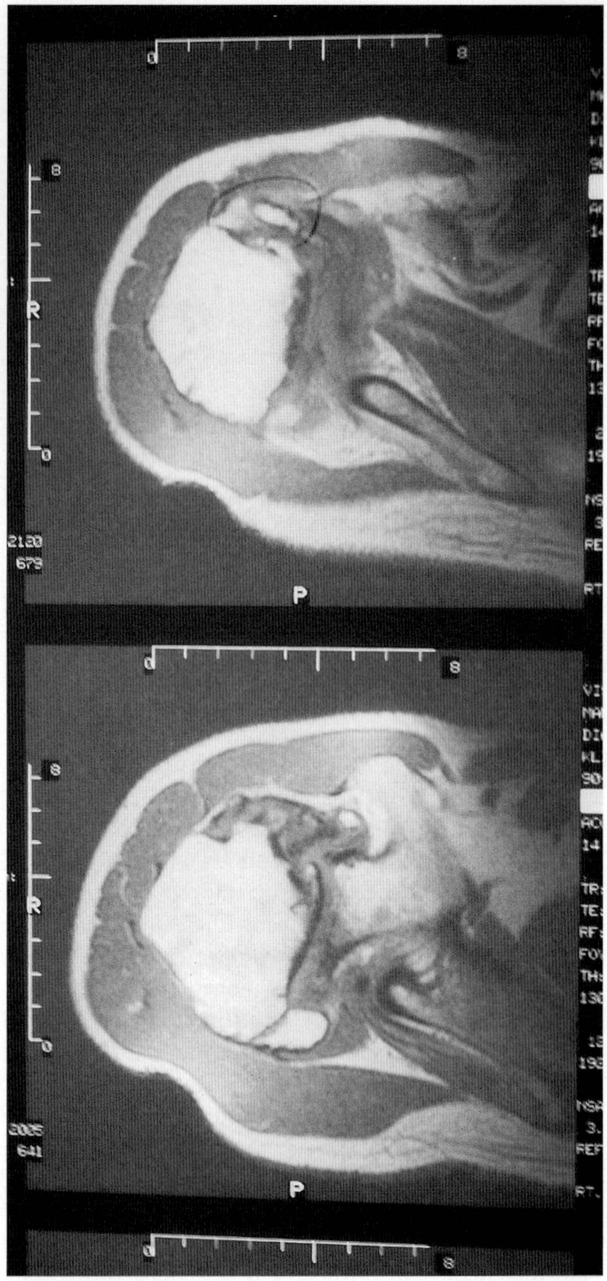

B

FIG. 3. Radiographic **(A)** and magnetic resonance images **(B)** demonstrating severe secondary arthritis developing after a Putti–Platt procedure. The magnetic resonance images also show stretching of the overtight anterior repair with a posteriorly extruded humeral head and glenoid defect,

may be activity related, but a frequent component is night pain, especially with recumbence. In the case of instability, the patients will often report an event of instability or recurrent instability, and many will complain of neurologic deficit in sensation or motor function.

Examination

On clinical examination, the patients often have some form of atrophy or wasting. After recurrent surgery, scars will be well recognized. Often, there will be a deformity where the anterior portion of the shoulder is flattened and rounded posteriorly because of posterior subluxation of the humeral head. In most cases, there will be significant reduction in the range of motion, especially rotation. They may have external rotation less than neutral, in addition to limited internal rotation. Rotator-cuff tests often will be normal, because these tendons are often spared, unless damaged as a result of the traumatic instability. Crepitation will often be noted on range of motion, and in some cases, a ''harmonic'' crepitation with active abduction will be found. This is the result of bone rubbing on bone.

Imaging

Imaging can be helpful in this group, especially if patients have had previous stabilization surgery. The standard radiographs include a true anteroposterior view in the plane of the scapula and some form of lateral view (either straight axillary or West Point). This is especially important to document posterior glenoid wear and erosion. Computerized tomography scans can be helpful in documenting posterior glenoid wear and in surgical decision making. Hardware that has previously been used can be documented on standard radiographs for position, preoperative planning, and for possible joint surface effect. In some cases, magnetic resonance imaging can be helpful in assessing a thickened anterior capsule and tendon repair often present in an overtightened Putti–Platt procedure. Magnetic resonance images also can be used to assess the glenoid articular cartilage wear posteriorly as well as posterior humeral head extrusion (Fig. 3).

Laboratory

In cases of revision surgery, we must always consider a work-up to rule out infection. If there is any clinical suspicion, tests such as an erythrocyte sedimentation rate, white blood cell count with differential, and aspiration arthrogram may be indicated.

TREATMENT

Few studies have evaluated treatment options for glenohumeral arthritis resulting from instability. Depending on the degree of involvement, four treatment options exist: arthroscopic debridement, open debridement and release, glenohumeral arthroplasty, and glenohumeral fusion.

Arthroscopic Debridement

If the arthritic changes are not too far advanced or if mechanical symptoms predominate, arthroscopic debridement is helpful. If the main problem is limitation of motion, arthroscopic debridement can provide an increase in motion for those with a large inferior humeral head osteophyte. Generally, however, the results are temporary. Recognizing this limitation, attempts have been made to use this modality in a serial fashion. Ogilvie-Harris and Wiley (62) evaluated 54 patients with osteoarthritis treated arthroscopically. After an average 3-year follow-up, two thirds of those with only mild arthritis had successful results. However, good results were obtained in only one third of the cases with more advanced disease. Ogilvie-Harris and D'Angelo (63) reviewed shoulder arthroscopy that was performed on 439 patients with all types of shoulder pathology over a 10-year period with a minimal follow-up of 1 year. Regarding arthritis, they concluded that arthroscopic debridement was useful for treating early osteoarthritis but was less useful in treating severe osteoarthritis. Ellman et al. (64) noted that more advanced degenerative disease gains little from arthroscopic intervention. They performed arthroscopic debridement on 18 patients with early degenerative arthritis simulating impingement syndrome. After a 6-month to 3-year period, pain gradually returned to the preoperative level in one; five reported only minor pain; and four had improvement. Green and Norris (65) studied 20 shoulders in 19 patients with an average age of 43 years who underwent arthroscopic treatment. Only six (26%) had subjective improvement, and this lasted an average of 8 months. Fourteen of these ultimately underwent arthroplasty at an average of 2.7 years later.

Open Debridement and Release

MacDonald et al. (66) reported 10 patients with an internal rotation contracture and pain after an anterior repair for recurrent dislocation. Six also had arthritic changes. All were treated with an anterior soft-tissue release and subscapularis lengthening. All patients had less pain and increased external rotation at follow-up. Young and Rockwood (45) had success with anterior release in these patients when the degenerative changes were not too far advanced. The patient with refractory pain and advanced glenohumeral arthrosis requires a total shoulder arthroplasty. Hawkins and Angelo (50) treated seven shoulders without surgery and four with release and lengthening of the anterior structures. Two had a total shoulder replacement in addition to the release. All four patients undergoing surgical treatment had reduced pain and improved motion after surgery. In a series of patients with osteoarthritis, Neer (67) treated four with open debridement, but all four continued to deteriorate. Cofield (68) stated that a limited synovectomy is reasonable if the cartilage thickness is at least one half of its normal thickness. He further noted that open synovectomy is preferred in the presence of bursal hypertrophy or rotator-cuff insufficiency.

When performing this procedure, one of the primary issues is to release and lengthen the subscapularis tendon and anterior capsule similar to the technique that was described for shoulder arthroplasty (Fig. 4; 69–73).

Arthroplasty

Typically, arthritic changes after instability will result in arthritic changes to both the humeral and glenoid surfaces. In these cases, total shoulder arthroplasty should be considered. In the less common instance, in which only the humeral head is involved, such as impression defects after recurrent instability, hemiarthroplasty can be considered. Cofield (70) reported that dislocation arthropathy is an indication for arthroplasty. Neer (71) reported a consecutive series of 273 total shoulder replacements; 26 were per-

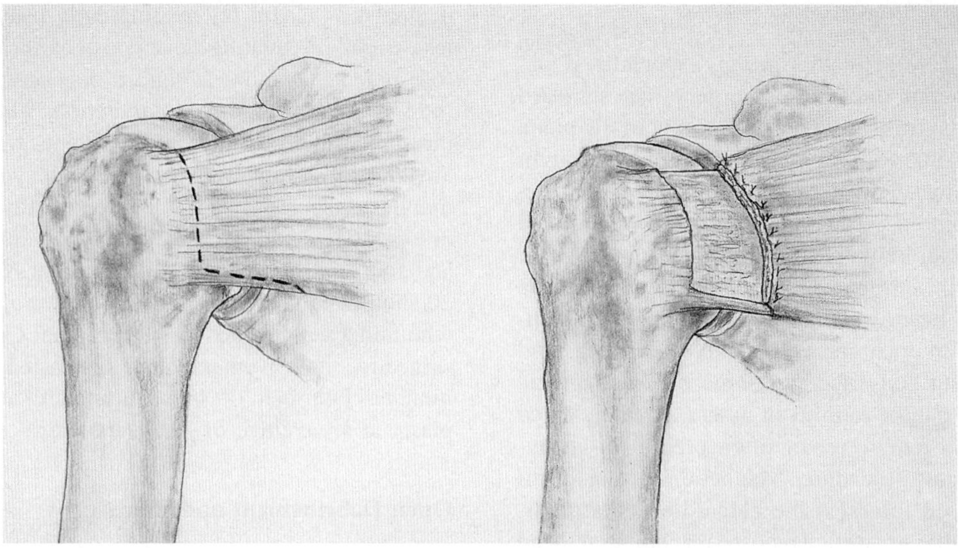

A B

FIG. 4. Example of a technique for releasing and lengthening the subscapularis tendon. The subscapularis tendon and capsule are divided obliquely **(A)**, and the resulting flaps are sewn end-to-end, effectively lengthening the tendon complex **(B)**.

formed because of arthritis caused by recurrent dislocation. They noted that instability repairs may excessively tighten the joint in one direction and cause a fixed subluxation in the direction opposite from the side of repair, leading to severe degenerative arthritis (71,74). In Neer's series (71) of 18 total shoulder replacements for arthritis resulting from instability, most of which had previous surgery, satisfactory to excellent results were observed in 17. They noted the importance of the soft tissues and capsule at the time of the initial surgery, including the need to lengthen the subscapularis tendon when it was contracted. Young and Rockwood (45) reviewed four patients who underwent Bristow procedures, developed arthritis, and underwent revision with total shoulder replacement. All four had relief of pain and a functional range of motion. Bigliani et al. (75) reported that 17 patients, who had osteoarthritis of the glenohumeral joint after surgery for glenohumeral instability, underwent prosthetic replacement. Thirteen men and four women with an average age of 43 years were studied. The interval from the initial instability repair to prosthetic replacement averaged 16 years. Before the operation, all patients had severe functional disability caused by pain and limited range of motion, especially external rotation. Twelve patients underwent total shoulder replacement, and five patients underwent humeral head replacement. At an average follow-up period of 3 years, 13 (77%) satisfactory results and four (23%) unsatisfactory results were obtained. Pain was relieved in 16 (94%) of the 17 patients. Range of motion improved by an average of 37 degrees of elevation and 53 degrees of external rotation. Previous surgery had distorted the anatomy, and special techniques were required to correct anterior soft-tissue contracture and to compensate for posterior glenoid bone loss.

In the treatment of glenohumeral arthritis after instability, the issue of hemiarthroplasty versus total shoulder arthroplasty is controversial and dependent on several variables beyond the scope of this chapter (76,77). In general, the glenoid surface should be neutralized and the soft-tissues balanced. Therefore, if the glenoid surface demonstrates concentric wear, a hemiarthroplasty may result in a satisfactory outcome, whereas patients with eccentric wear will require glenoid replacement with possible bone grafting to reestablish a neutral surface.

Arthrodesis

The final treatment option is arthrodesis of the glenohumeral joint (68,78–86). The reason for performing this procedure in patients with instability arthropathy is typically for the recurrent, disabling instability rather than for the arthritic component of their disease. The rare female patient that might belong in this category typically has multidirectional instability refractory to multiple and complex stabilization procedures. These patients often have significant arthropathy resulting from both the instability and the multiple stabilization procedures.

The position of fusion has varied, but approximately 40 degrees of internal rotation, 30 degrees of abduction, and 30 to 40 degrees of forward elevation is optimal. An intraoperative guide to confirm the position of fusion is to make certain that the hand can be placed to the mouth.

Unfortunately, the results of fusion in these patients are marginal because of the poor cosmesis and restricted motion. Arthrodesis is the final treatment option and should be carefully considered. Patients needing this intervention have extremely complex shoulder pathology.

SUMMARY

Glenohumeral arthritis is a documented complication of glenohumeral instability. Articular injury can occur at the initial traumatic event, at the time of reduction, or after repetitive subluxations. Associated soft-tissue injury such as rotator-cuff tear or contracture also may predispose to arthritis. The most common causes seem to be related to surgical complications or missed diagnosis.

Consideration should be given to proper treatment of recurrent instability to decrease the likelihood of articular damage and subsequent osteoarthritis.

REFERENCES

1. Samilson RL, Prieto V. Dislocation arthroplasty of the shoulder. *J Bone Joint Surg [Am]* 1983;65:456–460.
2. Soslowsky LJ, Flatow EL, Bigliani LU, Pawluk RJ, Ateshian GA, Mow VC. Quantitation of in situ contact areas of the glenohumeral joint: a biomechanical study. *J Orthop Res* 1992;10:524–533.
3. Flower WH. On pathologic changes produced in the shoulder joint by traumatic dislocation. *Trans Path Soc London* 1861;12: 179–200.
4. Eve FS. A case of subcoracoid dislocation of the humerus with the formation of an indentation on the posterior surface of the head. *Medico-Chirurg Trans Soc London* 1880;63:317–321.
5. Joessel D. Ueber die recidine der humerus-luxationen. *Dtsch Z Chir* 1880;13:167–184.
6. Hill HA, Sachs MD. The grooved defect of the humeral head: a frequently unrecognized complication of dislocations of the shoulder. *Radiology* 1940;35:690–700.
7. Kuster E. Ueber Habituelle Schulter Luxation. *Verh Dtsch Ges Chir* 1882;11:112–114.
8. Cramer F. Resection des Oberamkopfes wegen Habitueller Luxation (Nach einem im Arzlichen Verein zu Wiesbaden Gehaltenen Vortrage). *Berl Klin Wochenschr* 1882;19:21–25.
9. Löbker K. Einige Práparate van habitueller Schulterluxation. *Arch Klin Chir* 1887;34:658–667.
10. Schüller M. *Berl Klin Wochenschr* 1896;33:760.
11. Staffel F. *Verh Dtsch Ges Chir* 1895;24:651–656.
12. Franke GH. Dislocations of shoulder. *Dtsch Z Chir* 1898;48:399.
13. Hermodsson I. Rontgenologische Studein uber die Traumatischen und Habituellen Schultergelenk-Verrenkungen Nach Vorn und Nach Unten. *Acta Radiol Suppl* 1934;20:1–173.
14. Roberts A, Wickstrom J. Prognosis of posterior dislocation of the shoulder. *Acta Orthop Scand* 1971;42:328–337.
15. Cooper A. On the dislocation of the os humeri upon the dorsum scapula, and upon fractures near the shoulder joint. *Guy Hosp Rep* 1839;4: 265–284.
16. Malgaigne JF. *Traite des fractures et des luxations.* Paris: JB Balliere, 1855.
17. Bayley JIL, Kessel L. Posterior location of the shoulder: the clinical spectrum. *J Bone Joint Surg [Br]* 1978;60:440.
18. Bloom MH, Obata WG. Diagnosis of posterior dislocation of the shoulder with use of Velpeau and angle-up roentgenographic views. *J Bone Joint Surg [Am]* 1967;49:943–949.
19. Cautilli RA, Joyce MF, Mackell JV Jr. Posterior dislocation of the glenohumeral joint. *Jefferson Orthop* 1978;7:15–20.
20. Dorgan JA. Posterior dislocation of the shoulder. *Am J Surg* 1955;89: 890–900.
21. Hawkins RJ, Neer CS II, Pianta R, Mendoza FX. Missed posterior dislocations of the shoulder. Presented at the American Academy of Orthopaedic Surgery Annual Meeting, New Orleans, Louisiana, February, 1982.
22. Hawkins RJ, Neer CS II, Pianta RM, Mendoza FX. Locked posterior dislocation of the shoulder. *J Bone Joint Surg [Am]* 1987;69:9.
23. Heller KD, Forst J, Forst R, Cohen B. Posterior dislocation of the shoulder. *Arch Orthop Trauma Surg* 1994;113:228–231.
24. Hill NA, McLaughlin HL. Locked posterior dislocation simulating a frozen shoulder. *J Trauma* 1963;3:225–234.
25. Hippocrates. *Works of Hippocrates with an English translation.* London: William Heinemann, 1927.
26. Bardenheuer BA. Die Verletzungen Der Oberon Extremitaten. *Dtsch Chir* 1886;63:268–418.
27. Thomas TT. Habitual or recurrent anterior dislocation of the shoulder. *Am J Med Sci* 1909;137:229–246.
28. Thomas TT. Habitual or recurrent dislocation of the shoulder: forty-four shoulder operations in 42 patients. *Surg Gynecol Obstet* 1921;32: 291–299.
29. Albert E. Arthodese bei einer Habituellen Luxation der Schultergelenkes. *Klin Rundschau* 1898;2:281–283.
30. Hildebrand. Zur operativen behandlung der habituellen schulterluxation. *Arch Klin Chir* 1902;66:360–364.
31. Clairmont P, Ehrlich H. Ein Neues Operations-Verfahren zur Behandlung der Habituellen Schulterluxation Mittels Muskelplastik. *Verh Dtsch Ges Chir* 1909;38:79–103.
32. Finsterer H. Die operative behandlung der habituellen schulterluxation. *Dtsch Z Chir* 1917;141:354–497.
33. Nicola T. Acute anterior dislocation of the shoulder. *J Bone Joint Surg [Am]* 1949;31:153–159.
34. Nicola T. Anterior dislocation of the shoulder: role of the articular capsule. *J Bone Joint Surg* 1942;24:614–616.
35. Nicola T. Recurrent anterior dislocation of the shoulder. *J Bone Joint Surg* 1929;11:128–132.
36. Nicola T. Recurrent dislocation of the shoulder. *Am J Surg* 1953;8: 85–91.
37. Nicola T. Recurrent dislocation of the shoulder: its treatment by transplantation of the long head of the biceps. *Am J Surg* 1929;6:815.
38. Henderson MS. Habitual or recurrent dislocation of the shoulder. *Surg Gynecol Obstet* 1921;33:1–7.
39. Henderson MS. Tenosuspension operation for recurrent or habitual dislocation of the shoulder. *Surg Clin North Am* 1949;5:997–1007.
40. Gallie WE, LeMesurier AB. Recurring dislocation of the shoulder. *J Bone Joint Surg [Br]* 1948;30:9–18.
41. Bateman JE. Gallie technique for repair or recurrent dislocation of the shoulder. *Surg Clin North Am* 1963;43:1655–1662.
42. Perthes G. Uber operationen bei habitueller schulterluxation. *Dtsch Z Chir* 1906;85:199–222.
43. Bankart ASB. Recurrent or habitual dislocation of the shoulder joint. *Br Med J* 1923;2:1132–1133.
44. Bankart ASB. The pathology and treatment of recurrent dislocation of the shoulder joint. *Br J Surg* 1939;26:23–29.
45. Young DC, Rockwood CA Jr. Complications of a failed Bristow procedure and their management. *J Bone Joint Surg [Am]* 1991;73:969–981.
46. Zuckerman JD, Matsen FA III. Complications about the glenohumeral joint related to the use of screws and staples. *J Bone Joint Surg [Am]* 1984;66:175.
47. Sisk TD, Boyd HB. Management of recurrent anterior dislocation of the shoulder: DuToit-type or staple capsulorrhaphy. *Clin Orthop* 1974;103:150.
48. Rockwood CA Jr, Young DC. Complications and management of the failed Bristow shoulder reconstruction. *Orthop Trans* 1989;13:232.
49. Neer CS II. *Shoulder reconstruction.* Philadelphia: WB Saunders, 1990.
50. Hawkins RJ, Angelo RL. Glenohumeral osteoarthrosis: a late complication of the Putti-Platt repair. *J Bone Joint Surg [Am]* 1990;72: 1193–1197.
51. Norris TR. C-Arm fluoroscopic evaluation under anesthesia for glenohumeral subluxations. In: Bateman JE, Welsh RP, eds. *Surgery of the shoulder.* Philadelphia: BC Decker, 1984.
52. Hawkins RH, Hawkins RJ. Failed anterior reconstruction for shoulder instability. *J Bone Joint Surg [Br]* 1985;67:709–714.
53. Hindmarsh J, Lindberg A. Eden-Hybbinette's operation for recurrent dislocation of the humero-scapular joint. *Acta Orthop Scand* 1967;38: 459–478.
54. Solonen KA, Rokkanen P. The results of operative treatment for recurrent dislocation of glenohumeral joint. *Acta Orthop Scand* 1972;43:101–108.
55. Lindholm TS. Results of treatment for anterior recurrent dislocation of the shoulder joint with the Eden-Hybbinette operation. *Acta Orthop Scand* 1974;45:508–517.
56. Lombardo SJ, Kerlan RK, Jobe RW, Carter VS, Blazina ME, Shields CL Jr. The modified Bristow procedure for recurrent dislocation of the shoulder. *J Bone Joint Surg [Am]* 1976;58:256–261.

57. Hastings DE, Coughlin LP. Recurrent subluxation of the glenohumeral joint. *Am J Sports Med* 1981;9:352–355.
58. Norris TR, Bigliani LU, Harris E. Complications following the modified Bristow repair for shoulder instability. Presented at the American Shoulder and Elbow Surgeons 3rd Open Meeting, San Francisco, 1987.
59. Flatow EL, Soslowsky LJ, Ateshian GA, et al. Shoulder joint anatomy and the effect of subluxations and size mismatch on patterns of glenohumeral contact. *Orthop Trans* 1991;15:803.
60. Kinnett JG, Warren RF, Jacobs B. Recurrent dislocation of the shoulder after age fifty. *Clin Orthop* 1980;149:164–168.
61. Neer CS II, Craig EV, Fukuda H. Cuff-tear arthroplasty. *J Bone Joint Surg [Am]* 1983;65:1232–1244.
62. Ogilvie-Harris DJ, Wiley AE. Arthroscopic surgery of the shoulder. *J Bone Joint Surg [Br]* 1986;68:201–207.
63. Ogilvie-Harris DJ, D'Angelo G. Arthroscopic surgery of the shoulder. *Sports Med* 1990;9:120–128.
64. Ellman HE, Harris E, Kay SP. Early degenerative joint disease simulating impingement syndrome: arthroscopic findings. *Arthroscopy* 1992;8:482–487.
65. Green A, Norris TR. *Failed arthroscopic treatment of glenohumeral arthritis.* Williamsburg, VA: AESE, 1993.
66. MacDonald PB, Hawkins RJ, Fowler PJ, Miniaci A. Release of the subscapularis for internal rotation contracture and pain after anterior repair for recurrent dislocation of the shoulder. *J Bone Joint Surg* 1992;74:734–737.
67. Neer CS II. Replacement arthroplasty for glenohumeral osteoarthritis. *J Bone Joint Surg [Am]* 1974;56:1–13.
68. Cofield RH. Degenerative and arthritic problems of the glenohumeral joint. In: Rockwood CA, Matsen FA III, eds. *The shoulder.* Philadelphia: WB Saunders, 1990:678–749.
69. Cofield RH. Arthrodesis and resection arthroplasty of the shoulder. In: McCollister EC, ed. *Surgery of the musculoskeletal system.* New York: Churchill Livingstone, 1983:109–124.
70. Cofield RH. Unconstrained total shoulder prostheses. *Clin Orthop* 1983;173:97–108.
71. Neer CS II, Watson KC, Stanton FJ. Recent experience in total shoulder replacement. *J Bone Joint Surg [Am]* 1982;64:319–336.
72. Neer CS. Unconstrained shoulder arthroplasty. *Instr Course Lect* 1985;34:278–286.
73. Rockwood CA Jr. The technique of total shoulder arthroplasty. *Instr Course Lect* 1990;39:437–447.
74. Neer CS II, Foster CR. Inferior capsular shift for involuntary inferior and multidirectional stability of the shoulder: a preliminary report. *J Bone Joint Surg [Am]* 1980;62:897–908.
75. Bigliani LU, Weinstein DM, Glasgow MT, Pollock RG, Flatow EL. Glenohumeral arthroplasty for arthritis after instability surgery. *J Shoulder Elbow Surg* 1995;4:87–94.
76. Bell S, Gschwend N. Clinical experience with total arthroplasty and hemiarthroplasty of the shoulder using the Neer prosthesis. *Int Orthop* 1986;10:217.
77. Boyd AD Jr, Thomas WH, Scott RD, Sledge CG, Thornhill TS. Total shoulder arthroplasty versus hemiarthroplasty. *J Arthroplasty* 1990;5:329–336.
78. Barton NJ. Arthrodesis of the shoulder for degenerative conditions. *J Bone Joint Surg [Am]* 1972;54:1759.
79. Becker W. *The arthrodesis in the restoration of working ability.* Stuttgart: Georg Thieme, 1975:25.
80. Cofield RH. Shoulder arthrodesis and resection arthroplasty. *Instr Course Lect* 1985;34:268–277.
81. Davis JB, Cottrell GW. A technique for shoulder arthrodesis. *J Bone Joint Surg [Am]* 1962;44:657.
82. De Velasco Polo G, Cardoso Monterrubio A. Arthrodesis of the shoulder. *Clin Orthop* 1973;90:178.
83. Kalamchi A. Arthrodesis for paralytic shoulder: review of ten patients. *Orthopedics* 1978;1:204–208.
84. Richards RR, Beaton D, Hudson AR. Shoulder arthrodesis with plate fixation: function outcome analysis. *J Shoulder Elbow Surg* 1993;2:225–239.
85. Richards RR, Waddel JP, Hudson AR. Shoulder arthrodesis for the treatment of brachial plexus palsy. *Clin Orthop* 1985;198:250–258.
86. Wilde AH, Brems JJ, Boumphrey FS. Arthrodesis of the shoulder: current indications and operative technique. *Orthop Clin North Am* 1987;18:463–472.

The Unstable Shoulder,
edited by R.F. Warren, E.V. Craig, and D.W. Altchek.
Lippincott–Raven Publishers, Philadelphia © 1999.

CHAPTER 30

Instability After Prosthetic Arthroplasty

Keith Kenter and David M. Dines

Prosthetic shoulder replacement has proved to be a highly successful and predictable procedure (1–3) that challenges the surgeon to meet the functional demands placed on the shoulder. An equal balance between complete mobility and adequate stability must be accomplished, and it is no surprise that instability can occur after prosthetic shoulder arthroplasty.

The overall complication rate for unconstrained total shoulder arthroplasty in the patient without rheumatoid arthritis is 9% (4). Glenohumeral instability ranks second in frequency after only aseptic loosening of the glenoid component as a complication of total shoulder arthroplasty (5). The incidence of instability ranges from 0% (6–8) to 29% (9), with an average of 1.8% (10; Table 1).

Neer (20) initially reported his instability results from 48 cases of shoulder arthroplasty for osteoarthrosis. He described two cases of transient subluxation and three cases of recurrent dislocation. The two subluxation cases were successfully treated with muscle-strengthening therapy. Later, Neer et al. (11) reported on a larger series of 194 shoulder replacements. Thirteen cases in this series developed postarthroplasty instability; however, only four cases underwent revision surgery. Further, a review of 236 shoulder replacement arthroplasties performed at our institution revealed 10 cases in which revision surgery was needed for instability (12). Although each of these studies demonstrated the low rate of revision surgery for instability, the results from these reports emphasize that instability after shoulder arthroplasty is difficult to treat successfully. Thus, the prevention of postarthroplasty shoulder instability by proper positioning of the prosthesis and recognizing appropriate soft-tissue balance during the primary shoulder replacement is the cornerstone of managing this complication.

K. Kenter: Department of Orthopaedic Surgery, University of Missouri, Columbia, Missouri 65212.

D. M. Dines: Department of Orthopaedic Surgery, Albert Einstein College of Medicine; and The Hospital for Special Surgery, New York, New York 10021; and Department of Orthopaedic Surgery, Long Island Jewish Medical Center, Great Neck, New York 11201.

This chapter focuses on the complication of instability after unconstrained shoulder arthroplasty. Discussion of a classification system is presented to help organize the shoulder surgeon's evaluation when confronted with this complication. Finally, treatment options, based on the specific contributing pathologic factors, are addressed, with emphasis on the development of prosthetic instability during the chronology of the postoperative course.

CLASSIFICATION AND PATHOGENESIS

Normal glenohumeral stability is provided by a number of mechanisms that work in concert to ensure proper shoulder function, including the maintenance of adequate mobility. The loads placed on the shoulder are offset by passive, static, and dynamic constraints. Small loads are balanced by the bony anatomy (21), joint volume (22), and atmospheric pressures (23). Larger loads are offset by static constraints consisting of the capsuloligamentous complex and the labrum, as well as the dynamic properties of the rotator-cuff muscle group (5,22,24). Shoulder arthroplasty can disrupt these interactions, thus increasing the potential for glenohumeral instability.

Instability encompasses the continuum of the terms subluxation and dislocation. *Subluxation* refers to a partial or incomplete dislocation of the joint, maintaining some contact between the implanted humeral head and glenoid prosthesis. *Dislocation* is defined as complete displacement of the joint without any contact between the prosthetic components. Instability after an unconstrained shoulder replacement is usually classified based on the pathologic direction of the prosthetic humeral head in relation to the glenoid. These directions include superior, anterior, posterior, and inferior displacements. It also is possible to have combinations of these directions in some complex situations. Thus, by identifying the direction of displacement, an organized evaluation of the pathogenesis can be obtained to provide proper treatment options (Table 2).

TABLE 1. *Incidence of instability*

Author	Total	Anterior	Posterior	Inferior	Superior	NS
Amstutz (1988) 1	56	0	0	0	30	3
Arntz (1993) 14	18	1	0	0	0	0
Barrett (1987) 2	50	0	1	0	7[a]	0
Brenner (1989) 15	53	0	1	0	4	0
Clayton (1982) 16	22	1	1	0	0	0
Figgie (1992) 6	27	0	0	0	8[a]	0
Gristina (1987) 17	132	2	0	0	0	0
Hawkins (1989) 13	70	0	1	0	1	0
McCoy (1989) 7	29	0	0	0	0	0
McElwain (1987) 18	13	1	0	0	0	1
Moeckel (1993) 12	236	7	3	0	0	0
Neer (1982) 11	194	4	2	2	5	0
Pollock (1992) 8	30	0	0	0	0	0
Roper (1990) 19	25	0	0	0	1	2
Torchia (1994) 9	89	0	1	0	0	25
Totals	1,044	16	10	2	56	31

NS, Nonspecified direction.
[a] Not all patients were symptomatic, and instability diagnosed by radiographs only.

Superior Instability

Superior migration of the prosthetic humeral head is considered to be the most common form of instability after shoulder arthroplasty. It has been associated with dynamic muscle dysfunction and rotator-cuff rupture or failed repair (2,4,25,26). One of the primary functions of the rotator-cuff muscle group is to stabilize the humeral head in the glenoid fossa, thus resisting the shear forces of the deltoid. When this dynamic couple is absent or lost, the upward pull of the deltoid will exert a superior shear, resulting in a superior migration of the humeral head. Boyd et al. (25) demonstrated that the amount of superior migration is not directly related to the size of a rotator-cuff tear but is more dependent on poor preoperative rotator-cuff function.

TABLE 2. *Classification of instability after shoulder arthroplasty*

Superior	Rotator-cuff failure/deficiency Coracohumeral ligament failure Humeral head prosthesis above greater tuberosity Inferior placement of glenoid component Superior tilt of glenoid component
Anterior	Anterior glenoid bone loss (e.g., patient with RA) Excessive humeral prosthesis anteversion Subscapularis muscle rupture Coracohumeral ligament failure
Posterior	Posterior glenoid bone loss (e.g., patient with OA) Excessive humeral prosthesis retroversion Overtightened subscapularis muscle
Inferior	Settling of the humeral component Rotator-interval capsule defect Pseudosubluxation

OA, osteoarthritis; RA, rheumatoid arthritis.

In this situation, the humeral head articulates with the superior portion of the glenoid component. This leads to eccentric loads on the glenoid component, resulting in a tendency for micromotion in the prosthesis–cement–bone interface (2,27). This can produce a superior tilting of the glenoid component, a condition commonly referred to as a "rocking-horse" glenoid (Fig. 1). This phenomenon may occur in patients with osteoarthritis with rotator-cuff dis-

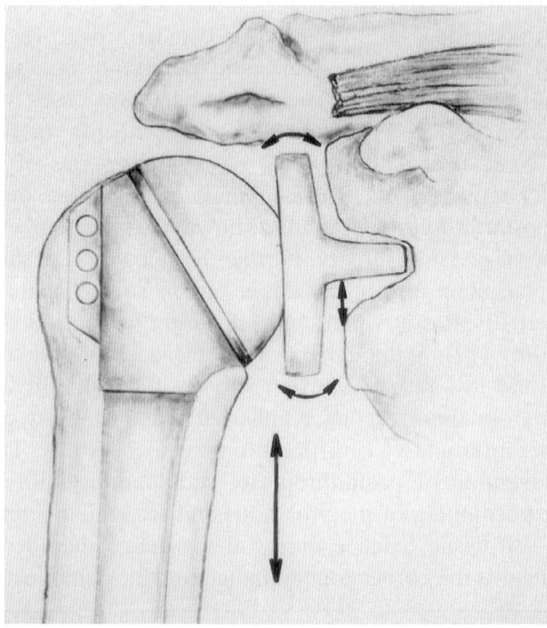

FIG. 1. Rotator-cuff deficiency and the production of a "rocking-horse" glenoid component. (From Bisson JL, Dines DM. Total shoulder arthroplasty. In: Craig EV, ed. *Textbook of orthopedic surgery.* Philadelphia: Williams & Wilkins, 1998, with permission.)

ease. McCoy et al. (7) demonstrated that patients with rheumatoid arthritis with rotator-cuff disease show no evidence of loose glenoid components. This may be a result of the limited demands placed on the shoulder arthroplasty in this patient population. Further, the disease involvement in patients with rheumatoid arthritis may result in lower shear forces placed on the glenoid component when compared with patients with osteoarthritis or those after trauma.

Another cause for superior instability after shoulder arthroplasty is the failure to restore the appropriate anatomic relation between the humerus and the scapula. This is most commonly associated with a proud implantation of the humeral component, resulting in a lengthened humerus (Fig. 2). The malposition of the glenoid component, either seated too inferior or placed with a superior tilt, will also result in superior instability of the shoulder arthroplasty (Fig. 3).

Anterior Instability

Anterior instability is most commonly associated with the disruption of the repaired subscapularis muscle, malposition of the humeral component, or dysfunction of the anterior deltoid (12,27). Rupture of the repaired subscapularis muscle is the most common cause of anterior instability after shoulder arthroplasty. Moeckel et al. (12) demonstrated this finding in

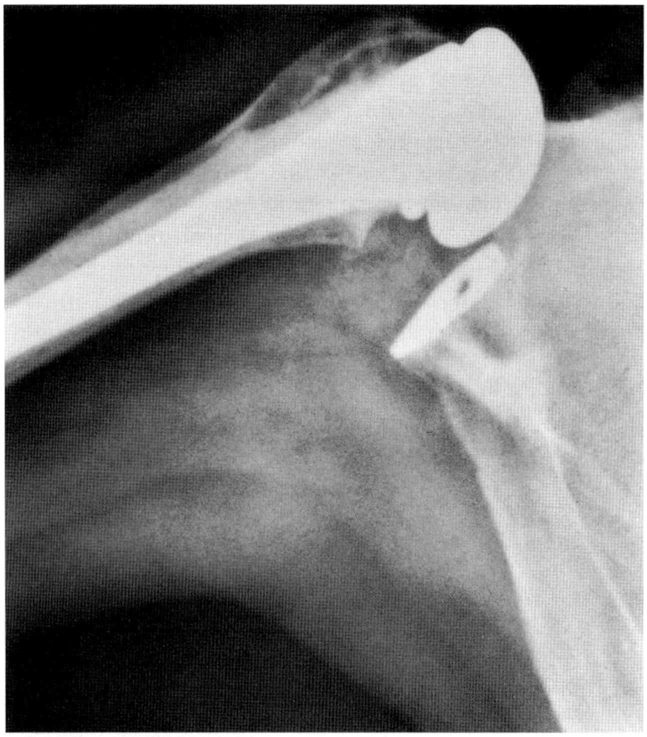

FIG. 3. Radiograph of a glenoid component placed inferior and with a superior tilt, leading to superior instability of the shoulder arthroplasty.

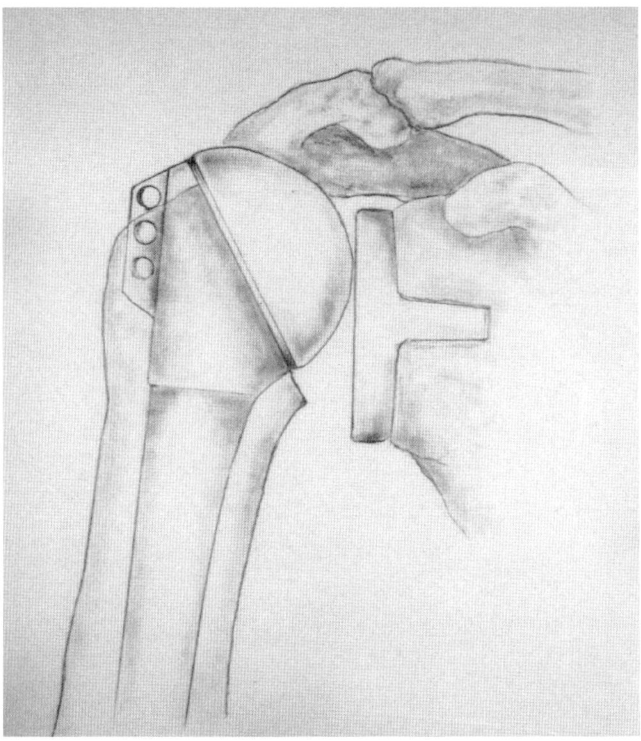

FIG. 2. Humeral component placed too high, resulting in superior migration of the prosthesis and impingement. (From Dines DM, Warren RF. Modular shoulder hemiarthroplasty for acute fractures: surgical considerations. *Clin Orthop* 1994;307:18–26, with permission.)

all seven cases of anterior instability after total shoulder arthroplasty at the time of revision surgery. Disruption of the subscapularis repair may be due to (a) a too tight repair from excessive plication of the muscle itself, (b) overstuffing the shoulder joint with a too large humeral head or a too thick glenoid component, (c) overaggressive postoperative rehabilitation, or (d) poor myofascial tissue quality, as seen with rheumatoid arthritis, for example.

Humeral-component malposition is another variable that may lead to anterior instability. This is commonly associated with a modular prosthesis. The prosthetic humeral head can act as a landmark to assist the shoulder surgeon for proper stem version. In a modular prosthesis, the prosthetic stem is placed in the humeral shaft without the modular head component. Thus, with an inexperienced shoulder surgeon, malposition of the humeral stem may occur. Importance must be placed on the proximal humeral cut. The cutting guide that is used will mark the correct anteversion for the humeral prosthesis. The placement of the humeral component fin 1 cm posterior to the bicipital groove can also orient the proper anteversion. Wirth and Rockwood (27) found from their series that decreased humeral-component retroversion (of 20 degrees or less) was present in all total shoulder replacements surgically explored for anterior instability. The version of the prosthetic components works in close concert with the surrounding soft tissues of the shoulder, and neither should be considered independent of the other.

Posterior Instability

As discussed with anterior instability, posterior instability after prosthetic shoulder arthroplasty is influenced by the close relation between component position and the surrounding soft tissues. Posterior instability is usually associated with a glenoid component of more than 20 degrees of retroversion or a humeral component in more than 45 degrees of retroversion (5). In 1989, Hawkins et al. (13) reported on eight complications of total shoulder arthroplasty. One of the complications was posterior dislocation resulting from improper retroversion of the humeral component. Of the 10 cases of instability after total shoulder arthroplasty from our institution, three were in the posterior direction (12). The factors involved in these three cases of posterior instability were excessive humeral retroversion, a retrotilted glenoid component (Fig. 4A and B), and soft-tissue imbalance caused by an overtightening of the subscapularis muscle.

Characteristic erosion patterns can be seen in patients with arthrosis of the glenohumeral joint. It is of utmost importance for the shoulder surgeon to recognize the pat-

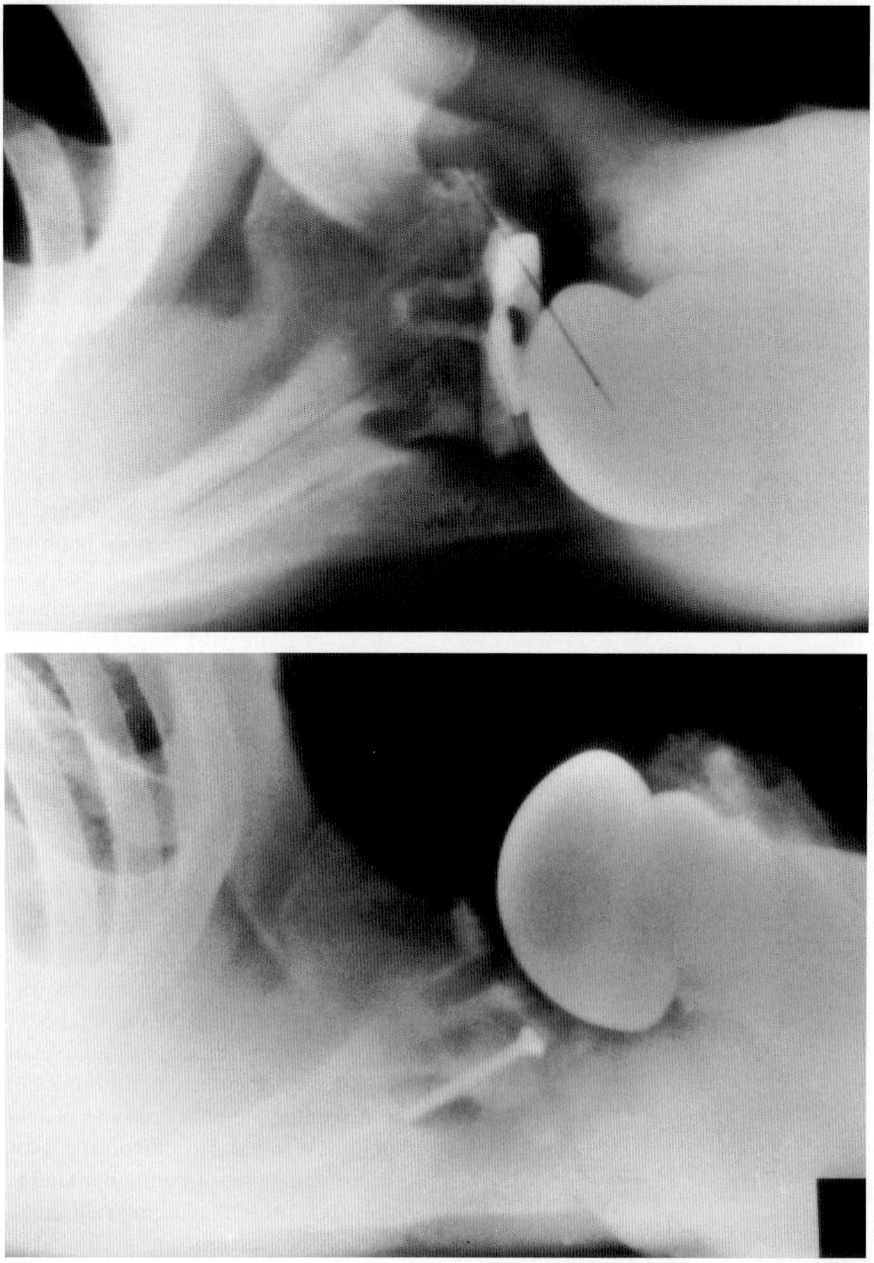

A

B

FIG. 4. Posterior instability of a total shoulder arthroplasty can be the result of a retrotilted glenoid **(A)**. During revision surgery, attention is directed toward correcting the glenoid component and placing it in a more neutral position **(B)**.

terns at the time of primary shoulder arthroplasty. For example, patients with rheumatoid arthritis have a central to anterior erosive pattern of the glenoid, whereas posterior glenoid erosion is commonly seen with degenerative osteoarthrosis. Failure to recognize this posterior glenoid deficiency can lead to a retrotilted glenoid component and thus a greater potential for postoperative posterior instability. This deficiency can be readily seen with proper axillary view radiographs. If the patient's arm cannot be placed in the proper position because of severe pain, then computerized tomography (CT) or magnetic resonance imaging (MRI) may be necessary.

Again, the same soft tissues as those discussed with anterior instability apply to posterior instability after shoulder arthroplasty. Overtightening of the subscapularis muscle can act as a driving force on the prosthetic humeral head in the posterior direction. This becomes particularly problematic in patients with underlying posterior capsular laxity because of the osteoarthritic condition. A large redundant posterior capsule alone can cause posterior instability. Plication of the posterior capsule by visualization through the anterior glenohumeral arthrotomy or by making a second incision through a posterior approach can prevent this potential complication. The capsule at the level of the rotator interval is another soft-tissue restraint that may influence posterior instability. An open rotator-interval capsule has been demonstrated to contribute to posterior translation in cadaveric shoulders (28).

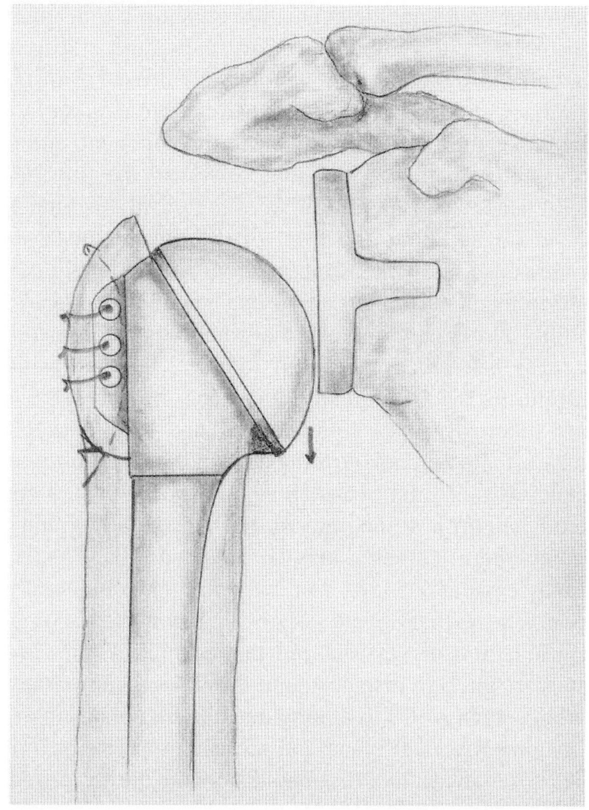

FIG. 5. Humeral component placed too low after a proximal humerus fracture, resulting in inferior instability. (From Dines DM, Warren RF. Modular shoulder hemiarthroplasty for acute fractures: surgical considerations. *Clin Orthop* 1994;307:18–26, with permission.)

Inferior Instability

True inferior instability after shoulder prosthetic replacement commonly occurs as a complication in the treatment of proximal humerus fractures. This is attributed to failure to restore proper humeral length when performing a hemiarthroplasty for three- and four-part fractures in which the normal anatomic landmarks are difficult to identify (Fig. 5; 29–31). The resultant resting tension of the deltoid and rotator-cuff muscles allows the inferior migration of the humeral head and subsequent weakness during arm elevation.

Another cause of inferior instability is insufficiency of the anterosuperior capsule and the rotator-interval capsule. Imbrication of the rotator-interval capsule has been shown to help minimize inferior translation (28).

Finally, pseudosubluxation, a temporary postoperative finding demonstrating inferior displacement of the prosthetic humeral head, is a common phenomenon identified on radiographs. It is thought to be influenced by the formation of an intracapsular hematoma, inhibition of the deltoid muscle resulting from axillary nerve dysfunction either by anesthetic agents or other neuropathy, or the loss of the negative intra-articular pressure by capsular venting (32).

PATIENT EVALUATION

As with any initial evaluation of a patient, a detailed history must first be obtained. Questions are asked regarding why the primary shoulder arthroplasty was performed, including the symptoms at that time, and the date when the prosthesis was implanted. Present symptoms and the nature of the current problem should be addressed, as well as the postoperative time when these symptoms developed. For example, in the case of anterior instability caused by failure of the repaired subscapularis muscle, a patient may explain that during the early postoperative period, there was an acute episode from the rehabilitation program that produced the current symptoms. If possible, a copy of the initial operative report should be obtained. This report may describe specific intraoperative findings or complications that can complement the history and help in making a current diagnosis of postarthroplasty instability.

Next, a methodical physical examination is performed to determine the direction of instability. Inspection of the surgical incision and the quality of muscle tone about the entire shoulder girdle is performed. Active and passive range-of-motion, muscle strength, and a detailed neurologic examination of the extremity are also recorded. Apprehension maneuvers and translation testing of the glenohumeral joint will be of benefit for the diagnoses of anterior or posterior instability. The sulcus test will assist in the diagnosis of inferior instability.

Plain film radiographic evaluation includes a true anteroposterior (glenoid view), an axillary view, and a scapular Y view of the shoulder. The glenoid view is used to inspect the superior–inferior relation between the humeral and glenoid components, the tilt of the glenoid component, and the relation between the greater tuberosity and the prosthetic humeral head. The superior curve of the prosthetic humeral head should be above the level of the greater tuberosity. This view also allows close inspection of the glenoid component to evaluate for loosening that may be secondary to instability. Internal- and external-rotation anteroposterior views may be needed adequately to assess the tuberosities. Nondisplaced and minimally displaced fractures of the greater tuberosity may go unnoticed and be a source of rotator-cuff dysfunction leading to superior instability. In difficult cases of inferior instability secondary to shortened humeral length, a scanogram or full-length radiograph of the contralateral humerus may be obtained (33). The axillary and scapular Y views can determine glenohumeral reduction. The axillary view also evaluates glenoid component orientation or version, and the scapular Y view will assist with inferior displacement. Additional radiographic modalities such as CT scanning and MRI have advantages for imaging the axial plane and are useful as preoperative studies to evaluate native glenoid version during primary shoulder arthroplasty (34). However, these modalities are limited by the amount of scatter produced from the implanted prosthetic components. The MRI has advantages in soft-tissue imaging and thus may be very useful, despite the implanted metal components, to evaluate the rotator cuff for disease. Frich and Moller (35) developed a plain film radiographic technique to determine version of the humeral component.

TREATMENT

Instability after shoulder prosthetic arthroplasty may be noticed intraoperatively immediately after implantation of the components, during the early postoperative period, or much later postoperatively after rehabilitation has been completed. As discussed, the pathogenesis of postarthroplasty shoulder instability usually relates to a soft-tissue imbalance or component malposition or both. Because there is a limited constraint in most shoulder components, stability is thus dependent on the soft-tissue envelope. This emphasizes the importance of intraoperatively assessing the range of motion and translation after a shoulder prosthesis has been implanted. The postoperative rehabilitation program must be within these limits defined in the operating room. Again, the cornerstone of treatment of this complication after prosthetic arthroplasty is prevention by recognizing these soft-tissue limitations.

Intraoperative Instability

Several preoperative conditions may potentiate instability of the initial shoulder arthroplasty. Glenoid erosion, excessive retroversion of the native humerus, fixed posterior dislocation, excessive anterior soft-tissue contractures, severe proximal humerus fractures, and neurogenic pathology are some of the more common preoperative conditions associated with postarthroplasty instability. Koch et al. (36) recently demonstrated poor functional results with superior migration of the humeral head component in patients with Parkinson's disease. If these conditions are not recognized, then the potential increases for intraoperative and very early postoperative instability.

As mentioned, patients with long-standing osteoarthrosis can have posterior glenoid deficiencies from erosive changes. Treatment of this problem is graduated, based on the severity of the glenoid deficiency. In situations with mild glenoid erosion that result in mild retroversion, the anterior aspect of the glenoid can be contoured with careful reaming to create a more neutral orientation (Fig. 6). Moderate glenoid deficiencies can be corrected by using custom glenoid components that are constructed posteriorly to

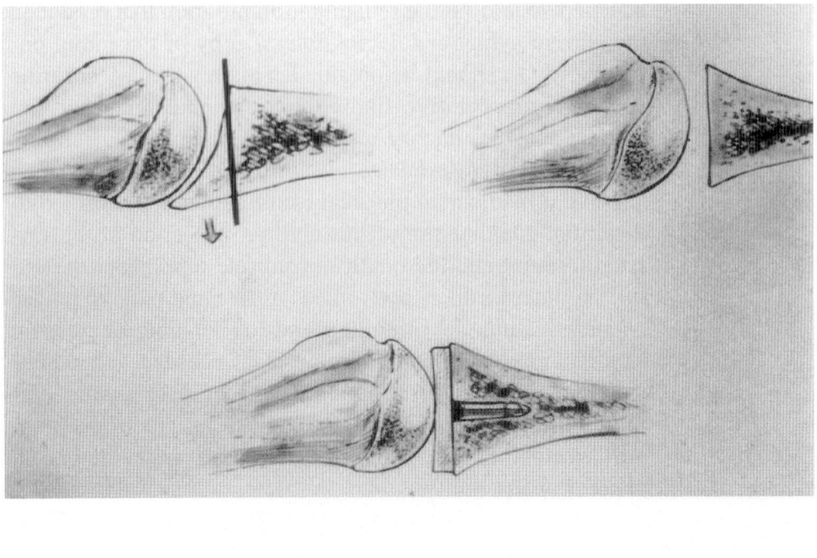

FIG. 6. Careful reaming of the anterior margin will allow a neutral position of the glenoid component.

counterbalance the bony deformity. Both mild and moderate glenoid deformities also can be offset by placing the humeral component in less retroversion (37). Cases with severe glenoid deficiency, most commonly seen in revision shoulder arthroplasty, will usually require the addition of bone graft (38). This can be accomplished with autologous iliac crest or with allograft. The bone graft is contoured to match the glenoid defect and fixed with screws (Fig. 7). The glenoid component is then cemented in place, as in primary shoulder arthroplasty. A custom-built glenoid prosthesis also can be used if bone is limited.

Excessive humeral retroversion or fixed posterior shoulder dislocation are other important preoperative factors that can cause intraoperative instability. These conditions produce a significant soft-tissue imbalance. Proper placement of the humeral component can minimize the risks of postarthroplasty instability; however, this complication is best avoided by proper soft-tissue balance. In the majority of these cases, there are tight anterior structures. Most significantly, the subscapularis muscle is contracted. Conversely, the posterior capsule is stretched because of the displaced humeral head. A methodical approach to this soft-tissue imbalance is paramount. The soft tissues can be adequately balanced by (a) release of the upper portion of the pectoralis major tendon from the humerus; (b) structural lengthening of the subscapularis muscle with a coronal Z-plasty or by removing the subscapularis muscle laterally with a piece of bone and then reattaching the complex medially around the prosthesis or, if present, into a bony defect (39,40; Fig. 8); (c) careful release, if needed, of the anterior capsule; and (d) posterior capsulorrhaphy (41).

Severe proximal humerus fractures can result in shortening of the humeral length at the time of shoulder prosthetic replacement and can be seen as intraoperative inferior instability. When present, the greater tuberosity serves as the anatomic landmark for the level of the prosthetic humeral head. The humeral head should sit just above the tip of the greater tuberosity. An extended deltopectoral approach is used without detaching the deltoid from the humerus. After the bone fragments have been removed, the proximal humerus is delivered, and the stem of a trial humerus is placed in the medullary canal of the humeral shaft. Appropriate humeral height is determined by applying gentle inferior traction on the arm and selecting a level of implant that will allow the superior portion of the humeral head to lie within the upper half of the glenoid (42). We routinely cement the stem to ensure maintenance of humeral length and rotation. It also is important that the size of the prosthetic head be small enough to allow the tuberosities to be reattached to the humeral shaft. Bone graft also may be needed to assist the union of the tuberosities to the humeral shaft (42).

Intraoperative evaluation of the implanted shoulder arthroplasty must be performed in a methodical fashion to recognize any potential instability. Our goals are to achieve 30% to 50% translation from the center of the contact point of the humeral head on the glenoid in both the anteroposterior and inferior directions. Motion must also be carefully assessed in the operating room and recorded in the operative note. The shoulder arthroplasty should have 30 to 40 degrees of external rotation. This documentation is important for rehabilitation limits during the early postoperative period.

Early Postoperative Instability

Factors that influence instability in the early postoperative period are the malposition of the components or soft-tissue failure. Usually, the patients have instability symptoms after an acute episode. Pseudosubluxation, a phenomenon described earlier, also can be identified during the early postoperative period. This generally is a self-limited condition and can be treated with immobilization and simple rehabilitation exercises. Other authors have treated other forms of early instability with immobilization with mixed results.

In his series of 194 patients, Neer (11) reported three of four shoulder arthroplasty dislocations treated successfully with closed reduction and immobilization. In this same series, all subluxation cases treated with the same nonoperative method had poor results (11). Later in 1988, Amstutz et al. (1) reported that 60% of the complications after shoulder arthroplasty that required revision surgery were attributable to instability. Half of Neer's subluxations reported in his large series were in the anterior direction. In our institution's series, we found that all cases of anterior in-

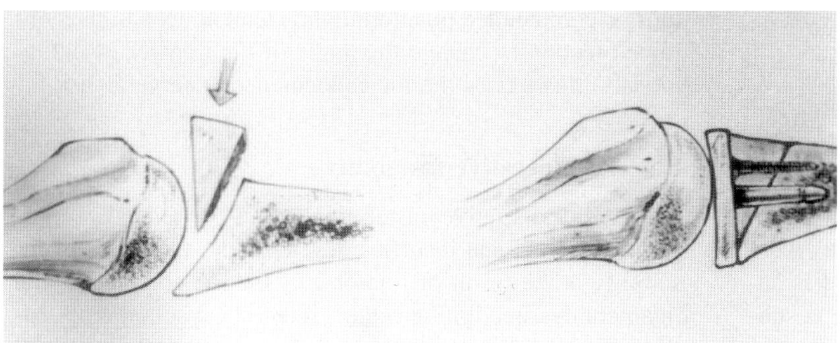

FIG. 7. Placement of a well-contoured bone graft can help to place the glenoid component in a neutral position. (From Moeckel BH, Altchek DW, Warren RF, Wickiewicz TL, Dines DM. Instability of the shoulder after arthroplasty. *J Bone Joint Surg [Am]* 1993;75:492–497, with permission.)

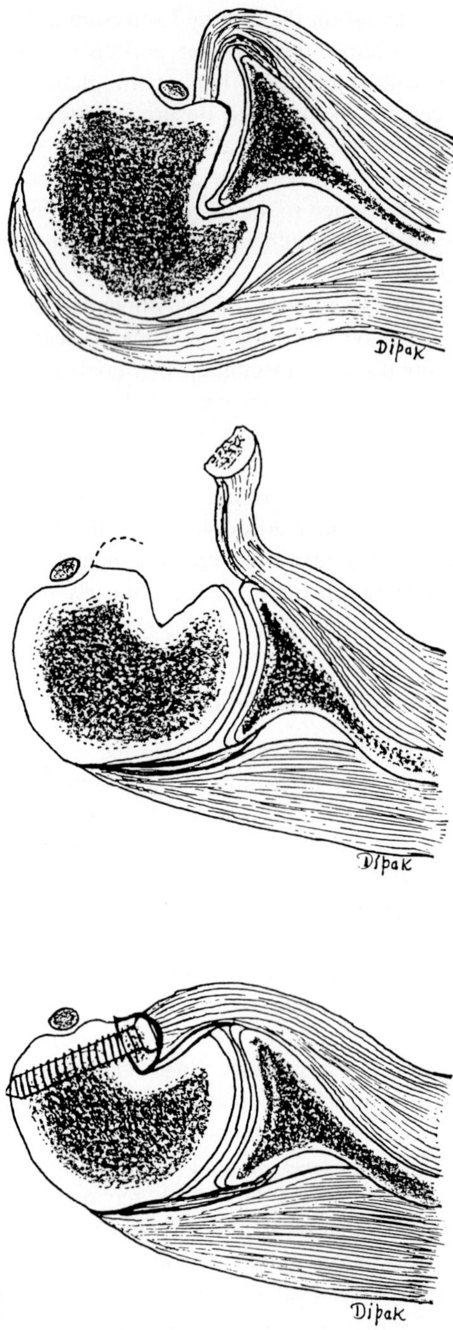

A

B

C

FIG. 8. A–C: Functional lengthening of a contracted subscapularis muscle by a medially placed transfer into a bony defect, which can be present in chronic posterior dislocations of the humeral head.

stability required revision surgery (12). Nonoperative treatment for anterior instability after shoulder arthroplasty is not successful. Of the seven anterior instability cases in our series, two were treated with initial physical therapy. Nonoperative treatment failed in these two cases, and they were subsequently surgically revised (12). We believe that anterior instability usually does not occur unless there is subscapularis tendon failure.

The treatment for this soft-tissue problem depends on first determining that the prosthetic components are in proper version. If there is excessive anteversion of either the humeral head or glenoid component, the repaired subscapularis will not be able to tolerate the abnormal anteriorly directed forces. Component revision is then necessary to correct the problem. We have used a modular head–neck prosthesis that offers an option for correction of humeral version without revising the stem. This is accomplished by changing the angle of the mortise stem in reference to the humeral head. Another factor that can result in abnormal forces on the repaired subscapularis tendon is overstuffing the shoulder joint. Too large a humeral head or too thick a glenoid component can cause this condition. Trial humeral heads can be placed on modular components to find the appropriate size at the time of revision surgery, and the avoidance of metal-backed glenoid components during primary arthroplasty can help to prevent this complication.

The management of anterior instability in the early postoperative period is surgical mobilization of the failed subscapularis tendon repair. When the tissue is well preserved, repeated repair of the tendon can be performed. It cannot be stressed enough that repair of a ruptured subscapularis tendon is technically demanding. Thus, the repair of the subscapularis at the time of primary shoulder arthroplasty is extremely important. If the tissue is tenuous, then augment the repair with nonabsorbable tape. In cases of recurrent instability or in salvage procedures, reconstruction of the subscapularis tendon has been described (12,43).

Moeckel et al. (12) demonstrated the use of an Achilles tendon allograft as a technique for reconstruction. The bone from the calcaneus is anchored to the base of the coracoid on the scapula, and the tendon is secured to the humerus at the anatomic subscapularis tendon insertion on the lesser tuberosity (Fig. 9). It is important to obtain proper tension of this graft, as it is with the primary repair of the native subscapularis. We like to position the shoulder at 60 degrees of abduction and at 30 to 40 degrees of external rotation at the time of repair or reconstruction. Another technique used to reconstruct an irreparable subscapularis is the transfer of the upper portion of the pectoralis major tendon (43). The tendon is transferred in a superolateral direction to a bony trough created just lateral to the bicipital groove. The vector for this transfer may be too anterior and result in excessive humeral head translations anteriorly. Some authors recommended positioning this tendon deep to the conjoined tendon to change the angle of the transfer (44). Obviously, this places the musculocutaneous nerve at risk.

Late Postoperative Instability

Late postoperative instability is mostly related to progressive soft-tissue insufficiency. Usually, this form of instability is the result of rotator-cuff failure, coracoacromial ligament dysfunction, or rotator-interval capsular laxity. Although some of this soft-tissue imbalance may be the result

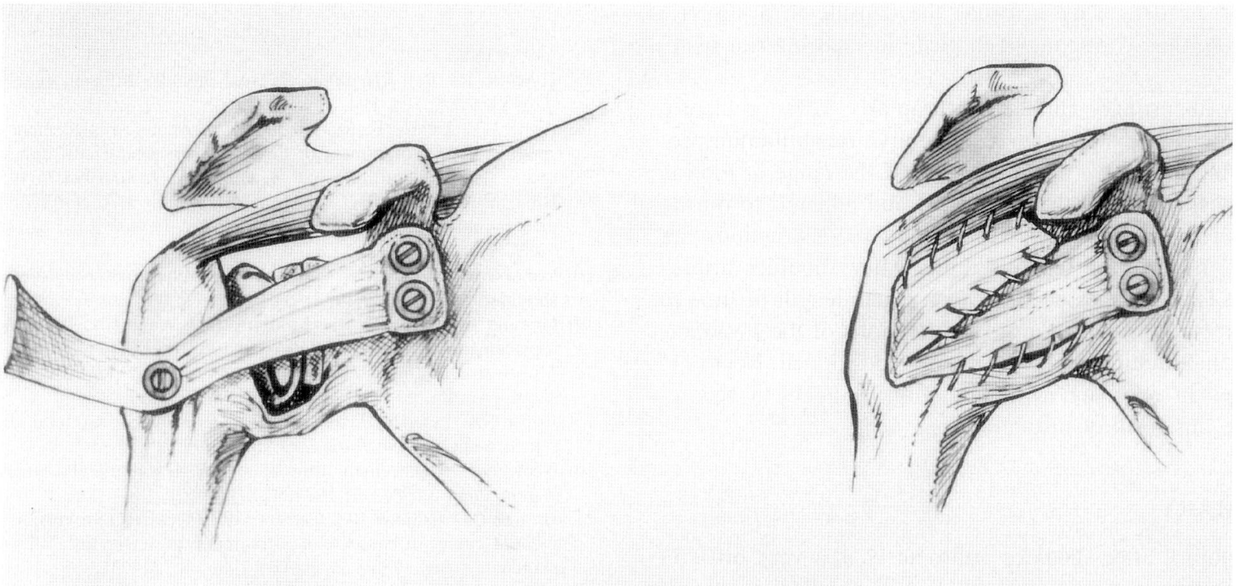

FIG. 9. The use of an Achilles tendon allograft for reconstruction of the subscapularis tendon. The excess allograft may be reflected upon itself, filling in other anterior defects. (From Moeckel BH, Altchek DW, Warren RF, Wickiewicz TL, Dines DM. Instability of the shoulder after arthroplasty. *J Bone Joint Surg [Am]* 1993;75:492–497, with permission.)

of unrecognized pathology at the time of shoulder arthroplasty, other important factors, such as joint diseases and the size of the implant, can play roles in this complication. Rheumatoid arthritis is a classic example of a disease process that may contribute to late postoperative instability after shoulder arthroplasty. The destructive nature of the inflammatory pathway results in a slow breakdown of the surrounding soft-tissue envelope. Also, the size of the prosthetic humeral head can indirectly influence the tension of the soft tissue, resulting in a loose soft-tissue envelope with an undersized implant and overtightening of tissue, as already demonstrated with a too large humeral head.

Progressive superior instability is most commonly seen in the late postoperative period after shoulder arthroplasty. This complication is attributed to rotator-cuff dysfunction. Management of this problem is very similar to the general treatment of rotator-cuff tendinopathy. Many of these patients will have impingement-like symptoms and will usually respond to nonoperative treatment. Boyd et al. (25) noted no increase in pain with superior migration of the prosthetic humeral head. If the shoulder is painful and function is severely impaired, then repair of the rotator-cuff tear is performed. If there is an irreparable rotator-cuff tear, then revision to a hemiarthroplasty with a larger humeral head (but not overstuffed) should be considered. The potential complication of glenoid loosening as a long-term result of superior migration of the humeral component is more problematic. In conversion to a hemiarthroplasty, the soft-tissue envelope must be meticulously balanced to avoid early anterior or posterior instability complications. Finally, the use of hooded glenoid components acting as a buttress to treat superior migration has not given satisfactory results, as loosening of these prostheses has developed.

Many patients with rotator-cuff tendinopathy after shoulder arthroplasty have had previous surgery for impingement symptoms. The quality of the coracoacromial ligament in these cases must be inspected carefully at the time of primary shoulder arthroplasty. A dysfunctional coracoacromial ligament is another cause of late postoperative anterosuperior instability (45). The incompetent arch fails to act as a restraint to anterosuperior instability. When the ligament is salvageable, repair to the acromion is performed to establish the anterosuperior buttress. If the coracoacromial ligament has been resected, then reconstruction with allograft tissue, with a technique similar to that described for subscapularis reconstruction, may be considered. Reconstruction of this ligament by mobilizing a 0.5 × 3-cm strip of conjoined tendon and transferring this laterally to the acromion has been described (41). However, the results of using this techniques are poor.

Last, the rotator-interval capsule has been demonstrated to play a role in posterior and inferior instability (28). Deficiencies in this capsular region or a dysfunctional coracohumeral ligament can be approached in a graduated fashion. For simple openings of the rotator-interval capsule, a primary closure is all that is needed to be successful. If the coracohumeral ligament at this region is repairable, then it can be incorporated into the capsular repair. Plication of the capsule, sometimes up to several centimeters, may be necessary to restore proper function. If the tissue quality is poor, then augmentation with nonabsorbable tape through the capsule and secured to the coracoid through drill holes may be needed. This suspends the capsule in a superior direction, thus correcting both posterior and inferior instability.

As with primary shoulder arthroplasty, revision arthroplasty must withstand the postoperative rehabilitation program. Intraoperative documentation of the range of motion and translation must be performed and adhered to during rehabilitation. Soft-tissue repairs and reconstructions are usually needed for late instability after shoulder arthroplasty. These tissues need an appropriate length of time to heal before stressing. Thus, modifications of the postoperative rehabilitation protocols must be developed. Neer (11) outlined an approach with limitation in goals to accommodate this form of instability.

SUMMARY

Instability after shoulder arthroplasty is a very difficult complication to treat successfully. A methodical approach, which includes a detailed history and physical examination, as well as appropriate radiographic modalities, is needed during the evaluation. A thorough understanding of soft-tissue balancing and proper component size and position cannot be overemphasized. The postoperative rehabilitation protocol must respect the documented range-of-motion limitations obtained intraoperatively. The cornerstone of management for this complication is prevention. However, surgical treatment options include appropriate balance of the soft-tissue envelope, revision of the components, and reconstruction of soft-tissue or bony deficiencies, sometimes with the use of allograft tissues.

REFERENCES

1. Amstutz HC, Thomas BJ, Kabo M, Jinnah RH, Dorey FJ. The DANA total shoulder arthroplasty. *J Bone Joint Surg [Am]* 1988;70:1174–1182.
2. Barrett WP, Franklin, JL, Jackins SE, Wyss CR, Matsen FA III. Total shoulder arthroplasty. *J Bone Joint Surg [Am]* 1987;69:865–872.
3. Cofield RH. Total shoulder arthroplasty with the Neer prosthesis. *J Bone Joint Surg [Am]* 1984;66:899–906.
4. Silliman J, Hawkins R. Complications following shoulder arthroplasty. In: Friedman R, ed. *Arthroplasty of the shoulder.* New York: Thieme, 1994:242–253.
5. Wirth MA, Rockwood CA Jr. Complications of total shoulder-replacement arthroplasty. *J Bone Joint Surg [Am]* 1996;78:603–616.
6. Figgie MP, Inglis AE, Figgie HE III, Sobel M, Burstein AH, Kraay MJ. Custom total shoulder arthroplasty in inflammatory arthritis: preliminary results. *J Arthroplasty* 1992;7:1–6.
7. McCoy SR, Warren RF, Bade HA III, Ranawat CS, Inglis AE. Total shoulder arthroplasty in rheumatoid arthritis. *J Arthroplasty* 1989;4:105–113.
8. Pollock RG, Deliz ED, McIlveen SJ, Flatow EL, Bigliani LU. Prosthetic replacement in rotator cuff-deficient shoulders. *J Shoulder Elbow Surg* 1992;1:173–186.
9. Torchia ME, Cofield RH. Long-term results of Neer total shoulder arthroplasty. *Orthop Trans* 1994–1995;18:977.
10. Cofield RH. Shoulder arthroplasty: current techniques. Instructional course lecture, American Academy of Orthopaedic Surgeons 64th Annual Meeting, San Francisco, 1997.
11. Neer CS II, Watson KC, Stanton FJ. Recent experience in total shoulder replacement. *J Bone Joint Surg [Am]* 1982;64:319–337.
12. Moeckel BH, Altchek DW, Warren RF, Wickiewicz TL, Dines DM. Instability of the shoulder after arthroplasty. *J Bone Joint Surg [Am]* 1993;75:492–497.
13. Hawkins RJ, Bell RH, Jallay B. Total shoulder arthroplasty. *Clin Orthop* 1989;242:188–194.
14. Arntz GT, Jackins S, Matsen FA III. Prosthetic replacement of the shoulder for the treatment of defects in the rotator cuff and surface of the glenohumeral joint. *J Bone Joint Surg [Am]* 1993;75:485–491.
15. Brenner BC, Ferlic DC, Clayton ML, Dennis DA. Survivorship of unconstrained total shoulder arthroplasty. *J Bone Joint Surg [Am]* 1989;71:1289–1296.
16. Clayton ML, Ferlic DC, Jeffers PD. Prosthetic arthroplasties of the shoulder. *Clin Orthop* 1982;164:184–191.
17. Gristina AG, Romano RL, Kammire GC, Webb LX. Total shoulder replacement. *Orthop Clin North Am* 1987;18(3):445–453.
18. McElwain JP, English M. The early results of porous-coated total shoulder arthroplasty. *Clin Orthop* 1987;218:217–224.
19. Roper BA, Paterson JMH, Day WH. The Roper-Day total shoulder replacement. *J Bone Joint Surg [Br]* 1990;72:694–697.
20. Neer CS II. Replacement arthroplasty for glenohumeral osteoarthritis. *J Bone Joint Surg [Am]* 1974;56:1–13.
21. Brewer BJ, Wubben RC, Carrera GF. Excessive retroversion of the glenoid cavity: a cause of non-traumatic posterior instability of the shoulder. *J Bone Joint Surg [Am]* 1986;68:724–731.
22. Matsen FA III, Thomas SC, Rockwood CA Jr. Glenohumeral instability. In: Rockwood CA Jr, Matsen FA III, eds. *The shoulder.* Philadelphia: WB Saunders, 1990:534–540.
23. Levick JR. Joint pressure-volume studies: their importance, design, and interpretation. *J Rheumatol* 1983;10:353–357.
24. Turkel SJ, Panio MW, Marshall JL, Girgis FG. Stabilizing mechanisms preventing anterior dislocation of the glenohumeral joint. *J Bone Joint Surg [Am]* 1981;63:1208–1217.
25. Boyd AD Jr, Aliabadi P, Thornhill TS. Postoperative proximal migration in total shoulder arthroplasty: incidence and significance. *J Arthroplasty* 1991;6:31–37.
26. Franklin JL, Barrett WP, Jackins SE, Matsen FA III. Glenoid loosening in total shoulder arthroplasty: association with rotator cuff deficiency. *J Arthroplasty* 1988;3:39–46.
27. Wirth MA, Rockwood CA Jr. Glenohumeral instability following shoulder arthroplasty. *Orthop Trans* 1995;19:459.
28. Harryman DT II, Sidles JA, Harris SL, Matsen FA III. The role of the rotator interval capsule in passive motion and stability of the shoulder. *J Bone Joint Surg [Am]* 1992;74:53–66.
29. Moeckel BH, Dines DM, Warren RF, Altchek DW. Modular hemiarthroplasty for fractures of the proximal humerus. *J Bone Joint Surg [Am]* 1992;74:884–889.
30. Dines DM, Altchek DW. Hemiarthroplasty techniques for proximal humerus fractures. *Comp Orthop* 1991;Jan/Feb:25–31.
31. Bisson JL, Dines DM. Total shoulder arthroplasty. In: Craig EV, ed. *Textbook of orthopedic surgery.* Philadelphia: Williams & Wilkins, 1998.
32. Warner JJP, Deng XH, Warren RF, Torzilli PA, O'Brien SJ. Superoinferior translation in the intact and vented glenohumeral joint. *J Shoulder Elbow Surg* 1993;2:99–105.
33. Gill GG. A simple roentgenographic method for the measurement of bone length; modification of Milwee's method of slit scanography. *J Bone Joint Surg* 1944;26:767–769.
34. Friedman RJ, Hawthorne KB, Genez BM. The use of computerized tomography in the measurement of glenoid version. *J Bone Joint Surg [Am]* 1992;74:1032–1037.
35. Frich LH, Moller BN. Retroversion of the humeral prosthesis in shoulder arthroplasty. Measurements of angle from standard radiographs. *J Arthroplasty* 1989;4:277–280.
36. Koch LD, Cofield RH, Ahlskog JE. Total shoulder arthroplasty in patients with Parkinson's disease. *J Shoulder Elbow Surg* 1997;6:24–28.
37. Neer CS II. Glenohumeral arthroplasty. In: Neer CS, ed. *Shoulder reconstruction.* Philadelphia: WB Saunders, 1990:181–185.
38. Neer CS II, Morrison DS. Glenoid bone-grafting in total shoulder arthroplasty. *J Bone Joint Surg [Am]* 1988;70:1154–1162.
39. McLaughlin HL. Posterior dislocation of the shoulder. *J Bone Joint Surg [Am]* 1952;34:584–590.

40. Hawkins RJ, Neer CS II, Pianta RM, Mendoza FX. Locked posterior dislocation of the shoulder. *J Bone Joint Surg [Am]* 1987;69:9–18.
41. Wirth MA, Rockwood CA Jr. Complications of shoulder arthroplasty. *Clin Orthop* 1994;307:47–69.
42. Dines DM, Warren RF. Modular shoulder hemiarthroplasty for acute fractures. Surgical considerations. *Clin Orthop* 1994;307:18–26.
43. Wirth MA, Selzer DG, Rockwood CA Jr. Pectoralis muscle transfer in patients with recurrent anterior glenohumeral instability. Presented at the Southern Medical Association 87th Annual Meeting, New Orleans, October, 1993.
44. Resch H, Povacz P. Pectoral major muscle transfer in case of irreparable chronic tear of subscapularis tendon. *J Shoulder Elbow Surg* 1997;6:224.
45. Field LD, Dines DM, Zabinski SJ, Warren RF. Hemiarthroplasty of the shoulder for rotator cuff arthropathy. *J Shoulder Elbow Surg* 1997;6:18–23.

Subject Index

Page numbers followed by f indicate figures and page numbers followed by t indicate tables.

T

V

W

X